P9-DOC-517

KOPPLE AND MASSRY'S NUTRITIONAL MANAGEMENT OF RENAL DISEASE

SECOND EDITION

KOPPLE AND MASSRY'S NUTRITIONAL MANAGEMENT OF RENAL DISEASE

SECOND EDITION

Editors

JOEL D. KOPPLE, M.D.

Professor of Medicine and Public Health
David Geffen School of Medicine at UCLA
UCLA School of Public Health
Los Angeles, California
Chief
Division of Nephrology and Hypertension
Harbor-UCLA Medical Center
Torrance, California

SHAUL G. MASSRY, M.D.

Professor of Medicine
Keck School of Medicine
University of Southern California
Los Angeles, California

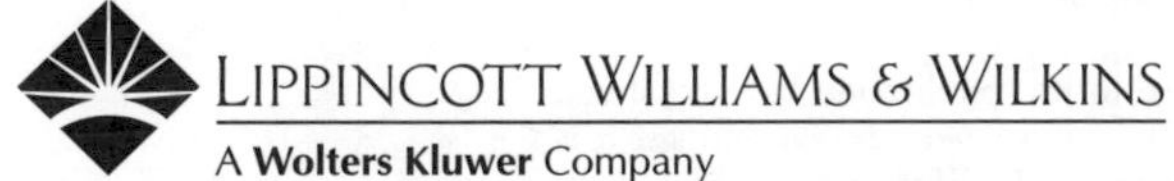

A **Wolters Kluwer** Company
Philadelphia • Baltimore • New York • London
Buenos Aires • Hong Kong • Sydney • Tokyo

Acquisitions Editor: Timothy Y. Hiscock
Developmental Editor: Lisa Consoli
Production Editor: Danielle Power
Manufacturing Manager: Benjamin Rivera
Cover Designer: Karen Quigley
Compositor: Maryland Composition
Printer: Maple Press

530 Walnut Street
Philadelphia, PA 19106 USA
LWW.com

Printed in the USA

Library of Congress Cataloging-in-Publication Data

Kopple and Massry's nutritional management of renal disease / [edited by] Joel D. Kopple, Shaul G. Massry.—2nd ed.
p.; cm.
Rev. ed. of: Nutritional management of renal disease. 1997.
Includes bibliographical references and index.
ISBN 0-7817-3594-7
1. Kidney—Disease—Diet therapy. 2. Chronic renal failure—Diet therapy. 3. Kidneys—Diseases—Nutritional aspects. 4. Chronic renal failure—Nutritional aspects. I. Title: Nutritional management of renal disease. II. Kopple, Joel D. III. Massry, Shaul G.
[DNLM: 1. Kidney Disease—diet therapy. 2. Nutrition. WJ 300 K83 2003]
RC903.N88 2003
616.6'10654—dc21

2003045801

---

10 9 8 7 6 5 4 3 2 1

To our wives Madelynn Kopple and Meira Massry; to our children David, Robin, Michael, Deborah, and Joshua Kopple; and Efrat, Ram, Raef, and Emma Cogan, Guy and Alexis, Yael, and Dina Massry and Kenneth Grudko; and to Jeffrey Alan Kopple

CONTENTS

CONTRIBUTING AUTHORS

Kevin C. Abbott, M.D. Director of Dialysis, Walter Reed Army Medical Center, Washington, D.C.

Magdalena Adeva-Andany, M.D. Nephrology Specialist, Department of Internal Medicine, Hospital Juan Canaléjo, La Coruna, Spain

George Bakris, M.D. Director, Hypertension Training Program, Rush Presbyterian–St. Luke's Medical Center, Chicago, Illinois

Rinaldo Bellomo, M.D. Professor, Department of Medicine, University of Melbourne; and Director of Intensive Care Research, Department of Intensive Care, Austin & Repatriation Medical Centre, Melbourne, Australia

Jonas Bergström, M.D., Ph.D. *(deceased)* Professor Emeritus, Baxter Novum and Renal Medicine, Karolinska Institute, Huddinge University Hospital, Stockholm, Sweden

Gianni Biolo, M.D. Department of Clinical, Morphological, and Technological Sciences, Division of Internal Medicine, University of Trieste, Trieste, Italy

Jerrilynn D. Burrowes, Ph.D., R.D., C.D.N. Assistant Professor, Department of Nutrition, C. W. Post Campus, Long Island University, Brookville, New York

Richard Casaburi, M.D., Ph.D. Professor, Department of Medicine, UCLA School of Medicine, and Chief, Division of Respiratory and Critical Care Physiology and Medicine, Harbor-UCLA Medical Center, Torrance, California

Vimal Chadha, M.D. Assistant Professor, Department of Pediatrics, Virginia Commonwealth University; and Chairman, Division of Pediatric Nephrology, Medical College of Virginia, Richmond, Virginia

Charles Chazot, M.D. Ancien Assistant Chef de Clinique a la Faculte, Nephrologie, Centre de Rein Artificiel, Tassin, France

David B. Cockram, Ph.D., R.D., L.D. Ross Products Division, Abbott Laboratories, Medical Nutrition Research and Development, Columbus, Ohio

Rita Cornelis, Ph.D. Research Director F.W.O., Department of Analytical Chemistry, University of Ghent, Ghent, Belgium

Laura Dertenois, M.D. Research Fellow, Department of Internal Medicine, Nephrology Division, University of Genoa, Genoa, Italy

Natale G. De Santo, M.D. Chair and Full Professor, Departments of Nephrology and Pediatrics, Second University of Naples, Naples, Italy

Annemieke Dhondt, M.D., Ph.D. Associate Professor, Department of Internal Medicine, and Dialysis Unit Supervisor, Renal Division, University Hospital of Ghent, Ghent, Belgium

Burl R. Don, M.D. Professor, Department of Medicine, University of California, Davis; and Director of Clinical Nephrology, University of California Davis Medical Center, Sacramento, California

Michael E. Falkenhain, M.D. Associate Professor of Medicine, Department of Nephrology, Ohio State University, Columbus, Ohio

Robert Nicholas Foley, M.D. Associate Professor, Department of Medicine, University of Minnesota; and Director, Nephrology Analytical Services, Minneapolis Medical Research Foundation, Hennepin County Medical Center, Minneapolis, Minnesota

Charles J. Foulks, M.D., F.A.C.P., F.A.C.N. Professor, Department of Medicine, Texas A&M University Health Science Center and College of Medicine; and Medical Director, Scott & White Clinic, Temple, Texas

Denis Fouque, M.D., Ph.D. Professor of Nephrology, University Claude Bernard Lyon 1; and Associate Chief, Division of Nephrology, Hôpital Edouard Herriot, Lyon, France

Harold A. Franch, M.D. Renal Division, Emory University School of Medicine, Atlanta, Georgia

Giacomo Garibotto, M.D. Associate Professor of Nephrology, Department of Internal Medicine, Nephrology Division, University of Genoa, Genoa, Italy

Gianfranco Guarnieri, M.D. Full Professor, Department of Internal Medicine, University of Trieste; and Chief, Clinica Medica Generale, Ospedale di Cattinara, Trieste, Italy

Judith A. Hartman, R.D. Division of Nephrology, The Ohio State University Medical Center, Columbus, Ohio

Lee Hebert, M.D. Department of Medicine, Ohio State University Medical Center, Columbus, Ohio

Olof Heimbürger, M.D. Division of Renal Medicine, Department of Clinical Science, Karolinska Institute; and Senior Physician, Department of Renal Medicine, Huddinge University Hospital, Stockholm, Sweden

Raimund Hirschberg, M.D. Professor, Department of Medicine, University of California, Los Angeles; and Attending Nephrologist, Department of Medicine, Harbor-UCLA Medical Center, Torrance, California

Walter H. Hörl, M.D. Department of Medicine III, Division of Nephrology and Dialysis, University of Vienna, Vienna, Austria

T. Alp Ikizler, M.D. Vanderbilt University Medical Center, Nashville, Tennessee

Kamyar Kalantar-Zadeh, M.D., M.P.H. Assistant Professor of Medicine and Pediatrics, Department of Medicine, UCLA School of Medicine; and Director of Outcome Research and Information, Department of Medicine, Division of Nephrology and Hypertension, Harbor-UCLA Medical Center, Torrance, California

George A. Kaysen, M.D. Chief, Division of Nephrology, University of California, Davis School of Medicine, Davis, California

Bertram L. Kasiske, M.D. University of Minnesota, Hennepin County Medical Center, Minneapolis, Minnesota

Saulo Klahr, M.D. John E. and Adaline Simon Professor of Medicine, Department of Internal Medicine, Washington University School of Medicine; and Physician, Department of Internal Medicine, Barnes-Jewish Hospital, St. Louis, Missouri

Joel D. Kopple, M.D. Professor of Medicine and Public Health, David Geffen School of Medicine at UCLA, UCLA School of Public Health, Los Angeles, California; and Chief, Division of Nephrology and Hypertension, Harbor-UCLA Medical Center, Torrance, California

Kiyoshi Kurokawa, M.D., M.A.C.P. Professor and Director, Institute of Medical Sciences, Tokai University, Bohseidai, Kangawa, Japan

Norbert Lameire, M.D. Professor of Medicine, Department of Internal Medicine, University of Ghent; and Renal Division, Department of Internal Medicine, University Hospital, Ghent, Belgium

Bengt Lindholm, M.D., Ph.D. Associate Professor, Baxter Novum and Renal Medicine, Karolinska Institute, Huddinge University Hospital, Stockholm, Sweden

Cathi Jackson Martin, R.D., C.S.R., L.D.N. Research Coordinator, Departments of Medicine and Nephrology, Vanderbilt University Medical Center, Nashville, Tennessee

Shaul G. Massry, M.D. Professor of Medicine, Keck School of Medicine, University of Southern California, Los Angeles, California

Linda M. McCann, R.D., C.S.R., L.D. Director of Nutrition, Satellite Healthcare, Mountain View, California

Rajnish Mehrotra, M.D., M.B.B.S. Assistant Professor of Medicine, Division of Nephrology and Hypertension, David Geffen School of Medicine and Research and Education Institute, and Director, Peritoneal Dialysis, Harbor-UCLA Medical Center, Torrance, California

William E. Mitch, M.D. Edward Randall Professor of Medicine, and Chairman, Department of Medicine, University of Texas, Galveston, Texas

Toshio Miyata, M.D., Ph.D. Professor, The Institute of Medical Sciences, Tokai University; and Professor, Department of Nephrology, Tokai University School of Medicine, Bohseidai, Kanagawa, Japan

Sharon M. Moe, M.D. Associate Professor of Medicine and Associate Dean for Research Support, Indiana University School of Medicine; and Director of Nephrology, Wishard Memorial Hospital, Indianapolis, Indiana

Nadia Pastorino, M.D. Department of Internal Medicine, Nephrology Division, University of Genoa, Genoa, Italy

Alessandra F. Perna, M.D., Ph.D. Researcher and Assistant Professor, Departments of Nephrology and Pediatrics, Second University of Naples, Naples, Italy

Lara Pupim, M.D., M.S.C.I. Research Assistant Professor, Department of Medicine, Vanderbilt University, Nashville, Tennessee

Ralph Rabkin, M.D., M.B.Ch.B., F.R.C.P. (Glasgow) Emeritus Professor, Departments of Medicine and Nephrology, Stanford University, Stanford, California; and Research Service, Veterans Administration, Palo Alto Health Care System, Palo Alto, California

Roberta Situlin, M.D. Department of Clinical, Morphological, and Technological Sciences, Division of Internal Medicine, University of Trieste, Trieste, Italy

M. Sivalingham, M.D.

Miroslaw Smogorzewski, M.D. Ph.D. Associate Professor, Division of Nephrology, Department of Medicine, Keck School of Medicine, University of Southern California, Los Angeles, California

Peter Stenvinkel, M.D., Ph.D. Associate Professor, Department of Renal Medicine, Department of Clinical Science, Karolinska Institute; and Senior Lecturer, Department of Renal Medicine, Huddinge University Hospital, Stockholm, Sweden

Gabriele Toigo, M.D. Associate Professor, Department of Internal Medicine, University of Trieste; and Chief, Geriatria, Ospedale Maggiore, Trieste, Italy

Raymond Vanholder, M.D., Ph.D. Professor, Faculty of Medicine, and Medical Doctor, Department of Internal Medicine, Nephrology Division, University Hospital of Ghent, Ghent, Belgium

Christoph Wanner, M.D. Professor, Department of Medicine, Nephrology Division, and Chief, University Clinic, Wuerzburg, Germany

Bradley A. Warady, M.D. Professor of Pediatrics, University of Missouri–Kansas City School of Medicine; and Chief, Section of Pediatric Nephrology and Director, Dialysis and Transplantation, Children's Mercy Hospital, Kansas City, Missouri

Mark E. Williams, M.D., F.A.C.P. Associate Clinical Professor, Joslin Diabetes Center, Harvard Medical School; and Beth Israel Deaconess Medical Center, Boston, Massachusetts

Jane Y. Yeun, M.D., F.A.C.P. Director, Fellowship Training Program, Department of Internal Medicine, Division of Nephrology, University of California, Davis, Sacramento, California; and Nephrology Section Chief, Department of Internal Medicine, Nephrology Section, Sacramento Veterans Administration Medical Center, Mather, California

Foreword to the First Edition

"Food is life"

This aphorism is an apt description of the theme of *Nutritional Management of Renal Disease*. In a collection of well-documented and contemporary essays by an outstanding group of recognized experts, Professors Kopple and Massry provide an elegant and complete cataloging of the relationships between nutrition and the kidney, both in health as well as in disease.

Quite appropriately, the majority of the contributions relate to the interactions between nutrient intake and acute and chronic renal failure. Nevertheless, fundamental principles, such as the influence of diet on normal renal function and blood pressure control, the assessment of nutritional disorders, and compliance with dietary recommendations are afforded appropriate coverage. Modification of the composition of nutrient, mineral, and trace element intake as aspects of the management approach to patients with nephrotic syndrome, renal insufficiency, or those receiving renal replacement therapy receives very careful and analytical attention. Attention to the nutritional management of children as well as adults with renal disease expands the breadth of reviews.

Physicians caring for patients with renal disease will be grateful for this compilation of information, presented in an easily read yet scholarly fashion. The answers to the frequently asked question, "Doctor, what should I do with my food intake to help my condition?" will be found in the well-written chapters of this monograph.

In this era of "evidence based" medicine, such a thorough and comprehensive review of a complex and often controversial topic is indeed very welcome, and long overdue. The international flavor of the contributing authors and the skillful editing carried out by Professors Kopple and Massry serve only to further enhance the value of this work. I plan to have this book at close hand when the need arises to counsel patients on the nutritional aspects of the management of renal disease. I am confident that other readers of this superb contribution will agree with this assessment.

Richard J. Glassock, M.D.
Professor and Chairman
Department of Internal Medicine
University of Kentucky
Lexington, Kentucky

Foreword

The second edition of *Nutritional Management of Renal Disease*, which is edited by Joel D. Kopple, M.D., and Shaul G. Massry, M.D., is an extremely important book for all physicians and other health care providers who deal with patients afflicted with either acute or chronic kidney failure. Whether or not there is an associated acute or chronic illness, patients with renal disease sustain many metabolic and nutritional abnormalities that affect their morbidity and mortality. Doctors Kopple and Massry have assembled a group of experts who are actively working in the field, thus assuring the most up-to-date information. The breadth of the book's content is outstanding, and virtually every aspect of the field of nutrition and metabolism in acute and chronic renal failure is covered in this excellent 37 chapter book.

As world leaders in the field, Doctors Kopple and Massry have the ability to combine superb scholarship, including extensive and pertinent referencing, with practical aspects that are important in the care of renal patients. Whether one is concerned with carbohydrate, lipid, or protein metabolism; uremic toxicity; oxidant or carbamyl stress; inflammation and malnutrition; calcium, phosphorus, and vitamin D metabolism; sodium and electrolyte perturbations; the importance of homocysteine, parathyroid hormone or carnitine; nutrition in adults or children on hemodialysis, continuous renal replacement therapy or renal transplantation, the physiologic or metabolic response to exercise training; and much more, this book should be an integral part of the library of physicians and other health care providers who desire to provide optimal care to their patients with kidney disease or acute or chronic renal failure.

Robert W. Schrier, M.D.
Professor of Medicine
University of Colorado
School of Medicine
Denver, Colorado

Foreword

Preface to the First Edition

In recent years, there has been a marked increase in scientific information and medical know-how in the field of nutritional disorders and nutritional therapy in patients with renal disease and those with acute or chronic renal failure. Methods for provision of nutritional therapy to these patients have expanded enormously. The potential importance of these developments is underscored by evidence indicating that markers of malnutrition strongly predict morbidity and mortality rates in patients with chronic renal failure.

These new developments and the increasing complexity of this field convinced us that a new compendium of information concerning nutrition and metabolism of individuals with renal disease or renal failure is timely and would be a useful addition to the literature. We have assembled a group of 53 experts from the United States and Europe to contribute 30 chapters to this book. Several chapters are devoted to scholarly reviews of the scientific literature concerning the nutritional and metabolic status of individuals with renal disease. These topics include protein, amino acid, carbohydrate, lipid, mineral, trace element, vitamin and carnitine metabolism, uremic toxicity, the causes of protein-calorie malnutrition in renal disease, the effects of protein-calorie malnutrition on renal function, methods of assessment of nutritional status, and the effect of nutritional and non-nutritional factors on the progression of chronic renal failure. These chapters emphasize the integral relationships between nutrition and the metabolic and clinical status of patients afflicted with renal disease or renal failure. Other contributions focus more on nutritional disorders and treatment of specific clinical conditions such as hypertension, chronic renal insufficiency, nephrotic syndrome, chronic dialysis, renal transplantation, and acute renal failure. Finally, the book contains chapters that review treatment with growth factors, exercise training, drug-nutrient reactions, the nutritional management of children with chronic renal failure or renal transplantation and such practical issues as continuous renal replacement therapy, attaining compliance to dietary prescription, and available food supplements and enteral nutrition preparations.

We have tried to make this book both a reference source for information on the derangements in nutrition and metabolism and a practical guide to the nutritional management of patients with renal disease. To this end, the authors of individual chapters were selected to have both scientific expertise and direct "hands on" experience with renal-related research and/or treatment of such patients.

We have attempted to organize this book so that each chapter stands by itself and provides the reader with a comprehensive understanding of the subject or management problem in question. In addition, topics in each chapter are cross-referenced to other chapters where the subject is discussed. We hope that the reader will find this book a scholarly yet practical resource for understanding and treating the nutritional disorders of the patient with renal disease or renal failure.

Appreciation is expressed to the staff at Williams & Wilkins and to our own secretarial and administrative staff for their efforts in bringing this book to fruition.

Joel D. Kopple
Shaul G. Massry

Preface to the First Edition

Preface

We are pleased to present the Second Edition of the book, *Nutritional Management of Renal Disease.* Many advances have occurred in the field of nutrition in nephrology since the publication of the first edition, and these advances have affected both the theoretical foundations of this discipline as well as specific methods of treatment in this field. Examples of these many changes include the following:

Our understanding of the pathogenesis and clinical consequences of nutritional disorders in individuals with renal disease and renal failure has increased enormously. The contribution of inflammation to malnutrition, morbidity, and mortality has become better defined. Moreover, the importance of managing cardiovascular disease and of controlling lipid metabolism, inflammation, and other risk factors for vascular disease for patients with chronic kidney disease or kidney failure has become much more evident. These advances have been associated with a much keener appreciation of the importance of encouraging a health enhancing lifestyle for these individuals. In this regard, our understanding of the benefits of exercise training for maintenance dialysis patients has become better defined. There have also been major improvements in methods of serum phosphorus control and in the prevention and treatment of hyperparathyroidism. In addition, the National Kidney Foundation Kidney Disease Dialysis Outcomes Quality Initiative (K/DOQI) *Clinical Practice Guidelines for Nutrition in Chronic Renal Failure* have been recently developed and published.

The use of more efficient methods of dialysis treatment—particularly the use of continuous renal replacement therapy—has become much more widespread for the management of patients who are critically ill and who have acute or chronic renal failure or other fluid, mineral, or nitrogen retaining states. Daily and longer-duration hemodialysis are becoming more frequently employed. Some of the benefits and hazards of using different growth factors for the treatment of acutely or chronically ill patients have become better defined. All of these advances, as well as others, have impelled us to develop the second edition of this book, and the nutritional issues relevant to these advances are discussed in detail in the appropriate chapters.

This book is designed to be both easily readable and, at the same time, to provide an extensively referenced work whereby the reader can seek out primary research data if he/she wishes to examine a subject more thoroughly. Most of the chapters in this book were not written by the editors, but rather by experts in specific fields. Authors are derived from 10 countries and from four continents: Asia, Australia, Europe, and North America.

We would like to express our appreciation and gratitude to these authors for the enormous effort that they have expended in bringing forth this book. Although we accept responsibility for any weaknesses in the organization and structure of the book, the credit for the scholarship and wisdom contained in this book rightfully belongs to the individual authors. We thank Lippincott Williams & Wilkins, and, in particular, their editors Tim Hiscock, Lisa Consoli, and Danielle Power for their superb technical support and encouragement that were so important for bringing this book to fruition.

Joel D. Kopple, M.D.
Shaul G. Massry, M.D.

KOPPLE AND MASSRY'S NUTRITIONAL MANAGEMENT OF RENAL DISEASE

SECOND EDITION

1

PROTEIN AND AMINO ACID METABOLISM IN RENAL DISEASE AND IN RENAL FAILURE

GIACOMO GARIBOTTO
NADIA PASTORINO
LAURA DERTENOIS

The mechanisms by which humans adapt their protein metabolism to nutritional and disease-associated conditions are finely tuned. However, substantial loss of lean body mass associated with organ dysfunction may be observed in several conditions, among which are renal diseases and renal failure. Weight loss, or decrease in lean body mass, commonly is observed in acute renal failure and nephrotic syndrome and, together with anorexia and weakness, when chronic uremia is advanced. Malnutrition has been attributed mainly to inadequate intake of nutrients and/or superimposed illnesses. However, a major question regards the effects that renal disease and its treatment(s) may have *per se* on amino acid and protein metabolism. In this review the major potential mechanisms for alterations in protein metabolism in renal diseases and renal failure are explored. Available evidence indicates that several factors that are intrinsic to renal diseases or are associated with different treatment modalities or comorbidities promote net protein catabolism in renal patients. These factors are different in patients at different stages of chronic renal failure (CRF) and modalities of treatments and act on different pathways of protein turnover and on different pools of visceral or somatic proteins.

INTRODUCTORY REMARKS AND METHODOLOGIC CONSIDERATIONS IN THE MEASURE OF WHOLE-BODY AND ORGAN PROTEIN TURNOVER

The body of a 70-kg man contains about 12 kg of protein and 200 to 250 g of free amino acids. Only 5 g of amino acids are present in the circulation, whereas about 130 g of the free amino acids are present intracellularly (1,2). Protein mainly is stored in skeletal muscle. The principal metabolic systems responsible for the maintenance of body protein and amino acid homeostasis are protein degradation, protein synthesis, amino acid oxidation (with production of CO_2), and amino acid synthesis of nonessential or conditionally essential amino acids (Fig. 1.1) (1,2). Changes in the rates of these metabolic processes cause adaptations in protein balance with the final effects on nitrogen (N) retention systems varying depending on the strength of the prevailing factor. (See Munro and Crim [1] and Young and Yu [2] for review.) In the human adult, despite the stability of body protein mass, body proteins turn over at a high rate. As much as 250 to 300 g of protein are degraded daily, and their constituent amino acids are in large part reutilized in protein synthesis. This fast and continuous catabolism and resynthesis of body protein accounts for about 70% to 80% of the turnover of free essential amino acids in the basal, postabsorptive state. The efficiency by which amino acids are recycled from protein breakdown is so high that, given the nutrient intake common in the Western countries, only 12 to 15 g of nitrogen are eliminated via urine daily, reflecting the net catabolism of about 70 to 90 g of protein (1, 2). These amino acids lost are to be replaced by the diet or synthesized by the body.

Conventionally, in humans protein metabolism and requirements have been investigated by the N balance technique. N balance is the net result of several metabolic reactions involved in the degradation and synthesis of protein, which does not give information on the processes of protein turnover. Rates of protein synthesis and degradation can be measured by determining amino acid incorporation into proteins or release from *in vivo* or isolated and perfused organs. Since the classic studies performed by Schoenheimer and coworkers in humans (3), a vast literature on protein metabolism both in the healthy and disease-associated conditions has been developed. Current techniques for the measure of protein turnover *in vivo* in humans are based on the isotopic dilution of a tracer (2,4). Different approaches to

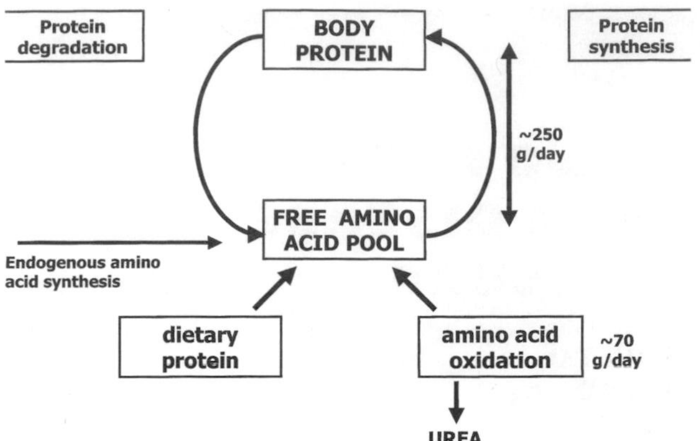

FIGURE 1.1. A schematic view of the major systems responsible for the maintenance of body protein homeostasis in humans.

the measurement of whole-body turnover that rely on several assumptions have been used (4). The major one is that the body amino acids consist of just two homogenous pools or compartments—one containing all the amino acids in proteins and the other containing the free amino acids in body fluids. By the most common approach, protein turnover rates (i.e., the rates of exchange of amino acids between these two compartments) are evaluated by introducing a labeled (either a radioactive or a stable isotope) amino acid into the free amino acid pool and studying its dilution by unlabeled amino acids from the degradation of endogenous or dietary proteins or its disappearance into oxidative pathways and synthesis. Because of its properties in the regulation of protein turnover, the essential amino acid L-leucine, labeled in the carboxyl position with ^{13}C or ^{14}C, has been studied the most. The decarboxylation of leucine is the first step of leucine degradation, and the produced $^{13}CO_2$ or $^{14}CO_2$ can be measured in the expired air (whole-body leucine oxidation).

The constant isotope infusion approach with whole-body sampling is easy to apply and requires only a few samples of arterial or arterialized blood. However, it yields no information on the individual roles of different components (i.e., tissue or organs) of the whole body. Therefore, it is difficult to extrapolate data obtained from whole-body sampling to protein metabolism in individual organs and tissues. To gain more information regarding the relative rates of protein turnover in specific organs and tissues, methods that combine the constant infusion of a tracer with the arteriovenous difference technique have been developed (5–7).

AMINO ACID AND PROTEIN METABOLISM IN THE HUMAN KIDNEY

Amino Acid Metabolism

The human kidney is actively involved in the homeostasis of body amino acid pools. This is achieved through the synthesis, degradation, filtration, reabsorption, and urinary excretion of amino acids. In the normal condition a great amount of amino acids (about 50 to 70 g/day) is filtered and almost completely (97% to 98%) reabsorbed by the proximal tubules (8,9).

Studies based on amino acid balance across the human kidney have shown that in the postabsorptive state there is a net renal uptake or release of several amino acids (9–12). Moreover, after the infusion of amino acids, the kidney plays a considerable role in their removal from blood (12). The kidney is the major organ for the disposal of glutamine from the arterial blood. Nitrogen derived from extracted glutamine is used for ammonia formation (1,10,11). Recent studies in humans indicate the occurrence of considerable organ specificity in the use of glutamine and alanine, the major gluconeogenic amino acids. Glutamine mainly is used by the kidney, whereas alanine mainly is used by the liver (13). Almost 80% of gluconeogenesis from body glutamine takes place in the kidney, and the production of glucose by the human kidney accounts for as much as 25% of glucose rate of appearance in the whole body. This amount is fairly matched by a similar amount of glucose used by the kidney itself (13). Therefore, in only a few situations does the kidney export glucose to other tissues (13).

The kidney also plays a major role in synthesis of nonessential amino acids, such as serine, tyrosine, and arginine, which are released into the renal veins and exported to other tissues (8–11). The magnitude of the net release or uptake of amino acids by the normal kidney can be understood if one considers that in a 70-kg man the daily net production of serine is approximately 3 to 4 g; it is approximately 1 g of tyrosine and approximately 2 g of arginine. Besides that, the kidney also releases smaller amounts (less than 1 g/day) of threonine, lysine, taurine, and leucine into the systemic circulation (10,11).

Some of the amino acids exported by the kidney are not newly synthesized but may derive from intrarenal peptide degradation. The release of serine may be an example of this process. In the postabsorptive state the human kidney takes up only small amounts of glycine (the precursor for serine synthesis) from the circulation, and there is no stoichiometry between the uptake of glycine and the release of serine (9–11). The intrarenal catabolism of glutathione, sarcosine, or other peptides or low–molecular-weight proteins could provide the kidney with precursors for net serine synthesis (8). It is noteworthy that in humans the kidney is the only organ that releases serine into the systemic circulation (8,10,11). The supply of serine from the kidney to other tissues is almost constant and persists during hyperaminoacidemia or metabolic acidosis (8,11).

Other amino acids are converted into the final product from a precursor that is taken up from the arterial blood. This takes place for tyrosine, the release of which has been reported to be lower (10) or strictly stoichiometric (14) with the uptake of phenylalanine. In the general, healthy population, tyrosine is not considered to be indispensable because it is produced from phenylalanine by the activity of phenylalanine hydroxylase, an enzyme located mainly in the liver, pancreas, and kidney (15). In animals the activity of the enzyme appears to be small in the kidney, suggesting a relatively minor role of this organ in the hydroxylation of phenylalanine (15). However, recent studies that have used stable tyrosine and phenylalanine isotopes to track the metabolic pathways of phenylalanine indicate that the human kidney plays a role greater than previously presumed in the metabolism of this amino acid (16,17). Actually, the phenylalanine hydroxylation activity across the kidney appears to be similar or even greater than that across the splanchnic area (17,18). According to Tessari et al. (16), hydroxylation accounts for more than two-thirds of renal phenylalanine disposal, indicating that the major fate of the phenylalanine taken up by the kidney is *de novo* formation of tyrosine. It is noteworthy that the release of tyrosine by the healthy kidney is similar in amounts to those deriving from protein breakdown in muscle (6,10,14,18). Tyrosine produced *"de novo"* in the kidney or released by protein breakdown by peripheral tissues is used by splanchnic organs for synthetic processes and/or for oxidation (16).

Another example of metabolic substrate interconversion in the human kidney is given by the conversion of citrulline, which is taken up by the arterial blood, into arginine. Arginine, in addition to its role in protein synthesis, plays multiple roles: it is the precursor of nitric oxide (NO), creatine, agmatine, and other polyamines and is an intermediate in the urea cycle. The net production of arginine within the kidney is as much as 10% to 12% of the total appearance of arginine within the body (3).

The kidney also is involved in the metabolism of sulfur amino acids. A net release of taurine and cysteine has been observed to occur in the renal vein (10,11). Homocysteine metabolism appears to be different in rat and human kidneys. Whereas in rats homocysteine is taken up actively by the kidney (19), no significant arteriovenous difference for free and protein-bound homocysteine has been shown to occur in humans (20).

The human kidney is also an important site for the catabolism of low–molecular-weight (molecular weight less than 50,000) plasma proteins and peptides (such as insulin, C-peptide, growth hormone [GH], leptin, and other peptide hormones) but not of intermediate–molecular-weight proteins, such as immunoglobulin G (molecular weight 160,000). Because the glomerulus allows the filtration only of those proteins with a molecular weight of less than 50,000, the catabolism of plasma proteins by the kidney seems to occur by glomerular filtration and subsequent tubular reabsorption. Dipeptides can be taken up into proximal tubule cells by an active-transport mechanism or are cleared in the brush border of the proximal tubule (8,21).

KIDNEY PROTEIN TURNOVER AND ITS RELATION TO WHOLE-BODY PROTEIN METABOLISM

During adult life, kidney size and protein content are maintained fairly constant, indicating that processes of protein synthesis and degradation within the kidney are regulated tightly. However, several changes in kidney protein turnover may occur in response to physiologic and pathologic stimuli (21). Amino acids, the substrates for protein synthesis, are provided to the kidney via several routes. Similarly to other organs, amino acids can reach the kidney cells via arterial blood flow. However, at variance with other organs, the tubule cells are provided with amino acids both from luminal and antiluminal sites (7,21,22). Moreover, an additional source of amino acids comes from the degradation of reabsorbed low–molecular-weight proteins filtered by the glomerulus. Data reported in 1999 suggest that kidney protein turnover is partly dependent on this process (22). Tessari et al. evaluated protein metabolism across the human kidney by ^{14}C-leucine kinetics (Fig. 1.2) (14). The rate of leucine appearance from the kidney (an index of protein degradation) was slightly higher than the rate of disposal. Oxidation of leucine by the kidney was high, representing about 55% of total disposal. Nonoxidative disposal of leucine, an index of protein synthesis, was markedly lower than the rate of appearance. Considering the net balance of leucine (and thereby of protein), these data show that in the postabsorptive state the human kidney is in a state of a negative balance. According to a compartmental model of leucine metabolism, leucine entering the renal cells is only 6% of arterial supply, with the largest portion of arterial delivery released into the renal vein. According to this model, the major portion of leucine appearance into the cell is derived from intrarenal protein degradation. These data suggest a greater dependency of kidney protein synthesis on the leucine supplied from endogenous protein breakdown than from arterial delivery. The high amount of CO_2 produced within

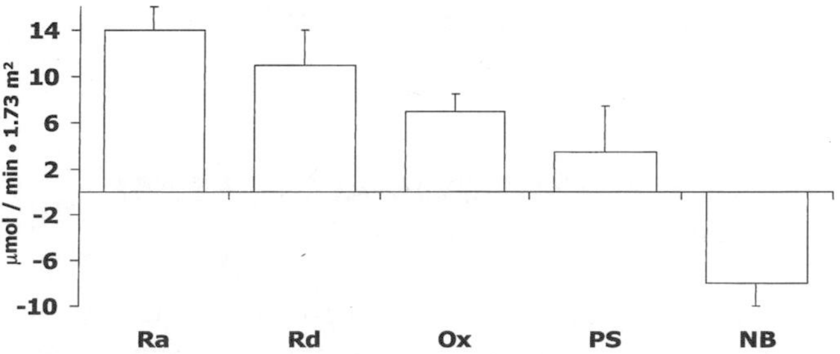

FIGURE 1.2. Leucine metabolism across the human kidney. Ra, rate of appearance (an expression of protein degradation); Rd, rate of disposal (protein synthesis + leucine oxidation); Ox, oxidation; PS, protein synthesis; NB, Net leucine (protein) balance. (From Tessari P, Garibotto G, Inchiostro S, et al. Kidney, splanchnic, and leg protein turnover in humans. Insight from leucine and phenylalanine kinetics. *J Clin Invest* 1996;98:1481–1492, with permission.)

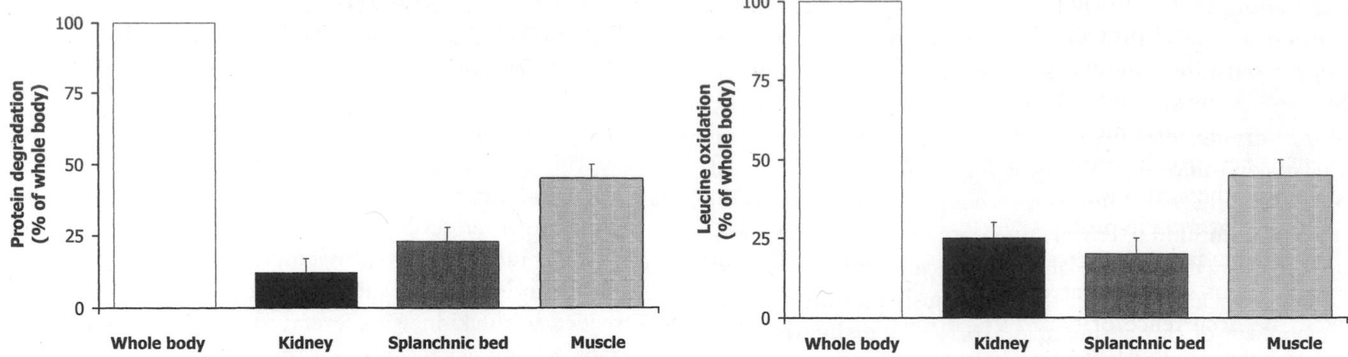

FIGURE 1.3. The contribution of individual organs to whole-body protein degradation and leucine oxidation. (From Gelfand RA, Glickman MG, Castellino P, et al. Measurement of L-[1-14C]leucine kinetics in splanchnic and leg tissues in humans. Effect of amino acid infusion. *Diabetes* 1988; 37:1365–1372, with permission; and Tessari P, Garibotto G, Inchiostro S, et al. Kidney, splanchnic, and leg protein turnover in humans. Insight from leucine and phenylalanine kinetics. *J Clin Invest* 1996;98:1481–1492, with permission.)

the kidney from leucine is derived partly from leucine released from endogenous proteolysis and partly from ketoisocaproic acid (the product of transamination of leucine) taken up from the arterial blood (14). Given the entity of the negative protein balance and leucine oxidation by the human kidney, it has been supposed that this is not the result of the catabolism of renal structural proteins; instead, it mainly is the result of degradation of filtered peptides and small-weight proteins (14,22).

Fig. 1.3 shows the individual roles of kidney, splanchnic organs, and muscle in whole-body protein degradation and leucine oxidation. Even if muscle fractional protein synthesis and oxidation, expressed per gram of tissue, are low (about 1% to 2%), the whole-muscle mass accounts for as much as 32% to 36% of whole-body protein degradation (Fig. 1.3) (6,14). Splanchnic organs make up about 22% of whole-body protein degradation. The percent contribution of the human kidney to whole-body protein degradation is approximately 10%. According to these results, the kidney plays a major role in leucine (hence in protein) catabolism because 25% of whole-body leucine oxidation takes place within the kidney versus 48% to 50% in muscle and 18% in splanchnic organs.

PROTEIN TURNOVER IN ACUTE RENAL FAILURE

Patients with acute renal failure (ARF) are frequently catabolic (23). ARF is often a complication of trauma, sepsis, or multiple organ failure, which on their own affect protein and amino acid metabolism and cause several alterations, including increased energy expenditure, loss of protein stores, malnutrition, susceptibility to infections, and impaired wound healing (24). However, studies in experimental models indicate that ARF *per se* can induce alterations in protein and amino acid metabolism that can contribute to wasting and dysfunction.

Protein and Amino Acid Metabolism in Uncomplicated Acute Renal Failure

It is interesting that, even if ARF as an isolated disease is common, there is no study dealing with the effect of uncomplicated ARF on protein turnover in humans and our current knowledge comes from studies performed in animals with experimental acute uremia. *In vitro* and *in vivo* studies in rats have shown that in ARF the rate of ureagenesis is accelerated (24,25) and is blocked only partially when animals are fed with glucose (26). Lacy (26) showed that the liver of acutely uremic rats removed from the perfusate had increased amounts of amino acids, when compared to sham-operated animals. Moreover, Frohlich et al. (27) observed that increased ureagenesis was associated with increased glucose production in the liver in rats with ARF. Initially, studies suggested that the degradation of endogenous liver proteins and/or amino acid could provide the substrates for both urea and glucose production. However, Bondy et al. found that the hepatic increase in urea synthesis in rats with ARF was prevented partially by adrenalectomy (28), suggesting that glucocorticoids are responsible for the increased net catabolism in ARF.

Specific changes in muscle-protein metabolism taking place in rats with ARF have been shown in different laboratories. Both Clark and Mitch (29,30) and Flugel-Link et al. (31) observed an increased release of amino acids from the isolated perfused hindquarter of rats with ARF. To study whether abnormal protein and carbohydrate metabolism are linked in ARF, the effects of insulin on net muscle-protein degradation and glucose uptake were measured in the perfused hindquarters of paired ARF and sham-operated rats (29). At an early stage of ARF glucose uptake was depressed significantly and muscle-protein degradation increased; moreover, rates of protein degradation were only partially responsive to the insulin's antiproteolytic effect (29). This indicates the occurrence of early, concurrent alterations in protein and glucose metabolism. However, after 48 hours of ARF, net protein breakdown increased further because protein synthesis also was depressed (29). Flugel-Link et al. observed that muscle-protein synthesis was not altered, but protein degradation was greater in the hindquarters of acute uremic versus sham-operated rats (31). These results indicated the occurrence of two different alterations that can cause catabolism in ARF: an increase in protein degradation (which appears to be the consequence of altered glucose metabolism and is stimulated by glucorticoids) and a decrease in protein synthesis.

The enhanced protein degradation in acutely uremic rats does not appear to be the result of increased muscle cathepsin B1, cathepsin D, or alkaline protease activities (31). Therefore, activation of lysosomal proteolysis by ARF also seems unlikely. The stimulation of Ca^{2+}-activated proteolysis also seems unlikely because inhibition of this pathway does not correct the accelerated proteolysis in the skeletal muscle of rats with ARF. In 1998, Price et al. provided several lines of evidence indicating that adenosine triphosphate (ATP) and ubiquitin-dependent proteolytic pathway are responsible for an increase in muscle-protein degradation in ARF (32). In addition, these authors observed that the activity of branched-chain ketoacid dehydrogenase (which is the rate-limiting enzyme for branched-chain amino acid [BCAA] oxidation and catabolism) was severalfold increased in skeletal muscle from acutely uremic rats.

There is also clear evidence from experimental studies in animals that acute uremia in muscle depresses amino acid uptake. Arnold and Holliday observed that both basal and insulin-stimulated uptake of α-amino-isobutyrric acid (a nonmetabolizable analogue of alanine) was diminished in muscle of rats with ARF (33). The occurrence of such a defect could aggravate net protein catabolism by decreasing muscle-protein synthesis and thereby causing loss of muscle proteins. More recently, Maroni et al. demonstrated that the insulin-response curve was altered in muscle of rats with ARF, with physiologic concentrations of insulin-stimulating methyl-aminoisobutyric acid (MeAIB) uptake staying normal, whereas both basal and maximal insulin-stimulated MeAIB uptake was lower in muscles from rats with ARF (34).

All these observations support the conclusion that the activation of ATP-dependent ubiquitin–proteasome proteolytic pathway and changes in amino acid transport and catabolism contribute to the accelerated loss of muscle observed in acutely uremic rats. Metabolic acidosis also can contribute to accelerating the catabolic processes because acidosis occurs commonly in patients with ARF not only because the elimination of H^+ is diminished, but also because there is an increase in net protein breakdown, with an increased production of H^+.

Protein and Amino Acid Metabolism in Trauma and Sepsis

In patients with trauma or sepsis, the picture is one of rapid muscle loss with an increased liver synthesis of acute-phase proteins (3,35). Studies of protein turnover in patients with injury have shown that whole-body protein degradation is stimulated, whereas whole-body protein synthesis is increased to a lesser degree (2,35). An increase in the activity of the ubiquitin–proteasome dependent proteolytic pathway has been shown to occur both in septic animals (36) and humans (37). Other proteolytic systems, such as the lysosomal and Ca^{2+}-activated systems, have been reported in patients with head trauma (38).

Sepsis and injury cause both hormone and immune responses, which can interact with the regulation of amino acid and protein metabolism. The hormone response to sepsis and injury is characterized by the release of counterregulatory hormones such as glucagon, cathecholamines, GH, and glucocorticoids (3,35), which can lead to loss of lean body mass. The immune response is represented mainly by the secretion of several proinflammatory cytokines, such as tumor necrosis factor (TNF), interleukin-6 (IL-6), and IL-1, which could cause catabolism (35,39). Some *in vitro* studies have shown that these cytokines *per se* are not able to provoke a direct catabolic event (35). Results from experiments in rats adrenalectomized or treated with mifepristone (RU 486) suggest that TNF exerts most of its catabolic effects on muscle-protein breakdown through the release of glucocorticoids, whereas IL-1 causes net catabolism through a mechanism not yet identified (35,40). It is worth noting that there is an interaction between the inflammatory and hormone responses, with some cytokines (such as IL-1) stimulating the synthesis of glucocorticoids via the hypothalamus. Glucocorticoids on their own may reduce the secretion of inflammatory cytokines in a feedback system that could protect the body from negative tissue levels of cytokine release (35,41).

Another possibility is that acute injury causes protein wasting by decreasing muscle-protein synthesis through the inhibition of some circulating growth factor(s). In response to infection or injection of proinflammatory cytokines, the plasma concentration of insulin like growth factor-1 (IGF-1) is markedly reduced (42), whereas that of plasma and muscle IGF-binding protein 1 (IGFBP-1) is increased dramatically (43). In human skeletal muscle cells, IGFBP-1 inhibits IGF-stimulated protein synthesis and overall rates of protein turnover (44).

Changes in amino acid metabolism caused by trauma or sepsis also can favor a catabolic response. Muscle is an important site for glutamine production, which is used for protein synthesis or exported to the splanchnic organs and cells of the immune system. The increased glutamine release in sepsis could induce a muscle glutamine depletion, which can depress protein synthesis (45). Moreover, sepsis can inhibit glutamine transport, with depletion of intracellular pools of this amino acid (46).

Is It Possible to Restrict Catabolism in ARF?

During catabolic injuries there is a loss of cell mass and fat, with progressive expansion of the extracellular fluid compartment. Although feeding catabolic patients can diminish the rate of protein and fat loss, it does not prevent the occurrence of a negative balance (47). Studies have shown significant losses of body proteins despite "adequate" or "supraadequate" energy diets (1,47,48). Progressive understanding of the mechanisms causing excessive protein metabolism in ARF, sepsis, and trauma has led to study of the effects of new therapeutic agents to restrict catabolism. Studies have evaluated the effects of inhibitors of proteolytic pathways or of growth factors. Clinical studies indicate that excessive whole-body or muscle net catabolism in patients with acute injury can be reversed by the administration of growth factors, such as GH, IGF-I, or both (49–51). (For extensive review of this issue, see Chapters 5, 30, and 32.)

Metabolic alterations leading to loss of lean body mass in ARF could overlap with those arising from net catabolism induced by the process of hemodialysis itself. It has been suggested that the type of dialyzer membrane used in patients with ARF may have an impact on clinical outcomes, such as sepsis, recovery of renal function, and death (52). In this regard biocompatible (synthetic) membranes appear to induce a less inflammatory response and may offer an advantage in these patients (52,53).

Chronic Renal Failure and End-Stage Renal Disease

Weight loss, with decreased lean and fat mass, may be observed frequently in patients undergoing maintenance hemodialysis (MHD) or peritoneal dialysis (PD) (54). Cross-sectional findings suggest that in patients with chronic renal disease, dietary protein and energy intakes, as well as nutritional indices, progressively decline as the glomerular filtration rate (GFR) decreases, with signs of protein and calorie malnutrition becoming overt when GFR is less than 10 mL/min (55). In a prospective analysis Ikizler et al. (56) observed that the decline in spontaneous protein intake progressed along with the decrease in renal function, with intakes less than 0.6 g/kg when creatinine clearance was less than 10 mL/min. Anorexia therefore plays an important role in malnutrition and likely can be a confounding factor in the evaluation of results from studies on protein turnover in patients with advanced CRF. Several factors, such as altered amino acid metabolism, acidosis, hormone alterations, dialytic treatment by itself, and a chronic inflammatory state, are considered to play individually different roles in the wasting syndrome of patients with end-stage renal disease (ESRD).

Alterations in Amino Acid Metabolism

Patients with CRF present several abnormalities in blood and, to a lesser degree, muscle amino acid profiles (18,56, 57). The plasma concentration of nonessential amino acids has been reported to be abnormally high, whereas that of several essential amino acids has been reported to be abnormally low (57,58). Moreover, the distribution of some amino acids between the extracellular and intracellular compartment is altered (58). Typical alterations in plasma amino acid levels in patients with moderately advanced CRF and nonreduced protein intakes are increased levels of citrulline, 1- and 3-methylhistidine, proline, glycine, and cysteine and homocysteine and decreased levels of valine, serine, and tyrosine (56,58–61). In patients with advanced CRF, plasma leucine levels also decline (18). The free tryptophan plasma level is in the normal range, but total tryptophan is decreased, owing to reduced binding to proteins (62). The abnormality in the pattern of plasma amino acids resembles that observed in malnutrition and can be aggravated further by low nutrient intake. However, BCAAs, mainly valine, are lower in plasma in patients with CRF than in controls with the same protein intake, indicating the occurrence of metabolic abnormalities induced by kidney failure *per se* (18,60).

The loss of metabolizing renal tissue can account for several of the amino acid abnormalities found in CRF. Some amino acids, such as 3-methylhistidine and 1-methylhistidine, increase in blood because of their reduced clearance. Moreover, in patients with CRF the synthesis of several amino acids newly generated within the kidney, such as arginine, serine, and tyrosine, is reduced (10). The abnormal arginine supply to tissues in uremia may have detrimental effects because arginine is the precursor for NO. A diminished availability of NO may be implicated in the genesis of hypertension and the function and integrity of endothelial cells, with implications for atherosclerotic processes (63). Moreover, NO is a mediator for several hormones, including IGF-I and GH, and a reduced NO availability could cause reduced hormone effects (64). However, a decrease in arginine levels is observed in patients with ESRD only during acute illnesses (65), suggesting the existence of sources of arginine other than the kidney. Lau et al. (66) have examined plasma kinetics of arginine and assessed the activity of the L-arginine–NO pathway in adults with ESRD before and after hemodialysis. In the postabsorptive state endogenous leucine and arginine fluxes were similar, whereas the citrulline fluxes were four to five times higher in patients with ESRD than in the healthy controls. This is intriguing and suggests organs other than the kidney are able to maintain the homeostasis of arginine in ESRD. If and to what extent NO production is inhibited in uremia is unclear, however. Other authors observed that total NO excretion and production are lower in uremic patients (67, 68).

In patients with moderate-advanced CRF the renal release of tyrosine is reduced and directly correlates with tyrosine blood levels, suggesting that the depressed production of tyrosine by the kidney plays a major role in decreasing blood levels of this amino acid in CRF (10). Some homeostatic phenomena both in the diseased kidney and splanchnic organs to restore tyrosine pools occur in patients with CRF (69). However, these are more accommodating than fully compensatory responses, which are not able to prevent tyrosine pools from being depleted in uremic patients. Tyrosine therefore can be considered a "conditionally essential" amino acid in patients with CRF (69).

The renal output of serine, as well as arterial and muscle levels of this amino acid, are reduced in CRF (10,60,61). Moreover, the forearm muscle does not take up serine from the arterial blood, contrary to the healthy condition (70). Whether this defect is the result of decreased levels of serine owing to defective renal synthesis or to a specific defect of transport of serine by muscle is unknown. Serine depletion may be a limiting factor for protein synthesis in circulating cells, as shown by *in vitro* studies (71).

In patients with CRF, a reduced release of valine and leucine from muscle is likely responsible for their reduced levels in blood (18,70). The release of valine from peripheral tissues is diminished even if compared to the release of phenylalanine, lysine, or tyrosine, which are markers of net protein breakdown (70). It is possible that an increased muscle degradation of valine, probably resulting from metabolic acidosis and/or an impaired glucose utilization, accounts for the low release of this amino acid from peripheral tissues. Studies in rats with CRF indicate that the correction of metabolic acidosis raises both plasma and muscle BCAA levels by decreasing the transamination and decarboxylation in muscle (72). Studies in humans are in agreement with these findings (73–75). During the course of CRF, abnormalities resulting from decreased nutrient intake overlap with those caused by acidosis, and the declining plasma valine levels have been reported as an index of poor nutrition and reduced lean body mass (76).

An abnormal pattern of sulphur plasma amino acids has been described in patients with CRF (77,78). Both free and protein-bound cysteine and homocysteine and cysteinsulphinic acid (CSA) have been reported to be high in plasma of uremic patients, whereas methionine is normal and taurine is low (77,79). In muscle, major alterations regard reduced pools of taurine and increased pools of methionine (79). The causes for the low muscle taurine levels are still unknown; an interesting possibility is an inhibition of CSA decarboxylase (79). In patients with CRF there is also a decreased fractional uptake of cysteine by peripheral tissues, and this alteration may be at least in part responsible for the increase in blood of the same amino acid (70). The consequences of the reduced intracellular taurine pools in renal patients are not known. Taurine may have a role as an antioxidant and in muscle contractility and is involved in a wide range of metabolic effects in the brain and retina (80).

Amino acids, besides protein constituents, serve multiple and diverse physiologic functions. It is possible that the abnormal cellular amino acid metabolism contributes to toxicity and to alterations of the immune and signal-transduction functions in renal patients. Moreover, uremic patients may have increased nutritional requirements for some amino acids, of which the synthesis by the kidney is decreased. It is worth noting that after the administration of amino acids orally (81) or intraperitonally (82) in patients with CRF or those undergoing continuous ambulatory peritoneal dialysis (CAPD), the uptake by muscle of tyrosine and leucine is low in relation to the composition of mixed-muscle protein. This suggests that a reduced supply of these amino acids increases protein requirements and decreases the efficient use of amino acid supplements. The use of specially designed amino acid supplements has been found to be associated with a more positive N balance (83) in patients with CRF. However, specific isotope–kinetics-based studies on the requirements for individual amino acids for patients with CRF or ESRD are not available.

PROTEIN METABOLISM IN CRF

Experimental Models of CRF

Most investigations on the effects of chronic uremia on protein metabolism have been performed in rats and include both *in vitro* and *in vivo* studies. In all studies, rats with CRF present abnormal protein turnover as expressed by decreased growth and increased muscle net release of essential amino acids and urea production (84–88). Garber et al. (85) found an increase in the release of glutamine and alanine from incubated muscle of rats with CRF, which suggested the occurrence of an increase in protein degradation. Moreover, protein synthesis was reduced. Harter et al. (86) showed an increase in the release of tyrosine and phenylalanine (amino acids that are not metabolized in muscle, and their release expresses net protein breakdown) from incubated muscle of rats with CRF in comparison with controls; muscle net protein breakdown was greater when rats ingested diets containing 10% casein, suggesting that a low-protein intake could increase muscle-protein catabolism in uremia. In starved uremic rats Holliday et al. found that protein synthesis declined to a greater extent than in controls (87); moreover, when rats were fed following a period of stress, muscle-protein synthesis was depressed again. Li and Wassner (88) observed that, in perfused hemicorpus preparations, uremic rats lost more weight than control rats; the accelerated weight loss resulted from lower rates of protein synthesis and higher rates of protein degradation. Moreover, changes in body lipid content correlated with the rate of protein degradation both in control and uremic rats, suggesting that protein degradation rates are linked to energy metabolism. In addition to the amount of protein in the diet, the amino acid composition of diets also can influence growth of uremic rats. Pennisi et al. (89) observed that a diet consisting of essential amino acids results in greater growth suppression and accelerated ureagenesis if compared to isonitrogenous diets composed of mixtures of essential and nonessential amino acids or casein.

The accelerated wasting observed in uremic rats has been attributed to excess parathyroid hormone (90) or defective 25(OH)D_3 synthesis (91). More recently, metabolic acidosis has been shown to play a major role in increasing protein degradation in uremic rats. (See Chapter 9 for an extensive review.) It has been found that the ATP-dependent, ubiquitin-requiring pathway is the most important pathway activated by acidosis (92). This proteolytic pathway has been found to be increased in muscle during sepsis, denervation, cancer, burns, and starvation (35). Thus the mechanisms being elucidated for acidosis appear relevant to the loss of body proteins in a variety of other catabolic states. Metabolic acidosis, besides its effects on increasing protein degradation, causes a resistance to the action of anabolic hormones, such as GH and IGF-I (93).

Whole-Body Protein Metabolism in Patients with CRF

Only in a few studies has whole-body protein turnover been measured in patients with CRF and results compared with those of healthy, adult individuals (Table 1.1). All studies included clinically stable patients, in which protein turnover was examined in the basal, postabsorptive state. On one hand, Goodship et al. (94), by using ^{15}N-,^{13}C-leucine, did not find any difference in whole-body protein synthesis, degradation, and amino acid oxidation in nonacidotic patients with moderately severe CRF (GFR 11.4 mL/min, range 8.7 to 21.4 mL/min) ingesting diets containing 1 g protein/kg and 32 kcal/kg. Similar data were obtained by Adey et al. (95) in patients with CRF and iothalamate clearances ranging from 8 to 60 mL/min. On the other hand, Castellino et al. (96), by using ^{14}C-leucine kinetics, reported decreased rates of synthesis, degradation, and leucine oxidation, with resultant reduced net protein catabolism in nonacidemic patients with CRF (creatinine clearance 24, range 10 to 43 mL/min) ingesting 1.1 g/protein/kg. In a longitudinal study, Lim et al. (97) evaluated protein turnover rates by ^{13}C-leucine kinetics in patients with advanced CRF before and after alkali treatment. When acidosis was treated, rates of protein turnover were lower than in control subjects. In this study patients had a 25% lower protein intake than control subjects. Overall, results from these studies indicate that in clinically stable patients with CRF in whom acidosis has been prevented, whole-body rates of protein degradation and synthesis are normal or lower than normal. Net protein balance (the result of the difference from synthesis and degradation) is either normal or decreased.

A few studies regard patients with ESRD—either patients undergoing MHD or PD—and their results are somewhat conflicting. Berkelhammer et al. (98) evaluated protein turnover by ^{13}C-leucine kinetics in robust patients undergoing MHD. Protein and calorie intake (about 1 g/kg and 30 to 40 kcal/kg, respectively) was similar in patients and controls. They observed that protein degradation was normal, but net protein balance was more negative than in controls because leucine oxidation was greater than in control subjects. It is noteworthy that patients had metabolic acidosis (mean HCO_3 = 17 mmol/L), and this could have

TABLE 1.1. WHOLE-BODY PROTEIN TURNOVER IN PATIENTS WITH CHRONIC RENAL FAILURE OR END-STAGE RENAL DISEASE AS COMPARED TO HEALTHY CONTROLS, IN THE POSTABSORPTIVE STATE

Author	Tracer	Degradation	Oxidation	Synthesis	Balance
Patients with chronic renal failure					
Castellino et al. (96)	^{14}C-leucine	Reduced	Reduced	Reduced	Less negative
Goodship et al. (94)	^{13}C-leucine	Normal	Normal	Normal	Similar to controls
Lim et al. (97)	^{13}C-leucine	Reduced	Reduced	Reduced	Less negative
Adey et al. (95)	^{13}C-leucine	Normal	Normal	Normal	Similar to controls
Patients undergoing maintenance hemodialysis					
Berkelammer et al. (98)	^{13}C-leucine	Normal	Increased	Decreased	More negative
Lau et al. (66)	^{13}C-leucine	Normal	Reduced	Normal	Less negative
Lim et al. (99)	^{13}C-leucine	Normal	—	—	—
Giordano et al. (100)	^{2}H-leucine	Increased	—	—	—
Patients undergoing continuous ambulatory peritoneal dialysis					
Goodship et al. (101)	^{13}C-leucine	Decreased	Decreased	Decreased	Less negative
Castellino et al. (102)	^{14}C-leucine	Decreased	Decreased	Decreased	Less negative

TABLE 1.2. EFFECTS OF TREATMENT OF METABOLIC ACIDOSIS ON WHOLE-BODY PROTEIN METABOLISM IN PATIENTS WITH CRF AND ESRD

Author	Tracer	Degradation	Oxidation	Synthesis	Condition
Reaich et al. (75)	^{13}C-leucine	Reduced	Reduced	Reduced	CRF
Lim et al. (97)	^{13}C-leucine	Reduced	Reduced	Unchanged	CRF
Graham et al. (104)	^{13}C-leucine	Reduced	Unchanged	Reduced	CAPD
Graham et al. (105)	^{13}C-leucine	Reduced	Unchanged	Reduced	MHD

CRF, chronic renal failure; ESRD, end-stage renal disease; CAPD, continuous ambulatory peritoneal dialysis; MHD, maintenance hemodialysis.

accounted for the increased rates of leucine oxidation. However, whole-body protein degradation, again by using ^{13}C-leucine kinetics, has been reported to be normal (99), and leucine oxidation is normal (99) or decreased (66) in nonacidemic patients undergoing MHD. In 2001 Giordano et al. (100), using ^{2}H-leucine, observed increased whole-body protein degradation in nonmalnourished, nonacidemic patients undergoing MHD.

Two studies are available on whole-body leucine turnover in patients treated with CAPD. Goodship et al. (101) demonstrated by the ^{14}C-leucine kinetics that leucine flux, leucine oxidation, and nonoxidative disposal were all lower in fed patients undergoing CAPD. Patients showed a lower net catabolism than controls. Because patients ingested a lower protein intake than controls, this might have influenced the results. In 1999 Castellino et al. (102) again observed a reduced overall protein turnover in patients undergoing CAPD in the postabsorptive state. Analogous to whole-body studies, muscle-protein turnover rates have been reported to be in the low-normal range in patients treated with CAPD (82).

In children with CRF, rates of whole-body protein degradation are related to bicarbonate levels, suggesting that acidosis plays a major role in increasing protein degradation (103). Table 1.2 summarizes the results of studies on the treatment of metabolic acidosis on protein metabolism in patients with CRF or ESRD. Reaich at al. (75) observed that correcting metabolic acidosis by administering $NaHCO_3$ for 4 weeks to patients with CRF was followed by a 28% to 29% decrease in protein degradation and leucine oxidation, with no change in rates of protein synthesis (Fig 1.4). Graham et al., in two sequential studies (104,105), evaluated the effects of treating metabolic acidosis in patients treated with MHD or PD, respectively. At the baseline, these patients presented values for protein degradation and synthesis that were elevated if compared to values reported in the literature in healthy subjects (3,4,106). A marked decrease in protein degradation and synthesis was observed after correction of acidemia. It is worth noting that no effect on leucine oxidation was observed; however, these subjects presented very low rates of basal leucine oxidation (about 9% of basal protein degradation).

Taken together, these studies indicate that whole-body protein turnover in patients with ESRD is altered variably. If metabolic acidosis occurs, an alteration in the mechanisms controlling protein balance is shown by an increase in leucine oxidation and/or protein degradation. In the absence of acidosis, the picture is that of whole-body protein turnover

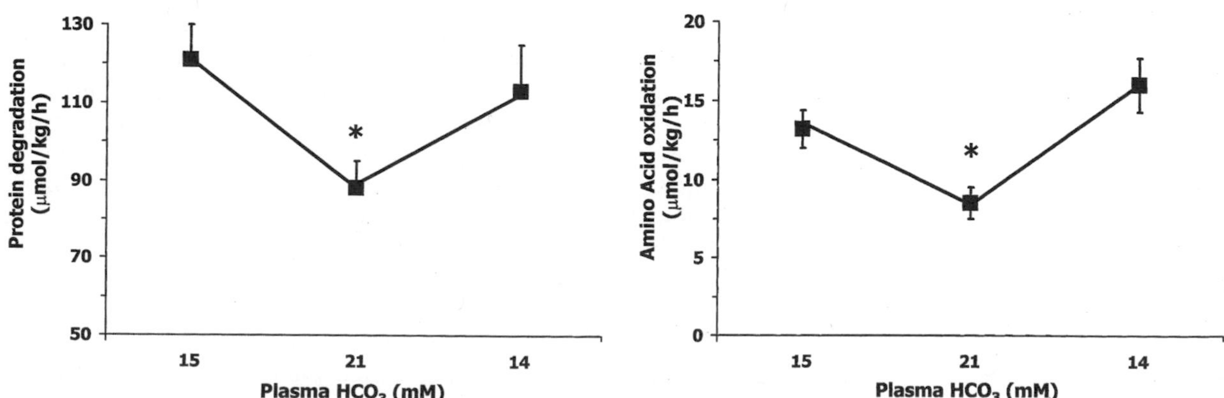

FIGURE 1.4. Rates of whole-body protein degradation (*left panel*) and leucine oxidation (*right panel*) in patients with chronic renal failure before and after 4 weeks of treatment with sodium bicarbonate or saline. (From Reaich D, Channon SM, Scrimgeour CM, et al. Correction of acidosis in humans with CRF decreases protein degradation and amino acid oxidation. *Am J Physiol* 1993; 265:E230–E235, with permission.)

parameters normal or lower than in the healthy condition. The reduced metabolic activity of the diseased kidney may account for the decrease in leucine oxidation and amino acid appearance. A decrease in nutrient intake also is postulated to decrease protein turnover rates. Moreover, hyperinsulinemia, commonly observed in patients with ESRD, mainly in patients undergoing PD, may account for reduced leucine appearance and oxidation rates (107).

Muscle Protein Turnover

Early studies examining net amino acid exchange across peripheral tissues in nonmalnourished patients with moderate-advanced CRF (creatinine clearance 10 to 30 mL/min) matched with controls eating similar diets (18,108) failed to show an increase in net muscle breakdown, at variance with data obtained in experimental models of uremia in animals. Also, Alvestrand et al. (109) observed that in patients treated with MHD the release of amino acids from the lower limb leg was not increased.

More recently, mixed muscle-protein synthesis and degradation have been evaluated by the measurement of the 3H-phenylalanine kinetics in patients with moderately advanced CRF (70). Patients were not malnourished, and protein intake was between 0.9 and 1.0 g/kg. Metabolic acidosis was observed in eight of nine patients (mean HCO_3 = 20 mmol/L). Net protein balance across the forearm was negative and was similar to controls because protein degradation was greater than protein synthesis. However, rates of muscle-protein turnover were greater than in control subjects, analogous to what was observed in whole-body protein turnover studies in patients with CRF and metabolic acidosis (104,105). Inverse correlations were observed between net protein balance and blood bicarbonate (and the ratio of protein synthesis to protein degradation and blood bicarbonate as well), suggesting that acidosis is responsible for the more negative protein balance (Fig 1.5). It is interesting that, when muscle-protein turnover was evaluated in patients with similar degrees of CRF but without acidemia, rates of muscle-protein turnover were similar to controls (110). These results are in accordance with observations in the whole body, showing that protein degradation is increased in patients with CRF with metabolic acidosis. Moreover, basal rates of synthesis and degradation of mixed-muscle proteins appear to be in the normal range if acidosis is corrected in nonmalnourished patients with CRF and unrestricted nutrient intakes.

The measurements of amino acid kinetics associated with the limb perfusion made in these studies represent the average of synthetic rates of all muscle proteins. In 2000 Adey et al. (95) measured the synthesis rate of myosin heavy chain in muscle biopsies obtained in patients with CRF and moderate renal impairment. Myosin heavy chain is the main contractile protein responsible for the conversion of ATP to mechanical energy as muscle contraction, and it contributes for ~20% to synthetic rates of mixed-muscle protein (111). Despite the finding that rates of whole-body ^{13}C-leucine turnover were similar to controls, the authors observed significantly lower synthetic rates of myosin heavy chain as well as mitochondrial protein, muscle cytochrome c-oxidase activity, and citrate synthase, suggesting that in CRF decreased energy availability is responsible for reduced protein synthesis rates (Fig 1.6).

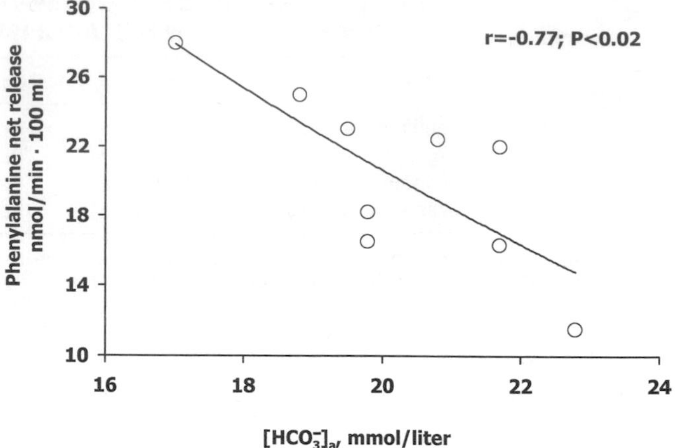

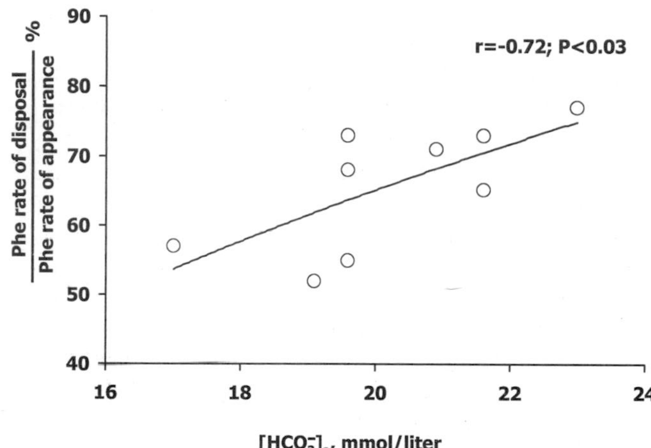

FIGURE 1.5. Relationships of forearm phenylalanine net release (*upper panel*) and the ratio protein synthesis/protein degradation (*lower panel*) to arterial HCO_3 in fasting patients with chronic renal failure ingesting unrestricted diets. (From Garibotto G, Russo R, Sofia A, et al. Skeletal muscle protein synthesis and degradation in patients with chronic renal failure. *Kidney Int* 1994; 45:1432–1439, with permission.)

Another possibility is that muscle-protein turnover in uremic patients is inhibited by some circulating factor(s) that accumulates in blood. Reduced bioavailability of IGF-1, resulting from increased serum-binding proteins, may play a role in decreasing muscle-protein synthesis. Recently, protein turnover of mixed-muscle proteins has been evaluated in a group of nonacidotic patients undergoing MHD with stabilized, chronic protein–calorie malnutrition, before and after the administration of recombinant human growth hormone (rhGH) for 6 weeks (112,113). In these

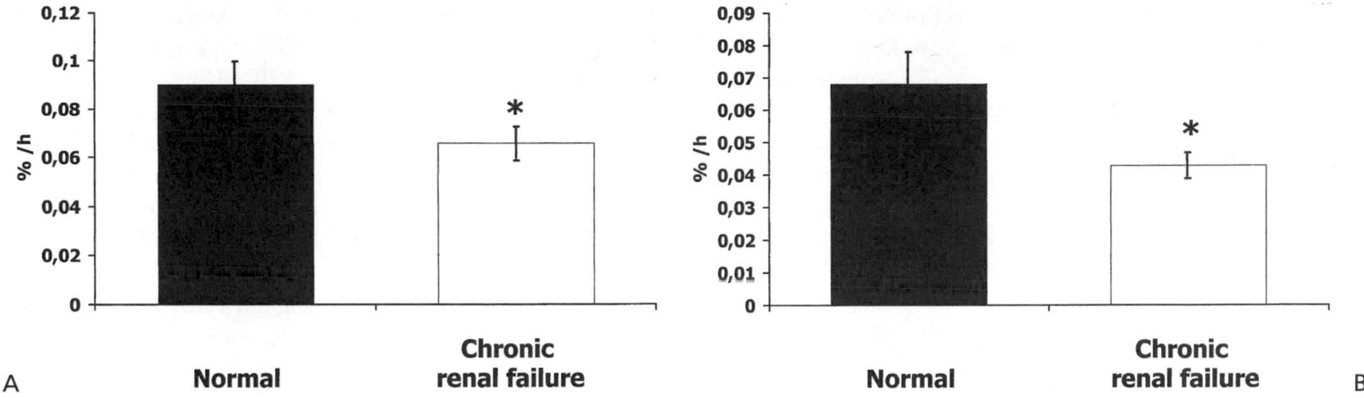

FIGURE 1.6. Fractional synthesis rate (FSR) of mixed-muscle protein **(A)** and myosin heavy chain **(B)** in patients with chronic renal failure (CRF) and normal control subjects. Patients with CRF have a lower FSR of mixed-muscle protein (* $p < 0.05$) and myosin heavy chain (* $p < 0.02$) than control subjects. (From Adey D, Kumar R, McCarthy JT, et al. Reduced synthesis of muscle proteins in chronic renal failure. *Am J Physiol Endocrinol Metab* 2000;278(2):E219–E225, with permission.)

patients, rates of forearm muscle-protein synthesis and degradation were in the lower range of the values recorded in normal healthy subjects (112). However, when patients were given rhGH, both muscle-protein synthesis and whole-body oxygen consumption increased (113). It interesting that changes in the rates of muscle-protein synthesis were related to variations in the changes in IGFBP-1 (which decreased in blood) and in the IGF-1/IGFBP-3 ratio (which increased in blood), suggesting the dependency of muscle-protein synthesis on the availability of "free" IGF-1 levels. Moreover, changes in resting expenditure were for a great part accounted for by the increased rates of muscle-protein synthesis. These results suggest the occurrence of a causal relationship between the observed changes in protein synthesis rates and energy metabolism (because protein synthesis is an energy-requiring process) and that both energy metabolism and protein synthesis can be increased by the administration of growth factors.

An emerging issue in studies on muscle perfusion is the role of vasculature, which in conjunction with hormonal effects plays an important role in the control of muscle metabolism and function (114). Besides reduced energy metabolism or reduced bioavailability of growth factors, a major factor causing wasting could be related to the changes in muscle structure and reduction of nutritive blood flow observed in patients with CRF (115).

In summary, available data suggest that metabolic acidosis and some unknown factor (including the reduced availability of IGF-1, changes in muscle blood flow, or reduced oxidative metabolism) have different, additive detrimental effects on muscle-protein metabolism in uremia by acting on different pathways of protein turnover and different pools of skeletal-muscle proteins.

Protein Repletion and Feeding

In the healthy condition of protein and energy balance there is no change in the size of body protein pools over days or weeks. However, in muscle as in other tissues, a diurnal cycle pattern in the size of protein pools occurs during the day (3), with protein saved during feeding and the same amount lost during overnight fasting. During feeding, increased availability of amino acids (mainly essential amino acids and BCAA) and increased insulin levels increase muscle-protein synthesis and decrease muscle-protein degradation, respectively.

If and to what extent CRF and ESRD affect whole-body or muscle-protein metabolism in the protein-fed state is unclear. Castellino et al. studied the combined effect of hyperaminoacidemia and hyperinsulinemia (i.e., a condition simulating a meal) on ^{14}C-leucine kinetics in patients with moderate-advanced CRF (96). They observed that during hyperaminoacidemia, whole-body protein synthesis was markedly diminished in comparison with healthy controls. This suggests that CRF *per se* may be associated with a lesser anabolic response to feeding. In 1999 the same authors (102) observed that whole-body protein synthesis, degradation, and amino acid oxidation were normal in patients undergoing CAPD evaluated in the same experimental setting. It is unclear if this may be the result of a more complete correction of protein abnormalities by PD or of other causes. An alteration in the postprandial use of amino acids has been shown in patients with ESRD as a result of type-1 diabetes (116).

A few studies have examined the effects of feeding on amino acid metabolism in muscle. In patients with CRF, the ingestion of a beef steak (69) or of an amino acid mixture (81) is followed by abnormalities in amino acid levels that are even more marked than those observed in the postabsorptive state. Nonessential amino acids predominate in the protein-fed amino acid pattern (69,81). The mechanisms for these alterations were explored by Deferrari et al. when they studied the splanchnic exchange of amino acids after the ingestion of an amino acid meal (69). In response to the meal, a reduced uptake by splanchnic organs was observed for those amino acids that increased more in arterial blood, especially nonessential amino acids. Complementing the altered splanchnic and arterial amino acid profile, an altered pattern of amino acid repletion in peripheral tissues was observed (81). A large percentage of the amino acids taken up by the leg during the absorptive period was no longer accounted for by BCAA; instead it was accounted for by nonessential amino acids (81). Therefore, these data indicate that in patients with CRF the primacy of BCAA in supplying N to peripheral tissues is overcome by the increase in arterial blood of nonessential amino acids. It is unknown whether the altered amino acid exchange in the protein-fed state has effects on muscle-protein metabolism. The imbalanced profile of amino acids taken up by peripheral tissues may affect protein synthesis because an appropriate pattern of amino acids is necessary to replenish N in muscle (117). In this regard leucine, isoleucine, and tyrosine uptake, relative to total amino acid uptake, were lower in patients and below their proportion in muscle protein (81). Therefore, the use of amino acids for muscle-protein synthesis may be less in patients with CRF in the protein-fed state.

Endocrine Abnormalities

Several hormonal derangements, including resistance to anabolic hormones (insulin, GH, IGF-1), hyperparathyroidism, hyperglucagonemia, and altered thyroid hormone and metabolism also are implicated as factors contributing to loss of lean body mass in patients with CRF. Insulin is a key regulating factor of protein metabolism for the conservation of lean body mass. Although the effects of insulin *per se* on protein synthesis are controversial, even small increases in blood insulin levels, well within the physiologic range, are associated with pronounced suppression of protein breakdown (3,4). A dose-response relationship has been shown to occur in human forearm skeletal muscle when insulin has been infused locally; an increase in the insulin level in the brachial artery to concentrations of about 30 μU/mL maximally suppresses (30% to 40%) protein degradation (118). A postreceptor defect in muscle responsiveness to insulin is the cause of insulin resistance with regard to glucose metabolism occurring in patients with CRF (119). However, it is not clearly understood whether insulin resistance regarding glucose metabolism also extends to the antiproteolytic action of this hormone. If so, it would contribute to the muscle wasting often found in uremic patients. Alvestrand et al. found that euglycemic hyperinsulinemia obtained by the insulin clamp technique in patients undergoing MHD was followed by a positive amino acid leg balance and a decline in intracellular amino acids that were similar to those seen in controls (109). Castellino et al. observed that during hyperinsulinemia, whole-body ^{14}C-leucine flux, leucine oxidation, and nonoxidative leucine disposal of patients with CRF (96) and patients treated with CAPD (102) are similar to the normal condition. Similar observations have been made in patients with CRF with metabolic acidosis by using ^{13}C-leucine kinetics (120). Although the results of these studies, in which insulin has been raised in the high physiologic level (i.e., at about 60 to 100 μU/mL), indicate that the effect of insulin on whole-body protein metabolism is not altered in uremic patients, it is nevertheless possible that subtle defects of insulin response occur at basal or low insulin levels. Both in normal subjects (70) and in patients with type II diabetes (121) basal rates of muscle-protein degradation as well as net proteolysis are inversely related to insulin levels, suggesting that an inhibitory action of basal insulin levels on protein degradation takes place. However, such a relationship has not been found in patients with CRF eating unrestricted diets and with mild acidosis (70), suggesting that the inhibitory effect of basal insulin on muscle-protein degradation is blunted partially by acidemia.

An increase in counter-regulatory hormones (cortisol, glucagon) could cause an increased catabolic response in patients with ESRD in conditions associated with fasting or subnormal energy intake. Plasma cortisol half-life is prolonged in patients with CRF, and basal and integrated 24-hour plasma cortisol often are elevated in patients treated with MHD; moreover, plasma-free cortisol is increased to a greater extent than total cortisol, indicating a reduction in binding to cortisol-binding protein. (See Sayegh and Lim [122] for a review.) In animals, glucorticoids are the primary effector of the catabolic response to acidosis (52), trauma, and sepsis (3,35). Although the catabolic effect of cortisol on protein metabolism in humans is well established, the quantitative importance of this response is unclear. From studies in which cortisol has been administered in healthy volunteers, the occurrence of hyperglycemia, with its attendant hyperinsulinemia, has been responsible for the tachyphylaxis to chronic cortisol infusion (123). In patients with CRF and a nonrestricted diet the degree of acidosis and serum cortisol levels are correlated with variations in muscle-protein balance (70). Moreover, it has been observed that reduced physical activity increases the catabolic response to cortisol in humans (124), and ESRD patients are often inactive.

Plasma glucagon levels are elevated in patients with renal insufficiency as a result of impaired glucagon degradation. In the healthy condition, glucagon appears to be able to stimulate protein degradation; however, these effects are counteracted by the basal insulin concentrations (125).

Clinical and experimental observations indicate that CRF *per se* is characterized by a resistance to GH and IGF-1 (126,127). Resistance to GH is responsible for the stunted growth of uremic children. Besides its stimulatory effects of growth and anabolism, circulating GH (and IGF-1) levels play an important role in the metabolic response to fasting by contributing to protein conservation (128). A resistance to GH and/or IGF-1, therefore, could account for a defective anabolism when patients are fed and/or to an increased catabolic response to fasting.

Increased levels of circulating GH-binding protein (129) and a decrease in liver GH-receptor messenger RNA (130) may be involved in the pathogenesis of GH resistance. It has been found that in rats with CRF there is also a direct resistance to IGF-1 in muscle (131).

Resistance to growth factors in CRF also may be the result of circulating inhibitors. The majority of circulating IGF-1 is bound to IGFBPs; because of its rapid changes in serum concentration, IGFBP-1 is assumed to modulate the free fraction of IGF-1 (132). Both children and adults with CRF present an increased IGF-binding capacity, owing to an increase in the levels of IGFBP-1 and IGFBP-2 (133, 134). The amount of these circulating inhibitors of IGF-1 increases in patients with CRF along with the decrease in GFR (135).

In summary, evidence coming from studies performed both in animals and humans indicates that CRF is associated with resistance to GH and IGF-1 action. The evidence of a resistance to the insulin's antiproteolytic action is lacking. Besides reduced growth in uremic children, clinical consequences of these alterations likely entail a decreased ability to maintain lean body mass in conditions characterized by low insulin availability and high stress, counter-regulatory hormones, such as during fasting and intercurrent illnesses.

Microinflammation

In recent years several investigators have shown that a significant percentage of chronic hemodialysis and PD patients have increased levels of proinflammatory cytokines (IL-1, IL-6, TNF-α), suggesting that a systemic inflammatory response is common in dialysis-treated patients. (See Chapter 13 for a review.) Moreover, cross-sectional studies suggest that inflammation is responsible for serologic and anthropometric evidence of malnutrition (136). Several visceral proteins that decrease in blood in response to malnutrition, such as albumin, prealbumin, transferrin, and retinal-binding protein, are also negative acute-phase proteins, and their liver synthesis is depressed by inflammation. (See Chapters 12 and 13 for a review.) The effects of a chronic inflammatory state on somatic proteins may be variable (35). In animal models of sepsis, inflammatory cytokines increase protein degradation via a process that involves glucocorticoids and activation of the ubiquitin pathway (35). TNF/cachectin has been studied most extensively and appears to play a clear role because its administration in the intact animal causes both anorexia and cachexia (137). However, this catabolic response may not be common to all tissues (138,139).

Accelerated whole-body rates of protein turnover are well-recognized features of acute infection (140). However, the response of protein turnover to subacute and chronic inflammation state is nonhomogeneous; some studies have shown an increase in whole-body protein turnover rates (141), and others have shown a decrease (142,143). In 2001 Paton et al. (144) studied whole-body protein turnover in patients affected by melioidiosis, a systemic gram-negative bacterial infection characterized by abscess formation and marked inflammatory response. Whole-body rates of protein turnover were increased, both in the fasted and fed state. However, these accelerated rates of protein turnover comprised almost equal increases in the rates of synthesis and catabolism so that the rate of oxidation and net protein catabolism were not different from those in control subjects. This contrasts with studies in the stressed state and in acute infections, where protein breakdown is increased more than protein synthesis, with an increase in net protein catabolism. The reasons for the variability in protein turnover in response to chronic infection is unknown and could be related to an attenuated response resulting from malnutrition (145) or variations in the inflammatory response and cytokine secretion. It also has been suggested that subacute or chronic infection may be distinguished from other stress states by an adaptive response that serves to limit oxidation and N loss (146). In this regard, it has been observed that protein oxidation is inversely related to body mass index (BMI) in patients with chronic infection (144), suggesting that an adaptive response to nutrient restriction is more successful in better-nourished patients. This is also consistent with the observation that obese subjects lose a lower proportion of lean mass than do lean people during starvation (146) and that in patients treated with MHD, a higher BMI is associated with lower mortality and morbidity rates (147). However, to what extent the microinflammatory state associated with uremia affects the individual determinants of protein turnover has not been studied specifically so far.

Effects of Low-Protein Diets on Protein Turnover in Patients with CRF

Humans are able to maintain lean body mass and body-protein balance over a broad range of dietary intakes of protein. Studies performed by whole-body, steady-state stable isotope infusions have shown that the human body responds to a reduced intake of proteins with integrated and adaptive metabolic changes involving a reduction in amino acid oxidation with more efficient use of amino acids deriving from protein degradation; a decrease in protein degradation; and, ultimately, a decrease in whole-body protein synthesis (106,148). Impaired ability to activate these mechanisms in patients with CRF would impair N conservation when nutrient intake is reduced. The understanding of how CRF affects the body's ability to respond to variations in nutrient intake is important because low-protein, high-calorie diets commonly are used in the conservative treatment of CRF.

Several N balance studies have shown that patients with advanced CRF can maintain neutral or slightly positive N balance with protein intakes as low as 0.55 to 0.60 g/kg. (See Lim and Kopple [149] for a review.) Indirect data suggest that the mechanisms by which protein turnover adapts to a low-protein intake can be impaired in the presence of metabolic acidosis. Williams et al. (150) evaluated the effects of low-protein diets on the urinary excretion of 3-methylhistidine (as an index of muscle catabolism) in adults with CRF before and after treatment of acidosis. Alkali treatment decreased 3-methylhistidine and N urinary excretion, suggesting that acidosis impairs nitrogen utilization and promotes muscle catabolism. Other studies indicate that when acidosis is corrected, the adaptation of protein metabolism to low-protein diets is unimpaired. Goodship et al. (94) observed that in nonacidotic patients with moderate CRF the adaptive response to a standard low-protein diet (0.6 g/kg/day) included both a normal decline in the rates of whole-body leucine oxidation and protein degradation. Bernhard et al. (151) studied the effects of low-protein diets (1.1 versus 0.71 g/kg) on ^{13}C-leucine kinetics in patients with moderate CRF. At the end of the 3-month low-protein period protein degradation decreased by about 8% and leucine oxidation decreased by 18%; nutritional status was unmodified. Taken together, these studies suggest that, under sufficient energy intake, a low-protein diet containing 0.6 to 0.7 g/kg protein is nutritionally safe during CRF.

Two studies indicate that protein metabolism and N balance adapt successfully in patients who are compliant to a very–low-protein diet (VLPD), supplemented with essential amino acids and keto acids. Masud et al. (152) administered a VLPD (0.28 g/protein/kg) supplemented with keto acids or amino acids in nonacidotic patients with CRF. When patients were studied 3 weeks after the start of the VLPD regimen, they found that body nitrogen balance was neutral and that this was achieved by a marked reduction in whole-body amino acid oxidation and postprandial inhibition of protein degradation. In a second study, Tom et al. (153) evaluated the long-term adaptive response of six patients with CRF to VLPD-supplemented diets. At the end of the study, rates of body N balance did not differ from basal values and so protein synthesis, degradation and amino acid oxidation, indicating that N balance was achieved by long-term suppression of amino acid oxidation and protein degradation (Fig 1.7).

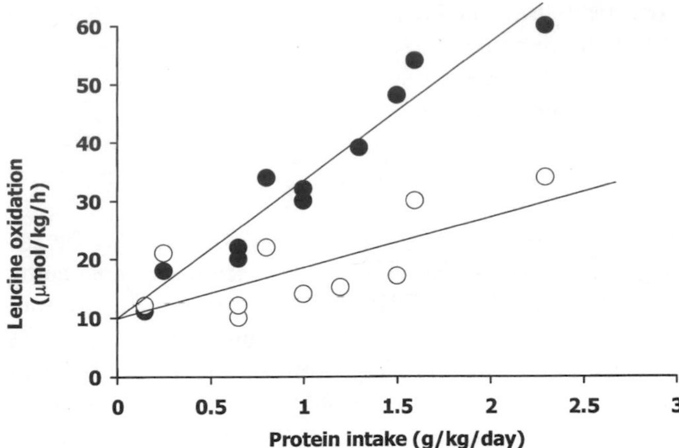

FIGURE 1.7. Relationships between rates of leucine oxidation and protein intake during fasting (*open circles*) and feeding (*solid circles*) in normal subjects and patients with chronic renal failure. (From Tom K, Young VR, Chapman T, et al. Long-term adaptive responses to dietary protein restriction in chronic renal failure. *Am J Physiol Endocrinol Metab* 1995;268:E668–E677, with permission.)

Effects of Hemodialysis on Protein Metabolism

The effects of dialysis on nutrition are multifaceted. On one hand, the "amount" of dialysis delivered appears to be an important factor that affects dietary intake and nutritional status of patients with ESRD (154). On the other hand, dialysis-related factors contribute to the increase of protein requirements with respect to the predialysis phase. A hemodialysis session may impair protein metabolism in different ways: (a) because of the associated losses of substrates, and (b) because of the promotion of net protein catabolism by the process itself.

During a hemodialysis session there are obligatory nutrient losses. Amino acid losses vary from 5 to 12 g (155, 156).

It is noteworthy that the amount of amino acids removed during one hemodialysis session is similar or greater than the amount of amino acids existent in extracellular fluids (about 5 to 6 g for a 70-kg man). However, plasma amino acid levels decline only by 20% to 50% after the hemodialysis session (155,156); actually, a study has documented an increase in plasma of some of the essential amino acids (157). Therefore, some other organ, such as skeletal muscle or the splanchnic bed, likely counterbalances this amino acid loss with an increase in efflux.

A few studies have evaluated the effects of hemodialysis on protein metabolism. The instability of ^{13}C-CO_2 during hemodialysis may cause the study on ^{13}C-leucine kinetics to be difficult to interpret. Lim et al. (99) studied whole-body ^{13}C-leucine turnover before and immediately after hemodialysis with nonbiocompatible (cuprophane) membranes. Hemodialysis was not associated with changes in whole-body protein degradation rates, but it caused a decrease in leucine oxidation and whole-body protein synthesis rates. More recently, Lau et al. studied ^{13}C-leucine kinetics during a study on the effects of hemodialysis (66) (polysulfone dialyzers) on arginine turnover. Also, these authors observed that rates of whole-body protein degradation did not increase during and 8 hours after hemodialysis. Lofberg et al. observed that one single session of hemodialysis lowers the ribosome content in skeletal muscle (157), suggestive of decreased protein synthesis. More recently, it has been shown that hemodialysis acutely decreases protein synthesis in muscle, as studied by the phenylalanine "flooding" dose technique (158). Taken together, these data suggest that the acute net catabolism induced by hemodialysis is not the result of an increase in protein degradation but of a decrease in protein synthesis, which likely occurs in muscle. The decrease in protein synthesis is possibly the result of a decrease of the amino acid availability to tissues during treatment, owing to the amino acid losses during the dialytic session. However, Lofberg showed no significant change in intracellular muscle amino acid concentrations during hemodialysis (158), suggesting that other factors may account for changes in protein synthesis.

Besides the acute effects of hemodialysis on reducing substrate availability and causing net protein catabolism, extensive reports in the literature suggest that activation of the alternate pathway of complement is an additional mechanism leading to malnutrition in dialysis patients (159,160). The exposure of whole blood to cellulosic membranes, such as cuprophane, results in leucocyte synthesis and release of IL-1 and TNF-α. These effects are late and likely can be detected when studies are more prolonged. Different filter materials can stimulate amino acid efflux from muscle to various extents. Gutierrez et al. demonstrated an increased efflux of amino acids from the lower limb after sham hemodialysis in healthy subjects using bioincompatible, but not biocompatible, membranes (160,161). The increased release of amino acids was observed at about 6 hours after the start of the dialysis—a time period consistent with the activation of monocytes and production of proinflammatory cytokines, with their subsequent action on skeletal muscle. Moreover, after sham dialysis with cuprophane there was an increase in leg release and arterial levels of 3-methylhistidine, which is suggestive of increased muscle-protein breakdown. These results support the conclusion that the biocompatibility of the membrane can affect favorably the nutritional status. Some clinical studies (162,163) are in keeping with this hypothesis.

Effects of PD on Protein Turnover

Despite substantial glucose absorption, loss of lean body mass, with preservation or increase in fat stores, may be even more prevalent in patients undergoing PD than in those treated with MHD (54). Patients undergoing PD present blood and tissue levels of essential amino acids that are even lower than those observed in patients undergoing MHD (164), which suggests a response of protein turnover to depletion or reduced release from tissue because of hyperinsulinemia. Goodship et al. (101) studied ^{14}C-leucine turnover and nutritional status in a control group and in 10 patients with CRF before the initiation of CAPD and after a 3-month treatment. The study was performed while patients were fed intermittently. Before initiating CAPD, protein intake was lower than in normal subjects, but it increased significantly after 3 months of treatment. Leucine oxidation was lower in CRF subjects than in controls, and the balance between protein synthesis and degradation was higher both before initiating CAPD and after 3 months of treatment. Leucine flux was lower in the uremic patients before treatment than after treatment with CAPD, although this difference did not reach statistical significance. More recently, Castellino et al. (102) measured whole-body ^{14}C-leucine turnover in combination with the euglycemic insulin-clamp technique with or without amino acid infusion in eight patients undergoing CAPD. Basal rates of protein degradation, leucine oxidation, and whole-body protein synthesis were reduced in patients as compared to controls. During the euglycemic hyperinsulinemia, leucine flux declined by about 32% and leucine net balance became less negative, similar to controls. When insulin was infused together with amino acids, protein synthesis rose and leucine balance became similarly positive in patients and controls. Taken together, data from these studies suggest that the response of protein turnover in patients undergoing CAPD is to activate mechanisms to minimize protein loss from the body. Whether this response is the result of nutrient depletion or of the concurrent hyperinsulinemia is not understood. Because the whole-body antiproteolytic response to insulin is preserved in patients undergoing CAPD and the anabolic response to insulin and amino acids is also normal, persisting hyperinsulinemia, in association with glucose delivery, could contribute to preservation of muscle mass. To evaluate if changes in substrate and insulin levels that occur during PD have effects on muscle-protein dynamics, Garibotto et al. (82) evaluated muscle-protein dynamics by the forearm-perfusion method associated with 3H-phenylalanine kinetics in acute, cross-over studies in which patients undergoing PD served as their own controls. Studies were performed in the basal state and during PD with dialysates containing dextrose alone or during PD with dialysates containing dextrose alone or dextrose and amino acids. PD with dextrose alone induced a two-fold to three-fold increase in insulin and a 20% to 25% decrease in amino acid, mainly BCAA, levels. PD caused an acute decrease in muscle-protein degradation, which was inversely related to insulin levels. Protein degradation declined maximally (by about 30%) when insulin levels were about 18 to 25 U/L, with no further decline thereafter (Fig. 1.8). These data are in accordance with the exquisite sensitivity of muscle-protein metabolism to insulin. Despite this decrease in protein degradation, there was not an anabolic effect because a concurrent decrease in muscle-protein synthesis was observed. The decrease in muscle-protein synthesis correlated with the decline in blood of several essential amino acids, suggesting that the removal of substrates for protein synthesis via peritoneal drainage associated with hyperinsulinemia blunts protein turnover. When muscle-protein turnover was evaluated with dialysates containing dextrose or dextrose and amino acids, both the decline in blood amino acids and

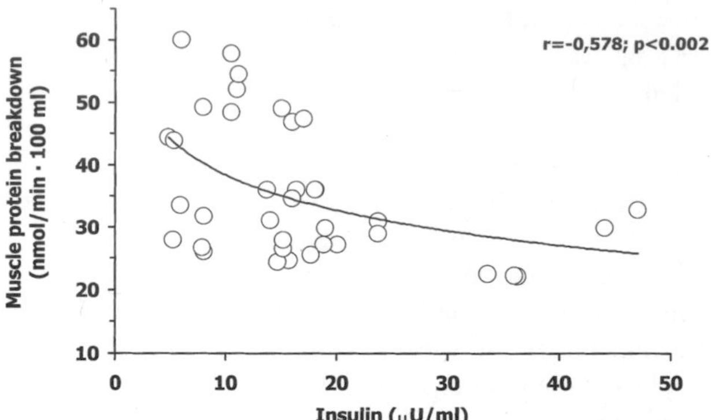

FIGURE 1.8. Relationships between rates of muscle-protein degradation and insulin levels during peritoneal dialysis. (From Garibotto G, Sofia A, Canepa A, et al. Acute effects of peritoneal dialysis with dialysates containing dextrose or dextrose and amino acids on muscle protein turnover in patients with chronic renal failure. *J Am Soc Nephrol* 2001;12:557–567, with permission.)

in muscle-protein synthesis was prevented and net protein balance across muscle was less negative.

These studies indicate that, in patients undergoing PD in the fasting state, the moderate hyperinsulinemia that occurs during PD with dextrose alone causes an antiproteolytic action that is obscured by a parallel decrease in amino acid availability for protein synthesis. However, the combined use of dextrose and amino acids results in a cumulative effect because of the suppression of muscle-protein degradation (induced by insulin) and the stimulation of muscle-protein synthesis (induced by amino acid availability). It is therefore possible that in patients treated with PD, when fasting or when nutrient intake is reduced, muscle mass could be better maintained by the combined use of dextrose and amino acids.

Protein Metabolism in the Nephrotic Syndrome and in Comorbidities Associated with ESRD

Protein Turnover in the Nephrotic Syndrome

Patients with nephrotic syndrome frequently present with protein-energy malnutrition, which often is obscured by edema (165). However, the mechanisms by which patients with nephrotic syndrome lose muscle mass are not fully understood (165). Turnover of albumin is increased greatly in the nephrotic syndrome. (For an extensive review, see Chapter 24.) Therefore, the need to continue to synthesize increased amounts of albumin could be a stimulus for the increase in degradation of body proteins. In addition, patients with nephrotic syndrome often have concurrent factors (acidosis, inflammation, anorexia, etc.) that may negatively affect protein metabolism.

Nephrotic rats gain weight at a rate significantly slower than normal rats (166) even if they are fed a high-protein diet. However, whole-body protein synthesis and degradation are not different between nephrotic and control rats, and leucine oxidation is decreased (167). This suggests that nephrotic rats can adapt to the continuous protein losses with a reduction in amino acid oxidation to conserve body proteins. Choi et al. (168) evaluated whether dietary-protein restriction causes protein catabolism in doxorubicin (Adriamycin) nephrosis. During the administration of a low-protein diet leucine oxidation and urinary urea nitrogen excretion in nephrotic rats decreased by 18% and 37%, respectively. Again, rates of whole-body protein synthesis and degradation did not differ between nephrotic and control rats. These studies suggest that nephrotic rats are able to conserve protein when protein intake is restricted and that moderate proteinuria does not increase protein catabolism. A few studies have evaluated the effects of the nephrotic syndrome on whole-body rates of protein synthesis and degradation in humans. Maroni et al. (169) reported that leucine flux, oxidation, and whole-body protein synthesis in nephrotic patients were not different from control subjects under similar dietary intakes. Lim et al. (170) observed a decrease in whole-body protein degradation and synthesis as studied by ^{13}C-leucine in nephrotic subjects; however, patients ingested lower amounts of proteins in comparison with control subjects (0.84 versus 1.17 g/kg, respectively). Rates of leucine oxidation were related to protein intake both in patients and controls, suggesting that the homeostatic response to nutrient deprivation is conserved in patients with the nephrotic syndrome. De Sain-van der Velden et al. (171) measured protein turnover by the use of ^{13}C-valine kinetics in nephrotic subjects ingesting about 0.8 g/protein/kg and compared their data to control subjects under similar diets. Patients had similar values of valine oxidation, synthesis, and flux. Zanetti et al. (172) also showed normal rates of whole-body protein degradation, but an increased rate of synthesis of albumin and fibrinogen, in patients with low-grade nephrotic proteinuria.

Taken together, these data suggest that in patients with nephrotic syndrome, whole-body protein degradation and synthesis are not increased and that mechanisms to reduce N losses are activated properly when N intake is reduced. These data also suggest that malnutrition in nephrotic patients is mainly the result of anorexia. To determine if nephrotic patients can adapt successfully to a protein-restricted diet, Maroni et al. (169) studied whole-body protein turnover and nitrogen balance in nephrotic patients when they received diets providing 1.6 g or 0.8 g/kg and 35 kcal/kg. Whole-body protein turnover was measured both during fasting and feeding by using intravenous ^{13}C-leucine and intragastric 2H3-leucine. Nitrogen balance was positive in both nephrotic and control subjects consuming either diet. Moreover, in both nephrotic and control subjects, anabolism was the result of a suppression of whole-body protein degradation and stimulation of protein synthesis during feeding. When protein intake was restricted the principal compensatory response was a decrease in amino acid oxidation, and this response was the same in both groups. With the low-protein diet, leucine oxidation rates were inversely proportional to proteinuria, suggesting that proteinuria is a stimulus to conserve dietary essential amino acids. Therefore, these data indicate that nephrotic patients activate normal responses to dietary protein restriction and feeding and that a diet providing 0.8 g of protein (plus 1 g protein per g of urinary proteins) and 35 kcal per kg per day maintains body N.

Aging and Protein Metabolism

In several Western countries, persons over age 65 years are expected soon to become the majority of those who will require maintenance dialysis therapy. Nutritional problems are common in elderly patients with ESRD and contribute to much of the debility and morbidity found in this group of dialysis patients (173). Low dietary intake and diminished muscle masses are common in older individuals and may cause low or even normal values of blood urea nitrogen and serum creatinine, even in the presence of advanced renal failure (174).

A decrease in body protein is a major characteristics of aging (175,176). It involves mainly muscle proteins and is associated with decreased muscle strength and functional impairment. Whole-body protein kinetics studies indicate that protein synthesis and degradation are similar in young and elderly adults when results are expressed per lean body mass (177,178). However, when muscle-protein metabolism has been studied specifically, the findings show deficits in muscle-protein synthesis with advancing age and suggest that these deficits are specific to certain muscle-protein components, such as myosin heavy chain and mitochondrial protein (179). In addition, in elderly subjects a decreased sensitivity of insulin action regarding protein metabolism, as well as a higher amino acid extraction by liver and gut during feeding, have been described (180). These alterations in protein metabolism resulting from senescence likely potentiate those caused by uremia.

Diabetic Nephropathy

Patients with CRF secondary to diabetes mellitus, which is the major cause of ESRD in several countries, have higher incidences of malnutrition as compared to nondiabetic subjects. Intercurrent illnesses, poor glycemic control, the high occurrence of nephrotic syndrome, gastroparesis, diabetic diarrhea, and underdialysis are possible causes of loss of muscle mass and functional impairment in subjects with diabetes. In addition to abnormalities resulting from uremia, patients with diabetes and uremia display multiple endocrine abnormalities, including lack of insulin or insulin resistance (type-2 diabetes) and increased cortisol, glucagons, and epinephrine, which *per se* could induce catabolism or cause an impairment in the response to low nutrient intakes (181). Therefore, wasting syndrome in patients with ESRD because of diabetes may occur as the result of the overlapping of abnormalities in the metabolic control of protein turnover that are individually peculiar to diabetes and uremia.

The anticatabolic effect of insulin is known for several years in patients with insulin-dependent diabetes mellitus (IDDM). Several investigators consistently have observed an increased rate of protein degradation and amino acid oxidation in insulin-withdrawn type-1 diabetic patients, an abnormality that is corrected only partially by insulin treatment (176). In view of these effects, it is possible that low-protein diets, which are used in patients with CRF resulting from diabetic nephropathy, are inadequate and cause loss of lean body mass. Only one study is available on this issue. Brodsky et al. (181) evaluated the effects of a low-protein diet (0.6 g/kg) on whole-body ^{13}C-leucine kinetics in six patients with IDDM and early nephropathy. A low-protein diet was accompanied by an initial decline in leucine oxidation, which returned to basal values by 12 weeks. Moreover, N balance persisted to be negative in the period of protein restriction. This issue is controversial because long-term studies failed to show evidence of change in anthropometric measures, serum albumin, and transferrin in IDDM patients undergoing long-term protein restriction (183,184).

A few studies (178,179) have explored protein metabolism in diabetic patients with ESRD. Luzi et al. measured whole-body protein turnover in type-1 IDDM patients receiving hemodialysis, and following kidney or combined kidney–pancreas transplantation, and compared results to normal controls (113,185). Fasting diabetic patients on hemodialysis presented reduced rates of whole-body proteolysis and protein synthesis, but leucine oxidation rates were comparable to healthy subjects (i.e., inadequately high). When amino acids were infused with insulin to simulate feeding, protein synthesis increased in controls, but there was no change in diabetic uremic patients. After kidney transplantation (185), protein turnover normalized; moreover, insulin sensitivity of protein metabolism was restored to normal, with the exception of leucine oxidation, which was not normally suppressed. Following kidney–pancreas transplantation both protein turnover and leucine oxidation normalized (113). Also, the anabolic effects of hyperinsulinemia and hyperaminoacidemia were restored after combined kidney–pancreas transplantation. Taken together, these data suggest that the defect in whole-body protein metabolism in IDDM patients treated with MDH is much more severe than that of both conditions alone and that when nephropathy develops additional defects take place in insulin's ability to stimulate protein synthesis when substrate availability is increased. Kidney transplant alone, although beneficial in terms of protein turnover, cannot completely revert the alterations caused by uremia and type-1

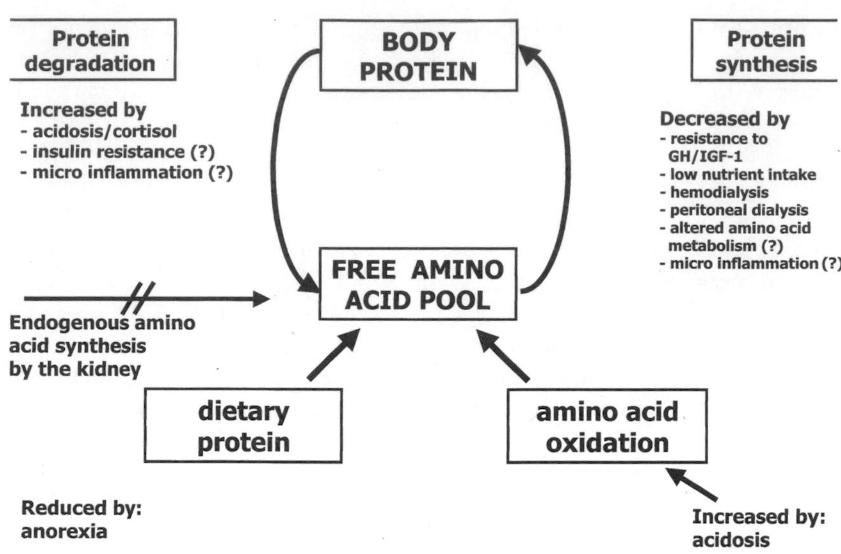

FIGURE 1.9. Overview of protein and amino acid metabolism in renal disease and renal failure.

diabetes, whereas kidney–pancreas graft achieves a normalization of protein metabolism. Despite the alterations in whole-body protein metabolism clearly outlined by these studies, there is no information on the effects of diabetic nephropathy on the determinants of muscle mass.

Although type-II noninsulin dependent diabetes mellitus (NIDDM) is far more common, its effects on protein metabolism have been studied far less frequently. In the absence of nephropathy, the picture is that of maintenance of lean body mass in the presence of hyperglycemia, in contrast with the fast protein wasting in decompensated type-1 IDDM. The presence of even limited amounts of circulating insulin is likely to prevent severe protein amino acid catabolic response. Most, but not all, studies show that despite the occurrence of significant impairment of insulin-mediated glucose metabolism, whole-body and muscle-protein turnover are normal in patients with type-2 diabetes mellitus. This gives support to the idea that there is a dissociation between the effects of insulin on glucose and amino acid metabolism. When diabetic nephropathy complicates type-2 NIDDM, the picture changes dramatically, with a great amount of patients with ESRD developing malnutrition. However, there is no information on the combined effects of type-2 diabetes and uremia on muscle-protein metabolism.

In conclusion, many factors contribute to net protein catabolism in patients with chronic renal disease and renal failure. These factors are illustrated in Fig. 1.9. The relative contributions of each of these processes may vary according to the stage of impairment of renal function, the modality of treatment for the renal disease, and the type of renal replacement therapy for patients with renal failure.

REFERENCES

1. Munro NH, Crim MC. Protein and amino acids. In: Shils ME, Olson JA, eds. *Modern nutrition in health and disease,* 8th ed. Baltimore: Williams & Wilkins, 1994:3–35.
2. Young VR, Yu Y. Protein and amino acid metabolism. In: Fischer JE, ed. *Nutrition and metabolism in the surgical patients* 2nd ed. Boston: Little, Brown, 1996:159–201.
3. Schoenheimer R, Rattner S, Rittenberg D. Studies in protein metabolism. X. The metabolic activity of body proteins investigated with L(-)leucine containing two isotopes. *J Biol Chem* 1939;130:703–732.
4. Bier DM. Intrinsically difficult problems; the kinetics of body proteins and amino acids in man. *Diabetes Metab Rev* 1989;5: 111–132.
5. Tessari P. Effects of insulin on whole body and muscle protein metabolism. *Diabetes Metab Rev* 1994;10:253–285.
6. Gelfand RA, Glickman MG, Castellino P, et al. Measurement of L-[1-14C]leucine kinetics in splanchnic and leg tissues in humans. Effect of amino acid infusion. *Diabetes* 1988;37: 1365–1372.
7. Deutz NE, Wagenmakers JM, Soeters P. Discrepancy between muscle and whole body protein turnover. *Curr Opinion Clin Nutr Metab Care* 1999;2:33–38.
8. Kuhlmann MK, Kopple JD. Amino acid metabolism in the kidney. *Sem Nephrol* 1990;10:445–457.
9. Fukuda S, Kopple JD. Uptake and release of amino acids by the normal dog kidney. *Min Electr Metab* 1980;3:237–247.
10. Tizianello A, Deferrari G, Gurreri G, et al. Renal metabolism of amino acids in subjects with normal renal function and in patients with renal insufficiency. *J Clin Invest* 1980;65: 1163–1173.
11. Tizianello A, Deferrari G, Garibotto G, et al. Renal ammoniagenesis in an early stage of metabolic acidosis in man. *J Clin Invest* 1982;69:240–250.
12. Brundin T, Wahren J. Renal oxygen consumption, thermogenesis, and amino acid utilization during i.v. infusion of amino acids in man. *Am J Physiol* 1994;67:E648–E655.
13. Stumvoll M, Perriello G, Meyer C, et al. Role of glutamine in human carbohydrate metabolism in kidney and other tissues. *Kidney Int* 1999;55:778–792.
14. Tessari P, Garibotto G, Inchiostro S, et al. Kidney, splanchnic, and leg protein turnover in humans. Insight from leucine and phenylalanine kinetics. *J Clin Invest* 1996;98:1481–1492.
15. Ayling JE, Pirson WD, Janabi JM, et al. Kidney phenylalanine hydroxylase from man and rat. Comparison with the liver enzyme. *Biochemistry* 1974;13:78–85.
16. Tessari P, Deferrari G, Robaudo C, et al. Phenylalanine

hydroxylation across the kidney in humans. *Kidney Int* 1999; 56:2168–2172.
17. Moller N, Meek S, Bigelow M, et al. The kidney is an important site for in vivo phenylalanine-to-tyrosine conversion: a metabolic role of the kidney. *Proc Natl Acad Sci USA* 2000;97: 1242–1246.
18. Tizianello A, Deferrari G, Garibotto G, et al. Abnormalities of amino acid and keto acid metabolism in renal failure. In: Davison D, ed. *Nephrology*. London: Baillière, 1988;1011–1019.
19. Bostom A, Brosnan JT, Hall B, et al. Net uptake of plasma homocysteine by the rat kidney in vivo. *Atherosclerosis* 1995; 116:59–62.
20. van Guldener C, Donker AJ, Jakobs C, et al. No net renal extraction of homocysteine in fasting humans. *Kidney Int* 1998; 54:166–169.
21. Rabkin R, Dahl DC. Factors controlling intracellular protein turnover in the kidney. *Semin Nephrol* 1990;10:472–480.
22. Garibotto G, Tessari P, Sacco P, et al. Amino acid metabolism, substrate availability and the control of protein dynamics in the human kidney. *J Nephrol* 1999;12:203–211.
23. Wesson D, Mitch WE, Wilmore DW. Nutritional considerations in the treatment of acute renal failure. In: Brenner JM, Lazarus BM, eds. *Acute renal failure.* Philadelphia: WB Saunders, 1983:618–642.
24. Persike EC, Addis T. Increased rate of urea formation following removal of renal tissue. *Am J Physiol* 1949;158:149.
25. Sellers A, Katz L, Marmorsten J. Effect of bilateral nephrectomy on urea formation in rat liver slices. *Am J Physiol* 1957;191: 345.
26. Lacy WW. Effects of acute uremia on amino acid uptake and urea production by perfused rat liver. *Am J Physiol* 1969;216: 1300.
27. Frohlich J, Scholmreich J, Hoppe-Seyler G, et al. The effect of acute uremia on gluconeogenesis in isolated perfused rat livers. *Eur J Clin Invest* 1974;4:453–459.
28. Bondy P, Engel F, Farrar B. The metabolism of amino acids and protein in the adrenalectomized-nephrectomized rat. *Endocrinology* 1949;44:476–482.
29. Clark AS, Mitch WE. Muscle protein turnover and glucose uptake in acutely uremic rats. Effects of insulin and the duration of renal insufficiency. *J Clin Invest* 1983;72(3):836–845.
30. Mitch WE. Amino acid release from the hindquarter and urea appearance in acute uremia. *Am J Physiol* 1982;241: E226–E232.
31. Flugel-Link RM, Salusky IB, Jones MR, et al. Protein and amino acid metabolism in posterior hemicorpus of acutely uremic rats. *Am J Physiol* 1983;244:E615–E623.
32. Price SR, Reaich D, Marinovic A, et al. Mechanisms contributing to muscle-wasting in acute uremia: activation of amino acid catabolism. *J Am Soc Nephrol* 1998;9:439–443.
33. Arnold WC, Holliday MA. Tissue resistance to insulin stimulation of amino acid uptake in acutely uremic rats. *Kidney Int* 1979;16:124–130.
34. Maroni BJ, Haesemeyer RW, Kutner MH, et al. Kinetics of system A amino acid uptake by muscle: effects of insulin and acute uremia. *Am J Physiol* 1990;258:F1304–F1310.
35. Hasselgren PO, Fischer JE. Counter-regulatory hormones and mechanisms in amino acid metabolism with special reference to the catabolic response in skeletal muscle. *Curr Opinion Clin Nutr Metab Care* 1999;2:9–14.
36. Tiao G, Fagan JM, Samuels N, et al. Sepsis stimulates nonlysosomal energy-dependent proteolysis and increases ubiquitin mRNA levels in rat skeletal muscle. *J Clin Invest* 1994;94: 2255–2264.
37. Tiao G, Hobler S, Wang JJ, et al. Sepsis is associated with increased mRNAs of the ubiquitin-proteasome proteolytic pathway in human skeletal muscle. *J Clin Invest* 1997;99:163–168.
38. Mansoor O, Beaufrere B, Boirie Y, et al. Increased mRNA levels for components of the lysosomal, Ca^{2+}-activated, and ATP-ubiquitin-dependent proteolytic pathways in skeletal muscle from head trauma patients. *Proc Natl Acad Sci USA* 1996;93: 2714–2718.
39. Del Rey A, Basedovsky HO. Metabolic and neuroendocrine effects of proinflammatory cytokines. *Eur J Clin Invest* 1992; 22:10–15.
40. Zamir O, O'Brien W, Thompson R, et al. Reduced muscle protein breakdown in septic rats following treatment with interleukin-1 receptor antagonist. *Int J Biochem* 1994;26: 943–950.
41. Langhans W, Hrupka B. Interleukins and tumor necrosis factor as inhibitors of food intake. *Neuropeptides* 1999;33:415–424.
42. Thissen JP, Underwood LE, Ketelslegers JM. Regulation of insulin-like growth factor-I in starvation and injury. *Nutr Rev* 1999;57:167–176.
43. Bentham J, Rodriguez-Arnao J, Ross RJ. Acquired growth hormone resistance in patients with hypercatabolism. *Horm Res* 1993;40:87–91.
44. Frost RA, Lang CH. Differential effects of insulin-like growth factor I (IGF-I) and IGF-binding protein-1 on protein metabolism in human skeletal muscle cells. *Endocrinology* 1999;140: 3962–3970.
45. Mac Lennan PA, Brown RA, Rennie MJ, et al. A positive relationship between protein synthetic rates and intracellular glutamine concentration in perfused rat skeletal muscle. *FEBS Letters* 1987;215:187–191.
46. Ardawi MSM, Majzoub MF. Glutamine metabolism in skeletal muscle of septic rats. *Metabolism* 1991;40:155–164.
47. Streat SJ, Beddoe AH, Hill GL. Aggressive nutritional support does not prevent protein loss despite fat gain in septic intensive care patients. *J Trauma* 1987;27:262–264.
48. Plank LD, Connolly AB, Hill GL. Sequential changes in metabolic response in severely septic patients during the first 23 days after the onset of peritonitis. *Ann Surg* 1988;208:143–149.
49. Ziegler TR, Lazarus JM, Young LS, et al. Effects of recombinant human growth hormone in adults receiving maintenance hemodialysis. *J Am Soc Nephrol* 1991;2:1130–1135.
50. Biolo G, Iscra F, Bosutti A, et al. Growth hormone decreases muscle glutamine production and stimulates protein synthesis in hypercatabolic patients. *Am J Physiol (Endocrinol Metab)* 2000;279:E323–E332.
51. Debroy MA, Wolf SE, Zhang XJ, et al. Anabolic effects of insulin-like growth factor in combination with insulin-like growth factor binding protein-3 in severely burned adults. *J Trauma* 1999;47:904–910.
52. Hakim RM, Wingard RL, Parker RA. Effect of the dialysis membrane in the treatment of patients with acute renal failure. *N Engl J Med* 1994;331:1338–1342.
53. Himmelfarb J, Tolkoff-Rubin N, Chandran P, et al. A multicenter comparison of hemodialysis membranes in the treatment of acute renal failure. *J Am Soc Nephrol* 1998;257–266.
54. Bergstrom J. Nutrition and mortality in hemodialysis. *J Am Soc Nephrol* 1996;6:1329–1341.
55. Kopple JD, Berg R, Houser H, et al. Nutritional status of patients with different levels of chronic renal failure. Modification of Diet in Renal Disease Study Group. *Kidney Int Suppl* 1989; 27:S184–S194.
56. Ikizler TA, Greene J, Wingard RL, et al. Spontaneous dietary protein intake during progression of chronic renal failure. *J Am Soc Nephrol* 1995;6:1386–1391.
57. Kopple JD. Abnormal amino acid and protein metabolism in uremia. *Kidney Int* 1978;14:340–349.

58. Alvestrand A, Furst P, Bergstrom J. Intracellular amino acids in uremia. *Kidney Int Suppl* 1983;16:S9–S16.
59. Tizianello A, Deferrari G, Garibotto G, et al. Branched-chain amino acid metabolism in chronic renal failure. *Kidney Int Suppl* 1983;24:S17–S22.
60. Kopple JD. Nutritional therapy in kidney failure. *Nutr Rev* 1981;39:193.
61. Bergstrom J, Alvestrand A, Furst P. Plasma and muscle free amino acids in maintenance hemodialysis patients without protein malnutrition. *Kidney Int* 1990;38:10–16.
62. Walser M, Hill SB. Free and protein-bound tryptophan in serum of untreated patients with chronic renal failure. *Kidney Int* 1993;44:1366–1371.
63. Kuhlencordt PJ, Gyurko R, Han F, et al. Accelerated atherosclerosis, aortic aneurysm formation, and ischemic heart disease in apolipoprotein E/endothelial nitric oxide synthase double-knockout mice. *Circulation* 2001;24(104):448–454.
64. Fryburg DA. NG-monomethyl-L-arginine inhibits the blood flow but not the insulin-like response of forearm muscle to IGF-I: possible role of nitric oxide in muscle protein synthesis. *J Clin Invest* 1996;97:1319–1328.
65. Suh H, Peresleni T, Wadhwa N, et al. Amino acid profile and nitric oxide pathway in patients on continuous ambulatory peritoneal dialysis: L-arginine depletion in acute peritonitis. *Am J Kidney Dis* 1997;29:712–719.
66. Lau T, Owen W, Yu YM, et al. Arginine, citrulline, and nitric oxide metabolism in end-stage renal disease patients. *J Clin Invest* 2000;105:1217–1225.
67. Schmidt RJ, Baylis C. Total nitric oxide production is low in patients with chronic renal disease. *Kidney Int* 2000;58: 1261–1266.
68. Wever R, Boer P, Hijmering M, et al. Nitric oxide production is reduced in patients with chronic renal failure. *Arterioscler Thromb Vasc Biol* 1999;19:1168–1172.
69. Tizianello A, Deferrari G, Garibotto G, et al. Abnormal amino acid metabolism after amino acid ingestion in chronic renal failure. *Kidney Int Suppl* 1987;22:S181–S185.
70. Garibotto G, Russo R, Sofia A, et al. Skeletal muscle protein synthesis and degradation in patients with chronic renal failure. *Kidney Int* 1994;45:1432–1439.
71. Galbraith RA, Buse MG. Effects of serine on protein synthesis and insulin receptors. *Am J Physiol* 1981;241:C167–C171.
72. Hara Y, May RC, Kelly RA, et al. Acidosis, not azotemia, stimulates branched-chain, amino acid catabolism in uremic rats. *Kidney Int* 1987;32:808–814.
73. Lofberg E, Wernerman J, Anderstam B, et al. Correction of acidosis in dialysis patients increases branched-chain and total essential amino acid levels in muscle. *Clin Nephrol* 1997;48: 230–237.
74. Kooman JP, Deutz NE, Zijlmans P, et al. The influence of bicarbonate supplementation on plasma levels of branched-chain amino acids in haemodialysis patients with metabolic acidosis. *Nephrol Dial Transplant* 1997;12:2397–2401.
75. Reaich D, Channon SM, Scrimgeour CM, et al. Correction of acidosis in humans with CRF decreases protein degradation and amino acid oxidation. *Am J Physiol* 1993;265:E230–E235.
76. Young GA, Swanepoel CR, Croft MR, et al. Anthropometry and plasma valine, amino acids, and proteins in the nutritional assessment of hemodialysis patients. *Kidney Int* 1982;21: 492–499.
77. Laidlaw SA, Smolin LA, Davidson WD, et al. Sulfur amino acids in maintenance hemodialysis patients. *Kidney Int* 1987; 32:S191.
78. Bergstrom J, Alvestrand A, Furst P, et al. Sulphur amino acids in plasma and muscle in patients with chronic renal failure: evidence for taurine depletion. *J Intern Med* 1989;226:1–7.
79. Suliman ME, Anderstam B, Lindholm B, et al. Total, free, and protein-bound sulphur amino acids in uraemic patients. *Nephrol Dial Transplant* 1997;12:2332–2338.
80. Huxtable RJ. Physiological actions of taurine. *Physiol Rev* 1982; 72:101–112.
81. Garibotto G, Deferrari G, Robaudo C, et al. Disposal of exogenous amino acids by muscle in patients with chronic renal failure. *Am J Clin Nutr* 1995;62:136–142.
82. Garibotto G, Sofia A, Canepa A, et al. Acute effects of peritoneal dialysis with dialysates containing dextrose or dextrose and amino acids on muscle protein turnover in patients with chronic renal failure. *J Am Soc Nephrol* 2001;12:557–567.
83. Alvestrand A, Ahlberg M, Furst P, et al. Clinical results of long-term treatment with a low protein diet and a new amino acid preparation in patients with chronic uremia. *Clin Nephrol* 1983; 19:67–72.
84. Wang M, Vyhmester J, Kopple JD, et al. Effect of protein intake on weight gain and plasma amino acid levels in uremic rats. *Am J Physiol* 1976;230:1455–1459.
85. Garber AJ. Skeletal muscle protein and amino acid metabolism in experimental chronic uremia in the rat: accelerated alanine and glutamine formation and release. *J Clin Invest* 1978;62: 623–632.
86. Harter HR, Karl IE, Klahr S, et al. Effect of reduced renal mass and dietary protein intake on amino acid release and glucose uptake by rat muscle in vitro. *J Clin Invest* 1979;64:513–523.
87. Holliday MA, Chantler C, MacDonnel R, et al. Effect of uremia on nutritionally-induced variations in protein metabolism. *Kidney Int* 1977;11:236–245.
88. Li JB, Wassner SJ. Protein synthesis and degradation in skeletal muscle of chronically uremic rats. *Kidney Int* 1986;29: 1136–1143.
89. Pennisi AJ, Wang M, Kopple JD. Effects of protein and amino acid diets in chronically uremic and control rats. *Kidney Int* 1978;13:472–479.
90. Garber AJ. Effects of parathyroid hormone on skeletal muscle and amino acid metabolism in the rat. *J Clin Invest* 1983;71: 1806–1821.
91. Harter HR, Birge SJ, Martin KJ, et al. Effects of vitamin D metabolites on protein catabolism of muscle from uremic rats. *Kidney Int* 1983;23:465–472.
92. Price SR, England BK, Bailey JL, et al. Acidosis and glucocorticoids concomitantly increase ubiquitin and proteasome subunit mRNAs in rat muscle. *Am J Physiol* 1994;267:C955–C960.
93. Kuemmerle N, Krieg RJ Jr, Latta K, et al. Growth hormone and insulin-like growth factor in non-uremic acidosis and uremic acidosis. *Kidney Int Suppl* 1997;58:S102–S105.
94. Goodship THJ, Mitch WE, Hoerr RA, et al. Adaptation to low-protein diets in renal failure: leucine turnover and nitrogen balance. *J Am Soc Nephrol* 1990;1:66–75.
95. Adey D, Kumar R, McCarthy JT, et al. Reduced synthesis of muscle proteins in chronic renal failure. *Am J Physiol Endocrinol Metab* 2000;278(2):E219–E225.
96. Castellino P, Solini A, Luzi L, et al. Glucose and amino acid metabolism in chronic renal failure: effect of insulin and amino acids. *Am J Physiol* 1992;262:F168–F176.
97. Lim VS, Yarasheski KE, Flanigan MJ. The effect of uremia, acidosis, and dialysis treatment on protein metabolism: a longitudinal leucine kinetic study. *Nephrol Dial Transplant* 1998;13: 1723–1730.
98. Berkelhammer CH, Baker JP, Leiter LA, et al. Whole body protein turnover in adult hemodialysis patients as measured by ^{13}C-leucine. *Am J Clin Nutr* 1987;46:778–783.
99. Lim VS, Bier DM, Flanigan MJ, et al. The effect of hemodialysis on protein metabolism. A leucine kinetic study. *J Clin Invest* 1993;91:2429–2436.

100. Giordano M, De Feo P, Lucidi P, et al. Increased albumin and fibrinogen synthesis in hemodialysis patients with normal nutritional status. *J Am Soc Nephrol* 2001;12:349–354.
101. Goodship TH, Lloyd S, Clague MB, et al. Whole-body leucine turnover and nutritional status in continuous ambulatory peritoneal dialysis. *Clin Sci* 1987;73:463–469.
102. Castellino P, Luzi L, Giordano M, et al. Effects of insulin and amino acids on glucose and leucine metabolism in CAPD patients. *J Am Soc Nephrol* 1999;10:1050–1058.
103. Boirie Y, Broyer M, Gagnadoux MF, et al. Alterations of protein metabolism by metabolic acidosis in children with chronic renal failure. *Kidney Int* 2000;58:236–241.
104. Graham KA, Reaich D, Channon SM, et al. Correction of acidosis in hemodialysis decreases whole-body protein degradation. *J Am Soc Nephrol* 1997;8:632–637.
105. Graham KA, Reaich D, Channon SM, et al. Correction of acidosis in CAPD decreases whole body protein degradation. *Kidney Int* 1996;49:1396–1400.
106. Motil KJ, Matthews DE, Bier DM, et al. Whole-body leucine and lysine metabolism: response to dietary protein intake in young men. *Am J Physiol* 1981;240:E712–E721.
107. Petrides AS, Luzi L, DeFronzo RA. Time-dependent regulation by insulin of leucine metabolism in young healthy adults. *Am J Physiol* 1994;267:E361–E368.
108. Deferrari G, Garibotto G, Robaudo C, et al. Leg metabolism of amino acid and ammonia in patients with chronic renal failure. *Clin Science* 1985;69:143–150.
109. Alvestrand A, DeFronzo RA, Smith D, et al. Influence of hyperinsulinemia on intracellular amino acids levels and amino acid exchange across splanchnic and leg tissues in uremia. *Clin Sci* 1988;74:155–162.
110. Garibotto G, Russo R, Sofia A, et al. Muscle protein turnover in CRF patients with metabolic acidosis or normal acid-base balance. *Miner Electrolyte Metab* 1996;22:58–61.
111. Balagopal P, Ljungqvist O, Nair KS. Skeletal muscle myosin heavy-chain synthesis rate in healthy humans. *Am J Physiol* 1997;272:E45–E50.
112. Garibotto G, Barreca A, Russo R, et al. Effects of recombinant human growth hormone on muscle protein turnover in malnourished hemodialysis patients. *J Clin Invest* 1997;99:97–105.
113. Garibotto G, Barreca A, Sofia A, et al. Effects of growth hormone on leptin metabolism and energy expenditure in hemodialysis patients with protein-calorie malnutrition. *J Am Soc Nephrol* 2000;11:2106–2113.
114. Clark MG, Colquhon EQ, Rattigan S, et al. Vascular and endocrine control of muscle metabolism. *Am J Physiol* 1995;268: E797–E803.
115. Bradley JR, Anderson JR, Evans DB, et al. Impaired nutritive skeletal muscle blood flow in patients with chronic renal failure. *Clin Sci* 1990;79:239–245.
116. Luzi L, Battezzati A, Perseghin G, et al. Combined pancreas and kidney transplantation normalizes protein metabolism in insulin-dependent diabetic-uremic patients. *J Clin Invest* 1994; 93:1948–1958.
117. Austin SA, Clemens MJ. The regulation of protein synthesis in mammalian cells by amino acid supply. *Biosci Report* 1981;1: 35–41.
118. Louard RJ, Fryburg DA, Gelfand RA, et al. Insulin sensitivity of protein and glucose metabolism in human forearm skeletal muscle. *J Clin Invest* 1992;90:2348–2354.
119. May RC. Effects of renal insufficiency on nutrient metabolism and endocrine function. In: Mitch WE, Klahr S, eds. *Nutrition and the kidney.* Boston: Little, Brown, 1993;35–47.
120. Reaich D, Gralun KA, Channon SM, et al. Insulin-mediated changes in protein degradation and glucose uptake after correction of acidosis in humans with CRF. *Am J Physiol* 1995;268: E121–E126.
121. Denne SC, Brechtel G, Johnson A, et al. Skeletal muscle proteolysis is reduced in non insulin-dependent diabetes mellitus and is unrelated to euglicemic hyperinsulinemia or intensive insulin therapy. *J Clin Endocrinol Metab* 1995;80:2371–2377.
122. Sayegh R, Lim VS. Endocrine disturbances. In: Daugirdas JT, Blake PG, Ing TS, eds. *Handbook of dialysis,* 3rd ed. Lippincott Williams & Wilkins, 2001;522–529.
123. Miyoshi H, Shulman G, Peters E, et al. Hormonal control of substrate cycling in humans. *J Clin Invest* 1988;81:1545–1555.
124. Ferrando AA, Stuart CA, Sheffield-Moore M, et al. Inactivity amplifies the catabolic response of skeletal muscle to cortisol. *J Clin Endocrinol Metab* 1999;84:3515–3521.
125. Wolfe RR, Durkot MJ, Allsop J, et al. Glucose metabolism in severely burned patients. *Metabolism* 1979;28:1031–1039.
126. Kopple JD, Ding H, Gao XL. Altered physiology and action of insulin-like growth factor-1 in skeletal muscle in chronic renal failure. *Am J Kidney Dis* 1995;26:248–255.
127. Fouque D, Peng SC, Kopple JD. Impaired metabolic response to recombinant Insulin-like Growth Factor-1 in dialysis patients. *Kidney Int* 1995;47:876–883.
128. Norrelund H, Nair KS, Jorgensen JO, et al. The protein-retaining effects of growth hormone during fasting involve inhibition of muscle-protein breakdown. *Diabetes* 2001;50:96–104.
129. Tonshoff B, Edén S, Weiser E, et al. Reduced hepatic growth hormone (GH) receptor gene expression and increased plasma GH binding protein in experimental uremia. *Kidney Int* 1994; 45:1085–1092.
130. Tonshoff B, Powell DR, Zhao D, et al. Decreased hepatic insulin-like growth factor (IGF)-I and increased IGF binding protein-1 and -2 gene expression in experimental uremia. *Endocrinology* 1997;138:938–946.
131. Ding H, Gao XL, Hirschberg R, et al. Impaired actions of insulin-like growth factor 1 on protein synthesis and degradation in skeletal muscle of rats with chronic renal failure. Evidence for a post-receptor defect. *J Clin Invest* 1996;97: 1064–1075.
132. Thissen JP, Ketelslegers JM, Underwood LE. Nutritional regulation of the insulin-like growth factors. *Endocr Rev* 1994;15: 80–101.
133. Lee PD, Conover CA, Powell DR. Regulation and function of insulin-like growth factor-binding protein-1. *Proc Soc Exp Biol Med* 1993;204:4–29.
134. Hokken-Koelega AC, Stijnen T, de Muinck Keizer-Schrama SM, et al. Placebo-controlled, double-blind, cross-over trial of growth hormone treatment in prepubertal children with chronic renal failure. *Lancet* 1991;338:585–590.
135. Frystyk J, Ivarsen P, Skjaerbaek C, et al. Serum-free insulin-like growth factor I correlates with clearance in patients with chronic renal failure. *Kidney Int* 1999;56:2076–2082.
136. Stenvinkel P, Heimburger O, Paultre F, et al. Strong association between malnutrition, inflammation and atherosclerosis in chronic renal failure. *Kidney Int* 1999;55:1899–1911.
137. Tracey KJ, Morgello S, Koplin B, et al. Metabolic effects of cachectin/tumor necrosis factor are modified by site of production. Cachectin/tumor necrosis factor-secreting tumor in skeletal muscle induces chronic cachexia, while implantation in brain induces predominantly acute anorexia. *J Clin Invest* 1990;86: 2014–2024.
138. Jepson MM, Pell JM, Bates PC, et al. The effects of endotoxaemia on protein metabolism in skeletal muscle and liver of fed and fasted rats. *Biochem J* 1986;235:329–336.
139. Long CL, Jeevanandam M, Kim BM, et al. Whole body protein synthesis and catabolism in septic man. *Am J Clin Nutr* 1977; 30:1340–1344.

140. Shaw JHF, Wildbore M, Wolfe RR. Whole body protein kinetics in severely septic patients: the response to glucose infusion and total parenteral nutrition. *Ann Surg* 1987;225:288–294.
141. Macallan DC, McNurlan MA, Milne E, et al. Whole body protein turnover and the response to nutrition in human immunodeficiency virus infection. *Am J Clin Nutr* 1995;61:816–826.
142. Selberg O, Suttman U, Meltzer A, et al. Effect of increased protein intake and nutritional status on whole body protein metabolism of AIDS patients with weight loss. *Metab Clin Exp* 1995;44:1159–1165.
143. Maccallan DC, McNurlan MA, Kurpad AV, et al. Whole body protein metabolism in human pulmonary tuberculosis and undernutrition: evidence for anabolic block in tuberculosis. *Clin Sci* 1998;94:321–331.
144. Paton NI, Angus B, Chaowagul W, et al. Protein and energy metabolism in chronic bacterial infection: studies in melioidosis. *Clin Sci* 2001;100:101–110.
145. Tomkins AM, Garlick PJ, Schofield WN, et al. The combined effect of infection and malnutrition on protein metabolism in children. *Clin Sci* 1983;65:313–324.
146. Forbes GB. Lean body mass fat interrelationships in humans. *Nutr Rev* 1987;45:225–231.
147. Kopple JD, Zhu X, Lew NL, et al. Body weight-for-height relationships predict mortality in maintenance hemodialysis patients. *Kidney Int* 1999;56:1136–1148.
148. Young VR. Kinetics of human acid metabolism: nutritional implications and some lessons. McCollum Award Lecture. *Am J Clin Nutr* 1987;46:709–725.
149. Lim VS, Kopple JD. Protein metabolism in patients with chronic renal failure: role of uremia and dialysis. *Kidney Int* 2000;58:1–10.
150. Williams B, Hattersley J, Layward E, et al. Metabolic acidosis and skeletal muscle adaptation to low protein diets in chronic uremia. *Kidney Int* 1991;40:779–786.
151. Bernhard J, Beaufrere B, Laville M, et al. Adaptive response to a low-protein diet in predialysis chronic renal failure patients. *J Am Soc Nephrol* 2001;12:1249–1254.
152. Masud T, Young VR, Chapman T, et al. Adaptive responses to very low protein diets: the first comparison of ketoacids to essential amino acids. *Kidney Int* 1994;45:1182–1192.
153. Tom K, Young VR, Chapman T, et al. Long-term adaptive responses to dietary protein restriction in chronic renal failure. *Am J Physiol Endocrinol Metab* 1995;268:E668–E677.
154. Schoenfeld PY, Henrt RR, Laird NM, et al. Assessment of nutritional status of the national cooperative dialysis study population. *Kidney Int* 1983;23:80–88.
155. Kopple JD, Swendseid ME, Shinaberger JH, et al. The free and bound amino acids removed by hemodialysis. *Trans Am Soc Artif Int Org* 1973;19:309–313.
156. Ikizler TA, Flakoll PJ, Parker R, et al. Amino acid and albumin losses during hemodialysis. *Kidney Int* 1994;46:830–837.
157. Lofberg E, Wernerman J, Noree LO, et al. Ribosome and free amino acid content in muscle during hemodialysis. *Kidney Int* 1991;39:984–989.
158. Lofberg E, Essen P, McNurlan M, et al. Effect of hemodialysis on protein synthesis. *Clin Nephrol* 2000;54:284–294.
159. Gutierrez A, Alvestrand A, Bergstrom J. Membrane selection and muscle protein catabolism. *Kidney Int Suppl* 1992;38:S86–S90.
160. Gutierrez A, Alvestrand A, Wahren J, et al. Effect of in vivo contact between blood and dialysis membranes on protein catabolism in humans. *Kidney Int* 1990;38:487–494.
161. Gutierrez A, Bergstrom J, Alvestrand A. Protein catabolism in sham hemodialysis: effects of different membranes. *Clin Nephrol* 1992;38:20–29.
162. Lindsay RM, Spanner E. A hypothesis: the protein catabolic rate is dependent upon the type and amount of treatment in dialyzed uremic patients. *Am J Kidney Dis* 1989;132:382–389.
163. Parker TF 3rd, Wingard RL, Husni L, et al. Effect of the membrane biocompatibility on nutritional parameters in chronic hemodialysis patients. *Kidney Int* 1996;49:551–556.
164. Lindholm B, Alvestrand A, Furst P, et al. Plasma and muscle free amino acids during continuous ambulatory peritoneal dialysis. *Kidney Int* 1989;35:12.
165. Guarnieri GF, Toigo G, Situlin R, et al. Nutritional state in patients on long-term low-protein diet or with nephrotic syndrome. *Kidney Int Suppl* 1989;27:S195–S200.
166. Kaysen GA. Albumin metabolism in the nephrotic syndrome: the effect of dietary protein intake. *Am J Kidney Dis* 1988;12:461–480.
167. Choi EJ, May RC, Bailey J, et al. Mechanisms of adaptation to proteinuria in adriamycin nephrosis. *Am J Physiol* 1993;265:F257–F263.
168. Choi EJ, Bailey J, May RC, et al. Metabolic responses to nephrosis: effect of a low-protein diet. *Am J Physiol* 1994;266:F432–F438.
169. Maroni BJ, Staffeld C, Young VR, et al. Mechanisms permitting nephrotic patients to achieve nitrogen equilibrium with a protein-restricted diet. *J Clin Invest* 1997;99:2479–2487.
170. Lim VS, Wolfson M, Yarasheski KE, et al. Leucine turnover in patients with nephrotic syndrome: evidence suggesting body protein conservation. *J Am Soc Nephrol* 1998;9:1067–1073.
171. de Sain-Van Der Velden MG, de Meer K, Kulik W, et al. Nephrotic proteinuria has no net effect on total body protein synthesis: measurements with (13)C valine. *Am J Kidney Dis* 2000;35:1149–1154.
172. Zanetti M, Barazzoni R, Garibotto G, et al. Plasma protein synthesis in patients with low-grade nephrotic proteinuria. *Am J Physiol* 2001;280:E591–E597.
173. Latos DL. Chronic dialysis in patients over age 65. *J Am Soc Nephrol* 1996;7:637–646.
174. Lindeman RD. Overview: renal physiology and pathophysiology of aging. *Am J Kidney Dis* 1990;16:275–282.
175. Timiras PS. Aging of the skeleton, joints and muscles. In: Timiras PD, ed. *Physiological basis of aging and geriatrics,* 2nd ed. Boca Raton: CRC Press, 1994;259–272.
176. Rothstein M. Altered proteins, errors and aging. In: Segal HL, Rothstein M, Bergamini P, eds. *Protein metabolism in aging.* New York: Wiley-Liss, Inc. 1990;3–14.
177. Gersovitz M, Bier D, Matthews D, et al. Dynamic aspects of whole body glycine metabolism. Influence of protein intake in young adult and elderly males. *Metabolism* 1980;29:1087–1094.
178. Robert JJ, Bier D, Schoeller D, et al. Effect of intravenous glucose on whole body leucine dynamics, studied with 1-^{13}C-leucine, in healthy, young and elderly adults. *J Gerontol* 1984;39:673–681.
179. Nair KS. Age-related changes in muscle. *Mayo Clin Proc* 2000;75S:S14–S18.
180. Boirie Y, Gachon P, Cordat N, et al. Differential insulin sensitivities of glucose, amino acid, and albumin metabolism in elderly men and women. *J Clin Endocrinol Metab* 2001;86:638–644.
181. Brodsky IG, Robbins DC, Hiser E, et al. Effects of low-protein diets on protein metabolism in insulin-dependent diabetes mellitus patients with early nephropathy. *J Clin Endocrinol Metab* 1992;75:351–357.
182. Bier DM. Protein metabolism in type II diabetes mellitus. In:

Nair KS, ed. *Protein metabolism in diabetes mellitus.* London: Smith Gordon, 1992;243–248.
183. Walker JD, Bending JJ, Dodds RA, et al. Restriction of dietary protein and progression of renal failure in diabetic nephropathy. *Lancet* 1989;2:1411–1415.
184. Zeller K, Whittaker E, Sullivan L, et al. Effect of restricting dietary protein on progression of renal failure in patients with insulin-dependent diabetes mellitus. *N Engl J Med* 1991;324: 78–84.
185. Battezzati A, Luzi L. Protein metabolism after B-cell function replacement in type I diabetes. In: Tessari P, Soeters P, Pittoni G, et al., eds. *Amino acid and protein metabolism in health and disease: nutritional implications.* London: Smith-Gordon, 1997; 141–147.

2

CARBOHYDRATE METABOLISM IN RENAL FAILURE

MARK E. WILLIAMS

Now widely recognized, abnormalities in glucose metabolism in uremia first were described 90 years ago (1–3). Among the many metabolic derangements now associated with uremia, the characteristic abnormalities of glucose metabolism are insulin resistance and carbohydrate intolerance (4). Insulin secretion, insulin metabolism, and insulin sensitivity all may be abnormal in the patient with uremia (5). Of these, insulin clearance predictably is impaired, insulin secretion is inadequate, and insulin sensitivity is reduced in the majority of individuals. As a result, insulin resistance is the dominant carbohydrate effect in uremia (6), unrelated to underlying diabetes mellitus. Factors affecting glycemia in the uremic patient are listed in Table 2.1.

By definition, insulin resistance is present when a given concentration of insulin is associated with a subnormal glucose response (7). Clinically, evidence for insulin resistance is found in the form of a normal fasting blood sugar in the presence of hyperinsulinemia, a blunted response to exogenous insulin, and a diminished effect of intravenous insulin to improve glucose uptake (8,9). The major site of reduced insulin-stimulated glucose transport in uremic patients occurs in peripheral tissues, primarily in skeletal muscle (10). In the complex action of insulin on muscle, several studies have determined that a postreceptor defect is present, although the pathogenesis is not certain. The characteristic feature of insulin resistance may be present early in the course of renal disease (11), and the majority of uremic individuals are affected to some extent (10,12). However, insulin secretion in the form of a diminished secretory response to glucose plays a contributing role (13). In many patients with chronic renal failure, insulin secretion is relatively unresponsive, and glucose intolerance or mild fasting hyperglycemia is the result. Although hyperglycemia is not severe, the long-term effects of hyperglycemia and hyperinsulinemia combined can be significant (14). Alternatively, other patients with uremia may do better at maintaining normoglycemia because of compensatory hyperinsulin production, so that normal blood glucose levels are maintained. It is likely that varying degrees of insulin resistance and insulin secretion result in a spectrum of abnormalities in glucose metabolism, with a delayed and diminished response to insulin, normal to high serum insulin values, and normal to elevated fasting blood sugar levels being the most common.

Several factors are becoming increasingly more recognizable as contributions to these abnormalities. They include uremia itself, hyperparathyroidism, vitamin D status, metabolic acidosis (15,16), and anemia (Table 2.2). This chapter will discuss these abnormalities, as well as hypoglycemia, monitoring glycemic control, the effect of dietary protein restriction on glucose metabolism, and the buildup of advanced glycation end products in uremia.

INSULIN RESISTANCE

In reality, insulin sensitivity is somewhat variable in patients with renal disease, just as in other disorders such as type 2 diabetes mellitus, obesity, or even normal subjects (11). Numerous studies have led to the conclusion that uremic insulin resistance appears to be restricted to defects in glucose uptake and muscle protein metabolism (1). The former is neither the result of suppressed insulin hormone secretion nor of failure of insulin to normally suppress hepatic glucose production (5). According to euglycemic hyperinsulinemic clamp studies in patients with renal disease, hepatic glucose uptake is normal and hepatic glucose production suppresses normally in uremia (17). Alternatively, the ability of insulin to stimulate peripheral glucose disposal by muscle and adipose tissue is markedly impaired (see later in this chapter). Although an increase in net proteolysis, the resultant be-

TABLE 2.1. MAJOR FACTORS CONTRIBUTING TO GLUCOSE METABOLISM IN UREMIA

Insulin resistance
Impaired insulin secretion
Reduced clearance of insulin
Poor nutrition
Diabetes mellitus

TABLE 2.2. POTENTIAL FACTORS IN INSULIN RESISTANCE OF UREMIA

Hyperparathyroidism
Accumulation of uremic toxins
Metabolic acidosis
Relative vitamin D deficiency
Anemia

tween protein synthesis and degradation, has been reported in uremia (18), the antiproteolytic action of insulin may be normal (12). Another insulin-mediated effect, enhancement of sodium pump activity leading to translocation of potassium into cells, has increased sensitivity to uremia (19).

Glucose transport, one of the major activities of insulin, is believed to be rate limiting for glucose uptake in peripheral tissues (12). Insulin binding creates a hormone-receptor interaction to enhance an insulin-signaling pathway where membrane and intracellular events lead to the biologic actions of the hormone, such as the flux of glucose into the cell (20). The transport of glucose into cells is mediated by specific glucose transporter proteins (Fig. 2.1). Insulin action at the cellular level is complex (10). However, it is known to include the following: activation of intrinsic tyrosine kinase activities found in the receptor intracellular β subunit portion, intracellular responses including generation of messengers for insulin, interiorization of the receptor-insulin complex within the cell, translocation of hexose transporter units into the plasma membrane from intracellular storage sites, and the downstream metabolic effects of the hormone (21,22).

Insulin initiates its actions by binding to the tetrameric membrane receptor (23). There is no evidence in type 2 diabetes mellitus, obesity, or uremia that altered receptor messenger RNA (mRNA) transcription occurs. The products of mRNA translation include a linear α and β sequence; the receptor for insulin consists of two extracellular α subunits, each linked to a transmembrane β subunit. Insulin initiates its action by low-affinity binding to the tetrameric membrane receptor. The insulin receptor is a member of the family of receptor tyrosine kinases. Following insulin binding, the receptor undergoes autophosphorylation on multiple tyrosine residues. Autophosphorylation is impor-

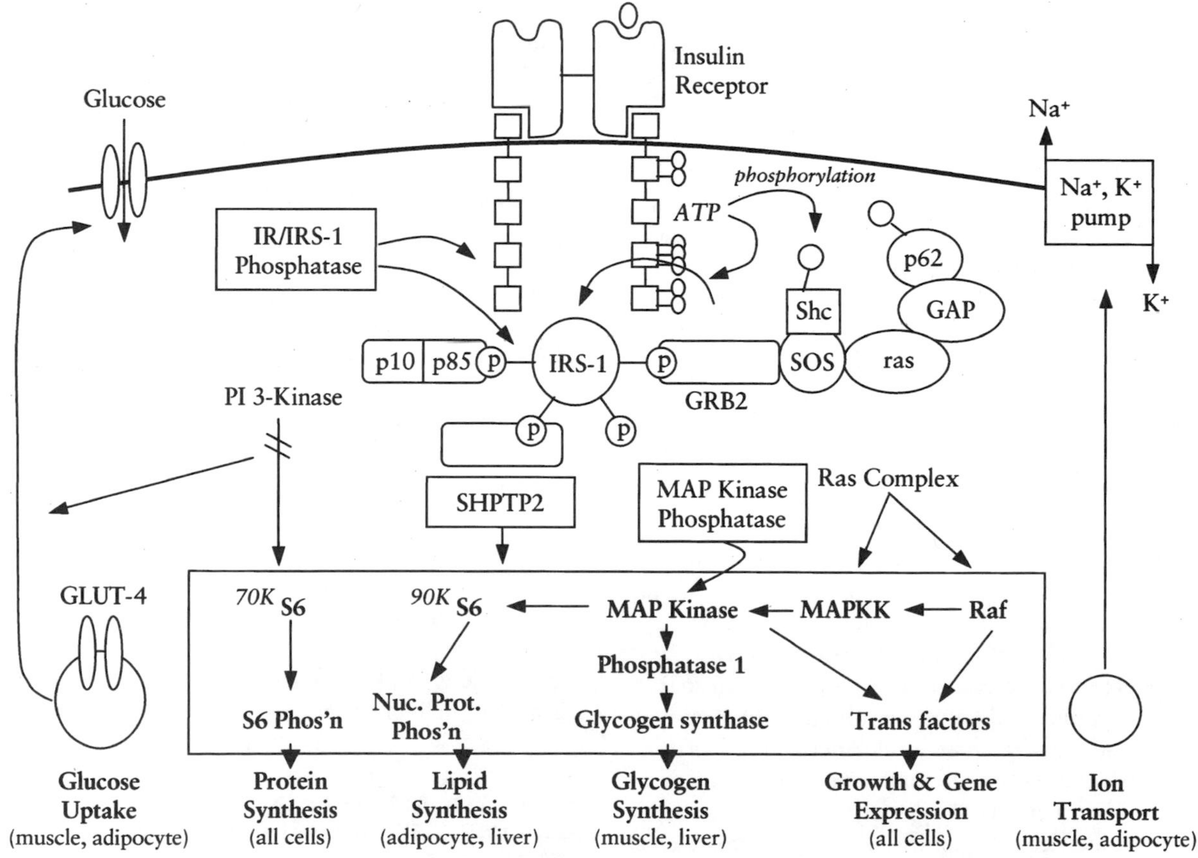

FIGURE 2.1. Schematic representation of the insulin receptor and activation of insulin-triggered cellular events in responsive tissues. In activating glucose transport and disposal pathways at the cellular level, insulin binds to the α subunit of its receptor, causing the β subunit to autophosphorylate and phosphorylate insulin receptor substrate-1, a cytoplasmic receptor. IRS-1 interacts with proteins such as PI-3-kinase. Activation of Glut-4, the glucose transporter, follows. Other complex signaling pathways are involved in glycogen synthesis and other cellular events.

tant in activation of receptor tyrosine kinase activity for other substrates, in addition to the actions of the hormone itself. The principal substrate of the activated receptor is the cytosolic protein, insulin receptor substrate-1 (IRS-1). The insulin-signaling pathway is central to the biologic actions of insulin and is itself a complex process known to include the phosphorylation cascade and generation of intracellular messengers for insulin. The IRS-1 substrate is linked to serine kinases, which act on enzymes like glycogen synthase, transcription factors, and other proteins to produce many of the final biologic effects of the hormone (Fig. 2.1). In muscle and adipose tissue, insulin stimulates glucose uptake by promoting translocation of an intracellular pool of glucose transporters to the plasma membrane. In the absence of continued insulin secretion, the cellular actions of the hormone dissipate in two ways: through dissociation of insulin from the receptor complex and through dephosphorylation of IRS-1 and the receptor kinase.

The cellular mechanisms by which uremia interferes with insulin action on glucose transport in target tissues remain uncertain (Table 2.3). Despite its importance, impaired insulin binding to its receptor or related effects on β-subunit phosphorylation and tyrosine kinase activity do not appear to account for insulin resistance in uremia (24). Reduced binding could result from a decreased number of available insulin receptors or from reduced receptor affinity for the hormone. However, in chronically uremic rats, insulin binding to its receptor is unaltered in skeletal muscle (25,26), liver (27), and adipocytes (28). The molecular mass of receptor also does not differ from the nonuremic state. Finally, tyrosine kinase activity is normal, not decreased, in receptors from liver, muscle, and adipocytes in uremic rats. Similar to the best-studied insulin-resistant state—type 2 diabetes mellitus—none of the possible insulin-receptor defects appear to be important in uremic insulin resistance.

The aforementioned data do suggest that the insulin resistance in uremia involves sites distal to the insulin receptor, from the generation of intracellular messengers for insulin (10) to glucose transport to effects of insulin on one of the intracellular enzymes involved in glucose metabolism itself (29). Several lines of evidence suggest that multiple defects are possible: (a) the release of small–molecular-weight intracellular mediators for insulin action following its binding to the receptor may be impaired; (b) uremia also may interfere with glucose action at the level of the glucose transport system. Changes in glucose transport expression, translocation, or activity may be required. Although several glucose transporters have been identified, the expression of glut-4, a major glucose transporter in striated muscle, is normal in muscle from uremic animals (24). However, related defects such as decreases in the insulin-stimulated transporter translocation to the cell surface (less recruitment) or a fractional decrease in transporter activity (less activation) may exist. Some differences might be related to polymorphism in the regulatory part of the transporter chain (3). The subsequent modulation of insulin by intracellular regulatory enzymes and intracellular pathways of glucose metabolism, including glucose oxidation and glucose storage, also could be impaired in uremia. Data suggest that the impairment in glucose storage via glycogen synthase activity is an important factor (30). Muscle glycogen synthesis is impaired to a lesser degree in uremia. Several studies have shown abnormalities in oxidative glucose metabolism in renal failure. It is different to quantitate insulin-mediated intracellular events directly in humans.

TABLE 2.3. POTENTIAL CELLULAR DEFECTS UNDERLYING UREMIC INSULIN RESISTANCE

Initial processing of insulin-receptor complexes
Generation of intracellular messengers
Phosphorylation of enzymes of metabolic pathways
Translocation of hexose transporter units
Glycogen synthase activity
Glucose oxidation

In the complex metabolic milieu of uremia, variations in insulin sensitivity may reflect interactions of multiple genetic and nongenetic factors; several etiologic factors in insulin resistance have been evaluated, primarily over the past decade, as reviewed by Alvestrand (12). Among the contributing factors are hyperparathyroidism, metabolic acidosis (15), cytokine activation (31), and anemia (32). In addition to these factors, buildup of a uremic toxin could account for the observed improvement in insulin-mediated glucose metabolism in tissues, associated with hemodialysis and peritoneal dialysis treatment (33,34). However, a recent study demonstrated diminished insulin sensitivity early in patients with renal disease (immunoglobulin A nephropathy and polycystic kidney disease), including a subset with essentially normal renal function tests (35) (Fig. 2.2). Another study demonstrated insulin resistance in adult patients with polycystic kidney disease with normal kidney function and no buildup of uremic toxins (36).

Among these potential etiologic factors, work done primarily in the past decade has focused attention on the interrelated roles of parathyroid hormone, 1,25-dihydroxy vitamin D, and calcium in uremic glucose intolerance. The characteristic uremic features of insulin resistance and relatively impaired insulin secretion have been evaluated. Similar to diabetes research, studies have used the plasma disappearance of glucose (glucose utilization), indirectly described as the glucose metabolic rate divided by plasma insulin levels, to relate these two features.

Conflicting evidence for a primary role of parathyroid hormone and uremic glucose intolerance has accrued over the past quarter century. Initially, insulin sensitivity, glucose utilization, or insulin secretion were noted to be affected by parathyroidectomy in uremic patients with secondary hyperparathyroidism (37). Subsequent studies generally re-

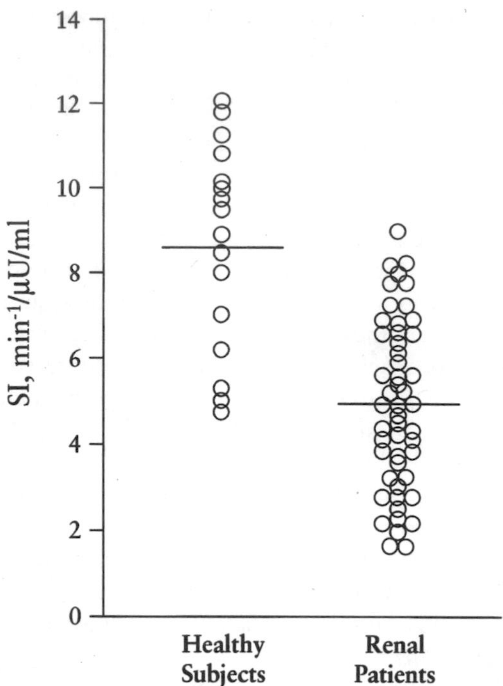

FIGURE 2.2. Insulin sensitivity index (SI), a calculated measure of the effect of insulin on glucose disappearance, in renal patients compared to healthy controls. SIs for renal subsets were 5.1 ± 0.7 (serum creatinine <1.3 mg%), 5.1 ± 0.7 (serum creatinine 1.3 to 3.0 mg%), and 4.7 ± 0.6 (serum creatinine >3 mg%), compared to 8.6 ± 0.8 (controls). (From Fliser D, Pacini G, Engelleiter R, et al. Insulin resistance and hyperinsulinemia are already present in patients with incipient renal disease. *Kidney Int* 1998;53: 1343–1347, with permission.)

ported that medical or surgical parathyroidectomy had no effect on insulin sensitivity, although glucose intolerance improved because of an increase in insulin secretion (see later in this chapter).

The amelioration of hyperparathyroidism by parathyroidectomy does not appear to affect insulin sensitivity (38). Even with control of hyperparathyroidism in uremia, animal and human studies showed persistent peripheral insulin resistance in uremia. By suppression of insulin secretion, inadequate control of excessive parathyroid secretion would be predicted to lead to ongoing glucose intolerance (39). In addition to these effects, 1,25-dihydroxy vitamin D administration is known to return insulin sensitivity toward normal, either directly or by reducing secondary hyperparathyroidism itself. Initial data supported a direct role for vitamin D deficiency in the pathogenesis of impaired glucose metabolism in uremia. Similar to the role of parathyroid hormone, vitamin D regulation of both insulin secretion and insulin sensitivity has been evaluated. Whereas most studies have examined the role of vitamin D in insulin secretion, two recent studies have followed the observation of Mak (40) that single pharmacologic doses of vitamin D may improve insulin resistance in patients undergoing hemodialysis. In a study that confirmed severe insulin resistance in a group of patients undergoing hemodialysis (sensitivity decreased by roughly half), Kautzky-Willer showed that 12 weeks of 1,25-dihydroxy vitamin D had a direct effect to improve insulin sensitivity to values similar to control groups, without any apparent changes in insulin secretion (41).

Similarly, one-alpha hydroxy vitamin D_3, a synthetic vitamin D analogue that undergoes 25-hydroxylation in the liver to 1,25-dihydroxycholecalciferol, improved insulin resistance (measured as the rate constant for plasma glucose disappearance) in 14 chronic hemodialysis patients by 33% after 4 weeks to a level similar to controls (38). In both studies, parathyroid hormone concentrations decreased (by roughly 25% to 50%), potentially accounting for the effect of vitamin D to improve insulin resistance.

This summary indicates that disturbances in the parathyroid/vitamin D axis may play a role in insulin sensitivity and glucose intolerance of uremia. Potential mechanisms in these complex pathophysiologic changes in parathyroid and vitamin D homeostasis remain incompletely understood. However, related changes in calcium balance and cytosolic calcium could provide one mechanism (42). In addition to these direct effects of parathyroid hormone or vitamin D, it is known that elevated cytosolic calcium in insulin target-tissue cells renders them resistant to insulin. The mechanism by which high levels of cytosolic calcium interfere with cellular insulin action appears to involve post-receptor stages of insulin action. Phosphorylation and de-phosphorylation of the primary insulin-sensitive substrates, glycogen synthase, and insulin-regulatable glucose transporter (Glut-4) have been evaluated. High levels of intracellular calcium inhibit phosphorylase phosphatase activity, preventing normal dephosphorylation of glycogen synthase and Glut-4 in response to insulin. Serum calcium levels are variable in uremia, depending in part on parathyroid and vitamin D status. Total serum calcium levels would be expected to rise with advanced hyperparathyroidism.

LOW PROTEIN DIET

Insulin resistance and glucose metabolism do not occur in total isolation in patients with uremia. In patients with and without diabetes, other metabolic relationships exist, among them protein metabolism. Patients with uremia—mainly those undergoing dialysis—have a high prevalence of protein malnutrition (44,45). Up to 67% of patients with end-stage renal disease are protein-malnourished. 60% have a serum albumin level below the lower limit of normal (46). The undernourished state is associated with significantly increased mortality risk (45). Protein malnutrition is frequently present even before dialysis therapy commences. A common contributing factor is anorexia. Spontaneous dietary protein intake decreases significantly as renal failure progresses (47). Furthermore, low protein diets are commonly prescribed for patients with renal failure to slow the progression of chronic renal failure.

The efficacy of dietary protein restriction in slowing the progression of either diabetic or nondiabetic kidney disease has been evaluated in several clinical trials (48). While these have not shown consistent benefit, pooling of the results in a meta-analysis concluded that dietary protein restriction was justified in patients with chronic renal disease and renal insufficiency (49). Fewer studies have been done in patients with diabetic kidney disease, and they have not routinely included the use of angiotensin-converting enzyme inhibitor therapy. Two small controlled trials have demonstrated a reduced rate of decline in glomerular filtration rate with a dietary protein restriction of 0.6 g/kg/day (50,51). However, data suggest that patients with diabetes and end-stage renal disease have more cachexia, slightly lower serum albumin levels, and poorer overall nutritional status than nondiabetic patients.

Beneficial effects of dietary protein restriction on glucose metabolism have been reported in patients with diabetes without uremia (52). Patients with diabetes may adapt differently than patients without diabetes to dietary protein restriction. Although nutritional recommendations for protein intake for individuals with diabetes are lacking (53), it is known that an average of 10% to 20% of daily caloric intake derives from protein. Low-protein diets may obligate increased carbohydrate rations to maintain sufficient caloric intake (54). Despite this, no worsening of carbohydrate metabolism results.

Glucose intolerance, secondary to uremia, may be reversed by treatment with a low-protein diet (55). Treatment with a dietary protein restriction and an amino acid/ketoacid supplement over 6 months increased insulin secretion and returned glucose metabolism to normal (56) in children with uremia. Rigalleau et al. (57) confirmed the improvement in insulin sensitivity and glucose disposal in adults. Whether the effect is specific to uremia, however, is unclear. Despite a high carbohydrate intake, glucose intolerance is improved, insulin levels are reduced, and reduced insulin resistance is observed in hyperinsulinemic–euglycemic clamp studies (58). Increased insulin sensitivity involves endogenous glucose production, glucose oxidative disposal, and glucose nonoxidative disposal, despite lower plasma insulin levels. Higher energy production rates result. Which factor associated with insulin resistance of uremia might be corrected by a low-protein diet is unknown.

Despite these beneficial effects on glucose metabolism, however, patients with diabetes may be at risk for increased protein malnutrition because of greater protein breakdown secondary to insulin deficiency (59). An increase in net proteolysis as a result of an imbalance between protein synthesis and degradation reported in uremic animals may be related to insulin resistance (18). Insulin, an important anabolic hormone, affects protein metabolism by inhibiting muscle proteolysis. Uremic resistance to insulin involves not only carbohydrate but also protein metabolism (48). Patients with diabetes placed on a low-protein diet experience maladaptive protein undernutrition, related to accelerated protein degradation and amino acid oxidation (60). As a result, dietary protein restriction should be used cautiously in diabetic patients with chronic kidney disease.

INSULIN HOMEOSTASIS IN UREMIA

Although insulin secretion is impaired in uremia, glucose intolerance in uremia is not primarily the result of reduced insulin secretion (10). Because some degree of insulin resistance is nearly universal, insulin responsiveness from β cells plays a decisive role in determining whether net glucose intolerance is present. Peripheral insulin resistance may occur in the presence of nonoral peripheral glucose uptake in uremia, and the highest insulin responses are seen in those patients who preserve normal glucose tolerance (12). Insulin secretion is known to be relatively impaired in chronic renal failure (14,61). However, as with the mechanism of insulin resistance in uremia, the mechanism of inhibition of insulin secretion is not adequately understood.

Stimulus-secretion coupling in the normal pancreatic β-cell, reviewed by Alvestrand et al. (13), involves an interplay among glucose metabolism, plasma membrane electrophysiology, potassium fluxes, and calcium homeostasis. Normally, glucose promotes a depolarization of β cells as a result of closing of glucose- and ATP-regulated potassium channels in the plasma membrane. The voltage-activated Ca^{2+} channels in the plasma membrane subsequently open. Release of insulin is initiated when calcium influxes and cytoplasmic calcium rises. Under conditions of experimental insulin resistance in animals, insulin secretion may increase as much as 10-fold above normal. Following weeks of hemodialysis, insulin secretion in humans with renal failure modestly increases (62).

Apart from pancreatic β cell insulin production, the normal role of the kidneys in the handling of insulin and insulin homeostasis is well established (17). In the presence of normal renal function, insulin undergoes combined filtration and tubular secretion by extraction from peritubular blood cells (63). Most then is retained by endocytosis and degraded in proximal tubular cells. Insulin is concentrated in the renal cortex, filtered at the glomerulus, reabsorbed proximally, and then metabolized to small breakdown products. Arteriovenous insulin concentrations fall by about one-third because of uptake of the hormone by normal kidneys (64). Overall, this renal process on a daily basis degrades roughly 25% of normally produced insulin. As renal function wanes, filtration and tubular secretion fall, leading to reduced renal insulin clearance. Uptake by the failing kidneys declines to less than 10%, related to decreased insulinase activity. The insulin half-life thus is prolonged. Decreased metabolic clearance rates of insulin have been demonstrated in undialyzed patients with chronic renal failure (6). Following weeks of dialysis, improvement occurs, suggesting a dialyzable factor that blunts insulin degradation by extrarenal tissues (13). Reduced renal degradation of exogenous insulin leads to increased insulin levels in the presence of chronic renal failure (35) and contributes to elevated basal insulin levels.

Glucose intolerance may not develop in chronic renal failure in the absence of parathyroid hormone (65). Although conflicting data exist in some studies, both experimental and clinical studies have shown that excessive secondary hyperparathyroidism is associated with impaired insulin secretion. Previous studies provided indirect evidence that the state of secondary hyperparathyroidism blunted insulin release. When serum parathyroid hormone is absent or normalized, the insulin-secretory response to hyperglycemia increases, in the absence of changes in peripheral insulin resistance (66). In uremic patients with uncontrolled hyperparathyroidism, insulin resistance coexists with a lack of the compensatory increase in insulin secretion in response to a glucose load. After parathyroidectomy, improved insulin responsiveness to a glucose load, without any change in insulin resistance, results in improved glucose tolerance (66). Similar indirect animal data in the uremic hyperparathyroid dog model show that parathyroidectomy results in greater insulin secretion and glucose tolerance (61). Direct supportive evidence was reported by Fadda et al. in a study of isolated pancreatic islets in the uremic rat model. Insulin release from isolated pancreatic islets from uremic rats was inhibited. Postparathyroidectomy, islet-cell insulin release was similar to control values (66).

As with other causes of impaired insulin secretion, the mechanisms by which parathyroid excess might blunt pancreatic insulin release in response to glucose is not understood. Acutely, parathyroid hormone stimulates calcium influx in diverse cell types, including heart, lung, and kidney. In the pancreas, calcium overloading may occur during chronic parathyroid exposure. A sustained increase in cytosolic calcium has been proposed as a cellular mechanism.

The same interplay of parathyroid hormone, vitamin D, and calcium, which affects insulin resistance, also applies to the aforementioned studies on insulin secretion. Not all clinical studies have supplemented patients with vitamin D, and none assessed the specific role of vitamin D. More recent data suggest that 1,25-dihydroxy vitamin D deficiency, independent of parathyroid hormone and calcium, contributes to the abnormalities in insulin secretion and glucose intolerance. Uremic patients with iatrogenic vitamin D deficiency on maintenance dialysis displayed glucose intolerance as a result of inhibition of insulin hypersecretion in conditions of insulin resistance. Repleted with vitamin D, patients with uremia became glucose tolerant and hyperinsulinemic, with a 50% increase in insulin secretion during hyperglycemic clamp studies (40). The improvement occurred without significant changes in serum parathyroid levels. Studies in vitamin D-deficient animals with normal renal function show that vitamin D repletion improves insulin secretion from intact animals, as well as from isolated perfused pancreas (67).

ADVANCED GLYCOSYLATION END PRODUCTS

In addition to the previously mentioned issues of glucose metabolism, of related importance is the accumulation of advanced glycosylation end products (AGEs) in uremia (68). Endogenous AGEs are heterogeneous late products of mainly glucose-protein interactions, which form chemically cross-linked molecules. Glucose reacts nonenzymatically with protein amino groups to initiate glycation and yield a variety of glycotoxins. AGEs are candidate pathogenetic factors for the secondary complications of diabetes mellitus (69). A growing body of evidence points to the contribution of AGEs to multiple diabetic complications, including renal and vascular disease (70–72). AGEs are produced by a reaction between sugars and proteins in patients with long-term hyperglycemia (Fig. 2.3A). AGE balance reflects ongoing production and removal by renal and extrarenal clearance mechanisms (Fig. 2.3B). Data suggest that rate of formation of AGEs is proportional to the blood glucose level, integrated over a sustained period (73,74). For example, the levels of Amadori products, formed at an intermediate stage in the biochemical pathway on numerous proteins, are elevated proportionate to the degree of hyperglycemia. Overall, the amount of glycosylated adducts that forms appears to vary directly with ambient glucose concentrations (72,76), although some studies have been unable to show a correlation between serum glucose and concurrent AGE levels (75). Vlassara et al. (77) attributed the increase in AGEs in tissues of diabetic patients to hyperglycemia. A correlation was found between levels of fructolysine, a mirror of hyperglycemia, and AGE levels in serum as well as in a variety of tissues (78).

Newer data suggest that AGE formation may result when hyperglycemia increases formation of reactive oxygen species (79). Although tissue AGE levels correlate with prevailing levels of glucose, glycated hemoglobin, and fructolysine, indicating a role for hyperglycemia, additional evidence suggests that other carbohydrates may act as glycating agents in humans. The rate of formation of some AGEs also may be dependent on the concentration of carbohydrate precursors.

Although a growing number of AGEs have had their structures identified and may become measured clinically (80,81), the exact structure of many others *in vivo* remains largely undefined. AGEs have been identified in hemoglobin, β-2 microglobulin, β-amyloid protein, and lens crystalline (82). AGEs have been localized by immunoassay to the characteristic lesions of atherosclerosis and glomerulosclerosis in patients with diabetes (82,83).

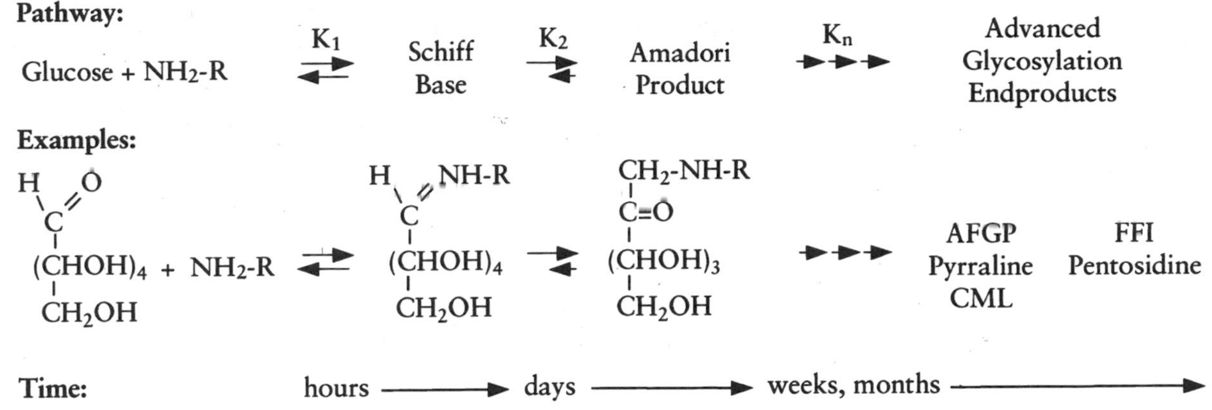

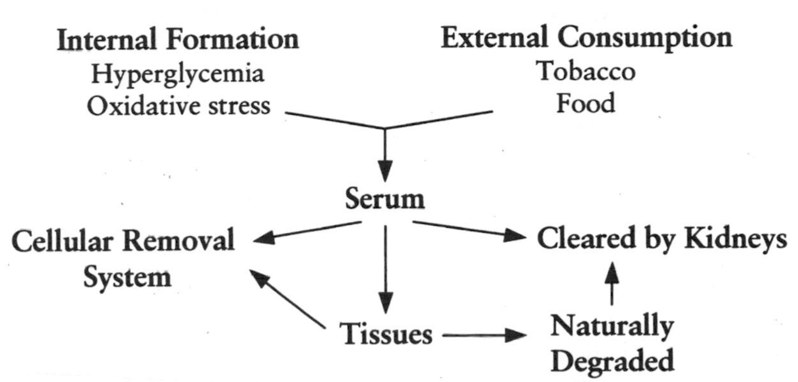

FIGURE 2.3. **A:** Schematic pathway for the formation of advanced glycosylation end products (AGEs) in the presence of hyperglycemia. Amadori products undergo a complex set of rearrangements to form AGEs, long-lived macromolecules that are glycosylated. **B:** Homeostasis (i.e., formation and clearance) of AGEs. Internal formation occurs as a result of hyperglycemia and, more recently described in uremia, oxidative stress.

Inhibitors of the AGE pathway are under development (84). In a growing group of AGE inhibitors, which inhibit AGE formation or their cross-linking, aminoguanidine can lower AGE levels in incubating plasma (85) and is known to retard the progression of diabetic complications in animal models (84). Preliminary results of a human trial of aminoguanidine (pimagedine) in type 1 patients with diabetic nephropathy have been reported (86–88).

Serum AGE levels appear to reflect the ongoing balance between production and removal of AGEs and AGE precursors. In addition to the level of glycemic control and glucose metabolism, renal function is a determinant of the level of AGEs in plasma and in tissues. AGE peptides accumulate in the circulation of diabetic and nondiabetic patients with uremia (80). The plasma levels of AGEs rise dramatically in uremia, although the highest serum AGE concentrations occur in patients with both diabetes mellitus and renal failure (89). Both glycosylated AGEs and small AGE breakdown products are filtered and reabsorbed by the kidneys (90). It is likely that uremia is associated not only with well-defined AGEs but also with AGE precursors.

The reasons for accumulation of individual AGEs and AGE products in uremia increasingly are understood. Because the kidneys play a major role in the clearance of some AGEs (90), diminished renal clearance likely plays a part (91). AGE levels correlate strongly with serum creatinine levels, and the half-life of AGEs is prolonged by renal failure. Several identified AGEs and AGE peptides are disposed of by glomerular filtration, tubular reabsorption, and catabolism. In patients undergoing hemodialysis and peritoneal dialysis, AGE levels are highly elevated regardless of their glycemic status (75). Dialytic clearance of AGEs, even of low molecular weight, is somewhat limited in both conventional hemodialysis and peritoneal dialysis. However, efficient removal of some AGE compounds has been demonstrated in high flux, high permeability hemodialysis

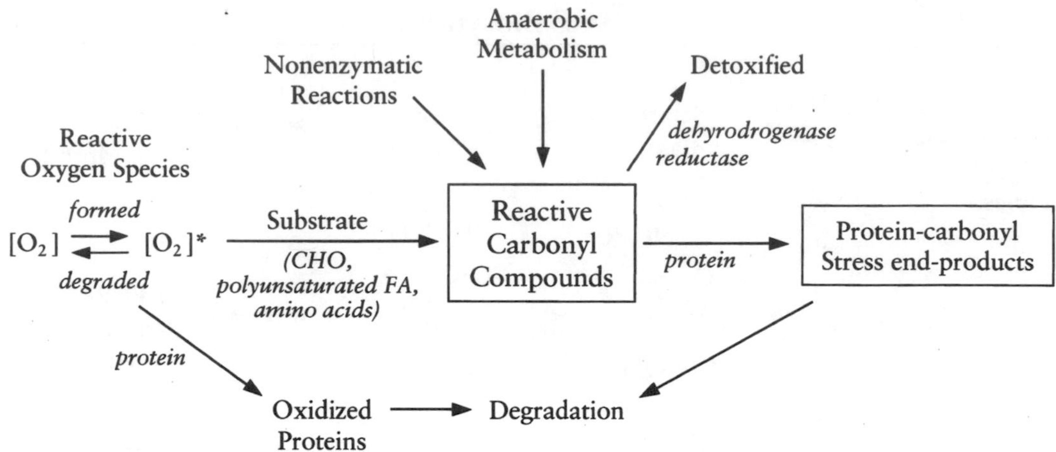

FIGURE 2.4. Proposed pathway leading to "carbonyl stress" in uremia, as a consequence of either increased production or decreased clearance, through detoxification or degradation mechanisms (see references 94 and 96). Carbonyl stress end product generation is enhanced in uremia by increased oxidative stress (i.e., increased formation of reactive oxygen species) and oxidation of carbohydrates, lipids, and amino acid substrates. (Modified from Miyata T, Ypersele de Strihou C, Kurokawa K, et al. Alterations in non-enzymatic biochemistry in uremia: origin and significance of "carbonyl stress" in long-term uremic complications. *Kidney Int* 1999;55:389–399, with permission.)

membranes (92). Shortly following a successful kidney transplant, serum AGE levels return to the range of diabetic patients who have normal renal function.

In addition to decreased renal clearance of some AGEs, however, uremia is associated with two alterations in the metabolic milieu that also result in their enhanced formation—insulin resistance and autoxidation of carbohydrates (70). Regarding the latter, AGEs are products of the combined processes of glycation and oxidation (93–95) (Fig. 2.4). AGEs therefore may accumulate as a result of increased formation in uremia not related to hyperglycemia. The formation of carbonyl compounds more broadly generated by other oxidation of carbohydrates has been termed "carbonyl stress" (96). Enhanced formation results from the accumulation of carbonyl precursors derived principally from carbohydrates. In addition to glycation, nonenzymatic oxidative processes take place *in vivo.* The importance of oxidative stress has been demonstrated in several studies, suggesting that AGEs are largely glycoxidation products and formed by oxidative degradation of sugars such as fructose or ribose or from the autooxidation of glucose itself.

Whether formed primarily by glycation or oxidation or both, AGEs may contribute, in important ways, to uremic toxicity (97,98), including dialysis-related amyloidosis, dyslipidemia, and atherosclerosis (70). AGEs which accumulate appear to be deposited irreversibly in many tissues, including kidney, vascular walls, and crystalline lens. In addition to altering the structure and function of tissue proteins, AGEs stimulate cellular responses through specific AGE receptors, have proinflammatory effects (99,100), and contribute to the generation of reactive oxygen intermediates. Infusion of preformed AGEs into healthy animals causes gene dysfunction, including those for cytokines, growth factors, and matrix proteins. Intracellular glycosylation by glucose or other intracellular sugars may occur on cellular or nuclear proteins, leading to defective signal transduction, activation of intracellular messages, gene dysfunction, and multiple cytokine release.

ROLE OF ABNORMAL CARBOHYDRATE METABOLISM IN UREMIC COMPLICATIONS

The higher prevalence of cardiovascular complications in uremic patients managed on chronic dialysis compared to similar age populations has been known for a quarter of a century (101). Despite advances in dialysis technology, the cardiovascular mortality rate in patients with end-stage renal disease is more than 20 times that of the general population. After statistical adjustment for age, gender, and the presence of diabetes mellitus, mortality resulting from cardiovascular causes remains more than 10 times higher in patients requiring dialysis. Multiple atherogenic risk factors for vascular occlusive disease are known to exist in the end-stage renal disease milieu (102). They include traditional risk factors (hypertension, dyslipidemia, smoking, and diabetes mellitus), and others more specifically associated with uremia (anemia, increased oxidative stress, hemodynamic overload, hyperhomocysteinemia, and AGEs). Other risk factors in uremia (inflammation, viral infections, uremic toxins, and dialysis incompatibility) have been proposed. In diabetes mellitus, multiple risk factors are involved in the development and progression of atherosclerotic occlusive disease (103). Compared to nondiabetic patients, individuals with diabetes have a heightened risk of developing coronary heart disease (104), as well as an increased risk of death from myocardial infarction or congestive heart failure.

The relationship between hyperglycemia and macrovascular disease has been shown in several prospective studies (105). Independent of other conventional risk factors, such as plasma lipid levels, hypertension, smoking, and insulin levels, the significance of hyperglycemia as a coronary risk factor has been shown by the United Kingdom Prospective Diabetes Study (UKPDS) (106). Even mild hyperglycemia places patients at risk for future macrovascular disease (107).

The role of glucose in atherosclerotic progression is postulated to be mediated through several mechanisms, including endothelial dysfunction, platelet dysfunction, lipid alterations to a more atherogenic profile, a procoagulant state, and increased formation of AGEs. The hyperglycemic state may accelerate atherogenesis through a number of processes, including endothelial injury, atherosclerotic plaque buildup, enhanced susceptibility to oxidation, and alterations in platelet function. Although glucose itself may be directly toxic to endothelial cells (108), an additional contribution may be made by the formation of AGEs in excess, associated with endothelial dysfunction, direct promotion of atherogenic plaque formation, and susceptibility of low-density lipoproteins to oxidation (77). Limited data suggest that AGE levels may be considered biomarkers of cardiovascular disease (109). In addition to glucose toxicity in diabetes mellitus, insulin resistance and hyperinsulinemia are thought to be involved in the development and progression of atherosclerosis; as with hyperglycemia, other factors associated with insulin resistance likely contribute to the risk of macrovascular disease related to insulin resistance. These include hyperlipidemia (110) and coagulation defects (111). Hyperinsulinemia also may contribute to cardiovascular risk through direct effects on the arterial vascular wall (112,113).

The association of insulin resistance and cardiovascular abnormalities in nondiabetic patients also has been well documented (114) and termed the "insulin resistance syndrome" (115). Independent of progression to overt diabetes, otherwise healthy individuals with hyperinsulinemia, initiated by insulin resistance, are at increased risk of ischemic coronary disease (116). Although insulin resistance, glucose intolerance, and hyperinsulinemia are common biochemical consequences of uremia, as described earlier, the relative importance of these compared to traditional and renal disease–related risk factors for macrovascular disease in nondiabetic uremic patients remains uncertain (117). For example, hypertension and dyslipidemia are almost universal in end-stage renal disease. Increased low-density lipoprotein levels are evident in the majority. Insulin enhances hepatic very-low-density lipoprotein triglyceride synthesis and may reduce the rate of metabolism of VLDL. Hyperinsulinemia may play a role in the decreased fibrinolytic activity characteristic of patients with chronic renal failure. In end-stage renal disease, AGE-modified macromolecules, metabolized in turn to low–molecular-weight peptide fragments, may circulate and form a class of atherogenic reactive intermediates. An interaction between glycation, oxidative stress, and inflammation in the vasculopathy of uremia was proposed in 2000 (100). Additional research is needed to clarify these relationships in the nondiabetic uremic patient.

HYPOGLYCEMIA

Another well-recognized disturbance of glucose metabolism in chronic renal failure is the development of hypoglycemia, which may occur in both diabetic and nondiabetic patients (118,119). Although hypoglycemia is far less common than glucose intolerance in patients with uremia (120), hypoglycemia is more common than generally appreciated (2). The risk of hypoglycemia is a deterrent to achieving glycemic control at current target levels in patients with diabetes. End-stage renal disease unrelated to diabetes is the second most frequent cause of hypoglycemia in hospitalized patients (1,121) and has a high mortality rate (121).

Although these abnormalities in insulin secretion, metabolism, and target organ sensitivity result in insulin resistance and a common state of glucose intolerance (20), renal insufficiency alternatively may affect the body's ability to maintain adequate blood sugar levels. For example, as chronic renal failure worsens, patients may develop improved carbohydrate tolerance. As with uremic carbohydrate intolerance, many factors appear to contribute to uremic hypoglycemia (Table 2.4). Among them are diminished caloric intake, impaired hepatic glycogenolysis, use of certain medications, prolonged insulin action, and impaired counterregulatory responses (122). Both improved glucose tolerance in diabetic patients and cases of overt hypoglycemia in both diabetic and nondiabetic patients with renal failure have been the subject of frequent reports (123,124). Patients with renal insufficiency who develop hypoglycemia need not have diabetes, although almost half of reported cases have had diabetic nephropathy (120). However, multiple contributing factors usually are present. Uremic hypoglycemia, however, is usually not "spontaneous" but has chronic renal failure as a contributing cause (124).

Hypoglycemia generally is defined as being below the lower limits of the fasting reference range of 72 mg/dL. "Spontaneous" hypoglycemia has been used synonymously with "uremic" hypoglycemia since first used by Block and

TABLE 2.4. FACTORS CONTRIBUTING TO UREMIC HYPOGLYCEMIA

Poor caloric intake
Impaired hepatic glycogenolysis
Defective renal gluconeogenesis
Diminished counterregulatory response
Certain medication use

Rubinstein 30 years ago to describe three patients with type 2 diabetes who suffered hypoglycemia during terminal renal failure (125). Most subsequent reports of cases were in the 1970s, including more than 30 cases in 16 published papers (124). In a 1991 review of the literature, Toth and Lee reported that only four of 36 cases lacked other factors such as other illnesses, malnutrition, or drugs that could have accounted for the hypoglycemia. Only a few cases had type 2 diabetes or known impaired glucose tolerance (124).

Among abnormalities in insulin and glucose metabolism associated with renal failure, the primary one detectable by laboratory evaluation is hyperinsulinemia. As noted earlier, the kidneys are the most important extrahepatic organs for degradation of insulin, although their contribution to insulin removal decreases with declining renal function. In the context of uremic peripheral insulin resistance, impaired renal degradation would serve to offset hyperglycemia in the absence of other factors. Some patients with uremic hypoglycemia do have inappropriately elevated insulin levels (not related to an insulinoma), but insulin levels generally have been reported as normal when measured (125). A second abnormality in insulin/glucose metabolism related to renal failure is defective renal gluconeogenesis. During starvation, the kidneys become a major source of glucose production through gluconeogenesis from precursor molecules. Not easily measured, the role of impaired renal gluconeogenesis in uremic patients remains uncertain. Other abnormalities also have been proposed or evaluated, including a defect in hepatic gluconeogenesis indirectly related to renal failure and impaired counterregulatory hormonal responses that normally would defend against hypoglycemia.

In order of importance, glucagon, epinephrine, cortisol, and growth hormone normally are secreted in response to hypoglycemia and serve to maintain the normoglycemic state. This protective response is known to be impaired in patients with diabetes mellitus (126). In uremic diabetic patients with hypoglycemia, deficiencies in glucagon and catecholamines are known to occur (127). In one study of nondiabetic patients undergoing chronic hemodialysis, insulin-induced hypoglycemia produced normal amounts of epinephrine compared to controls (122). However, responses of plasma adrenocorticotropic hormone, cortisol, and growth hormone were lacking. Regulation of pituitary and adrenal function is complicated by the presence of uremia, making its assessment difficult. Overtly impaired function is generally secondary to an abnormality unrelated to renal failure (124). Most uremic patients with "spontaneous" hypoglycemia have normal adrenal and thyroid function. In summary, whereas renal failure commonly predisposes to hypoglycemia, no defect specific to uremia generally is isolated, and one of the causes described later in this chapter generally is found. The term "spontaneous" hypoglycemia should be avoided in favor of uremic hypoglycemia until an underlying mechanism is better defined.

Hypoglycemia also may be nosocomial, secondary to a number of medications (128). In insulin-treated patients with diabetes, the use of insulin with prolonged duration of action is usually present. The need for exogenous insulin may be eliminated entirely in the diabetic patient with renal failure. Unusually severe, prolonged hypoglycemic reactions following treatment with oral hypoglycemic agents in renal failure have been noted for 40 years (129). Between 1% and 2% of sulfonylurea-treated patients develop severe hypoglycemia annually (130). Renal failure is a common risk factor for hypoglycemia in patients receiving sulfonylureas. Although early reports cited tolbutamide and related sulfonylureas, glyburide has become important as a cause of hypoglycemia. A recent Canadian study reported seven cases of hypoglycemia resulting from glyburide (glibenclamide in Europe) (131). Despite its short half-life, glyburide is prolonged in severe renal dysfunction, and two hepatic metabolites with hypoglycemic activity are excreted renally. Episodes generally occurred after months to years of glyburide therapy, although hypoglycemia occurred shortly after initiation of therapy in one patient. Predisposing factors in this and other studies have included reduced oral intake, previous hypoglycemia, and longer duration of diabetes. Chlorpropamide has been the most frequent sulfonylurea implicated in hypoglycemia in the presence of renal failure, related to the renal elimination of this long-acting agent.

Increased risk of hypoglycemia as a result of β-adrenergic–blocking drugs occurs in the presence of renal failure. The secretion of insulin and glucagon, glycogenolysis in muscle, and hepatic gluceoneogenesis are all modulated by sympathetic tone (132). Plasma glucose levels may be increased (inhibition of insulin release) or decreased (decreased glucagon release). The hypoglycemic action also is related to the diminished adrenergic response to hypoglycemia (120). Profound hypoglycemia may occur in patients undergoing chronic dialysis in the absence of diabetes (133). Another potent inducer of hypoglycemia in both therapeutic and toxic doses when renal function is normal—salicylates—may cause hypoglycemia at lower doses in renal failure. The hypoglycemic mechanism of salicylates remains controversial (134). Patients with severe renal failure also may be at risk for hypoglycemia secondary to the administration of propoxyphene (135) or sulfonamides (136). The latter are related structurally to sulfonylureas, and hypoglycemia may be related to hyperinsulinemia.

MONITORING GLYCEMIC CONTROL IN UREMIA

Monitoring of glycemia is a proven cornerstone for improving diabetes care (137). However, in addition to altering determinants of glycemic control, such as insulin kinetics, sensitivity to the hormone, and carbohydrate metabolism, uremia may alter the very measurement used to monitor integrated glycemic control. Whereas consistent glycemic control becomes progressively more difficult in uremia, the relationship between mean blood glucose levels and measured hemoglobin A1C also may be altered significantly (138).

Adequate glycemic control is present in uremia when the fasting blood sugar is less than 140 mg% and the glycosylated hemoglobin level is near 7%. Indices of glycemic control remain important when implementing changes in diabetes management. Compared to earlier stages of diabetes, however, evidence in favor of tight glycemic control in the patient with uremia has been less convincing (139). Chronic hyperglycemia can continue to have adverse effects on multiple organ systems in the patient with uremia and diabetes. Strict glycemic control during dialysis can minimize symptoms of gastroparesis, which has been noted to be predictive of hospitalization and mortality (140). Intradialytic weight-gain correlates with glycemic control in patients undergoing dialysis and may contribute to morbidity and mortality (141). Patients with poor glycemic control, which promotes increased thirst, gain more weight than those with good glycemic control and may suffer from intradialytic hypotension. Finally, a study of 226 patients with diabetes undergoing chronic dialysis showed that poor glycemic control was associated with increased morbidity from vascular and diabetic complications, malnutrition, and shortened patient survival (139). Rates of survival in those with good glycemic control exceeded those for all patients with diabetes, as reported by the U.S. Renal Data Systems (142). Hypoglycemic episodes were more common in the group with better glycemic control. However, duration of diabetes was not reported, and risk factors and comorbidities were not adequately analyzed. Strict control of hyperglycemia, therefore, is difficult and may not be popular in uremic or end-stage diabetic patients. Reasons commonly cited include lack of confidence about the ability to control cardiovascular and other organ system damage; fear of hypoglycemia, a common occurrence when glycemic management is aggressive; absent or atypical symptoms with hyperglycemia; and the questionable reliability of glycated hemoglobin levels in uremia.

Sequential measurement of A1C levels is accepted as the most accurate method of evaluating glycemic control in patients with diabetes. Glycosylated hemoglobin (HbA1C) informs the physician and the patient about the mean blood glucose levels over the previous 6 to 8 weeks and complements home blood monitoring by the patient. In the United States, a remarkably small percentage of diabetic patients with end-stage renal disease undergo regular glycosylated hemoglobin testing (143). Glycosylated hemoglobin results from the nonenzymatic posttranslational modification of hemoglobin A, the dominant hemoglobin component. Of the four glycosylated fractions of hemoglobin, glycohemoglobin methods most commonly measure hemoglobin A1C. The normal range of glycosylated hemoglobin in the laboratory is 4.5% to 7%. Several different laboratory methods exist for measuring A1C. Since completion of the Diabetes Control and Complications Trial, interest in standardization of these methods has grown.

It now is accepted that measurement of glycosylated hemoglobin may be less informative in the presence of uremia (2). Three pitfalls exist in interpreting A1C: (a) The labile changes in blood sugar levels, common in patients with uremia, may not be evident when this index of chronic glycemic control is used. (b) The reduced erythrocyte life span in untreated uremia may be expected to reduce levels of glycosylated hemoglobin. (c) False elevations of hemoglobin A1C may occur by some assays methods. In patients with uremia and diabetes, analytic interference occurs as a result of carbamylated hemoglobin when the assay is performed by techniques that separate the hemoglobin fractions by electrical charge. Carbamylated hemoglobin results when cyanate, a dissociation product of urea, combines in reaction with the amino group of hemoglobin in the presence of high blood urea concentrations. As reviewed by Tzamaloukas, methods for separating hemoglobin fractions based on electrical charge will not distinguish between glycosylated and carbamylated hemoglobin, which have similar electrical charges (138). Either column- and ion-exchange chromatography or agar gel electrophoresis should be used.

However, it also should be noted that the hemoglobin A1C fraction is relatively less affected by carbamylation than the other hemoglobin A1 fractions that undergo glycosylation (144). Other glycohemoglobin assays, including color imagery of thiobarbituric acid, borate-agarose affinity chromatography, and serum high-pressure liquid chromatography assays, will not be affected by uremia. Because A1C may not reflect blood glucose levels in patients with uremia accurately, alternative methods have been sought. Measurement of fructosamine, a glycosylated protein specifically assayed commercially, reflects glycemic control over a shorter period than hemoglobin A1C (2 to 3 weeks) and may be of value as an index of intermediate glycemic control (145). Unlike A1C, serum fructosamine levels do not appear to be affected by uremia. However, they are influenced not only by glucose control, but also by protein concentrations in the serum. A few studies have evaluated fructosamine levels in patients with uremia (146). Finally, in contrast to information mentioned previously, several studies have demonstrated a general reliance between blood glucose levels and glycosylated hemoglobin in patients with uremia, independent of whether the assay used was interfered with by carbamylation (138).

ACKNOWLEDGMENTS

I would like to acknowledge Caitlin Sparks for her assistance in the preparation and completion of this manuscript.

REFERENCES

1. Mujais SK, Fadda G. Carbohydrate metabolism in end-stage renal disease. *Semin Dial* 1989;2:46–53.
2. Mak RH. Impact of end-stage renal disease and dialysis on glycemic control. *Semin Dial* 2000;13:4–8.
3. DeFronzo RA, Andres K, Edgar P, et al. Carbohydrate metabolism in uremia: a review. *Medicine* 1973;52:469–481.
4. Hampers CL, Soeldoner JS, Doak PB, et al. Effects of chronic renal failure and hemodialysis on carbohydrate metabolism. *J Clin Invest* 1966;45:1719–1731.
5. DeFronzo RA, Smith D, Alvestrand A. Insulin action in uremia. *Kidney Int* 1983;24(S16):S102–S124.
6. DeFronzo RA, Tobin J, Rowe JW, et al. Glucose intolerance in uremia. *J Clin Invest* 1978;62:425–435.
7. Moller DE, Flier JS. Insulin resistance -mechanisms, syndromes, and implications. *N Engl J Med* 1991;325:938–948.
8. DeFronzo RA, Alvestrand A, Smith D, et al. Insulin resistance of uremia. *J Clin Invest* 1981;67:563–572.
9. Bergman RN, Finegood DT, Ader M. Assessment of insulin sensitization in vivo. *Endocr Rev* 1985;6:45–53.
10. Hager SR. Insulin resistance in uremia. *Am J Kidney Dis* 1989; 14:272–276.
11. Fliser D, Pacini G, Engelleiter R, et al. Insulin resistance and hyperinsulinemia are already present in patients with incipient renal disease. *Kidney Int* 1998;53:1343–1347.
12. Alvestrand A. Carbohydrate and insulin metabolism in renal failure. *Kidney Int* 1997;52(S62):S48–S52.
13. Alvestrand A, Mujagic M, Wajngot A, et al. Glucose intolerance in uremic patients: The relative contributions of impaired beta-cell function and insulin resistance. *Clin Nephrol* 1989;31: 175–183.
14. Mak RHK, Bettinelli A, Turner C, et al. The influence of hyperparathyroidism on glucose metabolism in uremia. *J Clin Endocrinol Metab* 1985;60:229–233.
15. Reaid D, Channon SM, Scrimgeous CM, et al. Correction of acidosis in humans with chronic renal failure decreases protein degradation and amino acid oxidation. *Am J Physiol* 1993;265: E230–E235.
16. Mak RHK. Insulin resistance but IgF-1 sensitivity in chronic renal failure. *Am J Physiol* 1996;271:F114–119.
17. Adrogue HJ. Glucose homeostasis and the kidney. *Kidney Int* 1992;42:1266–1271.
18. Garibotto G, Russo R, Sofia A, et al. Skeletal muscle protein synthesis and degradation in patients with chronic renal failure. *Kidney Int* 1994;45:1432–1439.
19. Goecke IA, Bonilla S, Marusic ET, et al. Enhanced insulin sensitivity in extrarenal potassium handling in uremic rats. *Kidney Int* 1991;39:39–43.
20. Mak RHK. Renal disease, insulin resistance, and glucose intolerance. *Diabetes Rev* 1994;2:19–28.
21. Luo RZ, Beniac DR, Fernandes A, et al. Quaternary structure of the insulin-insulin receptor complex. *Science* 1991;285: 1077–1084.
22. White MF, Kahn CR. The insulin signaling pathway. *J Biol Chem* 1994;269:1–8.
23. Olefsky JM. The insulin receptor: a multifunctional protein. *Diabetes* 1990;39:1008–1016.
24. Friedman JE, Dohm GL, Elton CW, et al. Muscle insulin resistance in uremic humans: glucose transport, glucose transporter, and insulin receptor. *Am J Physiol* 1991;261:E87–E94.
25. Cecchin FO, Ittoop M, Sinha K, et al. Insulin resistance in uremia: insulin receptor kinase activity in liver and muscle from chronic uremic rats. *Am J Physiol* 1988;254(4 Part 1): E394–E401.
26. Contreras I, Caro JF, Aveledo L, et al. In chronic uremia, insulin activates receptor kinase but not pyruvate dehydrogenase. *Nephron* 1992;61:77–81.
27. Kaufman JM, Caro JF. Insulin resistance in uremia: characterization of insulin action, binding, and processing in isolated hepatocytes from chronic uremic rats. *J Clin Invest* 1983;71: 698–708.
28. Truglia JA, Hayes GR, Lockwood DH. Intact adipocyte insulin receptor phosphorylation and in vitro tyrosine kinase activity in animal models of insulin resistance. *Diabetes* 1988;37:147–153.
29. Smith D, DeFronzo RA. Insulin resistance in uremia mediated by post-binding defects. *Kidney Int* 1982;22:54–60.
30. Castellino P, Solino A, Luzi L, et al. Glucose and amino acid metabolism in chronic renal failure: effects of insulin and amino acids. *Am J Physiol* 1992;262:F168–174.
31. Pereira BJG, Shapiro L, King AJ. Plasma levels of Il-1B, TNF-alpha, and their specific inhibitors in undialyzed chronic renal failure, CAPD, and hemodialysis patients. *Kidney Int* 1994;45: 890–896.
32. Borisova AM, Djambuzova A, Todoma K, et al. Effects of erythropoietin on the metabolic state and peripheral insulin sensitivity in diabetic patients on hemodialysis. *Nephrol Dial Transplant* 1993;8:93–95.
33. McCobb ML, Izzo MS, Lockwood DH. Characterization and partial purification of a factor from uremic human serum that induces insulin resistance. *J Clin Invest* 1985;75:391–397.
34. Foss MC, Gouveia LM, Moyses NM, et al. Effect of hemodialysis on peripheral glucose metabolism of patients with chronic renal failure. *Nephron* 1996;73:48–53.
35. Eidemak I, Felt-Rasmussen B, Kanstrup IL, et al. Insulin resistance and hyperinsulinemia in mild to moderate progressive chronic renal failure and its association with aerobic work capacity. *Diabetologia* 1995;38:565–572.
36. Vareesangthip K, Tong P, Wilkenson R, et al. Insulin resistance in adult polycystic disease. *Kidney Int* 1997;52:503–508.
37. Amend WJ Jr, Steinberg SM, Lowrie EG, et al. The influence of serum calcium parathyroid hormone upon glucose metabolism in uremia. *J Lab Clin Med* 1975;86:435–444.
38. Gunal AI, Celiker H, Celebi H, et al. Intravenous alfacalderol improves insulin resistance in hemodialysis patients. *Clin Nephrol* 1997;48:109–113.
39. Graf H, Prager P, Kovarik J, et al. Glucose metabolism and insulin sensitivity in patients on chronic hemodialysis. *Metabolism* 1995;34:974–997.
40. Mak RHK. Intravenous 1,25 dihydroxycholecalciferol corrects glucose intolerance in hemodialysis patients. *Kidney Int* 1992; 41:1049–1054.
41. Kautzky-Willer A, Pacini G, Barnas U, et al. Intravenous calcitriol normalizes insulin sensitivity in uremic patients. *Kidney Int* 1995;47:200–206.
42. Lu KC, Shieh SD, Lin SH, et al. Hyperparathyroidism, glucose tolerance, and platelet intracellular free calcium in chronic renal failure. *Q J Med* 1994;87:359–365.
43. Draznin B. Cytosolic calcium and insulin resistance. *Am J Kidney Dis* 1993;27(S3):32–38.
44. Owen WF, Lew NL, Liu Y, et al. The urea reduction ratio and serum albumin concentration as predictors of mortality in patients undergoing hemodialysis. *N Engl J Med* 1993;329: 1001–1008.
45. Goldwasser P, Mittman N, Antignani A, et al. Predictors of mortality on hemodialysis. *J Am Soc Nephrol* 1993;3: 1613–1622.
46. Obrador GT, Ruthazer R, Arora P, et al. Prevalence of factors associated with sub-optimal care before initiation of dialysis in the United States. *J Am Soc Nephrol* 1999;10:1793–1800.
47. Ikizer TA, Greene JH, Wingard RL, et al. Spontaneous dietary

protein intake during progression of chronic renal failure. *J Am Soc Nephrol* 1995;6:1386–1391.
48. Mitch WE. Dietary protein restriction in patients with chronic renal failure. *Kidney Int* 1991;40:326–341.
49. Pedrini MT, Levey AS, Lau J, et al. The effect of dietary protein restriction on the progression of diabetic and nondiabetic renal diseases: a meta-analysis. *Ann Intern Med* 1996;124:627–632.
50. Zeller K, Whittaker E, Sullivan L, et al. Effect of restricting dietary protein and progression of renal failure in patients with insulin-dependent diabetes mellitus. *N Engl J Med* 1991;324:78–84.
51. Walker JD, Bending JJ, Dodds RA, et al. Restriction of dietary protein and progression of renal insufficiency. *Lancet* 1989;2:1411–1416.
52. Larriviere F, Chrisson JL, Schiffin A, et al. Effects of dietary protein restriction on glucose and insulin metabolism in normal and diabetic patients. *Metabolism* 1994;43:461–467.
53. American Diabetes Association. Position statement. Nutrition recommendations and principles for people with diabetes mellitus. *Diabetes Care* 1997;20(S1):S14–S17.
54. Rigalleau V, Aparicio M, Gin H. Effects of low-protein diet on carbohydrate metabolism and energy expenditure (Review). *J Ren Nutr* 1998;8:175–178.
55. Snyder D, Pulido LB, Kagan A. Dietary reversal of the carbohydrate intolerance of uremia. *Procedures of the European Dialysis and Transplantation Association* 1968;5:205–211.
56. Mak RHK, Turner C, Thompson T, et al. The effects of low protein diet with amino acid/ketoacid supplements on glucose metabolism in children with uremia. *J Clin Endocrinol Metab* 1986;63:985.
57. Rigalleau V, Combe C, Blanchetier V, et al. Low protein diet in uremia: Effects on glucose metabolism and energy production rate. *Kidney Int* 1997;51:1222–1227.
58. Gin H, Aparicio M, Potaux L, et al. Low protein and low phosphorus diets in patients with chronic renal failure: influence on glucose tolerance and tissue insulin sensitivity. *Metabolism* 1987;36:1080–1085.
59. Brodsky IG, Robbins DC, Hiser E, et al. Effects of low-protein diets on protein metabolism in insulin-dependent diabetes mellitus patients with early nephropathy. *J Clin Endocrinol Metab* 1992;75:351–357.
60. Umplesby AM, Bouroujerdi FA, Brown PM, et al. The effect of metabolic control on leucine metabolism in type 1 (insulin-dependent) diabetic patients. *Diabetologia* 1986;29:131–141.
61. Akmal M, Massry SG, Goldstein DA, et al. Role of parathyroid hormone in the glucose intolerance of chronic renal failure. *J Clin Invest* 1985;75:1037–1044.
62. Lowrie EG, Soeldman JS, Hampers CL, et al. Glucose metabolism and insulin secretion in uremic, predialysis, and normal subjects. *J Lab Clin Med* 1970;76:603–612.
63. Rubenstein AH, Spitz I. Role of the kidney in insulin metabolism and excretion. *Diabetes* 1968;17:161–169.
64. Chamberlain MJ, Stimmler L. The renal handling of insulin. *J Clin Invest* 1967;46:911–921.
65. Mak RHK, Turner C, Haycock GB, et al. Secondary hyperparathyroidism and glucose intolerance in children with uremia. *Kidney Int* 1983;24(S16):S128–S133.
66. Fadda GZ, Akmal M, Premdas FH, et al. Insulin release from pancreatic islets: Effects of CRF and excess PTH. *Kidney Int* 1988;33:1066–1072.
67. Kadowski S, Norman AW. Dietary vitamin D is essential for normal insulin secretion from the perfused rat pancreas. *J Clin Invest* 1984;73:759–766.
68. Singh R, Barden A, Mori T, et al. Advanced glycation end products: a review. *Diabetologia* 2001;44:129–146.
69. Striker G. Glucose toxicity. *Kidney Int* 2001;59:799–800.
70. Raj DSC, Choudhury D, Welbourne TC, et al. Advanced glycation end products: A nephrologist's perspective. *Am J Kidney Dis* 2000;35:365–380.
71. Brownlee M. Negative consequences of glycation. *Metabolism* 2000;49(S1):9–13.
72. Bucala R, Vlassara H. Advanced glycosylation end products in diabetic renal and vascular disease. *Am J Kidney Dis* 1995;26:875–888.
73. Brownlee M, Vlassara H, Cerami A. Nonenzymatic glycosylation and the pathogenesis of diabetic complications. *Ann Intern Med* 1984;101:527–537.
74. Berg TJ, Dahl-Jorgensen K, Torjesen PH, et al. Increased serum levels of advanced glycation end products (AGEs) in children and adolescents with insulin-dependent diabetes mellitus. *Diabetes Care* 1997;20:1606–1608.
75. Papanastasiou P, Grass L, Rodela H, et al. Immunological quantification of advanced glycosylation end-products in the serum of patients on hemodialysis or CAPD. *Kidney Int* 1994;46:216–222.
76. Shimoike T, Inoguchi T, Umeda F, et al. The meaning of serum levels of advanced glycosylation end products in diabetic nephropathy. *Metabolism* 2000;49:1030–1035.
77. Vlassara H. Protein glycation in the kidney: role in diabetes and aging. *Kidney Int* 1996;49:1795–1802.
78. Dyer DG, Dunn JA, Thorpe SR, et al. Accumulation of Maillard reaction products in skin collagen in diabetes and aging. *J Clin Invest* 1993;91:2463–2469.
79. Nishikawa T, Edelstein D, Brownlee M. The missing link: a single unifying mechanism for diabetic complications. *Kidney Int* 2000;58(S77):S26–S30.
80. Makito Z, Vlassara H, Cedrami A, et al. Immunochemical detection of advanced glycation end products in vivo. *J Biol Chem* 1992;267:5133–5138.
81. Degenhardt TP, Grass L, Reddy S, et al. The serum concentration of the advanced glycation end-product N-(carboxymethyl) lysine is increased in uremia. *J Clin Invest* 1997;52:1064–1067.
82. Niwa T, Katsuzaki T, Miyasski S, et al. Immunohistochemical detection of imidazolone, a novel advanced glycation end product, in kidneys and aortas of diabetic patients. *J Clin Invest* 1997;99:1272–1280.
83. Miyata S, Monnier VM. Advanced glycated end-products in diabetic tissue using monoclonal antibody to pyrraline. *J Clin Invest* 1992;89:1102–1112.
84. Soulis-Liparota T, Cooper M, Papazoglou P, et al. Retardation by aminoguanidine of development of albuminuria, mesangial expansion, and tissue fluorescence in streptozocin-induced diabetic rat. *Diabetes* 1991;40:1328–1334.
85. Miyata T, Ueda Y, Yamada Y, et al. Accumulation of carbonyls accelerates the formation of pentosidine, an advanced glycation end product. *J Am Soc Nephrol* 1998;9:2349–2356.
86. Cattran D, Williams M, Wuerth JP, et al. Pimagedine (PG) reduces progression of retinopathy and lowers lipid levels in patients with type 1 diabetes mellitus (DM). *J Am Soc Nephrol* 1999;10:179A.
87. Whittier F, Spinowitz B, Wuerth JP, et al. Pimagedine (PG) safety profile in patients with type 1 diabetes mellitus (DM). *J Am Soc Nephrol* 1999;10:184A.
88. Williams ME, Wuerth JP, and for the Action 1 Investigator Group. Pimagedine (PG) slows progression of nephropathy and retinopathy and lowers lipid levels in patients with type 1 diabetes mellitus (DM). Diabetes mellitus: molecular mechanisms, genetics, and prospects for new therapy. Ketones symposium. 2000.
89. Williams ME. Dam (AGE) in diabetic ESRD: role of advanced glycosylation. *Semin Dial* 1996;9:1–4.
90. Miyata T, Ueda Y, Horie K, et al. Renal catabolism of advanced

glycation end products: the fate of pentosidine. *Kidney Int* 1998; 53:416–422.

91. Dawnay A, Millar DJ. The pathogenesis and consequences of AGE formation in uremia and its treatment. *Cell Mol Biol* 1998; 44:1081–1094.
92. Henle T, Deppisch R, Beck W, et al. Advanced glycated end-products (AGE) during haemodialysis treatment: discrepant results with different methodologies reflecting the heterogeneity of AGE compounds. *Nephrol Dial Transplant* 1999;13: 1968–1975.
93. Baynes JW, Thorpe SR. Role of oxidative stress in diabetic complications. A new perspective on an old paradigm. *Diabetes* 1999;48:1–9.
94. Miyata T, Wada Y, Cai Z, et al. Implications of an increased oxidative stress in the formation of advanced glycation end products in patients with end-stage renal failure. *Kidney Int* 1997;51:1170–1180.
95. Bucala R, Makita Z, Koschinsky T, et al. Lipid advanced glycosylation: pathway for lipid oxidation in vivo. *Proc Natl Acad Sci USA* 1993;90:1434–1438.
96. Miyata T, Ypersele de Strihou C, Kurokawa K, et al. Alterations in non-enzymatic biochemistry in uremia: origin and significance of "carbonyl stress" in long-term uremic complications. *Kidney Int* 1999;55:389–399.
97. Makita J, Radoff S, Rayfield EJ, et al. Advanced glycosylation end products in patients with nephropathy. *N Engl J Med* 1991; 325:836–842.
98. Miyata T, Inagi R, Iida Y, et al. Involvement of beta-2-microglobulin modified with advanced glycation end-products in the pathogenesis of hemodialysis-associated amyloidosis. *J Clin Invest* 1994;93:521.
99. Schwedler S, Schinzel R, Vaith P, et al. Inflammation and advanced glycation end products in uremia: simple coexistence, potentiation, or causal relationship? *Kidney Int* 2001;59: S32–S36.
100. Kaysen G. The microinflammatory state in uremia: causes and potential consequences. *J Am Soc Nephrol* 2001;12:1549–1557.
101. Lindner A, Charra B, Sherrard DJ, et al. Accelerated atherosclerosis in prolonged maintenance hemodialysis. *N Engl J Med* 1974;290:667–671.
102. Kasiske BL. The kidney in cardiovascular disease. *Ann Intern Med* 2001;134:707–709.
103. Gerstein HC, Mann JFE, Yi Q, et al. Albuminuria and risk of cardiovascular events, death, and heart failure in diabetic and nondiabetic individuals. *JAMA* 2001;286:421–426.
104. Stack AG, Bloembergen WC. Prevalence and clinical correlation of coronary artery disease among new dialysis patients in the United States: a cross sectional study. *J Am Soc Nephrol* 2001; 12:1516–1523.
105. Abu-Lebdeh HS, Hodge DO, Nguyen TT. Predictors of macrovascular disease in patients with type 2 diabetes mellitus. *Mayo Clin Proc* 2001;76:707–712.
106. Turner RC, Millns H, Neil HA, et al. Risk factors for coronary artery disease in noninsulin dependent diabetes mellitus: United Kingdom Prospective Diabetes Study (UKPDS: 23). *BMJ* 1998; 316:823–828.
107. Hadden M, Schmechel H, Schwanebeck U, et al. Predictors of coronary heart disease and death in NIDDM: the Diabetes Intervention Study experience. *Diabetologia* 1997;40(S2): S123–S124.
108. Stehouwer CDA, Fischer RF, Weng Y, et al. Endothelial dysfunction precedes development of micro albuminuria. *Diabetes* 1995;44:561–568.
109. Sugiyama S, Miyata T, Ueda Y, et al. Plasma levels of pentosidine in diabetic patients: an advanced glycation end product. *J Am Soc Nephrol* 1998;9:1681–1688.
110. Reaven GM, Chen YD, Jeppesen J, et al. Insulin resistance and hyperinsulinemia in individuals with small, dense, low density lipoprotein particles. *J Clin Invest* 1993;92:141–146.
111. Meigs JB, Mittleman MA, Nathan DM, et al. Hyperinsulinemia, hyperglycemia, and impaired hemostasis: the Framingham offspring study. *JAMA* 2000;283:221–227.
112. Zavaroni I, Sonora E, Pagliara M, et al. Risk factors for coronary artery disease in healthy persons with hyperinsulinemia and normal glucose tolerance. *N Engl J Med* 1989;334:374–379.
113. Despres JP, Lamarche B, Margie P, et al. Hyperinsulinemia as an independent risk factor for ischemic heart disease. *N Engl J Med* 1996;334:952–956.
114. Haffner SM, Stern MP, Housed HP, et al. Cardiovascular risk factors in confirmed prediabetic individuals. Does the clock for coronary heart disease start ticking before the onset of clinical diabetes? *JAMA* 1990;263:2893–2897.
115. Reaven GM. Role of insulin resistance in human disease (Syndrome X): an expanded definition. *Annu Rev Med* 1993;44: 121–128.
116. Pyorala M, Miettinen H, Laakso M, et al. Hyperinsulinemia predicts coronary heart disease risk in healthy middle-aged men. *Circulation* 1998;98:398–405.
117. Williams ME. What are the clinically important consequences of ESRD-Associated Endocrine Dysfunction? *Semin Dial* 1997; 10(1):16–18.
118. Peltzman SJ, Agarwal BN. Spontaneous hypoglycemia in end-stage renal failure. *Nephron* 1977;19:131–139.
119. Bansal VK, Brooks MH, York JC, et al. Intractable hypoglycemia in a patient with renal failure. *Arch Intern Med* 1997;139: 101–102.
120. Arem R. Hypoglycemia associated with renal failure. *Endocrinol Metab Clin North Am* 1989;18:103–121.
121. Haviv YS, Sharkia M, Safadi R. Hypoglycemia in patients with renal failure. *Ren Fail* 2000;22:219–223.
122. Ramirez G, Brueggemeyer C, Ganguly A. Counterregulatory hormonal response to insulin-induced hypoglycemia in patients on chronic hemodialysis. *Nephron* 1988;49:231–236.
123. Frizell M, Larsen R, Field JB. Spontaneous hypoglycemia associated with chronic renal failure. *Diabetes* 1973;22:493–498.
124. Toth EL, Lee DW. Spontaneous/uremic hypoglycemia is not a distinct entity: substantiation from a literature review. *Nephron* 1991;58:325–329.
125. Block MB, Rubinstein AH. Spontaneous hypoglycemia in diabetic patients with renal insufficiency. *JAMA* 1970;213: 1863–1866.
126. Cryer PE, Gerich JE. Glucose counterregulation, hypoglycemia, and intensive insulin therapy in diabetes mellitus. *N Engl J Med* 1985;313:232–241.
127. Borden G, Reichard GA, Hoeldtke RD, et al. Severe insulin-induced hypoglycemia associated with deficiencies in the release of counterregulatory hormones. *N Engl J Med* 1981;305: 1200–1205.
128. Williams ME, Roshan B. Role of the new oral hypoglycemic drugs in the diabetic patient with ESRD. *Semin Dial* 1999;12: 25–31.
129. Heikinheimo R. Severe prolonged hypoglycemia following tolbutamide and carbutamide treatment. *Diabetes* 1965;14: 606–608.
130. Krepinsky J, Ingram AJ, Clase CM. Prolonged sulfonylurea-induced hypoglycemia in diabetic patients with end-stage renal disease. *Am J Kidney Dis* 2000;35:500–505.
131. Rydberg T, Johnson A, Roder M, et al. Hypoglycemic activity of glyburide (glibenclamide) metabolites in humans. *Diabetes Care* 1994;17:1026–1030.
132. Grajower MM, Walter L, Albin J. Hypoglycemia in chronic

hemodialysis patients: association with propranolol use. *Nephron* 1980;26:126–129.

133. Zarate A, Gelfand M, Novello A, et al. Propranolol-associated hypoglycemia in patients on maintenance hemodialysis. *Int J Artif Organs* 1984;4:130–134.
134. Pandit MK, Burke J, Gustafson AB, et al. Drug-induced disorders of glucose tolerance. *Ann Intern Med* 1993;118:529–539.
135. Almirall J, Montoliu J, Torras A, et al. Propoxyphene-induced hypoglycemia in a patient with chronic renal failure. *Nephron* 1989;53:273–275.
136. Arem R, Garber AJ, Field JB. Sulfonamide-induced hypoglycemia in chronic renal failure. *Arch Intern Med* 1983;143:827–829.
137. Goldstein DE, Little RR, Lorenz RA, et al. Tests of glycemia in diabetes. *Diabetes Care* 1985;18:876–905.
138. Tzamaloukas AH. The use of glycosylated hemoglobin in dialysis patients. *Semin Dial* 1998;11:141–143.
139. Tzamaloukas AH, Murata GH, Zager PG, et al. The relationship between glycemic control and morbidity and mortality for diabetics on dialysis. *ASAIO J* 1993;39:880–885.
140. Eisenberg B, Murata GH, Tzamaloukas AH. Gastroparesis in diabetics on chronic dialysis: clinical and laboratory associations and predictive features. *Nephron* 1995;70:296–300.
141. Ifudu O, Dulin AL, Friedman EA. Interdialytic weight gain correlates with glycosylated hemoglobin in diabetic hemodialysis patients. *Am J Kidney Dis* 1994;23:686–691.
142. U. S. Renal Data System. *USKDS 1991 Annual data report: atlas of end-stage renal disease in the United States.* Bethesda, MD: National Institutes of Health, National Institute of Diabetes and Digestive and Kidney Diseases, 1991;E56–57.
143. U. S. Renal Data System. *USKDS 2000 Annual data report: atlas of end-stage renal disease in the United States.* Bethesda, MD: National Institutes of Health, National Institute of Diabetes and Digestive and Kidney Diseases, 2000;148.
144. Engbaek F, Christensen SE, Jespersen B. Enzyme immunoassay of hemoglobin A1c: analytical characteristics and clinical performance for patients with diabetes mellitus, with and without uremia. *Clin Chem* 1989;35:93–97.
145. Shoji T, Tabata T, Nishizawa M, et al. Clinical availability of serum fructosamine in diabetic patients with uremia. *Nephron* 1989;51:338–343.
146. Ghacha R, Sinha AK, Karkar AM. HbA1c and serum fructosamine as markers of the chronic glycemic state in type 2 diabetic hemodialysis patients. *Dial Transplant* 2001;30:214–264.

3

ALTERED LIPID METABOLISM AND SERUM LIPIDS IN RENAL DISEASE AND RENAL FAILURE

CHRISTOPH WANNER

To understand dyslipidemia in states of impairment of kidney function and kidney failure it is advantageous to understand some aspects of lipid metabolism. In general, all five major lipoproteins (chylomicrons, very-low-density lipoproteins [VLDL], low-density lipoproteins [LDL], intermediate-density lipoproteins [IDL], and high-density lipoproteins [HDL]) consist of lipids (cholesterol, triglyceride, and phospholipid) and apolipoproteins. The apolipoproteins (A-I, A-II, B-48, B-100, C-I, C-II, C-III, and E) are found in different distributions among the various lipoproteins and serve as cofactors for enzymes and as ligands for receptors. Chylomicrons, the largest lipoprotein particles, are almost absent in the fasting state. They are formed in the intestinal epithelial cells, and their main lipid content—triglyceride—is synthesized from reesterifcation of dietary monoglycerides and fatty acids. Triglycerides represent 90% of chylomicrons and are hydrolyzed by lipoprotein lipase (LPL) present in adipose and vascular tissue. This reaction requires the presence of apoprotein C-II (apoC-II). The residual particles or chylomicron remnants usually are removed rapidly by the liver via the interaction of apoE and its receptor, which is located on hepatocytes. In addition to dietary-derived chylomicrons, the liver has the capacity to produce endogenous lipoproteins from excess hepatocyte cholesterol and triglycerides. These lipids are synthesized and secreted as triglyceride-rich VLDLs. The triglycerides present in VLDLs gradually are removed by LPL (with apoC-II acting as a cofactor), resulting serially in IDLs and then in a smaller, denser particle consisting almost entirely of cholesterol esters. Therefore, IDLs (also named VLDL remnants) represent a transition step in the lipolysis of VLDL to LDLs, the main cholesterol-carrying lipoprotein in man, which accounts for 70% of circulating cholesterol (Fig. 3.1).

HDLs are the most abundant lipoprotein particles in human plasma, although they only carry approximately 20% of the circulating cholesterol. In humans, two main subclasses are recognized: HDL2 and HDL3. Nascent HDL, primarily derived from the liver, is released into the plasma as an empty container with the ability to attract free cholesterol to its surface. Subsequently, via the action of lecithin cholesterol acyltransferase (LCAT), cholesterol is esterified and moves into the interior of HDL. Cholesterol-loaded HDL particles with apoE subsequently are catabolized in the liver, releasing cholesterol esters for hydrolysis and excretion in the bile. These events are thought to prevent accumulation of cholesterol in a variety of peripheral cells and thus provide a means of reverse cholesterol transport. In addition, cholesterol ester transfer protein (CETP) can transfer cholesterol esters from HDL to a variety of lipoproteins, primarily VLDL and chylomicron remnants, providing another pathway for cell cholesterol removal. Thus, lipoprotein metabolism is a complex process involving a variety of regulatory proteins (apoproteins), cell receptors, and particle dimensions thought to be important in the orderly assimilation of lipids. The characteristics of the various lipoproteins as well as their lipid and apolipoprotein composition in healthy people are given in Table 3.1.

In recent years another apolipoprotein, the so-called lipoprotein(a) [Lp(a)] has become important for patients with renal disease because high levels appear to be especially atherogenic in this patient population. Apolipoprotein(a) [apo(a)] is a structural protein for Lp(a). Apo(a) exhibits a high homology to plasminogen and an extreme size polymorphism, with the apo(a) isoproteins ranging in size from 420 to 840 kD. Inherited in an autosomal codominant fashion, the apo(a) isoprotein is an important factor determining plasma Lp(a) concentrations, with an inverse correlation between the size of apo(a) isoprotein and the plasma Lp(a) concentration. The distribution of plasma Lp(a) levels is skewed highly toward lower concentrations, with more than two-thirds of the population having levels lower than 20 mg/dL. High plasma concentrations of Lp(a) (>30 mg/dL) are associated with the risk of premature coronary atherosclerosis, cerebrovascular atherosclerosis, and saphenous vein bypass graft stenosis (1).

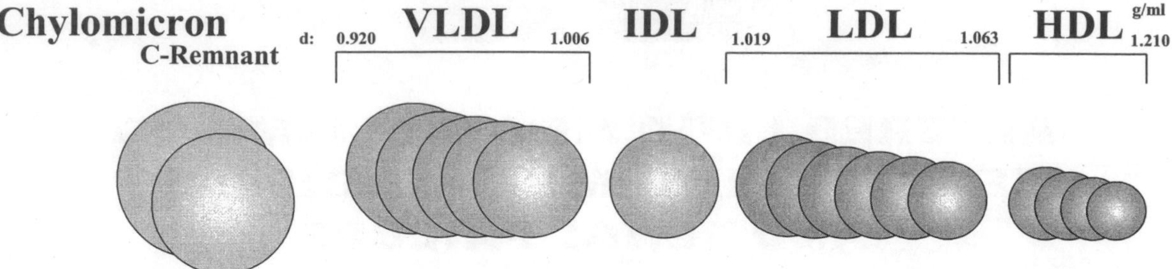

FIGURE 3.1. Classification of major lipoprotein particle-density classes.

TABLE 3.1. LIPOPROTEIN CLASSES OF HUMAN PLASMA

					Composition (% mass)				
	Density	Electrophoretic Mobility	Particle Diameter	Apolipoproteins	TG	FC	CE	PL	Pr
Chylomicrons	<0.95	—	>1,000	AI,AIV,B-48,C,E	90	1	2	5	2
VLDL	<1.006	pre-β	55	B-100,C,E	54	7	13	16	10
IDL	1.006–1.019	pre-β-β	25	B-100,C,E	20	9	34	20	17
LDL	1.019–1.063	β	20	B-100	4	9	34	20	17
Lp(a)	1.080–1.100	pre-β	24	B-100,(a)	3	9	36	18	34
HDL$_2$	1.063–1.125	α	11	AI,AII,E,C	5	5	13	35	42
HDL$_3$	1.125–1.210	α	9	AI,AII,E,C	3	3	15	23	56

TG = triglycerides; FC = free cholesterol (unesterified); CE = cholesteryl ester; PL = phospholipid; Pr = protein.

DYSLIPIDEMIA IN RENAL DISEASE AND RENAL FAILURE

The most characteristic patterns of serum lipids in patients with kidney disease and kidney failure are summarized in Table 3.2.

Nephrotic Syndrome

The dyslipidemia of the nephrotic syndrome is present in 70% to 90% of the patients and can occur in several forms. The most common (50%) is combined hyperlipidemia with an increase in serum total and LDL cholesterol and serum triglycerides (2–4). One-third of the patients have an exclusive elevation of LDL cholesterol; a less common pattern is elevated triglycerides alone (4%). Therefore, nephrotic patients with normal kidney function also may have an increase in plasma triglycerides, which can develop in the early course of the disease. Changes in the composition of lipoprotein particles also have been described with cholesterol enrichment in IDL but not LDL (5,6). The levels of HDL cholesterol may be low, normal, or high, and the level of HDL2 is reduced (2,7,8). High levels could be the result of high serum Lp(a) contaminating the HDL samples when the cholesterol is assayed. Therefore, the inconsistent results of HDL are most likely the consequence of selection criteria. HDL has been quantified in the urine in patients with nephrotic syndrome (9), and changes in the composition of urinary HDL have been ascribed to the effect of tubular catabolism on filtered lipoprotein (7). The reason why pa-

TABLE 3.2. COMMON LIPOPROTEIN ABNORMALITIES IN RENAL DISEASE

Renal Abnormality	Chylomicron Remnants	VLDL	IDL	LDL	HDL	Lp(a)[a]
Nephrotic syndrome	—	↑	↑↑	↑↑↑	↔–↓	↑↑↑
CRF	—	↑	↑	↓	↓	↑
Hemodialysis	↑↑	↑↑	↑↑	↓	↓	↑↑
CAPD	?	↑	↑↑	↑	↔	↑↑↑
Transplantation	—	↑	—	↑	↔	↔
Atherogenicity	+	+	+++	+++	Protective	++

VLDL, very-low-density lipoprotein; IDL, intermediate-density lipoprotein; LDL, low-density lipoprotein; HDL, high-density lipoprotein; Lp(a), lipoprotein(a); CRF, chronic renal failure; CAPD; continuous ambulatory peritoneal dialysis.
[a]Elevated in most but not all patients.

tients with the nephrotic syndrome present different accumulations of triglycerides and cholesterol has not been fully elucidated but includes many factors such as genetic apolipoprotein phenotypes, concomitant drug therapy, and the catabolic state of the individual. In contrast to nephrotic patients with normal kidney function, the presence of uremia leads to further changes, whereas diabetes mellitus does not affect the pattern of hyperlipoproteinemia (10).

In general, changes in plasma apoliprotein concentrations parallel the changes in lipoproteins. ApoB and E are increased, and apoA-I reflects HDL cholesterol levels. Levels of all three apoCs are increased, although there is no change in the apoC-II/C-III ratio (3). Markedly elevated Lp(a) concentrations have been found in the majority of patients with proteinuria (11,12) and the nephrotic syndrome (13), even when compared to controls of the same apo(a) isoform (14). On average, Lp(a) levels are elevated sixfold in patients with severe nephrotic syndrome (14). It is likely that the nephrotic syndrome results directly in elevation of Lp(a) because Lp(a) concentrations are reduced substantially when remission of the nephrotic syndrome is induced (14). Recent data suggest that the kidney is responsible for the metabolism of Lp(a) (15).

Mechanisms of Hyperlipidemia in the Nephrotic Syndrome

Not all patients with nephrotic syndrome have increased lipid levels, and those with elevations in VLDL have decreased fractional clearance rates (decreased catabolism) rather than increased synthesis (16). Two separate processes conspire to impede removal of triglyceride-rich lipoproteins. One is an abnormality in VLDL that decreases its ability to bind to endothelial surfaces in the presence of saturating LPL (17). This defect in VLDL function, and presumably structure, is a result of proteinuria (18). The second defect is an inability of LPL to bind effectively to the vascular endothelium (Fig. 3.2) (19).

Chronic Renal Failure

Patients with moderate proteinuria and progressive impairment of kidney function can be distinguished from those with nephrotic syndrome and normal kidney function. A detailed analysis by Samuelsson et al. (20) showed that the dyslipoproteinemia in early renal insufficiency has the same qualitative characteristics as that in advanced renal failure. Dyslipidemia already can be detected at the early stages of kidney insufficiency (20–22) and can be characterized better by abnormalities in the apolipoprotein than in the lipid profile (20). The main metabolic abnormality appears to be a delayed catabolism of triglyceride-rich lipoproteins resulting in increased concentrations of apoB-containing triglyceride-rich lipoproteins in VLDL and IDL and reduced levels of HDL. The hallmark of the altered apolipoprotein profile is considered to be a decreased apoA-I/apoC-III ratio (20). Quantitatively, there may be differences among patients because the extent of dyslipidemia in patients without nephrotic disease does not seem to depend on the urinary albumin excretion rate. The variation in urinary albumin excretion rate accounts for only 7% of the variation in cholesterol at nonnephrotic levels (23). Clearly, many other factors are involved in the regulation of serum cholesterol, and this is reflected in the wide variation in concentrations between and within populations. Dyslipidemia should not be seen as an isolated phenomenon; it should be seen in the context of cardiovascular disease. At all stages of kidney disease the patient's cardiovascular risk should be formally assessed and documented at presentation and at 6 monthly intervals thereafter. Risk assessment includes modifiable risk

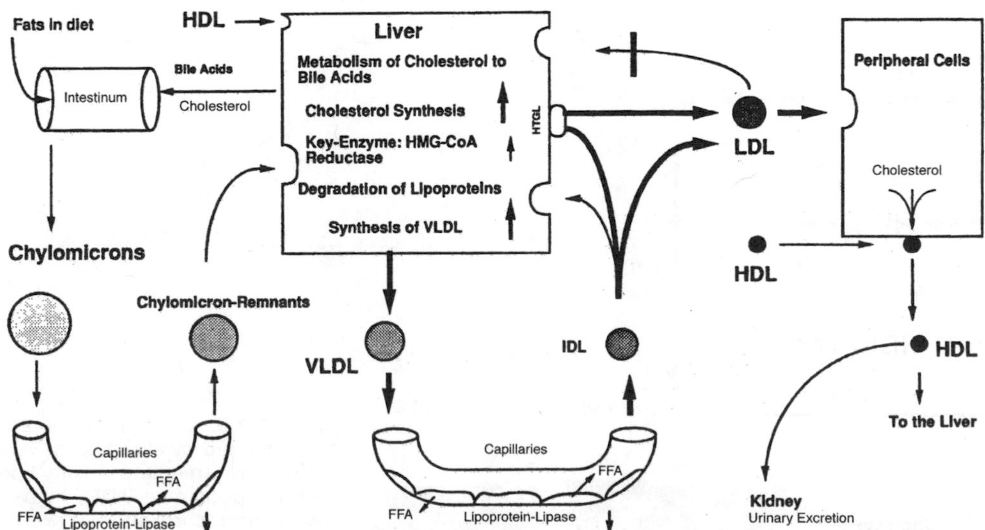

FIGURE 3.2. Schematic representation of lipoprotein metabolism in the nephrotic syndrome.

factors such as cigarette smoking, hyperglycemia, dyslipidemia, and hypertension. There is strong evidence from studies in the general population that cigarette smoking, glucose intolerance or poor diabetes control, hypertension, family history of vascular disease, and current or past history of vascular disease each independently may contribute to the risk of vascular disease (24–26). Inclusion of a medical record history of vascular disease as a mortality case-mix factor is recommended to quantitate the presence of vascular disease and to estimate complications and outcome (27).

Hemodialysis

The prevalence of dyslipidemia in end-stage renal disease (ESRD) is greater than in the general population (28,29). Patients undergoing hemodialysis exhibit a characteristic dyslipidemia consisting of hypertriglyceridemia and low HDL cholesterol levels (30–39). VLDL cholesterol typically is increased; however, levels of total and LDL cholesterol usually are normal or even may be low (40–44). This pattern further translates into the most characteristic feature of the ESRD-associated dyslipidemia represented by an accumulation of triglyceride-rich lipoproteins (VLDL remnants) (32) and IDLs (39,41). Furthermore, qualitative changes take place in LDL with a predominance of the small dense LDL (sdLDL) phenotype (Fig. 3.3) (44–48). The overall pattern is described best by an accumulation of apolipoprotein B-containing triglyceride-rich lipoprotein particles containing C-III and (a) or by lipoprotein Bc particles (37,38,49–51). A defect in postprandial chylomicron remnant clearance has been described as well (32,52).

Atherogenicity of Dyslipidemia

Growing evidence suggests that all of the components of this type of dyslipidemia (elevated VLDL remnants, IDL, sdLDL, low-HDL cholesterol) are independently atherogenic (53–55). Together they represent a set of lipoprotein abnormalities that, in addition to elevated LDL cholesterol, promote atherosclerosis. Triglycerides are linked physiologically to sdLDL and low-HDL concentrations, and it is likely that the increased sdLDL contributes to the atherogenic risk for hypertriglyceridemia (56–58). Atherogenic levels of sdLDL were found in patients with ESRD with triglycerides greater than 177 mg/dL (44). The accumulation of these lipoprotein particles contributes to a so-called atherogenic lipoprotein phenotype. A similar type of dyslipidemia also is seen in the general population and is called atherogenic dyslipidemia, which frequently occurs in patients with premature coronary heart disease and appears, in the absence of elevated LDL cholesterol, to be an independent atherogenic lipoprotein phenotype (59). Most patients with atherogenic dyslipidemia are insulin resistant, and many also have an elevated serum apolipoprotein B.

Several theories have been proposed regarding the cause of the increased atherogenicity. The primary metabolic defect is believed to be defective catabolism of triglyceride-rich lipoproteins (primarily VLDL) by the enzymes lipoprotein lipase (60) and hepatic lipase (61). Lipid peroxidation products are elevated in plasma (62) but appear not to be generated during hemodialysis (63). A defect in cholesterol transport has been reported (64), probably as a result of alterations in CETP and LCAT activities (65–67). With respect to mechanisms for sdLDL accumulation, the suggested causes include (a) decreased affinity for the LDL receptor (68) with increased clearance via the scavenger receptor (69); (b) increased susceptibility to oxidation and glycation, partly as a result of longer residence time in the circulation (70); (c) increased transcapillary permeability and filtration by the endothelium because of smaller size of the particles (71); and (d) greater affinity for binding to extracellular matrix such as arterial wall proteoglycans (72).

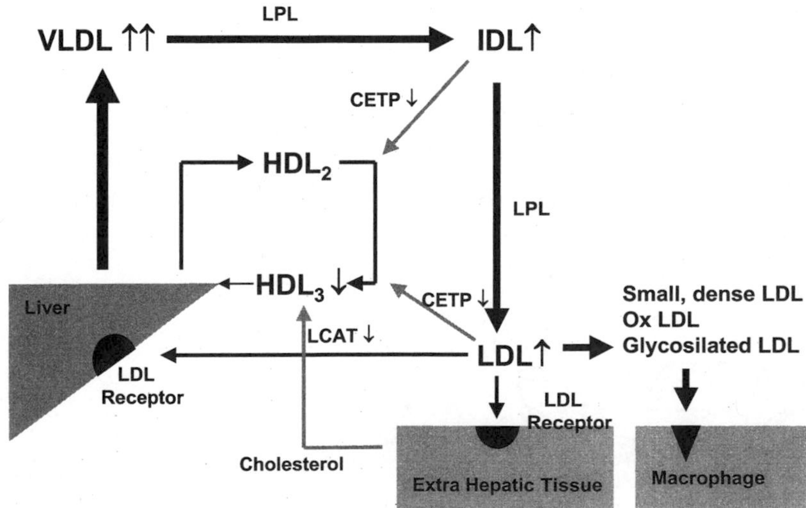

FIGURE 3.3. Lipoprotein metabolism in uremia is characterized by elevation of very-low-density lipoprotein, intermediate-density lipoprotein, and low-density lipoprotein (LDL); high-density lipoprotein metabolism is impaired as well. The accumulation of LDL leads to its modification and consequently requires uptake via scavenger receptors.

Assessment of the Atherogenic Risk by Serum Lipid Determination

The finding of an increased prevalence of atherogenic levels of VLDL remnants (28,73,74), IDL cholesterol (73,75,76) and sdLDL (40–43), in the context of normal plasma total and LDL cholesterol, highlights the need to look beyond the basic assessment of plasma concentrations of total and LDL cholesterol when assessing the cardiovascular risk posed by dyslipidemia in the hemodialysis population. However, measurements of these atherogenic lipoproteins currently are not available for routine laboratory evaluation. There is a strong correlation between plasma triglycerides and sdLDL concentrations, highlighting the physiologic role of triglycerides in sdLDL formation and its possible use as a surrogate marker. Triglyceride levels greater than 177 mg/dL (2 mmol/L), used to identify patients with sdLDL, had a sensitivity of 86% and a specificity of 79% (40). Peroxidative modification, particularly VLDL, also takes place in patients undergoing hemodialysis (77,78).

Continuous Ambulatory Peritoneal Dialysis

In patients with continuous ambulatory peritoneal dialysis (CAPD), qualitative lipoprotein abnormalities are similar to those found in patients undergoing hemodialysis, and most of the mechanisms that alter lipoprotein metabolism are probably also the same (79,80). Quantitatively, these patients have higher plasma cholesterol, triglyceride, LDL cholesterol, and apoB levels than patients undergoing hemodialysis (81–84). This additional increase is most likely the result of two additional factors (85): (a) The loss of considerable amounts of protein (7 to 14 g/day) into the peritoneal dialysate (86) and (b) excessive absorption of glucose (150 to 200 g/day) from the dialysis fluid. Whether protein loss triggers mechanisms that are operative in the nephrotic syndrome or whether hyperinsulinemia, through induction of advanced glycosylation of apoB, results in impaired receptor-mediated clearance of lipoproteins, remains to be established. However, the glucose load may increase triglyceride synthesis in hypertriglyceridemic patients, thereby contributing to a further increase in the concentration of triglyceride-rich lipoproteins (81,87–89). An interesting study in normolipidemic patients has shown that patients with CAPD appear to have less pronounced abnormalities of cholesterol transport than patients undergoing hemodialysis (90). This may be because of an increased clearance of unknown inhibitory factors, resulting in a better control of uremic lipoprotein metabolism and leading to decreased concentrations of such factors. Whether CAPD is more advantageous than hemodialysis with regard to the possible long-term effects of dyslipoproteinemia in renal failure remains to be clarified. However, CAPD patients also exhibit higher levels of Lp(a) than patients undergoing hemodialysis (91–93), which may outweigh other positive conditions.

Lipid Abnormalities After Kidney Transplantation

Dyslipidemia commonly is found in patients after renal transplantation and is associated with cardiovascular complications and graft atherosclerosis. Correlations have been found with cyclosporine and steroids as the major causes of lipid abnormalities. Distinct changes in serum lipid concentrations and lipoprotein composition related to immunosuppressive therapy can be demonstrated. Tacrolimus, another immunosuppressant, does not affect total and LDL cholesterol levels and engenders a smaller increase in triglyceride levels compared to cyclosporine (10% to 15% increase). The effects on HDL cholesterol are similar to the effects of cyclosporine on HDL (94). Posttransplant dyslipidemia is qualitatively and quantitatively dependent on age, gender, body weight and type, and dose of immunosuppressive agents (95). Although some former studies focused mainly on elevation of serum cholesterol, recent data emphasize an increase in serum triglycerides, LDL, and VLDL as major factors for cardiovascular disease. Alterations in size and density contribute to configurational changes of lipoproteins. Small and dense LDL exhibit reduced receptor-specific uptake and therefore bear increased atherogenicity. This corresponds with the finding that hypertriglyceridemia is considered to be an independent risk factor for cardiovascular disease. Because of the multiplicity of other cardiovascular risk factors, dyslipidemia also may accelerate the development of arteriosclerosis in a preinjured vascular endothelium. Immunosuppression withdrawal protocols have been used successfully to control pronounced hyperlipidemia in immunologically stable patients.

Kidney transplant recipients suffer a high morbidity and mortality as a result of premature cardiovascular disease (96). Two studies have shown higher serum cholesterol and triglyceride values in patients with ischemic heart disease as compared to those without ischemic heart disease (95,97). Vathsala et al. (98) reported a 36-month follow-up in 500 patients treated with cyclosporine and prednisone. They found that cardiovascular or cerebrovascular episodes occurred in 9.4% of patients and were significantly more common in hyperlipidemic (15.4%) than in normolipidemic (5.2%) subjects. A retrospective study demonstrated significantly higher concentrations of total cholesterol; triglycerides; and apolipoproteins B, C-II, C-III, and E in 25 patients with cardiovascular events as compared to 29 patients without cardiovascular events (99). A significant association was found between smoking and the proportion of patients with hypertension among those with cardiovascular disease. Massy et al. (100) found significantly higher serum triglyceride concentrations, but not cholesterol levels, in patients with ischemic heart disease. Whenever studies in patients with renal functional impairment find a significant rise in apoB-containing triglyceride-rich lipoprotein particles, the presence of partially delipidized lipoproteins or so-called remnant lipoproteins can be suspected. Indeed, Quaschning et al. (101) demonstrated an enrichment of triglycerides in VLDL and LDL in 218 patients with stable graft function. Triglyceride enrichment in LDL indicates that there is the accumulation of sdLDL, which are known to bear enhanced atherosclerotic risk. These lipoprotein particles also are considered to be of particular importance in the progression of renal injury.

THE VASCULAR RISK IN KIDNEY PATIENTS

The best available data are those from dialysis patients documented in registries. They show that cardiovascular disease is the leading cause of morbidity and mortality in hemodialysis patients; cardiac disease accounts for 44% of overall mortality (102,103). Approximately 22% of these deaths from cardiac causes are attributed to acute myocardial infarction. In patients who survive a myocardial infarction, the mortality from cardiac causes is 59.3% at 1 year, 73% at 2 years, and 89.9% at 3 years (104). Similar abysmal long-term prognosis has been reported from the Strasbourg region (France) for patients with type 2 diabetes mellitus starting dialysis (105). After adjusting for age, gender, race, and diagnosis of diabetes, mortality from cardiovascular disease is far greater in patients undergoing hemodialysis than in the general population. The risk ranges from 500-fold in individuals aged 25 to 35 to fivefold in individuals older than age 85 years (106). The excess risk of vascular disease is the result, at least in part, of an increased prevalence of conditions that are recognized as risk factors for vascular disease in the general population ("traditional" risk factors), and further to hemodynamic and metabolic factors characteristic of chronic kidney disease ("kidney disease–related") risk factors (107). However, vascular damage is developed during the progressive course of kidney disease and long before renal replacement starts.

Therefore, all kidney patients should be considered to be at the greatest risk of developing vascular disease. Measures to prevent vascular disease should not be based on the presence or absence of prior vascular disease or other risk factors; instead, it should be assumed that the risk for vascular disease is already sufficient enough to warrant the most aggressive management.

THE ROLE OF LIPOPROTEINS IN ATHEROSCLEROSIS OF PATIENTS WITH RENAL DISEASE

Nephrotic Syndrome

There is also no reason to doubt that the severe, persistent elevation of LDL, IDL, and Lp(a), regardless of cause, represents a highly atherogenic condition. The degree to which it increases the risk for coronary heart disease in patients with nephrotic disease remains uncertain. Relatively little and conflicting information has been published on the risk of atherosclerotic vascular disease (108–110). All of these studies were retrospective and flawed by small numbers, selection bias, and lack of control for other atherosclerotic risk factors (such as smoking, hypertension, and steroid therapy). Some studies include patients with minimal-change disease, who would most likely not remain nephrotic and hence not remain at risk for the long-term complications of hyperlipidemia. According to Ordonez et al. (111), the relative risk of myocardial infarction, after adjustment for hypertension and smoking, is 5.5, and the relative risk of coronary death is 2.8. The data were obtained in a series of patients (n = 142) matched with healthy subjects and followed prospectively for 5.6 and 1.2 years, respectively. Unfortunately, the cholesterol level data were insufficient to analyze the risk by specific lipid levels or by duration of hyperlipidemia. Until now, no study has been carried out identifying dyslipidemia as a major factor for cardiovascular complication in patients with nephritic disease, nor has a regression study been performed. This is because of the low prevalence of the nephrotic syndrome and the large number of patients required to show a significant reduction in coronary events following lipid-lowering therapy (112).

Hemodialysis and CAPD

Dyslipidemia and Atherosclerotic Vascular Disease

Lipid abnormalities have been suggested as a major cause of vascular disease in patients undergoing hemodialysis, and reviews have focused on the subject of renal failure, dialysis and dyslipidemia (113–115). A number of studies have examined the relationship between various lipid parameters and the presence of clinically apparent atherosclerosis in individuals receiving hemodialysis therapy (25,113, 116–118). These trials have been cross-sectional in nature, including only small numbers of patients, and have failed in part to distinguish atherosclerosis-related events from other forms of cardiovascular disease. Studies also have failed to control for other risk factors and have assessed only total plasma lipid levels rather than the lipoprotein disturbances that characterize the uremic dyslipidemia. It is therefore not surprising that the conclusions have been conflicting (119). In the largest and longest study to date, 419 dialysis patients were followed prospectively over a 21-year period during which time 49% died of cardiovascular disease and 23% experienced fatal or nonfatal ischemic events. Smoking, hypertension, and hypertriglyceridemia were identified as independent risk factors for ischemic cardiovascular disease (120). In contrast, several smaller cross-sectional studies have failed to find an association between elevated triglycerides and complications resulting from vascular disease (119). However, in a group of 196 patients with diabetes receiving hemodialysis, elevated cholesterol levels with high LDL to HDL ratios were associated with an increased risk of cardiac death during a 45-month follow-up period. Hypercholesterolemia was more common in the patients with diabetes than in matched nondiabetic dialyzed controls (121). Lipid measurements were done when patients commenced renal replacement therapy. In this respect it is worth noting that serum cholesterol concentrations decline with time on dialysis (122). Most cross-sectional studies with longitudinal follow-up also have failed to demonstrate that plasma total- and LDL cholesterol and triglycerides are associated with increased cardiovascular mortality in patients undergoing hemodialysis (123). There are no longitudinal studies reported for large numbers of patients followed from the start of dialysis that could delineate the degree of cardiac risk associated with the various lipid abnormalities prevalent in chronic uremia.

The Paradox of Cholesterol in Hemodialysis Patients

Prospective observational studies in the general population have shown that the relation between the risk of coronary-artery disease and blood cholesterol is roughly log-linear. However, inverse associations were observed among hemodialysis patients between blood cholesterol and all-cause (124) or cardiovascular (125) mortality. The relationship between serum cholesterol and mortality has been described as "J-shaped," and the risk of death is 4.3 times greater in hemodialysis patients with serum cholesterol less than 100 mg/dL (2.6 mmol/L) than in those with values between 200 and 250 mg/dL (5.2 to 6.5 mmol/L) (124). This phenomenon is known as reverse risk factors or reverse causality (see Chapter 11). Concomitant chronic illnesses that induce a compensatory decrease in cholesterol synthesis also are associated with an increased risk of death, producing artifactual negative associations between cholesterol and mortality (126,127). This effect may limit the extent to which standard observational studies can identify the true impact of serum cholesterol on the development of vascular disease in such populations (128).

Assessment of Risk by Measuring Lp(a)

Individual physician decisions are mandatory to define long life expectancy on renal replacement therapy. Cardiovascular risk calculations in the general population are done in decade intervals. A consistent elevation in plasma Lp(a) has been observed in patients undergoing hemodialysis in large case-controlled studies (129–136). The plasma Lp(a) level turned out to be an independent risk factor for cardiovascular disease in some (137–141), but not all, cross-sectional studies (142,143). In a large prospective study, an association of high plasma Lp(a) concentrations with vascular disease was demonstrated (136). In contrast, another prospective study found no difference in Lp(a) concentrations between survivors and nonsurvivors in a group of 412 patients with diabetes undergoing hemodialysis and peritoneal dialysis (144). In a recent prospective study, although Lp(a) was significantly associated with the risk of all-cause cardiovascular mortality by univariate Cox regression analysis, it was not an independent risk factor in multivariate analysis (123).

An increase in plasma Lp(a) has been identified only in patients exhibiting high–molecular-weight (HMW) apo(a) isoforms (131), but this has not been confirmed by others in different ethnic populations (132,133). Low–molecular-weight (LMW) apo(a) isoforms were independent and better predictors for coronary artery disease in a prospective follow-up of more than 400 patients over a period of 5 years (142). In large prospective studies the LMW apo(a) isoforms also predicted the risk for vascular disease (145) and the risk for carotid atherosclerosis (146). It appears that the Lp(a) plasma concentration and the apo(a) size play a synergistic role in advanced atherosclerosis (147). Increased plasma-free apo(a) fragments appear to account for only a small proportion of increased Lp(a) (148,149). No association was found between plasma apo(a) fragments and carotid artery plaques assessed by ultrasound in a recent cross-sectional study (150). Inflammation and nutrition affect the metabolism and the plasma concentrations of Lp(a) (151, 152). For unknown reasons, inflammation affected only HMW apo(a) isoforms (123). Therefore, it is proposed that Lp(a) should be measured in patients with a long life expectancy being treated with renal replacement therapy at 6-month intervals to quantitate risk for subsequent cardiovascular disease. In young patients with a long life expectancy being treated with renal replacement therapy and a Lp(a) of more than 30 mg/dL, the apolipoprotein(a) isoform should be determined.

Age and Lipid Lowering

Because cholesterol and LDL cholesterol levels are normal in most patients undergoing hemodialysis, coupled with the lack of long-term lipid-reducing studies in this population, the debate continues about the role of lipid-reducing therapy in ESRD, particularly about who should be targeted (153). Most patients undergoing hemodialysis today are of older age. Trials with statins have included sizable numbers of older people, mostly in the age range of 65 to 75 years. In these trials, older people showed a significant risk reduction with statin therapy (154). Thus, no hard-and-fast age restrictions appear necessary when selecting people with established coronary heart disease for LDL-lowering therapy. However, concomitant illness, general health status, and social issues may influence treatment decisions and may suggest a more conservative approach. Further studies and research in patients with uremia are required to assess the risk posed by abnormal lipoprotein particles in this population and the role of lipid-reducing agents in a population with dyslipidemia and the atherogenic lipoprotein phenotype rather than hyperlipidemia (155,156).

RELATION OF DYSLIPIDEMIA TO PROGRESSION OF RENAL DAMAGE

Chronic Progressive Kidney Disease

In experimental animal models, hyperlipidemia has been implicated in causing direct renal injury (157). In animal models, treatment of hyperlipidemia has led to an improvement of glomerular injury in nondiabetic and diabetic renal disease (158–161). It has been shown that altered serum lipoproteins interact with structures of the glomerulus (162, 163). LDL particles modified by glycosylation and oxidation exhibited enhanced binding to glycosaminoglycans of the glomerular basement membrane, causing increased permeability of the basement membrane. In addition, deposition of modified altered LDL particles in the mesangium may induce chemotactic signals for macrophages and stimulate mesangial cell proliferation. The preferential scavenger receptor-mediated uptake of modified LDL by monocytes/macrophages has been considered to cause the formation of glomerular and mesangial foam cells (157). Other mechanisms include mesangial expansion by accumulation of apoB and apoE, leading to a reduction in glomerular filtration surface area, an alteration in renal cortical tissue lipids, alterations in membrane fluidity and function induced by disturbances in fatty acids concentrations, and alterations in glomerular hemodynamics.

In humans with diabetic nephropathy, hyperlipidemia has been identified as a risk factor for a more rapid rate of decline in glomerular filtration rate and increased mortality (164,165). Most noteworthy, an increased plasma concentration of triglyceride-rich apoB-containing lipoproteins has been found to be linked to a more rapid decrease in renal function, and the combination of dyslipoproteinemia and hypertension appears to act synergistically to indicate a more rapid decline of renal function. Patients with type 1 diabetes with a serum cholesterol level greater than 7 mmol/L (270 mg/dL) show a more rapid decline of glomerular filtration rate than patients with a plasma cholesterol lower than 7 mmol/L (164). In a follow-up study multivariate analysis revealed that angiotensin converting enzyme (ACE) inhibitor (enalapril) therapy associated with a lower serum cholesterol concentration was superior to β-blocker (metoprolol) therapy associated with higher cholesterol concentrations in preventing deterioration of renal function in type 1 patients with diabetic nephropathy (163). Recently, high triglycerides and low-HDL cholesterol could be identified as strong predictors of more rapid progression of microalbuminuria in patients with type 2 diabetes with well-controlled blood pressure.

Several uncontrolled preliminary studies in small numbers of patients with diabetes and proteinuria suggested that treatment with a statin stabilizes or improves renal function (166). Further prospective long-term studies involving a large number of patients are required to prove or disprove the relevance of cholesterol-lowering therapy in retarding progression of diabetic nephropathy.

Kidney Transplantation

Animal Experiments and Histology

High cholesterol diets accelerate coronary artery disease of rat and rabbit cardiac allografts as well as vascular injury in a rat aorta allograft model in the absence or presence of immunosuppression (167–169). Oxidized lipoproteins are important in the pathogenesis of systemic atherosclerosis, but the antioxidant probucol failed to reduce vascular injury in rabbit aorta allograft while cholesterol levels were kept constant with diet (170). Cardiac allograft vasculopathy in rats was reduced by statin treatment (171).

The vascular lesions seen in chronic rejection and those that characterize systemic atherosclerosis often show similarities. Macrophages, foam cells, T cells, and proliferating smooth-muscle cells can be demonstrated in the vascular lesions. Apolipoprotein A-I, A-II, and B deposits have been detected in the vascular lesions from chronically rejecting renal allografts. At present, it is not clear whether vascular lipoprotein deposition is a passive phenomenon and the result rather than the cause of vascular injury. Oxidatively modified lipoproteins may play an important role in the pathogenesis of atherosclerosis. Tanabe et al. (172) investigated whether oxidized lipoproteins are present in arteries of rejecting kidneys. Using a monoclonal antibody to detect oxidized LDL, four of the five individuals with serum cholesterol greater than 240 mg/dL had evidence for oxidized LDL in the vascular intima. In contrast, none of the five patients with cholesterol of less than 240 mg/dL exhibited oxidized LDL in allograft arteries (172). Thus it is possible that oxidatively modified lipoproteins play a role in the pathogenesis of chronic allograft vasculopathy.

Observational Studies

Several investigators have found that transplant recipients with hyperlipidemia are more likely to have chronic rejection. Isoniemi et al. (173) examined risk factors among 98 renal allograft recipients who survived with a functioning allograft for at least 2 years. Levels of total and LDL cholesterol as well as triglycerides were correlated with subsequent chronic declines in renal function. Because proteinuria was not measured in this study, it is possible that patients already had graft injury that caused the high lipid levels. Dimeny et al. (174) demonstrated pretransplant levels of serum cholesterol that predicted late graft failure. Pretransplant cholesterol levels also correlated with acute rejection episodes during the first 6 months of follow-up after transplantation, and acute rejection initially was a strong risk factor for graft failure in the long run (175). Because most of these patients were treated with cyclosporine, it is interesting to speculate whether serum lipid levels influenced the biologic effects of cyclosporine. Cyclosporine binds to lipoproteins, and patients with lower plasma lipid and lipoprotein levels might have higher free cyclosporine drug levels. If the free fraction of cyclosporine is important for cell uptake, then plasma lipid and lipoprotein levels could influence the immunosuppressive and toxic effects of cyclosporine. Indeed, cyclosporine toxicity appears to be more common in patients with low plasma lipid levels (176).

Massy et al. (177) examined the relationship between posttransplant lipid levels and graft loss to chronic rejection in a cohort of patients who survived at least 6 months with a functioning allograft. Only 250 of the 706 patients of this cohort ever received cyclosporine, and most of these patients had cyclosporine electively withdrawn 1 year after transplantation (178). Using time-dependent covariates in a multivariate Cox proportional hazards analysis, Massy et al. (177) found that serum triglycerides, but not cholesterol, were independent risk factors for graft loss caused by chronic rejection. It remained unclear in this investigation whether treatment with statins had influenced these findings. The Cox model may have selected triglycerides as potent candidates for chronic graft failure after cholesterol-lowering treatment. However, the findings of Quaschning et al. (101) also demonstrated the abundance of triglyceride-rich lipoprotein particles in a large number of stable renal transplant recipients. These lipoprotein particles are potent candidates for the progression of renal insufficiency. Whether the lack of effect of serum cholesterol, in contrast to the findings of others (173,174), could be because few of the patients received long-term cyclosporine therapy remains speculative.

There is also evidence for an increased prevalence of oxidized lipoproteins after renal transplantation. Ghanem et al. (179) demonstrated that LDL particles were smaller in renal transplant recipients as compared to healthy controls. sdLDL particles exhibit a greater tendency to become oxidized. This was confirmed by showing that the lag time for copper oxidation of LDL was reduced in transplant recipients (179). In this study, monoclonal antibodies to oxidized LDL were also higher in transplant recipients compared to controls. It appears that oxidized LDL is particularly common in renal transplant recipients. Similarly, renal transplant recipients with histologically confirmed chronic rejection had increased plasma levels of malondialdehyde, an end product of lipid peroxidation (180).

SCREENING FOR DYSLIPIDEMIA

All patients should have total cholesterol, triglycerides, and HDL cholesterol measured at presentation, 3 months after beginning hemodialysis treatment, and every 6 months thereafter. LDL cholesterol should be calculated by the Friedewald formula when triglycerides are less than 400 mg/dL (4.56 mmol/L). For triglycerides between 400 and 800 mg/dL (4.56 to 9.12 mmol/L), direct LDL measurements should be done.

Evidence suggests that each of the aforementioned dyslipidemias is associated with vascular disease in the general population, and treatment may reduce the risk of vascular disease (24,25). Measurements are readily available in most clinical chemistry laboratories. As a result of biologic and laboratory variation in cholesterol and triglyceride measurements, a reliable assessment of these parameters in each individual requires at least three measurements carried out on three separate samples (25,26). Because of further variations in extracorporeal treatment modalities, only a complete plasma lipid profile should be ordered each time dyslipidemia assessment is recommended. Changes in therapy or other conditions that may affect dyslipidemia may make more frequent measurements necessary (24,181).

The Friedewald formula is valid in patients undergoing dialysis and is sufficiently accurate ($r = 0.95$ to 0.97 calculated LDL versus measured LDL) (182) to allow the determination of LDL cholesterol in the vast majority of patients (182).

[Friedewald LDL cholesterol = total cholesterol − (HDL cholesterol + triglyceride/5)] (26).

Approximately 20% of patients undergoing hemodialysis have total triglycerides above 400 mg/dL (4.56 mmol/L) (182). As in other forms of primary or secondary hyperlipoproteinemias, other methods should be used to measure LDL cholesterol when triglycerides are above 400 mg/dL. Direct LDL measurement, lipoprotein electrophoresis, or analytic ultracentrifugation (rarely available) should be performed. When triglycerides are more than 800 mg/dL (9.12 mmol/L), LDL measurement is not recommended. All blood collections for lipid screening should be performed, whenever possible, on patients in the fasting state. When screening for dyslipidemia is done in patients undergoing hemodialysis, blood should be drawn immediately before or at least 12 hours after a regularly scheduled hemodialysis treatment.

Patients should have a complete lipid profile measured every 6 weeks during the initiation phase of lipid lowering intervention. When target levels have been met, the frequency can be reduced to every 4 to 6 months. There is some evidence that the hemodialysis procedure acutely alters lipid levels, in particular triglyceride and free fatty acid levels (183). Because most studies linking dyslipidemias to vascular disease have measured lipid levels prior to the hemodialysis procedure, screening should be done at this time. Changes in therapy or other conditions that may affect dyslipidemias may make more frequent measurements necessary. Blood obtained from either fasting or nonfasting individuals can be used for total cholesterol and HDL cholesterol analysis (181). Any patient with elevated LDL cholesterol or other forms of dyslipidemia (elevated total cholesterol and triglycerides and/or low HDL cholesterol) should undergo clinical or laboratory assessment to rule out other secondary causes such as glucose intolerance, hypothyroidism, obstructive liver disease, alcohol abuse, or drugs that decrease HDL cholesterol.

Additional secondary disorders include drugs that increase LDL cholesterol and decrease HDL cholesterol (progestins or anabolic steroids) (184,185). It is particularly important to mention anabolic steroids, which may be used for treatment of renal anemia in countries where erythropoietin is not widely available as a result of economic constraints. The use of anabolic steroids and the benefits of raising hematocrit should be weighed against the potential risk of developing several forms of dyslipidemia and possible deteriorating vascular disease (184). Although in one study Lp(a) decreased, the patients' serum triglycerides increased; also, in most women receiving nandrolone decanoate, mild hirsutism and voice change are experienced (186). Antihypertensive or immunosuppressive medications (corticosteroids) may cause secondary dyslipidemia.

Screening for dyslipidemia should not be performed after surgery or during conditions that may acutely affect the lipid profile. Patients without any comorbid conditions and a low total cholesterol (<150 mg/dL; 3.9 mmol/L) should be investigated for possible nutritional deficits. Such comorbid conditions include acute infection; diarrhea; a vascular accident, such as myocardial infarction; or a situation associated with the reduction of food intake. In patients admitted to the hospital for a major coronary event, LDL cholesterol levels should be measured on admission or within 24 hours (24). This value can be used for treatment decisions. LDL cholesterol levels that begin to decline in the first few hours after a vascular event are significantly decreased by 24 to 48 hours and may remain low for many weeks. Thus, the initial (>24 hours) LDL cholesterol level obtained in the hospital may be substantially less than usual for the patient. Infection is accompanied by an acute phase reaction.

Activated acute phase and high levels of circulating cytokines, such as interleukin-6, lower cholesterol levels (187, 188). Low or declining serum cholesterol concentrations are predictive of increased mortality risk (124,125,189–191). Hypocholesterolemia is associated with chronic protein-energy deficits and/or the presence of comorbid conditions, including inflammation. Cholesterol is influenced by the same comorbid conditions, such as inflammation, that affect other nutritional markers (e.g., serum albumin) (192).

TREATMENT GUIDELINES

General Remarks

Guidelines on detection, evaluation, and treatment of high blood cholesterol in adults are available from United States (24) and European expert panels (25,26) as well as from many national societies. These guidelines are evidence-based and were developed for the general population in a rigorous manner. It is possible that trial results from the general population may not be applicable to patients with kidney disease or those being treated with kidney replacement therapy. There are no randomized controlled interventional trials in patients with kidney disease or in patients receiving renal replacement therapy that show that the treatment of dyslipidemias reduces the incidence of vascular disease. It is possible that in some subpopulations of patients undergoing hemodialysis, treatment of dyslipidemias may not be as safe or as effective at reducing the incidence of vascular disease as it is in the general population. Additional randomized, placebo-controlled trials are needed urgently; it is the author's belief that the use of placebo treatment arms is justified in the context of an appropriately designed trial, even when lipid levels fall within the treatment thresholds recommended by guidelines.

In principle, patients should be treated according to the recommendations of the expert panels of the joint European societies on prevention of coronary heart disease or the National Cholesterol Education Program (NCEP) (24–26). A high-risk strategy should be applied using the recommendations targeting patients with known cardiovascular disease. Similar to diabetes, ESRD is considered to be a coronary risk equivalent. In the absence of data from randomized trials, it can only be assumed that the interventions recommended by the various guidelines will similarly reduce vascular disease in patients with kidney disease and being treated with kidney replacement therapy. Although the concept of accelerated atherosclerosis has become widely accepted since it was first published by Lindner et al. in 1974 (193), it should be noted that all recommendations of lipid-lowering treatment is done in the absence of evidence that the risk of cardiovascular death is reduced by lowering lipid levels in individuals with kidney disease or kidney failure.

Treatment Aspects

Patients with elevated LDL cholesterol (100 to 129 mg/dL; 2.6 to 3.4 mmol/L) should be treated to achieve LDL cholesterol of less than 100 mg/dL. Treatment beyond LDL cholesterol lowering should be initiated in patients with triglycerides of 180 mg/dL or more (2.0 mmol/L). Research from experimental animals, laboratory investigations, epidemiology, and genetic forms of hypercholesterolemia indicate that elevated LDL cholesterol is a major cause of vascular disease (194). In addition, recent clinical trials robustly show that LDL cholesterol–lowering therapy reduces the risk of vascular disease in the general population (188,195). For these reasons one may decide to extrapolate, at least in part, these data to the high-risk group of patients with kidney disease and to adopt elevated LDL cholesterol as the primary target of cholesterol-lowering therapy. However, targeting LDL cholesterol alone may not be appropriate because elevated LDL cholesterol is not the feature of lipid abnormalities complicating uremia.

Patients with chronic kidney disease automatically are considered to have coronary heart disease equivalents and therefore are at the highest risk for developing vascular disease. They should have no major contraindications to therapy and no illness that makes prevention and/or treatment of vascular disease unlikely to be beneficial. Lipid-lowering drugs should be administered to achieve LDL cholesterol and non-HDL cholesterol target levels irrespective of whether symptomatic ischemic heart disease is present. LDL cholesterol levels higher than 100 mg/dL (2.6 mmol/L) and non-HDL cholesterol higher than 130 mg/dL (3.4 mmol/L) are treatment initiation thresholds for drug therapy.

There is little evidence suggesting that the risk attributable to LDL cholesterol is similar in patients undergoing hemodialysis and in the general population, but efficacy and safety of treatment for LDL cholesterol with a statin are identical (196,197). In general, the action points for drug treatment are based primarily on risk–benefit considerations. LDL-lowering therapy greatly reduces risk for major coronary events and stroke and yields highly favorable cost-effectiveness ratios. Those at increased risk are likely to get greater benefit (198–200). Action points for recommended management based on therapeutic efficacy are checked against currently accepted standards for cost effectiveness. Based on the current literature, patients undergoing hemodialysis are likely to achieve cost-effectiveness ratios via a reduction of morbidity and subsequent hospitalization episodes (201–204). However, the latter remains to be demonstrated.

Diet and Exercise

In patients with LDL cholesterol of 100 to 129 mg/dL (2.6 to 3.4 mmol/L) or triglycerides of more than 180 mg/dL (2.0 mmol/L), therapeutic lifestyle changes (TLC) should be initiated whenever possible. Patients with dyslipidemia should have dietary interviews and/or diaries focusing on the type and amount of fat ingested. Dietary interviews should be repeated at yearly intervals when target lipid levels are not with drug therapy. TLCs include (a) reduced intakes of saturated fat and cholesterol, (b) increased physical activity, and (c) weight control (24). However, patients undergoing hemodialysis already are subject to specific food and fluid-intake restrictions. The introduction of a diet restricted in saturated fatty acids might add nutritional difficulties, and the patients may be at a greater risk of developing protein-energy malnutrition. Some patients may benefit from replacement of saturated fat with nonsaturated fat dietary sources, but these patients should be selected carefully (205). In nonrenal patients, diets rich in polyunsaturated fatty acids of fish-oil origin (omega-3) increase the removal of triglyceride-rich lipoprotein remnants and reduce postprandial plasma lipoproteins (206). Eicosapentanoic acid reduces plasma remnant lipoproteins and prevents *in vivo* peroxidation of LDL in patients undergoing dialysis (207). When patients are selected for dietary therapy, physicians should refer them to qualified dietitians and nutritionists at all stages of dietary intervention.

Patients being treated with hemodialysis usually are less physically active than healthy sedentary controls, and this difference is pronounced in older individuals (208). There is an association between physical activity and nutritional status (208). Exercise training, if tolerated and maintained over long periods, may improve the dyslipidemia as well as the glucose tolerance in selected patients (209–211). Whether inactivity increases or exercise reduces mortality in maintenance dialysis patients is not known.

Weight control may be appropriate in early renal failure but is risky in patients with advanced stages of renal failure because of its danger of causing malnutrition. Optimization of body weight should best be done together with a moderate increase in physical activity. As a result of altered body composition in the uremic state, optimization of body weight should be preferred over reduction of body weight. Patients undergoing hemodialysis normally have a reduced mean subcutaneous fat area/body mass index (BMI) and an increased visceral fat area/BMI (212). Visceral fat accumulation occurs irrespective of BMI and is associated with serum triglycerides (212). Weight-for-height is a strong predictor of 12-month mortality in male and female patients undergoing hemodialysis. An inverse relationship between mortality rates and weight-for-height percentiles is highly significant for patients within the lower 50th percentile of body weight for height (213). Low BMI is associated with increased risk of hospitalization and mortality. For every one unit increase in BMI over 27.5 and up to 30, the relative risk of dying is reduced by 30% (214,215). It may be of importance for patients to have excess amounts of body fat and other nutrients on which they may draw in cases of inflammatory catabolic conditions (216).

Pharmacotherapy

Nephrotic Syndrome

The first therapeutic strategy to reduce serum lipids is the reduction of proteinuria. Serum total and LDL cholesterol concentration and Lp(a) levels are inversely correlated with serum albumin as well as proteinuria (217–219). Reduction in proteinuria induced by ACE inhibitors reduces serum Lp(a) and cholesterol and is used as an adjuvant to standard lipid-lowering therapy (220,221). In that context one may say that ACE-inhibitors are excellent lipid-lowering drugs in patients with proteinuria. Nevertheless, lipid-lowering therapy with statins is almost always necessary to adequately correct excessive cholesterol elevations. The bile acid–binding resins cholestyramine and colestipol (222,223), the fibric acid gemfibrozil (224), and probucol (225) have all demonstrated limited effects in short-term trials. Today the largest number of patients have been treated by statins (226), which are by far the most effective LDL cholesterol–lowering agents. Because of their good tolerance and low side effects, they currently represent the treatment of choice. Fish oil is a potent triglyceride-lowering agent. However, conflicting findings of increased LDL cholesterol concentrations and decreased HDL/LDL cholesterol ratios, the high number of capsules required for treatment, and the low tolerance does not make fish oil a favorite treatment. Because a sizable portion of patients with nephrotic disease have combined hyperlipidemia, the question of combined therapy arises. An effective drug combination is an HMG-CoA (hydroxy-methyl-glutaryl coenzyme A) reductase inhibitor and a fibric acid. However, the combination increases the risk for myopathy in patients without nephrotic syndrome and never has been tested specifically in nephrotic patients. Therefore, combination therapy should not be used in patients with the nephrotic syndrome.

Treatment for Hypercholesterolemia in Chronic Kidney Disease, Hemodialysis, and CAPD Patients

If after 3 months of TLC LDL cholesterol is more than 100 mg/dL (2.6 mmol/L), treatment with a statin should be initiated. If the LDL cholesterol goal is not achieved after 6 weeks of treatment, the dose of the statin should stepwise be increased and a lipid profile should be repeated after another 6 weeks. If the LDL cholesterol goal is not achieved with TLC and optimal treatment with a statin, additional measures should be considered.

Statins are the most effective drugs for lowering LDL cholesterol in patients undergoing hemodialysis (196,197, 227) and generally should be the first agents of choice. If LDL cholesterol is still more than 100 mg/dL (2.6 mmol/L) despite optimal treatment with a statin and diet, additional LDL cholesterol–lowering drug classes and agents should be considered (228). Nicotinic acid and its derivatives lower LDL cholesterol by 5% to 25% but are likely to cause side effects such as flushing, hyperglycemia, upper-gastrointestinal distress, and hepatotoxicity (24). Studies investigating the effect of nicotinic acid in patients undergoing hemodialysis are sparse (229–231). Bile acid sequestrants lower LDL cholesterol by 15% to 30%. They cause gastrointestinal distress and constipation when not taken with considerable amounts of fluids. They are contraindicated in dysbetalipoproteinemias including triglycerides higher than 180 mg/dL (2 mmol/L) (24) and are likely to further plasma triglycerides further. Therefore, nicotinic acid and bile acid sequestrants are not preferred treatments in patients undergoing hemodialysis. Sevelamer hydrochloride, a non-absorbed hydrogel of cross-linked polyallylamine hydrochloride, is available as a phosphate binder. Short-term favorable effects on the lipid profile have been observed, with a 20% to 30% decrease in LDL cholesterol, a 5% to 18% increase in HDL cholesterol, and no change in triglyceride concentrations, presumably related to the binding of bile acids by the compound (232–234). Liver function tests should be done at 6-week intervals. Monitoring of serum creatine kinase is mandatory only if muscle symptoms develop. Without a baseline serum value, creatine kinase values are not always conclusive in patients undergoing dialysis, so myopathy may be diagnosed clinically before laboratory assessment. The dosage of statins is usually the same as in the normal population.

Treatment for Hypertriglyceridemia in Chronic Kidney Disease, Hemodialysis, and CAPD Patients

Patients with triglycerides of more than 180 to 499 mg/dL (2.0 to 5.7 mmol/L) after 3 months of TLC should be treated with a statin to achieve a non-HDL cholesterol of less than 130 mg/dL. Patients with very high triglycerides (≥500 mg/dL) should be treated with a fibric-acid analogue with the dose adjusted according to renal function. In patients with triglycerides of more than 800 mg/dL (9 mmol/L) resistant to any intervention, the administration of fish oil and/or a changing to LMW heparin as anticoagulant during hemodialysis therapy should be considered. Aside from optimizing body weight and increased physical activity, drug therapy should be initiated to achieve non-HDL cholesterol goals. The finding that elevated triglycerides are an independent cardiovascular risk factor in some studies suggests that some triglyceride-rich lipoproteins are atherogenic (235,236). The latter are partially degraded VLDL, commonly called remnant lipoproteins. VLDL cholesterol can be a target of cholesterol-lowering therapy.

Adult treatment panel III identified the sum of LDL + VLDL cholesterol (termed non-HDL cholesterol, [total cholesterol − HDL cholesterol]) as a secondary target of therapy in patients with high triglycerides (180 to 499 mg/dL;2.0 to 5.7 mmol/L) (24). The goal for non-HDL cholesterol in patients with high triglycerides can be set at 30 mg/dL greater than that for LDL cholesterol on the premise that a VLDL cholesterol 30 mg/dL or less is normal. Therefore, the non-HDL goal should be less than 130 mg/dL (3.4 mmol/L). These target levels are more stringent and thus may have greater impact than the higher target levels suggested previously in patients undergoing hemodialysis (26,237). Non-HDL cholesterol has been demonstrated to remain one of the strongest predictors for intima media thickness in 897 patients undergoing hemodialysis as demonstrated by multivariate Cox regression analysis (238). Non-HDL cholesterol also has turned out to predict aortic atherosclerosis, determined by pulse-wave Doppler ultrasonography in a cohort of 205 patients undergoing hemodialysis (75). Therefore non-HDL cholesterol is an independent factor affecting arterial-wall thickening (intima media thickness) and stiffness (pulse-wave velocity) (75,238). Fibric-acid analogues are effective in lowering serum triglycerides and raising HDL cholesterol. The most common adverse effects of drug therapy are myositis and rhabdomyolysis (239). These adverse effects, however, can be minimized by adjusting the dose of the drugs according to the degree of renal function (240,241). Gemfibrozil, a fibric-acid analogue, is well tolerated, and the parent drug does not exhibit a tendency for accumulation and toxicity. Gemfibrozil has been shown to reduce cardiovascular mortality in the Veterans Affairs High-Density Lipoprotein Cholesterol Intervention Trial study, a large-scale secondary prevention study, by reducing triglycerides and increasing HDL cholesterol without affecting LDL cholesterol (242). However, gemfibrozil is not available in all countries or, by regulation in these countries, it is contraindicated in chronic renal insufficiency or if serum creatinine is more than 6 mg/dL and/or creatinine clearance is less than 15 mL/min. Although the third Adult Treatment Panel (ATP III) listed severe renal disease among the absolute contraindications for the use of fibric acids (24) the advice of this author is, based on several reports from the literature (243–245) together with several other investigators, that gemfibrozil can be administered safely in a dose of 600 mg/day. A pronounced lengthening of the plasma decay of fenofibric acid was observed in both hemodialysis and peritoneal dialysis patients. Fenofibrate therefore should be used with great caution, if at all, in dialysis patients (246).

The ATP III report does not specify a goal for increasing HDL but concedes that treatment of patients with isolated low HDL (<40 mg/dL, 1.0 mmol/L) is reserved for people with coronary heart disease risk equivalents (24). Low HDL cholesterol is a strong independent predictor of cardiovascular disease (247). Interesting new data demonstrate that HDL in an inflammatory milieu may change to a proinflammatory molecule (248) lacking effects that protect LDL from being oxidized (249,250). Similar findings were observed in patients undergoing hemodialysis (251). Apolipoprotein A-I, the major structural protein in HDL, exists in its free form in serum (252,253). Clearly, HDL composition and HDL antioxidant capacity are altered in patients undergoing hemodialysis (254). Although clinical trial results suggest that increasing HDL will reduce risk, the evidence is insufficient to specify a goal of therapy in the renal population. Therefore, the present working group felt that more research is needed on HDL and inflammation before recommendations for increasing HDL can be given.

Eicosapentanoic acid reduces plasma lipids (255–258) and remnant lipoproteins and prevents *in vivo* peroxidation of LDL in maintenance dialysis patients (207). Only one study of this question received negative results. More importantly, n-3 fatty acids from fish oil do not introduce a clinically important risk of bleeding, although doubling of bleeding time is apparent (259). Adjuvant therapy using LMW heparin for anticoagulation during hemodialysis or the use of polysulfone or polyamide high-flux dialysis has been shown to ameliorate hypertriglyceridemia in some but not all patients (260–263). Treatment of renal anemia with erythropoietin in patients undergoing hemodialysis lowered serum total cholesterol and triglycerides (264).

Combining a fibric-acid analogue with a statin should be avoided because of the high risk of rhabdomyolysis. Statins are effective and safe drugs to reduce LDL cholesterol (196,197) and are the agents of first choice. Myositis may occur in rare cases, particularly when high doses and/or combination therapy (statin and fibric-acid analogues) are used. There are no studies in patients undergoing hemodialysis on the safety and efficacy of combination therapy.

Treatment Options for Elevated Lp(a)

Other than hormonal therapies, such as adrenocorticotropic hormone (265,266), D-thyroxine (267), and nandrolone (186), no effective treatments to reduce plasma Lp(a) in patients undergoing hemodialysis treatment or in the general population are currently available. Two small studies described a reduction in plasma Lp(a) with the use of nicotinic acid in patients undergoing hemodialysis (230,231). Consequently, there are no large-scale interventional trials available investigating the effects of such treatments on cardiovascular disease in these patients. The use of anabolic steroids raises the hematocrit but is also associated with the development of dyslipidemia. The overall effect on the cardiovascular system in subjects with normal kidney function is not beneficial, although plasma Lp(a) concentrations may be lowered.

Treatment by Extracorporeal LDL Cholesterol Removal

LDL apheresis is a treatment modality for the secondary prevention of coronary events and may be considered after organ transplantation in situations when primary or secondary hyperlipidemias fail to respond to maximal drug therapy or a switch in immunosuppressive drugs. Because Lp(a) appears to have adverse biologic consequences in patients with renal failure (268) or patients under immunosuppression, and Lp(a) can be removed effectively, this therapy may be useful for selected patients with documented progressive vascular disease.

Treatment of Patients After Kidney Transplantation

Statins have been proven to effectively lower serum total and LDL cholesterol concentrations in renal transplant recipients. They are the drugs of choice in patients requiring lipid-lowering treatment. Cardiovascular complications are currently the most frequent causes of death among renal transplant recipients, and chronic rejection is the most important cause of long-term allograft loss. Vascular lesions seen in chronic rejection and those that characterize systemic atherosclerosis share similarities. Although evidence from prospective controlled interventional studies is lacking for prevention of cardiovascular complications, it is reasonable to adopt the recommendations of the joint European societies on prevention of coronary heart disease (25,26) or the NCEP ATP-III guidelines (24). These guidelines also can be used for initial classification, risk-factor assessment, and treatment initiation and to approach the target cholesterol level when drug therapy is considered. It is likely that effective control of serum lipids and lipoproteins may achieve a similar beneficial reduction in absolute mortality in renal transplant recipients as has already been demonstrated in individuals without kidney disease.

Almost all patients under immunosuppression after kidney transplantation exceed an absolute coronary artery disease risk of 20% over 10 years. They are considered to be in the highest risk group for developing a premature cardiovascular event with an even higher prevalence of lipid abnormalities. Although no event has taken place in most patients at the time of transplantation and shortly thereafter, so-called primary prevention is not routinely administered to patients. However, terms such as "primary prevention" are no longer appropriate because the cumulative incidence of coronary risk factors usually exceeds those that can be assessed by coronary risk charts. In addition, endothelial-dependent vasodilation is impaired in nearly all patients; this justifies using the target cholesterol levels that are valid for patients treated for the secondary prevention of cardiovascular disease. Guidelines suggest that in the presence of further risk factors for cardiovascular disease (endothelial dysfunction is already one) factor LDL cholesterol levels of more than 100 mg/dL (2.7 mmol/L) are a treatment initiation threshold for drug therapy. In the absence of risk factors, an LDL cholesterol level up to 130 mg/dL may be acceptable.

Therefore patients with a renal transplant are definitively considered as a high-risk population when lipid-lowering pharmacologic intervention is considered. When treatment options are evaluated with caution, most of the lipid-lowering drugs are safe and effective. Drug treatment is necessary in a considerable number of patients to control lipid disorders because dyslipidemia in renal transplant recipients is not particularly responsive to modification of dietary fat.

Cholesterol Reduction, Statins, and the Cytochrome P-450 System

Statins are the most effective drugs for reducing total and LDL cholesterol levels in transplant recipients and generally should be the first choice among pharmacologic agents in patients requiring treatment for hypercholesterolemia. The hydrophilic statins, such as pravastatin and fluvastatin, should be distinguished from the lipophilic agents, lovastatin and simvastatin, with regard to toxicity and active metabolite accumulation (269). Furthermore, lovastatin, simvastatin, and the synthetic statin atorvastatin are metabolized by cytochrome P-450 3A4 (CYP3A4). Because myositis, rhabdomyolysis, or other complications may occur, maximal doses of drugs in the latter group should be avoided, whereas pravastatin and fluvastatin have been administered at high doses over prolonged periods without adverse effects. The ALERT study has randomized more than 2,000 patients after kidney transplantation to either fluvastatin or placebo. Recently fluvastatin, metabolized mainly via CYP2C9, was increased to 80 mg/day without adverse effects in patients who have not met target cholesterol levels. In respect to effects of statins on HDL cholesterol, no recommendation has been given yet.

However, drug–drug interactions are not necessarily always deleterious. Drugs with the potential to produce interactions mediated by CYP3A4 include the calcium channel blocker diltiazem, which is used to save costs by cyclosporine immunosuppression. It has been argued that activation of the CYP3A4 enzyme pathway—for example, by a glass of grapefruit juice at breakfast—will lead to further reductions in cholesterol and coronary heart disease (269). Such potential interactions should be taken in mind, and a careful approach is mandatory to avoid harmful side effects to the patients.

Use of Statins to Maintain Kidney Transplants

Two randomized controlled clinical trials have demonstrated that statins reduced the severity of angiographic coronary artery disease and improved patient survival following cardiac transplantation (270,271). If the pathogenesis of allograft vasculopathy in renal and cardiac transplant recipients is similar, statins may hold promise for preventing and/or treating chronic renal allograft rejection as well. However, the mechanism whereby statins improve survival in heart transplant recipients is still not entirely clear. It is possible that statins have a direct, immunosuppressive effect. If so, the effect may require the presence of cyclosporine because there is no evidence that statins are immunosuppressive in normal individuals. Alternatively, the reduction in lipids caused by statins may increase the immunosuppressive effect of cyclosporine. At present, the best therapeutic approach for chronic rejection ultimately may be a combination therapy of lipid lowering and appropriate immunosuppression (271,272).

Lipid Lowering with Fibrates After Kidney Transplantation

In the few patients in whom hypertriglyceridemia and low HDL cholesterol are the leading lipid abnormalities, fibric-acid derivatives are appropriate. Combination therapy should not be administered in high doses of the various medicines.

REFERENCES

1. Kronenberg F, Steinmetz A, Kostner GM, et al. Lipoprotein(a) in health and disease. *Crit Rev Clin Lab Sci* 1996;33:495–543.
2. Joven J, Villabona C, Vilella E, et al. Abnormalities of lipoprotein metabolism in patients with the nephrotic syndrome. *N Engl J Med* 1990;323:579–584.
3. Ohta T, Matsuda I. Lipid and apolipoprotein levels in patients with nephrotic syndrome. *Clin Chim Acta* 1981;117:133–143.
4. Gherardi E, Rota E, Calandra S, et al. Relationship among the concentrations of serum lipoproteins and changes in their chemical composition in patients with untreated nephrotic syndrome. *Eur J Clin Invest* 1977;7:563–570.
5. Krämer-Guth A, Nauck M, Pavenstädt H, et al. Preferential uptake of intermediate-density lipoproteins from nephrotic patients by human mesangial and liver cells. *J Am Soc Nephrol* 1994;5:1081–1090.
6. Krämer A, Nauck M, Pavenstädt H, et al. Receptor-mediated uptake of IDL and LDL from nephrotic patients by glomerular epithelial cells. *Kidney Int* 1993;44:1341–1351.
7. Short CD, Durrington PN, Mallick NP, et al. Serum and urinary high-density lipoproteins in glomerular disease with proteinuria. *Kidney Int* 1986;29:1224–1228.
8. Appel GB, Blum CB, Chien S, et al. The hyperlipidemia of the nephrotic syndrome. *N Engl J Med* 1985;312:1544–1548.
9. Jüngst D, Caselmann WH, Kutschera P, et al. Relation of hyperlipidemia in serum and loss of high density lipoproteins in urine in the nephrotic syndrome. *Clin Chim Acta* 1987;168:159–167.
10. Joven J, Villabona C, Viletta E. Pattern of hyperlipoproteinemia in human nephrotic syndrome: Influence of renal failure and diabetes mellitus. *Nephron* 1993;64:565–569.
11. Karadi I, Romics L, Palos G, et al. Lp(a) lipoprotein concentration in serum of patients with heavy proteinuria of different origin. *Clin Chem* 1989;35:2121–2123.
12. Thomas ME, Freestone A, Varghese Z, et al. Lipoprotein(a) in patients with proteinuria. *Nephrol Dial Transplant* 1992;7: 597–601.
13. Stenvinkel P, Berglund L, Heimbürger O, et al. Lipoprotein (a) in nephrotic syndrome. *Kidney Int* 1993;44:1116–1123.
14. Wanner C, Rader D, Bartens W, et al. Elevated plasma lipoprotein(a) in patients with the nephrotic syndrome. *Ann Intern Med* 1993;119:263–269.
15. Kronenberg F, Trenkwalder E, Lingenhel A, et al. Renovascular arteriovenous differences in Lp[a] plasma concentrations suggest removal of Lp[a] from the renal circulation. *J Lipid Res* 1997; 38:1755–1763.
16. de Sain-van der Velden MG, Kaysen GA, Barrett HA, et al. Increased VLDL in nephrotic patients results from a decreased catabolism while increased LDL results from increased synthesis. *Kidney Int* 1998;53:994–1001.
17. Kaysen GA, Pan X-M, Couser WG, et al. Defective lipolysis persists in hearts of rats with Heymann nephritis in the absence of nephrotic plasma. *Am J Kidney Dis* 1993;22:128–134.
18. Davies RW, Staprans I, Hutchison FN, et al. Proteinuria, not altered albumin metabolism, affects hyperlipidemia in the nephrotic rat. *J Clin Invest* 1990;86:600–605.
19. Shearer GC, Kaysen GA. Proteinuria and plasma compositional changes contribute to defective lipoprotein catabolism in the nephrotic syndrome by separate mechanisms. *Kidney Int* 2001; 37(Suppl 2):S119–S122.
20. Samuelsson O, Attmann PO, Knight-Gibson C, et al. Lipoprotein abnormalities without hyperlipidemia in moderate renal insufficiency. *Nephrol Dial Transplant* 1991;9:1580–1585.
21. Attmann PO, Alaupovic P. Lipid and apolipoprotein profiles of uremic dyslipoproteinemia—Relation to renal function and dialysis. *Nephron* 1991;57:401–410.
22. Grützmacher P, März W, Peschke B, et al. Lipoproteins and apolipoproteins during the progression of chronic renal disease. *Nephron* 1988;50:103–111.
23. Warick GL, Fox JG, Boulton-Jones JM. The relationship between urinary albumin excretion rate and serum cholesterol in primary glomerular disease. *Clin Nephrol* 1994;41:135–137.
24. Executive Summary of the Third Report of the National Cholesterol Education Program (NCEP) Expert Panel on Detection, Evaluation, and Treatment of High Blood Cholesterol in Adults (Adult Treatment Panel III). *JAMA* 2001;285:2486–2497.
25. Wood D, De Backer G, Faergeman O, et al. and members of the Second Joint Task Force of European and other Societies on Coronary Prevention. Prevention of coronary heart disease in clinical practice. *Eur Heart J* 1998;19:1434–1503.
26. Pyorala K, Wood D. Prevention of coronary heart disease in clinical practice. European recommendations revised and reinforced. *Eur Heart J* 1998;19:1413–1415.
27. Farias MA, McClellan W, Soucie JM, et al. A prospective comparison of methods for determining if cardiovascular disease is a predictor of mortality in dialysis patients. *Am J Kidney Dis* 1994;23:382–388.
28. Kasiske BL. Hyperlipidemia in patients with chronic renal disease. *Am J Kidney Dis* 1998;32:S142–S156.
29. Brunzell JD, Albers JJ, Haas LB, et al. Prevalence of serum lipid abnormalities in chronic hemodialysis. *Metabolism* 1977;26: 903–910.
30. Pedro BJ, Senti M, Rubies PJ, et al. When to treat dyslipidaemia of patients with chronic renal failure on haemodialysis? A need to define specific guidelines [see comments]. *Nephrol Dial Transplant* 1996;11:308–313.
31. Lacour B, Roullet JB, Beyne P, et al. Comparison of several atherogenicity indices by the analysis of serum lipoprotein composition in patients with chronic renal failure with or without haemodialysis, and in renal transplant patients. *J Clin Chem Clin Biochem* 1985;23:805–810.
32. Cheung AK, Wu LL, Kablitz C, et al. Atherogenic lipids and lipoproteins in hemodialysis patients. *Am J Kidney Dis* 1993; 22:271–276.
33. Rapoport J, Aviram M, Chaimovitz C, et al. Defective high-density lipoprotein composition in patients on chronic hemodialysis. A possible mechanism for accelerated atherosclerosis. *N Engl J Med* 1978;299:1326–1329.
34. Rubies-Prat J, Espinel E, Joven J, et al. High-density lipoprotein cholesterol subfractions in chronic uremia. *Am J Kidney Dis* 1987;9:60–65.
35. Atger V, Duval F, Frommherz K, et al. Anomalies in composition of uremic lipoproteins isolated by gradient ultracentrifugation: relative enrichment of HDL in apolipoprotein C-III at the expense of apolipoprotein A-I. *Atherosclerosis* 1988;74:75–83.
36. Joven J, Rubies-Prat J, Espinel E, et al. Apoprotein A-I and

high density lipoprotein subfractions in patients with chronic renal failure receiving hemodialysis. *Nephron* 1985;40: 451–454.
37. Parsy D, Dracon M, Cachera C, et al. Lipoprotein abnormalities in chronic haemodialysis patients. *Nephrol Dial Transplant* 1988;3:51–56.
38. Senti M, Romero R, Pedro BJ, et al. Lipoprotein abnormalities in hyperlipidemic and normolipidemic men on hemodialysis with chronic renal failure. *Kidney Int* 1992;41:1394–1399.
39. Joven J, Vilella E, Ahmad S, et al. Lipoprotein heterogeneity in end-stage renal disease. *Kidney Int* 1993;43:410–418.
40. Attman PO, Alaupovic P. Lipid and apolipoprotein profiles of uremic dyslipoproteinemia—relation to renal function and dialysis. *Nephron* 1991;57:401–410.
41. Oi K, Hirano T, Sakai S, et al. Role of hepatic lipase in intermediate-density lipoprotein and small, dense low-density lipoprotein formation in hemodialysis patients. *Kidney Int* 1999;56 Suppl 71:S227–S228.
42. Attman PO, Samuelsson O, Alaupovic P. Lipoprotein metabolism and renal failure. *Am J Kidney Dis* 1993;21:573–592.
43. Oda H, Keane WF. Lipid abnormalities in end stage renal disease. *Nephrol Dial Transplant* 1998;13 Suppl 1:45–49.
44. Deighan CJ, Caslake MJ, McConnell M, et al. Atherogenic lipoprotein phenotype in end-stage renal failure: origin and extent of small dense low-density lipoprotein formation. *Am J Kidney Dis* 2000;35:852–862.
45. Quaschning T, Schomig M, Keller M, et al. Non-insulin-dependent diabetes mellitus and hypertriglyceridemia impair lipoprotein metabolism in chronic hemodialysis patients. *J Am Soc Nephrol* 1999;10:332–341.
46. Rajman I, Harper L, McPake D, et al. Low-density lipoprotein subfraction profiles in chronic renal failure. *Nephrol Dial Transplant* 1998;13:2281–2287.
47. O'Neal D, Lee P, Murphy B, et al. Low-density lipoprotein particle size distribution in end-stage renal disease treated with hemodialysis or peritoneal dialysis. *Am J Kidney Dis* 1996;27: 84–91.
48. Ambrosch A, Domroese U, Westphal S, et al. Compositional and functional changes of low-density lipoprotein during hemodialysis in patients with ESRD. *Kidney Int* 1998;54:608–617.
49. Attman PO, Samuelsson OG, Moberly J, et al. Apolipoprotein B-containing lipoproteins in renal failure: the relation to mode of dialysis. *Kidney Int* 1999;55:1536–1542.
50. Wakabayashi Y, Okubo M, Shimada H, et al. Decreased VLDL apoprotein CII/apoprotein CIII ratio may be seen in both normotriglyceridemic and hypertriglyceridemic patients on chronic hemodialysis treatment. *Metabolism* 1987;36:815–820.
51. Kandoussi AM, Hugue V, Parra HJ, et al. Apolipoprotein AI and apolipoprotein B containing particle analysis in normolipidemic hemodialyzed patients: evidence of free apolipoprotein E. *Am J Nephrol* 1996;16:287–292.
52. Weintraub M, Burstein A, Rassin T, et al. Severe defect in clearing postprandial chylomicron remnants in dialysis patients. *Kidney Int* 1992;42:1247–1252.
53. Stampfer MJ, Krauss RM, Ma J, et al. A prospective study of triglyceride level, low-density lipoprotein particle diameter, and risk of myocardial infarction. *JAMA* 1996;276:882–888.
54. Gardner CD, Fortmann SP, Krauss RM. Association of small low-density lipoprotein particles with the incidence of coronary artery disease in men and women. *JAMA* 1996;276:875–881.
55. Griffin BA, Freeman DJ, Tait GW, et al. Role of plasma triglyceride in the regulation of plasma low density lipoprotein (LDL) subfractions: relative contribution of small, dense LDL to coronary heart disease risk. *Atherosclerosis* 1994;106:241–253.
56. Foley RN, Parfrey PS, Sarnak MJ. Clinical epidemiology of cardiovascular disease in chronic renal disease. *Am J Kidney Dis* 1998;32:S112–S119.
57. Austin MA, Mykkanen L, Kuusisto J, et al. Prospective study of small LDLs as a risk factor for non-insulin dependent diabetes mellitus in elderly men and women. *Circulation* 1995;92: 1770–1778.
58. Austin MA, King MC, Vranizan KM, et al. Atherogenic lipoprotein phenotype. A proposed genetic marker for coronary heart disease risk. *Circulation* 1990;82:495–506.
59. Hulthe J, Bokemark L, Wikstrand J, et al. The metabolic syndrome, LDL particle size, and atherosclerosis: the Atherosclerosis and Insulin Resistance (AIR) study. *Arterioscler Thromb Vasc Biol* 2000;20:2140–2147.
60. Arnadottir M, Thysell H, Dallongeville J, et al. Evidence that reduced lipoprotein lipase activity is not a primary pathogenetic factor for hypertriglyceridemia in renal failure. *Kidney Int* 1995; 48:779–784.
61. Applebaum-Bowden D, Goldberg AP, Hazzard WR, et al. Postheparin plasma triglyceride lipases in chronic hemodialysis: evidence for a role for hepatic lipase in lipoprotein metabolism. *Metabolism* 1979;28:917–924.
62. Lucchi L, Banni S, Botti B, et al. Conjugated diene fatty acids in patients with chronic renal failure: evidence of increased lipid peroxidation? *Nephron* 1993;65:401–409.
63. Schettler V, Wieland E, Verwiebe R, et al. Plasma lipids are not oxidized during hemodialysis. *Nephron* 1994;67:42–47.
64. Hsia SL, Perez GO, Mendez AJ, et al. Defect in cholesterol transport in patients receiving maintenance hemodialysis. *J Lab Clin Med* 1985;106:53–61.
65. Bories PC, Subbaiah PV, Bagdade JD. Lecithin: cholesterol acyltransferase activity in dialyzed and undialyzed chronic uremic patients. *Nephron* 1982;32:22–27.
66. Jung K, Neumann R, Precht K, et al. Lecithin: cholesterol acyltransferase activity, HDL-cholesterol and apolipoprotein A in serum of patients undergoing chronic haemodialysis. *Enzyme* 1980;25:273–275.
67. Mendez AJ, Perez GO, Hsia SL. Defect in cholesteryl ester transport in serum of patients with uremia receiving maintenance hemodialysis: increased inhibitor activity for cholesteryl ester transfer. *J Lab Clin Med* 1988;111:677–683.
68. Horkko S, Huttunen K, Kesaniemi YA. Decreased clearance of low-density lipoprotein in uremic patients under dialysis treatment. *Kidney Int* 1995;47:1732–1740.
69. Nigon F, Lesnik P, Rouis M, et al. Discrete subspecies of human low density lipoproteins are heterogeneous in their interaction with the cellular LDL receptor. *J Lipid Res* 1991;32:1741–1753.
70. de Graaf J, Hak-Lemmers HL, Hectors MP, et al. Enhanced susceptibility to in vitro oxidation of the dense low density lipoprotein subfraction in healthy subjects. *Arterioscler Thromb* 1991;11:298–306.
71. Packard CJ, Shepherd J. Lipoprotein heterogeneity and apolipoprotein B metabolism. *Arterioscler Thromb Vasc Biol* 1997;17: 3542–3556.
72. Anber V, Griffin BA, McConnell M, et al. Influence of plasma lipid and LDL-subfraction profile on the interaction between low density lipoprotein with human arterial wall proteoglycans. *Atherosclerosis* 1996;124:261–271.
73. Oda H, Yorioka N, Okushin S, et al. Remnant-like particle cholesterol may indicate atherogenic risk in patients on chronic hemodialysis. *Nephron* 1997;76:7–14.
74. Nestel PJ, Fidge NH, Tan MH. Increased lipoprotein-remnant formation in chronic renal failure. *N Engl J Med* 1982;307: 329–333.
75. Shoji T, Nishizawa Y, Kawagishi T, et al. Intermediate-density lipoprotein as an independent risk factor for aortic atherosclero-

sis in hemodialysis patients. *J Am Soc Nephrol* 1998;9: 1277–1284.
76. Nishizawa Y, Shoji T, Emoto M, et al. Reduction of intermediate density lipoprotein by pravastatin in hemo- and peritoneal dialysis patients. *Clin Nephrol* 1995;43:268–277.
77. Daerr WH, Windler ET, Greten H. Peroxidative modification of very-low-density lipoproteins in chronic hemodialysis patients [letter]. *Nephron* 1993;63:230–231.
78. McEneny J, Loughrey CM, McNamee PT, et al. Susceptibility of VLDL to oxidation in patients on regular haemodialysis. *Atherosclerosis* 1997;129:215–220.
79. Lindholm B, Norbeck HE. Serum lipids and lipoproteins during continuous ambulatory peritoneal dialysis. *Acta Med Scand* 1986;220:143–151.
80. Thomas ME, Moorhead JF. Lipids in CAPD: A review. *Contrib Nephrol* 1990;85:92–99.
81. Sniderman A, Cianflone K, Kwiterovich PO Jr, et al. Hyperapobetalipoproteinemia: The major dyslipoproteinemia in patients with chronic renal failure treated with chronic ambulatory peritoneal dialysis. *Atherosclerosis* 1987;65:257–264.
82. Ramos JM, Heaton A, McGurk JG, et al. Sequential changes in serum lipids and their subfractions in patients receiving continuous ambulatory peritoneal dialysis. *Nephron* 1983;35: 20–23.
83. Roncari DAK, Breckenridge WC, Khanna R, et al. Rise in high-density lipoprotein cholesterol in some patients treated with CAPD. *Perit Dial Bull* 1988;1:136–141.
84. Boeschoten EW, Zuyderhoudt FMJ, Krediet RT, et al. Changes in weight and lipid concentrations during CAPD treatment. *Perit Dial Bull* 1988;19:8–13.
85. Morrison G. Metabolic effects of continuous ambulatory peritoneal dialysis. *Ann Rev Med* 1989;40:163–172.
86. Saku K, Sasaki J, Naito S, et al. Lipoprotein and apolipoprotein losses during continuous ambulatory peritoneal dialysis. *Nephron* 1989;51:220–224.
87. Lameire N, Matthys D, Matthys E, et al. Effect of long-term CAPD on carbohydrate and lipid metabolism. *Clin Nephrol* 1988;30:S53–S58.
88. Breckenridge WC, Roncari DAK, Khanna R, et al. The influence of continuous ambulatory peritoneal dialysis on plasma lipoproteins. *Atherosclerosis* 1992;45:249–258.
89. Haas LB, Wahl PW, Sherrard DJ. A longitudinal study of lipid abnormalities in renal failure. *Nephron* 1983;33:145–159.
90. Dieplinger H, Schoenfeld PY, Fielding CJ. Plasma cholesterol metabolism in end-stage renal disease. *J Clin Invest* 1986;77: 1071–1083.
91. Shoji T, Nishizawa Y, Nishitani H, et al. High serum lipoprotein(a) concentration in uremic patients treated with continuous ambulatory peritoneal dialysis. *Clin Nephrol* 1992;38:271–276.
92. Anwar N, Bhatnager D, Short CD, et al. Serum lipoprotein(a) concentrations in patients undergoing continuous ambulatory peritoneal dialysis. *Nephrol Dial Transplant* 1993;8:71–74.
93. Webb AT, Reaveley DA, O'Donnell M, et al. Lipoprotein(a) in patients on maintenance haemodialysis and continuous ambulatory peritoneal dialysis. *Nephrol Dial Transplant* 1993;8: 609–613.
94. Taylor DO, Barr ML, Radovanovic B, et al. A randomized multicenter comparison of tacrolimus and cyclosporine immunosuppressive regimens in cardiac transplantation: decreased hyperlipidemia and hypertension with tacrolimus. *J Heart Lung Transplant* 1999;18:335–345.
95. Kasiske BL. Risk factors for accelerated atherosclerosis in renal transplant recipients. *Am J Med* 1988,84:985–992.
96. Raine AEG. Hypertension and ischaemic heart disease in renal transplant recipients. *Nephrol Dial Transplant* 1995;10(Suppl 1):95–100.
97. Heule H, Keusch G, Uhlschmid G, et al. Kardiovaskuläre Krankheiten nach Nierentransplantation: eine Analyse prädisponierender Faktoren. *Schweiz Med Wochenschr* 1981;111:709–716.
98. Vathsala A, Weinberg RB, Schoenberg L, et al. Lipid abnormalities in cyclosporine-prednisolone-treated renal transplant recipients. *Transplantation* 1989;48:37–43.
99. Abdulmassih Z, Chevalier A, Bader C, et al. Role of lipid disturbances in the atherosclerosis of renal transplant patients. *Clin Transplant* 1992;6:106–113.
100. Massy ZA, Chadefaux-Vekemans B, Chevalier A, et al. Hyperhomocysteinaemia: a significant risk factor for cardiovascular disease in renal transplant recipients. *Nephrol Dial Transplant* 1994;9:1103–1108.
101. Quaschning T, Mainka T, Nauck M, et al. Immunosuppression enhances atherogenicity of lipid profile after transplantation. *Kidney Int* 1999;56(Suppl 71):S235–S237.
102. Causes of death. USRDS. United States Renal Data System. *Am J Kidney Dis* 1997;30:S107–S117.
103. The USRDS Dialysis Morbidity and Mortality Study: Wave 2. United States Renal Data System. *Am J Kidney Dis* 1997;30: S67–S85.
104. Herzog CA, Ma JZ, Collins AJ. Poor long-term survival after acute myocardial infarction among patients on long-term dialysis [see comments]. *N Engl J Med* 1998;339:799–805.
105. Chantrel F, Enache I, Bouiller M, et al. Abysmal prognosis of patients with type 2 diabetes entering dialysis [see comments]. *Nephrol Dial Transplant* 1999;14:129–136.
106. Foley RN, Parfrey PS, Sarnak MJ. Clinical epidemiology of cardiovascular disease in chronic renal disease. *Am J Kidney Dis* 1998;32:S112–S119.
107. Parfrey PS, Foley RN. The clinical epidemiology of cardiac disease in chronic renal failure. *J Am Soc Nephrol* 1999;10: 1606–1615.
108. Berlyne GM, Mallick NP. Ischemic heart disease as a complication of nephrotic syndrome. *Lancet* 1969;2:399–400.
109. Curry RC, Roberts WC. Status of the coronary arteries in the nephrotic syndrome. *Am J Med* 1977;63:183–192.
110. Wass V, Cameron JS. Cardiovascular disease and the nephrotic syndrome: The other side of the coin. *Nephron* 1981;27:58–61.
111. Ordonez JD, Hiatt R, Killebraw E, et al. The increased risk of coronary heart disease associated with nephrotic syndrome. *Kidney Int* 1993;44(3):638–642.
112. Thomas ME, Harris KPG, Ramaswamy C, et al. Simvastatin therapy of hypercholesterolemic patients with nephrotic syndrome of significant proteinuria. *Kidney Int* 1993;44: 1124–1129.
113. Hahn R, Oette K, Mondorf H, et al. Analysis of cardiovascular risk factors in chronic hemodialysis patients with special attention to the hyperlipoproteinemias. *Atherosclerosis* 1983;48: 279–288.
114. Avram MM, Fein PA, Antignani A, et al. Cholesterol and lipid disturbances in renal disease: the natural history of uremic dyslipidemia and the impact of hemodialysis and continuous ambulatory peritoneal dialysis. *Am J Med* 1989;87:55N–60N.
115. Attman PO. Hyperlipoproteinaemia in renal failure: pathogenesis and perspectives for intervention. *Nephrol Dial Transplant* 1993;8:294–295.
116. Ponticelli C, Barbi G, Cantaluppi A, et al. Lipid abnormalities in maintenance dialysis patients and renal transplant recipients. *Kidney Int* 1978;13:72–78.
117. D'Elia JA, Weinrauch LA, Gleason RE, et al. Preliminary screening of the relationship of serum lipids to survival of chronic dialysis patients. *Ren Fail* 1993;15:203–209.
118. Kimura K, Saika Y, Otani H, et al. Factors associated with calcification of the abdominal aorta in hemodialysis patients. *Kidney Int* 1999;56 Suppl 71:S238–S241.

119. Ma KW, Greene EL, Raij L. Cardiovascular risk factors in chronic renal failure and hemodialysis populations. *Am J Kidney Dis* 1992;19:505–513.
120. Kates DM, Haas L, Brunzell J, et al. Risk factors for cardiovascular disease in end-stage renal failure patients: A 21 year study. *J Am Soc Nephrol* 1995 (abstract).
121. Tschope W, Koch M, Thomas B, et al. Serum lipids predict cardiac death in diabetic patients on maintenance hemodialysis. Results of a prospective study. The German Study Group Diabetes and Uremia. *Nephron* 1993;64:354–358.
122. Lapuz M, Avram MM, Lustig A, et al. Fall of cholesterol with time on dialysis: impact on atherogenicity. *ASAIO Trans* 1989; 35:258–260.
123. Zimmermann J, Herrlinger S, Pruy A, et al. Inflammation enhances cardiovascular risk and mortality in hemodialysis patients. *Kidney Int* 1999;55:648–658.
124. Lowrie EG, Lew NL. Death risk in hemodialysis patients: the predictive value of commonly measured variables and an evaluation of death rate differences between facilities. *Am J Kidney Dis* 1990;15:458–482.
125. Degoulet P, Legrain M, Reach I, et al. Mortality risk factors in patients treated by chronic hemodialysis. Report of the Diaphane collaborative study. *Nephron* 1982;31:103–110.
126. Corti MC, Guralnik JM, Salive ME, et al. Clarifying the direct relation between total cholesterol levels and death from coronary heart disease in older persons. *Ann Intern Med* 1997;126: 753–760.
127. Ritz E. Why are lipids not predictive of cardiovascular death in the dialysis patient? *Miner Electrolyte Metab* 1996;22:9–12.
128. Baigent C, Burbury K, Wheeler D. Premature cardiovascular disease in chronic renal failure. *Lancet* 2000;356:147–152.
129. Dieplinger H, Lackner C, Kronenberg F, et al. Elevated plasma concentrations of lipoprotein(a) in patients with end-stage renal disease are not related to the size polymorphism of apolipoprotein(a). *J Clin Invest* 1993;91:397–401.
130. Irish AB, Simons LA, Savdie E, et al. Lipoprotein(a) levels in chronic renal disease states, dialysis and transplantation. *Aust N Z J Med* 1992;22:243–248.
131. Kronenberg F, Konig P, Neyer U, et al. Multicenter study of lipoprotein(a) and apolipoprotein(a) phenotypes in patients with end-stage renal disease treated by hemodialysis or continuous ambulatory peritoneal dialysis. *J Am Soc Nephrol* 1995;6: 110–120.
132. Hirata K, Kikuchi S, Saku K, et al. Apolipoprotein(a) phenotypes and serum lipoprotein(a) levels in maintenance hemodialysis patients with/without diabetes mellitus. *Kidney Int* 1993; 44:1062–1070.
133. Auguet T, Senti M, Rubies PJ, et al. Serum lipoprotein(a) concentration in patients with chronic renal failure receiving haemodialysis: influence of apolipoprotein (a) genetic polymorphism. *Nephrol Dial Transplant* 1993;8:1099–1103.
134. Fiorini F, Masturzo P, Mij M, et al. Lipoprotein(a) levels in hemodialysis patients: relation to glucose intolerance and hemodialysis duration. *Nephron* 1995;70:500–501.
135. Webb AT, Reaveley DA, O'Donnell M, et al. Lipoprotein (a) in patients on maintenance haemodialysis and continuous ambulatory peritoneal dialysis. *Nephrol Dial Transplant* 1993;8: 609–613.
136. Cressman MD, Heyka RJ, Paganini EP, et al. Lipoprotein(a) is an independent risk factor for cardiovascular disease in hemodialysis patients. *Circulation* 1992;86:475–482.
137. Docci D, Manzoni G, Bilancioni R, et al. Serum lipoprotein(a) and coronary artery disease in uremic patients on chronic hemodialysis. *Int J Artif Organs* 1994;17:41–45.
138. Koda Y, Nishi S, Suzuki M, et al. Lipoprotein(a) is a predictor for cardiovascular mortality of hemodialysis patients. *Kidney Int* 1999;56 Suppl 71:S251–S253.
139. Webb AT, Reaveley DA, O'Donnell M, et al. Lipids and lipoprotein(a) as risk factors for vascular disease in patients on renal replacement therapy. *Nephrol Dial Transplant* 1995;10: 354–357.
140. Docci D, Manzoni G, Baldrati L, et al. Serum lipoprotein(a) as an independent cardiovascular risk factor for patients undergoing chronic hemodialysis [letter]. *Nephron* 1995;69: 195.
141. del Cura J, Gil PA, Borque L, et al. Lipoprotein (a) in chronic renal failure patients undergoing hemodialysis: does it have an independent role in the development of further cardiovascular complications? [letter]. *Nephron* 1993;65:644–645.
142. Bachmann J, Tepel M, Raidt H, et al. Hyperhomocysteinemia and the risk for vascular disease in hemodialysis patients. *J Am Soc Nephrol* 1995;6:121–125.
143. Koch M, Kutkuhn B, Trenkwalder E, et al. Apolipoprotein B, fibrinogen, HDL cholesterol, and apolipoprotein(a) phenotypes predict coronary artery disease in hemodialysis patients. *J Am Soc Nephrol* 1997;8:1889–1898.
144. Koch M, Kutkuhn B, Grabensee B, et al. Apolipoprotein A, fibrinogen, age, and history of stroke are predictors of death in dialysed diabetic patients: a prospective study in 412 subjects. *Nephrol Dial Transplant* 1997;12:2603–2611.
145. Kronenberg F, Neyer U, Lhotta K, et al. The low molecular weight apo(a) phenotype is an independent predictor for coronary artery disease in hemodialysis patients: a prospective follow-up. *J Am Soc Nephrol* 1999;10:1027–1036.
146. Kronenberg F, Kathrein H, Konig P, et al. Apolipoprotein(a) phenotypes predict the risk for carotid atherosclerosis in patients with end-stage renal disease. *Arterioscler Thromb* 1994;14: 1405–1411.
147. Marcovina SM, Koschinsky ML. Lipoprotein(a) concentration and apolipoprotein(a) size: A synergistic role in advanced atherosclerosis? *Circulation* 1999;100:1151–1153.
148. Mooser V, Marcovina SM, Wang J, et al. High plasma levels of apo(a) fragments in Caucasians and African-Americans with end-stage renal disease: implications for plasma Lp(a) assay. *Clin Genet* 1997;52:387–392.
149. Trenkwalder E, Gruber A, Konig P, et al. Increased plasma concentrations of LDL-unbound apo(a) in patients with end-stage renal disease. *Kidney Int* 1997;52:1685–1692.
150. Kronenberg F, Trenkwalder E, Sturm W, et al. LDL-unbound apolipoprotein(a) and carotid atherosclerosis in hemodialysis patients. *Clin Genet* 1997;52:377–386.
151. Yang WS, Kim SB, Min WK, et al. Atherogenic lipid profile and lipoprotein(a) in relation to serum albumin in haemodialysis patients. *Nephrol Dial Transplant* 1995;10:1668–1671.
152. Kario K, Matsuo T, Kobayashi H, et al. High lipoprotein (a) levels in chronic hemodialysis patients are closely related to the acute phase reaction. *Thromb Haemost* 1995;74:1020–1024.
153. Wheeler DC. Cardiovascular disease in patients with chronic renal failure. *Lancet* 1996;348:1673–1674.
154. Grundy SM, Cleeman JI, Rifkind BM, et al. Cholesterol lowering in the elderly population. Coordinating Committee of the National Cholesterol Education Program. *Arch Intern Med* 1999;159:1670–1678.
155. Baigent C, Wheeler DC. Should we reduce blood cholesterol to prevent cardiovascular disease among patients with chronic renal failure? *Nephrol Dial Transplant* 2000;15:1118–1119.
156. Wheeler DC. Should hyperlipidaemia in dialysis patients be treated? *Nephrol Dial Transplant* 1997;12:19–21.
157. Schlöndorff D. Cellular mechanisms of lipid injury in the glomerulus. *Am J Kidney Dis* 1993;22:279–285.
158. Kasiske BL, O'Donnell MC, Cleary MP, et al. Treatment of

hyperlipidemia reduces glomerular injury in obese Zucker rats. *Kidney Int* 1988;33:667–672.
159. Harris KPG, Purkerson ML, Yates J, et al. Lovastatin ameliorates the development of glomerulosclerosis and uremia in experimental nephrotic syndrome. *Am J Kidney Dis* 1990;15:16–23.
160. Kasiske BL, O-Donnell MP, Garvis WJ, et al. Pharmacologic treatment of hyperlipidemia reduces glomerular injury in rat 5/6 nephrectomy model of chronic renal failure. *Circ Res* 1998;62:367–374.
161. Schmitz PH, Kasiske BL, O'Donnell MP, et al. Lipids and progressive renal injury. *Semin Nephrol* 1989;9:354–369.
162. Lee HS, Lee JS, Koh HI, et al. Intraglomerular lipid deposition in routine biopsies. *Clin Nephrol* 1991;36:67–75.
163. Sato H, Suzuki S, Ueno M, et al. Localization of apolipoprotein(a) and B-100 in various renal diseases. *Kidney Int* 1993;43:430–435.
164. Samuelsson O, Aurell M, Knight-Gibson C, et al. Apolipoprotein-B-containing lipoproteins and the progression of renal insufficiency. *Nephron* 1993;63:279–285.
165. Mulec H, Johnson SA, Wiklund O, et al. Cholesterol: A renal risk factor in diabetic nephropathy? *Am J Kidney Dis* 1993;22:196–201.
166. Mulec H, Johnson A, Björck S. Relationship between serum cholesterol and diabetic nephropathy. *Lancet* 1990;1:1537–1538.
167. Laden AM. Experimental atherosclerosis in rat and rabbit allografts. *Arch Pathol* 1972;93:240–245.
168. Alonso DR, Starek PK, Minick CR. Studies on the pathogenesis of atheroarteriosclerosis induced in rabbit cardiac allografts by the synergy of graft rejection and hypercholesterolemia. *Am J Pathol* 1977;87:415–442.
169. Tanaka H, Sukhova GK, Libby P. Interaction of the allogeneic state and hypercholesterolemia in arterial lesion formation in experimental cardiac allografts. *Arterioscler Thromb* 1994;14:734–745.
170. Meiser BM, Wenke K, Thiery J, et al. Simvastatin decreases accelerated graft vessel disease after heart transplantation in an animal model. *Transplant Proc* 1993;25:2077–2079.
171. Anderson HO, Holm P, Nordestgaard BG, et al. Effect of the antioxidant probucol on transplant arteriosclerosis in aorta-allografted rabbits. *J Mol Cell Cardiol* 1995;27:1561–1571.
172. Tanabe S, Ueda M, Han YS, et al. Presence of oxidized LDL in transplant arteriosclerotic lesions obtained from renal transplant recipients. *Transplant Proc* 1998;30:116–118.
173. Isoniemi H, Numinen M, Tikkanen M, et al. Risk factors predicting chronic rejection of renal allograft. *Transplantation* 1994;57:68–72.
174. Dimeny E, Wahlberg J, Lithell H, et al. Hyperlipidaemia in renal transplantation: Risk factor for long-term graft outcome. *Eur J Clin Invest* 1995;25:574–583.
175. Dimeny E, Tufvesion G, Lithell H, et al. The influence of pretransplant lipoprotein abnormalities on the early results of renal transplantation. *Eur J Clin Invest* 1993;23:572–579.
176. De Groen PC, Aksamit AJ, Rakela J, et al. Central nervous system toxicity after liver transplantation: The role of cyclosporine and cholesterol. *N Engl J Med* 1987;317:861–866.
177. Massy ZA, Guijarro C, Wiederkehr MR, et al. Chronic renal allograft rejection: Immunologic and nonimmunologic risk factors. *Kidney Int* 1996;49:518–524.
178. Heim-Duthoy KL, Chitwood KK, Tortorice KL, et al. Elective cyclosporine withdrawal one year after renal transplantation. *Am J Kidney Dis* 1994;24:846–853.
179. Ghanem H, van den Dorpel MA, Weimar W, et al. Increased low density lipoprotein oxidation in stable kidney transplant recipients. *Kidney Int* 1996;49:488–493.
180. Cristol JP, Maggi MF, Vela C, et al. Lipid metabolism and oxidative stress in renal transplantation: Implications for chronic rejection. *Transplant Proc* 1996;28:2820–2821.
181. National Heart, Lung, and Blood Institute. NIH publication No 95-3045. *Recommendations regarding public screening for measuring blood cholesterol.* Bethesda, MD: NHLBI, 1995.
182. Nauck M, Kramer-Guth A, Bartens W, et al. Is the determination of LDL cholesterol according to Friedewald accurate in CAPD and HD patients? *Clin Nephrol* 1996;46:319–325.
183. Ingram AJ, Parbtani A, Churchill DN. Effects of two low-flux cellulose acetate dialysers on plasma lipids and lipoproteins—a cross-over trial. *Nephrol Dial Transplant* 1998;13:1452–1457.
184. Mottram DR, George AJ. Anabolic steroids. *Baillieres Best Pract Res Clin Endocrinol Metab* 2000;14:55–69.
185. Stone NJ. Secondary causes of hyperlipidemia. *Med Clin North Am* 1994;78:117–141.
186. Teruel JL, Lasuncion MA, Rivera M, et al. Nandrolone decanoate reduces serum lipoprotein(a) concentrations in hemodialysis patients. *Am J Kidney Dis* 1997;29:569–575.
187. Bologa RM, Levine DM, Parker TS, et al. Interleukin-6 predicts hypoalbuminemia, hypocholesterolemia, and mortality in hemodialysis patients. *Am J Kidney Dis* 1998;32:107–114.
188. LaRosa JC, He J, Vupputuri S. Effect of statins on risk of coronary disease: a meta-analysis of randomized controlled trials. *JAMA* 1999;282:2340–2346.
189. Goldwasser P, Mittman N, Antignani A, et al. Predictors of mortality in hemodialysis patients. *J Am Soc Nephrol* 1993;3:1613–1622.
190. Piccoli GB, Quarello F, Salomone M, et al. Are serum albumin and cholesterol reliable outcome markers in elderly dialysis patients? *Nephrol Dial Transplant* 1995;10 Suppl 6:72–77.
191. Iseki K, Kawazoe N, Fukiyama K. Serum albumin is a strong predictor of death in chronic dialysis patients. *Kidney Int* 1993;44:115–119.
192. Cano N, Costanzo-Dufetel J, Calaf R, et al. Prealbumin-retinol-binding-protein-retinol complex in hemodialysis patients. *Am J Clin Nutr* 1988;47:664–667.
193. Lindner A, Charra B, Sherrard DJ, et al. Accelerated atherosclerosis in prolonged maintenance hemodialysis. *N Engl J Med* 1974;290:697–701.
194. LaRosa JC, Hunninghake D, Bush D, et al. The cholesterol facts. A summary of the evidence relating dietary fats, serum cholesterol, and coronary heart disease. A joint statement by the American Heart Association and the National Heart, Lung, and Blood Institute. The Task Force on Cholesterol Issues, American Heart Association. *Circulation* 1990;81:1721–1733.
195. Ross SD, Allen IE, Connelly JE, et al. Clinical outcomes in statin treatment trials: a meta-analysis. *Arch Intern Med* 1999;159:1793–1802.
196. Wanner C, Horl WH, Luley CH, et al. Effects of HMG-CoA reductase inhibitors in hypercholesterolemic patients on hemodialysis. *Kidney Int* 1991;39:754–760.
197. Robson R, Collins J, Johnson R, et al. Effects of simvastatin and enalapril on serum lipoprotein concentrations and left ventricular mass in patients on dialysis. The Perfect Study Collaborative Group. *J Nephrol* 1997;10:33–40.
198. Jonsson B, Johannesson M. Cost-benefit analysis of lipid lowering therapy. *Eur Heart J* 1997;18:165–166.
199. Jonsson B, Johannesson M, Kjekshus J, et al. Cost-effectiveness of cholesterol lowering. Results from the Scandinavian Simvastatin Survival Study (4S). *Eur Heart J* 1996;17:1001–1007.
200. Pearson TA. Lipid-lowering therapy in low-risk patients. *JAMA* 1998;279:1659–1661.
201. Ikizler TA, Wingard RL, Harvell J, et al. Association of morbidity with markers of nutrition and inflammation in chronic he-

modialysis patients: a prospective study. *Kidney Int* 1999;55: 1945–1951.

202. Ridker PM, Rifai N, Lowenthal SP. Rapid reduction in C-reactive protein with cerivastatin among 785 patients with primary hypercholesterolemia. *Circulation* 2001;103:1191–1193.
203. Ridker PM, Rifai N, Pfeffer MA, et al. Long-term effects of pravastatin on plasma concentration of C-reactive protein. The Cholesterol and Recurrent Events (CARE) Investigators. *Circulation* 1999;100:230–235.
204. Ridker PM, Rifai N, Pfeffer MA, et al. Inflammation, pravastatin, and the risk of coronary events after myocardial infarction in patients with average cholesterol levels. Cholesterol and Recurrent Events (CARE) Investigators. *Circulation* 1998;98: 839–844.
205. Gokal R, Mann JI, Oliver DO, et al. Dietary treatment of hyperlipidemia in chronic hemodialysis patients. *Am J Clin Nutr* 1978;31:1915–1918.
206. Weintraub MS, Zechner R, Brown A, et al. Dietary polyunsaturated fats of the W-6 and W-3 series reduce postprandial lipoprotein levels. Chronic and acute effects of fat saturation on postprandial lipoprotein metabolism. *J Clin Invest* 1988;82: 1884–1893.
207. Ando M, Sanaka T, Nihei H. Eicosapentanoic acid reduces plasma levels of remnant lipoproteins and prevents in vivo peroxidation of LDL in dialysis patients. *J Am Soc Nephrol* 1999; 10:2177–2184.
208. Johansen KL, Chertow GM, Ng AV, et al. Physical activity levels in patients on hemodialysis and healthy sedentary controls. *Kidney Int* 2000;57:2564–2570.
209. Harter HR, Goldberg AP. Endurance exercise training. An effective therapeutic modality for hemodialysis patients. *Med Clin North Am* 1985;69:159–175.
210. Goldberg AP, Hagberg JM, Delmez JA, et al. Metabolic effects of exercise training in hemodialysis patients. *Kidney Int* 1980; 18:754–761.
211. Goldberg AP, Geltman EM, Gavin JR III, et al. Exercise training reduces coronary risk and effectively rehabilitates hemodialysis patients. *Nephron* 1986;42:311–316.
212. Odamaki M, Furuya R, Ohkawa S, et al. Altered abdominal fat distribution and its association with the serum lipid profile in non-diabetic haemodialysis patients. *Nephrol Dial Transplant* 1999;14:2427–2432.
213. Kopple JD, Zhu X, Lew NL, et al. Body weight-for-height relationships predict mortality in maintenance hemodialysis patients. *Kidney Int* 1999;56:1136–1148.
214. Fleischmann E, Teal N, Dudley J, et al. Influence of excess weight on mortality and hospital stay in 1346 hemodialysis patients [see comments]. *Kidney Int* 1999;55:1560–1567.
215. Hakim RM, Lowrie E. Obesity and mortality in ESRD: is it good to be fat? *Kidney Int* 1999;55:1580–1581.
216. Wood D. European and American recommendations for coronary heart disease prevention. *Eur Heart J* 1998;19 Suppl A: A12–A19.
217. Jüngst D, Caselmann WH, Kutschera PM, et al. Relation of hyperlipidemia in serum and loss of high density lipoproteins in urine in the nephritic syndrome. *Clin Chim Acta* 1987;168: 159–167.
218. Kaysen GA, Gambertoglio J, Felts J, et al. Albumin synthesis, albuminuria and hyperlipidemia in the nephrotic syndrome. *Kidney Int* 1987;31:1368–1376.
219. Wanner C, Bartens W, Nauck M, et al. Lipoprotein(a) in patients with the nephrotic syndrome: Influence of immunosuppression and proteinuria. *Miner Electrolyte Metab* 1996;118: 246–254.
220. Keilani T, Schlueter WA, Levin ML, et al. Improvement of lipid abnormalities associated with proteinuria using fosinopril, an angiotensin-converting enzyme inhibitor. *Ann Intern Med* 1993;118:246–254.
221. Gansevoort RT, Heeg JE, Dikkeschei FD, et al. Symptomatic antiproteinuric treatment decreases serum lipoprotein(a) concentration in patients with glomerular proteinuria. *Nephrol Dial Transplant* 1994;9:244–250.
222. Valeri A, Gelfand J, Blum C, et al. Treatment of the hyperlipidemia of the nephrotic syndrome: A controlled trial. *Am J Kidney Dis* 1986;6:388–396.
223. Rabelink AJ, Hene RJ, Erkelens DW, et al. Effects of simvastatin and cholestyramine on lipoprotein profile in hyperlipidaemia of nephrotic syndrome. *Lancet* 1988;2:1335–1338.
224. Groggel GC, Cheung AK, Ellis-Benigni K, et al. Safe and effective treatment of the hyperlipidemia of nephrotic syndrome with gemfibrozil. *Kidney Int* 1989;36:266–271.
225. Bridgeman JF, Rosen SM, Thorp JM. Complications during clofibrate treatment of nephrotic syndrome hyperlipoproteinaemia. *Lancet* 1972;2:506–509.
226. Fried LF, Orchard TJ, Kasiske BL. Effect of lipid reduction on the progression of renal disease: a meta-analysis. *Kidney Int* 2001;59:260–269.
227. Fiorini F, Patrone E, Castelluccio A. Clinical investigation on the hypolipidemic effect of simvastatin versus probucol in hemodialysis patients. *Clin Ter* 1994;145:213–217.
228. Massy ZA, Ma JZ, Louis TA, et al. Lipid-lowering therapy in patients with renal disease. *Kidney Int* 1995;48:188–198.
229. Saika Y, Kodama N, Kimura K, et al. Plasma nicotinic acid levels in hemodialysis patients after the administration of niceritrol. *Nippon Jinzo Gakkai Shi* 1999;41:430–435.
230. Shoji T, Nishizawa Y, Kawasaki K, et al. Effects of the nicotinic acid analogue niceritrol on lipoprotein Lp(a) and coagulation-fibrinolysis status in patients with chronic renal failure on hemodialysis. *Nephron* 1997;77:112–113.
231. Nakahama H, Nakanishi T, Uyama O, et al. Niceritrol reduces plasma lipoprotein(a) levels in patients undergoing maintenance hemodialysis. *Ren Fail* 1993;15:189–193.
232. Chertow GM, Burke SK, Dillon MA, et al. Long-term effects of sevelamer hydrochloride on the calcium x phosphate product and lipid profile of haemodialysis patients. *Nephrol Dial Transplant* 1999;14:2907–2914.
233. Chertow GM, Burke SK, Lazarus JM, et al. Poly[allylamine hydrochloride] (RenaGel): a noncalcemic phosphate binder for the treatment of hyperphosphatemia in chronic renal failure. *Am J Kidney Dis* 1997;29:66–71.
234. Slatopolsky EA, Burke SK, Dillon MA. RenaGel, a nonabsorbed cal. *Kidney Int* 1999;55:299–307.
235. Hodis HN. Triglyceride-rich lipoprotein remnant particles and risk of atherosclerosis. *Circulation* 1999;99:2852–2854.
236. Byrne CD. Triglyceride-rich lipoproteins: are links with atherosclerosis mediated by a procoagulant and proinflammatory phenotype? *Atherosclerosis* 1999;145:1–15.
237. Rubies-Prat J, Reverter JL, Senti M, et al. Calculated low-density lipoprotein cholesterol should not be used for management of lipoprotein abnormalities in patients with diabetes mellitus. *Diabetes Care* 1993;16:1081–1086.
238. Shoji T, Kawagishi T, Emoto M, et al. Additive impacts of diabetes and renal failure on carotid atherosclerosis. *Atherosclerosis* 2000;153:257–258.
239. Langer T, Levy RI. Acute muscular syndrome associated with administration of clofibrate. *N Engl J Med* 1968;279:856–858.
240. Grutzmacher P, Scheuermann EH, Siede W, et al. Lipid lowering treatment with bezafibrate in patients on chronic haemodialysis: pharmacokinetics and effects. *Klin Wochenschr* 1986;64: 910–916.
241. Pelegri A, Romero R, Senti M, et al. Effect of bezafibrate on lipoprotein (a) and triglyceride-rich lipoproteins, including in-

termediate-density lipoproteins, in patients with chronic renal failure receiving haemodialysis. *Nephrol Dial Transplant* 1992; 7:623–626.

242. Rubins HB, Robins SJ, Collins D, et al. Gemfibrozil for the secondary prevention of coronary heart disease in men with low levels of high-density lipoprotein cholesterol. Veterans Affairs High-Density Lipoprotein Cholesterol Intervention Trial Study Group. *N Engl J Med* 1999;341:410–418.
243. Irish AB, Thompson CH. The effects of gemfibrozil upon the hypercoagulable state in dyslipidaemic patients with chronic renal failure. *Nephrol Dial Transplant* 1996;11:2223–2228.
244. Evans JR, Forland SC, Cutler RE. The effect of renal function on the pharmacokinetics of gemfibrozil. *J Clin Pharmacol* 1987; 27:994–1000.
245. Pasternack A, Vanttinen T, Solakivi T, et al. Normalization of lipoprotein lipase and hepatic lipase by gemfibrozil results in correction of lipoprotein abnormalities in chronic renal failure. *Clin Nephrol* 1987;27:163–168.
246. Desager JP, Costermans J, Verberckmoes R, et al. Effect of hemodialysis on plasma kinetics of fenofibrate in chronic renal failure. *Nephron* 1982;31:51–54.
247. Boden WE. High-density lipoprotein cholesterol as an independent risk factor in cardiovascular disease: assessing the data from Framingham to the Veterans Affairs High-Density Lipoprotein Intervention Trial. *Am J Cardiol* 2000;86:19L–22L.
248. Van Lenten BJ, Hama SY, de Beer FC, et al. Anti-inflammatory HDL becomes pro-inflammatory during the acute phase response. Loss of protective effect of HDL against LDL oxidation in aortic wall cell cocultures. *J Clin Invest* 1995;96:2758–2767.
249. Navab M, Berliner JA, Subbanagounder G, et al. HDL and the inflammatory response induced by LDL-derived oxidized phospholipids. *Arterioscler Thromb Vasc Biol* 2001;21:481–488.
250. Gowri MS, Van der Westhuyzen DR, Bridges SR, et al. Decreased protection by HDL from poorly controlled type 2 diabetic subjects against LDL oxidation may be due to the abnormal composition of HDL. *Arterioscler Thromb Vasc Biol* 1999; 19:2226–2233.
251. Morena M, Cristol JP, Dantoine T, et al. Protective effects of high-density lipoprotein against oxidative stress are impaired in haemodialysis patients. *Nephrol Dial Transplant* 2000;15: 389–395.
252. Neary RH, Gowland E. The effect of renal failure and haemodialysis on the concentration of free apolipoprotein A-1 in serum and the implications for the catabolism of high-density lipoproteins. *Clin Chim Acta* 1988;171:239–245.
253. Duval F, Frommherz K, Atger V, et al. Influence of end-stage renal failure on concentrations of free apolipoprotein A-1 in serum. *Clin Chem* 1989;35:963–966.
254. Al Saady NM, Leatham EW, Gupta S, et al. Monocyte expression of tissue factor and adhesion molecules: the link with accelerated coronary artery disease in patients with chronic renal failure. *Heart* 1999;81:134–140.
255. Hamazaki T, Nakazawa R, Tateno S, et al. Effects of fish oil rich in eicosapentaenoic acid on serum lipid in hyperlipidemic hemodialysis patients. *Kidney Int* 1984;26:81–84.
256. Bilo HJ, Homan van der Heide JJ, Gans RO, et al. Omega-3 polyunsaturated fatty acids in chronic renal insufficiency. *Nephron* 1991;57:385–393.
257. Rolf N, Tenschert W, Lison AE. Results of a long-term administration of omega-3 fatty acids in haemodialysis patients with dyslipoproteinaemia. *Nephrol Dial Transplant* 1990;5: 797–801.
258. Rylance PB, Gordge MP, Saynor R, et al. Fish oil modifies lipids and reduces platelet aggregability in haemodialysis patients. *Nephron* 1986;43:196–202.
259. Donnelly SM, Ali MA, Churchill DN. Effect of n-3 fatty acids from fish oil on hemostasis, blood pressure, and lipid profile of dialysis patients. *J Am Soc Nephrol* 1992;2:1634–1639.
260. Seres DS, Strain GW, Hashim SA, et al. Improvement of plasma lipoprotein profiles during high-flux dialysis. *J Am Soc Nephrol* 1993;3:1409–1415.
261. de Precigout V, Higueret D, Larroumet N, et al. Improvement in lipid profiles and triglyceride removal in patients on polyamide membrane hemodialysis. *Blood Purif* 1996;14:170–176.
262. Goldberg IJ, Kaufman AM, Lavarias VA, et al. High flux dialysis membranes improve plasma lipoprotein profiles in patients with end-stage renal disease. *Nephrol Dial Transplant* 1996;11 Suppl 2:104–107.
263. Blankestijn PJ, Vos PF, Rabelink TJ, et al. High-flux dialysis membranes improve lipid profile in chronic hemodialysis patients. *J Am Soc Nephrol* 1995;5:1703–1708.
264. Pollock CA, Wyndham R, Collett PV, et al. Effects of erythropoietin therapy on the lipid profile in end-stage renal failure. *Kidney Int* 1994;45:897–902.
265. Arnadottir M, Berg AL, Kronenberg F, et al. Corticotropin-induced reduction of plasma lipoprotein(a) concentrations in healthy individuals and hemodialysis patients: relation to apolipoprotein(a) size polymorphism. *Metabolism* 1999;48: 342–346.
266. Arnadottir M, Berg AL, Dallongeville J, et al. Adrenocorticotrophic hormone lowers serum Lp(a) and LDL cholesterol concentrations in hemodialysis patients. *Kidney Int* 1997;52: 1651–1655.
267. Bommer C, Werle E, Walter-Sack I, et al. D-thyroxine reduces lipoprotein(a) serum concentration in dialysis patients. *J Am Soc Nephrol* 1998;9:90–96.
268. Wanner C, Bartens W. Lipoprotein(a) in renal patients: is it a key factor in the high cardiovascular mortality. *Nephrol Dial Transplant* 1994;1066–1068.
269. Wanner C, Krämer-Guth A, Galle J. Use of HMG-CoA reductase inhibitors after kidney and heart transplantation. *Bio Drugs* 1997;8:387–393.
270. Cockcroft JR, Wilkinson IB. Cholesterol reduction, statins and the cytochrome P-450 system. *Eur Heart J* 2000;21: 1555–1556.
271. Kobashigawa JA, Katznelson S, Laks H, et al. Effect of pravastatin on outcomes after cardiac transplantation. *N Engl J Med* 1995;333:621–627.
272. Wenke K, Meiser B, Thiery J, et al. Simvastatin reduces graft vessel disease and mortality after heart transplantation. *Circulation* 1997;96:1398–1402.
273. Wanner C, Bartens W, Galle J. Clinical utility of antilipidemic therapies in chronic renal allograft failure. *Kidney Int* 1995; 48(Suppl 52):S60–S62.
274. Kasiske BL. Role of circulating lipid abnormalities in chronic renal allograft rejection. *Kidney Int* 1999;56(Suppl 71): S28–S30.

4

UREMIC TOXICITY

BENGT LINDHOLM
OLOF HEIMBÜRGER
PETER STENVINKEL
JONAS BERGSTRÖM

The state of uremia affects virtually all organ tissues and functions of the body; therefore, the metabolic and nutritional derangements are prominent features of the uremic syndrome. The word *uremia* is derived from two ancient Greek words: *ouron* means urine and *haima* means blood. Literally, uremia is urine in the blood. Thus, the term uremia implies that accumulation of excretory products such as urea in the blood results in the toxic condition of uremia. However, it is obvious that this definition is too narrow to cover all aspects of the uremic syndrome. A definition that comes closer to reality and emphasizes all aspects of loss of renal cell mass and functions therefore is suggested: "Uremia is a toxic syndrome caused by severe glomerular insufficiency, associated with disturbances in tubular and endocrine functions of the kidney. It is characterized by retention of toxic metabolites, associated with changes in volume and electrolyte composition of the body fluids and excess or deficiency of various hormones."

The primary event in urine formation is the glomerular ultrafiltration process. The ultrafiltrate is reduced in volume and modified as to composition by the metabolic activity of the tubular cells. The final urine, which is the end result of these processes, contains urea and other nitrogenous metabolites in high concentration and has an appropriate volume and electrolyte composition to maintain homeostasis. Clearly, the development of the uremic state is primarily the consequence of severe glomerular insufficiency, which is a prerequisite for retention of toxic, nitrogenous metabolites.

The sieving properties of the glomerular filter permits compounds with a molecular weight of up to 58,000 daltons (Da) or higher to be filtered and eliminated from the blood. Consequently, compounds within a very wide molecular-weight spectrum are retained in the body fluids in conditions with reduced glomerular filtration, provided that they are not eliminated by other routes.

The long-term survival of patients with end-stage renal disease (ESRD) undergoing maintenance hemodialysis (HD) is strong evidence that some of the most important uremic toxins are dialyzable through artificial membranes with a molecular size cutoff of less than 10,000 Da. However, the presence of a variety of residual symptoms and the high mortality in patients undergoing dialysis indicates that there may be toxic compounds accumulating in uremia that are either not removed at all or are insufficiently removed by standard dialysis (1–3).

Severe glomerular insufficiency, however, always is associated with secondary disturbances in tubular functions, which may explain such aspects of uremia as hyperkalemia and metabolic acidosis. Disturbances in intermediary metabolism as a result of loss of metabolizing tubular cells, as well as impaired synthesis of hormones produced by the kidneys (erythropoietin, calcitriol) and impaired catabolism of peptide hormones, also are involved in the symptomatology of the uremic syndrome. It may be impossible to separate such disturbances from direct effects of toxic compounds retained as a consequence of reduced renal function.

UREMIC SYMPTOMS AND SIGNS

Symptoms and signs that commonly are observed in uremia are presented in Table 4.1. Particularly striking are the neurologic signs and symptoms including mental changes, fatigue, muscle twitching, stupor, convulsions, coma, and symptomatic peripheral neuropathy. The gastrointestinal symptoms such as anorexia and vomiting may be associated with stomatitis, glossitis, gastritis, pancreatitis, and enterocolitis.

Cardiovascular symptoms including heart failure, hypertension (disorders closely connected with salt and water retention), pericarditis, left ventricle hypertrophy, cardiac arythmias, cardiomyopathy, endothelial dysfunction and atherosclerosis are also common features of the uremic syndrome (Chapters 10 and 13). Other typical changes in fluid and electrolyte balance are hyperkalemia (Chapter 18), metabolic acidosis (Chapter 9), hyperphosphatemia, and distur-

TABLE 4.1. UREMIC SYMPTOMS AND SIGNS

Central nervous system	*Cardiovascular system*
Stupor	Pericarditis
Coma	Cardiomyopathy
Insomnia	Hypertension
Tremor	Arteriosclerosis
Asterixis	Heart failure
Myoclonus	Arrhythmias
Cramps	Edema—overhydration
Fatigue	Endothelial dysfunction
Confusion	
Electroencephalogram changes	*Respiratory system*
	Pneumonitis—"uremic lung"
	Pulmonary edema
Peripheral nerves	
Numbness, paresthesia	*Skin*
Restless legs	Dry skin
Sensory loss	Pruritus
Muscle weakness	Pigmentation
Pareses	Bleeding
Autonomous neuropathy	Retarded wound healing
Hypotension	
	Musculoskeletal system
Gastrointestinal tract	Osteodystrophy
Anorexia	Osteomalacia
Nausea, vomiting	Pain and fractures
Hiccup	Carpal tunnel syndrome
Stomatitis	Amyloidosis
Gastritis	Myopathy
Parotitis	Muscle weakness and wasting
Colitis	
Bleeding	*Endocrine and metabolic changes*
Fetor uremicus	Hyperparathyroidism
	Glucose intolerance
Hematologic and immunologic	Lipid abnormalities
Anemia	Amino acid disturbances
Granulocyte dysfunction	Oxidative stress
Lymphocyte dysfunction	Malnutrition
Immunodeficiency	Hypoalbuminemia
Infection susceptibility	Muscle wasting
Malignancies	Growth retardation
Inflammation	Impotence
	Reduced libido
	Hypothermia

bances in calcium homeostasis (Chapter 17). Decreased production and increased destruction of red cells result in anemia (Chapter 22). Impaired hemostasis leads to bleeding from the mucous membranes in the skin (caused by a defect in platelet aggregation), and fibrinolysis is inhibited as well. Pruritus and hyperpigmentation of the skin in chronic uremia also are encountered frequently.

The immunologic response is impaired in patients with uremia, and the susceptibility to infections may be increased. However, inflammatory parameters including proinflammatory cytokines often are elevated and may contribute to the malnutrition, inflammation, and atherosclerosis (MIA) syndrome, which is associated with increased mortality (see section on proinflammatory cytokines later in this chapter and Chapter 13).

Disturbances in calcium and phosphorus metabolism give rise to uremic osteodystrophy causing conditions such as osteomalacia, osteosclerosis, osteitis fibrosa with bone pain, and fractures. In children, retardation of growth also can occur. (See Chapter 17 and Chapter 29.)

A number of changes in intermediary metabolism also are encountered in patients with uremia, including abnormalities in protein and amino acid metabolism (Chapter 1) as well as in carbohydrate (Chapter 2) and lipid metabolism (Chapter 3). Other consequences of renal failure are the loss of endocrine functions of the kidney, insufficient production of erythropoietin contributing to renal anemia (Chapter 22), and lack of active vitamin D (calcitriol) leading to deficient intestinal calcium absorption and osteodystrophy (Chapter 17). Moreover, the normal kidney has an important role in catabolizing various peptide hormones, and loss of these abilities may lead to endocrine disturbances.

Cell-membrane transport is abnormal in uremia. The active sodium efflux is inhibited and the transmembrane potential of skeletal muscle cells is decreased in patients with severe uremia (4,5), signifying inhibition of the electrogenic sodium pump or increased membrane permeability for sodium. This abnormality is reversed by adequate dialysis (6).

In summary, uremia seems to affect practically all organs and tissues of the body; mucous and serous membranes are affected, various transport phenomena in the cell membranes are inhibited, and intermediary metabolic processes are impaired. These alterations are responsible for or contribute to the nutritional problems in patients with renal disease.

TOXIC EFFECTS OF UREMIC PLASMA OR SERUM

Indirect evidence of uremic toxicity has been obtained from bioassay studies *in vivo* and *in vitro* that showed that plasma, serum, ultrafiltrate, and dialysate from patients with uremia affect numerous biologic processes. There are only a few *in vivo* bioassays of uremic toxicity. Infusion of uremic ultrafiltrate to normal rats results in lowering of intestinal calcitriol receptor number and increased receptor messenger RNA (mRNA) levels similar to those found in uremic rats (7). A study in the rat demonstrates that intraperitoneal ingestion of a middle-molecular fraction of ultrafiltrate obtained at the beginning of the first dialysis treatment in patients with chronic renal failure (CRF), as well as the same fraction from normal urine, inhibits appetite (8). This effect was obtained only for the fraction 1000–5000 dalton, which inhibited both sucrose intake and protein intake in a dose-dependent manner. These results suggest that toxic compounds in the middle-molecular weight fraction, which normally are excreted in urine, accumulate in the plasma in uremia and suppress food intake.

There is experimental evidence that dialyzable molecules

play a role for development of uremic symptoms. In rats with renal failure, uremic encephalopathy quantified by electroencephalogram has been demonstrated to be attenuated by peritoneal dialysis (PD) (9). Progressive loss of nephrons in rats with CRF may be retarded by PD, suggesting that a circulating uremic toxin is involved in the advancement of glomerulosclerosis (10).

There are numerous *in vitro* studies of uremic toxicity. Uremic sera inhibits *in vitro* erythropoiesis (11–13), lymphocyte transformation and proliferation (14), natural killer cell activity (15), and mononuclear phagocytes (16). Platelet-activating–factor synthesis is inhibited by uremic ultrafiltrate, and this effect appears to be associated with an inhibition of phospholipase A2 and acetyltransferase activity (17). Uremic toxins accumulating in the plasma of patients with renal failure not only affect essential neutrophil functions and thereby the unspecific immune response but also influence neutrophil survival by modulating the rate of apoptotic cell death (18). Uremic serum reduces inotropy and induces arrhythmias in cultured cardiac myocytes (19). Plasma from patients with uremia depresses nerve-mediated smooth-muscle contraction (20).

A variety of metabolic processes *in vitro* are impaired in the presence of uremic plasma or serum. Glucose utilization and glycolysis are inhibited (Chapter 2). There also is inhibition of protein synthesis, mitochondrial metabolism, uncoupling of phosphorylation (21), inhibition of fibrinolysis, and lipolysis. Production of apolipoprotein A-1 is inhibited by uremic serum and its subfractions (22).

Several transmembrane transport systems in a variety of cells also are inhibited *in vitro* in the presence of uremic serum or ultrafiltrate. These include transport of sodium in cell membranes (23), calcium in mitochondria (24), erythrocyte membrane in calcium pumps (25), uric acid in liver slices (26), hippuric-acid derivatives in kidney tissue (27), and amino acids in muscle (28). The nuclear uptake of calcitriol receptor is inhibited by uremic ultrafiltrate (29), suggested to play a role in calcitriol resistance of patients with renal failure.

In vitro inhibition of several enzymes also has been reported. Among these are lipoprotein lipase (30), xanthine oxidase (26), phenylalanine hydroxylase (31), Na^+, K^+-ATPase in brain, red cells and aortic strips (32–34), thiopurine methyltransferase (35), δ-amino levulinic-acid synthetase (36), and transketolase in red cells (37) and nervous tissue (38). However, no inhibition was found in erythrocytes by other investigators (39). Tranketolase inhibition has been suggested to play a role in peripheral neuropathy of uremia. The effects of uremic serum on transmembrane transport mechanisms and transport enzymes (Na^+, K^+-ATPase) are of special interest in view of Bricker's (40) hypothesis that a humoral factor, produced as a result of homeostatic adaptation to sodium retention and which decreases tubular sodium reabsorption, might be important in uremia by inhibiting transmembrane transport in other cells as well. In conclusion, there is evidence that a variety of clinical disturbances, such as anemia; immunologic deficiency; bleeding tendency; disorders of protein, carbohydrate, and lipid metabolism; and various membrane-transport disturbances may be related to toxins or inhibitors present in plasma or other body fluids in patients with uremia.

DEFINITION OF A UREMIC TOXIN

For a substance to be defined as a uremic toxin, a necessary criterion is that it is present in increased concentrations in body fluids and/or tissues in patients with renal failure. Correlations have been sought between the appearance of certain uremic signs and the concentration of one or more particular substances in plasma. However, such correlations, if found, are no proof that one specific substance is responsible because a great number of substances excreted by the kidneys accumulate simultaneously as renal function deteriorates. Therefore, additional criteria have to be applied before a substance is defined as a uremic toxin.

Substances known to be present in raised concentration in patients with uremic signs and symptoms have been given to humans or experimental animals or added to various tissues, cells, or enzymes *in vitro* to prove whether they exert toxic effects. Many of these experiments are open to criticism because the concentrations used were often much higher than those encountered in the blood of patients with uremia. Another criticism of the *in vitro* experiments is that they reflect only acute toxicity and therefore will be inadequate for assessing chronic toxicity, which occurs in uremia. Even when investigations are performed correctly, with the compound present in concentrations comparable to those found in patients with uremia, it may be doubtful if these *in vitro* effects relate to *in vivo* toxicity.

It is possible that a number of compounds, each of which present in a concentration too low to be toxic, may act synergistically to produce toxic effects. There is also evidence that when certain compounds, known to accumulate in uremia, are present together in the medium, they may induce *in vitro* toxic effects that are not found when these compounds are present alone. In normal rats single doses of cresole, putrescine, methylguanidine, and acetoin had no effect on oxygen consumption, but some combinations of these substances reduced oxygen consumption significantly (41). These studies raise the question of whether testing of some uremic compounds has to be made in a "uremic" environment. Also, most studies on uremic toxins assume their presence in blood, whereas intracellular and local uremic toxin levels are less well investigated. For example, local uremic toxins present in the gastrointestinal tract were found to influence insulin resistance, based on the effects of an oral adsorbent in rats with renal insufficiency (42).

Criteria to be fulfilled by a uremic toxin may be summarized as follows:

1. The compound should be chemically identified. Specific and accurate quantitative analysis in biologic fluids should be possible.
2. The plasma level and/or tissue concentrations of the compound should be higher in patients with uremia than in patients without uremia.
3. High concentrations should be related to specific uremic symptoms that are ameliorated or disappear when the concentration is reduced.
4. When studying toxicity of specific compounds in human subjects, experimental animals, and/or in an appropriate *in vitro* system, the concentrations used should be comparable to those found in the body fluids and/or tissues of patients with uremia.

Applying these stringent criteria it is evident that among the numerous compounds known to be retained in patients with uremia, only a few have toxic effects proved to be of clinical relevance. Many of these compounds are suspected toxins (Table 4.2).

TABLE 4.2. UREMIC TOXINS

Established	Suspected
Water	Magnesium
Sodium	Sulfate
Potassium	Trace elements
Hydrogen ions	Creatinine
Inorganic phosphate	Methylguanidine
Urea	Guanidinosuccinic acid
Cyanate	Other guanidines
Oxalic acid	Methylated arginines
Parathyroid hormone	Amino acids
β_2-microglobulin	Homocysteine
	ADMA
	Phenols
	Indoles
	Amines
	RCOs
	Uric acid
	Pseudouridine
	Myoinositol
	Acid mucopolysaccharides
	Middle molecules
	AGEs
	ALEs
	AOPPs
	ACEs
	Various peptide hormones
	Natriuretic factors
	Complement factors
	GIPs
	DIPs
	Leptin
	Proinflammatory cytokines

ADMA, asymmetric dimethylarginine; RCOs, reactive carbonyl compounds; AGEs, advanced glycation end products; ALEs, advanced lipoxidation end products; AOPPs, advanced oxidized protein products; ACEs, advanced carbamoylated end products; GIPs, granulocyte-inhibiting protein; DIPs, degranulation-inhibiting protein.

FACTORS THAT INFLUENCE UREMIC TOXICITY

Dialysis Treatment

Patients undergoing dialysis still exhibit uremic symptoms. Many continue to suffer from residual symptoms and endocrine and metabolic disturbances, as well as morbidity induced by the therapeutic procedures, such as cardiovascular instability, enhanced protein catabolism, malnutrition, infection, inflammation, biomaterial incompatibility, and psychologic disturbances.

The aim of dialysis treatment is to normalize the volume and composition of the body fluids and attempt to remove as efficiently as possible some uremic toxins. Efficacy of removal by various blood-purification modalities is governed mainly by three properties of these substances: molecular size, the degree of plasma protein binding, and their intercompartmental distribution.

Diffusive transport as used in dialysis treatment favors the elimination of small molecular compounds such as urea and creatinine, but larger molecules also are removed, especially when using synthetic high-flux membranes or the peritoneal membrane, which have larger average poor sizes than low-flux cellulose membranes. For elimination of larger molecules convective transport with high-flux membranes, as used in hemofiltration and hemodiafiltration, is advantageous because larger molecules are eliminated with the same efficacy (clearance) as small molecules up to a molecular size where the sieving properties of the membrane become rate-limiting. Larger pore size, however, has little effect on the removal of protein-bound toxins (43).

Small, Middle, and Large Molecules

Commonly, uremic retention products are subdivided according to molecular size because this property plays a pivotal role regarding how efficiently they are removed by dialysis, "small" molecules having a molecular weight of less than 500 (or 350) Da, "middle" molecules having a molecular weight between 500 (350) to 5,000 Da, and "large" molecules having a molecular weight higher than 5,000 Da. This subdivision, of course, is arbitrary, considering that the uremic retention products represent a continuous spectrum of molecular sizes.

Protein Binding

Several small molecular size solids may behave anomalously in dialysis treatment because they are to a varying extent protein bound, which reduces or prevents diffusive transport, thus making them appear much larger than their actual molecular weight (44). This can hamper their dialytic removal (45). Serum albumin is the major protein for transporting several metabolic products and drugs. Several compounds retained in uremia also exert a displacement effect on albumin binding of the amino acid tryptophan and of several drugs with affinity to albumin (e.g., phenytoin and digoxine) (46). This displacement phenomenon may become clinically important by increasing the bioavailability of such drugs, thereby carrying a risk of drug intoxication if the dosage is not appropriately reduced. Protein-bound uremic solutes include, for example, 3-carboxy-4-methyl-5-propyl-2-furanpropionic acid, indoxyl sulfate, hippuric acid, homocysteine (Hcy), and p-cresol (45). Protein-bound, and lipophilic, uremic solutes are important uremic toxins that differ in their dialytic behavior from urea and other water-soluble uremic compounds.

Protein Intake

It is a common clinical experience that treatment with a low-protein diet lessens uremic signs and symptoms, especially gastrointestinal symptoms. It also results in a reduction in blood urea concentration. It can be concluded that at least some of the uremic toxins are products of protein and amino acid metabolism. Also, other constituents in food may result in the formation of uremic toxins (43).

Intestinal Bacterial Flora

The bacterial flora of the gut appears to be involved in the pathogenesis of uremic toxicity. It has been shown that germ-free rats with acute uremia survive longer than those with normal intestinal flora (47,48). A toxic role by the bacterial flora in the gut is further supported from observations that patients with severe uremia showed marked clinical improvement of asterixis, myoclonus, and mental alertness following "sterilization" of the bowel with broad-spectrum antibiotics (49). Abnormal colonization of the small intestine by both anaerobic and aerobic bacteria has been reported (50). In fact, several metabolites retained in uremic plasma arise from bacterial activity in the intestinal tract (*vide infra*).

TOXICITY OF INORGANIC SUBSTANCES IN UREMIA

Homeostatic control of water, inorganic ion, and acid–base balance mainly is accomplished by the kidneys. When renal function deteriorates, the kidneys are unable to exert full homeostatic control, resulting in disturbances in water and electrolyte metabolism. Water and electrolyte abnormalities contribute to the toxic symptomatology in the majority of patients with uremia and, if left unattended, may lead to a fatal outcome. With the advent of improved diagnostic methods, a better understanding of the principles of fluid and electrolyte balance, and more effective therapeutic regimens (ion-exchange resins, diuretics, dialysis), the problems of water and electrolyte disturbances in uremia can be mastered to the extent that they only rarely are the direct cause of death.

The abnormalities of water and electrolyte metabolism in uremia will be reviewed briefly with emphasis on toxic effects. For a more complete review of the subject, see Chapter 18.

Water

Water overload may be either approximately isotonic, as in most edematous conditions, or hypotonic, as in water intoxication. A patient with oliguric acute renal failure is especially prone to develop water intoxication as a result of excessive water intake caused by inappropriate thirst or by iatrogenic infusion of an excess of low-electrolyte or electrolyte-free solutions. Water excess in patients with renal failure may produce edema, heart failure, and hypertension (see Chapter 10 and Chapter 18). In water intoxication a variety of signs and symptoms such as mental confusion, restlessness, twitching, muscle cramps, convulsions, and coma may occur. These probably are related to osmotic water transport into the central nervous system, resulting in brain edema.

Sodium

Sodium retention is a cardinal feature of both acute and chronic renal failure and may give rise to hypertension, pulmonary edema, heart failure, and peripheral edema (Chapter 10 and Chapter 18). Patients with near-end-stage renal failure usually can maintain sodium homeostasis as fractional sodium reabsorption is decreased in surviving nephrons. This partially compensates for the decrease in glomerular filtration of sodium, although the ability to regulate sodium excretion in relation to the sodium intake is impaired. Several factors have been suggested to contribute to the adaptation of fractional sodium reabsorption in chronic uremia; among them is that the secretion of a potential natriuretic hormone may cause general toxic effects on solute transport in the body cells by inhibiting Na+, K+AT-Pase (40). Serum samples obtained from patients undergoing HD contained substance(s) that inhibited Na, K-ATPase *in vitro* and acutely caused alterations in myocyte relaxation and calcium metabolism (51). This may contribute to the diastolic dysfunction in patients with uremia.

Potassium

In renal insufficiency, failure to excrete potassium may result in hyperkalemia, caused by oral intake or parenteral administration of potassium or following release of potassium from the tissues during endogenous catabolism. The risk of potassium intoxication is particularly high in patients with acute oliguric posttraumatic renal failure with rapid tissue breakdown; severe hyperkalemia is rarely present when the urinary volumes are adequate, and it is potentiated by metabolic acidosis because potassium moves out of the cells as pH decreases. In addition, several drugs commonly used in patients with ESRD may contribute to hyperkalemia, such as angiotensin converting enzyme (ACE) inhibitors, ACE receptor blockers, amiloride, and spironolactone.

Progressive hyperkalemia is attended by neuromuscular and cardiovascular disturbances with typical ECG changes, ultimately leading to ventricular fibrillation and cardiac arrest (Chapter 18).

Hydrogen Ions

A common feature of renal failure is metabolic acidosis, resulting from the inability to excrete excess metabolically generated hydrogen ions. Severe and prolonged metabolic acidosis results in major disturbances and a number of fundamental metabolic and physiologic processes, causing central nervous system disorders, hyperventilation, hyperkalemia, and abnormalities in energy and metabolism. Metabolic acidosis in patients with renal failure has adverse effects on bone mineral metabolism. It may directly induce dissolution of bone and also alter bone metabolism by stimulating osteoblast-mediated bone resorption, inhibiting osteoblast-mediated bone formation, and altering the serum concentrations or biologic actions of parathyroid hormone and vitamin D. These effects are in review. Correction of acidosis in patients undergoing HD may forestall the development of hyperparathyroid bone disease (54).

From the nutritional point of view it is of interest that metabolic acidosis is an important stimulus for net protein catabolism, as evident from studies in experimental animals and in humans (55–57). In rats, protein degradation in muscle is stimulated by metabolic acidosis by mechanisms that require cortisol (58,59). Experiments in rats with CRF demonstrate that acidosis, rather than uremia, appears to enhance muscle-protein catabolism (60). This effect seems to be mediated by the stimulation of skeletal muscle branched-chain ketoacid decarboxylation, which increases the catabolism of the branched-chain amino acids (valine, leucine, and isoleucine) that mainly are metabolized in muscle tissue (61). Acidosis stimulates proteolysis in muscle by inducing the transcription of genes encoding for enzymes participating in the adenosine triphosphate (ATP)-dependent cytosolic ubiquitin–proteasome proteolytic pathway (62).

In nondialyzed patients with chronic uremia, the correction of metabolic acidosis improves the nitrogen balance and reduces urea appearance and muscle proteolysis (63, 64). In dogs studies using a constant infusion of ^{14}C-leucine, acute metabolic acidosis elicited an increase in leucine flux and leucine oxidation, as compared to controls (65). Studies in normal subjects, using a continuous infusion of ^{13}C-leucine, have demonstrated that total-body protein breakdown and apparent leucine oxidation are higher during acidosis than during alkalosis (66,67). In nondialyzed patients with CRF, the correction of acidosis reduced protein degradation and leucine oxidation (68). A study in normal subjects demonstrates that metabolic acidosis reduces the synthesis rate of albumin significantly (69). Intracellular concentration in muscle of valine (one of the branched-chain amino acids) is low in patients undergoing HD, and the levels correlate with the predialysis standard bicarbonate level, which varied between 18 and 24 mmol/L, suggesting that even slight and intermittent acidosis may stimulate the catabolism of valine in muscle, resulting in a valine depletion that potentially may limit protein synthesis (70). Correction of acidosis may prevent acidosis-related protein wasting (57,71,72) and restores low muscle concentration of branched-chain amino acids to normal levels (73). However, the clinical importance of metabolic acidosis in uremia as a risk factor for the development of malnutrition is far from settled. A better understanding of this problem would require prospective studies of groups of malnourished patients with acidosis in whom acid–base balance is corrected.

Phosphate

Phosphate is known to accumulate in patients with renal insufficiency. The plasma concentration increases when the glomerular filtration rate (GFR) falls below 25% of normal. The role of phosphate retention in causing increased parathyroid activity early in the course of renal failure and its contribution to various clinical and biochemical abnormalities observed in patients with uremia is reviewed in Chapter 17. Restriction of dietary phosphate or removal of phosphate by oral calcium carbonate administration or other phosphate binders prevents deterioration of renal function in the remnant kidney model of CRF in the rat presumably by prevention of renal calcification (74–76).

A high inorganic phosphate concentration in plasma carries the risk of calcium phosphate deposits in organs and tissues and vascular calcification (77,78), and although a high phosphate concentration in plasma may reflect high dietary protein intake, a high serum phosphate level is associated with increased mortality (78,79). The development of cardiovascular calcification has been suggested as one mechanism by which an increased phosphorous concentration or an increased calcium–phosphorous product results in increased cardiovascular mortality (79).

Magnesium

It is well established that the serum magnesium concentration is increased in most patients with severe renal insufficiency. Toxic manifestations in the form of vomiting, malaise, hypotension, decreased reflexes, arrhythmias, and cardiac arrest have been observed after magnesium salt administration to patients with renal failure.

Sulfate

Inorganic sulfate excreted by the kidneys is derived mostly from oxidation of sulfur-containing amino acids. The plasma concentration of sulfate is increased in uremia proportional to acidosis, creatinine, and inorganic phosphate concentrations and inversely proportional to the GFR (80). Patients undergoing HD have increased plasma levels of sulfate, which are reduced by the dialysis treatment (81,82).

There is little evidence that sulfate is toxic; when sulfate concentration increases, it partly "replaces" the chloride ion in the extracellular fluid. It has been speculated whether sulfate *may* be involved in the pathogenesis of renal osteodystrophy, possibly by complex formation with calcium in the gut or in plasma (80). The sweat sulfate concentration is increased in CRF (83), and it has been suggested that unstable calcium sulfate complexes deposited in the skin could be a significant factor in dialysis-related pruritus (83).

Trace Elements

Heavy metals and other trace elements are normal constituents of food and drinking water. Some of them are essential, but some can be harmful. In patients with uremia, accumulation of trace elements has to be expected because of reduced renal excretion. In addition, excessive uptake from dialysis fluid, dialysis equipment, or medications may occur. High concentrations of aluminum, arsenic, chromium, copper, cobalt, silicon, and other trace elements have been observed in uremic plasma and/or tissues. The accumulation and toxicity of trace elements in uremia is discussed in detail in Chapter 19.

Water, sodium, potassium, hydrogen ions, and phosphate are established uremic toxins. However, magnesium, sulfate, and trace elements are to be regarded as suspected uremic toxins (Table 4.2).

ORGANIC COMPOUNDS OF LOW MOLECULAR WEIGHT

Urea

The chemical theory of the pathogenesis of the uremic syndrome begins with Prévost and Dumas (84), who discovered in 1821 that removal of the kidneys leads to an increase in blood urea concentration. However, already in 1831 Richard Bright (85) had questioned the role of urea as a uremic toxin.

Urea is quantitatively the most important end product of nitrogen metabolism in mammals and accounts for about 85% of the urinary nitrogen excretion. The urea concentration increases in the body fluids when GFR is reduced. The blood concentration of urea, however, also is dependent on the nitrogen intake and the balance between endogenous protein synthesis and breakdown. Thus, in conditions of hypercatabolism (e.g., after severe trauma and in sepsis), the urea production rate is grossly increased.

Evidence implicating urea as a toxic substance in uremia was brought forward by a number of investigators who administered urea to experimental animals or to normal subjects. Urea injections shortened the survival of acutely uremic rats (86). However, it may not be possible to distinguish toxic effects of urea from side effects such as dehydration, osmotic diuresis, or water shifts between extracellular and intracellular fluid.

More relevant are clinical experiments where urea was added to dialysis fluid. Nephrectomized dogs maintained by PD may develop severe toxic symptoms including coma at a blood urea concentration of 370 to 480 mg/dL (62 to 80 mmol/L) (87). In contrast, dogs whose ureters had been transplanted into the ileum remained virtually free of toxic symptoms, even when the blood urea concentration rose to 800 mg/dL (133 mmol/L) (88). Dogs subjected to PD against high concentrations of urea 1 g/dL (167 mmol/L) or potassium isocyanate 15 mg/dL (1.9 mmol/L) in the dialysis fluid showed shortened survival compared with dogs dialyzed without these additions (89). Isocyanate, which may be derived spontaneously from urea, may contribute to the uremic syndrome by carbamoylation reactions with free amino acids and proteins (*vide infra*).

Patients with acute renal failure dialyzed against a solution containing sufficient urea to prevent a change in the blood urea concentration showed the same degree of clinical improvement in the uremic syndrome during dialysis as patients in whom urea was removed (90). Chronic patients with uremia treated with HD improved despite maintaining the plasma urea concentration in the range 200 to 300 mg/dL (33 to 50 mmol/L) but the hemorrhagic diathesis persisted. At higher concentrations, however, toxic symptoms occurred such as headache, vomiting, and fatigue (91). In similar experiments in patients with CRF, high concentrations of urea in the blood were associated with malaise, lethargy, pruritus, headache, vomiting, and bleeding tendencies (92). In these patients the lowest plasma concentrations of urea, at which symptoms began to appear, were 200 to 300 mg/dL (33 to 50 mmol/L). When urea loading was stopped, headache and vomiting subsided quickly. Furthermore, addition of urea to the dialysis fluid in uremic subjects caused glucose intolerance (93).

Overall, there is little evidence that high blood urea concentrations are harmful in patients undergoing dialysis, provided that they are dialyzed adequately. On the contrary, several studies demonstrate that low urea concentrations are associated with reduced survival, presumably because low urea levels reflect a low protein intake, thus being an index of malnutrition (57,94–98). The results of the National Cooperative Dialysis Study, a nationwide multicenter study performed in the United States (99), may appear contradictory. In this study two groups of patients with low time-averaged concentration (TAC) of urea and long or short dialysis times, respectively, and two groups of patients with high TAC of urea and long or short dialysis times, respectively, were studied for 24 to 52 weeks (99). The two groups of patients with high TAC values had a larger number of treatment failures and more deaths in the poststudy phase than did the two groups with a low TAC. However, in this study high and low TAC were obtained by adjusting the dose of dialysis and the protein intake was normalized and did not differ between the groups, implying that the groups with high TAC were underdialyzed with regard to small molecules. Unfortunately, these results have been misinterpreted to imply that blood urea levels reflect adequacy of dialysis, so that in underdialyzed patients with low protein intake and low urea levels the dose of dialysis is not adjusted appropriately.

In a retrospective analysis of laboratory data from more than 12,000 patients undergoing HD a low blood urea nitrogen (BUN) level, presumably reflecting a low protein intake, was associated with an increased risk of death. However, mortality also increased when BUN was excessively high, presumably as a sign of underdialysis (96). The results of the ongoing Hemodialysis Study hopefully may provide additional information about the role of urea as a uremic toxin (100).

Urea Removal and Adequacy of Dialysis

A more appropriate estimation of the dose of dialysis regarding the removal of small molecules is obtained by calculating an estimation of Kt/Vurea, where K = urea clearance (in milliliters per minute), t = length of dialysis (in minutes), V = distribution volume of urea (in milliliters). Kt/Vurea may be modified to include the effects of ultrafiltration and of residual renal function (101). A simpler expression of the dose of dialysis for small molecules is the urea reduction rate (i.e., the ratio between predialysis minus postdialysis concentration and the predialysis concentration of urea) (102).

It should be apparent from the foregoing discussion about blood or serum urea levels and clinical outcome in patients undergoing dialysis that urea is a "surrogate molecule" for a uremic toxin. When using Kt/Vurea or urea reduction rate as a measure for the dose of dialysis, one assumes that the most relevant uremic toxins are small molecules that are removed by dialysis in a similar manner as urea; this, however, may not be correct (*vide infra* about middle molecules). The observation that patients treated with continuous ambulatory peritoneal dialysis (CAPD) seem to thrive and survive at considerably lower Kt/Vurea than patients undergoing HD contradicts this assumption as well as the observation that patients treated with low-volume predilution hemofiltration (i.e., using convective transport for solute removal) have been reported to have superior survival and rehabilitation compared with patients undergoing HD despite very low total clearance of small molecules (103). Thus, accumulation of solutes other than urea may correlate better with toxic uremic symptoms and the "residual uremic syndrome" in patients undergoing dialysis (104).

In Vitro *Effects of Urea*

Numerous *in vitro* studies have been performed using different test systems and media containing high concentrations of urea. A number of enzyme systems are inhibited by urea but only at concentrations that are much higher than those occurring in patients with uremia. For a more detailed review of *in vitro* studies of urea see Bergström and Wehle (1). However, urea in concentrations of 1 to 100 mmol/L have been shown to inhibit acetylcholine-induced relaxation of rabbit thoracic aortic rings in a concentration-dependent manner, suggesting that urea interferes with endothelium-derived nitric oxide (NO) production (105).

Urea and Structural Protein Changes

One indirect way by which urea might induce toxicity is by inducing *carbamoylation* of proteins (106). Cyanate, spontaneously transformed from urea, increases as renal function decreases. Acting as a potential toxin, the active form of cyanate, isocyanic acid, carbamoylates amino acids, proteins, and other molecules, changing their structure, charge, and function. The resulting *in vivo* carbamoylation can modify the molecular activity of enzymes, cofactors, hormones, low-density lipoproteins (LDLs), antibodies, receptors, and transport proteins. Carbamoylated molecules can block, enhance, or be excluded from metabolic pathways, thereby influencing the fate of noncarbamoylated molecules. Although not an "all-or-none" phenomenon, urea-derived cyanate and its actions are contributing causes of toxicity in uremia. One such end product is carbamoylated hemoglobin, and it has been demonstrated that the proportion of carbamoylated to total hemoglobin is increased in renal failure (107,108) and that it is a positive correlation between TAC and carbamoylated hemoglobin levels in patients undergoing HD (109). Carbamoylation of total plasma protein and albumin has been found to be increased in renal failure (110–112). The levels of carbamoylated plasma protein were correlated to blood urea concentrations (113). It has been suggested that carbamoylated hemoglobin or plasma protein might be used as a time-integrated urea-derived index of adequate dialysis (107, 109).

Isocyanic acid, $HN=C=O$, the active form of cyanate, reacts irreversibly with multiple lysine sites within a protein forming ϵ-amino-carbamoyl-lysine (ϵ-N-C-lysine) as well as with the nonprotonated amino group of amino acids, forming α-aminocarbamoyl-amino acids (CAAs) from free amino acids (FAAs) (106). When cyanate molecules are consumed because of these reactions, new molecules are formed because of the equilibrium between urea and cyanate. Reversible carbamoylation occurs at the hydroxyl (OH) group of tyrosine, serine, or threonine and the sulfhydryl group of cysteine.

Structural modification by carbamoylation has been in the reduced ligand binding to albumin in uremia (42, 110–112,114). *In vitro* studies show that carbamoylation has an inhibiting effect on actin polymerization. It was suggested that this results in loss of ordered filament structure and shape of the lens fiber cells, thus predisposing to cataract development (115). It is interesting that administration of cyanate for sickle cell disease results in cataracts and peripheral neuropathy (106). LDL that was mildly carbamoylated *in vitro* had lower plasma clearance than unmodified LDL in normal humans. Similarly, LDL isolated from patients with uremia had a reduced plasma clearance after injection in rabbits (116). It may be speculated that the decreased *in vivo* clearance of LDL may contribute to the accelerated atherosclerosis in patients with uremia. Using a polyclonal antibody it has been demonstrated that urea-derived cyanate forms homocitrulline (ϵ-N-C-lysine) in leukocyte proteins in patients with renal failure being treated with PD and that cyanate added *in vitro* to normal polymorphonuclear leukocytes strongly inhibit bactericidal superoxide release (108,117). It was suggested that altered function of leukocytes may result in part from posttranslational modification of proteins by carbamoylation. Increased carbamoylation of tyrosine with formation of N-carbamoyl-tyrosine also has been observed in patients with renal failure, associated with low plasma tyrosine levels. The concentration of carbamoylated tyrosine varied in patients undergoing CAPD in parallel with blood urea (117). Carbamoylation not only alters the activity of various enzymes and hormones and changes the binding, transport, and excretion of LDL; the decrease in the anabolically active FAAs pool by carbamoylation forming CAAs (118) also contributes in part to decreased protein synthesis muscle wasting and anemia in uremia (119).

In conclusion, there is overwhelming evidence that the extreme accumulation of urea in uremia exerts toxic effects. Clinically high concentrations may induce headache, fatigue, nausea, vomiting, glucose intolerance, and bleeding tendency. In addition, urea is one of the few substances that exerts *in vitro* toxic effects at concentrations found in the blood of patients with uremia. However, it should be emphasized that severe uremic gastrointestinal, cardiovascular, mental, and neurologic changes are not observed in patients dialyzed against high urea concentrations (90). The case for protein carbamoylation having a role in uremic toxicity needs to be defined. Obviously it is not possible to explain the wide spectrum of uremic symptoms and signs by urea intoxication only. Urea should be considered a "mild" uremic toxin, and its role in the pathophysiology of uremia is not well defined.

Creatinine

Creatinine, which is nonenzymatically produced from the creatine pool in skeletal muscle but also to some extent is generated from exogenous creatine present in meat, is the major *guanidine* compound retained in patients with diminished GFR. Creatinine routinely is determined in plasma or serum as a measure of impairment of renal function, and it might be expected that a variety of uremic symptoms correlate with the plasma creatinine level; this, however, implies an effective relationship rather than a causal one. In fact, high serum creatinine levels correlate with low mortality in patients undergoing HD, presumably because the creatinine generation rate reflects the size of the muscle mass (96). Creatinine seems to be relatively nontoxic. Large amounts of creatinine have been fed to healthy subjects without any adverse effects (120,121), and animals also tolerate large doses (122).

There is a possibility that metabolites of creatinine formed by bacteria in the gut might be absorbed, accumulating in the body fluids of patients with uremia. In patients with decreased renal function, extrarenal clearance of creatinine is increased (123,124). A larger quantity of creatinine is excreted into the gut and metabolized than in normal subjects (125), which may account for the fact that a portion of endogenously formed creatinine is not found in either the urine or as an increased body pool. The following metabolites have been identified: 1-methylhydantoin, creatine, sarcosine, monomethylamine, glyoxylate–glycolate, and methylguanidine (126).

Guanidines (Other Than Creatinine)

Guanidines in high concentrations inhibit a wide variety of enzymes of biologic interest. Guanidine derivatives are potent inhibitors of mitochondrial respiration *in vitro* (127) and interfere with mitochondrial calcium transport (128). The first evidence of accumulation of guanidines (other than creatinine) in uremia came in 1915, when Foster (129) extracted a toxic base from uremic blood that, when injected into guinea pigs, caused dyspnea, convulsions, coma, and death. Subsequently, this material has been identified as guanidine. Later, numerous studies confirmed that guanidine or guanidinelike compounds are elevated in uremia and hypertension. Guanidino compounds such as methylguanidine and guanidinosuccinic acid are neuroexcitatory agents and perhaps may contribute to the etiology of uremic encephalopathy (130). Uremic concentrations of guanidine compounds, guanidine-succinate, guanidine-proprionate, and guanidine-butyrate inhibit neutrophil superoxide production *in vitro*, and this may compromise host-defense function (131).

Methylguanidine

For many years investigators have been interested in the role of methylguanidine (MG) as a uremic toxin. MG is provided by a diet rich in broth or in boiled beef, which contain large amounts of MG formed from the oxidation of creatinine during boiling. Endogenous production of MG occurs by conversion from creatinine and from arginine (132). Biosynthesis of MG from creatinine takes place in several organs (133). Results from studies using isolated hepatocytes suggest that MG is synthetized from creatine by hepatic microsomes, at least two enzymes are involved (134), and the reaction is stimulated by superoxide radicals (135). In rats with renal failure the conversion of MG from creatinine was found to be considerably higher than in normal rats (136). In the chemical conversion of creatinine into MG, creatol (5-hydroxycreatinine) is an intermediate metabolite (137). Creatol has been isolated from uremic urine and suggested to be a uremic toxin (138). Low-protein diet and essential amino acid supply decrease the serum concentration and urinary excretion of MG in CRF (139), presumably as a result of decreased turnover of arginine. The increase in urinary excretion of MG in uremia is related to the plasma creatinine concentration, which suggests increased production (140).

Specific methods for determination of MG and other guanidines using ion-exchange chromatography or high-performance liquid chromatography (HPLC) (141–143) show that in most patients with uremia MG levels in plasma are below 3 μmol/L. In dogs with acute or CRF changes in plasma methylguanidine paralleled changes in creatinine. The renal clearance of methylguanidine exceeds that of creatinine, suggesting that methylguanidine undergoes tubular secretion (144). There is evidence from tissue determinations in experimental animals, from observations in postdialysis rebound and from injections of labeled MG, that MG, which is a strongly basic compound, accumulates preferentially in the intracellular fluid compartment (140). It is possible that the toxic effects of MG may be obtained despite relatively low plasma concentrations because the toxicity might be exerted within the cells where the concentrations are much higher.

Infusion of MG into dogs caused a syndrome resembling uremia with anorexia, vomiting, diarrhea, pruritus, anemia, altered glucose tolerance, high plasma fibrinogen levels, reduced fibrinolytic activity, defective calcium absorption, stomach and duodenal ulceration, hemorrhage, convulsions, and semi-coma (145). MG inhibits the NO pathway in macrophages (146) and induces relaxation in contraction-stimulated aortic rings (105). However, the concentrations of MG used were considerably higher than those found in uremic sera.

Guanidinosuccinic Acid

Guanidinosuccinic acid (GSA) appears in much higher concentrations both in the plasma and urine of patients with uremia than in normal plasma and urine, suggesting increased production. GSA also concentrates in cerebrospinal fluid to up to 100 times higher levels than in controls (147, 148), reaching levels about 10 to 20 μmol/L. Low-protein diet and essential amino acids diminished the serum concentration and urinary excretion of GSA in CRF (139). Hemodialysis removes GSA as well as other guanidine compounds, and this temporarily may decrease the inhibition of erythrocyte transketolase activity in patients undergoing HD (149).

GSA is formed in the liver by transamidation of arginine to aspartic acid. This is in agreement with the concept that renal failure leads to suppression of glycine amidinotransferase, resulting in a decrease of GAA formation and the transfer of the amidino group of arginine to aspartic acid. A metabolic relationship between urea and GSA was suggested on basis of the strong correlation between serum urea concentration and GSA urinary excretion (148,278). The glycine amidinotransferase activity in the kidney of rabbits with CRF has been reported to be reduced (150). The excretion of GAA is decreased in uremia despite an elevation in plasma concentration (151).

Infusion of GSA to normal rats resulted in suppression of calcitriol synthesis at concentrations similar to those present in uremic ultrafiltrate (152). Behavioral toxicity of intraperitoneally injected GSA was observed in mice, resulting in electrocorticographic changes and convulsions (145, 153). In conclusion, GSA has been reported to exert a variety of toxic effects *in vitro,* but its role as uremic toxin is not clear.

Methylated Arginine Metabolites

Some methylated arginine metabolites such as N-monomethyl-arginine (NMMA), asymmetric dimethyl-arginine (ADMA), and symmetric dimethyl-arginine (SDMA) are present in increased concentrations in plasma of patients with uremia compared to normal subjects (154,155). NMMA and ADMA but not SDMA are competitive inhibitors of the NO pathway and may interfere with regulation of vascular tone by inhibiting vasodilation, thereby contributing to endothelial dysfunction (156). Vallance et al. (157) reported that plasma concentrations of dimethylated arginines are increased in patients with uremia to a level that blocks NO-induced vasodilation and speculated that ADMA might have a role in hypertension of patients with ESRD. However, a study using an alternative analytical technique demonstrates that the plasma concentrations of NMMA and ADMA, although higher in patients with uremia than in controls, were about 10-fold lower than earlier reported (158). Tracer studies in the rat with labeled SDMA indicate that it is a major precursor of endogenous dimethylamine, a putative uremic toxin (159). In a prospective study of 225 patients treated with HD, ADMA (but not SDMA) was shown to be a strong and independent predictor of both overall mortality and cardiovascular outcomes in multivariate analysis (160).

Other Guanidines

A number of other guanidine compounds have been found in increased concentrations in serum from patients with uremia. They include guanidine, guanidinobutyric acid, guanidinopropionic acid, taurocyamine, α-ketogammaguanidinovaleric acid, and homoarginine (147,148).

Guanidinopropionic acid has been reported to inhibit glucose-6-phosphate dehydrogenase *in vitro* (161), and it inhibits lymphocyte proliferation (162). Glycocyamine (and creatinine and creatine) added to postdialysis uremic plasma has been reported to reduce insulin binding to its receptors in erythrocytes (163). High doses of guanidine have been shown to induce alterations in transaminase pattern of liver, kidney, and muscle in the rat (164).

In conclusion, various guanidine compounds accumulate in patients with uremia. However, most *in vitro* and *in vivo* toxic effects have been observed at much higher concentrations than are found in patients with uremia. The role of guanidines as uremic toxins is still not well defined.

Products of Nucleic-Acid Metabolism

Uric Acid and Other Purine Derivates

Uric acid, the end product of purine metabolism in primates, normally is excreted in the urine, but to some extent it also is converted by bacteria in the gut. Moderate hyperuricemia frequently occurs early in the course of chronic renal disease but becomes marked only in the terminal stage of uremia. Functional adaptation of the residual nephrons in CRF results in increased urate excretion per nephron because of both decreased tubular reabsorption and increased tubular secretion.

Hyperuricemia in advanced renal failure only rarely results in manifest gout unless there is a predisposition to this clinical syndrome. Patients with uremic pericarditis have been found to have uric-acid concentrations in the blood exceeding those in patients with uremia without pericarditis, but it is not clear whether there is a causal relationship. Intravenous infusion of 0.5 to 2 g (3 to 12 mmol) uric acid in normal humans raised the serum level as high as 22.4 mg/dL (1.33 mmol/L) without any toxic effects (165). Urate ions are essentially freely filterable, and protein binding does not significantly impair dialyzance (166). Increased concentrations of inosine, xantine, and hypoxantine have been observed in adults and children with uremia (167,168).

It has been demonstrated that purine derivates (urate and theophylline) suppress calcitriol synthesis in rats and inhibit receptor-binding affinity for DNA (169). In patients with renal failure treatment with allopurinol suppresses plasma uric-acid concentration and increases calcitriol concentrations (170).

Pyridine Derivatives

Products of pyridine metabolism also have been isolated from HD fluid and estimated in uremic plasma. Higher plasma levels of *pseudouridine* have been found in patients with uremia than in normal subjects (171,172). The concentration of pseudouridine, and to a lesser extent cytidine, is elevated in cerebrospinal fluid of children with uremia, and it was suggested that elevated pseudouridine might have a role in uremic encephalopathy (168). Pseudouridine excretion is impaired in renal failure, and increased tubular reabsorption contributes to its retention (172). A fraction isolated from urine that inhibits glucose utilization *in vitro* in rat diaphragm has been shown to consist of pseudouridine (173).

Amino Acids, Dipeptides, and Tripeptides

Numerous abnormal amino acid concentrations in plasma have been found in patients with uremia (see Chapter l). Among consistent findings are high concentrations of several nonessential amino acids, decreased concentrations of essential amino acids, and a decreased ratio of phenylalanine/tyrosine and of valine/glycine. These changes are probably not the result of reduced urinary excretion of amino acids, but more likely are caused by nutritional inadequacy or by toxic changes in protein metabolism. Several posttranscriptionally modified amino acids such as hydroxyproline, hydroxylysine, 1-methylhistidine, and 3-methylhistidine are not reused for protein synthesis and accumulate in patients with uremia as a result of impaired renal excretion. There is, however, no evidence that they exert any toxic effects.

Amino acids (free, conjugated, and protein bound) are exposed to an abnormal environment in the patient with uremia and may undergo a variety of alterations such as carbamoylation, glycation, nitration, and oxidation, which may contribute to metabolic and nutritional abnormalities. Carbamoylation of free amino acids may account, in part, for the lower than normal levels of free amino acids in patients with uremia (118).

Tryptophan, which is largely bound to plasma protein (albumin), is abnormally low in uremia despite a normal or raised free tryptophan concentration (174); a low free tryptophan concentration, however, was found in nondialyzed patients on a low-protein diet (175). This reduced binding appears to be part of a more general abnormality in uremia because albumin binding of a number of drugs, such as diphenylhydantoin, digitoxin, and sulphonamides, also is reduced, probably because of competitive binding by other metabolites retained in uremia. Increased muscle intracellular concentrations of nonprotein tryptophan are reported to be present in chronic patients with renal failure (176).

Amino acids used in protein synthesis are of the L-configuration, whereas D-amino acids rarely occur in proteins. However, D-amino acids are detected in microorganisms and some of them may accumulate in stable proteins as a result of *in vivo* racemization. Most free D-amino acids are present in plasma and are excreted in the urine. The total plasma concentrations of D-amino acids, D-phenylalanine and D-tyrosine, are elevated in renal failure, presumably because of depletion of D-amino acid oxidase (177). Whether they exert any toxic effects needs further investigation.

Plasma β-aminoisobutyric acid levels are elevated in uremic plasma, but there is no correlation with plasma levels of urea, creatinine, and uric acid (178). Mice given pharmacologic doses of β-aminoisobutyric acid showed twitching and cramps, and some of them died, at plasma levels that were a hundred times higher than those encountered in patients with uremia.

δ-aminolevulinic acid, a precursor of heme synthesis, is elevated in plasma cerebrospinal fluid, saliva; and erythrocytes from patients with CRF (179). Its urinary excretion is reduced, in keeping with lessened production.

Determination of amino acids and related compounds before and after hydrolysis of deproteinized plasma have revealed the presence of several conjugated amino acids. The concentration of bound amino acids is higher in uremic than in normal plasma (180,181). Some of them may represent dipeptides, whereas others may be of a larger molecular size (see later in this chapter). Much higher concentrations of β-aspartylglycine have been detected in uremic sera than in normal sera; toxicity has been assessed in mice with acute renal failure receiving 1 g/kg body weight, resulting in alterations of behavior, low activity, and low response to stimuli, such as sound and shaking, an hour after the injection (182). In view of the high doses required to obtain toxic symptoms *in vivo,* toxicity in patients with uremia is not substantiated.

Sulfur Amino Acids

The sulfur-containing amino acids—Hcy, cysteine–homocysteine, and cystathionine—have been shown to accumulate in patients with uremia (181–187). Hcy has attracted particular interest because elevated plasma levels are associated with accelerated arteriosclerosis in the general population (see Chapter 7).

The tripeptide glutathione serves as a sulfhydryl buffer and plays a key role in detoxification by reaction with hydrogen peroxide and organic peroxides. Oxidized glutathione levels have been found to be elevated in plasma from CRF patients (as were the levels of malondialdehyde), indicating that patients with uremia are exposed to increased oxidative stress (188).

Methylesterification of erythrocyte-membrane proteins, a reaction involved in recognition of repair of specifically damaged proteins, is impaired in uremia, which is accompanied by a significant increase in intracellular s-adenosylhomocysteine, a potent inhibitor of methyltransferase (189). Erythrocyte-membrane protein methylesterification was found to be reduced in patients with uremia and particularly evident for cytoskeletal component ankyrin, which is known to be involved in membrane stability and integrity. The s-adenosylhomocysteine levels in red blood cells was sevenfold higher in patients with uremia than in normal controls. Based on these data it was suggested that the structural damages accumulating in erythrocyte-membrane proteins are not repaired adequately, which could contribute to the state of disrupted red blood cell function in uremia. It also was reported that formation of s-adenosylhomocysteine from Hcy appears to be increased significantly in erythrocytes *in vitro* when Hcy concentration comparable to the plasma levels in patients with uremia was added to the incubation medium (190).

Homocysteine

In patients with CRF, where atherosclerotic complications are a leading cause of death, elevated plasma Hcy levels occur more frequently than any other conventional risk factor (191). The prevalence of hyperhomocysteinemia is 85% to 100% among patients with advanced CRF and patients being treated with maintenance dialysis (192–194). Hyperhomocysteinemia in CRF is associated with various abnormalities in the concentration of other sulfur amino acids and their metabolites, such as elevated plasma levels of s-adenosylmethionine, s-adenosylhomocysteine, cystathionine, cysteine, cysteinesulfinic acid, inorganic sulfate and glutathione (low levels), and low plasma and muscle taurine levels (190,195–199).

The mechanisms by which plasma total Hcy (tHcy) levels increase in CRF are not fully understood. Possible causes include accumulation of toxic compounds that inhibit metabolism (200), reduced renal clearance, impaired degradation by the kidneys, deficiencies or altered metabolism of vitamins (B_6, folate, B_{12}), and/or abnormally high requirements for these vitamins (201,202). Folate is an important determinant of plasma tHcy and folate deficiency, which may be present in unsupplemented patients with uremia and may contribute additionally to the high prevalence of hyperhomocysteinemia. Aside from the removal of water-soluble vitamins by dialysis in patients with CRF, there are several other causes of vitamin deficiency, including reduced dietary intake, effects of unidentified uremic toxins, and use of medications that may decrease absorption or activity of specific vitamins (see Chapter 7).

Hcy exists in plasma as protein-bound and free forms. More than 70% of plasma tHcy is protein bound, with albumin being the main Hcy binding protein (184). A correlation between plasma tHcy and serum albumin has been reported in CRF in different studies and may be related to the high albumin binding of Hcy (192,203–206). Moreover, plasma tHcy also showed a negative correlation with subjective global nutritional assessment score (high values denote malnutrition), suggesting that malnutrition influences the tHcy plasma levels (192). Stepwise multiple regression analysis revealed that normalized protein equivalent of nitrogen appearance (an indicator of protein intake, based on urea appearance) was an independent predictor of plasma tHcy levels in patients undergoing HD (192,204), indicating that the protein (methionine) intake is a determinant of plasma tHcy in CRF. Thus, nutritional status and serum albumin levels in CRF may play independent roles as determinants of plasma tHcy concentration. This should be taken into consideration when evaluating the role of Hcy as a risk factor for cardiovascular disease (CVD).

Hyperhomocysteinemia is present in the vast majority of patients treated with HD, but patients with CRF with CVD had lower tHcy levels (192). However, the prevalence of hypoalbuminemia, low protein intake, and malnutrition may be more prevalent in the patients with CVD than in those without. Thus, the association between CVD, malnutrition, and hypoalbuminemia partly may explain why plasma Hcy levels were lower in patients with CRF and CVD (192). This apparently paradoxical relationship between tHcy levels and CVD in patients undergoing dialysis does not rule out the possibility that hyperhomocysteinemia is a risk factor for CVD in CRF, considering that even mild hyperhomocysteinemia appears to be a risk factor in the general population and that there is, as yet, no known threshold for the atherogenicity of plasma tHcy levels. Hence, almost all patients may have had longstanding elevated plasma tHcy levels within a range that makes them prone to develop atherosclerosis, whereas other cardiovascular risk factors such as malnutrition, hypoalbuminemia, inflammation, and diabetes mellitus, which lower tHcy, may confound the relationship between CVD and the absolute levels of tHcy. It also is possible that hyperhomocysteinemia is not particularly harmful but that it interacts with other atherogenic factors (e.g., within the redox thiol system), thereby enhancing the risk of CVD (see Chapter 7).

In conclusion, Hcy probably may act as a uremic toxin both by inducing vascular disease and by being a precursor of the highly toxic metabolites such as s-adeninehomocysteine, which perhaps have several effects in biosynthesis, modification, or regulation of various metabolic pathways. However, the final proof that Hcy is a uremic toxin still is lacking.

Aliphatic Amines

Aliphatic amines are formed by bacterial action in the gut: 3-methylamine (TMA) from lecithine and choline and l-methylamine (MMA) from sarcosine, creatinine, and homomethylguanidine. Both TMA and MMA may act as precursors of 2-methylamine (DMA).

Total aliphatic amines, MMA, DMA, TMA and trimethylamine-N-oxide are elevated in uremic plasma, and the concentrations are decreased by dialysis (207–209). The "burden" of uremic toxins was estimated by measuring plasma levels and urinary excretion of dimethylamines and trimethylamines before and after renal transplantation (207), and it was concluded that there is significant intracellular sequestration in renal disease. Patients with severe uremia have increased duodenal concentrations of DMA (49). Sterilization of the gut with broad-spectrum antibiotics decreases the blood concentrations of DMA and TMA with clinical improvement of asterixis, myoclonus, and mental alertness. It was suggested that potentially toxic metabolites in the small intestine may have appreciable nutritional and toxic sequelae in uremia. High duodenal amine levels are associated with abnormal colonization of the small intestine by both anaerobic and aerobic bacteria (50). Aliphatic amines (MA, DMA, ethanolamine, propylamine, isobutylamine, and butylamine) are highly elevated in the gastric juice of patients with acute renal failure, and it was suggested that these amines may induce an activation of the antral G cells, resulting in hypergastrinemia (210).

Aromatic Amines

Aromatic amines are degradation products of the aromatic amino acids (phenylalanine and tyrosine) and are formed by decarboxylation. High concentrations of free and conjugated aromatic amines have been observed in uremic plasma.

Polyamines

Putrescine, spermidine, and spermine are widely distributed in the human body. They are strongly basic, low–molecular-weight compounds that appear to be a universal prerequisite for growth (211). Putrescine, spermidine, and spermine are formed in animal tissues; cadaverine and putrescine also are formed by intestinal bacteria by decarboxylation of lysine and ornithine in the intestine. The urinary excretion of polyamines is increased in cancer patients and in patients with infections. Free polyamines in plasma, expressed as spermine equivalents, are elevated in children and adult patients with uremia, and these elevated concentrations persist following institution of dialysis therapy (212).

The free spermidine concentration is much higher in cells than in plasma. Higher red cell levels of spermidine were found in patients with uremia compared to normal controls, whereas the spermine concentrations were not different (213).

Spermine has been identified as an *in vitro* inhibitor of erythropoiesis in patients with CRF (214,215). Spermine, spermidine, and putrescine exert a significant effect on erythroid colony formation than on granulocyte-macrophage colony formation, and putrescine inhibited the bioactivity of erythropoietin noncompetitively (216). Polyamines (such as spermine, spermidine, putrescine, and cadaverin) have been suggested to play a role in uremic inhibition of erythropoiesis (13). Spermidin–protein conjugates from patients undergoing HD affect etythropoiesis (215). The data suggest that polyamines are uremic toxins that are involved in the anemia of end-stage renal failure. A hypothesis was brought forward that the raised polyamine level in chronic dialysis patients possibly could contribute to accelerated cardiovascular disease observed in patients undergoing dialysis by stimulating proliferation of arterial smooth-muscle cells, a central process in atherogenesis (217).

Indoles

Largely as a result of bacterial action in the gut, tryptophan is deaminated and decarboxylated, giving rise to a number of metabolites (tryptamine, indoleacetic acid, skatole, skatoxyl, indole, indoxyl, indican, and others). By action of tryptophan hydroxylase and tryptophan pyrrolase, a number of biologically active compounds are produced, including 5-hydroxytryptamine (serotonin).

Various indoles have been found in increased concentrations in plasma or in dialysates of patients with uremia (218). These compounds are readily removed by dialysis (219,220). Some of these are carcinogenic pyrolysis products (3-amino-1,4-dimethyl-5H-pyrido-4,3-b-indole [Trp-P-1] and 3-amino-1-methyl-5H-pyrido-4,3-b-indole [Trp-P-2]), which are detected in red cells as well. The carcinogen levels per gram of hemoglobin were elevated significantly. These products have inhibiting effects on platelet function, monoamine oxidase, and dopamine metabolism and are potential uremic toxins (221–224). High concentrations of indoleacetic acid and N-acetyltryptophan suggest increased transamination of tryptophan and a possible defect in renal amino acid acylase in uremia. The concentration of 5-hydroxyindoleacetic acid in brain tissue is high in uremic rats (225). Increased levels of lipofuscin derived from 3-hydroxyanthranilic acid are present in patients with CRF (226).

Low single doses of indole given intraperitoneally to normal rats reduced oxygen consumption, but neither uremic serum nor indole (or cresol, putrescine, methylguanidine, or acetoine) had any effects *in vitro* on tissue respiration (41). Indoxyl (and a furan fatty acid) in concentrations present in the serum of patients with uremia inhibits thyroxine hepatocyte transport in uremia (227).

Indoxyl sulfate, which is strongly albumin bound and inhibits binding of drugs (228), can be removed by oral sorbent base or carbon, as demonstrated in experimental uremic rats (218,229). Indoxyl sulfate also seems to stimulate the progression of glomerulosclerosis in the rat, and a low-protein diet and an oral sorbent reduced the serum levels and the progression (218,230). Indoxyl sulfate is removed also by CAPD (231).

Phenols

Phenols, phenolic acid, and their conjugates have been found in increased concentrations in uremic plasma, cerebrospinal fluid, and dialysate, and it has been suggested that they play a primary role in the pathogenesis of the uremic syndrome (232). Phenols, phenol acids, and their conjugates are formed as a result of the deamination, decarboxylation, and oxidation of the aromatic amino acids tyrosine and phenylalanine. Some of them are products of bacterial action in the gut. Phenolic compounds are conjugated in the liver with glucuronic or sulphuric acid.

Using more specific methods the plasma concentration of several phenolic compounds has been reported to be elevated in renal failure. These include phenol; cresol (233); hippuric acid (234–239); hexachlorobenzene, 1.1-di(4-Chlorophenyl)-2.2-dichloroethane (240); p-hydroxybenzoic acid and p-hydroxyphenylacetic acid (241); o-hydroxyhippuric acid (240); 3- and 4-hydroxyhippuric acid (242) and paraaminohippuric acid (234); phenylacetylglutamine (235); and the norepinephrine metabolites, dihydroxyphenylglycol and vanillylmandelic acid (243). Several of these studies demonstrate that phenols are removed by dialysis treatment. Phenols such as hippuric acid and p-cresol behave like a larger molecule during HD as a result of protein binding (244). It also has been demonstrated that an oral sorbent decreases the serum concentration of phenol and cresol in uremic rats (245). High concentrations of hydroxyphenylacetic acid have been observed in nerves of patients with uremia (246). Hippuric acid and paraaminohippuric acid have been suggested as suitable markers of uremic toxicity (234).

Several *in vitro* studies point to a toxic role of phenols in uremia and suggest that conjugated phenols are toxic as well (247). In a study of the effect of several uremic metabolites on phagocyte-reactive species production, only p-cresol had a significant effect at concentrations similar to those in uremic plasma (248). In conclusion, there is evidence that phenolic compounds retained in uremia may exert toxic effects, especially on membrane transport and metabolism, and that these effects may occur at concentrations present in uremic plasma.

Carbohydrate Derivatives

Myoinositol is a member of the vitamin B complex. It is a natural constituent of food and is synthesized in muscle, liver, brain, and kidneys. The major pathway for myoinositol catabolism requires initial oxidation to D-glycuronate in the renal cortex. In patients with renal failure, the concentration in plasma, cerebrospinal fluid, and cauda equina nerves of myoinositol and urinary excretion of myoinositol are elevated (246,249), suggesting that the production is increased or catabolism is decreased.

Concentrations of erythritol, mannitol, and sorbitol also have been found to be markedly elevated in serum from patients undergoing HD (249). The mannitol concentration in red cells and cerebrospinal fluid also is increased in uremia (250). A relationship was demonstrated between the increase in sorbitol in cerebrospinal fluid and signs of peripheral neuropathy in nondialyzed patients with uremia (250).

The significance is unknown. Metabolites of vitamin C, ascorbic acid-2-sulfate, and ascorbic acid-2-O-β-glucuronide have been identified in uremic plasma (251,252). A double conjugate of glucuronidate and o-hydroxyhippuric acid also has been found to accumulate in patients with uremia (253,254).

3-deoxyglucosone, a potent protein cross-linking intermediate of the Maillard reaction, is present in elevated concentrations in uremic serum (255), and it was suggested that 3-deoxyglucosone may be responsible for uremic complications by promoting the formation of advanced glycosylation end products (256). It should be noted that 3-deoxyglucosone and other reactive aldehydes are found in high concentrations in heat-sterilized glucose-based PD solutions (257).

Maltose and isomaltose appear in elevated concentrations in uremic serum and accumulate further in patients undergoing CAPD receiving a dialysis solution with polyglucose as the osmotic agent (258,259). No toxicity was observed over periods up to 3 months with polyglucose (259). However, mild skin rash is reported to occur in some patients (260).

Several sialylic compounds have been isolated from uremic ultrafiltrate (261), but their role as uremic toxins remains undefined. Several furancarboxylic acids accumulate in renal failure and may act as inhibitors of ligand binding to albumin in uremia (262,263). In conclusion, various carbohydrate derivatives as well as amines, indoles, and phenols all belong to the group of suspected uremic toxins (Table 4.2).

Oxalic Acid

Oxalic acid concentrations are elevated in uremia, with plasma concentrations varying proportionate to plasma urea concentrations (264–271). Patients with end-stage renal failure may have calcium oxalate kidney stones (272), and calcium oxalate crystal deposits have been found in various organs and tissues, most prominent in the myocardium, thyroid gland, kidneys, synovia cartilage, bone, skin, blood vessels, and periodontum (273,274).

It is plausible that calcium oxalate microcrystals may be casually related to CVD and osteoarthritis of patients with ESRD and may be a contributing factor to the progression of CRF. Serum calcium oxalate supersaturation is a consequence of oxalate retention rather than increased local production of oxalate in CRF patients (275). Hemodialysis reduces the plasma oxalate concentration by about 60% (264,265,269,270). Patients being treated with CAPD or HD appear to have about the same plasma oxalate levels (269). Attempts have been made to reduce serum oxalate in patients undergoing dialysis by supplementation of diet with high doses of pyridoxine. The rationale for this being that pyridoxine (vitamin B_6) is the coenzyme for amino transferase, which catalyzes the transamination of glyoxylate to glycine; if this pathway is impaired, the glyoxylate is oxidized to oxalate. The results, however, are conflicting (266,276,277), and high-dose pyridoxine supplementation did not decrease plasma oxalate concentration in a population of patients undergoing HD (271).

High doses of ascorbic acid (vitamin C) (800 mg per day), which is a precursor of oxalate, causes an elevation of plasma oxalate in patients undergoing HD (278), whereas routine supplementation with 100 mg per day has no such effect. Consequently, administration of vitamin C should be restricted to doses necessary to correct vitamin C deficiency.

Oxalic acid suppresses replication and migration of human endothelial cells (524) and inhibits thrombocyte aggregation (279). However, it is not known if these findings have any relevance to uremic toxicity *in vivo*.

In conclusion, the evidence is overwhelming that oxalate is involved in the symptomatology of renal failure by causing secondary oxalosis with calcium oxalate deposition in several organs. Oxalate is by definition a uremic toxin.

Other Metabolites

The organic-acid fraction of hemofiltrates of patients with uremia separated in the form of methyl esters by gas chromatography and mass spectrometry yielded a similar pattern of organic-acid methylates as found in urine from normal individuals. More than 80 different organic compounds were identified (e.g., aromatic acids, aliphatic acids, dicarboxylic acids, phenols, amines, indoles, purines, pyridines, carbohydrates), and nine unknown compounds also were characterized according to their mass spectrometric data (280). N-phenylacetyl-α-amino glutarimide was present in hemofiltrate at levels 50 to 100 times higher than in urine, and the reduction in hemofiltrate concentration with time during treatment was far more rapid than for the other compounds (280).

Serum levels of succinic acid, adipic acid, 3-methyladipic acid, pimelic acid, azelaic acid, and 2.4-dimethyladipic acid also are increased considerably in uremic plasma (281). Xanthopterin, a metabolic end product of the nonconjugated pterins dihydrobiopterin and tetrahydrobiopterin, is elevated in serum and red cells from patients undergoing HD (282). Its protein binding is reduced in renal failure, and it is removed by HD. Because xantopterin is known to inhibit cell growth *in vitro,* it has been suggested to have a toxic role in uremia (282).

Uremic red blood cells have been reported to show increased susceptibility to *in vitro* lipid oxidation (see later in this chapter). Malondialdehyde, which is a secondary breakdown product of unsaturated fatty-acid peroxides, is elevated in patients with CRF (283,284). Malondialdehyde was suggested to be a putative uremic toxin, associated with lipid peroxidation and reduced red cell survival (283,284).

Oxidative Stress and Formation of "End Products"

Uremia is associated with increased oxidative stress, resulting in the production of reactive carbonyl compounds (RCOs) (285) from the metabolism of carbohydrates, lipids, and amino acids. These RCOs react with protein residues forming advanced glycation end products (AGEs) and advanced lipoxidation end products (ALEs) (*vide infra*). Miyata et al. have used the term "carbonyl stress" (285) to describe the excess oxidative formation of carbonyl groups (aldehydes and ketones) in patients with CRF (286,287). Examples of RCOs formed from carbohydrates and ascorbate are glyoxal, methylglyoxal, arabinose, glycoaldehyde, 3-deoxyglucosone, and dehydroascorbate. They react nonenzymatically with protein amino acid groups yielding AGEs such as carboxy methyl-lysine, pentosidine, pyrrotine, imidazolone, and other compounds. Lipid peroxidation of polyunsaturated fatty acids results in metabolites such as malondialdehyde, 4-hydroxynonenal, and other aldehydes as well as acrolein. The myeloperoxidase catalyzed metabolism of hydroxy-amino acids also results in formation of highly reactive aldehydes. The excess oxidant stress in uremia results in oxidative modification in plasma proteins, in particular in albumin (288,289). Increased oxidative stress may act synergetically with uremia to cause carbamoylation of lens proteins, leading to cataract, which is overrepresented in patients with uremia.

Oxidative stress and interactions between NO and reactive oxygen species (ROS) leads to generation of highly reactive and cytotoxic byproducts such as peroxynitrate, which can attack DNA, lipids, and proteins. Peroxynitrate reacts with tyrosine to produce nitrotyrosine. Alternatively, ROS can activate tyrosine to form tyrosol, a radical that may oxidize NO to produce nitrotyrosine. Increased tyrosine nitration of the brain has been demonstrated in rats with renal insufficiency (290).

The low plasma albumin concentration in patients with uremia, and the oxidation of albumin, will decrease plasma antioxidant defenses and increase the likelihood of oxidant stress-induced tissue injury and CVD in these patients. Accumulation of RCOs and "carbonyl stress" in uremia appear to be important components of uremic toxicity, and these compounds are strongly suspected to be uremic toxins. Antioxidant therapy rather than dialysis therapy alone may alleviate these manifestations of uremic toxicity.

MIDDLE MOLECULES AS UREMIC TOXINS

The Middle Molecule Hypothesis

The hypothesis that molecules with a larger molecular size than urea and creatinine might be uremic toxins stems from observations by Scribner and his group in Seattle that suggested that PD, despite less efficiency with regard to dialysis of small molecules, was superior to HD in controlling neuropathy (291), presumably because the peritoneal membrane was more leaky and thus more effective at removing middle molecules (MMs) than the HD membranes (292). The observation that prolongation of dialysis time could arrest or reverse peripheral neuropathy independently of the predialysis values of urea and creatinine also suggested a toxic role of larger molecules than urea and creatinine (293).

These clinical findings formed the basis for the square meter-hour hypothesis (294). This hypothesis relates the efficiency of dialysis to the numbers of hours of dialysis per week and the active membrane surface area. It later was suggested that the term square meter-hour hypothesis should be changed to MM hypothesis (295). Numerous attempts were made to prove or disprove the hypothesis by applying various dialysis strategies specially designed to increase or decrease the presumed level of the MMs in body fluids and relate these changes to the symptomatology of the patient or to the *in vitro* toxicity of plasma or dialysate. Overall, the results were inconclusive. No direct determinations of MMs in plasma were performed in most of these studies.

Based on vitamin B_{12}-clearance studies for various dialyzers and dialysate flow rates, assuming the renal clearance of endogenous MMs to be equal to GFR (endogenous creatinine clearance), a dialysis index was devised that expresses the weekly clearance of MMs (dialysis clearance plus renal clearance) in relation to the minimum "safe" clearance, which was assumed to be 30 L/wk for a standard patient with a body surface area of 1.73 m^2, based on clinical observations (296).

In an attempt to define the adequacy of dialysis and to assess the relative importance of small molecules and MMs as uremic toxins, a prospective randomized multicenter study, the National Cooperative Dialysis Study, was performed in the United States (297). One hundred fifty-one patients were randomly assigned to one of four different dialysis schedules for at least 24 weeks, resulting in either a low or high time-averaged blood urea concentration. The highest morbidity was found in patients with a high average blood urea concentration on a short dialysis schedule, but patients with a high urea concentration on a long dialysis schedule also had higher morbidity than groups of patients with a low average urea concentration on a long or short dialysis schedule. The results emphasize that underdialysis with regard to small molecules is harmful, but they do not exclude a role for MMs in morbidity of patients undergoing HD because length of dialysis seemed to be an independent predictor of the outcome (298).

The MM hypothesis had a great impact on dialyzer and membrane technology and dialysis strategies even before any MMs had been measured in patients undergoing dialysis. More permeable membranes were developed in response to the MM hypothesis, and MM removal (*in vitro* B_{12} and inulin clearances) is taken into consideration when designing new dialyzers. Some of the advantages of treatment modalities such as hemofiltration, hemodiafiltration, CAPD, and charcoal hemoperfusion have been ascribed to efficient removal of MMs.

Larger molecules are removed more efficiently by convective transport than by diffusive transport (299). However, Keshaviah et al. (300), comparing high-efficiency HD and hemofiltration, could find no difference in symptomatology, including nerve-conduction velocity, that could be ascribed to the more efficient removal of MM by hemofiltration. A subsequent report on a larger number of patients is confirmatory in demonstrating that short, high-efficiency HD with presumably adequate MM removal does not result in deterioration of peripheral-nerve function or other toxic effects. Somatic neuropathy of clinical importance now is rare in patients undergoing HD despite shorter dialysis times, perhaps because of improved membrane technology and dialyzer design together with improved control of hyperparathyroidism and better nutrition.

It is well established that patients treated with CAPD may survive and thrive equally well as patients treated with HD despite their average weekly clearance of urea in relation to body mass (Kt/Vurea) being lower than in patients undergoing dialysis. Note, however, that the concept of Kt/Vurea is entirely different in CAPD and HD because K, t, and V differ between the two modalities (301–304). Furthermore, serum urea concentration is stable in CAPD but fluctuates in HD patients. Protein intake (estimated from protein catabolic rate [PCR] by using urea kinetics) is correlated with Kt/Vurea both in HD and CAPD. Note that this partly may be the result of mathematic coupling. However, the relationship between PCR and K/Vurea is different in patients undergoing HD, so that the patients undergoing CAPD require considerably lower Kt/Vurea for the same PCR than the patients undergoing HD and also that with increasing Kt/Vurea the increase in PCR is larger in CAPD than in HD patients (305). This has been explained in favor of MM playing a more important role for uremic anorexia than small molecules, assuming that MM removal is relatively more efficient with CAPD than with HD (305). In fact, direct measurements have shown that patients treated with CAPD have significantly lower levels of MM in plasma than patients undergoing HD (305,306).

Determination and Characterization of MMs

Evidence for the existence of peptidic substances with MM characteristics was brought forward by Cristol et al. (307) in 1938—long before the MM hypothesis was developed. Subsequently, a large number of studies have demonstrated that MM fractions that contain peptides or conjugated amino acids accumulate in plasma or ultrafiltrate from patients with uremia (253,306,308–312), but only a few of these compounds have been fully chemically characterized. Some of these compounds have been characterized as glucuronide conjugates of amino acids (253,308,313).

Several groups have used gel-permeation chromatography of plasma, serum, dialysate, ultrafiltrate, and urine for separation of one or more fractions in the MM-weight range that, in general, were detected by ultraviolet (UV) absorption at different wavelengths (314,315). Most of these studies showed that MMs are present in higher concentrations in uremic than in normal plasma or serum. However, some acidic and other compounds isolated in the gel filtration fraction have lower molecular weights than originally thought (253,308,316).

The MM fractions isolated by soft–gel-permeation chromatography represent a complex mixture of compounds, presumably with different molecular weights, different generation rates, different optical densities, and different biologic activities. Some groups have attempted to separate and characterize the uremic MM fractions obtained by gel filtration further by applying ion-exchange chromatography (310,317–320), electrophoretic methods (315,321,322), and paper or thin-layer chromatography (323).

HPLC affords faster separation, better resolution, and higher sensitivity than conventional liquid chromatography on soft gels. The principles of gel permeation, ion-exchange, reversed-phase, and ion-pair chromatography all can be performed in the HPLC mode. Several groups have used HPLC for separation and isolation of MM compounds (316, 324–330). In one study using HPLC no less than 100 MM peaks were separated (324).

Some MM compounds have been isolated in pure form, and their molecular structures have been identified. For preparation and concentration of larger amounts of material in the MM range, membrane technology has been applied successfully. Reverse osmosis with subsequent lyophilization, followed by desalting procedures, has been used for isolation of peptidic compounds that exhibit toxicity *in vitro* (331,332). Abiko et al. (310), using ultrafiltration, gel-filtration, and ion-exchange chromatography, were able to isolate and characterize five peptides from plasma ultrafiltrate of severely ill patients with uremia.

Using high-voltage electrophoresis, isotachophoresis, mass spectrometry, and enzymatic hydrolysis one of the compounds of a MM fraction (7c) was identified to be glucuronyl-O-hydroxyhippurate (i.e., a conjugate between glucuronic acid and glycine) (253,308). The molecular weight is 371, which is much lower than would have been expected from the behavior in gel-permeation chromatography. This study also showed that this compound is not only an endogenous metabolite that accumulates in uremic plasma but also can be formed from ingested salicylic acid by conjugation with glucuronic acid and glycine (330). Using HPLC and nuclear magnetic resonance (NMR), it later was confirmed that glucuronyl-OH-hippurate is an endogenous metabolite found in normal urine and accumulating in uremic plasma (313). A conjugate of glucuronic acid with o-hydroxybenzoic acid also was identified from uremic plasma and normal urine (254). A glutamine-rich compound was isolated by HPLC and identified as phenylacetyl-glutamine. It subsequently was synthesized (333).

The Necker group in Paris has partly identified a MM compound called b4-2, which appears to be a carbohydrate with neurotoxic properties (334). The b4-2 solute is a glucuronide with a molecular weight of 568. Sialyl compounds in the range between 500 and 2,000 Da is another class of compounds that are found in normal urine but are usually not detectable in serum (261).

Toxic Effects of Crude MM Fractions

Numerous studies of toxic effects of MM have been performed using crude MM fractions isolated by various chromatographic and electrophoretic methods. Among effects reported are the following: inhibition of proliferation of undifferentiated cell lines (332,335) and hematopoietic cell lines (331,336), depression of several immunologic functions (337,338), neurotoxicity (339), polymerization of tubulin (340), increased osmotic fragility of erythrocytes and increased hemolysis (337,341), decreased granulocyte mobility and phagocytosis (342), cardiotoxicity (343), inhibition of platelet aggregation (344,345), blunted effect of somatomedin and insulin on sulfate uptake in cartilage (346), inhibition of glucose utilization (347), insulin resistance (311), inhibition of protein synthesis and amino acid transport (28), inhibition of mitochondrial storage of calcium (348), and reduced binding of drugs to plasma protein (349).

A factor within the molecular-weight range of 750 to 900 has been shown to inhibit osteoclast mitogenesis and could have a potential role in regulation of bone growth and remodeling (350). A 500 to 2,000 dalton subfraction of uremic plasma inhibits apolipoprotein A-1 production by a human hepatoma cell line (22). Degradation peptidic products in uremic plasma containing the RGDS sequence have been found in elevated concentration in uremic ultrafiltrate (351). The material showed an inhibitory effect on fibrinogen binding to control platelets, and it was concluded that these products might be involved in the bleeding defect of uremia.

In most of the aforementioned bioassay studies, MM fractions were present in the medium in approximately the same concentrations as found in uremic plasma. The results suggest that MMs cause or contribute to many symptoms and signs of uremia such as anemia, susceptibility to infection, immunologic incompetence, bleeding, neuropathy, glucose intolerance, and lipid changes. However, many of these studies lack appropriate controls, namely corresponding MM fractions isolated from nonuremic individuals. Furthermore, most *in vitro* experiments only measure acute toxic effects and do not necessarily reflect long-term metabolic effects present in chronically uremic patients. It is also unclear to what extent *in vitro* studies with crude MM fractions using isolated tissues, cell cultures, or enzyme preparations reflect uremic toxicity *in vivo* (i.e., the clinical relevance may be questioned).

A few experimental studies have been reported in which MM fractions were injected or infused into experimental animals. A MM fraction of uremic ultrafiltrate, isolated by membrane filtration, has been demonstrated to inhibit ingestions of orally infused carbohydrate and protein solutions in a dose dependent manner in conscious, free-moving rats (8). MM fractions, derived from uremic plasma ultrafiltrate or normal urine, act in the splanchnic region and/or brain to inhibit food intake; this effect is specific for ingestive behavior, whereas these fractions did not affect the display of sexual behavior (352). These findings lend support to the supposition that one or more MM compounds are causing uremic anorexia.

Clinical Studies of MMs

In most studies of accumulation and elimination of MMs in renal failure, nonspecific methods have been used that measure quantitatively the UV absorption of fractions isolated by gel-permeation chromatography alone or in combination with ion-exchange chromatography. Such studies have shown that the excretion rate for separate fractions or "peaks" varies greatly from patient to patient, suggesting that the generation rate may vary considerably (317).

Most of the UV-absorbing peaks of MMs in plasma are low or absent when the creatinine clearance is higher than 15 mL/min, but they become elevated exponentially as renal function is deteriorated further (353). The renal clearance of different MM fractions, isolated by gel-permeation chromatography, followed by ion-exchange chromatography is higher than, or similar to, the creatinine clearance or inulin clearance (353,354). When compared with inulin clearance, clearance of these fractions is about the same, thus indicating no tubular reabsorption or secretion of these MMs in patients with uremia (354). Similar results were observed in experiments using the isolated rat kidney perfused with uremic hemofiltrated media (i.e., either a clearance of MM similar to GFR or, at low perfusate concentration, evidence of tubular secretion) (355).

"Sick" patients with uremia (such as those with infection, pericarditis, peripheral neuropathy, malnutrition, and severe fluid retention) tend to have higher MMs in plasma than patients free of these complications (356–359). Higher generation rates of MMs in the "sick" patients than in the asymptomatic patients may explain this difference in part (356,358,359). However, there is a considerable overlap of MM levels between "sick" and asymptomatic patients, and it is not possible to correlate the levels of different MM fractions with specific uremic symptoms (360).

Some support of MM involvement in uremic neurotoxicity comes from the observation of a significant degree of inverse correlation between crude MM accumulation and motor nerve-conduction velocity in patients with uremia (361). Correlations have been found between the plasma levels of immunoreactive parathyroid hormone (PTH) and MMs (358,362). This is of interest because PTH has been suggested to be a general uremic toxin and it has been speculated that toxic effects of PTH are mediated by MMs (362).

Several investigators have found that dialysis treatment reduces the plasma concentration of MMs recovered in the dialysis fluid in some studies (318,363). In patients kept on stable HD schedules there is a negative correlation between the plasma concentration of MM fractions with molecular weight around 1,000 Da and dialysis index of MMs (363), but other MM fractions show no significant correlation to dialysis index. The reduction of plasma MM concentrations by standard HD is of the same order of magnitude as the reduction of the concentration of urea and creatinine, despite the higher molecular weights of the MMs. An explanation for this may be that the distribution volume from which these MMs are extracted is limited, approximating extracellular fluid volume.

Comparison of MM measurements in patients in a carefully controlled study of long (7.5 hours) versus short (3.6 hours) HD revealed higher MM levels on short dialysis. The differences were, however, relatively small, indicating that the MMs have a higher dialyzance and therefore a smaller size than what was proposed for MMs separated by gel filtration (>1,000 Da) (318). These results might imply that the MM solutes measured have a higher dialyzance and therefore smaller size than the 1,000 to 2,000 Da proposed for uremic MMs isolated by gel filtration. This conclusion is in agreement with the recent results of the chemical characterization of such MMs (253,308,334).

The elimination of MM substances by a cuprophane dialyzer was found to be sufficiently effective to prevent excessive increases of the plasma level of MMs in stable patients undergoing short-term regular dialysis treatment (353).

Patients undergoing CAPD have been shown to have lower plasma MM levels than patients being treated with intermittent HD (306), confirming the concept that CAPD is a more efficient dialytic method for MM removal. In patients undergoing CAPD, there was a good correlation between the appearance rate of different MM fractions (called 7a, 7b, and 7c) and the protein intake or the urea appearance rate, indicating that a major part of the fractions are products of protein catabolism (1).

Hemoperfusion using activated carbon reduces the concentration of MMs (364–366). It has been claimed that MM removal by hemoperfusion is more efficient than by HD (366); this was, however, not confirmed by others (364, 365). Following renal transplantation, uremic MMs disappear from plasma more rapidly than urea and creatinine (367), presumably because not only the elimination rate but also the generation rate decreases.

In conclusion, there is strong indirect evidence that compounds in the MM-weight range that accumulate in uremia are toxic. However, because most of these compounds are still not fully identified, their role as uremic toxins remains undefined.

ADVANCED GLYCOSYLATION END PRODUCTS

Circulating reducing sugars such as glucose react nonenzymatically with proteins (the Maillard reaction) to initiate a posttranscriptional modification process known as advanced glycosylation (287). Schiff bases are formed by interaction of the reducing sugar with free amino groups, and in the course of days these are rearranged to form Amadori products. Such reversible products slowly are transformed into irregularly cross-linked AGEs, the formation of which have been implicated in the structural and functional alterations of collagen and other long-lived proteins in diabetes and aging (368). AGEs also may be formed by glycosylation of phospholipids, which initiates lipid oxidation with formation of oxidized LDL (369). Circulating levels of oxidized LDL were elevated in patients with diabetes and correlated significantly with lipid AGE levels (369), supporting the concept that AGE oxidation plays an important role in initiating lipid oxidation *in vivo*.

AGEs have attracted interest as potential uremic toxins that may be involved in vascular problems, capillary basement-membrane thickening, and diminished resilience of extracellular matrix and macrophage dysfunction (370). Immunochemical studies indicate that tissue AGEs that form *in vivo* appear to contain a common immunologic epitope (371,372). In patients with diabetes who required HD, the levels of AGE peptides were five times higher than in normal subjects. AGEs also have been identified in β-2-microglobulin amyloid deposits obtained from patients undergoing dialysis (see section on β-2-microglobulin amyloidosis). Conventional HD reduced serum creatinine by 75%, whereas the level of low-molecular AGE peptides fell by only 24%; high-flux dialysis was far more efficient for their removal (372). CAPD patients have about the same AGE peptide levels as patients treated with conventional HD. The AGE normalizes rapidly after renal transplantation.

Pentosidin, which is a fluorescent, bifunctional condensation product of arginine, lysine, and ribose, is formed through the Maillard reaction, which binds strongly to collagen and other proteins. It accumulates in human tissues with age, and its accumulation is enhanced in uremia and diabetes (373–376). Long-term glycosylation of proteins with hexoses leads to pentosidine formation, which requires the presence of oxygen (374). Five-carbon sugars contributing to pentosidine formation could be formed from larger sugars by oxidative fragmentation or from trioses, tetroses, and ketoses by condensation and/or reverse aldol reactions (374).

Odetti et al. (376) quantified pentosidine in serum and erythrocytes using HPLC and found moderately elevated serum levels in patients with diabetes and very high serum and erythrocyte levels in uremia. Takahashi et al. (377) reported that most of the pentosidine in serum is protein bound, requiring hydrolysis of protein to obtain it in free form. The total pentosidine serum level was on average almost 20 times higher than in controls. These observations and the findings that pentosidine is very high in collagen (373) and erythrocytes (376) from patients with uremia suggest that it accumulates because of lack of renal function, presumably because of accumulation of pentosidine precursors, the nature of which is not known. It has been suggested that pentosidine may be a molecular marker for the cumulative damage to proteins in diabetes, aging, and uremia (374). However, the clinical relevance of elevated tissue and plasma levels of pentosidine in patients with renal failure is not established.

During PD, AGEs also may form locally in the peritoneal membrane as a result of reaction with glucose and reactive aldehydes in the form of glucose degradation products (GDPs) present in PD solutions. GDPs are formed during heat sterilization of the PD solution, and new solutions with reduced aldehyde levels have been developed. Although it generally is assumed that glucose and GDPs in the PD solutions mainly have local effects, and not systemic effects, GDPs may contribute to the anorexia caused by PD solutions (378).

The role of AGEs as uremic toxins is not defined, and it is not known if AGEs contribute to increased morbidity and mortality in patients with ESRD. However, AGEs should be considered as suspected uremic toxins.

THE TRADE-OFF HYPOTHESIS

According to the trade-off hypothesis, which was originated by Bricker (40) in 1972, certain humoral factors that may exert toxic effects accumulate in uremia, not as a consequence of reduced renal excretion but because of homeostatic adaptation to the reduced GFR.

Natriuretic Factors

Bricker (40) postulated that a natriuretic hormone, which is stimulated by volume expansion, accounts for decreased fractional reabsorption of sodium in chronic uremia when the glomerular filtration falls. In the end stage of renal failure natriuretic hormone activity is assumed to be excessively high, exerting an inappropriate (toxic) effect on the active transport of sodium and other substances in all body cells.

Elevated plasma concentrations of substances that show digoxinelike activity and inhibit Na, K-ATP-ase have been demonstrated in patients with uremia (379,380). The concentration was not different before and after HD because of strong binding to serum proteins (380). A dialyzable factor was demonstrated to be present in deproteinized plasma from patients with renal failure; it had an inhibiting effect on Na, K-ATP-ase activity *in vitro* but seemed to have no demonstrable role in sodium homeostasis (381). A uremic toxin fraction in the MM range (300 to 2,000 Da) was demonstrated to be more abundant in uremic than in normal erythrocytes (382).

A nonpeptidic, nondigitalislike natriuretic hormone with a molecular weight of 360 was reported to have a strong and rapid effect on sodium transport in various *in vitro* systems (383). When given to intact rats it produces profound natriuresis but little or no kaliuresis. To what extent any of the natriuretic factors identified exert toxic effects on various cells and tissues *in vivo* in patients with uremia remains enigmatic.

Parathyroid Hormone

An example of a trade-off effect is the increased secretion of PTH seen in uremia. The increase of plasma PTH occurs in part as a consequence of phosphate retention, which by decreasing ionized calcium stimulates the parathyroid glands to increase PTH secretion. This in turn tends to lower the phosphate threshold and to increase phosphate excretion, thereby creating a new steady state with normal plasma phosphate and calcium but elevated PTH secretion. In end-stage renal failure the PTH secretion is elevated to an extent that toxic effects are encountered. An important consequence of the increased PTH levels in uremia is the development of bone disease, characterized by osteitis fibrosa. For that reason PTH is by definition a uremic toxin.

PARATHYROID HORMONE AS A GENERAL UREMIC TOXIN

PTH may have several additional toxic effects in uremia, some of which are mediated by increased calcium entry into cells and by exaggerated stimulation of adenosine monophosphate (see Chapter 8). The following uremic manifestations can be induced by excessive plasma levels of PTH: encephalopathy, neuropathy, dialysis dementia, bone disease (Chapter 17), aseptic necrosis, soft-tissue calcification, soft-tissue necrosis, myopathy, pruritus, hypertension, cardiomyopathy, carbohydrate intolerance, hyperlipidemia, anemia, sexual dysfunction, and protein wasting.

PTH has attracted attention as a factor that might interfere with blood pressure regulation and cardiovascular function in uremia. Hypertension is common in primary hyperparathyroidism. Long-term infusion of PTH to normal subjects elicits hypertension (384). In rats with CRF, parathyroidectomy significantly decreases the blood pressure response to calcium infusion, suggesting that the presence of

PTH plays a permissive role for the hypertensive action of hypercalcemia (385).

Myocardial hypertrophy with increased heart calcium content is seen in subtotally nephrectomized rats and is not normalized by parathyroidectomy (386). In another study on subtotally nephrectomized rats the myocardial ATP and phosphocreatine content, the mitochondrial oxygen consumption, and the mitochondrial and myofibrillar creatine phosphokinase activities were decreased, and the myocardial calcium content and calcium uptake increased (387).

Hyperparathyroidism is associated with weakness and wasting; whether this is a specific effect of PTH has been debated (388). Garber found that PTH induces muscle-protein breakdown *in vitro* (389). However, Wassner and Li did not observe any effect of PTH on glucose uptake, protein synthesis, and degradation or amino acid release in rat muscle perfused *in vitro* either with or without insulin (390). Proximal muscle weakness and impaired respiratory muscle strength were reported to improve after parathyroidectomy in a uremic patient (391).

The anemia of CRF also has been suggested to be aggravated by hyperparathyroidism. Improvement of anemia has been observed in patients with renal failure after parathyroidectomy (392).

It has been reported that PTH inhibits erythropoiesis *in vitro*, an effect that can be overcome by adding erythropoietin to the medium (393). However, in a group of patients with varying degrees of renal failure, multivariate analysis showed that plasma PTH itself was not a significant predictor of hematocrit levels or serum inhibition of erythroid progenitor cell growth (394). Adding PTH or its fragments to the medium had no effect on *in vitro* erythropoiesis (394). Similar results have been reported by other investigators (395). One study demonstrates that patients undergoing dialysis with elevated serum PTH had a reduced number of CD4 lymphocytes and high CD8 lymphocytes, compared with patients with normal PTH, suggesting that PTH might have an immunosuppressive effect on T-cell immunity (396).

Increased osmotic fragility of erythrocytes and shortened erythrocyte survival also have been reported to be consequences of secondary hyperparathyroidism (397), which might contribute to the anemia of renal failure. The increased osmotic fragility induced by PTH seems to be mediated by stimulation of Ca-ATPase (398). PTH also decreases red blood cell deformability, an effect that requires the presence of calcium and can be inhibited by the calcium channel blocker verapamil (399). PTH has been reported to accelerate the erythrocyte sedimentation rate, an effect that also seems to be calcium dependent (400).

PTH seems to play a role in the glucose intolerance of renal failure. By using clamp techniques it can be demonstrated that parathyroidectomy can prevent glucose intolerance in dogs with CRF without affecting insulin resistance (401), indicating that PTH in CRF interferes with the ability of the β cells to augment insulin secretion appropriately in response to the insulin-resistant state. In adolescents and young adults the glucose metabolic rate (hyperglycemic clamp) correlates negatively with the PTH level in plasma but improves after parathyroidectomy, with higher insulin concentrations during hyperglycemia but without any effect on insulin sensitivity (402). Improved glucose tolerance and insulin secretion without a change in insulin resistance also is seen in children with uremia after correction of secondary hyperparathyroidism by phosphate restriction and oral phosphate binders (403). Decreased lipid metabolism also has been associated with hyperparathyroidism in CRF (404).

In conclusion, PTH appears to play a role in soft-tissue and organ calcification, metabolic abnormalities of protein, carbohydrate and lipid metabolism, and a variety of other changes seen in patients with uremia including anemia and heart and skeletal muscle dysfunction. PTH is to be considered an established uremic toxin.

HIGH–MOLECULAR-WEIGHT PEPTIDES AND PROTEINS

The normal kidney excretes proteins of a molecular mass less than 50,000 by both luminal and contraluminal uptake in the proximal tubular cells, where they are degraded. It therefore would not be surprising if chronic uremia with lack of renal tissue would lead to accumulation of biologically active and potentially toxic compounds with a higher molecular weight than middle molecules. Some low–molecular-weight proteins appearing in increased concentrations in renal failure are α2-microglobulin (β2-M), α1-icroglobulin, β2-microglobulin, leptin, lysozyme, retinal-binding protein, β2-glucoprotein, amylase, and ribonuclease (RNase). High-molecular proteins such as granulocyte-inhibiting protein, degranulation-inhibiting protein, and complement factors as well as proinflammatory cytokines with a molecular weight of more than 15,000 isolated from normal and uremic urine or from uremic plasma ultrafiltrate or dialysate have been shown to exert several adverse effects *in vitro*.

Thus, *in vitro* studies suggest a role for high–molecular-weight compounds in causing uremic toxicity. Considering the fact that such compounds are not readily removed by conventional dialysis treatment and that patients with uremia can be kept alive and thriving on intermittent dialysis, it initially was believed that these are not major uremic toxins. This has, however, proved to be wrong in light of recent findings that chronic accumulation of β2-M may cause a new form of amyloidosis in patients hemodialyzed for more than 6 to 8 years. Furthermore, the annual mortality rate in patients undergoing dialysis is still as high as 10% to 20%, indicating that dialysis treatment is inadequate in correcting uremia and its consequences.

Also, there are not only quantitative but also qualitative changes of peptides and proteins in uremia. One prominent feature of uremia is the progressive and irreversible alteration of proteins because of nonenzymatic modification of amino acids by carbamoylation, forming advanced carbamoylated end products (ACEs) (106), AGEs (405), ALEs (405), and advanced oxidation protein products (AOPPs) (406). Oxidation of albumin is enhanced in the presence of uremic toxins (407). Some of these alterations are part of the aging process, but these degenerative changes are largely accelerated in uremia.

Thus, peptides and proteins are modified by low-molecular compounds accumulating in uremia. Isocyanic acid, spontaneously formed from urea, results in carbamoylation and development of ACEs (106). Glucose and other carbohydrates undergo oxidative and nonoxidative reactions yielding metabolites that are linked with amino groups of several proteins forming AGEs (405). Lipids including polyunsaturated fatty acids undergo lipid peroxidation, forming malondialdehyde and other lipid peroxidation products, modifying proteins into ALEs (405). Oxidative stress, and reactive carbonyl compounds accumulating in uremia, result in AOPPs (408). These changes result in impaired biologic functions of peptides and proteins, and thus may contribute to the uremic syndrome. The possible detrimental role of proinflammatory cytokines in the development of the MIA syndrome (409–415), which is associated with most premature deaths in patients undergoing dialysis, has emerged as a major new field in regard to uremic toxins (see later in this chapter and Chapter 13).

β2-Microglobulin and Dialysis-Related Amyloidosis

Introduction

β2-M first was isolated from human urine and characterized by Berggård and Beam in 1968 (416). It is a small globular protein with a molecular weight of 11,815. β2-M is present on the plasma membranes of all mammalian cells, except erythrocytes and thrombocytes. It constitutes the light (invariable) chain of the major histocompatibility complex (human leukocyte antigen, or HLA, class I). When the HLA complex is degraded, β2-M is separated from the heavy chain and transferred to the extracellular fluid—a phenomenon called "shedding."

The normal serum concentration of β2-M is 1.0 to 2.5 mg/L. The renal elimination of β2-M is reduced in patients with renal failure; the serum level of β2-M correlates directly with the serum creatinine level and inversely with the GFR. The serum β2-M concentration in patients undergoing dialysis can be elevated up to 50-fold (i.e., to about 50 mg/L or more), but if residual renal function is present the concentration is lower (417,418).

More than 95% of circulating β2-M in patients with uremia is in monomeric form, but the occurrence of complex formations of β2-M with circulating macromolecules as glycoproteins and immunoglobulins also has been demonstrated (419).

β-2-Microglobulin Amyloidosis

Since 1975, several authors have reported an abnormally high incidence of carpal tunnel syndrome (CTS) in chronic HD patients, a complication that is in general only observed after more than 6 years of dialysis and seems to increase with the time on dialysis. It also has been noted that patients with CTS exhibit signs and symptoms in joints, especially in the shoulder. Destructive arthropathy and bone lesions include generalized arthritis, scapulohumeral periarthritis, and arthropathy with joint effusions. The main symptoms include inflammation with stiffness and spontaneous fractures.

Joint symptoms first appear after 7 to 10 years of HD treatment and often coincide with the CTS symptoms. The symptoms are more common in patients who are older than 40 years of age on admission for HD and seem to occur earlier after start of dialysis treatment with increasing age. The incidence of arthropathy is particularly high in centers where patients have been treated for 10 years or more. In 1985, Gejyo et al. (418) showed that the main constituent of free amyloid deposits found in CTS and in dialysis arthropathy is β2-M. The percentage of patients who require surgery for CTS increases greatly, from very low for those being treated with HD for less than 8 years, to 50% for those treated for 14 years, to 100% for those treated for 20 years (418).

Pathogenesis

Several studies have been made to identify additional factors that may be of importance for the development of β2-M amyloidosis (1,417,418,420). Among factors implicated to be of pathophysiologic importance are structural modifications of the β2-M molecule; AGEs; free radicals; cytokines; deposition of iron, calcium, and aluminum. Membrane bioimcompatibility also has been suggested to be of importance. It has been demonstrated that the β2-M from most of the amyloid fibrils isolated from connective tissue of patients treated with HD consists of acidic β2-M, and that acidic β2-M from the urine of patients treated with HD but not β2-M from normal subjects has brown color and fluorescence, which is characteristic for AGEs formed by the Maillard reaction. The acidic β2-M as well as the amyloid fibrils reacted with anti-AGE antibody. Niwa et al. reported that AGEs are present both in the amyloid deposits from patients with uremia and in infiltrating macrophages surrounding the amyloid deposits (421).

Elimination of β2-M

The major site of breakdown of β2-M is the kidney, where it is filtered in the glomeruli and reabsorbed and degraded in the proximal tubular cells. Extrarenal catabolism contributes only about 3% of the total elimination of β2-M.

Hemodialysis membranes of regenerated cellulose (cuprophane) are almost impermeable to β2-M, and thus do not contribute to its removal. Synthetic membranes for HD, hemofiltration and hemodiafiltration—the high-flux membranes—have larger pore sizes and higher molecular-weight cutoffs and are more efficient and more suitable for removal of larger molecules such as β2-M, especially if used in the hemofiltration mode. An additional factor contributing to the elimination of β2-M when using such membranes is the adsorption of circulating β2-M onto the membrane (422).

Using the same polysulfone membrane for HD and hemofiltration, it was shown that β2-M was removed more efficiently by convective than by diffusive transport (423–429). By using a high-flux, biocompatible acrylonitrile membrane for dialysis, about 500 mg β2-M per week is eliminated (425) (i.e., insufficient amounts compared to the production of β2-M in healthy subjects, which is in the order of about 1,500 mg per week). During hemofiltration, about 1,000 mg/week of β2-M may be eliminated (i.e., still less than the daily production but considerably more than with HD) (429), thus being potentially beneficial for preventing or delaying the onset of amyloidosis.

CAPD eliminates 140 to 320 mg per week of β2-M (430). Thus, PD clears β2-M better than HD with cuprophane. The β2-M plasma levels in CAPD patients have been reported to be about the same in patients undergoing HD (427,431), but most reports document lower levels of β2-M than in patients on HD (432,433).

The development of β2-M amyloidosis has been observed most persistently in long-term HD patients who also constitute the largest group of patients being treated with renal replacement therapy. Considering that dialysis with low-flux membranes are impermeable to β2-M, one might expect that treatment by methods that remove β2-M might be better, resulting in either delayed onset or, at best, reduction of amyloid deposits and its related symptoms.

In conclusion, β2-M has been recognized as the major precursor protein of dialysis-related amyloidosis in long-term dialysis treatment. β2-M and, in particular, AGE-modified β2-M, should be recognized as an established uremic toxin.

Leptin

The discovery of the *ob* gene product leptin (16 kD) has increased our understanding of the physiologic system that regulates eating behavior. Recent studies have demonstrated that most, but not all, patients with ESRD have inappropriately high leptin levels (434,435). It has been speculated that leptin may be a uremic toxin that mediates anorexia and wasting (436). Serum-free leptin levels are elevated, whereas serum-bound leptin levels remain stable in patients with ESRD (437). Besides regulating appetite, leptin also may play a role in insulin metabolism, sodium handling, hematopoiesis, and bone formation in patients with ESRD (438).

As the kidneys clear other polypeptide hormones, it seems reasonable to surmise that leptin also accumulates in the case of renal failure as a result of reduced renal clearance. Indeed, the kidney is the principal site of elimination of circulating leptin in healthy subjects (439). Moreover, an inverse correlation between leptin and GFR has been demonstrated in patients with various degrees of renal failure (440), and in rats bilateral nephrectomy reduces plasma leptin clearance by 80% (441). Recent *in vivo* studies in rats show that uptake and degradation of leptin by renal tissue is the main mechanism of elimination (442). The important role of the kidney in leptin metabolism is underscored further by the fact that renal transplantation normalizes leptin levels (443).

Not all patients with ESRD have elevated leptin levels (444), and some patients even have low leptin levels, suggesting that other tissues such as splanchnic organs contribute to leptin removal (445). Moreover, because patients with ESRD have lower leptin mRNA levels than controls, this could suggest that decreased plasma leptin clearance is a part of the efferent feedback loop that down-regulates the expression of the *ob* gene in hyperleptinemic ESRD patients (440). However, other factors associated with ESRD, such as hyperinsulinemia and inflammation, may affect leptin levels (438). It also should be pointed out that female gender and obesity are important factors that affect serum leptin levels in patients with ESRD (438).

Although there is as yet no direct evidence that increased levels of leptin cause anorexia, some indirect evidence suggests that leptin may mediate anorexia in patients with ESRD (436,446,447). Moreover, it has been shown that high levels of serum leptin relative to fat mass might be associated with weight loss in patients undergoing HD (448), and increasing serum leptin levels are associated with a loss of lean body mass in patients treated with CAPD (449). However, because others find no association between the leptin concentration and recent change in weight or nutritional status in ESRD (435,450), the question if elevated serum leptin levels cause anorexia is open.

Taken together, although hyperleptinemia is a common phenomenon in patients with ESRD, it is not a ubiquitous finding. Moreover, although some indirect evidence suggests that elevated leptin levels might cause anorexia, not all studies have found such a relationship. Accordingly, on the basis of the present amount of knowledge, leptin can be regarded only as a suspected uremic toxin.

Granulocyte-Inhibiting Proteins and Degranulation-Inhibiting Proteins

The group of Hörl et al. (451) isolated from uremic ultrafiltrate a uremic polypeptide (GIP I) with inhibiting effects on glucose uptake, chemotaxis, oxidative metabolism, and intracellular bacterial killing and speculated that this protein might be responsible for the leukocyte dysfunction commonly seen in patients with uremia. The protein has a molecular weight of 28,000 Da and shows strong homology with a 10,000 Da-protein representing the variable part of the kappa-light chain of patients suffering from rheumatoid arthritis or β-cell lymphoma and other kappa-light chains. Later the same group has isolated a second granulocyte inhibitor protein (GIP II) with a molecular weight of approximately 9,500 Da that cross-reacts with assays for intact β2-M. Also, this peptide has inhibitory effects on oxidative metabolism and glucose uptake in granulocytes.

Another protein with inhibitory effect on release of lactoferrin, collagenase, and gelatinase from granulocytes with a molecular weight of about 14,000 Da, called degranulation-inhibiting protein (DIP I), also was purified from uremic ultrafiltrates (451). Finally, the same group identified a fourth protein, DIP II, identified as complement factor D (452). It is still unclear to what extent these newly isolated polypeptides cause or contribute to increased sensitivity to infection in patients with uremia.

Complement Factors

Highly elevated plasma levels of the immunosuppressive complement fragment Ba with a molecular weight of 33,000 Da have been observed in patients undergoing regular dialysis, presumably because renal catabolism of this small-molecular protein is impaired (453). Factor D, an essential enzyme in the alternative pathway of complement activation also is increased tenfold in serum of patients with end-stage renal failure (454). It was speculated whether this might lead to enhanced formation of C5a during dialysis or whether it could be beneficial by increasing the solubilization of immune precipitates. The possible role of complement components as uremic toxins and, in particular, their potential role as mediators of microinflammation was reviewed in 2001 (455).

Proinflammatory Cytokines

Most premature deaths in patients with ESRD are associated with the presence of the MIA syndrome, which is an important part of the residual uremic syndrome, although it is in part caused by coexisting comorbidity (409,410,412, 414,415,456,457). Inflammation, as evidenced by elevated C-reactive protein (CRP) (412,458) or proinflammatory cytokine (459,460) levels, has been shown to predict malnutrition and cardiovascular and/or total mortality in patients with ESRD with or without ongoing dialysis treatment. The prevalence of elevated CRP (>8 to 10 mg/L) in predialysis and dialysis patient populations is high and ranges between 30% and 50% (461). The role of inflammation in malnutrition, morbidity, and mortality in patients with CRF is discussed in Chapter 13.

The causes of inflammation in patients with ESRD are probably multifactorial. However, because the prevalence of inflammation is high already at the predialysis stage (411, 462), it is evident that factors unrelated to the dialysis procedure, such as comorbidity and decreased renal clearance of proinflammatory cytokines, contribute. Available studies suggest that the proinflammatory cytokine system activity is elevated in patients with ESRD (460,463), and several lines of evidence suggest that decreased renal clearance might play an important role. At first, strong positive correlations between GFR and various cytokines have been found in undialyzed patients at various stages of ESRD (462). Second, lower urinary soluble interleukin-6 receptor (SIL-6R) excretion has been documented in patients with ESRD compared with controls (464). Finally, animal experiments have shown that the plasma half-life of IL-1α was increased after nephrectomy, suggesting that the kidneys are the main organs through which IL-1α is excreted (465). However, as the half-life of various cytokines is short and local tissue cytokine inactivation may be the most important pathway of cytokine degradation, more research is needed to determine the relative importance of the kidney in cytokine clearance.

Nevertheless, as data have suggested that accumulation of tumor necrosis factor-α (TNF-α) may contribute to the development of neurologic, hematologic, and nutritional complications in uremia, it has been suggested that TNF-α indeed may be considered as a uremic toxin (466). It is notable that many symptoms and findings prevalent in the uremic syndrome, such as anorexia, fatigue, depression, weight loss, decreased gastric emptying, and intestinal bleeding, are known to be associated with elevated levels of proinflammatory cytokines (467). It is interesting that data have demonstrated that on a per gram basis proinflammatory cytokines are more anorexigenic than leptin and that proinflammatory cytokines produce anorexia of greater magnitude with far lower doses (468).

The MIA syndrome has strong links with oxidative stress, which may cause inflammation. It also has links with endothelial dysfunction, as discussed in Chapter 13.

In conclusion, proinflammatory cytokines, such as IL-6 and TNF-α, are elevated in patients with ESRD, in part because of decreased renal clearance, but it is not yet known whether elevated levels of cytokines are the consequence of uremia or the result of comorbidities such as cardiovascular disease, infection, and systemic diseases. Moreover, it has not yet been determined whether anticytokine therapies including removal of cytokines will reduce any specific uremic symptoms. Accordingly, on the basis of the present knowledge, proinflammatory cytokines could be regarded as suspected but not as established uremic toxins.

GENERAL CONCLUSIONS

The emphasis in the quest for the uremic toxins has shifted from small–molecular-weight inorganic and organic compounds during the 1960s and before, to middle molecules during the 1970s and to PTH and β2-M and other low–molecular-weight proteins during the 1980s. During the last decade, the research has more and more focused on high–molecular-weight proteins as well as on alterations in amino acids, peptides, and proteins and formation of various end products such as AGEs.

During the past decades, considerable effort and time have been spent by scientists on the isolation and identification of toxic substances that cause various uremic symptoms. However, despite impressive advances within this research, it remains to be found which compounds cause the most typical and clinically important uremic manifestations, such as anorexia, neurologic disturbances, and low-grade inflammation. Uremia is a syndrome with multifactorial pathogenesis, and we are still far from a complete understanding of all aspects of uremic toxicity. Further research hopefully will elucidate the basic mechanisms involved in uremic toxicity, resulting in the development of improved diagnostic methods and more efficient therapeutic methods to remove uremic toxins and prevent their accumulation.

ACKNOWLEDGMENTS

This chapter is a revised version of the chapter on uremic toxicity by Jonas Bergström in the previous edition of this book (469), which contains a larger number of earlier references. Jonas Bergström started to revise this chapter but died on August 17, 2001. We the coauthors are grateful for the inspiration and teaching of this truly great nephrologist, scientist, mentor, and friend.

We thank Ms. M. Johansson, Dr. A.R. Tony Qureshi, and Dr. E. Garcia-Lopez for valuable assistance in the preparation of this chapter.

REFERENCES

1. Bergström J, Wehle B. Clinical implications of middle and larger molecules. In: Nissenson A, Fine R, Gentile D, eds. *Clinical dialysis.* Norwalk, CT: Appleton & Lange, 1995:204–234.
2. Vanholder R, De Smet R, Lameire NH. Redesigning the map of uremic toxins. *Contrib Nephrol* 2001;133:42–70.
3. Horl WH. Uremic toxins: new aspects. *J Nephrol* 2000;13 Suppl 3:S83–S88.
4. Cunningham JN Jr, Carter NW, Rector FC Jr, et al. Resting transmembrane potential difference of skeletal muscle in normal subjects and severely ill patients. *J Clin Invest* 1971;50(1):49–59.
5. Bilbrey GL, Carter NW, White MG, et al. Potassium deficiency in chronic renal failure. *Kidney Int* 1973;4(6):423–430.
6. Cotton JR, Woodard T, Carter NW, et al. Resting skeletal muscle membrane potential as an index of uremic toxicity. A proposed new method to assess adequacy of hemodialysis. *J Clin Invest* 1979;63(3):501–506.
7. Patel SR, Ke HQ, Hsu CH. Regulation of calcitriol receptor and its mRNA in normal and renal failure rats. *Kidney Int* 1994;45(4):1020–1027.
8. Anderstam B, Mamoun AH, Sodersten P, et al. Middle-sized molecule fractions isolated from uremic ultrafiltrate and normal urine inhibit ingestive behavior in the rat. *J Am Soc Nephrol* 1996;7(11):2453–2460.
9. Lipman JJ, Lawrence PL, DeBoer DK, et al. Role of dialysable solutes in the mediation of uremic encephalopathy in the rat. *Kidney Int* 1990;37(3):892–900.
10. Motojima M, Nishijima F, Ikoma M, et al. Role for "uremic toxin" in the progressive loss of intact nephrons in chronic renal failure. *Kidney Int* 1991;40(3):461–469.
11. Wallner SF, Vautrin RM, Kurnick JE, et al. The effect of serum from patients with chronic renal failure on erythroid colony growth in vitro. *J Lab Clin Med* 1978;92(3):370–375.
12. Mitelman M, Levi J, Djaldetti M. Functional activity of uremic erythroblast incubated in autologous and homologous plasma. *Blut* 1979;38(6):467–471.
13. Macdougall IC. Role of uremic toxins in exacerbating anemia in renal failure. *Kidney Int Suppl* 2001;78:S67–S72.
14. Donati D, Degiannis D, Raskova J, et al. Uremic serum effects on peripheral blood mononuclear cell and purified T lymphocyte responses. *Kidney Int* 1992;42(3):681–689.
15. Asaka M, Iida H, Izumino K, et al. Depressed natural killer cell activity in uremia. Evidence for immunosuppressive factor in uremic sera. *Nephron* 1988;49(4):291–295.
16. Wessel-Aas T. The effect of serum and plasma from haemodialysis patients on human mononuclear phagocytes cultured in vitro. *Acta Pathol Microbiol Scand [C]* 1981;89(6):345–351.
17. Wratten ML, Tetta C, De Smet R, et al. Uremic ultrafiltrate inhibits platelet-activating factor synthesis. *Blood Purif* 1999;17(2-3):134–141.
18. Cohen G, Rudnicki M, Horl WH. Uremic toxins modulate the spontaneous apoptotic cell death and essential functions of neutrophils. *Kidney Int Suppl* 2001;78:S48–S52.
19. Weisensee D, Low-Friedrich I, Riehle M, et al. In vitro approach to 'uremic cardiomyopathy.' *Nephron* 1993;65(3):392–400.
20. Matsumoto A, Yamasaki M, Yonemura K, et al. Depression of nerve-mediated smooth muscle contractions in vitro by plasma of an anephric rabbit and uremic patients. *Jpn J Physiol* 1981;31(6):947–956.
21. Delaporte C, Gros F, Anagnostopoulos T. Inhibitory effects of plasma dialysate on protein synthesis in vitro: influence of dialysis and transplantation. *Am J Clin Nutr* 1980;33(7):1407–1410.
22. Kamanna VS, Kashyap ML, Pai R, et al. Uremic serum subfraction inhibits apolipoprotein A-I production by a human hepatoma cell line. *J Am Soc Nephrol* 1994;5(2):193–200.
23. Kramer HJ, Gospodinov D, Kruck F. Functional and metabolic studies on red blood cell sodium transport in chronic uremia. *Nephron* 1976;16(5):344–358.
24. Russell JE, Avioli LV. The effect of chronic uremia on intestinal mitochondrial activity. *J Lab Clin Med* 1974;84(3):317–326.
25. Lindner A, Gagne ER, Zingraff J, et al. A circulating inhibitor of the RBC membrane calcium pump in chronic renal failure. *Kidney Int* 1992;42(6):1328–1335.
26. White AG, Nachev P. Uremic inhibition of purine uptake by rat hepatic slices. *Am J Physiol* 1975;228(2):436–440.
27. Orringer EP, Weiss FR, Preuss HG. Azotaemic inhibition of organic anion transport in the kidney of the rat: mechanisms and characteristics. *Clin Sci* 1971;40(2):159–169.
28. Cernacek P, Spustova V, Dzurik R. Inhibitor(s) of protein synthesis in uremic serum and urine: partial purification and rela-

tionship to amino acid transport. *Biochem Med* 1982;27(3): 305–316.

29. Patel SR, Ke HQ, Vanholder R, et al. Inhibition of nuclear uptake of calcitriol receptor by uremic ultrafiltrate. *Kidney Int* 1994;46(1):129–133.
30. Yukawa S, Tone Y, Sonobe M, et al. Study on the inhibitory effect of uremic plasma on lipoprotein lipase. *Nippon Jinzo Gakkai Shi* 1992;34(9):979–985.
31. Young GA, Parsons FM. Impairment of phenylalanine hydroxylation in chronic renal insufficiency. *Clin Sci* 1973;45(1): 89–97.
32. Sohn HJ, Stokes GS, Johnston H. An Na, K ATPase inhibitor from ultrafiltrate obtained by hemodialysis of patients with uremia. *J Lab Clin Med* 1992;120(2):264–271.
33. Deray G, Pernollet MG, Devynck MA, et al. Plasma digitalislike activity in essential hypertension or end-stage renal disease. *Hypertension* 1986;8(7):632–638.
34. Stokes GS, Willcocks D, Monaghan J, et al. Measurement of circulating sodium-pump inhibitory activity in uraemia and essential hypertension. *J Hypertens Suppl* 1986;4(6):S376–S378.
35. Pazmino PA, Sladek SL, Weinshilboum RM. Thiol S-methylation in uremia: erythrocyte enzyme activities and plasma inhibitors. *Clin Pharmacol Ther* 1980;28(3):356–367.
36. Yalouris AG, Lyberatos C, Chalevelakis G, et al. Effect of uremic plasma on mouse liver delta-aminolevulinic acid synthetase activity. *Clin Physiol Biochem* 1986;4(6):368–371.
37. Kuriyama M, Mizuma A, Yokomine R, et al. Erythrocyte transketolase activity in uremia. *Clin Chim Acta* 1980;108(2): 169–177.
38. Sterzel RB, Semar M, Lonergan ET, et al. Relationship of nervous tissue transketolase to the neuropathy in chronic uremia. *J Clin Invest* 1971;50(11):2295–2304.
39. Warnock LG, Cullum UX, Stouder DA, et al. Erythrocyte transketolase activity in dialysis patients with neuropathy. *Biochem Med* 1974;10(4):351–359.
40. Bricker NS. On the pathogenesis of the uremic state. An exposition of the "trade-off hypothesis." *N Engl J Med* 1972;286(20): 1093–1099.
41. Hohenegger M, Vermes M, Esposito R, et al. Effect of some uremic toxins on oxygen consumption of rats in vivo and in vitro. *Nephron* 1988;48(2):154–158.
42. Okada K, Takahashi Y, Okawa E, et al. Relationship between insulin resistance and uremic toxins in the gastrointestinal tract. *Nephron* 2001;88(4):384–386.
43. Dhondt A, Vanholder R, Van Biesen W, et al. The removal of uremic toxins. *Kidney Int Suppl* 2000;76:S47–S59.
44. Powell D, Bergström J, Dzurik R, et al. Toxins and inhibitors in chronic renal failure. *Am J Kidney Dis* 1986;7(4):292–299.
45. Vanholder R, De Smet R, Lameire N. Protein-bound uremic solutes: the forgotten toxins. *Kidney Int Suppl* 2001;78: S266–S270.
46. Gulyassy PF, Bottini AT, Stanfel LA, et al. Isolation and chemical identification of inhibitors of plasma ligand binding. *Kidney Int* 1986;30(3):391–398.
47. Einheber A, Carter D. The role of the microbial flora in uremia. I. Survival times of germfree, limited-flora, and conventionalized rats after bilateral nephrectomy and fasting. *J Exp Med* 1966;123(2):239–250.
48. Carter D, Einheber A, Bauer H, et al. The role of the microbial flora in uremia. II. Uremic colitis, cardiovascular lesions, and biochemical observations. *J Exp Med* 1966;123(2):251–266.
49. Simenhoff ML, Saukkonen JJ, Burke JF, et al. Amine metabolism and the small bowel in uraemia. *Lancet* 1976;2(7990): 818–821.
50. Simenhoff ML, Saukkonen JJ, Burke JF, et al. Bacterial populations of the small intestine in uremia. *Nephron* 1978;22(1-3): 63–68.
51. Periyasamy SM, Chen J, Cooney D, et al. Effects of uremic serum on isolated cardiac myocyte calcium cycling and contractile function. *Kidney Int* 2001;60(6):2367–2376.
52. Bushinsky DA. The contribution of acidosis to renal osteodystrophy. *Kidney Int* 1995;47(6):1816–1832.
53. Kraut JA. The role of metabolic acidosis in the pathogenesis of renal osteodystrophy. *Adv Ren Replace Then* 1995;2(1):40–51.
54. Lefebvre A, de Vernejoul MC, Gueris J, et al. Optimal correction of acidosis changes progression of dialysis osteodystrophy. *Kidney Int* 1989;36(6):1112–1118.
55. Bergström J, Wang T, Lindholm B. Factors contributing to catabolism in end-stage renal disease patients. *Miner Electrolyte Metab* 1998;24(1):92–101.
56. Kopple JD. Pathophysiology of protein-energy wasting in chronic renal failure. *J Nutr* 1999;129(I S Suppl):247S–251S.
57. Lim VS, Kopple JD. Protein metabolism in patients with chronic renal failure: role of uremia and dialysis. *Kidney Int* 2000;58(1):1–10.
58. May RC, Kelly RA, Mitch WE. Metabolic acidosis stimulates protein degradation in rat muscle by a glucocorticoid-dependent mechanism. *J Clin Invest* 1986;77(2):614–621.
59. May RC, Kelly RA, Mitch WE. Mechanisms for defects in muscle protein metabolism in rats with chronic uremia. *J Clin Invest* 1987;79:1099–1103.
60. Hara Y, May RC, Kelly RA, et al. Acidosis, not azotemia, stimulates branched-chain, amino acid catabolism in uremic rats. *Kidney Int* 1987;32(6):808–814.
61. May RC, Hara Y, Kelly RA, et al. Branched-chain amino acid metabolism in rat muscle: abnormal regulation in acidosis. *Am J Physiol* 1987;252(6 Pt 1):E712-E718.
62. Mitch WE, Medina R, Grieber S, et al. Metabolic acidosis stimulates muscle protein degradation by activating the adenosine triphosphate-dependent pathway involving ubiquitin and proteasomes. *J Clin Invest* 1994;93(5):2127–2133.
63. Papadoyannakis NJ, Stefanidis CJ, McGeown M. The effect of the correction of metabolic acidosis on nitrogen and potassium balance of patients with chronic renal failure. *Am J Clin Nutr* 1984;40(3):623–627.
64. Williams B, Hattersley J, Layward E, et al. Metabolic acidosis and skeletal muscle adaptation to low protein diets in chronic uremia. *Kidney Int* 1991;40(4):779–786.
65. Rodriguez NR, Miles JM, Schwenk WF, et al. Effects of acute metabolic acidosis and alkalosis on leucine metabolism in conscious dogs. *Diabetes* 1989;38(7):847–853.
66. Straumann E, Keller U, Kury D, et al. Effect of acute acidosis and alkalosis on leucine kinetics in man. *Clin Physiol* 1992; 12(1):39–51.
67. Reaich D, Channon SM, Scrimgeour CM, et al. Ammonium chloride-induced acidosis increases protein breakdown and amino acid oxidation in humans. *Am J Physiol* 1992;263(4 Pt 1):E735–E739.
68. Reaich D, Channon SM, Scrimgeour CM, et al. Correction of acidosis in humans with CRF decreases protein degradation and amino acid oxidation. *Am J Physiol* 1993;265(2 Pt 1): E230–E235.
69. Ballmer PE, McNurlan MA, Hulter HN, et al. Chronic metabolic acidosis decreases albumin synthesis and induces negative nitrogen balance in humans. *J Clin Invest* 1995;95(1):39–45.
70. Bergström J, Alvestrand A, Furst P. Plasma and muscle free amino acids in maintenance hemodialysis patients without protein malnutrition. *Kidney Int* 1990;38:108–114.
71. Graham KA, Reaich D, Channon SM, et al. Correction of acidosis in CAPD decreases whole body protein degradation. *Kidney Int* 1996;49(5):1396–1400.

72. Boirie Y, Broyer M, Gagnadoux MF, et al. Alterations of protein metabolism by metabolic acidosis in children with chronic renal failure. *Kidney Int* 2000;58(1):236–241.
73. Lofberg E, Wernerman J, Bergström J. Branched-chain amino acids in muscle increase during correction of acidosis in hemodialysis (HD) patients (Abstract). *J Am Soc Nephrol* 1993;4.
74. Ibels LS, Alfrey AC, Haut L, et al. Preservation of function in experimental renal disease by dietary restriction of phosphate. *N Engl J Med* 1978;298(3):122–126.
75. Loghman-Adham M. Role of phosphate retention in the progression of renal failure. *J Lab Clin Med* 1993;122(1):16–26.
76. Nakamura M, Suzuki H, Ohno Y, et al. Oral calcium carbonate administration ameliorates the progression of renal failure in rats with hypertension. *Am J Kidney Dis* 1995;25(6):910–917.
77. Braun J, Oldendorf M, Moshage W, et al. Electron beam computed tomography in the evaluation of cardiac calcification in chronic dialysis patients. *Am J Kidney Dis* 1996;27(3):394–401.
78. Goodman WG, Goldin J, Kuizon BD, et al. Coronary-artery calcification in young adults with end-stage renal disease who are undergoing dialysis. *N Engl J Med* 2000;342(20):1478–1483.
79. Block GA, Hulbert-Shearon TE, et al. Association of serum phosphorus and calcium x phosphate product with mortality risk in chronic hemodialysis patients: a national study. *Am J Kidney Dis* 1998;31(4):607–617.
80. Michalk D, Klare B, Manz F, et al. Plasma inorganic sulfate in children with chronic renal failure. *Clin Nephrol* 1981;16(1): 8–12.
81. Koopman BJ, Jansen G, Wolthers BG, et al. Determination of inorganic sulfate in plasma by reversed-phase chromatography using ultraviolet detection and its application to plasma samples of patients receiving different types of haemodialysis. *J Chromatogr* 1985;337(2):259–266.
82. Gutierrez R, Oster JR, Schlessinger FB, et al. Serum sulfate concentration and the anion gap in hemodialysis patients. *ASAIO Trans* 1991;37(2):92–96.
83. Cole DE, Boucher MJ. Increased sweat sulfate concentrations in chronic renal failure. *Nephron* 1986;44(2):92–95.
84. Prévost JL, Dumas JA. Examen du sang et de son action dans les divers phenomenes de la vie (Examination of the blood and its action in the different phenomena of life). *Ann Chim Phys* 1821;23:90.
85. Bright R. *Reports of medical cases, selected with a view of illustrating the symptoms and cure of diseases by reference to morbid anatomy.* London: Longman Rees Orme Brown Green, 1831.
86. Levine S, Saltzman A. Are urea and creatinine uremic toxins in the rat? *Ren Fail* 2001;23(1):53–59.
87. Grollman EF, Grollman A. Toxicity of urea and its role in the pathogenesis of uremia. *J Clin Invest* 1959;38:749.
88. Bollman JL, Mann FC. Nitrogenous constituents of blood following transplantation of ureters into different levels of intestine. *Proc Soc Exp Biol Med* 1927;24:923.
89. Gilboe DD, Javid MJ. Breakdown products of urea and uremic syndrome. *Proc Soc Exp Biol Med* 1964;115:633.
90. Merrill JP, Legrain M, Hoigne R. Observations on the role of urea in uremia. *Am J Med* 1953;14:519.
91. Johnson WJ, Hagge WW, Wagoner RD, et al. Effects of urea loading in patients with far advanced renal failure. *Mayo Clin Proc* 1972;47:21–29.
92. Hutchings RH, Hegstrom RM, Scribner BH. Glucose intolerance in patients on long-term intermittent dialysis. *Ann Intern Med* 1966;65:275.
93. Hutchings RH, Hegstrom RM, Scribner BH. Two years experience with periodic hemodialysis in the treatment of chronic uremia. *Trans Am Soc Artif Intern Organs* 1962;8:266.
94. Degoulet P, Legrain M, Reach I, et al. Mortality risk factors in patients treated by chronic hemodialysis. *Nephron* 1982;31: 103–110.
95. Shapiro JI, Argy WP, Rakowski TA, et al. The unsuitability of BUN as a criterion for prescription dialysis. *Trans Am Soc Artif Intern Organs* 1983;29:129–134.
96. Lowrie EG, Lew NL. Death risk in hemodialysis patients: the predictive value of commonly measured variables and an evaluation of death rate differences between facilities. *Am J Kidney Dis* 1990;15(5):458–482.
97. Bergström J. Nutrition and adequacy of dialysis in hemodialysis patients. *Kidney Int* 1993;43(Suppl 41):S261–S267.
98. Acchiardo SR, Moore LW, Latour PA. Malnutrition as a main factor in morbidity and mortality of hemodialysis patients. *Kidney Int* 1983;24 [Suppl 16]:S199–S203.
99. Lowrie EG, Laird NM, Henry RR. Protocol for the National Cooperative Dialysis Study. *Kidney Int Suppl* 1983;13: S11–S18.
100. Gotch FA. Kt/V is the best dialysis dose parameter. *Blood Purif* 2000;18(4):276–285.
101. Daugirdas JT. Second generation logarithmic estimates of single-pool variable volume Kt/V: an analysis of error. *J Am Soc Nephrol* 1993;4(5):1205–1213.
102. Owen WF Jr, Lew NL, Liu Y, et al. The urea reduction ratio and serum albumin concentration as predictors of mortality in patients undergoing hemodialysis. *N Engl J Med* 1993;329(14): 1001–1006.
103. Schaefer K, Asmus G, Quellhorst E, et al. Optimum dialysis treatment for patients over 60 years with primary renal disease. Survival data and clinical results from 242 patients treated either by haemodialysis or haemofiltration. *Proc Eur Dial Transplant Assoc Eur Ren Assoc* 1985;21:510–523.
104. Depner TA. Uremic toxicity: urea and beyond. *Semin Dial* 2001;14(4):246–251.
105. Sorrentino R, Sorrentino L, Pinto A. Effect of some products of protein catabolism on the endothelium-dependent and -independent relaxation of rabbit thoracic aorta rings. *J Pharmacol Exp Ther* 1993;266(2):626–633.
106. Kraus LM, Kraus AP Jr. Carbamoylation of amino acids and proteins in uremia. *Kidney Int Suppl* 2001;78:S102–107.
107. Fluckiger R, Harmon W, Meier W, et al. Hemoglobin carbamylation in uremia. *N Engl J Med* 1981;304(14):823–827.
108. Kraus LM, Miyamura S, Pecha BR, et al. Carbamoylation of hemoglobin in uremic patients determined by antibody specific for homocitrulline (carbamoylated epsilon-N-lysine). *Mol Immunol* 1991;28(4-5):459–463.
109. Kwan JT, Carr EC, Neal AD, et al. Carbamylated haemoglobin, urea kinetic modeling and adequacy of dialysis in haemodialysis patients. *Nephrol Dial Transplant* 1991;6(1):38–43.
110. Bachmann K, Valentovic M, Shapiro R. A possible role for cyanate in the albumin binding defect of uremia. *Biochem Pharmacol* 1980;29(11):1598–1601.
111. Dengler TJ, Robertz-Vaupel GM, Dengler HJ. Albumin binding in uraemia: quantitative assessment of inhibition by endogenous ligands and carbamylation of albumin. *Eur J Clin Pharmacol* 1992;43(5):491–499.
112. Calvo R, Carlos R, Erill S. Effects of carbamylation of plasma proteins and competitive displacers on drug binding in uremia. *Pharmacology* 1982;24(4):248–252.
113. Oimomi M, Matsumoto S, Hatanaka H, et al. Determination of carbamylated plasma protein and its clinical application to renal failure. *Nephron* 1985;40(4):405–406.
114. Erill S, Calvo R, Carlos R. Plasma protein carbamylation and decreased acidic drug protein binding in uremia. *Clin Pharmacol Ther* 1980;27(5):612–618.
115. Kuckel CL, Lubit BW, Lambooy PK, et al. Methylisocyanate

and actin polymerization: the in vitro effects of carbamylation. *Biochim Biophys Acta* 1993;1162(1-2):143–148.
116. Horkko S, Huttunen K, Kervinen K, et al. Decreased clearance of uraemic and mildly carbamylated low-density lipoprotein. *Eur J Clin Invest* 1994;24(2):105–113.
117. Kraus LM, Elberger AJ, Handorf CR, et al. Urea-derived cyanate forms epsilon-amino-carbamoyl-lysine (homocitrulline) in leukocyte proteins in patients with end-stage renal disease on peritoneal dialysis. *J Lab Clin Med* 1994;123(6):882–891.
118. Kraus LM, Jones MR, Kraus AP Jr. Essential carbamoyl-amino acids formed in vivo in patients with end-stage renal disease managed by continuous ambulatory peritoneal dialysis: isolation, identification, and quantitation. *J Lab Clin Med* 1998; 131(5):425–431.
119. Kraus LM, Kraus AP Jr. The search for the uremic toxin: the case for carbamoylation of amino acids and proteins. *Wien Klin Wochenschr* 1998;110(15):521–530.
120. Rose WC, Dimmitt FW. Experimental studies on creatine and creatinine. VII. The fate of creatine and creatinine when administered to man. *J Biol Chem* 1916;26:345.
121. Shannon JA. The renal excretion of creatinine in man. *J Clin Invest* 1935;14:403.
122. Mason MF, Resnik H, Mino AS, et al. Mechanism of experimental uremia. *Arch Intern Med* 1937;60:312.
123. Mitch WE, Collier VU, Walser M. Creatinine metabolism in chronic renal failure. *Clin Sci (Colch)* 1980;58(4):327–335.
124. Hankins DA, Babb AL, Uvelli DA, et al. Creatinine degradation. II: Mathematical model including the effect of extra-renal removal rates. *Int J Artif Organs* 1981;4(2):68–71.
125. Jones JD, Burnett PC. Creatinine metabolism in humans with decreased renal function: creatinine deficit. *Clin Chem* 1974; 20(9):1204–1212.
126. Jones JD, Brunett PC. Creatinine metabolism and toxicity. *Kidney Int Suppl* 1975(3):294–298.
127. Davidoff F. Effects of guanidine derivatives on mitochondrial function. I. Phenethylbiguanide inhibition of respiration in mitochondria from guinea pig and rat tissues. *J Clin Invest* 1968; 47(10):2331–2343.
128. Davidoff F. Effects of guanidine derivatives on mitochondrial function. II. Reversal of guanidine-derivative inhibition by free fatty acids. *J Clin Invest* 1968;47(10):2344–2358.
129. Foster NB. The isolation of a toxic substance from the blood of uremic patients. *Trans Assoc Am Physicians* 1915;30:305.
130. De Deyn PP, D'Hooge R, Van Bogaert PP, et al. Endogenous guanidino compounds as uremic neurotoxins. *Kidney Int Suppl* 2001;78:S77–S83.
131. Hirayama A, Noronha-Dutra AA, Gordge MP, et al. Uremic concentrations of guanidino compounds inhibit neutrophil superoxide production. *Kidney Int Suppl* 2001;78:S89–S92.
132. Yokozawa T, Fujitsuka N, Oura H. Studies on the precursor of methylguanidine in rats with renal failure. *Nephron* 1991; 58(1):90–94.
133. Nagase S, Aoyagi K, Narita M, et al. Biosynthesis of methylguanidine in isolated rat hepatocytes and *in vivo*. *Nephron* 1985; 40(4):470–475.
134. Nagase S, Aoyagi K, Sakamoto M, et al. Biosynthesis of methylguanidine in the hepatic microsomal fraction. *Nephron* 1992; 62(2):182–186.
135. Nagase S, Aoyagi K, Narita M, et al. Active oxygen in methylguanidine synthesis. *Nephron* 1986;44(4):299–303.
136. Yokozawa T, Fujitsuka N, Oura H. Production of methylguanidine from creatinine in normal rats and rats with renal failure. *Nephron* 1990;56(3):249–254.
137. Nakamura K, Ienaga K, Yokozawa T, et al. Production of methylguanidine from creatinine via creatol by active oxygen species: analyses of the catabolism in vitro. *Nephron* 1991;58(1):42–46.
138. Nakamura K, Ienaga K. Creatol (5-hydroxycreatinine), a new toxin candidate in uremic patients. *Experientia* 1990;46(5): 470–472.
139. Ando A, Orita Y, Nakata K, et al. Effect of low protein diet and surplus of essential amino acids on the serum concentration and the urinary excretion of methylguanidine and guanidinosuccinic acid in chronic renal failure. *Nephron* 1979;24(4): 161–169.
140. Orita Y, Ando A, Tsubakihara Y, et al. Tissue and blood cell concentration of methylguanidine in rats and patients with chronic renal failure. *Nephron* 1981;27(1):35–39.
141. De Deyn PP, Marescau B, Swartz RD, et al. Serum guanidino compound levels and clearances in uremic patients treated with continuous ambulatory peritoneal dialysis. *Nephron* 1990;54(4): 307–312.
142. De Deyn P, Marescau B, Lornoy W, et al. Guanidino compounds in uraemic dialysed patients. *Clin Chim Acta* 1986; 157(2):143–150.
143. De Deyn PP, Robitaille P, Vanasse M, et al. Serum guanidino compound levels in uremic pediatric patients treated with hemodialysis or continuous cycle peritoneal dialysis. Correlations between nerve conduction velocities and altered guanidino compound concentrations. *Nephron* 1995;69(4):411–417.
144. Brooks DP, Rhodes GR, Woodward P, et al. Production of methylguanidine in dogs with acute and chronic renal failure. *Clin Sci (Colch)* 1989;77(6):637–641.
145. D'Hooge R, Pei YQ, Marescau B, et al. Convulsive action and toxicity of uremic guanidino compounds: behavioral assessment and relation to brain concentration in adult mice. *J Neurol Sci* 1992;112(1-2):96–105.
146. MacAllister RJ, Whitley GS, Vallance P. Effects of guanidino and uremic compounds on nitric oxide pathways. *Kidney Int* 1994;45(3):737–742.
147. De Deyn PP, Marescau B, Cuykens JJ, et al. Guanidino compounds in serum and cerebrospinal fluid of non-dialyzed patients with renal insufficiency. *Clin Chim Acta* 1987;167(1): 81–88.
148. Marescau B, De Deyn PP, Qureshi IA, et al. The pathobiochemistry of uremia and hyperargininemia further demonstrates a metabolic relationship between urea and guanidinosuccinic acid. *Metabolism* 1992;41(9):1021–1024.
149. Pietrzak I, Baczyk K. Erythrocyte transketolase activity and guanidino compounds in hemodialysis patients. *Kidney Int Suppl* 2001:S97–101.
150. Tofuku Y, Muramoto H, Kuroda M, et al. Impaired metabolism of guanidinoacetic acid in uremia. *Nephron* 1985;41(2): 174–178.
151. Levillain O, Marescau B, de Deyn PP. Guanidino compound metabolism in rats subjected to 20% to 90% nephrectomy. *Kidney Int* 1995;47(2):464–472.
152. Patel S, Hsu CH. Effect of polyamines, methylguanidine, and guanidinosuccinic acid on calcitriol synthesis. *J Lab Clin Med* 1990;115(1):69–73.
153. D'Hooge R, Pei YQ, Marescau B, et al. Behavioral toxicity of guanidinosuccinic acid in adult and young mice. *Toxicol Lett* 1992;64–65 Spec No:773–777.
154. Kielstein JT, Boger RH, Bode-Boger SM, et al. Asymmetric dimethylarginine plasma concentrations differ in patients with end-stage renal disease: relationship to treatment method and atherosclerotic disease. *J Am Soc Nephrol* 1999;10(3):594–600.
155. Wahbi N, Dalton RN, Turner C, et al. Dimethylarginines in chronic renal failure. *J Clin Pathol* 2001;54(6):470–473.
156. Morris ST, McMurray JJ, Spiers A, et al. Impaired endothelial function in isolated human uremic resistance arteries. *Kidney Int* 2001;60(3):1077–1082.
157. Vallance P, Leone A, Calver A, et al. Accumulation of an endog-

enous inhibitor of nitric oxide synthesis in chronic renal failure. *Lancet* 1992;339(8793):572–575.

158. Anderstam B, Katzarski K, Bergström J. Serum levels of NG, NG-dimethyl-L-arginine, a potential endogenous nitric oxide inhibitor in dialysis patients. *J Am Soc Nephrol* 1997;8(9): 1437–1442.
159. Kimoto M, Tsuji H, Ogawa T, et al. Detection of NG,NG-dimethylarginine dimethylaminohydrolase in the nitric oxide-generating systems of rats using monoclonal antibody. *Arch Biochem Biophys* 1993;300(2):657–662.
160. Zocalli C, Bode-Boger SM, Mallamaci F, et al. Plasma concentration of asymmetrical dimethylarginine and mortality in patients with end-stage renal disease: a prospective study. *Lancet* 2001;358(9299):2113–2117.
161. Gurreri G, Ghiggeri G, Salvidio G, et al. Effects of hemodialysis on guanidinopropionic acid metabolism. *Nephron* 1986;42(4): 295–297.
162. Shainkin-Kestenbaum R, Winikoff Y, Dvilansky A, et al. Effect of guanidino-propionic acid on lymphocyte proliferation. *Nephron* 1986;44(4):295–298.
163. Rocic B, Breyer D, Granic M, et al. The effect of guanidino substances from uremic plasma on insulin binding to erythrocyte receptors in uremia. *Horm Metab Res* 1991;23(10): 490–494.
164. Ramanjaneyulu PS, Indira K, Rao SV. Guanidine induced alterations in tissue transaminase patterns in the rat. *Biochem Mol Biol Int* 1993;31(6):1177–1180.
165. Folin O, Berglund H, Deriek C. The uric acid problem. An experimental study of animals and man including gouty subjects. *J Biol Chem* 1924;60:361.
166. Farrell PC, Ward RA, Hone PW. Uric acid: binding levels of urate ions in normal and uraemic plasma, and in human serum albumin. *Biochem Pharmacol* 1975;24(20):1885–1887.
167. Severini G, Aliberti LM. Liquid-chromatographic determination of inosine, xanthine, and hypoxanthine in uremic patients receiving hemodialysis treatment. *Clin Chem* 1987;33(12): 2278–2280.
168. Gerrits GP, Monnens LA, De Abreu RA, et al. Disturbances of cerebral purine and pyrimidine metabolism in young children with chronic renal failure. *Nephron* 1991;58(3):310–314.
169. Hsu CH, Patel SR, Young EW, et al. Effects of purine derivatives on calcitriol metabolism in rats. *Am J Physiol* 1991;260(4 Pt 2):F596–601.
170. Vanholder R, Patel S, Hsu CH. Effect of uric acid on plasma levels of 1,25(OH)2D in renal failure. *J Am Soc Nephrol* 1993; 4(4):1035–1038.
171. Schoots AC, Gerlag PG, Mulder AW, et al. Liquid-chromatographic profiling of solutes in serum of uremic patients undergoing hemodialysis and chronic ambulatory peritoneal dialysis (CAPD); high concentrations of pseudouridine in CAPD patients. *Clin Chem* 1988;34(1):91–97.
172. Dzurik R, Lajdova I, Spustova V, et al. Pseudouridine excretion in healthy subjects and its accumulation in renal failure. *Nephron* 1992;61(1):64–67.
173. Lajdova I, Spustova V, Mikula J, et al. Isolation of an additional inhibitor of glucose utilization in renal insufficiency: pseudouridine. *J Chromatogr* 1990;528(1):178–183.
174. Saito A, Niwa T, Maeda K, et al. Tryptophan and indolic tryptophan metabolites in chronic renal failure. *Am J Clin Nutr* 1980;33(7):1402–1406.
175. Cemacek P, Becvarova H, Gerova Z, et al. Plasma tryptophan level in chronic renal failure. *Clin Nephrol* 1980;14(5): 246–249.
176. Qureshi AR, Lindholm B, Garcia E, et al. Tryptophan and its metabolites in patients on continuous ambulatory peritoneal dialysis and following renal transplantation. *Nephrol Dial Transplant* 1994;9(7):791–796.
177. Young GA, Kendall S, Brownjohn AM. d-Amino acids in chronic renal failure and the effects of dialysis and urinary losses. *Amino Acids* 1994;6:283–293.
178. Gejyo F, Kinoshita Y, Ikenaka T. Elevation of serum levels of beta-aminoisobutyric acid in uremic patients and the toxicity of the amino acid. *Clin Nephrol* 1977;8(6):520–525.
179. Gorchein A, Webber R. delta-Aminolaevulinic acid in plasma, cerebrospinal fluid, saliva and erythrocytes: studies in normal, uraemic and porphyric subjects. *Clin Sci (Colch)* 1987;72(1): 103–112.
180. Frimpter GW, Thompson DD, Luckey EH. Conjugated amino acids in plasma of patients. *J Clin Invest* 1961;40:1208.
181. Gejyo F, Ito G, Kinoshita Y. Identification of N-monoacetylcystine in uraemic plasma. *Clin Sci (Colch)* 1981;60(3):331–334.
182. Wilcken DE, Gupta VJ. Sulphur containing amino acids in chronic renal failure with particular reference to homocystine and cysteine-homocysteine mixed disulphide. *Eur J Clin Invest* 1979;9(4):301–307.
183. Janssen MJ, van den Berg M, Stehouwer CD, et al. Hyperhomocysteinaemia: a role in the accelerated atherogenesis of chronic renal failure? *Neth J Med* 1995;46(5):244–251.
184. Ueland PM, Refsum H. Plasma homocysteine, a risk factor for vascular disease: plasma levels in health, disease, and drug therapy. *J Lab Clin Med* 1989;114(5):473–501.
185. Massy ZA, Chadefaux-Vekemans B, Chevalier A, et al. Hyperhomocysteinaemia: a significant risk factor for cardiovascular disease in renal transplant recipients. *Nephrol Dial Transplant* 1994;9(8):1103–1108.
186. Chauveau P, Chadefaux B, Coude M, et al. Hyperhomocysteinemia, a risk factor for atherosclerosis in chronic uremic patients. *Kidney Int Suppl* 1993;41:S72–S77.
187. Bachmann J, Tepel M, Raidt H, et al. Hyperhomocysteinemia and the risk for vascular disease in hemodialysis patients. *J Am Soc Nephrol* 1995;6(1):121–125.
188. Costagliola C, Iuliano G, Menzione M, et al. Systemic human diseases as oxidative risk factors in cataractogenesis. II. Chronic renal failure. *Exp Eye Res* 1990;51(6):631–635.
189. Pema AF, Ingrosso D, Zappia V, et al. Enzymatic methyl esterification of erythrocyte membrane proteins is impaired in chronic renal failure. Evidence for high levels of the natural inhibitor S-adenosylhomocysteine. *J Clin Invest* 1993;91(6): 2497–2503.
190. Perna AF, Ingrosso D, De Santo NG, et al. Mechanism of erythrocyte accumulation of methylation inhibitor S-adenosylhomocysteine in uremia. *Kidney Int* 1995;47(1):247–253.
191. Bostom AG, Lathrop L. Hyperhomocysteinemia in end-stage renal disease: prevalence, etiology, and potential relationship to arteriosclerotic outcomes. *Kidney Int* 1997;52(1):10–20.
192. Suliman ME, Qureshi AR, Barany P, et al. Hyperhomocysteinemia, nutritional status, and cardiovascular disease in hemodialysis patients. *Kidney Int* 2000;57(4):1727–1735.
193. Bostom AG, Shemin D, Lapane KL, et al. High dose-B-vitamin treatment of hyperhomocysteinemia in dialysis patients. *Kidney Int* 1996;49(1):147–152.
194. van Guldener C, Janssen MJ, Lambert J, et al. Folic acid treatment of hyperhomocysteinemia in peritoneal dialysis patients: no change in endothelial function after long-term therapy. *Perit Dial Int* 1998;18(3):282–289.
195. Suliman ME, Divino Filho JC, Barany P, et al. Effects of high-dose folic acid and pyridoxine on plasma and erythrocyte sulfur amino acids in hemodialysis patients. *J Am Soc Nephrol* 1999; 10(6):1287–1296.
196. Ross EA, Koo LC, Moberly JB. Low whole blood and erythro-

cyte levels of glutathione in hemodialysis and peritoneal dialysis patients. *Am J Kidney Dis* 1997;30(4):489–494.
197. Ceballos-Picot I, Witko-Sarsat V, Merad-Boudia M, et al. Glutathione antioxidant system as a marker of oxidative stress in chronic renal failure. *Free Radic Biol Med* 1996;21(6):845–853.
198. Alvestrand A, Furst P, Bergström J. Plasma and muscle free amino acids in uremia: influence of nutrition with amino acids. *Clin Nephrol* 1982;18(6):297–305.
199. Bergström J, Alvestrand A, Furst P, Lindholm B. Sulphur amino acids in plasma and muscle in patients with chronic renal failure: evidence for taurine depletion. *J Intern Med* 1989;226(3): 189–194.
200. Suliman M, Anderstam B, Bergström J. Evidence of taurine depletion and accumulation of cysteinsulfinic acid in chronic dialysis patients. *Kidney Int* 1996;50:1713–1717.
201. Descombes E, Hanck AB, Fellay G. Water soluble vitamins in chronic hemodialysis patients and need for supplementation. *Kidney Int* 1993;43(6):1319–1328.
202. Jennette JC, Goldman ID. Inhibition of the membrane transport of folates by anions retained in uremia. *J Lab Clin Med* 1975;86(5):834–843.
203. Hultberg B, Andersson A, Sterner G. Plasma homocysteine in renal failure. *Clin Nephrol* 1993;40(4):230–235.
204. Suliman ME, Lindholm B, Barany P, et al. Hyperhomocysteinemia in chronic renal failure patients: relation to nutritional status and cardiovascular disease. *Clin Chem Lab Med* 2001;39(8): 734–738.
205. Fodinger M, Mannhalter C, Wolfl G, et al. Mutation (677 C to T) in the methylenetetrahydrofolate reductase gene aggravates hyperhomocysteinemia in hemodialysis patients. *Kidney Int* 1997;52(2):517–523.
206. Vychytil A, Fodinger M, Wolfl G, et al. Major determinants of hyperhomocysteinemia in peritoneal dialysis patients. *Kidney Int* 1998;53(6):1775–1782.
207. Ihle BU, Cox RW, Dunn SR, et al. Determination of body burden of uremic toxins. *Clin Nephrol* 1984;22(2):82–89.
208. Baba S, Watanabe Y, Gejyo F, et al. High-performance liquid chromatographic determination of serum aliphatic amines in chronic renal failure. *Clin Chim Acta* 1984;136(1):49–56.
209. Bell JD, Lee JA, Lee HA, et al. Nuclear magnetic resonance studies of blood plasma and urine from subjects with chronic renal failure: identification of trimethylamine-N-oxide. *Biochim Biophys Acta* 1991;1096(2):101–107.
210. Lichtenberger LM, Gardner JW, Barreto JC, et al. Accumulation of aliphatic amines in gastric juice of acute renal failure patients. Possible cause of hypergastrinemia associated with uremia. *Dig Dis Sci* 1993;38(10):1885–1888.
211. Janne J, Poso H, Raina A. Polyamines in rapid growth and cancer. *Biochim Biophys Acta* 1978;473(3-4):241–293.
212. Saito A, Takagi T, Chung TG, et al. Serum levels of polyamines in patients with chronic renal failure. *Kidney Int Suppl* 1983; 16:S234–S237.
213. Swendseid ME, Panaqua M, Kopple JD. Polyamine concentrations in red cells and urine of patients with chronic renal failure. *Life Sci* 1980;26(7):533–539.
214. Radtke HW, Rege AB, LaMarche MB, et al. Identification of spermine as an inhibitor of erythropoiesis in patients with chronic renal failure. *J Clin Invest* 1981;67(6):1623–1629.
215. Galli F, Beninati S, Benedetti S, et al. Polymeric protein-polyamine conjugates: a new class of uremic toxins affecting erythropoiesis. *Kidney Int Suppl* 2001;78:S73–S76.
216. Kushner D, Beckman B, Nguyen L, et al. Polyamines in the anemia of end-stage renal disease. *Kidney Int* 1991;39(4): 725–732.
217. Bagdade JD, Subbaiah PV, Bartos D, et al. Polyamines: an unrecognised cardiovascular risk factor in chronic dialysis? *Lancet* 1979;1(8113):412–413.
218. Niwa T, Ise M. Indoxyl sulfate, a circulating uremic toxin, stimulates the progression of glomerular sclerosis. *J Lab Clin Med* 1994;124(1):96–104.
219. Manabe S, Suzuki M, Kusano E, et al. Elevation of levels of carcinogenic tryptophan pyrolysis products in plasma and red blood cells of patients with uremia. *Clin Nephrol* 1992;37(1): 28–33.
220. Lagana A, Liberti A, Morgia C, et al. Determination of indican and tryptophan in normal and uraemic patients by high-performance liquid chromatography with a new electrochemical detector. *J Chromatogr* 1986;378(1):85–93.
221. Ishikawa S, Manabe S, Yanagisawa H, et al. Inhibitory effects of tryptophan pyrolysis products on human platelet aggregation through inhibition of prostaglandin endoperoxide synthetase. *Food Chem Toxicol* 1987;25(11):829–835.
222. Manabe S, Kanai Y, Ishikawa S, et al. Carcinogenic tryptophan pyrolysis products potent inhibitors of type A monoamine oxidase and the platelet response to 5-hydroxytryptamine. *J Clin Chem Clin Biochem* 1988;26(5):265–270.
223. Ichinose H, Ozaki N, Nakahara D, et al. Effects of heterocyclic amines in food on dopamine metabolism in nigro-striatal dopaminergic neurons. *Biochem Pharmacol* 1988;37(17): 3289–3295.
224. Kanai Y, Wada O, Manabe S. Antagonism of gamma-aminobutyric acid A receptor-mediated responses by amino-gamma-carbolines. *J Pharmacol Exp Ther* 1990;252(3):1269–1276.
225. Hegstrand LR, Hine RJ. Variations of brain histamine levels in germ-free and nephrectomized rats. *Neurochem Res* 1986;11(2): 185–191.
226. Hegedus ZL, Frank HA, Steinman TI, et al. Increased levels of serum lipofuscin derived from 3-hydroxyanthranilic acid in patients with chronic renal failure. *Arch Int Physiol Biochim* 1987;95(5):457–463.
227. Lim CF, Bernard BF, de Jong M, et al. A furan fatty acid and indoxyl sulfate are the putative inhibitors of thyroxine hepatocyte transport in uremia. *J Clin Endocrinol Metab* 1993;76(2): 318–324.
228. Dasgupta A, Malik S. Fast atom bombardment mass spectrometric determination of the molecular weight range of uremic compounds that displace phenytoin from protein binding: absence of midmolecular uremic toxins. *Am J Nephrol* 1994;14(3): 162–168.
229. Niwa T, Miyazaki T, Hashimoto N, et al. Suppressed serum and urine levels of indoxyl sulfate by oral sorbent in experimental uremic rats. *Am J Nephrol* 1992;12(4):201–206.
230. Niwa T, Ise M, Miyazaki T. Progression of glomerular sclerosis in experimental uremic rats by administration of indole, a precursor of indoxyl sulfate. *Am J Nephrol* 1994;14(3):207–212.
231. Niwa T, Yazawa T, Kodama T, et al. Efficient removal of albumin-bound furancarboxylic acid, an inhibitor of erythropoiesis, by continuous ambulatory peritoneal dialysis. *Nephron* 1990; 56(3):241–245.
232. Wardle EN, Wilkinson K. Free phenols in chronic renal failure. *Clin Nephrol* 1976;6(2):361–364.
233. Niwa T. Phenol and p-cresol accumulated in uremic serum measured by HPLC with fluorescence detection. *Clin Chem* 1993;39(1):108–111.
234. Schoots AC, Dijkstra JB, Ringoir SM, et al. Are the classical markers sufficient to describe uremic solute accumulation in dialyzed patients? Hippurates reconsidered. *Clin Chem* 1988; 34(6):1022–1029.
235. Zimmerman L, Jornvall H, Bergström J. Phenylacetylglutamine and hippuric acid in uremic and healthy subjects. *Nephron* 1990; 55(3):265–271.

236. Liebich HM, Bubeck JI, Pickert A, et al. Hippuric acid and 3-carboxy-4-methyl-5-propyl-2-furanpropionic acid in serum and urine. Analytical approaches and clinical relevance in kidney diseases. *J Chromatogr* 1990;500:615–627.
237. Schoots AC, De Vries PM, Thiemann R, et al. Biochemical and neurophysiological parameters in hemodialyzed patients with chronic renal failure. *Clin Chim Acta* 1989;185(1):91–107.
238. Vanholder RC, De Smet RV, Ringoir SM. Assessment of urea and other uremic markers for quantification of dialysis efficacy. *Clin Chem* 1992;38(8 Pt 1): 1429–1436.
239. Rutten GA, Schoots AC, Vanholder R, et al. Hexachlorobenzene and 1,1-di(4-chlorophenyl)-2,2-dichloroethene in serum of uremic patients and healthy persons: determination by capillary gas chromatography and electron capture detection. *Nephron* 1988;48(3):217–221.
240. Suh B, Lee HW, Hong SY, et al. A new HPLC analytical method for o-hydroxyhippuric acid in uremic serum. *J Biochem Biophys Methods* 1986;13(4-5):211–220.
241. Niwa T, Ohki T, Maeda K, et al. A gas chromatographic-mass spectrometric assay for nine hydroxyphenolic acids in uremic serum. *Clin Chim Acta* 1979;96(3):247–254.
242. Liebich HM, Pickert A, Tetschner B. Gas chromatographic and gas chromatographic-mass spectrometric analysis of organic acids in plasma of patients with chronic renal failure. *J Chromatogr* 1984;289:259–266.
243. Hoeldtke RD, Israel BC, Cavanaugh ST, et al. Effect of renal failure on plasma dihydroxyphenylglycol, 3-methoxy-4-hydroxyphenylglycol, and vanillylmandelic acid. *Clin Chim Acta* 1989; 184(2):195–196.
244. Lesaffer G, De Smet R, Lameire N, et al. Intradialytic removal of protein-bound uraemic toxins: role of solute characteristics and of dialyser membrane. *Nephrol Dial Transplant* 2000;15(1): 50–57.
245. Niwa T, Ise M, Miyazaki T, et al. Suppressive effect of an oral sorbent on the accumulation of p-cresol in the serum of experimental uremic rats. *Nephron* 1993;65(1):82–87.
246. Niwa T, Asada H, Maeda K, et al. Profiling of organic acids and polyols in nerves of uraemic and non-uraemic patients. *J Chromatogr* 1986;377:15–22.
247. Wardle EN. How toxic are phenols? *Kidney Int Suppl* 1978(8): S13–S15.
248. Vanholder R, De Smet R, Waterloos MA, et al. Mechanisms of uremic inhibition of phagocyte reactive species production: characterization of the role of p-cresol. *Kidney Int* 1995;47(2): 510–517.
249. Niwa T, Tohyama K, Kato Y. Analysis of polyols in uremic serum by liquid chromatography combined with atmospheric pressure chemical ionization mass spectrometry. *J Chromatogr* 1993;613(1):9–14.
250. Pitkanen E, Bardy A, Pasternack A, et al. Plasma, red cell and cerebrospinal fluid concentrations of mannitol and sorbital in patients with severe chronic renal failure. *Ann Clin Res* 1976; 8(6):368–373.
251. Gallice PM, Monti JP, Braguer DL, et al. Identification of an ascorbic acid metabolite among "uremic middle molecules." *Clin Chem* 1990;36(7):1369–1372.
252. Gallice P, Sarrazin F, Polverelli M, et al. Ascorbic acid-2-0-beta-glucuronide, a new metabolite of vitamin C identified in human urine and uremic plasma. *Biochim Biophys Acta* 1994; 1199(3):305–310.
253. Zimmerman L, Jornvall H, Bergström J, et al. Characterization of a double conjugate in uremic body fluids. *FEBS Lett* 1981; 129(2):237–240.
254. Gallice P, Monti JP, Crevat A, et al. A compound from uremic plasma and from normal urine isolated by liquid chromatography and identified by nuclear magnetic resonance. *Clin Chem* 1985;31(1):30–34.
255. Niwa T, Takeda N, Miyazaki T, et al. Elevated serum levels of 3-deoxyglucosone, a potent protein-cross-linking intermediate of the Maillard reaction, in uremic patients. *Nephron* 1995; 69(4):438–443.
256. Inagi R, Miyata T, Yamamoto T, et al. Glucose degradation product methylglyoxal enhances the production of vascular endothelial growth factor in peritoneal cells: role in the functional and morphological alterations of peritoneal membranes in peritoneal dialysis. *FEBS Lett* 1999;463(3):260–264.
257. Linden T, Forsback G, Deppisch R, et al. 3-Deoxyglucosone, a promoter of advanced glycation end products in fluids for peritoneal dialysis. *Perit Dial Int* 1998;18(3):290–293.
258. Mistry CD, Fox JE, Mallick NP, et al. Circulating maltose and isomaltose in chronic renal failure. *Kidney Int Suppl* 1987;22: S210–S214.
259. Mistry CD, Gokal R. Single daily overnight (12-h dwell) use of 7.5% glucose polymer (Mw 18700; Mn 7300) +0.35% glucose solution: a 3-month study. *Nephrol Dial Transplant* 1993;8(5):443–447.
260. Queffeulou G, Lebrun-Vignes B, Wheatley P, et al. Allergy to icodextrin. *Lancet* 2000;356(9223):75.
261. Brunner H, Weisshaar G, Friebolin H, et al. Isolation of unusually composed sialyl-compounds from hemofiltrate. *Int J Artif Organs* 1989;12(12):755–761.
262. Mabuchi H, Nakahashi H. Determination of 3-carboxy-4-methyl-5-propyl-2-furanpropanoic acid, a major endogenous ligand substance in uremic serum, by high-performance liquid chromatography with ultraviolet detection. *J Chromatogr* 1987; 415(1):110–117.
263. Niwa T, Takeda N, Maeda K, et al. Accumulation of furancarboxylic acids in uremic serum as inhibitors of drug binding. *Clin Chim Acta* 1988;173(2):127–138.
264. Boer P, van Leersum L, Hene RJ, et al. Plasma oxalate concentration in chronic renal disease. *Am J Kidney Dis* 1984;4(2): 118–122.
265. Ramsay AG, Reed RG. Oxalate removal by hemodialysis in end-stage renal disease. *Am J Kidney Dis* 1984;4(2):123–127.
266. Morgan SH, Maher ER, Purkiss P, et al. Oxalate metabolism in end-stage renal disease: the effect of ascorbic acid and pyridoxine. *Nephrol Dial Transplant* 1988;3(1):28–32.
267. Prenen JA, Dorhout Mees EJ, Boer P. Plasma oxalate concentration and oxalate distribution volume in patients with normal and decreased renal function. *Eur J Clin Invest* 1985;15(1): 45–49.
268. Wolthers BG, Meijer S, Tepper T, et al. The determination of oxalate in haemodialysate and plasma: a means to detect and study "hyperoxaluria" in haemodialysed patients. *Clin Sci (Colch)* 1986;71(1):41–47.
269. McConnell KN, Rolton HA, Modi KS, et al. Plasma oxalate in patients with chronic renal failure receiving continuous ambulatory peritoneal dialysis or hemodialysis. *Am J Kidney Dis* 1991;18(4):441–445.
270. Marangella M, Petrarulo M, Mandolfo S, et al. Plasma profiles and dialysis kinetics of oxalate in patients receiving hemodialysis. *Nephron* 1992;60(1):74–80.
271. Costello JF, Sadovnic MC, Smith M, et al. Effect of vitamin B6 supplementation on plasma oxalate and oxalate removal rate in hemodialysis patients. *J Am Soc Nephrol* 1992;3(4): 1018–1024.
272. Oren A, Husdan H, Cheng PT, et al. Calcium oxalate kidney stones in patients on continuous ambulatory peritoneal dialysis. *Kidney Int* 1984;25(3):534–538.
273. Hoffman GS, Schumacher HR, Paul H, et al. Calcium oxalate

microcrystalline-associated arthritis in end-stage renal disease. *Ann Intern Med* 1982;97(1):36–42.

274. Reginato AJ, Ferreiro Seoane JL, Barbazan Alvarez C, et al. Arthropathy and cutaneous calcinosis in hemodialysis oxalosis. *Arthritis Rheum* 1986;29(11):1387–1396.
275. Worcester EM, Nakagawa Y, Bushinsky DA, et al. Evidence that serum calcium oxalate supersaturation is a consequence of oxalate retention in patients with chronic renal failure. *J Clin Invest* 1986;77(6):1888–1896.
276. Balcke P, Schmidt P, Zazgomik J, et al. Effect of vitamin B6 administration on elevated plasma oxalic acid levels in haemodialysed patients. *Eur J Clin Invest* 1982;12(6):481–483.
277. Tomson CR, Channon SM, Parkinson IS, et al. Effect of pyridoxine supplementation on plasma oxalate concentrations in patients receiving dialysis. *Eur J Clin Invest* 1989;19(2): 201–205.
278. Ono K. Secondary hyperoxalemia caused by vitamin C supplementation in regular hemodialysis patients. *Clin Nephrol* 1986; 26(5):239–243.
279. Camici M, Evangelisti L, Raspolli-Galletti M. The effect of oxalic acid on the aggregability of human platelet rich plasma. *Prostaglandins Leukot Med* 1986;21(1):107–110.
280. Pinkston D, Spiteller G, Von Henning H, et al. High resolution gas chromatography mass spectrometry of the methyl esters of organic acids from uremic hemofiltrates. *J Chromatogr* 1981; 223(1):1–19.
281. Niwa T, Ohki T, Maeda K, et al. Pattern of aliphatic dicarboxylic acids in uremic serum including a new organic acid, 2,4-dimethyladipic acid. *Clin Chim Acta* 1979;99(1):71–83.
282. Bakir AA, Shaykh M, Williams RH, et al. A study of xanthopterin in chronic renal failure. *Am J Nephrol* 1992;12(4): 224–228.
283. Miyata T, Fu MX, Kurokawa K, et al. Autoxidation products of both carbohydrates and lipids are increased in uremic plasma: is there oxidative stress in uremia? *Kidney Int* 1998;54(4): 1290–1295.
284. Hirayama A, Nagase S, Gotoh M, et al. Hemodialysis does not influence the peroxidative state already present in uremia. *Nephron* 2000;86(4):436–440.
285. Miyata T, Sugiyama S, Saito A, et al. Reactive carbonyl compounds related uremic toxicity ("carbonyl stress"). *Kidney Int Suppl* 2001;78:S25–S31.
286. Miyata T, Akhand AA, Kurokawa K, et al. Reactive carbonyl compounds as uremic toxins. *Contrib Nephrol* 2001(133): 71–80.
287. Miyata T, Kurokawa K, Van Ypersele De Strihou C. Advanced glycation and lipoxidation end products: role of reactive carbonyl compounds generated during carbohydrate and lipid metabolism. *J Am Soc Nephrol* 2000;11(9):1744–1752.
288. Himmelfarb J, McMonagle E. Albumin is the major plasma protein target of oxidant stress in uremia. *Kidney Int* 2001; 60(1):358–363.
289. Himmelfarb J, McMonagle E. Manifestations of oxidant stress in uremia. *Blood Purif* 2001;19(2):200–205.
290. Deng G, Vaziri ND, Jabbari B, et al. Increased tyrosine nitration of the brain in chronic renal insufficiency: reversal by antioxidant therapy and angiotensin-converting enzyme inhibition. *J Am Soc Nephrol* 2001;12(9):1892–1899.
291. Tenckhoff H, Curtis FK. Experience with maintenance peritoneal dialysis in the home. *Trans Am Soc Artif Intern Organs* 1970;16:90–95.
292. Scribner BH. Discussion. *Trans Am Soc Artif Intern Organs* 1965;11:29.
293. Jebsen RH, Tenckhoff H, Honet JC. Natural history of uremic polyneuropathy and effects of dialysis. *N Engl J Med* 1967; 277(7):327–333.
294. Babb AL, Popovich RP, Christopher TG, et al. The genesis of the square meter-hour hypothesis. *Trans Am Soc Artif Intern Organs* 1971;17:81–91.
295. Babb AL, Farrell PC, Uvelli DA, et al. Hemodialyzer evaluation by examination of solute molecular spectra. *Trans Am Soc Artif Intern Organs* 1972;18(0):98–105, 122.
296. Babb AL, Strand MJ, Uvelli DA, et al. Quantitative description of dialysis treatment: a dialysis index. *Kidney Int Suppl* 1975(2): 23–29.
297. Parker TF, Laird NM, Lowrie EG. Comparison of the study groups in the National Cooperative Dialysis Study and a description of morbidity, mortality, and patient withdrawal. *Kidney Int Suppl* 1983(13):S42–S49.
298. Henderson LW. Of time, TACurea, and treatment schedules. *Kidney Int Suppl* 1988;24:S105–S106.
299. De Francisco AL, Gordillo J, Cotorruelo JG, et al. Influence of dialysis membranes on the convective transport of middle molecules. *Int J Artif Organs* 1986;9(6):421–426.
300. Keshaviah P, Collins A. Rapid high-efficiency bicarbonate hemodialysis. *ASAIO Trans* 1986;32(1):17–23.
301. Clark WR, Ronco C. Reconciling differences in effective solute removal between intermittent and continuous therapies. *Semin Dial* 2001;14(4):289–293.
302. Henderson LW. Critical interpretation of adequacy parameters in peritoneal dialysis and hemodialysis. *Perit Dial Int* 1999;19 Suppl 2:538–544.
303. Henderson LW, Clark WR, Cheung AK. Quantification of middle molecular weight solute removal in dialysis. *Semin Dial* 2001;14(4):294–299.
304. Clark WR, Henderson LW. Renal versus continuous versus intermittent therapies for removal of uremic toxins. *Kidney Int Suppl* 2001;78:S298–303.
305. Bergström J, Lindholm B. Nutrition and adequacy of dialysis. How do hemodialysis and CAPD compare? *Kidney Int Suppl* 1993;40:S39–50.
306. Osada J, Gea T, Sanz C, et al. Evaluation of dialysis treatment in uremic patients by gel filtration of serum. *Clin Chem* 1990; 36(11):1906–1910.
307. Cristol P, Jeanbrau E, Monnier P. La polypeptidemie en pathologie renale. *J Med Franc* 1938;27:24.
308. Zimmerman L, Jornvall H, Bergström J, et al. Characterization of middle molecule compounds. *Artif Organs* 1981;4 Suppl: 33–36.
309. Gallice P, Fournier N, Crevat A, et al. Separation of one uremic middle molecules fraction by high performance liquid chromatography. *Kidney Int* 1983;23(5):764–766.
310. Abiko T, Onodera I, Sekino H. Characterization of an acidic tripeptide in neurotoxic dialysate. *Chem Pharm Bull (Tokyo)* 1980;28(5):1629–1633.
311. McCaleb ML, Izzo MS, Lockwood DH. Characterization and partial purification of a factor from uremic human serum that induces insulin resistance. *J Clin Invest* 1985;75(2):391–396.
312. Kaplan B, Gotfried M, Ravid M. Amino acid containing compounds in uremic serum-search for middle molecules by high performance liquid chromatography. *Clin Nephrol* 1986;26(2): 66–71.
313. Monti JP, Gallice P, Crevat A, et al. Identification by nuclear magnetic resonance and mass spectrometry of a glucuronic acid conjugate of o-hydroxybenzoic acid in normal urine and uremic plasma. *Clin Chem* 1985;31(10):1640–1643.
314. Grof J, Menyhart J. Molecular weight distribution, diffusibility and comparability of middle molecular fractions prepared from normal and uremic sera by different fractionation procedures. *Nephron* 1982;30(1):60–67.
315. Gallice PM, Crevat AD, Berland YF. Scaling up in isolation of

medium-size uraemic toxins. *J Chromatogr* 1991;539(2): 449–453.
316. Schoots AC, Mikkers FE, Claessens HA, et al. Characterization of uremic "middle molecular" fractions by gas chromatography, mass spectrometry, isotachophoresis, and liquid chromatography. *Clin Chem* 1982;28(1):45–49.
317. Furst P, Zimmerman L, Bergström J. Determination of endogenous middle molecules in normal and uremic body fluids. *Clin Nephrol* 1976;3(2):178–188.
318. Chapman GV, Farrell PC. Uremic middle molecules: separation and quantitation. *Artif Organs* 1981;4 Suppl:160–165.
319. Chapman GV, Ward RA, Farrell PC. Separation and quantification of the "middle molecules" in uremia. *Kidney Int* 1980; 17(1):82–88.
320. Faguer P, Man NK, Cueille G, et al. Improved separation and quantification of the "middle molecule" b4-2 in uremia. *Clin Chem* 1983;29(4):703–707.
321. Mikkers F, Ringoir S, De Smet R. Analytical isotachophoresis of uremic blood samples. *J Chromatogr* 1979;162(3):341–350.
322. Zimmerman L, Baldesten A, Bergström J, et al. Isotachophoretic separation of middle molecule peptides in uremic body fluids. *Clin Nephrol* 1980;13(4):183–188.
323. Menyhart J, Grof J. Many hitherto unknown peptides are principal constituents of uremic "middle molecules." *Clin Chem* 1981;27(10):1712–1716.
324. Saito A, Kanazawa I, Chung TG, et al. Analytical study for separation of middle molecules. *Artif Organs* 1981;4 Suppl: 13–16.
325. Mabuchi H, Nakahashi H. Analysis of small peptide in uremic serum by high-performance liquid chromatography. *J Chromatogr* 1982;228:292–297.
326. Mabuchi H, Nakahashi H. Systematic separation of medium-sized biologically active peptides by high-performance liquid chromatography. *J Chromatogr* 1981;213(2):275–286.
327. Mabuchi H, Nakahashi H. Medium-sized peptides in the blood of patients with uremia. *Nephron* 1983;33(4):232–237.
328. Navarro J, Grossetete MC, Defrasne A, et al. Isolation of an immunosuppressive fraction in ultrafiltrate from uremic sera. *Nephron* 1985;40(4):396–400.
329. Saito A, Suzuki I, Chung TG, et al. Separation of an inhibitor of erythropoiesis in "middle molecules" from hemodialysate from patients with chronic renal failure. *Clin Chem* 1986; 32(10):1938–1941.
330. Zimmerman L, Bergström J, Jornvall H. A method for separation of middle molecules by high performance liquid chromatography: application in studies of glucuronyl-o-hydroxyhippurate in normal and uremic subjects. *Clin Nephrol* 1986;25(2): 94–100.
331. Brunner H, Mann H, Essers U, et al. Preparative isolation of middle molecular weight fractions from the hemofiltrate of patients with chronic uremia. *Artif Organs* 1978;2(4):375–377.
332. Ehrlich K, Holland F, Turnham T, et al. Osmotic concentration of polypeptides from hemofiltrate of uremic patients. *Clin Nephrol* 1980;14(1):31–35.
333. Zimmerman L, Egestad B, Jornvall H, et al. Identification and determination of phenylacetylglutamine, a major nitrogenous metabolite in plasma of uremic patients. *Clin Nephrol* 1989; 32(3):124–128.
334. Cueille G, Man NK, Sausse A, et al. Characterization of subpeak b4.2, middle molecule. *Artif Organs* 1981;4 Suppl:28–32.
335. Delaporte C, Gros F, Jonsson C, et al. In vitro cytotoxic properties of plasma samples from uremic patients. *Clin Nephrol* 1982; 17(5):247–253.
336. Gutman RA, Huang AT. Inhibitor of marrow thymidine incorporation from sera of patients with uremia. *Kidney Int* 1980; 18(6):715–724.
337. Ota K, Sanaka T, Agishi T, et al. Influence of uremic middle molecules on blood cells. *Artif Organs* 1980;4(2):113–115.
338. Navarro J, Contreras P, Touraine JL, et al. Effect of middle molecules on immunological functions. *Artif Organs* 1981;4 Suppl:76–81.
339. Kumegawa M, Hiramatsu M, Yamada T, et al. Effects of intermediate-sized molecular components in uremic sera on nerve tissues in vitro. *Brain Res* 1980;198(1):234–238.
340. Braguer D, Chauvet-Monges AM, Sari JC, et al. Inhibition in vitro of the polymerization of tubulin by uremic middle molecules: corrective effect of isaxonine. *Clin Nephrol* 1983; 20(3):149–154.
341. Leber HW, Debus E, Grulich U, et al. Potential role of middle molecular compounds in the development of uremic anemia. *Artif Organs* 1981;4 Suppl:63–67.
342. Cichocki T, Hanicki Z, Klein A, et al. Influence of middle-molecular-weight solutes from dialysate on the migration rate of leukocytes. *Kidney Int* 1980;17(2):231–236.
343. Bernard P, Crest M, Rinaudo JB, et al. A study of the cardiotoxicity of uremic middle molecules on embryonic chick hearts. *Nephron* 1982;31(2):135–140.
344. Bazilinski N, Shaykh M, Dunea G, et al. Inhibition of platelet function by uremic middle molecules. *Nephron* 1985;40(4): 423–428.
345. Mabuchi H, Nakahashi H. Isolation and partial characterization of platelet aggregation inhibitors in the blood of dialyzed patients. *Nephron* 1983;35(2):112–115.
346. Phillips LS, Fusco AC, Unterman TG, et al. Somatomedin inhibitor in uremia. *J Clin Endocrinol Metab* 1984;59(4): 764–772.
347. Dzurik R, Spustova V. Metabolic actions of middle molecules. *Artif Organs* 1981;4 Suppl:59–62.
348. Fournier N, Gallice P, Crevat A, et al. Action on mitochondrial calcium metabolism of an ionophorous compound isolated from uremic plasma or normal urine. *Artif Organs* 1985;9(1):22–27.
349. Kinniburgh DW, Boyd ND. Isolation of peptides from uremic plasma that inhibit phenytoin binding to normal plasma proteins. *Clin Pharmacol Ther* 1981;30(2):276–280.
350. Andress DL, Howard GA, Birnbaum RS. Identification of a low molecular weight inhibitor of osteoblast mitogenesis in uremic plasma. *Kidney Int* 1991;39(5):942–945.
351. Walkowiak B, Michalak E, Borkowska E, et al. Concentration of RGDS-containing degradation products in uremic plasma is correlated with progression in renal failure. *Thromb Res* 1994; 76(2):133–144.
352. Mamoun AH, Sodersten P, Anderstam B, et al. Evidence of splanchnic-brain signaling in inhibition of ingestive behavior by middle molecules. *J Am Soc Nephrol* 1999;10(2):309–314.
353. Asaba H. Uremic middle molecules. Accumulation, renal excretion and elimination by extra-corporeal treatment. *Scand J Urol Nephrol Suppl* 1982;67:1–65.
354. Lustenberger N, Schindhelm K, Nordmeyer C, et al. Renal handling of middle molecules in uremic patients and in the isolated rat kidney. *Artif Organs* 1981;4 Suppl:110–114.
355. Schindhelm K, Schlatter E, Schurek HJ, et al. The isolated perfused rat kidney and uraemic middle molecules. *Contrib Nephrol* 1980;19:191–200.
356. Asaba H, Alvestrand A, Bergström J, et al. Uremic middle molecules in non-dialyzed azotemic patients: relation to symptoms and clinical biochemistries. *Clin Nephrol* 1982;17(2):90–95.
357. Man NK, Cueille G, Zingraff J, et al. Uremic neurotoxin in the middle molecular weight range. *Artif Organs* 1980;4(2): 116–120.
358. Oules R, Emond C, Claret G, et al. Middle molecule accumulation in uremia: an "extra uremic factor." *Artif Organs* 1981;4 Suppl:177–183.

359. Valek A, Spustova V, Lopot F, et al. Can plasma concentration of middle molecules contribute to assessment of adequate dialysis treatment? *Artif Organs* 1986;10(1):37–44.
360. Asaba H, Alvestrand A, Furst P, et al. Clinical implications of uremic middle molecules in regular hemodialysis patients. *Clin Nephrol* 1983;19(4):179–187.
361. Djukanovic LJ, Mimic-Oka JI, Potic JB. The effects of hemodialysis with different membranes on middle molecules and uremic neuropathy. *Int J Artif Organs* 1989;12(1):11–19.
362. Frohling PT, Kokot F, Cernacek P, et al. Relation between middle molecules and parathyroid hormone in patients with chronic renal failure. *Miner Electrolyte Metab* 1982;7(1):48–53.
363. Asaba H, Furst P, Oules R, et al. The effect of hemodialysis on endogenous middle molecules in uremic patients. *Clin Nephrol* 1979;11(5):257–266.
364. Winchester JF, Apiliga MT, Kennedy AC. Short-term evaluation of charcoal hemoperfusion combined with dialysis in uremic patients. *Kidney Int Suppl* 1976(7):S315–S319.
365. Oules R, Asaba H, Neuhauser M, et al. The removal of uremic small and middle molecules and free amino acids by carbon hemoperfusion. *Trans Am Soc Artif Intern Organs* 1977;23: 583–590.
366. Chang TM, Lister C. Middle molecules in hepatic coma and uremia. *Artif Organs* 1981;4 Suppl:169–172.
367. Asaba H, Bergström J, Furst P, et al. The effect of renal transplantation on middle molecules in plasma and urine. *Clin Nephrol* 1977;8(2):329–334.
368. Brownlee M, Cerami A, Vlassara H. Advanced glycosylation end products in tissue and the biochemical basis of diabetic complications. *N Engl J Med* 1988;318(20):1315–1321.
369. Bucala R, Makita Z, Koschinsky T, et al. Lipid advanced glycosylation: pathway for lipid oxidation *in vivo*. *Proc Natl Acad Sci U S A* 1993;90(14):6434–6438.
370. Ritz E, Deppisch R, Nawroth P. Toxicity of uraemia—does it come of AGE? *Nephrol Dial Transplant* 1994;9(1):1–2.
371. Makita Z, Vlassara H, Cerami A, et al. Immunochemical detection of advanced glycosylation end products in *vivo*. *J Biol Chem* 1992;267(8):5133–5138.
372. Makita Z, Radoff S, Rayfield EJ, et al. Advanced glycosylation end products in patients with diabetic nephropathy. *N Engl J Med* 1991;325(12):836–842.
373. Sell DR, Monnier VM. End-stage renal disease and diabetes catalyze the formation of a pentose-derived crosslink from aging human collagen. *J Clin Invest* 1990;85(2):380–384.
374. Sell DR, Nagaraj RH, Grandhee SK, et al. Pentosidine: a molecular marker for the cumulative damage to proteins in diabetes, aging, and uremia. *Diabetes Metab Rev* 1991;7(4):239–251.
375. Monnier VM, Sell DR, Nagaraj RH, et al. Maillard reaction-mediated molecular damage to extracellular matrix and other tissue proteins in diabetes, aging, and uremia. *Diabetes* 1992; 41 Suppl 2:36–41.
376. Odetti P, Fogarty J, Sell DR, et al. Chromatographic quantitation of plasma and erythrocyte pentosidine in diabetic and uremic subjects. *Diabetes* 1992;41(2):153–159.
377. Takahashi M, Kushida K, Kawana K, et al. Quantification of the cross-link pentosidine in serum from normal and uremic subjects. *Clin Chem* 1993;39(10):216–225.
378. Zheng ZH, Sederholm F, Anderstam B, et al. Acute effects of peritoneal dialysis solutions on appetite in non-uremic rats. *Kidney Int* 2001;60(6):2392–2398.
379. Kramer HJ, Pennig J, Klingmuller D, et al. Digoxin-like immunoreacting substance(s) in the serum of patients with chronic uremia. *Nephron* 1985;40(3):297–302.
380. Dasgupta A, Peng Y. Dialyzability and binding of digoxin-like immunoreactive factors (DLIF) with serum macromolecules in uremic patients on hemodialysis. *Life Sci* 1991;49(22): 1603–1609.
381. Stokes GS, Norris LA, Marwood JF, et al. Effect of dialysis on circulating Na,K ATPase inhibitor in uremic patients. *Nephron* 1990;54(2):127–133.
382. Gallice P, Lai E, Brunet P, et al. In vivo accumulation of sodium pump inhibitor by normal and uremic erythrocytes. *Int J Artif Organs* 1993;16(3):120–122.
383. Bricker NS, Zea L, Shapiro M, et al. Biologic and physical characteristics of the non-peptidic, non-digitalis-like natriuretic hormone. *Kidney Int* 1993;44(5):937–947.
384. Hulter HN, Melby JC, Peterson JC, et al. Chronic continuous PTH infusion results in hypertension in normal subjects. *J Clin Hypertens* 1986;2(4):360–370.
385. Iseki K, Massry SG, Campese VM. Effects of hypercalcemia and parathyroid hormone on blood pressure in normal and renal-failure rats. *Am J Physiol* 1986;250(5 Pt 2):F924–F929.
386. Rambausek M, Ritz E, Mall G, et al. Myocardial hypertrophy in rats with renal insufficiency. *Kidney Int* 1985;28(5):775–782.
387. el-Belbessi S, Brautbar N, Anderson K, et al. Effect of chronic renal failure on heart. Role of secondary hyperparathyroidism. *Am J Nephrol* 1986;6(5):369–375.
388. Kopple JD, Cianciaruso B, Massry SG. Does parathyroid hormone cause protein wasting? *Contrib Nephrol* 1980;20: 138–148.
389. Garber AJ. Effects of parathyroid hormone on skeletal muscle protein and amino acid metabolism in the rat. *J Clin Invest* 1983;71(6):1806–1821.
390. Wassner SJ, Li JB. Lack of an acute effect of parathyroid hormone within skeletal muscle. *Int J Pediatr Nephrol* 1987;8(1): 15–20.
391. Gomez-Fernandez P, Sanchez Agudo L, Miguel JL, et al. Effect of parathyroidectomy on respiratory muscle strength in uremic myopathy. *Am J Nephrol* 1987;7(6):466–469.
392. Szucs J, Mako J, Merey J. Blood requirement and subtotal parathyroidectomy in patients with chronic renal failure treated with hemodialysis. *Clin Nephrol* 1983;19(3):134–136.
393. Meytes D, Bogin E, Ma A, et al. Effect of parathyroid hormone on erythropoiesis. *J Clin Invest* 1981;67(5):1263–1269.
394. McGonigle RJ, Wallin JD, Husserl F, et al. Potential role of parathyroid hormone as an inhibitor of erythropoiesis in the anemia of renal failure. *J Lab Clin Med* 1984;104(6): 1016–1026.
395. Lutton JD, Solangi KB, Ibraham NG, et al. Inhibition of erythropoiesis in chronic renal failure: the role of parathyroid hormone. *Am J Kidney Dis* 1984;3(5):380–384.
396. Angelini D, Carlini A, Giusti R, et al. Parathyroid hormone and T-cellular immunity in uremic patients in replacement dialytic therapy. *Artif Organs* 1993;17(2):73–75.
397. Akmal M, Telfer N, Ansari AN, et al. Erythrocyte survival in chronic renal failure. Role of secondary hyperparathyroidism. *J Clin Invest* 1985;76(4):1695–1698.
398. Levi J, Malachi T, Djaldetti M, et al. Biochemical changes associated with the osmotic fragility of young and mature erythrocytes caused by parathyroid hormone in relation to the uremic syndrome. *Clin Biochem* 1987;20(2):121–125.
399. Bogin E, Earon Y, Blum M. Effect of parathyroid hormone and uremia on erythrocyte deformability. *Clin Chim Acta* 1986; 161(3):293–299.
400. Earon Y, Blum M, Bogin E. Effect of parathyroid hormone and uremic sera on the autoagglutination and sedimentation of human red blood cells. *Clin Chim Acta* 1983;135(3):253–262.
401. Akmal M, Massry SG, Goldstein DA, et al. Role of parathyroid hormone in the glucose intolerance of chronic renal failure. *J Clin Invest* 1985;75(3):1037–1044.
402. Mak RH, Bettinelli A, Turner C, et al. The influence of hyper-

parathyroidism on glucose metabolism in uremia. *J Clin Endocrinol Metab* 1985;60(2):229–233.
403. Mak RH, Turner C, Haycock GB, et al. Secondary hyperparathyroidism and glucose intolerance in children with uremia. *Kidney Int Suppl* 1983;16:S128–S133.
404. Nishizawa Y, Miki T, Okui Y, et al. Deranged metabolism of lipids in patients with chronic renal failure: possible role of secondary hyperparathyroidism. *Jpn J Med* 1986;25(1):40–45.
405. Miyata T, Saito A, Kurokawa K, et al. Advanced glycation and lipoxidation end products: reactive carbonyl compounds-related uraemic toxicity. *Nephrol Dial Transplant* 2001;16 Suppl 4: 8–11.
406. Witko-Sarsat V, Friedlander M, Capeillere-Blandin C, et al. Advanced oxidation protein products as a novel marker of oxidative stress in uremia. *Kidney Int* 1996;49(5):1304–1313.
407. Wratten ML, Sereni L, Tetta C. Oxidation of albumin is enhanced in the presence of uremic toxins. *Ren Fail* 2001;23(3-4):563–571.
408. Witko-Sarsat V, Friedlander M, Capeillere-Blandin C, et al. Advanced oxidation protein products as a novel marker of oxidative stress in uremia. *Kidney Int* 1996;49:1304–1313.
409. Bergström J, Lindholm B. Malnutrition, cardiac disease, and mortality: an integrated point of view [editorial]. *Am J Kidney Dis* 1998;32(5):834–841.
410. Stenvinkel P, Heimbürger O, Lindholm B, et al. Are there two types of malnutrition in chronic renal failure? Evidence for relationships between malnutrition, inflammation and atherosclerosis (MIA syndrome). *Nephrol Dial Transplant* 2000;15(7): 953–960.
411. Stenvinkel P, Heimbürger O, Paultre F, et al. Strong associations between malnutrition, inflammation and atherosclerosis in chronic renal failure. *Kidney Int* 1999;55:1899–1911.
412. Zimmermann J, Herrlinger S, Pruy A, et al. Inflammation enhances cardiovascular risk and mortality in hemodialysis patients. *Kidney Int* 1999;55(2):648–658.
413. Bologa RM, Levine DM, Parker TS, et al. Interleukin-6 predicts hypoalbuminemia, hypocholesterolemia, and mortality in hemodialysis patients. *Am J Kidney Dis* 1998;32:107–114.
414. Ikizler TA, Wingard RL, Harvell J, et al. Association of morbidity with markers of nutrition and inflammation in chronic hemodialysis patients: a prospective study. *Kidney Int* 1999;55(5): 1945–1951.
415. Owen WF, Lowrie EG. C-reactive protein as an outcome predictor for maintenance hemodialysis patients. *Kidney Int* 1998; 54(2):627–636.
416. Berggård I, Beam AG. Isolation and properties of a low molecular weight beta-2-globulin occurring in human biological fluids. *J Biol Chem* 1968;243(15):4095–4103.
417. Charra B, Calemard E, Laurent G. Chronic renal failure treatment duration and mode: their relevance to the late dialysis periarticular syndrome. *Blood Purif* 1988;6(2):117–124.
418. Gejyo F, Homma N, Maruyama H, et al. Beta 2-microglobulin-related amyloidosis in patients receiving chronic hemodialysis. *Contrib Nephrol* 1988;68:263–269.
419. Gorevic PD, Casey TT, Stone WJ, et al. Beta-2 microglobulin is an amyloidogenic protein in man. *J Clin Invest* 1985;76(6): 2425–2429.
420. Drueke T, Touam M, Zingraff J. Dialysis-associated amyloidosis. *Adv Ren Replace Ther* 1995;2(1):24–39.
421. Niwa T, Miyazaki S, Katsuzaki T, et al. Immunohistochemical detection of advanced glycation end products in dialysis-related amyloidosis. *Kidney Int* 1995;48(3):771–778.
422. Cheung AK, Chenoweth DE, Otsuka D, et al. Compartmental distribution of complement activation products in artificial kidneys. *Kidney Int* 1986;30(1):74–80.
423. Floge J, Granolleras C, Bingel M, et al. Beta 2-microglobulin kinetics during haemodialysis and haemofiltration. *Nephrol Dial Transplant* 1987;1(4):223–228.
424. Floege J, Bartsch A, Schulze M, et al. Clearance and synthesis rates of beta 2-microglobulin in patients undergoing hemodialysis and in normal subjects. *J Lab Clin Med* 1991;118(2): 153–165.
425. Zingraff J, Beyne P, Urena P, et al. Influence of haemodialysis membranes on beta 2-microglobulin kinetics: in vivo and in vitro studies. *Nephrol Dial Transplant* 1988;3(3):284–290.
426. Simon P, Cavarle YY, Ang KS, et al. Long-term variations of serum beta 2-microglobulin levels in hemodialysed uremics according to permeability and bioincompatibility of dialysis membranes. *Blood Purif* 1988;6(2):111–116.
427. Blumberg A, Burgi W. Behavior of beta 2-microglobulin in patients with chronic renal failure undergoing hemodialysis, hemodiafiltration and continuous ambulatory peritoneal dialysis (CAPD). *Clin Nephrol* 1987;27(5):245–249.
428. Kaiser JP, Hagemann J, von Herrath D, et al. Different handling of beta 2-microglobulin during hemodialysis and hemofiltration. *Nephron* 1988;48(2):132–135.
429. Floege J, Granolleras C, Deschodt G, et al. High-flux synthetic versus cellulosic membranes for beta 2-microglobulin removal during hemodialysis, hemodiafiltration and hemofiltration. *Nephrol Dial Transplant* 1989;4(7):653–657.
430. Sethi D, Murphy CM, Brown EA, et al. Clearance of beta-2-microglobulin using continuous ambulatory peritoneal dialysis. *Nephron* 1989;52(4):352–355.
431. Ballardie FW, Kerr DN, Tennent G, et al. Haemodialysis versus CAPD: equal predisposition to amyloidosis? *Lancet* 1986; 1(8484):795–796.
432. Tielemans C, Dratwa M, Bergmann P, et al. Continuous ambulatory peritoneal dialysis vs haemodialysis: a lesser risk of amyloidosis? *Nephrol Dial Transplant* 1988;3(3):291–294.
433. Sethi D, Brown EA, Gower PE. CAPD, protective against developing dialysis-associated amyloid? *Nephron* 1988;50(1):85–86.
434. Stenvinkel P, Heimbürger O, Lonngvist F. Serum leptin concentrations correlate to plasma insulin concentrations independent of body fat content in chronic renal failure. *Nephrol Dial Transpl* 1997;12:1321–1325.
435. Merabet E, Dagogo-Jack S, Coyne DW, et al. Increased plasma leptin concentrations in end-stage renal disease. *J Clin Endocrinol Metab* 1997;82:847–850.
436. Young GA, Woodrow G, Kendall S, et al. Increased plasma leptin/fat ratio in patients with chronic renal failure: a cause of malnutrition. *Nephrol Dial Transpl* 1997;12:2318–2323.
437. Widjaja A, Kielstein JT, Horn R, et al. Free serum leptin but not bound leptin concentrations are elevated in patients with end-stage renal disease. *Nephrol Dial Transplant* 2000;15(6): 846–850.
438. Stenvinkel P. Leptin and its clinical implications in chronic renal failure. *Mineral Electrol Metab* 1999;25:298–302.
439. Sharma K, Considine RV, Michael B, et al. Plasma leptin is partly cleared by the kidney and is elevated in hemodialysis patients. *Kidney Int* 1997;51(6):1980–1985.
440. Nordfors L, Lonnqvist F, Heimbürger O, et al. Low leptin gene expression and hyperleptinemia in chronic renal failure. *Kidney Int* 1998;54(4):1267–1275.
441. Cumin F, Baum HP, Levens N. Leptin is cleared from the circulation primarily by the kidney. *Int J Obesity* 1996;20: 1120–1126.
442. Zeng J, Patterson BW, Klein S, et al. Whole body leptin kinetics and renal metabolism in vivo. *Am J Physiol* 1997;273: E1102–E1106.
443. Kokot F, Adamczak M, Wiecek A. Plasma leptin concentration in kidney transplant patients at the early posttransplant period. *Nephrol Dial Transpl* 1998;13:2276–2280.

444. Eggertsen G, Heimbürger O, Stenvinkel P, et al. Influence of variation at the apolipoprotein E locus on lipid and lipoprotein levels in CAPD patients. *Nephrol Dial Transplant* 1997;12(1): 141–144.
445. Garibotti G, Russo R, Franceschini R, et al. Inter-organ leptin exchange in humans. *Biochem & Biophys Res Commun* 1998; 247:504–509.
446. Daschner M, Tonshoff B, Blum WF, et al. Inappropriate elevation of serum leptin levels in children with chronic renal failure. *J Am Soc Nephrol* 1998;9:1074–1079.
447. Johansen KL, Mulligan K, Tai V, et al. Leptin, body composition, and indices of malnutrition in patients on dialysis. *J Am Soc Nephrol* 1998;9:1080–1084.
448. Odamaki M, Furuya R, Yoneyama T, et al. Association of the serum leptin concentration with weight loss in chronic hemodialysis patients. *Am J Kidney Dis* 1999;33:361–368.
449. Stenvinkel P, Lindholm B, Lonngvist F, et al. Increases in serum leptin during peritoneal dialysis are associated with inflammation and a decrease in lean body mass. *J Am Soc Nephrol* 2000; 11:1303–1309.
450. Dagogo-Jack S, Ovalle F, Geary B, et al. Hyperleptinaemia in patients with end-stage renal disease treated by peritoneal dialysis. *Perit Dial Int* 1998;18:34–40.
451. Haag-Weber M, Mai B, Cohen G, et al. GIP and DIP: a new view of uraemic toxicity. *Nephrol Dial Transplant* 1994;9(4): 346–347.
452. Balke N, Holtkamp U, Horl WH, et al. Inhibition of degranulation of human polymorphonuclear leukocytes by complement factor D. *FEBS Lett* 1995;371(3):300–302.
453. Oppermann M, Kurts C, Zierz R, et al. Elevated plasma levels of the immunosuppressive complement fragment Ba in renal failure. *Kidney Int* 1991;40(5):939–947.
454. Pascual M, Paccaud JP, Macon K, et al. Complement activation by the alternative pathway is modified in renal failure: the role of factor D. *Clin Nephrol* 1989;32(4):185–193.
455. Deppisch RM, Beck W, Goehl H, et al. Complement components as uremic toxins and their potential role as mediators of microinflammation. *Kidney Int Suppl* 2001;78:S271–S277.
456. Riella MC. Malnutrition in dialysis: malnourishment or uremic inflammatory response? *Kidney Int* 2000;57(3):1211–1232.
457. Stenvinkel P, Heimbürger O, Paultre F, et al. Strong association between malnutrition, inflammation, and atherosclerosis in chronic renal failure. *Kidney Int* 1999;55(5):1899–1911.
458. Yeun JY, Levine RA, Mantadilok V, et al. C-reactive protein predicts all-cause and cardiovascular mortality in hemodialysis patients. *Am J Kidney Dis* 2000;35(3):469–476.
459. Bologa RM, Levine DM, Parker TS, et al. Interleukin-6 predicts hypoalbuminemia, hypocholesterolemia, and mortality in hemodialysis patients. *Am J Kidney Dis* 1998;32:107–114.
460. Kimmel PL, Phillips TM, Simmens SJ, et al. Immunological function and survival in hemodialysis patients. *Kidney Int* 1998; 54:236–244.
461. Stenvinkel P. Malnutrition and chronic inflammation as risk factors for cardiovascular disease in chronic renal failure. *Blood Purif* 2001;19:143–151.
462. Panichi V, Migliori M, De Pietro S, et al. C reactive protein in patients with chronic renal diseases. *Ren Fail* 2001;23(3-4): 551–562.
463. Pereira BJG, Shapiro L, King AV, et al. Plasma levels of IL-β, TNF-α and their specific inhibitors in undialyzed chronic renal failure, CAPD and hemodialysis patients. *Kidney Int* 1994;45: 890–896.
464. Memoli B, Postiglione L, Cianciaruso B, et al. Role of different dialysis membranes in the release of interleukin-6 soluble receptor in uremic patients. *Kidney Int* 2000;58:417–424.
465. Poole S, Bird TA, Selkirk S, et al. Fate of injected interleukin 1 in rats: Sequestration and degradation in the kidney. *Cytokine* 1990;2:416–422.
466. Espinosa M, Aguilera A, Auxiliarda BM, et al. Tumour necrosis factor alpha as uremic toxin: correlation with neuropathy, left ventricular hypertrophy, anemia, and hypertriglyceridemia in peritoneal dialysis patients. *Adv Perit Dial* 1999;15:82–86.
467. Kotler DP. Cachexia. *Ann Intern Med* 2000;133:622–634.
468. Kaibara A, Moshyedi A, Auffenberg T, et al. Leptin produces anorexia and weight loss without inducing an acute phase response or protein wasting. *Am J Physiol* 1998;43: R1518–R1525.
469. Bergström J. Uremic toxicity. In: Kopple JD, Massry SG, eds. *Nutritional management of renal disease,* 1st ed. Baltimore: Williams & Wilkins, 1997:97–190.

5

OXIDANT STRESS

WALTER H. HÖRL

Under physiologic conditions there is an equilibrium between prooxidant and antioxidant systems. A shift to the prooxidant side results in a state of oxidative stress. The antioxidants are classified as lipophilic (e.g., vitamin E, ubiquinone, carotenoids) or hydrophilic (e.g., ascorbate, uric acid) and the glutathione system (reduced and oxidized glutathione molecules, glutathione peroxidase, glutathione reductase). Intracellular superoxide dismutase and catalase also count as part of the enzymatic primary antioxidant defense system. This system reacts with oxygen radicals and hydrogen peroxide and catalyzes their detoxification (1).

OXIDATIVE STRESS AND CHRONIC KIDNEY DISEASES

Increased oxidative stress and impaired antioxidative defense mechanisms have been reported in patients with glomerular diseases (2). Reactive oxygen species (ROS) generated within the kidney by invading macrophages and leukocytes are important mediators in renal disease. ROS and neutrophil respiratory burst are produced by kidney glomerular cells in passive Heymann nephritis. In this model, which mimics membranous glomerulonephritis, a high concentration of hydrogen peroxide can be found in the glomerular basement membrane (3). Puromycin aminonucleoside nephritis, which resembles lesions observed in minimal-change nephritis, is associated with a rapid but temporary increase in hydroxyl radicals and hydrogen peroxide in the initial phase followed by a late increase in superoxide anion and hydroxyl radicals (4). Experimental immunoglobulin A nephritis and antiglomerular basement membrane antibody disease (equivalent to the human focal segmental necrotizing glomerulonephritis) also seem to be triggered by ROS (5,6). In noninflammatory renal injury such as the remnant kidney rat, which is a model of chronic renal failure, increased ROS synthesis has been described (7). In rats with remnant kidney–induced chronic renal failure, catalase seems to be more vulnerable to reactive oxygen intermediates than superoxide dismutase and glutathione peroxidase (GSH-Px) (8). Antioxidative therapies such as α-tocopherol or probucol either prevented or reversed the high protein excretion in experimental glomerulonephritis models; they also prevented or reversed damage secondary to oxidation (9–13). Administration of vitamin E was shown to reduce proteinuria in 10 out of 11 children with focal segmental glomerulosclerosis (14). Probucol therapy resulted in a decrease of proteinuria in seven out of 13 patients with different forms of glomerulonephritis treated for 24 weeks (15). We reported on the reduction of proteinuria in patients with idiopathic membranous nephropathy, treated with the oxygen radical scavenger probucol (16). We were able to demonstrate a distinct probucol-mediated effect with a slight to moderate reduction of proteinuria in most patients and partial remission in four of 15 treated patients.

An association between abnormal lipid metabolism and progression of glomerular and tubulointerstitial renal disease has been suggested over the last 15 years. Atherosclerosis and glomerulosclerosis may have some common lipoprotein-mediated pathogenic mechanisms. Oxidized low-density lipoproteins (LDL) may contribute to atherosclerosis and reduced relaxation in response to vasodilators. Oxidized LDL induces vasoconstriction in the isolated perfused rat kidney as a result of inactivation of nitric oxide (NO) by reactive oxygen species. Free radical scavengers provide protection against oxidized LDL-induced renal vasoconstriction (17). Chronic NO synthase inhibition in experimental animals causes hypertension, renal vascular injury, and proteinuria (18). Although NO can scavenge superoxide (O_2) and inhibits O_2 production, NO deficiency increases O_2 activity (19,20).

Vitamin E and selenium deficiencies induce renal injury in intact rat kidneys (21). However, vitamin E supplementation reduces glomerulosclerosis in the remnant kidney model (22) and alleviates renal injury but not hypertension in rats with chronic NO synthase inhibition (23), suggesting that oxidants were involved in the pathogenesis of vasculitis and proteinuria. Infusion of H_2O_2 into the renal artery resulted in a 50-fold increase in urinary protein excretion without any change in arterial pressure (24). Inhibition of xanthine oxidase causes marked reduction in proteinuria in

Heymann nephritis or aminonucleoside-induced nephrosis (25). Angiotensin II stimulates O_2 production in vascular (26) and renal (27) cells, whereas all of the effects of chronic NO-synthase inhibition are prevented by angiotensin II type 1 (AT1) receptor blockade (28). Recent findings of Onozato et al. (29) indicate a pathogenic role for AT1 receptors in the development of oxidative damage in the kidney during early diabetes mellitus; an angiotensin-converting enzyme (ACE) inhibitor or an angiotensin receptor blocker prevents these changes.

Annuk et al. (30) investigated the relationship between oxidative stress and endothelium-dependent vasodilation in patients with chronic renal failure. They found a lower GSSG/GSH (oxidized glutathione/reduced glutathione) ratio in patients with chronic renal failure as compared to healthy subjects. Endothelium-dependent vasodilatation was positively correlated with total antioxidative activity and GSH (reduced glutathione) but negatively correlated with GSSG, GSSG/GSH ratio, and diene conjugates. It was concluded that impaired endothelium vasodilation function and oxidative stress are related in patients with chronic renal failure (30).

Spontaneously hypertensive rats exhibit an increase in oxyradical production in and around microvascular endothelium. Data of Suzuki et al. (31) suggest that xanthine oxidase accounts for a putative source of oxyradical generation that is associated with an increasing arteriolar tone in this form of hypertension.

Oxidative stress is also a major cause of diabetic nephropathy (32,33). Oxidative stress accompanying the early onset of diabetes increases the kidney's susceptibility to develop diabetic nephropathy (34). Patients with diabetic nephropathy show higher oxidative stress than patients without renal complications (35). It has been suggested that activation of the transcription factor NF (nuclear factor)-kappaB is an initiating, amplifying, and perpetuating mechanism that converts disease-associated oxidative stress into cellular dysfunction relevant in renal diseases of various etiology (36).

Advanced glycation end products (AGEs) and oxidative stress may play an important role in the pathogenesis of diabetic nephropathy (33). Chronic administration of AGE albumin to nondiabetic rats led to activation of collagen, laminin, and transforming growth factor β (TGF-β) genes as well as proteinuria and glomerular changes similar to those seen in diabetic nephropathy (37,38). Short-term infusion of AGE albumin into normal mice resulted in the appearance of malondialdehyde (MDA) determinants in the vessel wall, activation of the pleotropic transcription factor NF-kappaB, and induction of heme oxygenase messenger RNA (39). Rats rendered diabetic with streptozotocin exhibited increased vascular permeability in intestine, skin, and kidneys. Complete inhibition of hyperpermeability in the skin and gut, and 90% in the kidneys, was obtained by administration of soluble receptor for AGE (RAGE). A role for free radicals was demonstrated in AGE–RAGE-mediated vascular hyperpermeability by using antioxidants (40).

Plasma levels of F2-isoprostanes, specific markers for lipid peroxidation, are elevated in patients with diabetes (41). Oxidation of glucose results in production of protein-reactive ketoaldehydes, hydrogen peroxide, and highly reactive oxidants, which may contribute to protein fragmentation and cross-linking in diabetes (42). Oxidation of unsaturated fatty-acid residues occurs during the formation of AGE phospholipids, which is inhibited by aminoguanidine. Attendant lipid peroxidation also is suppressed this way (43).

Increased oxidant stress may contribute to the increased risk of coronary heart disease in patients with nephrotic syndrome by means of hyperlipidemia and/or hypoalbuminemia. Dogra et al. (44) found significantly lower plasma oxygen radical absorbance capacity (ORAC) in patients with nephrotic syndrome as compared to controls. Plasma albumin was significantly positively correlated with plasma ORAC. Increased oxidative stress and subsequent activation of the transcription factor NF-kappaB has been linked to diabetic nephropathy in patients with type 1 and type 2 diabetes mellitus. However, treatment with the antioxidant thioctic acid (α-lipoic acid) for 3 years (600 mg/day) resulted in a decrease of oxidative stress in plasma samples by 48% and of transcription factor NF-kappaB–binding activity in peripheral blood mononuclear cells by 38% (45). However, the increase in glycoxidation and lipoxidation products in plasma and tissue proteins of patients with chronic diseases such as diabetes, rheumatoid arthritis, or atherosclerosis may occur without the necessity of oxidative stress (46). Chemical modification of proteins by carbohydrates and lipids in diabetes also may be caused by carbonyl stress.

Radiographic contrast agents may cause deterioration in renal function because of reactive oxygen species. Prophylactic oral administration of the antioxidant acetylcysteine, along with hydration, prevents the reduction in renal function induced by radiographic contrast agents in patients with chronic renal failure (47).

OXIDATIVE STRESS IN DIALYSIS PATIENTS

Oxidative stress in patients with chronic renal failure is maintained by immunologic and biochemical processes (48), metabolic acidosis (49), and hemodialysis therapy (50). Hemodialysis-induced oxidative stress may be mitigated by the use of biocompatible dialysis membranes (51). Patients with end-stage renal disease have higher levels of MDA and 4-hydroxynonenal, indicating increased lipid peroxidation (52). Oxidative stress is an atherosclerotic risk factor resulting from generation of oxidized LDL (53). In patients undergoing hemodialysis, generation of ROS at each dialysis session (54) is combined with a chronic deficiency in the major antioxidant systems (55,56). Potential oxidative stress-inducing factors include aging (57), inflammation (58,59), diabetes mellitus (60), and iron overload (61). Markers of lipid peroxidation such as TBARS (thiobarbituric acid reactive substances) and of protein oxidation such as AOPPs (advanced oxidation protein products) and protein carbonyls are increased significantly in patients undergoing hemodialysis. In contrast, erythrocyte copper zinc-dependent superoxide dismutase (CuZn-SOD), plasma GSH-Px, and glutathione reductase (GSSG-Red) activities and plasma ubiquinol and ascorbate levels were markedly decreased in hemodialysis patients as compared to healthy subjects. Inflammatory status and duration of dialysis treatment were found to be the most important factors associated with oxidative stress in patients undergoing hemodialysis, whereas age, diabetes, or iron overload did not influence oxidative markers or plasma and erythrocyte antioxidant systems (62). Disturbances in the antioxidant systems with a significant increase in erythrocyte GSH-Px and GSSG-Red activities and a significant decrease in the erythrocyte total level of GSH and plasma GSH-Px activity occur from the early stage of chronic renal failure. The alterations in the antioxidant system gradually increase with the degree of chronic renal failure, increase further in patients being treated with peritoneal dialysis, and are greatest in patients undergoing hemodialysis (63). Mezzano et al. (64) studied the relationships of inflammatory proteins and plasma homocysteine with markers of oxidative stress such as TBARS and AOPP in patients with chronic renal failure. They found no significant correlations between homocysteine and TBARS, AOPP, von Willebrand factor, adhesion molecules, soluble thrombomodulin, thrombin–antithrombin complexes, prothrombin fragments, or indices of activation of fibrinolysis. In contrast, acute-phase proteins showed significant, positive correlations with most markers of oxidative stress, endothelial dysfunction, and hemostatic activation.

Phagocyte function is suppressed during dialysis with cuprophane, which activates complement (65,66). In contrast, the activity of polymorphonuclear leukocytes (PMNLs) is unaltered when hemodialysis is conducted with non–complement-activating dialyzer membranes. In a prospective study, Vanholder et al. (67,68) found that during the first 12 weeks after starting hemodialysis, the glycolytic response and reactive oxygen production were substantially lower in patients treated with cuprophane as compared to those dialyzed with polysulfone membranes. Complement activation by cuprophane suppresses phagocytotic response both acutely and chronically. Himmelfarb et al. (69–71) found less granulocyte oxygen species production in response to exposure to *Staphylococcus aureus* during hemodialysis with complement-activating membranes as compared to non–complement-activating membranes. Rosenkranz et al. (72) observed significantly higher production of reactive oxygen intermediates by PMNL during hemodialysis with cuprophane as compared to polysulfone membranes. There are reports from several other groups showing both suppression and enhancement of neutrophil oxygen radical production by dialyzer membranes (73,74).

Jackson et al. (75) assessed the effect of a single episode of hemodialysis on antioxidant status in 22 patients. The increased total antioxidant capacity of serum, almost entirely the result of relatively high serum urate, decreased markedly after hemodialysis (398 ± 15 versus 136 ± 12 mmol/L). There was also a significant reduction of ascorbate and lipid corrected tocopherol, whereas thiol groups increased after dialysis. Tepel et al. (76) found significantly higher spontaneous and stimulated ROS production in lymphocytes from patients with end-stage renal disease as compared to healthy subjects. Regular hemodialysis sessions using biocompatible membranes had no effect on the elevated intracellular ROS in these patients. Nevertheless, hemodialysis therapy with biocompatible membranes results in the release of phosphatidylcholine hydroperoxide from activated neutrophils (77). Daschner et al. (78) estimated the lipid peroxidation products, MDA and hexanal, and lipophilic antioxidants and GSH in children undergoing pediatric hemodialysis and peritoneal dialysis. Plasma hexanal and antioxidants were normal in both groups of patients, whereas MDA was elevated and decreased after hemodialysis by 88%. GSH decreased slightly during hemodialysis. These data argue against a general increase in lipid peroxidation in uremia (78,79). A new hemodialytic method that incorporates liposomes and antioxidants to remove hydrophobic uremic toxins and minimize free radical–mediated damage has been described. Significant reduction of oxidation products as well as significantly greater removal of platelet-activating factor and bilirubin compared to conventional hemodialysis has been observed (79).

Vascular access protheses of patients treated by hemodialysis are subjected to excess oxidative stress. Weiss et al. (80) found a positive correlation between oxidative stress markers and the neointima of native arteriovenous fistulae or the pseudointima of the polytetrafluoroethylene grafts. TGF-β was associated with proliferation or repair in both native fistulae and grafts. Oxidative stress or injury increases production of TGF-β (81,82).

Heparin reduces PMNL superoxide production (83–85) and protects endothelial cells from ROS (86). Sela et al. (87) measured the rate of PMNL superoxide release and the plasma levels of oxidized glutathione both before and after dialysis in the presence and absence of heparin. The difference between the rates of superoxide release before and after dialysis was significantly smaller in the presence of heparin. Oxidized glutathione increased significantly during hemodialysis therapy in the absence of heparin. This increase, however, was not significant in the presence of heparin. Thus, anticoagulation by heparin may reduce hemodialysis-induced oxidative stress. Regional citrate anticoagulation, however, is more effective than anticoagulation with heparin at reducing PMNL degranulation and the release of myeloperoxidase (88).

Treatment with ACE inhibitors increases antioxidant defenses in animal experiments (89,90) and in patients undergoing hemodialysis (91). ACE inhibitor therapy caused greater predialytic content of red blood cell (RBC) glutathione and higher selenium-dependent GSH-Px activity and plasma B-carotene concentrations as compared to patients undergoing hemodialysis without ACE inhibitors. ACE inhibitor–induced accumulation of bradykinin may result in NO release, triggering an increase in antioxidant defense levels (91).

Nakayama et al. (92) compared plasma ascorbic acid and dehydroascorbic acid levels between patients undergoing maintenance hemodialysis and healthy subjects. Older patients (>55 years) undergoing hemodialysis had significantly lower mean total plasma ascorbic acid than the younger ones, whereas plasma dehydroascorbic acid levels were significantly higher in the elderly hemodialysis patients. There was an inverse correlation between patient age and ascorbic acid levels. There was also a correlation between patient age and dehydroascorbic levels as well as between patient age and lipid peroxide level (92). Ascorbic acid is oxidized to dehydroascorbic acid, which may be a biomarker of oxidative stress. Using this parameter, a greater oxidative stress in elderly than in younger hemodialysis patients was observed. The study of Nguyen-Khoa et al. (62), however, showed no difference between oxidative stress parameters of hemodialysis patients older or younger than age 70 years. Morena et al. (93) found a significant reduction in plasma vitamin C levels in patients undergoing regular hemodiafiltration (HDF) as compared to healthy subjects. The presence of oxidative stress in HDF patients was demonstrated by a significant increase in MDA and AOPP levels, and a decrease in GSH-Px activity. There was, however, no difference in plasma vitamin E between HDF patients and healthy subjects (93). Cigarette smoking increases plasma-circulating products of lipid peroxidation. Because smokers undergoing regular hemodialysis have lower vitamin C levels than nonsmokers, patients undergoing hemodialysis with vitamin C deficiency may by more susceptible to oxidative tissue damage caused by smoking (94).

MDA-modified proteins accumulate in the plasma of patients with end-stage renal disease. MDA is derived from the oxidation of polyunsaturated fatty acids. The MDA and other lipid-modified proteins are called *advanced lipidoxidation end products* (ALEs) (95).

Formation of AGEs and ALEs occurs from the interaction between proteins and reactive carbonyl compounds (RCOs) derived from carbohydrates and lipids. RCO production in uremia is mainly the result of oxidative stress and decreased renal clearance (96). Reduced renal function increases the serum pentosidine level in patients with uremia (97,98). The "carbonyl stress" is associated with long-term complications of patients with end-stage renal disease such as dialysis-related amyloidosis or atherosclerosis (96). In addition, uremia causes oxidant-mediated protein alterations (58,99,100).

Protein damage mediated by ROS results in oxidation of amino acid residues such as tyrosine. When dityrosine is formed, protein aggregation, cross-linking, and fragmentation occur. These dityrosine-containing cross-linked protein products were designated AOPPs (58,99). AOPPs were found in very high concentrations in the plasma of dialysis patients. Because patients treated with peritoneal dialysis and patients with preterminal renal failure also have significantly higher AOPP levels than healthy subjects, it was concluded that uremia induces a significant oxidative stress (58, 99). The accumulation of AOPPs starts at an early stage of chronic renal failure and gradually increases with the progression of renal failure. There is an inverse relationship between AOPP levels and creatinine clearance. A close relationship between AOPPs and AGE-pentosidine has been observed. Human serum albumin (HSA) exposed to chlorinated oxidants (HOCl) resulted in AOPP–HSA formation. Myeloperoxidase released during hemodialysis is a major factor contributing to AOPP formation. Myeloperoxidase and chlorinated oxidant-induced lipoprotein byproducts are present in atherosclerotic lesions (101,102). These data suggest that AOPPs may play a role in the development of atherosclerosis (103).

Plasmalogens are a phospholipid subclass found in cell membranes and plasma lipoproteins. They work as an endogenous antioxidant. The reduced content of serum plasmalogen phospholipids observed in patients undergoing maintenance hemodialysis also suggests increased oxidative stress (104).

AGEs may lead to progression of atherosclerosis by free oxygen radical production followed by a release of inflammatory cytokines (105,106), such as interleukin-6, ultimately leading to the production of C-reactive protein by the liver. Carboxymethyllysine (CML), generated by the myeloperoxidase-H_2O_2-chloride system of activated phagocytes, may play an important role in tissue damage at sites of inflammation as encountered in atherosclerosis. CML also is formed during lipid peroxidation or glucose autoxidation (107,108). It is suggested that the processes contribute synergistically to the tissue damage observed in patients with diabetes mellitus and/or chronic kidney disease (109). However, high serum AGE and CML levels in patients undergoing hemodialysis are not linked to increased mortality. Moreover, high serum AGEs overcome partly the negative impact of the acute-phase response on mortality in patients undergoing hemodialysis (110).

OXIDATIVE STRESS AND RENAL ANEMIA

Plasma levels of lipid peroxidation products correlate with the severity of renal anemia. A decrease in RBC count is associated with a deficiency of both reduced glutathione (111) and of the activity of enzymes that metabolize lipid peroxidation products; this results in diminished antioxidative capacity of blood in patients with uremia. Correction of renal anemia by recombinant human erythropoietin (rhuEPO) results in a decrease in MDA levels. Furthermore, 4-hydroxynonenal concentrations were doubled in hemodialysis patients with hemoglobin values of more than 10 g/dL, but they increased fourfold in those with hemoglobin of less than 10 g/dL. In addition, availability of antioxidants, reflected by enhanced superoxide dismutase and GSH-Px activities, increases after correction of renal anemia (112). These data suggest that the anemic state itself contributes to free radical production (113).

Erythrocyte membrane lipid peroxidation occurs in patients with chronic renal failure (114). In predialysis patients, erythrocyte susceptibility to lipid peroxidation is accelerated as compared to that in maintenance hemodialysis patients. The positive correlation between erythrocyte TBARS concentration and erythrocyte GSH-Px activity in patients with end-stage renal disease who are not undergoing hemodialysis suggests a compensatory increase in erythrocyte GSH-Px activity in response to oxidative stress (115). Mimic-Oka et al. (116) found an increase in the antioxidant-enzyme activities (glutathione peroxidase, superoxide dismutase) with the progression of chronic renal insufficiency. This increase was abolished in patients undergoing maintenance hemodialysis. It was suggested that the enhanced antioxidant enzyme activities could be a protective mechanism for the cells because of hyperproduction of free radicals in chronic renal failure. The lowering of RBC antioxidant activity in patients undergoing regular hemodialysis may contribute to the increased oxidative damage in uremia (116).

Serum albumin inhibits peroxidation of erythrocyte membrane lipids. Persistent hypoalbuminemia worsens the serum antioxidant activity, contributing to increased oxidative cell damage in uremia (115). Antioxidant capacity of blood in patients with end-stage renal disease is reduced due to the following:

1. Loss of water-soluble antioxidants during hemodialysis
2. Consumption by free radical formation
3. Renal anemia

Exogenous reduced glutathione administration resulted in improved RBC survival in patients undergoing hemodialysis (117). Correction of renal anemia by rhuEPO or novel erythropoiesis stimulating protein therapy also improves the antioxidant system. The erythrocytes represent a major component of the antioxidant capacity of the blood through the following:

1. Enzymes such as superoxide dismutase and catalase
2. The glutathione system
3. Regeneration of consumed redox equivalents via glutathione reductase and the oxidative pentose phosphate pathway
4. Cell proteins and low–molecular-weight antioxidants in the erythrocyte membrane (1)

Ludat et al. (118) compared MDA, GSH, and GSSG levels in hemodialysis patients with hematocrit of less than 30%, 30% to 39% and 40%. MDA levels were significantly lower in the group with normal hematocrit as compared to the two other groups. GSH and GSSG whole-blood levels in hemodialysis patients with hematocrit of 40% and 30% to 39% were significantly higher than in hemodialysis patients with hematocrit of less than 30%.There was also an inverse correlation between plasma 4-hydroxynonenal and the hemoglobin values in hemodialysis (119). Therefore, a substantial part of the oxidative stress in patients with end-stage renal disease is probably the result of renal anemia. However, treatment of renal anemia effectively may reduce oxidative stress in these patients.

Lipid peroxidation of the RBC membrane may result in resistance to erythropoietin due to enhanced hemolysis caused by oxidative stress. Gallucci et al. (120) investigated the degree of RBC-membrane oxidative damage in patients undergoing hemodialysis who failed to respond to maximal rhuEPO therapy. RBC MDA, reticulocyte count, plasma-free hemoglobin and serum lactate dehydrogenase were significantly higher, whereas plasma haptoglobin was significantly lower in these patients as compared to patients undergoing hemodialysis who showed a good response to standard rhuEPO therapy or to patients undergoing hemodialysis who needed no rhuEPO treatment.

Lipid peroxidation of the RBC membrane by free radicals and consequent impaired RBC deformability and splenic sequestration may be involved in the aging and lysis of RBCs. Thus, oxidative stress may contribute to the shortened survival of RBCs. Significant RBC production was observed with rhuEPO treatment. There was, however, no significant improvement in the RBC oxidative sensitivity, RBC deformability, splenic RBC volume, slow-mixing splenic RBC volume, and the intrasplenic RBC transit time with rhuEPO therapy (121). Correction of renal anemia by rhuEPO enhances oxidative stress on RBCs (122,123). Turi et al. (124) reported the prooxidant effect of rhuEPO therapy on the glutathione redox system and hemoglobin oxidation in children being treated with maintenance hemodialysis. Adjuvant vitamin E therapy alleviates the oxidative stress of rhuEPO. The high ratio of GSSG/GSH (an indicator of oxidative stress) and the level of carboxyhemoglobin (an indicator of hemolysis) decreased with vitamin E therapy (15 mg/kg per day per os). Furthermore, the combination of rhuEPO and vitamin E therapy increased hemoglobin and hematocrit values significantly earlier than rhuEPO treatment without vitamin E (125). Data of Taccone-Gallucci et al. (126) also showed that vitamin E supplementation has a sparing effect on the rhuEPO dosage requirement in patients undergoing hemodialysis.

OXIDATIVE STRESS AND IRON THERAPY

Intravenous iron supplementation may contribute to increased free radical production (52). Redox-active iron is a potent prooxidant. Hydroxyl radical and lipid alkoxyl radical are formed by the Fenton reaction. These reactive oxygen species trigger iron-induced lipid peroxidation in the presence of hydrogen peroxide or lipid hydroperoxides (126–130). Vitamin E is a potent antioxidant that inhibits lipid peroxidation (131,132). Roob et al. (133) showed that a single dose of vitamin E (1,200 U) attenuates lipid peroxidation in maintenance hemodialysis patients receiving intravenous iron. The acutely generated oxidant stress from administration of 100 mg iron sucrose and rhuEPO can be prevented by a single oral dose of melatonin (0.3 mg/kg) (134).

The mortality rate from cardiovascular disease of patients undergoing maintenance hemodialysis is estimated to be five to 20 times that of the general population (135), probably as a result, at least in part, of this population's enhanced oxidative stress (136–138). *In vivo* studies showed that iron overload may result in cardiomyopathy, manifested by ventricular arrhythmias and heart failure (139). Alterations of GSH-Px activity and increases in cytotoxic aldehyde concentrations in the heart may contribute to iron-induced heart failure (139). Extracellular hydroxyl radical formation is not responsible for iron-mediated cardiotoxicity (140). This does not, however, exclude that myocardial iron toxicity is the result of free radical damage generated intracellularly. Experimental data demonstrate that vitamin E (α-tocopherol) completely inhibits mitochondrial iron toxicity without affecting iron uptake or release. In contrast, the mild cardioprotective effect of ascorbate occurs in association with decreased cellular iron uptake (141).

OXIDATIVE STRESS AND VITAMIN E

Vitamin E is the main lipophilic antioxidant in humans (114,140) and reduces oxidative damage in RBCs (142, 143), platelets (144), and peripheral blood mononuclear cells (145,146). Adjuvant therapy with antioxidants such as α-tocopherol, ascorbic acid, and α-lipoic acid improves kidney function in animals and patients with diabetic nephropathy and the nephrotic syndrome (37,38,147,148). Vitamin E inhibits high–glucose-induced excessive collagen production by mesangial cells in culture (149). Oral supplementation of patients undergoing hemodialysis with vitamin E significantly decreased LDL susceptibility to copper-induced oxidation *in vitro* (150), increased LDL α-tocopherol content by 94% (151), and improved LDL clearance from the circulation and reduced the MDA content of LDL (152). Vitamin E suppressed 5-lipoxygenase-mediated oxidative stress in peripheral blood mononuclear cells of hemodialysis patients undergoing hemodialysis (153). In the study of Boaz et al. (154), 196 patients undergoing maintenance hemodialysis with preexisting cardiovascular disease received either 800 IU/day vitamin E or placebo for a median 519 days. A total of 16% assigned to vitamin E and 36% assigned to placebo had a primary endpoint (myocardial infarction, ischemic stroke, peripheral vascular disease, and/or unstable angina). No significant differences in the secondary endpoints (total mortality and cardiovascular disease mortality) were detected (154).

Regular hemodialysis treatment with cellulose-membrane dialyzers modified with vitamin E was associated with reduced LDL-MDA and oxidized LDL. Slowing of atherosclerosis progression also has been observed (155). Vitamin E-coated hemophane dialyzer membranes displayed a high biocompatibility similar to the synthetic polyamide dialyzer in terms of its effect on lymphocyte function. The vitamin E-coated dialyzer exerted, however, an additional suppressive effect on the overproduction of proinflammatory cytokines (156). In contrast, Dhondt et al. (157) found that other indices of membrane bioincompatibility, such as lymphocyte counts and expression of the leukocyte surface molecules CD11b, CD11c, and CD45, are altered more profoundly with a vitamin E-modified cellulose membrane as compared to the standard low-flux polysulfone membranes.

Shimazu et al. (158) measured superoxide anion radical producing ability of PMNLs, plasma hydroxyl radical producing ability, and superoxide anion radical scavenging activity in hemodialysis patients treated with a vitamin E-modified dialysis membrane. After 6 months, activation of PMNLs and activities of the oxidative stress parameters were attenuated by the antioxidant effects of the vitamin E-modified multilayer membrane. In patients undergoing hemodialysis, treatment with a vitamin E-modified dialyzer resulted in a more effective antioxidant defense than daily peroral administration of 400 mg vitamin E. The modified dialyzer with vitamin E led to a significant increase of serum vitamin E (33%) and plasma total antioxidant capacity and to a significant decrease of plasma MDA (159). MDA–LDL from patients undergoing hemodialysis disappears more slowly from the circulation as compared to LDL from healthy subjects. Treatment of these patients with α-tocopherol at doses of 600 mg/day for 2 weeks results in normal MDA concentrations in LDL (160).

One-month treatment with a vitamin E-modified multilayer membrane increased plasma vitamin E by 84.3% and RBC vitamin E by 76.7%. The increase in vitamin E was associated with an antiapoptotic effect in PMNLs and a hypostimulatory action on the PMNL respiratory burst (161).

Hemodialysis impairs endothelial function in patients with end-stage renal disease, probably by increasing oxidative stress. Miyazaki et al. (162) showed that a single session of hemodialysis using a noncoated dialyzer significantly impairs flow-mediated vasodilation associated with increased plasma levels of oxidized LDL. In contrast, hemodialysis with a vitamin E-coated membrane prevented dialysis-induced endothelial dysfunction and the increase in oxidized LDL.

OXIDATIVE STRESS AFTER TRANSPLANTATION

Long-term immunosuppression with cyclosporin A is associated with interstitial fibrosis of the kidney. Antioxidant therapy concurrent with cyclosporin A administration in rats resulted in the inhibition of cyclosporin-induced lipid peroxidation and interstitial fibrosis (163). However, antioxidant deficiency, which exposes tissues to free radical injury and lipid peroxidation, leads to marked tubulointerstitial fibrosis of the kidney (21). Cyclosporin causes an increase in plasma hydroperoxides from cholesterol esters and triglycerides as well as an increase in plasma peroxynitrile levels (164). Kandoussi et al. (165) found a significant increase in auto-antibodies directed against MDA–CDL and Cu^{2+}-oxidized LDL 1 year after renal transplantation in patients being treated with immunosuppression with cyclosporin. The values remained high during the second and the third year following transplantation. There was a significant correlation between cyclosporin trough levels and Ca^{2+}-oxidized LDL auto-antibodies. Antioxidant capacity of the urine of renal transplant recipients may predict early graft function (166). Long-term cyclosporin therapy may be associated with renal interstitial fibrosis. Antioxidant therapy concurrent with cyclosporin A administration in rats resulted in inhibition of cyclosporin-induced lipid peroxidation and a striking reduction in cyclosporin-induced chronic interstitial fibrosis and renal dysfunction (167).

Ischemia–reperfusion-induced renal injury is the most common cause of acute renal failure (168). Oxygen-derived free radical species have been implicated in the pathogenesis of this process (169,170). The endogenous scavenger superoxide dismutase (SOD) is depleted rapidly during ischemia and reperfusion, particularly the cytoplasmic copper-zinc form (171,172). SOD expression can be increased by delivery of the SOD gene to the kidney by intravenous injection. SOD gene transduction minimizes ischemia–reperfusion-induced acute renal failure (173).

Prostaglandins are known to inhibit hepatic injury from various causes including ischemia reperfusion (174–176). Prostaglandin E_1 exerts its cytoprotective effect in tert-butyl hydroperoxide-induced hepatic injury partly by inhibiting Ca^{2+}-calpain-μ-mediated mechanisms (177). Excessive oxidative stress and a lack of glutathione are associated with bronchiolitis obliterans syndrome after heart–lung transplantation (178). Iron may aggravate ROS-induced airway injury and the development of the bronchiolitis obliterans following lung transplantation (179).

Taurine protects liver from ischemia reoxygenation. The addition of taurine to perfusion and storage solutions or taurine supplementation of the donor has been recommended to protect transplanted organs (180). N-acetylcysteine also appears to have cytoprotective effects. It has been shown that this substance attenuates the increase in α-glutathione 5-transferase and circulating adhesion molecules after reperfusion of the donor liver (181). Dopamine induces the expression of the protective enzyme heme oxygenase 1 on cultured endothelial cells by an oxidative mechanism. These data may explain the significant improvement of long-term organ survival of the retrieved kidney after administration of dopamine to the organ donors (182).

REFERENCES

1. Grune T, Sommerburg O, Siems WG. Oxidative stress in anemia. *Clin Nephrol* 2000;53(Suppl 1):S18–S22.
2. Turi S, Nemeth I, Torkos A, et al. Oxidative stress and antioxidant defense mechanism in glomerular disease. *Free Radic Biol Med* 1997;22:161–168.
3. Neale TJ, Ullrich R, Ojha P, et al. Reactive oxygen species and neutrophil respiratory burst cytochrome b^{558} are produced by kidney glomerular cells in passive Heymann nephritis. *Proc Natl Acad Sci U S A* 1993;90:3645–3649.
4. Gwinner W, Landmesser U, Brandes RP, et al. Reactive oxygen species and antioxidant defense in puromycin aminonucleoside glomerulopathy. *J Am Soc Nephrol* 1997;8:1722–1731.
5. Kuemmerle NB, Chan W, Krieg RJ Jr, et al. Effects of fish oil and alpha-tocopherol in immunoglobulin A nephropathy in the rat. *Pediatr Res* 1998;43:791–797.
6. Boyce NW, Tipping PG. Holdsworth SR. Glomerular macrophages produce reactive oxygen species in experimental glomerulonephritis. *Kidney Int* 1989;35:778–782.
7. Aiello S, Noris M, Todeschini M, et al. Renal and systemic nitric oxide synthesis in rats with renal mass reduction. *Kidney Int* 1997;52:171–181.
8. Van den Branden C, Ceyssens B, Craemer D, et al. Antioxidant enzyme gene expression in rats with remnant kidney induced chronic renal failure. *Exp Nephrol* 2000;8:91–96.
9. Lee HS, Jeong JY, Kim BC, et al. Dietary antioxidant inhibits lipoprotein oxidation and renal injury in experimental focal segmental glomerulosclerosis. *Kidney Int* 1997;51:1151–1159.
10. Modi KS, Schreiner GF, Purkerson ML, et al. Effects of probucol in renal function and structure in rats with subtotal kidney ablation. *J Lab Clin Med* 1992;120:310–317.
11. Trachtman H, Schwob N, Maesaka J, et al. Dietary vitamin E supplementation ameliorates renal injury in chronic puromycin aminonucleoside nephropathy. *J Am Soc Nephrol* 1995;5:1811–1819.
12. Trachtman H, Del Pizzo R, Futterweit S, et al. Taurine attenuates renal disease in chronic puromycin aminonucleoside nephropathy. *Am J Physiol* 1992;262:F117–F123.
13. Hahn S, Kuemmerle NB, Chan W, et al. Glomerulosclerosis in the remnant kidney rat is modulated by dietary α-tocopherol. *J Am Soc Nephrol* 1998;9:2089–2095.
14. Tahzib M, Frank R, Gauthier B, et al. Vitamin E treatment of focal segmental glomerulosclerosis: results of an open-label study. *Pediatr Nephrol* 1999;13:649–652.
15. Ogawa M, Ueda S, Anzai N, et al. Decrease of urine protein

after treatment with probucol in patients with mild glomerulonephritis and arteriosclerosis. *Nephron* 1995;70:376–377.
16. Haas M, Mayer G, Wirnsberger G, et al. Antioxidant treatment of therapy-resistant idiopathic membranous nephropathy with probucol: A pilot study. *Wien Klin Wochenschr* 2002;114: 143–147.
17. Rahman MM, Varghese Z, Fuller BJ, et al. Renal vasoconstriction induced by oxidized LDL is inhibited by scavengers of reactive oxygen species and L-arginine. *Clin Nephrol* 1999;51: 98–107.
18. Zatz R, Baylis C. Chronic nitric oxide inhibition model six years on. *Hypertension* 1998;32:958–964.
19. Darley-Usmar V, Wiseman H, Halliwell B. Nitric oxide and oxygen radicals: A question of balance. *FEBS Lett* 1995;369: 131–135.
20. Clancy RM, Leszczynska-Piziak J, Abramson SB. Nitric oxide, an endothelial cell relaxation factor, inhibits neutrophil superoxide anion production via a direct action on the NADPH oxidase. *J Clin Invest* 1992;90:1116–1121.
21. Nath KA, Salahudeen AK. Induction of renal growth and injury in the intact rat kidney by dietary deficiency of antioxidants. *J Clin Invest* 1990;86:1179–1192.
22. Van den Branden C, Verelst R, Vamecq J, et al. Effect of vitamin E on antioxidant enzymes, lipid peroxidation products and glomerulosclerosis in the rat remnant kidney. *Nephron* 1997;76: 77–81.
23. Attia DM, Verhagen AMG, Stroes ES, et al. Vitamin E alleviates renal injury, but not hypertension during chronic nitric oxide synthase inhibition in rats. *J Am Soc Nephrol* 2001;12: 2585–2593.
24. Yoshioka T, Ichikawa I, Fogo A. Reactive oxygen metabolites cause massive, reversible proteinuria and glomerular sieving defect without apparent ultrastructural abnormality. *J Am Soc Nephrol* 1991;2:902–912.
25. Gwinner W, Plasger J, Brandes RP, et al. Role of xanthine oxidase in passive Heymann nephritis in rats. *J Am Soc Nephrol* 1999;10:538–544.
26. Laursen J, Rajagopalan S, Galis Z, et al. Role of superoxide in angiotensin II-induced but not catecholamine-induced hypertension. *Circulation* 1997;95:588–593.
27. Hannken T, Schroeder R, Stahl RAK, et al. Angiotensin II-mediated expression of $p27^{Kip1}$ and induction of cellular hypertrophy in renal tubular cells depend on the generation of oxygen radicals. *Kidney Int* 1998;54:1923–1933.
28. Verhagen AMG, Braam B, Boer P, et al. Losartan-sensitive renal damage caused by chronic NOC inhibition does not involve increased renal angiotensin II concentrations. *Kidney Int* 1999; 56:222–231.
29. Onozato ML, Tojo A, Goto A, et al. Oxidative stress and nitric oxide synthase in rat diabetic nephropathy: effects of ACEI and ARB. *Kidney Int* 2002;61:186–194.
30. Annuk M, Zilmer M, Lind L, et al. Oxidative stress and endothelial function in chronic renal failure. *J Am Soc Nephrol* 2001; 12:2747–2752.
31. Suzuki H, DeLano FA, Parks DA, et al. Xanthine oxidase activity associated with arterial blood pressure in spontaneously hypertensive rats. *Proc Natl Acad Sci U S A* 1998;95:4754–4759.
32. Ha H, Kim KH. Role of oxidative stress in the development of diabetic nephropathy. *Kidney Int* 1995;51:S18–S21.
33. Salahudeen AK, Kanji V, Reckelhoff JF, et al. Pathogenesis of diabetic nephropathy: a radical approach. *Nephrol Dial Transplant* 1997;12:664–668.
34. Kakkar R, Mantha SV, Radhi J, et al. Antioxidant defense system in diabetic kidney: a time course study. *Life Sci* 1997;60: 667–679.
35. Borcea V, Nourooz-Zadeh J, Wolff SP, et al. Alpha-lipoic acid decreases oxidative stress even in diabetic patients with poor glycemic control and albuminuria. *Free Radic Biol Med* 1999; 26:1495–1500.
36. Bierhaus A, Schiekofer S, Andrassy M, et al. The role of oxidative stress and subsequent NF-kappaB activation in renal disease. *Kidney Blood Press Res* 1999;22:299–305.
37. Cohen MP, Hud E, Wu VY. Amelioration of diabetic nephropathy by treatment with monoclonal antibodies against glycated albumin. *Kidney Int* 1994;45:1673–1679.
38. Vlassara H. Recent progress on the biologic and clinical significance of advanced glycosylation end products. *J Lab Clin Med* 1994;124:19–30.
39. Yan SD, Schmidt AM, Anderson GM, et al. Enhanced cellular oxidant stress by the interaction of advanced glycation end products with their receptors/binding proteins. *J Biol Chem* 1994; 269:9889–9897.
40. Wautier JL, Zoukorian C, Chappey O, et al. Receptor mediated endothelial dysfunction in diabetic vasculopathy: sRAGE blocks hyperpermeability. *J Clin Invest* 1996;97:238–243.
41. Gopaul NK, Anggard EE, Mallet AL, et al. Plasma 8-epi PGE (2 alpha) levels are elevated in individuals with non-insulin dependent diabetes mellitus. *FEBS Lett* 1995;368:225–229.
42. Hunt JV, Wolff SP. Oxidative glycation and free radical production: a causal mechanism of diabetic complications. *Free Radic Res Commun* 1991;12–13 Pt 1:115–123.
43. Bucala R, Makita Z, Koschinsky T, et al. Lipid advanced glycosylation: pathway for lipid oxidation in vivo. *Proc Natl Acad Sci U S A* 1993;90:6434–6438.
44. Dogra G, Ward N, Croft KD, et al. Oxidant stress in nephrotic syndrome: comparison of F2-isoprostanes and plasma antioxidant potential. *Nephrol Dial Transplant* 2001;16:1626–1630.
45. Hofmann MA, Schiekofer S, Isermann B, et al. Peripheral blood mononuclear cells isolated from patients with diabetic nephropathy show increased activation of the oxidative-stress sensitive transcription for NF-kappaB. *Diabetologia* 1999;42:222–232.
46. Baynes JW, Thorpe SR. Role of oxidative stress in diabetic complications: a new perspective on an old paradigm. *Diabetes* 1999;48:1–9.
47. Tepel M, van der Giet M, Schwarzfeld C, et al. Prevention of radiographic-contrast-induced in renal function by acetylcysteine. *N Engl J Med* 2000;343:180–184.
48. Baud L, Ardaillou R. Reactive oxygen species: production and role in the kidney. *Am J Physiol* 1986;251:F765–F776.
49. Roselaar SE, Nazhat NB, Winyard PG, et al. Detection of oxidants in uremic plasma by electron spin resonance spectroscopy. *Kidney Int* 1995;48:199–206.
50. Westhuyzen J, Adams CE, Fleming SJ. Evidence for oxidative stress during in vitro dialysis. *Nephron* 1995;70:49–54.
51. Dasgupta A, Hussain S, Ahmad S. Increased lipid peroxidation in patients on maintenance hemodialysis. *Nephron* 1992;60: 56–59.
52. Loughrey CM, Young IS, Lightbody JM, et al. Oxidative stress in hemodialysis. *Q J Med* 1994;87:679–683.
53. Maggi E, Bellazzi R, Falaschi F, et al. Enhanced LDL oxidation in uremic patients: an additional mechanism for accelerated atherosclerosis. *Kidney Int* 1994;45:876–883.
54. Nguyen AT, Lethias C, Zingraff J, et al. Hemodialysis membrane induced activation of phagocyte oxidative metabolism detected in vivo and in vitro within microamounts of whole blood. *Kidney Int* 1985;28:158–167.
55. Paul JL, Sall ND, Soni T, et al. Lipid peroxidation abnormalities in hemodialyzed patients. *Nephron* 1993;64:106–109.
56. Ceballos-Picot I, Witko-Sarsat V, Merad-Boudia M, et al. Glutathione antioxidant system as a marker of oxidative stress in chronic renal failure. *Free Radic Biol Med* 1996;21:845–853.
57. Olivieri O, Stanzial AM, Girelli D, et al. Selenium status, fatty

acids, vitamins A and E, and aging: the Nove study. *Am J Clin Nutr* 1994;60:510–517.
58. Witko-Sarsat V, Friedlander M, Nguyen-Khoa T, et al. Advanced oxidation protein products as novel mediators of inflammation and monocyte activation in chronic renal failure. *J Immunol* 1998;161:2524–2532.
59. Zimmermann J, Herrlinger S, Pruy A, et al. Inflammation enhances cardiovascular risk and mortality in hemodialysis patients. *Kidney Int* 1999;55:648–658.
60. Miyata T, Maeda K, Kurokawa K, et al. Oxidation conspires with glycation to generate noxious advanced glycation end products in renal failure. *Nephrol Dial Transplant* 1997;12:255–258.
61. Delmas-Beauvieux MC, Combe C, Peuchant E, et al. Evaluation of red blood cell lipoperoxidation in hemodialysed patients during erythropoietin therapy supplemented or not with iron. *Nephron* 1995;69:404–410.
62. Nguyen-Khoa T, Massy ZA, de Bandt JP, et al. Oxidative stress and haemodialysis: role of inflammation and duration of dialysis treatment. *Nephrol Dial Transplant* 2001;16:335–340.
63. Ceballos-Picot I, Witko-Sarsat V, Merad-Boudia M, et al. Glutathione antioxidant system as a marker of oxidative stress in chronic renal failure. *Free Radic Biol Med* 1996;21:845–853.
64. Mezzano D, Pais EO, Aranda E, et al. Inflammation, not hyperhomocysteinemia, is related to oxidative stress and hemostatic and endothelial dysfunction in uremia. *Kidney Int* 2001;60: 1844–1850.
65. Vanholder R, Ringoir S. Infectious morbidity and defects of phagocytic function in end-stage renal disease: A review. *J Am Soc Nephrol* 1993;3:1541–1554.
66. Ward RA. Phagocytic cell function as an index of biocompatibility. *Nephrol Dial Transplant* 1994;9(Suppl 2):46–56.
67. Vanholder R, Ringoir S, Dhondt A, et al. Phagocytosis in uremic and hemodialysis patients: A prospective and cross sectional study. *Kidney Int* 1991;39:320–327.
68. Vanholder R, Ringoir S. Polymorphonuclear cell function and infection in dialysis. *Kidney Int Suppl* 1992;38:S91–S95.
69. Himmelfarb J, Gerard NP, Hakim RM. Intradialytic modulation of granulocyte C5a receptors. *J Am Soc Nephrol* 1991;2: 920–926.
70. Himmelfarb J, Lazarus JM, Hakim RM. Reactive oxygen species production by monocytes and polymorphonuclear leukocytes during hemodialysis. *Am J Kidney Dis* 1991;17:271–276.
71. Himmelfarb J, Ault KA, Holbrook D, et al. Intradialytic granulocyte reactive oxygen species production: A prospective, crossover trial. *J Am Soc Nephrol* 1993;4:178–186.
72. Rosenkranz AR, Templ E, Traindl O, et al. Reactive oxygen product formation by human neutrophils as an early marker for biocompatibility of dialysis membranes. *Clin Exp Immunol* 1994;98:300–305.
73. Nguyen AT, Lethias C, Zingraff J, et al. Hemodialysis membrane-induced activation of phagocyte oxidative metabolism detected in vivo and in vitro within microamounts of whole blood. *Kidney Int* 1985;28:158–167.
74. Cristol JP, Canaud B, Rabesandratana H, et al. Enhancement of reactive oxygen species production and cell surface markers expression due to haemodialysis. *Nephrol Dial Transplant* 1994; 9:389–394.
75. Jackson P, Loughrey CM, Lightbody JM, et al. Effect of hemodialysis on total antioxidant capacity and serum antioxidants in patients with chronic renal failure. *Clin Chem* 1995;41: 1135–1138.
76. Tepel M, Echelmeyer M, Otie NN, et al. Increased intracellular reactive oxygen species in patients with end-stage renal failure: effect of hemodialysis. *Kidney Int* 2000;58:867–872.
77. Sanaka T, Higuchi C, Shinobe T, et al. Lipid peroxidation as an indicator of biocompatibility in haemodialysis. *Nephrol Dial Transplant* 1995;10(Suppl 3):34–38.
78. Daschner M, Lenhartz H, Botticher D, et al. Influence of dialysis on plasma lipid peroxidation products and antioxidant levels. *Kidney Int* 1996;50:1268–1272.
79. Wratten ML, Sereni L, Tetta C. Hemolipodialysis attenuates oxidative stress and removes hydrophobic toxins. *Artif Organs* 2000;24:685–690.
80. Weiss MF, Scivittaro V, Anderson JM. Oxidative stress and increased expression of growth factors in lesions of failed hemodialysis access. *Am J Kidney Diss* 2001;37:970–980.
81. Barcellos-Hoff M, Dix TA. Redox mediated activation of latent transforming growth factor-beta 1. *Mol Endocrinol* 1996;10: 1077–1083.
82. Leonarduzzi G, Scavazza A, Biasi F, et al. The lipid peroxidation end product 4-hydroxy-2,3-nonenal up-regulates transforming growth factor beta expression in the macrophage lineage: a link between oxidative injury and fibrosclerosis. *FASEB J* 1997;11: 851–857.
83. Laghi-Pasini F, Pasqui AL, Ceccatelli L, et al. Heparin inhibition of polymorphonuclear leukocyte activation in vitro: a possible pharmacological approach to granulocyte mediated vascular damage. *Thromb Res* 1984;35:527–537.
84. Cairo MS, Allen J, Higgins C, et al. Synergistic effect of heparin and chemotactic factor on polymorphonuclear leukocyte aggregation and degranulation. *Am J Pathol* 1983;113:67–74.
85. Leculier C, Couprie N, Adeleine P, et al. The effects of high molecular weight and low molecular weight heparins on superoxide ion production and degranulation by human polymorphonuclear leukocytes. *Thromb Res* 1993;69:519–531.
86. Hiebert L, Liu JM. Protective action of polyelectrolytes on endothelium. *Semin Thromb Hemost* 1991;17:42–46.
87. Sela S, Shurtz-Swirski R, Shapiro G, et al. Oxidative stress during hemodialysis: effect of heparin. *Kidney Int* 2001;59(Suppl 78):S159–S163.
88. Bos JC, Grooteman MPC, van Houte AJ, et al. Low polymorphonuclear cell degranulation during citrate anticoagulation: a comparison between citrate and heparin dialysis. *Nephrol Dial Transplant* 1997;12:1387–1393.
89. de Cavanagh EMV, Inserra F, Ferder L, et al. Superoxide dismutase and glutathione peroxidase activities are increased by enalapril and captopril in mouse liver. *FEBS Lett* 1995;361:22–24.
90. de Cavanagh EMV, Fraga CG, Ferder L, et al. Enalapril and captopril enhance antioxidant defenses in mouse tissues. *Am J Physiol* 1997;272:R514–R518.
91. de Cavanagh EMV, Ferder L, Carrasquendeo F, et al. Higher levels of antioxidant defenses in enalapril-treated versus non-enalapril-treated hemodialysis patients. *Am J Kidney Diss* 1999; 34:445–455.
92. Nakayama H, Akiyama S, Inagaki M, et al. Dehydroascorbic acid and oxidative stress in haemodialysis patients. *Nephrol Dial Transplant* 2001;16:574–579.
93. Morena M, Cristol JP, Bosc JY, et al. Convective and diffuse losses of vitamin C during haemodiafiltration session: a contributive factor to oxidative stress in haemodialysis patients. *Nephrol Dial Transplant* 2002;17:422–427.
94. Lim PS, Wang NP, Lu TC, et al. Evidence for alterations in circulating low-molecular-weight antioxidants and increased lipid peroxidation in smokers on hemodialysis. *Nephron* 2001; 88:127–133.
95. Miyata T, van Ypersele de Strihou C, Kurokawa K, et al. Alterations in non-enzymatic biochemistry in uremia: Origin and significance of "carbonyl stress" in long-term uremic complications. *Kidney Int* 1999;55:389–399.
96. Miyata T, Saito A, Kurokawa K. Reactive carbonyl compounds

related uremic toxicity ("carbonyl stress"). *Kidney Int Suppl* 2001;78:S25–S31.
97. Sugiyama S, Miyata T, Ueda Y, et al. Plasma level of pentosidine, an advanced glycation end product, in diabetic patients. *J Am Soc Nephrol* 1998;9:1681–1688.
98. Jadoul M, Ueda Y, Yasuda Y, et al. Influence of hemodialysis membrane type on pentosidine plasma level, a marker of "carbonyl stress." *Kidney Int* 1999;55:2487–2492.
99. Witko-Sarsat V, Descamps-Latscha B. Advanced oxidation protein products: Novel uraemic toxins and pro-inflammatory mediators in chronic renal failure? *Nephrol Dial Transplant* 1997; 12:1310–1312.
100. Himmelfarb J, McMonagle E, McMenamin E. Plasma protein thiol oxidation and carbonyl formation in chronic renal failure. *Kidney Int* 2000;58:2571–2578.
101. Daugherty A, Dunn JL, Rateri DL, et al. Myeloperoxidase, a catalyst for lipoprotein oxidation, is expressed in human atherosclerotic lesions. *J Clin Invest* 1994;94:437–444.
102. Anderson MM, Hazen SL, Hsu FF, et al. Human neutrophils employ the myeloperoxidase-hydrogen peroxide chloride system to convert hydroxyamino acids into glycoaldehyde, 2-hydroxypropanal, and acrolein. A mechanism for the generation of highly reactive alpha-hydroxy and alpha, beta-unsaturated aldehydes by phagocytes at sites of inflammation. *J Clin Invest* 1997; 99:424–432.
103. Witko-Sarsat V, Nguyen-Khoa T, Jungers P, et al. Advanced oxidation protein products as a novel molecular basis of oxidative stress in uraemia. *Nephrol Dial Transplant* 1999;14(Suppl 1):76–78.
104. Brosche T, Platt D, Knopf B. Decreased concentrations of serum phospholipid plasmalogens indicate oxidative burden of uraemic patients undergoing haemodialysis. *Nephron* 2002;90: 58–63.
105. Raj DS, Choudhury D, Welbourne TC, et al. Advanced glycation end products: a nephrologist's perspective. *Am J Kidney Dis* 2000;35:365–380.
106. Bierhaus A, Hofmann MA, Ziegler R, et al. AGEs and their interaction with AGE-receptors in vascular disease and diabetes mellitus. I. The AGE concept. *Cardiovasc Res* 1998;37: 586–600.
107. Fu MX, Requena JR, Jenkins AJ, et al. The advanced glycation end product, Nepsilon-(carboxymethyl)lysine, is a product of both lipid peroxidation and glycoxidation reactions. *J Biol Chem* 1996;271:9982–9986.
108. Thornalley PJ. Pharmacology of methylglyoxal: formation, modification of proteins and nucleic acids, and enzymatic detoxification—a role in pathogenesis and antiproliferative chemotherapy. *Gen Pharmacol* 1996;27:565–573.
109. Meng J, Sakata N, Imanaga Y, et al. Carboxymethyllysine in dermal tissues of diabetic and nondiabetic patients with chronic renal failure: relevance of glycoxidation damage. *Nephron* 2001; 88:30–35.
110. Schwedler SB, Metzger T, Schinzel R, et al. Advanced glycation end products and mortality in hemodialysis patients. *Kidney Int* 2000;62:301–310.
111. Costagliola C, Romano L, Sorice P, et al. Anemia and chronic renal failure. The possible role of the oxidative state of glutathione. *Nephron* 1989;52:11–14.
112. Canestrari F, Buoncristiani U, Galli F. Redox state, antioxidative activity and lipid peroxidation in erythrocytes and plasma of chronic ambulatory peritoneal dialysis patients. *Clinica Chimica Acta* 1995;234:127–136.
113. Sommerburg O, Grune T, Hampl H, et al. Does long-term treatment of renal anemia with recombinant erythropoietin influence oxidative stress in hemodialyzed patients? *Nephrol Dial Transplant* 1998;13:2583–2587.
114. Taccone-Gallucci M, Giardini O, Lubrano R, et al. Red blood cell lipid peroxidation in predialysis chronic renal failure. *Clin Nephrol* 1987;27:238–241.
115. Soejima A, Matsuzawa N, Miyake N, et al. Hypoalbuminemia accelerates erythrocyte membrane lipid peroxidation in chronic hemodialysis patients. *Clin Nephrol* 1999;51:92–97.
116. Mimic-Oka J, Simic T, Ekmescic V, et al. Erythrocyte glutathione peroxidase and superoxide dismutase activities in different stages of chronic renal failure. *Clin Nephrol* 1995;44:44–48.
117. Usberti M, Lima G, Arisi M, et al. Effects of exogenous reduced glutathione on the survival of red blood cells in hemodialyzed patients. *J Nephrol* 1997;10:261–265.
118. Ludat K, Sommerburg O, Grune T, et al. Oxidation parameters in complete correction of renal anemia. *Clin Nephrol* 2000; 53(Suppl 1):530–535.
119. Sommerburg O, Grune T, Hampl H, et al. Does treatment of renal anemia with recombinant erythropoietin influence oxidative stress in hemodialysis patients? *Clin Nephrol* 2000;53(Suppl 1):S23–S29.
120. Gallucci MT, Lubrano R, Meloni LC, et al. Red blood cell membrane lipid peroxidation and resistance to erythropoietin therapy in hemodialysis patients. *Clin Nephrol* 1999;52: 239–245.
121. Zachee P, Ferrant A, Daelemans R, et al. Oxidative injury to erythrocytes, cell rigidity and splenic hemolysis in hemodialyzed patients before and during erythropoietin treatment. *Nephron* 1993;65:288–293.
122. Linde T, Sandhagen B, Danielson BG, et al. Impaired erythrocyte fluidity during treatment of renal anaemia with erythropoietin. *J Intern Med* 1992;231:601–606.
123. Cristol JP, Bose JY, Badiou S, et al. Erythropoietin and oxidative stress in haemodialysis: beneficial effects of vitamin E supplementation. *Nephrol Dial Transplant* 1997;12:2312–2317.
124. Turi S, Nemeth I, Varga I, et al. The effect of erythropoietin on the cellular defence mechanism of red blood cells in children with chronic renal failure. *Pediatr Nephrol* 1992;6:536–541.
125. Nemeth I, Turi S, Haszon I, et al. Vitamin E alleviates the oxidative stress of erythropoietin in uremic children on hemodialysis. *Pediatr Nephrol* 2000;14:13–17.
126. Taccone-Gallucci M, Lubrano R, Meloni C, et al. Malondialehyde content of cell membrane is the most important marker of oxidative stress in haemodialysis patients. *Nephrol Dial Transplant* 1998;13:2711–2712.
127. Linpisarn S, Satoh K, Mikami T, et al. Effects of iron on lipid peroxidation. *Int J Hematol* 1991;54:181–188.
128. Minotti G, Aust SD. Redox cycling of iron and lipid peroxidation. *Lipids* 1992;27:219–226.
129. Khoschsorur G, Bratschitsch G, Roob JM, et al. Iron-induced lipid peroxidation in whole blood in vitro as determined by malondialdehyde and luminol-enhanced chemiluminescence: implications for iron supplementation to iron-depleted patients. *Med Sci Res* 1997;25:389–391.
130. Brown KE, Knudsen CA. Oxidized heme proteins in an animal model of hemochromatosis. *Free Radical Biol Med* 1998;24: 239–244.
131. Dieber-Rotheneder M, Puhl H, Waeg G, et al. Effect of oral supplementation with D-alpha-tocopherol on the vitamin E content of human low density lipoproteins and resistance to oxidation. *J Lipid Res* 1991;32:1325–1332.
132. Winklhofer-Roob BM, Ziouzenkova O, Puhl H, et al. Impaired resistance to oxidation of low density lipoprotein in cystic fibrosis: improvement during vitamin E supplementation. *Free Radical Biol Med* 1995;19:725–733.
133. Roob JM, Khoschsorur G, Tiran A, et al. Vitamin E attenuates oxidative stress induced by intravenous iron in patients on hemodialysis. *J Am Soc Nephrol* 2000;11:539–549.

134. Herrera J, Nava M, Romero F, et al. Melatonin prevents oxidative stress resulting from iron and erythropoietin administration. *Am J Kidney Dis* 2001;37:750–757.
135. Ritz E, Koch M. Morbidity and mortality due to hypertensive patients with renal failure. *Am J Kidney Dis* 1993;21(Suppl 2): 113–118.
136. Zima T, Haragsim L, Stipek S, et al. Lipid peroxidation on dialysis membranes. *Biochem Mol Biol Int* 1993;29:531–537.
137. Toborek M, Wasik T, Drozdz M, et al. Effect of hemodialysis in lipid peroxidation and antioxidant system in patients with chronic renal failure. *Metabolism* 1992;41:1229–1232.
138. Loughrey CM, Young IS, Lightbody JH, et al. Oxidative stress in hemodialysis. *Q J Med* 1994;87:679–683.
139. Bartfay WJ, Butany J, Lehotay DC, et al. A biochemical, histochemical and electron microscopic study on the effects of iron-loading on the hearts of mice. *Cardiovasc Pathol* 1999;8: 305–314.
140. Watts JA, Ford MD, Leonova E. Iron-mediated cardiotoxicity develops independently of extracellular hydroxyl radicals in isolated rat hearts. *J Toxicol Clin Toxicol* 1999;37:19–28.
141. Link G, Konijn AM, Hershko C. Cardioprotective effects of alpha-tocopherol, ascorbate, deferoxamine, and deferiprone: mitochondrial function in cultures, iron-loaded heart cells. *J Lab Clin Med* 1999;133:179–188.
142. Burton GW, Joyce A, Ingold KU. First proof that vitamin A is major lipid-soluble, chain-breaking antioxidant in human blood plasma. *Lancet* 1982;2:327 (letter).
143. Giardini O, Taccone-Gallucci M, Lubrano R. Effects of alpha tocopherol administration on red blood cell membrane lipid peroxidation in hemodialysis patients. *Clin Nephrol* 1984;21: 174–177.
144. Taccone-Gallucci M, Lubrano R, Del Principe D, et al. Platelet lipid peroxidation in haemodialysis patients: effects of vitamin E supplementation. *Nephrol Dial Transplant* 1989;4:975–978.
145. Taccone-Gallucci M, Giardini O, Ausiello C, et al. Vitamin E supplementation in hemodialysis patients: effects on peripheral blood mononuclear cell lipid peroxidation and immune response. *Clin Nephrol* 1986;25:81–86.
146. Lubrano R, Taccone-Gallucci G, Mannarino O, et al. Vitamin E supplementation and oxidative status of peripheral blood mononuclear cells and lymphocyte subset in hemodialysis patients. *Nutrition* 1992;8:94–97.
147. Brownlee M. Glycation products and the pathogenesis of diabetic complications. *Diabetes Care* 1992;15:1835–1843.
148. Schmidt AM, Vianna M, Gerlach M, et al. Isolation and characterization of two binding proteins for advanced glycosylation end products from bovine lung which are present on the endothelial cell surface. *J Biol Chem* 1992;267:14987–14997.
149. Trachtman H. Vitamin E prevents glucose-induced lipid peroxidation and increased collagen production in cultured rat mesangial cells. *Microvasc Res* 1994;47:232–239.
150. Panzetta O, Cominacini L, Garbin U, et al. Increased susceptibility of LDL to in vitro oxidation in patients on maintenance hemodialysis: effects of fish oil and vitamin E administration. *Clin Nephrol* 1995;44:303–309.
151. Islam KN, O'Byrne D, Devaraj S, et al. Alpha-tocopherol supplementation decreases the oxidative susceptibility of LDL in renal failure patients on dialysis therapy. *Atherosclerosis* 2000; 150:217–224.
152. Yukawa S, Hibino A, Maeda T, et al. Effect of alpha-tocopherol on in vitro and in vivo metabolism of low density lipoprotein in hemodialysis patients. *Nephrol Dial Transplant* 1995; 10(Suppl 3):1–3.
153. Maccarrone M, Meloni C, di Villahermosa SM, et al. Vitamin E suppresses 5-lipoxygenase-mediated oxidative stress in peripheral blood mononuclear cells of hemodialysis patients regardless of administration route. *Am J Kidney Dis* 2001;37:964–969.
154. Boaz M, Smetana S, Weinstein T, et al. Secondary prevention with antioxidants of cardiovascular disease in endstage renal disease (SPACE): randomised placebo-controlled trial. *Lancet* 2000;356:1213–1218.
155. Mune M, Yukawa S, Kishino M, et al. Effect of vitamin E on lipid metabolism and atherosclerosis in ESRD patients. *Kidney Int* 1999;71 (Suppl):S126–S129.
156. Girndt M, Lengler S, Kaul H, et al. Prospective crossover trial of the influence of vitamin E-coated dialyzer membranes on T-cell activation and cytokine induction. *Am J Kidney Dis* 2000; 35:95–104.
157. Dhondt A, Vanholder R, Glorieux G, et al. Vitamin E-bonded cellulose membrane and hemodialysis bioincompatibility: absence of an acute benefit on expressions of leukocyte surface molecules. *Am J Kidney Dis* 2000;36:1140–1146.
158. Shimazu T, Ominato M, Toyama K, et al. Effects of a vitamin E-modified dialysis membrane on neutrophil superoxide anion radical production. *Kidney Int* 2001;59(Suppl 78):S137–S143.
159. Mydlik M, Derzsiova K, Racz O, et al. A modified dialyzer with vitamin E and antioxidant defense parameters. *Kidney Int* 2001;78:S144–S147.
160. Yukawa S, Hibino A, Maeda T, et al. Effect of alpha-tocopherol on in vitro and in vivo metabolism of low-density lipoproteins in haemodialysis patients. *Nephrol Dial Transplant* 1995; 10(Suppl 3):1–3.
161. Galli F, Rovidati S, Chiarantini L, et al. Bioreactivity and biocompatibility of a vitamin E-modified multi-layer hemodialysis filter. *Kidney Int* 1998;54:580–589.
162. Miyazaki H, Matsuoka H, Itabe H, et al. Hemodialysis impairs endothelial function via oxidative stress: effects of vitamin E-coated dialyzer. *Circulation* 2000;101:1002–1006.
163. Wang C, Salahudeen AK. Lipid peroxidation accompanies cyclosporine nephrotoxicity: effects of vitamin E. *Kidney Int* 1995; 49:927–934.
164. Calo L, Semplicini A, Davis PA, et al. Cyclosporin-induced endothelial dysfunction and hypertension: are nitric oxide system abnormality and oxidative stress involved? *Transpl Int* 2000; 13(Suppl 1):S413–418.
165. Kandoussi AM, Glowacki F, Duriez P, et al. Evolution pattern of auto-antibodies against oxidized low-density lipoproteins in renal transplant recipients. *Nephron* 2001;89:303–308.
166. Shoskes DA, Shahed AR, Kim S, et al. Oxidant stress and antioxidant capacity in urine of renal transplant recipients predict early graft function. *Transplant Proc* 2001;33:984.
167. Soulis T, Cooper ME, Vranes D, et al. Effects of aminoguanidine in preventing experimental diabetic nephropathy are related to the duration of treatment. *Kidney Int* 1996;50: 627–634.
168. Padanilam BJ, Lewington AJ. Molecular mechanisms of cell death and regeneration in acute ischemic renal injury. *Curr Opin Nephrol Hyperten* 1999;8:15–19.
169. McCord JM. Oxygen-derived free radicals in postischemic tissue injury. *N Engl J Med* 1985;312:159–163.
170. Paller MS. Free radicals-mediated postischemic injury in renal transplantation. *Ren Fail* 1992;14:257–260.
171. Singh I, Gulati S, Orak JK, et al. Expression of antioxidant enzymes in rat kidney during ischemia-reperfusion injury. *Mol Cell Biochem* 1993;125:97–104.
172. Davies SJ, Reichardt-Pascal SY, Vaugham D, et al. Differential effect of ischemia-reperfusion injury on anti-oxidant enzyme activity in the rat kidney. *Exp Nephrol* 1995;3:348–354.

173. Yin M, Wheeler MD, Connor HD, et al. Cu/Zn-superoxide dismutase gene attenuates ischemia-reperfusion injury in the rat kidney. *J Am Soc Nephrol* 2001;12:2691–2700.
174. Sikujara O, Monden M, Toyoshima K, et al. Cytoprotective effect of prostaglandin I2 on ischemia-induced hepatic cell injury. *Transplantation* 1983;36:238–243.
175. Gove CD, Hughes RD, Kmiec Z, et al. In vivo and in vitro studies on the protective effects of 9beta-methylcalbacyclin, a stable prostacyclin analogue, in galactosamine-induced hepatocellular damage. *Prostaglandins Leukot Essent Fatty Acids* 1990; 40:73–77.
176. Nakano H, Monden M, Umeshita K, et al. Cytoprotective effect of prostaglandin I2 analogues on superoxide-induced hepatocyte injury. *Surgery* 1994;116:883–889.
177. Kishimoto SI, Sakon M, Umeshita K, et al. The inhibitory effect of prostaglandin E1 on oxidative stress-induced hepatocyte injury evaluated by calpain-n-mu activation. *Transplantation* 2000;69:2314–2319.
178. Behr J, Maier K, Braun B, et al. Evidence for oxidative stress in bronchiolitis obliterans syndrome after lung and heart-lung transplantation. *Transplantation* 2000;69:1856–1860.
179. Reid D, Snell G, Ward C, et al. Iron overload and nitric oxide-derived oxidative stress following lung transplantation. *Heart Lung Transplant* 2001;20:840–849.
180. Wettstein M, Häussinger D. Taurine attenuates cold ischemia-reoxygenation injury in rat liver. *Transplantation* 2000;69: 2290–2296.
181. Weigand MA, Plachky J, Thies JC, et al. N-acetylcysteine attenuates the increase in alpha-glutathione 5-transferase and circulating ICAM-1 and VCAM-1 after reperfusion in humans undergoing liver transplantation. *Transplantation* 2001;72: 694–698.
182. Berger SP, Hunger M, Yard BA, et al. Dopamine induces the expression of heme oxygenase-1 by human endothelial cells in vitro. *Kidney Int* 2000;58:2314–2319.

6

CARBONYL STRESS IN UREMIA

TOSHIO MIYATA
KIYOSHI KUROKAWA

Cardiovascular complications are undoubtedly important factors influencing the mortality of patients undergoing long-term dialysis treatment. Actual cardiovascular mortality in patients undergoing dialysis exceeds the expected mortality estimated on the basis of traditional risk factors, suggesting the existence of other unknown factor(s) that accelerate cardiovascular complications in uremia.

The accumulation in uremic circulation of uremic toxins or metabolites has been implicated for the development of atherosclerotic lesions in uremia. The field of uremic toxins has expanded markedly during the last decade. Most studies on uremic toxins have focused on disorders of enzymatic biochemistry. Attention has turned to progressive, nonenzymatic biochemistry. In this chapter, we focus on the carbonyl-amine chemistry in uremia, which results in two types of irreversible alterations of proteins: advanced glycation through the Maillard reaction and advanced lipoxidation derived from lipid peroxidation. We discuss chemistry of various reactive carbonyl compounds (RCOs) accumulating in the serum ("carbonyl stress"); their pathobiochemistry, particularly in relation to atherosclerosis; and, finally, the contribution of nutrition to carbonyl stress.

INCREASED ADVANCED GLYCATION END PRODUCTS AND OTHER PROTEIN MODIFICATIONS

The Maillard reaction, a nonenzymatic process, is initiated when proteins are exposed to glucose or other carbohydrates. It generates first reversible Schiff base adducts; then more stable Amadori rearrangement products; and, eventually, the irreversible advanced glycation end products (AGEs) (1). The role of AGEs in human pathology initially was highlighted in diabetes with hyperglycemia: AGEs levels are correlated with those of fructoselysine (2), a surrogate marker of prevailing plasma glucose concentration, and also with the severity of diabetic complications (3), a finding supporting their clinical relevance.

Of interest, AGEs accumulate in patients with uremia to a much greater extent than in patients with diabetes. Plasma levels of two well-known AGEs—pentosidine (4) and carboxymethyllysine (CML) (5)—in patients undergoing hemodialysis by far exceed those in normal or diabetic subjects. Other AGE adducts also accumulate in uremia such as glyoxal-lysine dimmer, methylglyoxal-lysine dimmer, and imidazolone (6,7). Among patients undergoing dialysis, diabetics and nondiabetics had similar plasma pentosidine and CML levels (4,5). Neither pentosidine nor CML correlated with fructoselysine levels in uremic subjects. It thus became clear that factor(s) other than hyperglycemia are critical for AGE formation in uremia. The fact that more than 90% of plasma pentosidine and CML are bound to albumin (4,5) suggests that its accumulation does not result from a decreased renal clearance of AGE-modified proteins.

The second approach to irreversible protein modification in uremia derives from studies of lipid metabolism, especially lipid peroxidation. Proteins are modified not only by carbohydrates but also by lipids. For instance, proteins modified by malondialdehyde accumulate in plasma proteins of patients undergoing hemodialysis (5). Malondialdehyde and other lipid peroxidation product–modified proteins are called the advanced lipoxidation end products (ALEs) (8).

Uremia thus is characterized by irreversible nonenzymatic protein modifications by AGEs/ALEs. In patients with renal failure, lipid peroxidation and advanced glycation of plasma proteins or skin collagens increase in close relation to each other (5,9).

"CARBONYL STRESS"

Both AGEs and ALEs are formed by carbonyl amine chemistry between protein residues and RCOs (8). These RCOs are produced constantly during the metabolism of carbohydrates, lipids, and amino acids (10–12). Recent studies confirm the accumulation of various RCOs derived from both carbohydrates and lipids in uremic plasma and suggest that they are indeed precursors of AGEs and ALEs (8,13,14). The prevailing plasma pentosidine level, for example, is shown to mirror the level of its RCOs precursor (13). The accumulation in uremic plasma of various RCOs derived from either carbohydrates or lipids as well as the subsequent carbonyl modification of proteins suggest that chronic uremia may be characterized as a state of "carbonyl stress" (14). AGEs/ALEs are therefore not markers of hyperglycemia, hyperlipemia in uremia but represent carbonyl stress and RCO accumulation.

Two competing but not mutually exclusive hypotheses should be considered to account for the cause of carbonyl stress (14): an increased generation or a decreased detoxification of RCOs. First, the production of RCOs is increased by oxidative stress. Several reports point to the existence of an increased oxidative stress in uremia (15). The uremic oxidative stress is worsened further during hemodialysis treatment (i.e., activation of complement and neutrophils) and generation of reactive oxygen species. A causal role of the oxidative stress in AGE and ALE formation is supported by the correlation existing in uremic serum between pentosidine and oxidative markers, such as dehydroascorbate (oxidized ascorbate) (16) and advanced oxidation protein products (17).

However, recent studies have shown that several RCOs derived from nonoxidative chemistry also are increased in uremia, suggesting the simultaneous involvement of nonoxidative chemistry in the genesis of uremic carbonyl stress. For example, the levels of 3-deoxyglucosone (18) and methylglyoxal (19), and of their protein adducts, all of which are formed independently from oxidative reactions, are increased in plasma proteins of patients undergoing hemodialysis.

The alternative hypothesis therefore is proposed: the RCO increase in uremia is derived from a decreased removal of RCOs. RCOs are detoxified by several enzymatic pathways, such as the glyoxalase pathway (20). Reduced glutathione and nicotinamide adenine dinucleotide phosphate, or NAD(P)H, contribute to their activity. RCOs such as methylglyoxal and glyoxal react reversibly with the thiol group of glutathione and subsequently are detoxified by glyoxalases I and II into D-lactate and glutathione. NAD(P)H also replenishes glutathione by increasing the activity of glutathione reductase. Decreased levels of glutathione and NAD(P)H therefore can result in augmented levels of a wide range of RCOs. It is of interest to know in this context that the glutathione concentration in red blood cells and the serum activity of glutathione-dependent enzymes are reduced significantly in uremia (21).

There has been little evidence that the RCO-detoxification mechanism might influence *in vivo* RCO formation and therefore serum AGE levels. A patient has been identified in whom a deficiency of glyoxalase I was associated with unusually elevated levels of AGEs (pentosidine and CML) and of their precursors (22). The cause of this deficiency remains unknown. Nevertheless, the association of very low levels of glyoxalase I with strikingly elevated levels of AGEs and RCO precursors implicates the glyoxalase detoxification system in the actual level of AGEs *in vivo*.

Mechanism that regulates carbonyl stress is another issue of interest. Superoxide dismutase (SOD) and glutathione peroxidase are antioxidant enzymes involved in the metabolism of hydrogen peroxide, which accelerates carbonyl stress (12,23). It is worth noting that glutathione peroxidase activities correlated inversely with pentosidine levels in uremic plasma (21). However, the plasma extracellular-SOD levels correlated with the pentosidine levels. These data suggest a link of altered redox regulation by antioxidant enzymes to an increased carbonyl stress. Furthermore, recent observation gives a new perspective in the regulation of AGE production by linking it to the prevailing effect of nitric oxide (NO) (24). NO effectively inhibits the pentosidine generation *in vitro*. It is best explained by the ability of NO to scavenge carbon-centered radicals and hydroxyl radicals, and consequently to suppress the formation of RCOs and pentosidine. NO might be therefore implicated in the atherogenic and inflammatory effects of carbonyl stress.

CLINICAL CONSEQUENCES OF CARBONYL STRESS

It remains to be demonstrated whether carbonyl stress is the passive result of long-term accumulation of vascular protein modifications or, alternatively, it plays an active role in the pathogenesis of atherosclerosis. Recent studies, however, support the active contribution of carbonyl stress in the atherogenesis.

The levels of AGEs in arterial tissues are higher in patients undergoing dialysis than in normal subjects (25). Both AGEs and ALEs are detectable by means of immunohistochemical approaches in the fatty streaks and in the thickened neointima of patients with uremia (26). Available evidence suggests that plasma levels of pentosidine are an independent variable of the presence of ischemic heart diseases and hypertension (27) and of left ventricular-wall thickness measured by echocardiography in patients undergoing hemodialysis (Zoccali C and Miyata T, unpublished observation).

In vitro, AGE-, and ALE-modified proteins initiate a range of cellular responses (28–32), including stimulation of monocyte chemotaxis and apoptosis, secretion of inflammatory cytokines from macrophages, proliferation of vascular smooth-muscle cells, stimulation of platelet aggregation, and production of vascular endothelial growth factor (VEGF) from endothelial cells. Independently of their AGE- and ALE-mediated effects, RCOs also interfere with various cellular functions and induce not only structural but also functional alterations of methylglyoxal increases of proteins. For example, exposure *in vitro* of cultured mesothelial and endothelial cells to messenger RNA and protein synthesis of VEGF (33). Repeated intraperitoneal loads of methylglyoxal, given to rats, also increase *in vivo* the peritoneal membrane expression of VEGF (33). Noteworthy in this context is the demonstration that, both in long-term peritoneal dialysis (PD) patients and in chronic uremic rat models (33,34), an increasing staining for AGEs, CML, and pentosidine is detected in peritoneal arterial walls, together with an augmented VEGF and basic fibroblast growth factor expression.

There are two major pathways, direct and indirect, through which carbonyl stress is sensed by cells and triggers a cascade of intracellular signal transduction. In the indirect pathway, the RCOs first interact with proteins or lipids in the physiologic environment surrounding the cells, which then undergo nonenzymatic glycation and lipoxidation resulting in the production of AGEs and ALEs. They bind with the receptor(s) on cell surfaces (e.g., receptor for AGE), thereby initiating intracellular signal transduction (35). By contrast, the direct pathway works before generation of AGEs and ALEs. The RCOs directly attack target molecules on cell surfaces or inside the cells, which initiates the subsequent signal transduction (36–40). For example, glyoxal and methylglyoxal possess two reactive carbonyl groups to make protein aggregates by cross-linking, which may amplify the signals for tyrosine phosphorylation of cellular proteins (36). In another model, the binding of 4-hydroxynonenal, a RCO-generated during lipid peroxidation, with epidermal growth factor receptor induces its clustering on the cell surface, thereby activating the mitogen activated protein family kinases (37). In vascular lesions, an increased oxidative stress, together with altered redox regulation and decreased RCO detoxification, may increase carbonyl stress, exacerbate endothelial dysfunction, and eventually lead to the development of atherosclerosis.

The consequences of carbonyl stress also have been implicated in other complications associated with uremia or long-term dialysis. First, renal failure is associated with resistance to the action of calcitriol (1.25 dihydroxivitamin D) (41), which partly is attributed to the inhibition by unknown uremic toxins of the interaction between the vitamin D receptor and vitamin D response elements (42). Patel et al. (43) demonstrated that RCOs capable of Schiff base formation with lysine residues of the vitamin D receptor inhibit its interaction with the vitamin D response element. Second, dialysis-related amyloidosis is a serious bone and joint destruction associated with uremia (44). Immunohistochemical and chemical analyses have indicated that B2-microglobulin amyloid deposits are modified by carbonyl stress (45–47). Third, the major problem associated with long-term PD is the progressive deterioration of the peritoneal membrane structure and function (i.e., ultrafiltration failure), which curtails its use in approximately 50% of patients within 5 years (48). Recent studies have cast a new light on its molecular mechanism (49). During PD, RCOs resulting both from glucose PD fluid and from uremic circulation enter the peritoneum (50), modify the peritoneal membrane (51), and initiate a number of cellular responses, leading to angiogenesis and vasodilation. The latter may increase the permeability for small solutes and glucose, stimulate glucose reabsorption, and result in faster than normal dissipation of the osmotic gradient across the peritoneal membrane with an eventual loss of ultrafiltration (49).

NUTRITION AND CARBONYL STRESS

The advanced glycation of proteins initially have been unraveled by food and nutrition biochemists. Various kinds of food indeed contain a significant amount of CML and pentosidine (52,53). Previous studies demonstrated that, although the modification of proteins with AGEs reduces the digestibility of proteins either by gaining resistance to the enzymatic digestion of proteases or by inhibiting digestive enzyme activity (53), a significant proportion of dietary AGEs are absorbed by the gastrointestinal tract into the circulation (54,55). He et al. demonstrated that approximately 10% of ingested AGE-modified ovalbumin was absorbed into the rat circulation (55). Of particular interest is the demonstration of a relationship between renal function and exogenous or food-derived AGE levels in the serum (54). Synthesized pentosidine was given orally to both normal and uremic rats, and their kinetics in the circulation was investigated. In normal rats, plasma pentosidine increased slightly and transiently to become undetectable at 6 hours. By contrast, in rats with 6/7 nephrectomy plasma pentosidine peaked at 3 hours and fell thereafter (calculated biologic half-life of 4.08 ± 1.68 h). In bilaterally nephrectomized rats, plasma pentosidine level peaked at 12 hours and decreased subsequently (calculated biologic half-life of 47.3 ± 10.2 h). The pathologic contribution of exogenous or food-derived AGEs still remains unknown.

Several lines of evidence have implicated the dietary contribution to the *in vivo* AGE accumulation. Dietary calorie restriction reduces the accumulation of tissue AGEs without affecting survival of the animals (56,57). Of note is the report by Sell et al. that longitudinal determination of the rates of pentosidine and CML formation predicts the individual longevity in mice and that calorie restriction retards this rate as compared to *ad libitum* feeding (58). Whether the same is true for humans is not known. More studies are required to elucidate the contribution of nutrition to the pathophysiology of carbonyl stress.

REFERENCES

1. Brownlee M, Cerami A, Vlassara H. Advanced glycosylation end products in tissue and the biochemical basis of diabetic complications. *N Engl J Med* 1988;318:1315–1321.
2. Dyer DG, Dunn JA, Thorpe SR, et al. Accumulation of Maillard reaction products in skin collagen in diabetes and aging. *J Clin Invest* 1993;91:2463–2469.

3. McCance DR, Dyer DG, Dunn IA, et al. Maillard reaction products and their relation to complications in insulin-dependent diabetes mellitus. *J Clin Invest* 1993;91:2470–2478.
4. Miyata T, Ueda Y, Shinzato T, et al. Accumulation of albumin-linked and free-form pentosidine in the circulation of uremic patients with end-stage renal failure: Renal implications in the pathophysiology of pentosidine. *J Am Soc Nephrol* 1996;7: 1198–1206.
5. Miyata T, Fu MX, Kurokawa K, et al. Autoxidation products of both carbohydrates and lipids are increased in uremic plasma: Is there oxidative stress in uremia? *Kidney Int* 1998;54:1290–1295.
6. Odani H, Shinzato T, Usami I, et al. Imidazolium crosslinks derived from reaction of lysine with glyoxal and methylglyoxal are increased in serum proteins of uremic patients: Evidence for increased oxidative stress in uremia. *FEBS Lett* 1998;427: 381–385.
7. Takayama F, Aoyama I, Tsukushi S, et al. Immunohistochemical detection of imidazolone and N^{ϵ}-(carboxymethyl)lysine in aortas of hemodialysis patients. *Cell Mol Biol* 1998;44:1101–1109.
8. Miyata T, van Ypersele de Strihou C, Kiyoshi Kurokawa, et al. Alterations in non-enzymatic biochemistry in uremia: Origin and significance of "carbonyl stress" in long-term uremic complications. *Kidney Int* 1999;55:389–399.
9. Meng I, Sakata N, Imanaga Y, et al. Evidence for a link between glycoxidation and lipoperoxidation in patients with chronic renal failure. *Clin Nephrol* 1999;51:280–289.
10. Wells-Knecht KJ, Zyzak DV, Litchfield JE, et al. Mechanism of autoxidative glycosylation: Identification of glyoxal and arabinose as intermediates in the autoxidative modification of protein by glucose. *Biochemistry* 1995;34:3702–3709.
11. Esterbauer H, Schuer RI, Zollner H. Chemistry and biochemistry of 4-hydroxynonenal, malondialdehyde and related aldehyde. *Free Radic Biol Med* 1991;11:81–128.
12. Anderson MM, Hazen SL, Hsu FE, et al. Human neutrophils employ the myeloperoxidase-hydrogen peroxide-chloride system to convert hydroxy-amino acids into glycolaldehyde, 2-hydroxypropanol, and acrolein: a mechanism for the generation of highly reactive cx-hydroxy and a, B-unsaturated aldehydes by phagocytes at sites of inflammation. *I Clin Invest* 1997;99:424–432.
13. Miyata T, Ueda Y, Yamada Y, et al. Carbonyl stress in uremia: Accumulation of carbonyls accelerate the formation of pentosidine, an advanced glycation end product. *J Am Soc Nephrol* 1998; 9:2349–2356.
14. Miyata T, Kurokawa K, Charles van Ypersele de Strihou. Advanced glycation and lipoxidation end products: Role of reactive carbonyl compounds generated during carbohydrate and lipid metabolism. *J Am Soc Nephrol* 2000;11:1744–1752.
15. Miyata T, Maeda K, Kurokawa K, et al. Oxidation conspires with glycation to create noxious advanced glycation end products in renal failure. *Nephrol Dial Transplant* 1997;12:255–258.
16. Miyata T, Wada Y, Cai Z, et al. Implication of an increased oxidative stress in the formation of advanced glycation end products in patients with end-stage renal failure. *Kidney Int* 1997;51: 1170–1181.
17. Witko-Sarsat V, Friedlander M, Capeillere-Blandin C, et al. Advanced oxidation protein products as a novel marker of oxidative stress in uremia. *Kidney Int* 1996;49:1304–1313.
18. Niwa T, Takeda N, Miyazaki T, et al. Elevated serum levels of 3 deoxyglucosone, a potent protein-cross-linking intermediate of the mallard reaction, in uremic patients. *Nephron* 1995;69: 438–443.
19. Odani H, Shinzato H, Matsumoto Y, et al. Increase in three a, B-dicarbonyl compound levels in human uremic plasma: Specific in vivo determination of intermediates in advanced Maillard reaction. *Biochem Biophys Res Commun* 1999;256:89–93.
20. Thomalley PJ. Advanced glycation and development of diabetic complications: Unifying the involvement of glucose, methylglyoxal and oxidative stress. *Endocrinol Metab* 1996;3:149–166.
21. Ueda Y, Miyata T, Hashimoto T, et al. Implication of altered redox regulation by antioxidant enzymes in the increased plasma pentosidine, an advanced glycation end product, in uremia. *Biochem Biophys Res Commun* 1998;245:785–790.
22. Miyata T, van Ypersele de Strihou C, Imasawa T, et al. Glyoxalase I deficiency is associated with an unusual level of advanced glycation end products in a hemodialysis patient. *Kidney Int* 2001; 60:2351–2359.
23. Nagai R, Ikeda K, Higashi T, et al. Hydroxyl radical mediates N-epsilon-(carboxymethyl)lysine formation from Amadori products. *Biochem Biophys Res Commun* 1997;234:167–172.
24. Asahi K, Ichimori K, Nakazawa H, et al. Nitric oxide inhibits the formation of advanced glycation and products. *Kidney Int* 2000;58:1780–1787.
25. Makita Z, Radoff S, Rayfield EJ, et al. Advanced glycosylation end products in patients with diabetic nephropathy. *N Engl J Med* 1991;325:836–842.
26. Miyata T, Ishikawa S, Asahi K, et al. 2-Isopropylidenehydrazono-4-oxo-thiazolidin-5-ylacetanilide (OPB-9195) inhibits the neointima proliferation of rat carotid artery following balloon injury: Role of glycoxidation and lipoxidation reactions in vascular tissue damage. *FEBS Letter* 1999;445:202–206.
27. Sugiyama S, Miyata T, Ueda Y, et al. Plasma level of pentosidine, an advanced glycation end product, in diabetic patients. *J Am Soc Nephrol* 1998;9:1681–1688.
28. Miyata T, Inagi R, Iida Y, et al. Involvement of 132-microglobulin modified with advanced glycation end products in the pathogenesis of hemodialysis-associated amyloidosis: Induction of human monocyte chemotaxis and macrophage secretion of tumor necrosis factor-a and interleukin 1. *J Clin Invest* 1994;93: 521–528.
29. Miyata T, Hori O, Zhang IH, et al. The receptor for advanced glycation endproducts mediates the interaction of AGE-132-microglobulin with human mononuclear phagocytes via an oxidant-sensitive pathway: Implication for the pathogenesis of dialysis-related amyloidosis. *J Clin Invest* 1997;98:1088–1094.
30. Hou FF, Miyata T, Boyce J, et al. β2-Microglobulin modified with advanced glycation end products delays monocyte apoptosis and induces differentiation into macrophage-like cells. *Kidney Int* 2001;59:990–1002.
31. Miyata T, Iida Y, Wada Y, et al. Monocyte/macrophage response to 62-microglobulin modified with advanced glycation end products. *Kidney Int* 1996;49:538–550.
32. Miyata T, Notoya K, Yoshida K, et al. Advanced glycation end products enhance osteoclast-induced bone resorption in cultured mouse unfractionated bone cells and in rats implanted with devitalized bone particles. *J Am Soc Nephrol* 1997;8:260–270.
33. Inagi R, Miyata T, Yamamoto T, et al. Glucose degradation product methylglyoxal enhances the production of vascular endothelial growth factor in peritoneal cells: Role in the pathogenesis of peritoneal membrane dysfunction in peritoneal dialysis. *FEBS Lett* 1999;463:260–264.
34. Combet S, Miyata T, Moulin P, et al. Vascular proliferation and enhanced expression of endothelial nitric oxide synthase in human peritoneum exposed to long-term peritoneal dialysis. *J Am Soc Nephrol* 2000;11:717–728.
35. Yan SD, Schmidt AM, Anderson GM, et al. Enhanced cellular oxidant stress by the interaction of advanced glycation end products with their receptors/binding proteins. *J Biol Chem* 1994; 269:9889–9897.
36. Ahkand AA, Kato M, Suzuki H, et al. Carbonyl compounds cross-link cellular proteins and activate protein-tyrosine kinase $p60^{c\text{-}src}$. *J Cellular Biochemistry* 1999;72:1–7.
37. Liu W, Ahkand AA, Kato M, et al. 4-Hydroxynonenal triggers

an epidermal growth factor receptor-linked signal pathway for growth inhibition. *J Cell Sci* 1999;112:2409–2417.

38. Liu W, Kato M, Akhand AA, et al. 4-Hydroxynonenal induces a cellular redox-related activation of the caspase cascade for apoptotic cell death. *J Cell Sci* 2000;113:635–641.
39. Du I, Suzuki H, Nagase F, et al. Methylglyoxal induces apoptosis in Jurkat leukemia T-cells by activating c-Jun N-terminal kinase. *J Cell Biochem* 2000;77:333–344.
40. Akhand AA, Hossain K, Mitsui H, et al. Glyoxal and methylglyoxal trigger distinct signals for MAP family kinases and caspase activation in human endothelial cells. *Free Radic Biol Med* 2001; 31:20–30.
41. Fukagawa M, Kaname S, Igarashi T, et al. Regulation of parathyroid hormone synthesis in chronic renal failure in rats. *Kidney Int* 1991;39:874–881.
42. Patel SR, Ke HQ, Vanholder R, et al. Inhibition of calcitriol receptor binding to vitamin D response elements by uremic toxins. *J Clin Invest* 1995;96:50–59.
43. Patel SR, Koenig YRJ, Hsu CH. Effect of glyoxylate on the function of the calcitriol receptor and vitamin D metabolism. *Kidney Int* 1997;52:39–44.
44. Miyata T, Jadoul M, Kurokawa K, et al. 132-Microglobulin in renal disease. *J Am Soc Nephrol* 1998;9:1723–1735.
45. Miyata T, Oda O, Inagi R, et al. 62-Microglobulin modified with advanced glycation end products is a major component of hemodialysis-associated amyloidosis. *J Clin Invest* 1993;92: 1243–1252.
46. Miyata T, Inagi R, Wada Y, et al. Glycation of human beta 2-microglobulin in patients with hemodialysis-associated amyloidosis: identification of the glycated sites. *Biochemistry* 1994;33: 12215–12221.
47. Niwa T, Miyazaki S, Katsuzaki T, et al. Immunohistochemical detection of advanced glycation end products in dialysis-related amyloidosis. *Kidney Int* 1995;48:771–778.
48. Krediet RT. The peritoneal membrane in chronic peritoneal dialysis. *Kidney Int* 1999;55:341–356.
49. Miyata T, Devuyst O, Kurokawa K, et al. Towards better dialysis compatibility: Advances in the biochemistry and pathophysiology of the peritoneal membranes. *Kidney Int* 2002;61:375–386.
50. Miyata T, Kurokawa K, van Ypersele de Strihou C. Advanced glycation and lipoxidation end products: Role of reactive carbonyl compounds generated during carbohydrate and lipid metabolism. *J Am Soc Nephrol* 2000;11:1744–1752.
51. Nakayama M, Kawaguchi Y, Yamada K, et al. Immunohistochemical detection of advanced glycosylation end products in the peritoneum and its possible pathophysiological role in CAPD. *Kidney Int* 1997;51:182–186.
52. Erbersdobler HF. Protein reactions during food processing and storage—their relevance to human nutrition. *Bibl Nutr Dieta* 1989;43:140–155.
53. O'Brien I, Morrissey PA. Nutritional and toxicological aspects of the Maillard browning reaction in foods. *Crit Rev Food Sci Nutr* 1989;28:211–248.
54. Miyata T, Ueda Y, Hone K, et al. Renal catabolism of advanced glycation end products: the fate of pentosidine. *Kidney Int* 1998; 53:416–422.
55. He C, Sabol J, Mitsuhashi T, et al. Inhibition of reactive products aminoguanidine facilitates renal clearance and reduces tissue sequestration. *Diabetes* 1999;48:1308–1315.
56. Lingelbach LB, Mitchell AE, Rucker RB, et al. Accumulation of advanced glycation endproducts in aging male Fischer 344 rats during long-term feeding of various dietary carbohydrates. *J Nutr* 2000;130:1247–1255.
57. Teillet L, Verbeke P, Gouraud S, et al. Food restriction prevents advanced glycation end product accumulation and retards kidney aging in lean rats. *J Am Soc Nephrol* 2000;11:1488–1497.
58. Sell DR, Kleinman NR, Monnier VM. Longitudinal determination of skin collagen glycation and glycoxidation rats predicts early death in C57BL/6NNIA mice. *FASEB J* 2000;14:146–156.

7

HOMOCYSTEINE

ALESSANDRA F. PERNA
NATALE G. DE SANTO

Homocysteine is an amino acid very similar to cysteine, except that it contains an additional methylene group in its side chain (1,2). Therefore, its name stresses the similarity with cysteine. Most importantly, however, homocysteine is a sulfur amino acid, with unique properties related to its molecule and to the formation of active derivatives (Fig. 7.1).

HOMOCYSTEINE METABOLISM

Homocysteine is not significantly contained in dietary constituents, is not considered to be an essential amino acid, and is not normally present in the backbone of endogenous proteins. Despite these negative statements, this amino acid is placed at the crossroads of an interesting and complicated metabolic pathway. At the beginning of this pathway we find methionine.

Methionine, an essential amino acid, is derived from the breakdown of proteins of dietary or endogenous origin. It is used for *de novo* protein biosynthesis, or can be enzymatically condensed with the adenosine moiety of adenosine triphosphate (ATP) to form S-adenosylmethionine (AdoMet), a sulfonium compound (Fig. 7.2). AdoMet donates its activated methyl group to many possible methyl acceptors in the transmethylation pathway. Transmethylations are widespread reactions, catalyzed by more than 40 different enzymes, which modify various methyl-accepting substrates, including small molecules (e.g., phosphatidylethanolamine and dopamine) and macromolecules (i.e., proteins, DNA, and RNA). Quantitatively, the most important reaction is the methylation of guanidinoacetate to form creatine, which consumes more than half of the available AdoMet. Several other small molecule methyltransferases are involved in detoxification, phospholipid biosynthesis, neurotransmitter and hormone biosynthesis, and metabolism. DNA methylation affects processes such as transcriptional regulation, chromatin structure, genome stability, and tumorigenesis (3,4). Protein methylation is involved in the repair of damaged proteins as well as other functions, as detailed later in this chapter.

The demethylated product of AdoMet is S-adenosylhomocysteine (AdoHcy), which represents a natural and potent competitive transmethylation inhibitor. AdoHcy is the only homocysteine precursor in a reversible reaction catalyzed by AdoHcy hydrolase. Inhibition of transmethylations does not ordinarily take place, due to rapid hydrolysis of toxic AdoHcy to homocysteine and adenosine. However, if homocysteine accumulates, hydrolysis slackens, and AdoHcy builds up, with the attending transmethylation inhibition (see reference 2 for a detailed review).

Homocysteine follows two pathways: transsulfuration or remethylation, with partitioning between the two depending on methionine intake, and AdoMet and AdoHcy concentrations (5). Transsulfuration commits homocysteine to conversion into cysteine through cystathionine (cystathionine β-synthase [CBS] catalyzes the rate-limiting step) and other sulfur-containing compounds (glutathione, taurine, H_2S, SO_4-). Remethylation consists in a methionine salvage pathway, which is important especially at times of methionine deficiency. Methionine synthase is the enzyme involved, which does not use ATP. The methyl group in the case of remethylation is donated by methyltetrahydrofolate (MTHF), the active circulating form of folic acid, which can be considered as a cosubstrate. In fact, the stoichiometry of the reaction requires one mole of MTHF per mole of methionine formed. MTHF is produced through methylenetetrahydrofolate reductase (MTHFR). An alternative reaction uses betaine as a methyl donor in the liver. Main cofactors involved in homocysteine metabolism are vitamin B_6 in transsulfuration (for both CBS and cystathioninase) and vitamin B_{12} in remethylation (methionine synthase). An additional enzyme, methionine synthase reductase, is important for regeneration of the methylcobalamin coenzyme necessary for methionine synthase activity (6).

HOMOCYSTINURIA: AN UNFORTUNATE EXPERIMENT OF NATURE WITH IMPLICATIONS REGARDING ATHEROSCLEROSIS

Homocystinuria is a group of inherited defects of enzymes relevant to homocysteine metabolism, leading to elevated

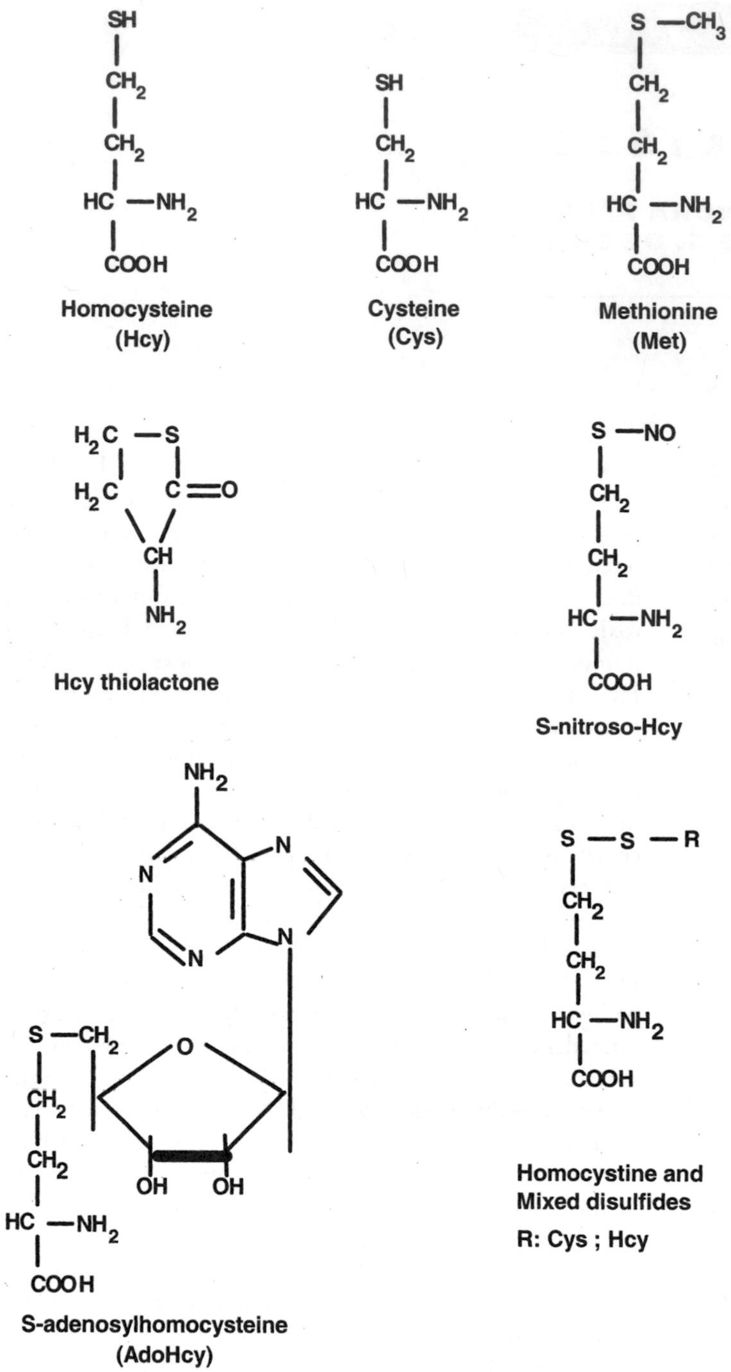

Homocysteine (Hcy)

Cysteine (Cys)

Methionine (Met)

Hcy thiolactone

S-nitroso-Hcy

S-adenosylhomocysteine (AdoHcy)

Homocystine and Mixed disulfides

R: Cys ; Hcy

FIGURE 7.1. In this figure, the most important homocysteine derivatives are depicted.

plasma homocysteine levels, usually in the severe range. Normal levels of fasting plasma homocysteine are considered to be between 8 and 10 μm in women and 10 and 12 μm in men. Moderate hyperhomocysteinemia is defined to be between 16 and 30 μm, intermediate is between 31 and 100 μm, and severe hyperhomocysteinemia is more than 100 μm (7).

Children affected by homocystinuria display distinct marfanoid features; in fact, the disease initially was classified among the inherited connective-tissue disorders. However, the cause of death in these young people (before therapy was implemented and outcomes were ameliorated substantially) was premature cardiovascular accidents (i.e., arterial or venous thrombosis, myocardial infarction, and stroke), and it was soon clear that high homocysteine in homocystinuria was the culprit in the genesis of cardiovascular disease (8). In fact, if CBS deficiency leads to increased homocysteine and methionine levels, defects of MTHFR or methionine synthase lead to increased levels of homocysteine, and not methionine, but the thromboatherosclerotic manifestations

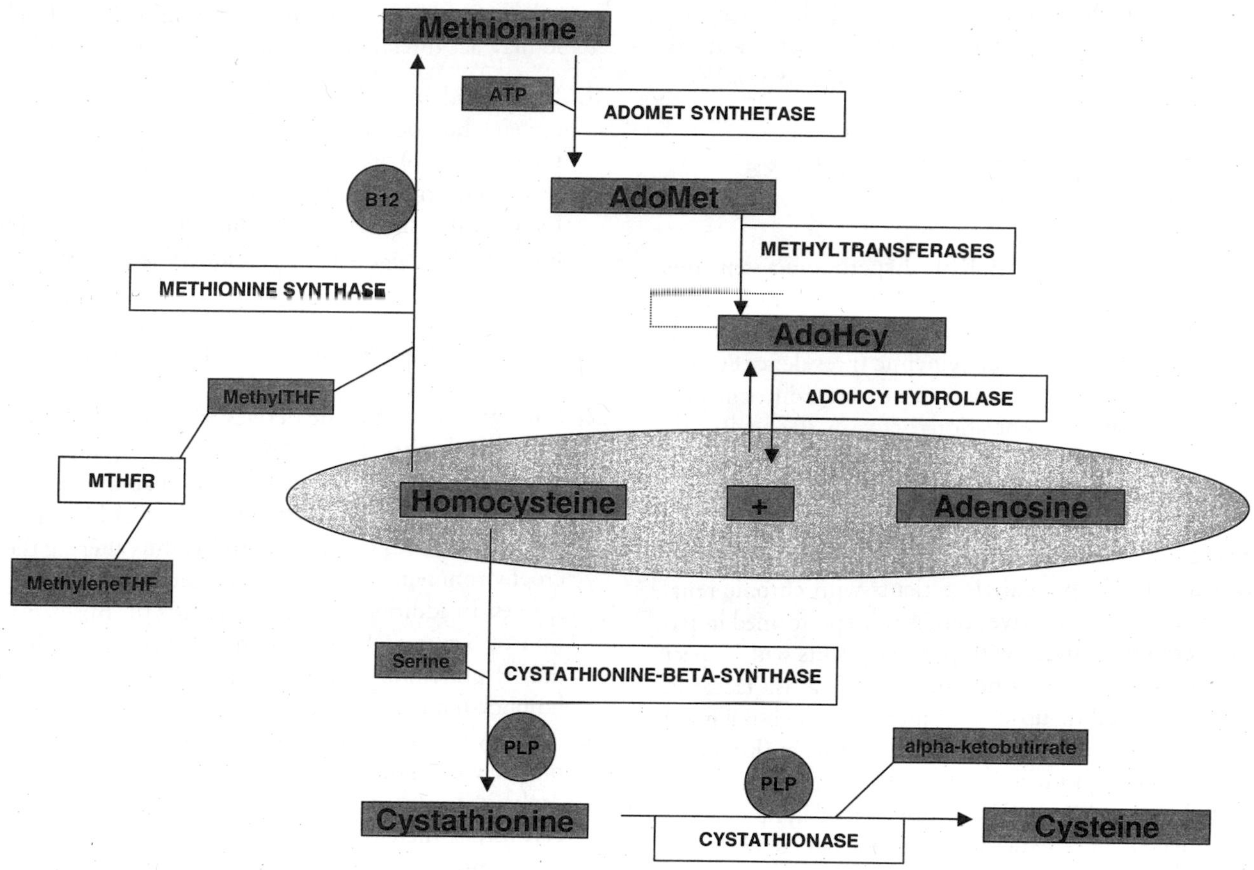

FIGURE 7.2. Metabolic pathways relative to homocysteine.

are identical to those of CBS deficiency. Therapy with vitamin B_6, folates and the like leads to significantly increased event-free survival rates (9). The attention of scientists therefore was drawn to homocysteine and its effects, and it was proposed that an increase in homocysteine levels could be linked to atherosclerosis (10).

THE GENERAL POPULATION

In the early 1990s, it was proposed that even moderate degrees of hyperhomocysteinemia present in the general population are associated with atherosclerotic cardiovascular disease and thrombophilia (11). Several prospective studies are available, and most support the notion that hyperhomocysteinemia is a causal risk factor. Large randomized, controlled intervention studies are under way, but three small intervention studies suggest that B vitamins have a protective effect. It also has been proposed that homocysteine has additive effects and acts synergistically with other risk factors (see reference 12 for review).

The methionine loading test (MLT) was developed to study the transsulfuration pathway in individuals heterozygous for CBS deficiency, and it also can be useful to identify subjects at higher risk for cardiovascular disease. It has been reported that a 2- to 4-hour MLT can uncover as many as 39% of individuals with homocysteine-related cardiovascular disease risk but with normal homocysteine levels (13). Although it initially was thought that MLT revealed only anomalies in enzymes of the transsulfuration pathway, it now is clear that it is sensitive to the remethylation pathway, at least in part. Therefore, an AdoMet increase brought about by MLT, even if it stimulates CBS and inhibits MTHFR, has to be handled by the remethylation pathway to some degree as well (14).

A thermolabile, less active variant of the MTHFR, arising from the C677T transition in the encoding gene, has been described, which can give rise to moderately increased homocysteine levels if folate intake is insufficient (15). About 10%, depending on the population considered, present this variant in the homozygous form, and heterozygous subjects are 20% to 30%. Possibly, there is a selective advantage in retaining this variant during evolution because it saves folates for thymidilate synthase and therefore DNA biosynthesis. Conflicting data are present in the literature concerning the association between the thermolabile variant and cardiovascular disease. For example, the prevalence of homozygous people is not different in the very old; thus its presence does not reduce longevity (16). It has been proposed that the C677T polymorphism represents a nutritional adaptation with health-promoting effects (12,17).

STUDIES IN CHRONIC RENAL FAILURE AND UREMIA

In chronic renal failure (CRF), hyperhomocysteinemia starts to appear when the glomerular filtration rate (GFR) decreases below 70 mL/min. Patients with uremia are almost constantly hyperhomocysteinemic (prevalence 80% to 95%). Hyperhomocysteinemia is of moderate-intermediate degree, with average concentrations between 20 and 40 μm. Levels depend on various factors, including if patients are on a standard vitamin supplementation as in some countries, or are not supplemented, and on their genetic background.

Hyperhomocysteinemia is associated with atherosclerotic arterial occlusion in predialysis patients with chronic renal failure (18). Two prospective studies were performed in patients undergoing dialysis, with positive results with respect to the hypothesis (i.e., that homocysteine is a risk factor in these patients). Follow-up was 17 months, which is a good length of time to observe cardiovascular events in this population given the high mortality rate (19,20). One prospective study in transplant patients showed that homocysteine was an independent predictor of cardiovascular events in men but not in women (21).

MECHANISMS OF HOMOCYSTEINE TOXICITY

Atherosclerosis is a form of chronic inflammation with reparative aspects similar to wound healing (22). Homocysteine seems to act on several of the mechanisms underlying atherosclerosis. Homocysteine may act as a toxin with respect to endothelial cells, can enhance vascular smooth-muscle cell proliferation, can increase platelet aggregation, and can act on the coagulation cascade and fibrinolysis, thus directly inducing or acting in a synergistic manner with other factors in determining the appearance of atherosclerosis. It activates coagulation factor V, X, and XII, along with decreased activation of protein C and cell-surface thrombomodulin and modulation of tissue plasminogen–activator binding to its endothelial receptor, annexin II, thus creating a prothrombotic environment (23).

Recently, induction of hyperhomocysteinemia in apoprotein E (ApoE)-null mice, a model of genetic susceptibility to atherosclerosis, accelerates the development of atherosclerotic lesions. In addition, several molecules involved in inflammation are increased. All these effects were suppressed with B-vitamin supplementation (24).

Knockout mice for the MTHFR gene, which display hyperhomocysteinemia, show developmental retardation and abnormal lipid deposition in the aorta (25). Homocysteine may act directly or through one of its derivatives.

1. In the oxidation of homocysteine, homocystine (homocysteine homodimer) or the mixed disulfides (homocysteine–cysteine) are generated along with hydrogen peroxide and other reactive oxygen species. This produces, for example, lipid peroxidation (26). We have shown, for example, that vitamin C and E administration to healthy individuals receiving a methionine load is able to prevent the alterations in endothelial cell function and coagulation caused by acute hyperhomocysteinemia (27).
2. S-nitroso-homocysteine derives from homocysteine oxidation with nitric oxide (NO). Thus, homocysteine acts as a NO scavenger, reducing its availability. Some evidence exists that homocysteine may affect NO synthesis and glutathione peroxidase activity, thus altering the microenvironment in the propagation of reactive oxygen species. In addition, evidence supports the misincorporation of S-nitroso-homocysteine in place of methionine during protein biosynthesis as a potential mechanism of homocysteine toxicity (28).
3. AdoHcy, the direct homocysteine precursor, may accumulate when homocysteine levels increase. AdoHcy hydrolysis, catalyzed by AdoHcy hydrolase, is reversible. Hydrolysis therefore may slow down if metabolites are not removed promptly, thus inducing an AdoHcy-mediated transmethylation inhibition (1,2).
4. Hcy thiolactone is a highly reactive anhydride that can occur as the result of a proofreading mechanism that impedes homocysteine misincorporation into proteins. Alternatively, homocysteine thiolactone can arise in a reaction that attaches homocysteine to initiator transfer RNA (tRNA). This homocysteine-tRNA then is methylated to methionine by a methylating factor. When methylation is deficient, the homocysteine-tRNA is hydrolyzed to produce homocysteine thiolactone (29,30).

CAUSES OF HYPERHOMOCYSTEINEMIA IN UREMIA

Theoretic possible causes of hyperhomocysteinemia in renal failure include the following: (a) impaired renal excretion, (b) reduced renal metabolism, (c) cofactor deficiency, and (d) inhibition of enzymes related to homocysteine metabolism by retained uremic toxins. It previously was thought that impaired renal excretion could be responsible, but it has been ascertained conclusively that homocysteine excretion is negligible. In fact, free homocysteine, non–protein-bound, is around 3.0 μm, depending on the study. For a normal GFR of 180 L/day, filtered homocysteine is then 540 μmol/day. However, tubular reabsorption plays an important role, in that it reabsorbs almost all of filtered homocysteine. Consequently, excreted homocysteine is only about 6 μmol/day. An algorithm postulating the complete and abrupt loss of renal filtration and absorption, in an individual weighing 70 kg, was developed. Assumptions are that homocysteine would have a distribution volume of 0.66 L/kg; that homocysteine freely equilibrates between extracellular and intracellular volume; and that unexcreted homocysteine is not metabolized in the body. The algorithm predicts that in 3 months, 12 μmol/L of homocysteine would accumulate in plasma (Perna AF and Ingrosso D, unpublished observation). This is not such a trivial amount, but the human body possesses a huge capacity for metabolizing homocysteine. In fact, homocysteine production is between 15 and 20 mmol/day, as judged by creatinine excretion.

Creatinine is a product of creatine, which is derived in turn from guanidinoacetate methylation. The AdoHcy produced in this transmethylation reaction originates from AdoMet. More than half of AdoMet in the body is consumed for creatine production. Homocysteine production then can be estimated from creatinine excretion. Homocysteine transport from the intracellular to the extracellular compartment is about 1.5 mmol/day, so most of it is metabolized intracellularly. The human body can metabolize about 6.8 μmol/kg/h of homocysteine and somewhat less in uremia (31). Therefore, it appears that, if renal function was abolished, consequent homocysteine accumulation could be prevented easily by its whole-body metabolic clearance, even if blunted in renal failure.

As for homocysteine metabolism in the renal parenchyma, results obtained in a rat model showed a 20% decrease of homocysteine in the renal vein with respect to the renal artery (32), but, in this experimental system, homocysteine is mostly present in its free non–protein-bound form. Van Guldener et al. instead measured homocysteine in the renal vein and renal artery of 20 patients with normal renal function undergoing a coronarography, and there was no significant difference (33).

No cofactor or cosubstrate is markedly deficient in uremia; not folates, which are actually higher in plasma and erythrocytes, nor vitamin B_6 or B_{12}, or betaine, or serine. Patients may be deficient, of course, in one or more cofactors. Dialysis treatment also can lead to removal of these substances.

We are left with the untested hypothesis that a uremic toxin may accumulate, leading to an impairment of one or more of the relevant enzymes of homocysteine metabolism. Supporting the role of retained uremic toxins are the following considerations:

1. In uremia, folates, a cosubstrate of methionine synthase, a key enzyme for homocysteine disposal even if used at high dosages, are not able to completely normalize homocysteine levels, suggesting that as-yet-unidentified uremic toxins may inhibit these enzymes (34).
2. Superflux dialyzers are able to reduce homocysteine levels in the long term. Conversely, conventional dialysis can reduce homocysteine levels up to a point because only free homocysteine is dialyzable, and most homocysteine is protein bound. A suggested explanation is that uremic toxins are dialyzed more efficiently by superflux dialyzers, thus easing the inhibition of the homocysteine-metabolizing enzymes (35).
3. Kidney transplant recipients are responsive to relatively high dosages of folates and normalize their plasma homocysteine levels after therapy (36).

CONSEQUENCES OF HYPERHOMOCYSTEINEMIA IN UREMIA

Patients with uremia have a high mortality rate, attributable mainly to cardiovascular disease: 9% per year, which is 30 times the risk in the general population. Even after age-adjustment, cardiovascular disease mortality remains 10 to 20 times higher than in the general population. This risk cannot easily be ascribed entirely to the presence of conventional risk factors or to the ones typical of the uremic state (e.g., hyperparathyroidism, hypertriglyceridemia). Hyperhomocysteinemia is the most prevalent among risk factors in these patients.

Uremia is a model of accelerated arteriosclerosis, and homocysteine is a risk factor in patients with uremia. Uremia is not a good model to study homocysteine and its link to arteriosclerosis, and in particular the effects of B-vitamin intervention on homocysteine levels, because of many confounding factors and a survivorship effect (37). However, it has been pointed out that any potential benefit of therapeutic intervention can very well exceed any hazard, given the high mortality rate of these patients (38). Therefore, to study the uremic model can be rewarding, despite any theoretical consideration.

Our laboratory has focused on one particular aspect of homocysteine toxicity—the link between homocysteine and hypomethylation. Additional evidence coming from other investigators in the field of uremia and other models of hyperhomocysteinemia is confirming its importance (39).

In fact, a consequence of the increased plasma levels of homocysteine in patients with uremia is an increase in the intracellular concentration of AdoHcy (40,41). This thioether is, as said earlier, the direct homocysteine precursor and the natural inhibitor of all AdoMet-dependent transmethylation reactions. The ratio [AdoMet]/[AdoHcy] is a good indicator of the normal flow of methyl groups transferred from the methyl donor to methyl acceptors within the cell. The increase of AdoHcy concentration in uremia, which is not paralleled by any increase of AdoMet concentration, gives way to a significant reduction of the [AdoMet]/[AdoHcy] ratio. This, in turn, causes a significant impairment of AdoMet-dependent membrane protein carboxyl methylation reaction, catalyzed by protein carboxyl methyltransferase (PCMT, EC 2.1.1.77).

This ubiquitous methylation reaction is involved in the repair of molecular damage, represented by L-isoaspartyl residues, spontaneously occurring in proteins through deamidation of labile asparagine residues. In the L-isoaspartyl residue, the regular alternation of nitrogen and carbon atoms in the peptide backbone is interrupted by the presence of an extra methylene group because the aspartyl is linked through its β-carbonyl to the subsequent residue in the peptide chain, which can result in the destabilization of protein local conformation:

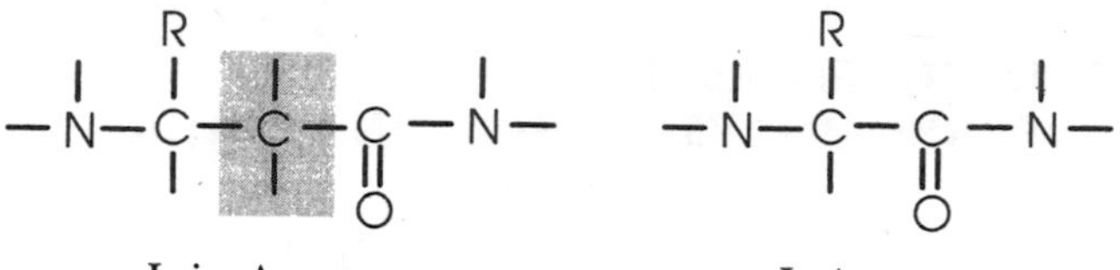

L-isoAsp L-Asp

The repair mechanism involves PCMT, and repeated cycles of methylation and demethylation allow the quantitative conversion of damaged L-isoaspartyl residues arising from asparagine degradation into normal L-aspartyl ones. Evidence confirmed the ability of this combined pathway to restore the biologic function of proteins thus inactivated. For example, enzymatic methyl esterification is able to restore, *in vitro*, a significant portion of the biologic activity of deamidated calmodulin. It is important to note that PCMT knockout mice die prematurely and large amounts of L-isoaspartyl–containing, isomerized proteins accumulate in tissues (42).

Characterization of methyl-accepting membrane protein species in chronic renal failure and hemodialysis patients show that the erythrocyte cytoskeletal component ankyrin (band 2.1), which connects spectrin and the integral membrane protein band 3 (AE1), is methylated (repaired) to a significantly lesser extent compared to normal.

We found that the reduction of the [AdoMet]/[AdoHcy] levels, measured by straightforward analytical procedures, is in good agreement with the degree of impairment of membrane protein repair. In fact, we measured the racemized and isomerized aspartyl residues (D-Asp + D-isoAsp), which appear as side products of the repair reaction. Proteins are cleaved by mild chemical and enzymatic digestion at 37°C using specific proteases. Accumulation of these residues in patients with end-stage renal disease is about one-third of controls, which, according to a computer simulation model corresponds to a residual PCMT activity of about 11% of normal. This degree of inhibition can lead to an up to 600-fold increase in L-isoaspartyl residues in erythrocyte proteins (43).

The final outcome is the inadequate repair of such structural alterations in erythrocyte membrane proteins, with the attending accumulation of damaged residues, in patients with chronic renal failure. Several crucial transmethylation-dependent processes, in addition to protein repair, in cells different from erythrocytes can be affected by a reduction in the [AdoMet]/[AdoHcy] ratio (44).

Homocysteine, at a concentration comparable to that present in patients with uremia, specifically inhibits, through AdoHcy accumulation, methylation of protein p21ras in cultured vascular endothelial cells. P21ras hypomethylation leads to reduced membrane association of this important regulator of cell cycle; thus, it may have important effects on atherosclerotic lesion formation through reduced endothelial cell proliferation (45).

It has been shown that an increase in plasma homocysteine is associated with parallel increases in plasma AdoHcy and to lymphocyte DNA hypomethylation, evaluated by HpaII digestion and 3H-dCTP-extension assay in women. Disruption of nonrandom DNA methylation pattern can lead to inappropriate gene expression and promotion of disease (46). It has been recently shown that DNA methylation is impaired in uremia. Folate treatment reverts this alteration in DNA methylation and also the consequent changes of gene expression in uremic/hyperhomocysteinemic patients (47).

We have shown that in plasma of patients with uremia, levels of damaged proteins (i.e., proteins containing the L-isoaspartyl residue mentioned earlier), are increased in uremia almost twofold. L-isoaspartyl residues in plasma proteins were quantitated using human recombinant PCMT. The major protein involved comigrated with serum albumin. Although hyperhomocysteinemia caused a redistribution of thiols bound to plasma proteins, this mechanism did not significantly contribute to the increase in isoaspartyl residues. Folate treatment can reduce, but not significantly, levels of damaged plasma proteins, meaning that other toxins besides homocysteine have a role in protein damage (48).

Van Guldener et al., using the powerful tool of stable isotope labeling of methionine, measured whole-body rates of methionine and homocysteine metabolism in fasting hemodialysis patients. They found significantly lower remethylation and transmethylation rates compared to controls (31).

Metabolic repercussions of folate administration, 15 mg/day per os for 2 months, are to increase the erythrocyte [AdoMet]/[AdoHcy] ratio to levels not significantly different from those detected in normal individuals (49). In fact, the folate-induced increase in methionine is handled by the cell through an increase in AdoMet biosynthesis.

In summary, hypomethylation is a consequence of high homocysteine in uremia. Transmethylation rates are lower in the body as a whole, and, in particular, protein repair is impaired.

THERAPY

Hyperhomocysteinemia could be ignored, pending the results of the intervention trials, which will be able to tell us if treatment is effective in terms of reducing cardiovascular risk, in general, and in uremia. Even screening for hyperhomocysteinemia is not recommended, with the exception of individuals with personal or familiar premature cardiovascular disease who do not present any of the traditional risk factors. The same considerations can be applied to patients with uremia. However, there is room for discussion, even in this era of evidence-based medicine, because in this particular group cardiovascular mortality is particularly high and screening is not necessarily expensive; therapy also is not always expensive, and it has very few side effects, at least in the case of folates. Possible means to lower homocysteine in uremia can include the following: (a) treat patients with cofactors, such as vitamin B_6 and vitamin B_{12}; (b) furnish folates, serine, and betaine, which can be considered cosubstrates; (c) treat with substances able to provide a higher concentration of free homocysteine in the circulation, such as N-acetylcysteine; and (d) improve dialysis and in general to have a kidney transplant.

Vitamin B_6 is not effective in these patients. No controlled study on the independent effects of vitamin B_{12} is available. N-acetylcysteine and betaine or serine seems to be equally ineffective (see reference 35 for review). Folates can reduce homocysteine levels by 30%, although not to normal levels. Utilized dosages are supraphysiologic (5 to 15 mg/day), and increasing dosages is not effective (34).

Folate deficiency results in the same hematologic picture as vitamin B_{12} deficiency. Therefore, therapy should be undertaken with both vitamins because utilization of folates alone would mask megaloblastosis produced by pernicious anemia, which would manifest itself only later with the severe and harder-to-heal neurologic deficits (50).

We have shown that metabolic repercussions of MTHF administration, 15 mg/day per os for 2 months, are to increase the [AdoMet]/[AdoHcy] ratio to levels not significantly different from those detected in normal individuals (49). Treatment with MTHF in patients undergoing hemodialysis significantly increases the [AdoMet]/[AdoHcy] ratio, indicating that the blockage in the normal flow of transmethylations is eased by treatment with MTHF. An increase in transmethylations therefore should induce a diminished accumulation of altered proteins, at least intracellularly, with relevant consequences in terms of protein function.

In conclusion, advantages of folate therapy are homocysteine reduction, whose reflections on cardiovascular risk remain to be established, but also prevent the alterations induced, at cellular level, by the decreased [AdoMet]/[AdoHcy] ratio, with possible metabolic reflections. In this respect, a case-control study indicated that plasma S-adenosylhomocysteine is a more sensitive marker of cardiovascular disease than plasma homocysteine (51).

REFERENCES

1. Perna AF. Homocysteine. In: Massry SG, Glassock RJ, eds. *Massry and Glassock's textbook of nephrology*, 4th ed. Philadelphia: Lippincott Williams and Wilkins, 2001;1258–1262.
2. Perna AF, Castaldo P, Ingrosso D, et al. Homocysteine, a new cardiovascular risk factor, is also a powerful uremic toxin. *J Nephrol* 1999;12:230–240.
3. Robertson KD, Wolffe AP. DNA methylation in health and disease. *Nature Reviews* 2000;1:11–19.
4. Chen RZ, Pettersson U, Beard C, et al. DNA hypomethylation leads to elevated mutation rates. *Nature* 1998;395:89–93.
5. Selhub J, Miller JW. The pathogenesis of homocysteinemia: interruption of the coordinate regulation by S-adenosylmethionine of the remethylation and transsulfuration of homocysteine. *Am J Clin Nutr* 1992;55:131–138.
6. Brown CA, McKinney KQ, Kaufmann JS, et al. A common polymorphism in methionine synthase reductase increases risk of premature coronary artery disease. *J Cardiovasc Risk* 2000;7:197–200.
7. Kang SS, Wong PWK, Malinow MR. Hyperhomocyst(e)inemia as a risk factor for occlusive vascular disease. *Ann Rev Nutr* 1992;12:279–298.
8. McCully KS. Vascular pathology of homocysteinemia: implications for the pathogenesis of atherosclerosis. *Am J Pathol* 1969;56:111–128.
9. Wilcken DEL, Wilcken B. The natural history of vascular disease in homocystinuria and the effects of treatment. *J Inherit Metab Dis* 1997;20:295–300.
10. Wilcken DEL, Wilcken B. The pathogenesis of coronary artery disease. A possible role for methionine metabolism. *J Clin Invest* 1976;57:1079–1082.
11. Clarke R, Daly L, Robinson K, et al. Hyperhomocysteinemia: an independent risk factor for vascular disease. *N Engl J Med* 1991;324:1149–1155.
12. Ueland PM, Refsum H, Beresford SAA, et al. The controversy over homocysteine and cardiovascular risk. *Am J Clin Nutr* 2000;72:324–332.
13. Bostom AG, Jacques PF, Nadeau MR, et al. Post-methionine load hyperhomocysteinemia in persons with normal fasting total plasma homocysteine: initial results from the NHLBI Family Heart Study. *Atherosclerosis* 1995;116:147–151.
14. Cattaneo M, Lombardi R, Lecchi A, et al. Is the oral methionine loading test insensitive to the remethylation pathway of homocysteine? *Blood* 1999;93:1118–1120.
15. Frosst P, Blom HJ, Milos R, et al. A candidate genetic risk factor for vascular disease: A common mutation in the methylenetetrahydrofolate reductase. *Nat Genet* 1995;10:111–113.
16. Brattström L, Zhang Y, Hurtig M, et al. A common methylenetetrahydrofolate reductase gene mutation and longevity. *Atherosclerosis* 1998;141:315–319.
17. Refsum H, Ueland PM. Recent data are not in conflict with homocysteine as a cardiovascular risk factor. *Curr Opin Lipidol* 1998;9:533–539.
18. Jungers P, Massy ZA, Khoa TN, et al. Incidence and risk factors of atherosclerotic cardiovascular accidents in predialysis chronic renal failure patients: a prospective study. *Nephrol Dial Transplant* 1997;12:2597–2602.
19. Bostom AG, Shemin D, Verhoef P, et al. Elevated fasting total plasma homocysteine levels and cardiovascular disease outcomes in maintenance dialysis patients. A prospective study. *Arterioscler Thromb Vasc Biol* 1997;17:2554–2558.
20. Moustapha A, Naso A, Nahlawi M, et al. Prospective study of hyperhomocysteinemia as an adverse cardiovascular risk factor in end-stage renal disease. *Circulation* 1998;97:138–141.

21. Massy ZA, Chadefaux-Vekemans B, Chevalier A, et al. Hyperhomocysteinemia: a significant risk factor for cardiovascular disease in renal transplant recipients. *Nephrol Dial Transplant* 1994;9: 1103–1108.
22. Ross R. Atherosclerosis: a defense mechanism gone awry. *Am J Pathol* 1993;143:987–1001.
23. Lentz SR. Mechanisms of thrombosis in hyperhomocysteinemia. *Curr Opin Hematol* 1998;5:343–349.
24. Hofmann MA, Lalla E, Lu Y, et al. Hyperhomocysteinemia enhances vascular inflammation and accelerates atherosclerosis in a murine model. *J Clin Invest* 2001;107:675–683.
25. Chen Z, Karaplis AC, Ackerman SL, et al. Mice deficient in methylenetetrahydrofolate reductase exhibit hyperhomocysteinemia and decreased methylation capacity, with neuropathology and aortic lipid deposition. *Hum Mol Genet* 2001;10:433–443.
26. Welch GN, Loscalzo J. Homocysteine and atherothrombosis. *N Engl J Med* 1998;338:1042–1050.
27. Nappo F, De Rosa N, Marfella R, et al. Impairment of endothelial functions by acute hyperhomocysteinemia and reversal by antioxidant vitamins. *JAMA* 1999;281:2113–2118.
28. Jakubowski H. Translational incorporation of S-nitrosohomocysteine into protein. *J Biol Chem* 2000;275:21813–21816.
29. Jakubowski H. Homocysteine thiolactone: metabolic origin and protein homocysteinylation in humans. *J Nutr* 2000;130: 377S–381S.
30. Antonio CM, Nunes MC, Refsum H, et al. A novel pathway for the conversion of homocysteine to methionine in eukariotes. *Biochem J* 1997;328:165–170.
31. van Guldener C, Kulik W, Berger R, et al. Homocysteine remethylation and methionine transmethylation are proportionally decreased in end-stage renal disease—a stable isotope study with L-[2H3-methyl-1-13C]methionine. *Kidney Int* 1999;56: 1064–1071.
32. Bostom AG, Brosnan JT, Hall B, et al. Net uptake of plasma homocysteine by the rat kidney in vivo. *Atherosclerosis* 1995; 116:59–62.
33. van Guldener C, Donker AJM, Jacobs C, et al. No net renal extraction of homocysteine in fasting humans. *Kidney Int* 1998; 54:166–169.
34. Sunder-Plassmann G, Fodinger M, Buchmayer H, et al. Effect of high dose folic acid therapy on hyperhomocysteinemia in hemodialysis patients: results of the Vienna multicenter study. *J Am Soc Nephrol* 2000;11:1106–1116.
35. Van Tellingen A, Grooteman MP, Bartels PC, et al. Long-term reduction of plasma homocysteine levels by super-flux dialyzers in hemodialysis patients. *Kidney Int* 2001;59:342–347.
36. Bostom AG, Shemin D, Gohh RY, et al. Treatment of mild hyperhomocysteinemia in renal transplant recipients versus hemodialysis patients. *Transplantation* 2000;69:2128–2131.
37. Bostom A, Culleton BF. Hyperhomocysteinemia in chronic renal disease. *J Am Soc Nephrol* 1999;10:891–900.
38. Baigent C, Burbury K, Wheeler D. Premature cardiovascular disease in chronic renal failure. *Lancet* 2000;356:147–152.
39. Dayal S, Bottiglieri T, Arning E, et al. Endothelial dysfunction and elevation of S-adenosylhomocysteine in cystathionine β-synthase-deficient mice. *Circ Res* 2001;88:1203–1209.
40. Perna AF, Ingrosso D, Zappia V, et al. Enzymatic methyl esterification of erythrocyte membrane proteins is impaired in chronic renal failure: evidence for high levels of the natural inhibitor S-adenosylhomocysteine. *J Clin Invest* 1993;91:2497–2503.
41. Perna AF, Ingrosso D, De Santo NG, et al. Mechanism of erythrocyte accumulation of methylation inhibitor S-adenosylhomocysteine in uremia. *Kidney Int* 1995;47:247–253.
42. Kim E, Lowenson JD, MacLaren DC, et al. Deficiency of a protein-repair enzyme results in the accumulation of altered proteins, retardation of growth, and fatal seizures in mice. *Proc Natl Acad Sci USA* 1997;94:6132–6137.
43. Perna AF, D'Aniello A, Lowenson JD, et al. D-aspartate content of erythrocyte membrane proteins is decreased in uremia: implications for the repair of damaged proteins. *J Am Soc Nephrol* 1997;8:95–104.
44. Perna AF, Ingrosso D, Galletti P, et al. Membrane protein damage and methylation reactions in chronic renal failure. *Kidney Int* 1996;50:358–366.
45. Wang H, Yoshizumi M, Lai K, et al. Inhibition of growth and p21ras methylation in vascular endothelial cells by homocysteine but not cysteine. *J Biol Chem* 1997;272(40):25380–25385.
46. Ping Y, Melnyk S, Pogribna M, et al. Increase in plasma homocysteine associated with parallel increases in plasma S-adenosylhomocysteine and lymphocyte DNA hypomethylation. *J Biol Chem* 2000;275:29316–29323.
47. Ingrosso D, Cimmino A, Perna AF, et al. Folate treatment and unbalanced methylation and changes of allelic expression induced by hyperhomocysteinaemia in patients with uremia. *Lancet* 2003; 361:1693–1699.
48. Perna AF, Castaldo P, De Santo NG, et al. Plasma proteins containing damaged L-isoaspartyl residues are increased in uremia: implications for mechanism. *Kidney Int* 2001;59: 2299–2308.
49. Perna AF, Ingrosso D, De Santo NG, et al. Metabolic consequences of folate-induced reduction of hyperhomocysteinemia in uremia. *J Am Soc Nephrol* 1997;8:1899–1905.
50. Herbert V, Bigauette J. Call for endorsement of a petition to the Food and Drug Administration to always add vitamin B-12 to any folate fortification or supplement. *Am J Clin Nutr* 1997;65: 572–573.
51. Kerins DM, Koury MJ, Capdevila A, et al. Plasma S-adenosylhomocysteine is a more sensitive indicator of cardiovascular disease than plasma homocysteine. *Am J Clin Nutr* 2001;74(6): 723–729.

8

CYTOSOLIC CALCIUM IN CHRONIC RENAL FAILURE, DIABETES MELLITUS, AND PHOSPHATE DEPLETION

SHAUL G. MASSRY
MIROSLAW SMOGORZEWSKI

Calcium ion is an important intracellular messenger controlling many cell functions such as growth, cell differentiation, membrane permeability, exocytosis, hormone secretion, synaptic activity, and gene expression (1). The calcium signals that regulate these functions are affected by the basal levels of intracellular concentration of calcium (cytosolic calcium $[Ca^{2+}]i$). Indeed, the calcium signal induced by a ligand is smaller when the basal levels of $[Ca^{2+}]i$ are elevated such as in human polymorphonuclear leukocytes (PMNLs) (2,3) and in rat pancreatic islets (4) and hepatocytes (5) (Fig. 8.1). In contrast, the elevation in the basal levels of $[Ca^{2+}]i$ in rat brain synaptosomes is associated with a greater calcium signal during their depolarization by KCl (6). A smaller or a greater calcium signal is associated with disturbed cell function; therefore, the maintenance of the basal levels of $[Ca^{2+}]i$ within the normal range is essential for the normal functioning of cells.

The basal levels of $[Ca^{2+}]i$ vary among various cells, among the same cells of various species (Table 8.1), and among a population of the same cell. In such populations of same cells, the levels of $[Ca^{2+}]i$ follow a Gaussian distribution, and such normal distribution is maintained but shifted to the right in disease settings associated with elevation in the levels of $[Ca^{2+}]i$ (Fig. 8.2) (2). Taken together, these observations suggest that the basal levels of $[Ca^{2+}]i$ are genetically determined.

The concentration of $[Ca^{2+}]i$ is four orders of magnitude lower than the extracellular concentration of calcium ion. This huge gradient favors the movement of calcium into the cell. Such an influx of calcium into cells is facilitated through calcium channels in the cell membrane. The latter also possesses two major transporting systems that facilitate the exit of calcium out of the cells; these are the Ca^{2+} ATPase and Na^{+}-Ca^{2+} exchanger. In addition, intracellular organelles such as endoplasmic reticulum, mitochondria, and nuclei possess pumps and channels that mediate release of calcium into cytosol and uptake of calcium from the cytosol into these organelles. Finally, a family of intracellular proteins (EF-hand family) (7,8) plays an important role in regulating the level of intracellular calcium. The most characterized of these proteins is calmodulin (9). The coordinated efforts of these channels, pumps, exchanger, and EF-hand family of proteins are responsible for maintaining the $[Ca^{2+}]i$ of each cell within a narrow normal range. When the functional integrity of these systems is deranged, an increase in the basal levels of $[Ca^{2+}]i$ may ensue.

TRANSPORT OF CALCIUM ACROSS THE CELL MEMBRANE

Calcium Channels

There are four types of calcium channels in the cell membrane. These include voltage-operated channels (VOC), receptor-operated channels (ROC), second messenger–operated channels (SMOC), and stretch-activated channels (SAC) (10). Any one cell therefore may possess many pathways for calcium influx.

There are several subtypes of VOC. Based on their voltage, time dependence, and pharmacologic properties, the VOC are classified as L, N, P, Q, R, and T types. The L-type calcium channels are high-voltage activated and strongly sensitive to a low concentration of dihydropyridine (DHP). The L-type calcium channels are present in neurons, cardiac myocytes, vascular smooth muscles, skeletal muscles, pancreatic beta cells, and other endocrine tissues. The L-type channels play an important role in the initiation of muscle contraction, in the facilitation of hormone and neurotransmitter release, and in calcium signal regulation of gene expression. The N-type calcium channels are also high-volt-

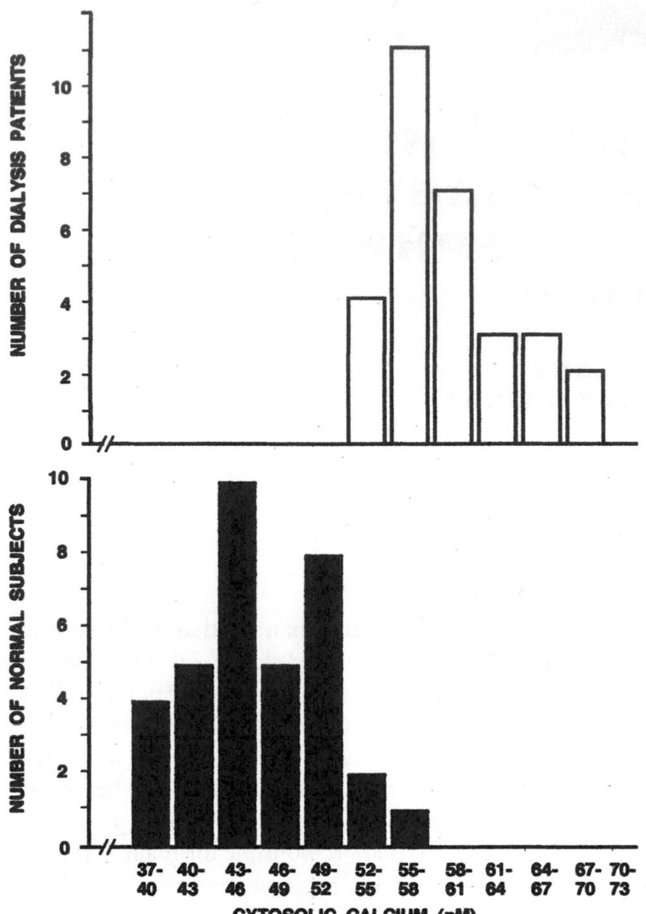

FIGURE 8.1. Frequency distribution of resting levels of $[Ca^{2+}]i$ of polymorphonuclear leukocytes from normal patients and patients undergoing dialysis. (From Alexiewicz JM, Smogorzewski M, Fadda GZ, et al. Impaired phagocytosis in dialysis patients: Studies on mechanisms. *Am J Nephrol* 1992;11:102–111, with permission.)

TABLE 8.1. LEVELS OF $[Ca^{2+}]i$ IN VARIOUS CELLS, RATS, HUMANS, AND OTHER ANIMALS

Cell Type	$[Ca^{2+}]i$ nM
Human PMNL	46 ± 0.74
Human B cells	80 ± 1.9
Human platelets	85 ± 5.0
Rat PMNL	108 ± 2.4
Rat pancreatic islet	82 ± 2.0
Rat hepatocytes	213 ± 1.3
Rat renal proximal tubular cells	160 ± 8.0
Rat cardiac myocytes	68 ± 0.8
Rat adipocytes	120 ± 4.3
Rat synaptosomes	345 ± 9.0
Rat thymocytes	60 ± 2.9
Rat skeletal muscle	56 ± 5.0
Rat vascular endothelium	71 ± 5.1

PMNL, polymorphonuclear leukocytes.
Data are presented as mean ± 1 standard error.

age activated but are insensitive to DHP. They are present primarily in presynaptic nerve terminals, neuronal bodies, and dendrites. The T-type channels are low-voltage activated and mildly sensitive to DHP. They are present in neurons and dendrites, and they display slow deactivation following sudden depolarization. For a more detailed discussion of VOC, the reader is referred to Tsien and Wheeler (11).

The ROCs are activated by binding of a ligand to its receptor on the cell membrane (12). The ion gating subunit is part of the receptor and is activated following the attachment of the ligand to the receptor (13). The activation of the ion gating subunit permits the influx of calcium into the cytosol. ROCs are present in many cells such as the N-methyl-D-aspartate receptor for glutamate in vertebrate neurons (14) and the adenosine triphosphate (ATP)-activated channels in smooth cardiac and skeletal muscles (15, 16), sensory neurons (17), macrophages (18), and exocrine glands (19).

The SMOCs are activated or modulated by second messengers generated intracellularly. These messengers include G proteins (20), protein kinase C (21), and IP_3 (22). Other SMOCs are activated by Ca^{2+} release; these channels are called Ca^{2+} release-activated channels (CRAC). This channel is highly selective for calcium (23). The SACs are involved in the regulation of cell volume, and they permit the influx of calcium as well as other ions (24).

Calcium Transport Out of Cells

The exit of calcium out of the cell is a critical process responsible for the maintenance of the Ca^{2+} gradient across the plasma membrane between the cytosol and the extracellular space. There are two transporting systems involved in this process and both require metabolic energy. These are the primary active plasma membrane Ca^{2+}ATPase (PMCA) and the secondary active Na^{+}-Ca^{2+} exchanger. The latter is driven by the sodium gradient generated by the Na^{+}-K^{+} ATPase.

The Ca^{2+} ATPase activity depends on ATP, which provides the energy for this calcium pump. There are two sites in the pump that interact with ATP. One of these sites has a high affinity for ATP (Km 1 − 2.5 μM), and the affinity for ATP of the other site is lower (Km 145 − 180 μM) (25). There are three human isoforms of PMCA (PMCA 1, 2, and 4) (25). The PMCA is stimulated by calmodulin (26); the latter decreases the Km of the pump for calcium from more than 30 to less than 1 μM and increases its V_{max} by as much as 10-fold (27).

The Na^{+}-Ca^{2+} exchanger (8,10,28) is an active calcium transporter that uses the electrochemical gradient of Na^{+} produced by the ATP-dependent Na^{+}-K^{+} ATPase. The exchanger transport three Na^{+} for one Ca^{2+}. The net direction of the exchange of these ions depends on the Na^{+} and Ca^{2+} gradients and on the transmembrane potential. The

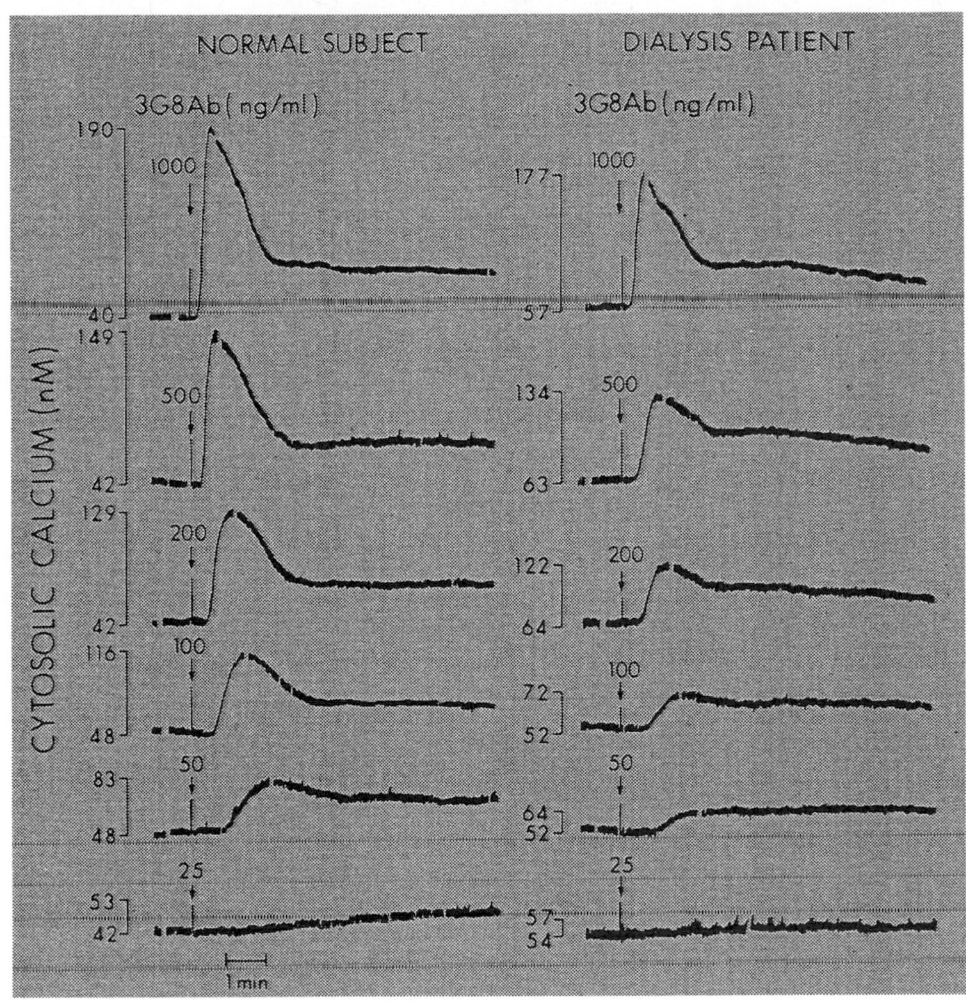

FIGURE 8.2. A study of the measurements of the resting levels of $[Ca^{2+}]i$ and the rise of $[Ca^{2+}]i$ in response to 3G8 monoclonal antibody (Ab) in polymorphonuclear leukocytes from a normal subject and a patients undergoing dialysis. (From Alexiewicz JM, Smogorzewski M, Fadda GZ, et al. Impaired phagocytosis in dialysis patients: Studies on mechanisms. *Am J Nephrol* 1992;11: 102–111, with permission.)

exchanger has a low affinity for Ca^{2+} but possesses high capacity for Ca^{2+} transport. This latter property assigns to the exchanger a dominant role in cells that are subjected to massive changes in intracellular calcium, such as cardiac myocytes; this is in comparison to the Ca^{2+}ATPase, which is more important in situations that require regulation of low changes in intracellular calcium. The Na^{+}-Ca^{2+} exchanger is present in almost all cells, but cardiac myocytes have a very high activity of the exchanger. Several isoforms of the Na^{+}-Ca^{2+} exchanger have been cloned.

INTRACELLULAR ORGANELLES AND INTRACELLULAR Ca^{2+} HOMEOSTASIS

Endoplasmic and Sarcoplasmic Reticulum

The endoplasmic reticulum (ER) and its counterpart in muscle, the sarcoplasmic reticulum (SR), play an important role in intracellular calcium homeostasis (8,29). They are organelles for calcium storage and release. The sarcoplasmic reticular calcium (SERCA)-ATPase mediates calcium uptake by the ER and SR. These organelles contain several calcium-binding proteins that operate as calcium stores. In addition, the ER and SR have receptors that activate calcium channels, permitting calcium release. These receptors include an IP_3 receptor (IP_3 R) and a ryanodine-cADP ribose receptor (RyR). The genes for these receptors have been cloned. The activation of these receptors stimulates an ROC that mediates the calcium release. These receptors are also Ca^{2+} sensitive. Therefore, once the receptors are activated with consequent release of calcium, this release would spread signals through a process of Ca^{2+}-induced Ca^{2+} release. Thus, the ER plays a critical role in Ca^{2+} signaling within the cell.

The Ca^{2+} stores of the ER are maintained by a process that couples the ER with plasma membrane. Depletion of ER from Ca^{2+} is sensed by Ca^{2+} channels in cell membrane resulting in calcium entry into the cell; this process is called *capacitated calcium entry* (CCE). The exact mechanisms responsible for this process are not defined, but it was proposed, among other things, that a calcium influx factor (CIF) may mediate CCE.

This discussion assigns an important role for the ER/SR

in the homeostasis of $[Ca^{2+}]i$; however, these cell organelles also play a paramount role in calcium signaling and other cell functions such as sterol synthesis, protein–protein interaction between ER/SR and plasma membrane, release of arachidonic acid, and apoptosis (29).

Mitochondria

The inner mitochondrial membrane possesses pathways for calcium uptake and calcium egress. The uptake of calcium by the mitochondria is mediated by a uniporter driven by electrochemical gradient (−180 mV inside). The egress pathways include sodium-dependent and sodium-independent ones. The Na^+-dependent pathway is a Ca^{2+}-$2Na^+$ exchanger, which transports one Ca^{2+} for $2Na^+$. The sodium-independent pathway is a Ca^{2+}-$2H^+$ exchanger, which transports one Ca^{2+} for $2H^+$ (8,30).

The potential capacity for Ca^{2+} uptake by the mitochondria is large and is about 10 times that of the Ca^{2+} egress. Therefore, the mitochondria can accumulate Ca^{2+} when the egress pathways are saturated. Thus, the mitochondria plays an important role in buffering Ca^{2+} during situations of high Ca^{2+} cellular overloads. The mitochondria provide the cell time to correct the condition of cellular Ca^{2+} overload by the cell through the utilization of the systems that facilitate pumping of calcium out of the cell.

Despite the large capacity of mitochondria to retain calcium loads, this property is not limitless. If the concentration of calcium in mitochondrial matrix reaches very high levels, damage of these cell organelles ensues with the final outcome being apoptosis and cell death.

CYTOSOLIC CALCIUM IN CHRONIC RENAL FAILURE

Chronic renal failure is associated with secondary hyperparathyroidism (31–33), and the blood levels of parathyroid hormone (PTH) begin to rise early in the course of renal failure (32,33) and continue to rise as renal failure progresses. These elevations in the blood levels of PTH in chronic renal failure (CRF) cause a sustained increase in the basal levels of $[Ca^{2+}]i$ of every cell. The mechanisms underlying the effect of chronic elevation in blood PTH on $[Ca^{2+}]i$ are complex and will be discussed in this chapter.

Acute Effects of Parathyroid Hormone on Cytosolic Calcium

Earlier studies showed that PTH enhances the entry of calcium into cells (34). Newer data demonstrated that PTH causes an acute rise in $[Ca^{2+}]i$ in many cells, including pancreatic islets, thymocytes, cardiac myocytes, hepatic cells, adipocytes, kidney cells, and osteoblasts (Table 8.2). This effect of PTH is receptor mediated and uses several cellular pathways (35), but these pathways are not uniform among these cells (Fig. 8.3) (35). In all these cells, PTH activates voltage-dependent and other calcium channels;

TABLE 8.2. THE EFFECTS OF PTH ON $[Ca^{2+}]i$ OF VARIOUS CELLS, THE CELLULAR PATHWAYS THAT ARE INVOLVED IN THIS ACTION OF PTH, AND THE SOURCE OF THE RISE IN $[Ca^{2+}]i$

	PTH				Cellular pathways				Source of Calcium	
Cell Type	1–84	1–34	Generation of cAMP	Inhibition by PTH Antagonist	Voltage-Dependent Calcium Channels	cAMP	G Protein(s)	Protein Kinase C	Extracellular	Intracellular
Cardiac myocytes	++	+	+	+	++	—	+	−	+	+
Pancreatic islets	++	+	+	+	+	+	+	+	+	−[a]
Thymocytes	++	−	+	+	+	+	+	+	+	−[a]
Hepatocytes	++	+	+	+	+	++	+	+	+	−[c]
Adipocytes	++	−	−	+	+	−	+	+	+	+
Renal cells	++	+	+	+	+	−[b]	+	+	+	+
Osteoblast[c]		+	+	+	+	+	+	+	+	+

PTH, parathyroid hormone; cAMP, cyclic adenosine monophosphate.
[a]PTH failed to increase $[Ca^{2+}]i$ in these cells when they were incubated in a free calcium media. It should be mentioned that cells incubated in free calcium media are calcium-depleted (low basal levels of $[Ca^{2+}]i$ and, therefore, mobilization of calcium from intracellular stores may be limited. However, other agonists were able to cause a rise in $[Ca^{2+}]i$ in cells incubated in calcium-free media when PTH failed to do so; examples include arginine vasopressin (AVP) and angiotensin if in hepatic cells and AVP in adipocytes. It seems, therefore, that if PTH raises $[Ca^{2+}]i$ by mobilizing intracellular calcium in these cells, such an action would depend on PTH-induced calcium influx, which is important in intracellular calcium mobilization (calcium–calcium release phenomenon); absence of such influx, when cells are incubated in a free calcium media, may impede intracellular calcium mobilization.
[b]cAMP pathway participates in the PTH-induced rise in $[Ca^{2+}]i$ of rabbit connecting tubular cells.
[c]The data on osteoblasts are derived from studies on rat osteosarcoma cell line UMR-106 and rat osteoblastlike cells ROS 17/2.8.

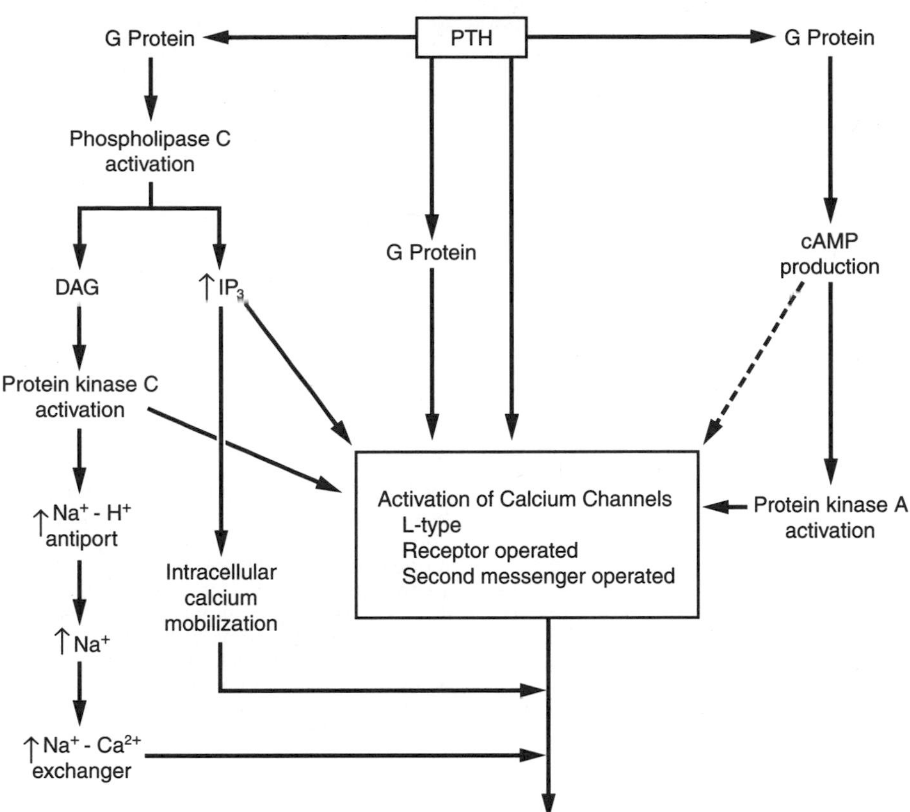

FIGURE 8.3. The potential cellular pathways through which parathyroid hormone (PTH) may mediate its action on $[Ca^{2+}]i$ of cells. DAG, Diacylglycerol. (From Fadda GZ, Massry SG. Impaired glucose-induced calcium signal in pancreatic islets in chronic renal failure. *Am J Nephrol* 1991;11:475–478, with permission.)

hence, the hormone-mediated calcium influx into cells is blunted or prevented by calcium channel blockers such as verapamil, nifedipine, or amlodipine.

It is of interest that some of these cells respond only to the intact molecule of PTH (PTH-(1-84)) (36), whereas in other cells the response to PTH-(1-84) is significantly greater than equimolar amounts of its aminoterminal fragment (PTH-(1-34)) (37). These observations suggest that the biologic activity of PTH assessed by calcium movement into cells resides not only in its aminoterminal fragment but in a bigger moiety containing the 1-34 amino acid sequence or in both the 1-34 fragment and another part of the carboxyterminal sequence of the hormone (35). Figure 8.4 shows a dose-response relationship between the rise in $[Ca^{2+}]i$ in rat hepatocytes and equimolar concentrations of PTH-(1-34) or PTH-(1-84), demonstrating the greater effect of the latter moiety of the hormone (37).

The aforementioned data indicate that the traditional (kidney and bone) and the nontraditional cells for PTH action must have the molecular machinery for the production of PTH receptors. Indeed, the messenger RNA (mRNA) for the PTH–PTH-related protein (PTH–PTHrP) receptor is present in the kidney, bone, heart, brain, spleen, aorta, ileum, skeletal muscle, lung, and testis (38,39). Thus, both physiologic and molecular evidence exist supporting the notion that almost all body organs are targets for PTH action; therefore, it is not surprising that chronic excess of PTH in CRF may exert a widespread deleterious effect on body function in uremia.

Chronic Effect of Parathyroid Hormone on Tissue Calcium Content and Basal Levels of $[Ca^{2+}]i$

Soft-tissue calcification is a common finding in patients with uremia, and increased calcium content was found in the cornea, skin, blood vessels, brain, peripheral nerves, heart, lungs, pancreas, liver, epididymal fat, and testis of patients and animals with renal failure (40). These abnormalities have been attributed, at least partly, to the state of secondary hyperparathyroidism of CRF because parathyroidectomy prevented the calcium accumulation in these tissues. These observations are consistent with the ability of PTH to augment entry of calcium into cells.

Newer data have shown that the increased calcium burden of the tissues in CRF also is associated with significant elevation of the basal levels of $[Ca^{2+}]i$ of various cells including brain synaptosomes, pancreatic islets, cardiac myocytes, hepatocytes, adipocytes, thymocytes, B cells, T cells, leukocytes, and platelets (41). An example of the changes

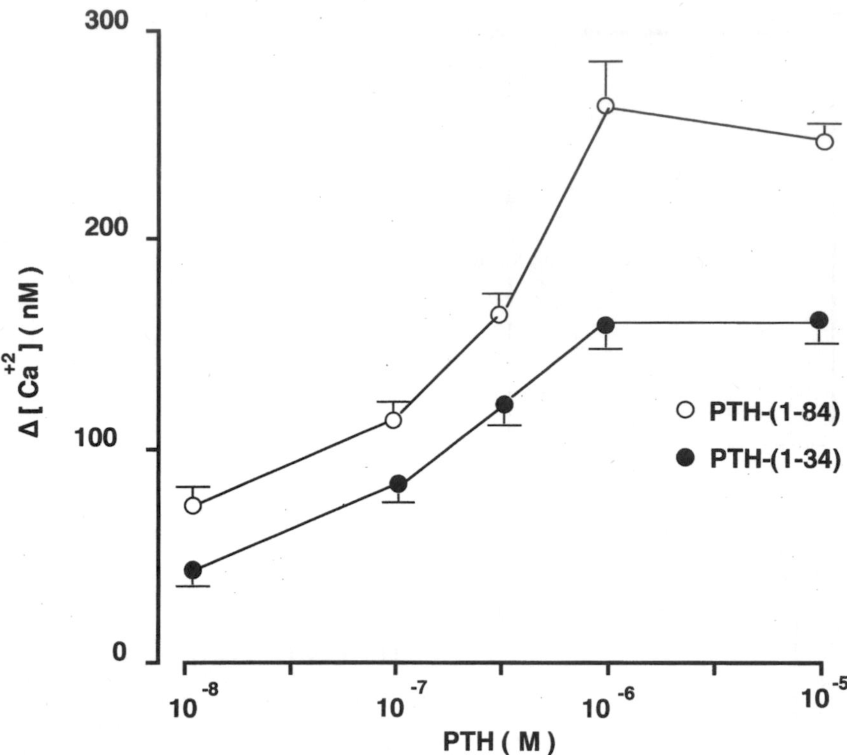

FIGURE 8.4. Dose-response relationship between the rise in [Ca^{2+}]i of rat hepatocytes and the concentration of parathyroid hormone (PTH). Each datum point is the mean of six to 12 studies, and brackets denote 1 SE. The changes in [Ca^{2+}]i were examined at 5 minutes after the exposure of hepatocytes to PTH. (From Klin M, Smogorzewski M, Khilnani H, et al. Mechanisms of PTH-induced rise in cytosolic calcium in adult rat hepatocytes. *Am J Physiol* 1994;267:G754–G763, with permission.)

in the basal levels of [Ca^{2+}]i of the cardiac myocytes of uremic rats is shown in Fig. 8.5. This chronic and sustained elevation in [Ca^{2+}]i of these cells is prevented or reversed by parathyroidectomy and/or by treatment with the calcium channel blocker verapamil. Again, these observations are in agreement with the property of PTH to augment entry of calcium into cells and with the finding that this action of the hormone uses voltage-dependent calcium channels that are blocked by verapamil.

Effect of Parathyroid Hormone on Phospholipids of Cell Membrane

PTH enhances phospholipid turnover in the kidney (43); affects phospholipid content of human red blood cells (44); and reduces total content of phospholipids, phosphatidylserine, phosphatidylethanolamine, and phosphatidylinositol in brain synaptosomes from rats with CRF (45). This latter effect is prevented by parathyroidectomy of the rats

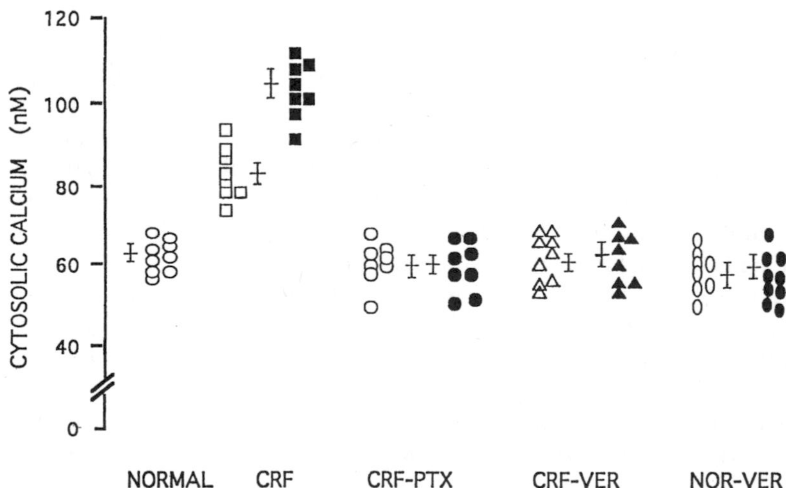

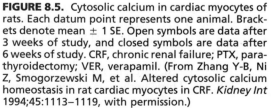

FIGURE 8.5. Cytosolic calcium in cardiac myocytes of rats. Each datum point represents one animal. Brackets denote mean ± 1 SE. Open symbols are data after 3 weeks of study, and closed symbols are data after 6 weeks of study. CRF, chronic renal failure; PTX, parathyroidectomy; VER, verapamil. (From Zhang Y-B, Ni Z, Smogorzewski M, et al. Altered cytosolic calcium homeostasis in rat cardiac myocytes in CRF. *Kidney Int* 1994;45:1113–1119, with permission.)

with CRF or by their treatment with verapamil. The action of PTH on phospholipid content of cell membrane may affect membrane fluidity, its permeability to ions, and the agonist/receptor interaction.

Mechanism of Sustained Elevation of Basal Levels of Cytosolic Calcium

Although PTH augments entry of calcium into cells, this action is not adequate to induce a sustained rise in $[Ca^{2+}]i$ because cells are endowed with powerful mechanisms that allow them to pump out excess calcium and/or buffer it by intracellular organelles (46). Therefore, the finding that the basal levels of $[Ca^{2+}]i$ of many cells are elevated in CRF indicates that the balance between calcium entry into cells, its extrusion out of cells, and/or its buffering within the cells is impaired.

As discussed earlier in this chapter, calcium extrusion from cells is regulated in major part, either directly or indirectly, by Ca^{2+}-ATPase, Na^+-Ca^{2+} exchanger, and Na^+-K^+-ATPase. The activities of Ca^{2+}-ATPase, Na^+-K^+-ATPase, and Na^+-Ca^{2+} exchanger of many cells are impaired in CRF (42).

It appears that the initial event leading to the sustained elevation of the basal level of $[Ca^{2+}]i$ in CRF is a PTH-induced augmentation of calcium entry into the cells, which would impair mitochondrial production of ATP. The subsequent decrease in ATP content of cells would impair the activities of Ca^{2+}-ATPase and Na^+-K^+-ATPase. The decrease in the phospholipid contents of cell membrane would contribute to the inhibition of the activity of Ca^{2+}-ATPase and Na^+-K^+-ATPase. The reductions in the activity of these two enzymes and of Na^+-Ca^{2+} exchanger lead to a decrease in calcium extrusion out of the cells. Such an effect in the face of a continued PTH-induced increase in calcium entry would result in calcium accumulation in the cells and to an increase in their basal levels of $[Ca^{2+}]i$. The latter would further inhibit mitochondrial oxidation and ATP production. Thus, a vicious circle develops until a new steady state is achieved with a low ATP content, a reduced V_{max} of Ca^{2+}-ATPase and Na^+-K^+-ATPase, a decreased activity of Na^+-Ca^{2+} exchanger, and elevation in the basal levels of $[Ca^{2+}]i$ (Fig. 8.6).

The formulation presented in Fig. 8.6 implies a sequence of events that occurs over time during the progression of CRF. The chronology of the events depicted in Fig. 8.6 was studied in pancreatic islets of rats during the evolution of CRF over a period of 6 weeks (47). The data of this study are shown in Fig. 8.7. The serum levels of PTH begin to rise during the first week of CRF. The V_{max} of

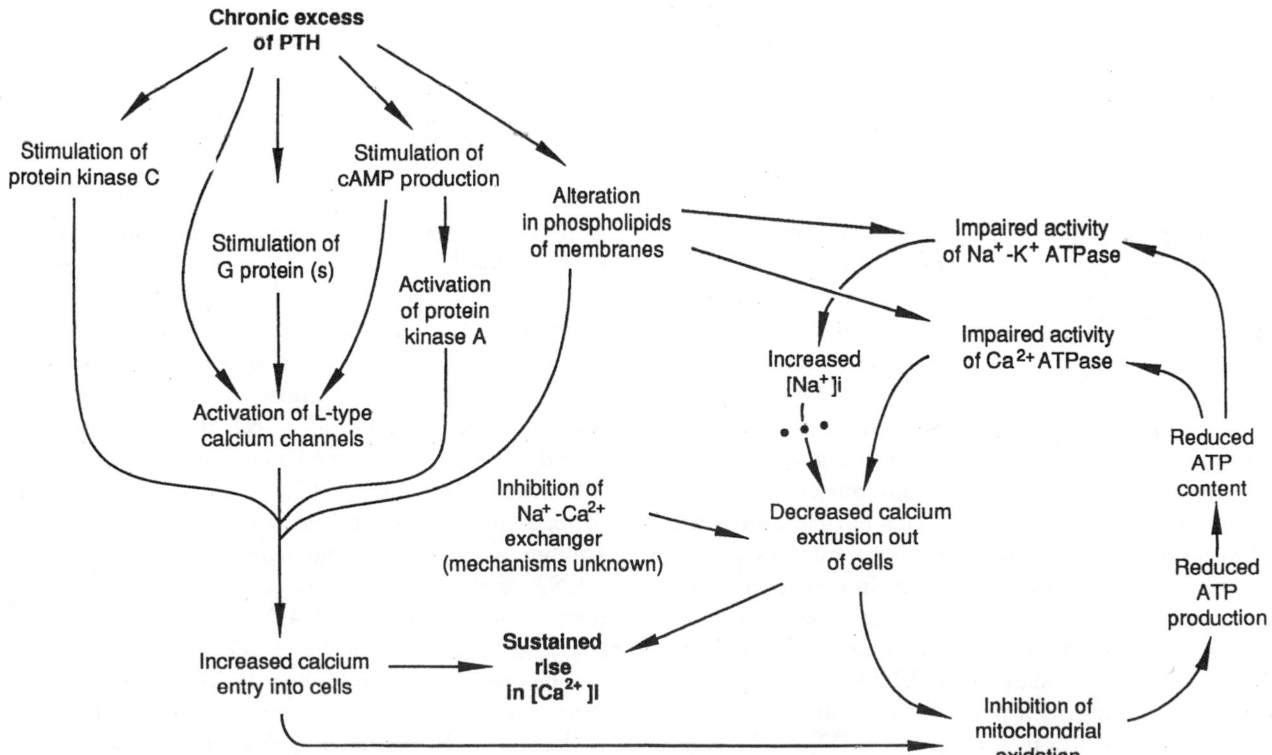

FIGURE 8.6. A schematic presentation of the sequence of events that lead to the elevation in the basal levels of $[Ca^{2+}]i$ in cells exposed to chronic excess of parathyroid hormone (PTH). (From Massry SG, Smogorzewski M. The mechanisms responsible for the PTH-induced rise in cytosolic calcium in various cells are not uniform. *Miner Elect Metab* 1995;21:13–28, with permission.)

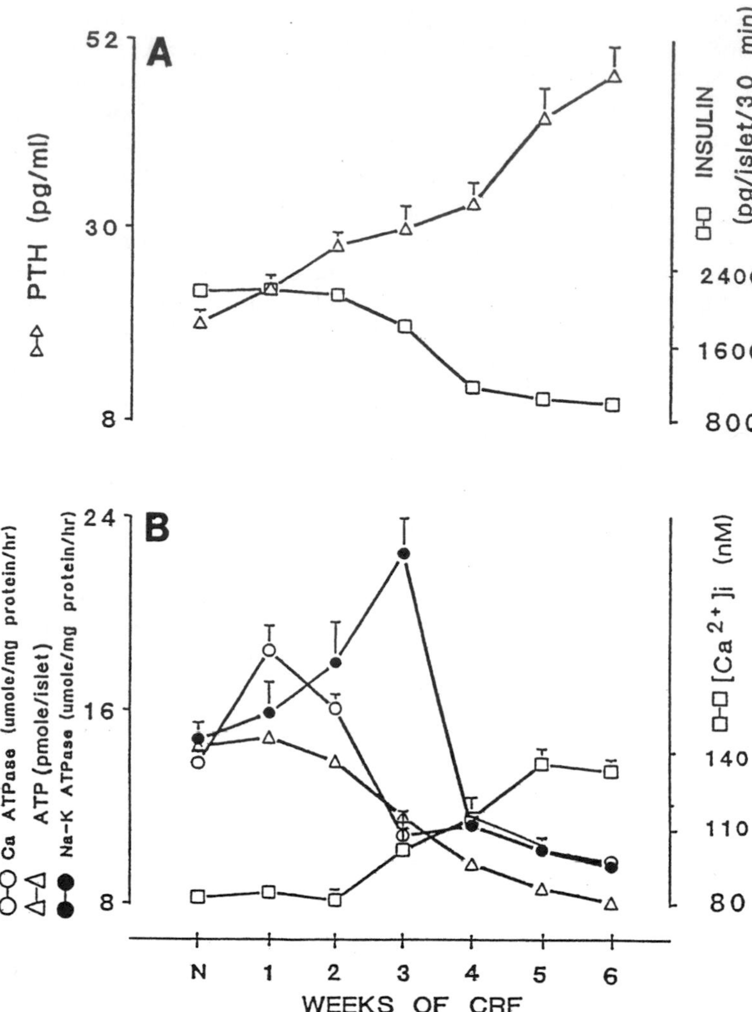

FIGURE 8.7. The chronologic relationship between the various parameters studied during the evolution of chronic renal failure over a period of 6 weeks in rat pancreatic islets. (From Levi E, Fadda GZ, Thanakitcharu P, et al. Chronology of cellular events leading to derangements in function of pancreatic islets in chronic renal failure. *J Am Soc Nephrol* 1992;3:1139–1146, with permission.)

Ca^{2+}-ATPase was higher during weeks 1 to 2, and of Na^{+}-K^{+}-ATPase during weeks 1 to 3 of CRF, but both activities fell to low levels thereafter. At week 3 of CRF, the ATP content started to fall, and the basal level of $[Ca^{2+}]$i began to rise. Thus, these data support the formulation shown in Fig. 8.6 and indicate that as serum levels of PTH begin to rise, calcium entry into islets is augmented. This in turn will stimulate the activity of Ca^{2+}-ATPase and the Na^{+}-Ca^{2+} exchanger, and calcium extrusion out of the islets is increased. As a result, $[Ca^{2+}]$i remains normal during the first 2 weeks of CRF. An activation of Na^{+}-Ca^{2+} exchanger may result in accumulation of sodium into islet, an event that would activate the Na^{+}-K^{+}-ATPase. As calcium entry is augmented further by the progressive rise in serum PTH levels, mitochondrial oxidation and ATP production would be reduced, resulting in lower ATP content. This fall in ATP causes a reduction in the V_{max} of Ca^{2+}-ATPase and Na^{+}-K^{+}-ATPase. Therefore, calcium extrusion out of the islets is reduced; consequently, $[Ca^{2+}]$i rises. This latter change was associated with the impairment in the function of the islets as manifested by a decrease in insulin secretion.

It is of interest that the sequence of events described in Fig. 8.7 does not continue but stabilizes at a new steady state. This may be the result of downregulation of the PTH receptors in CRF, an adaptive process that would protect the cells from further actions of the high blood levels of PTH and consequent continued accumulation of calcium, which eventually may lead to cell death. Indeed, studies have demonstrated that the PTH–PTHrP receptor mRNA is downregulated in CRF (48,49), an event that would lead to reduced receptor synthesis and hence a decrease in the number of receptors. The reduction in the amount of mRNA of the PTH–PTHrP receptors was found in both the traditional (kidney) (48,49) and the nontraditional organs (e.g., liver [49] and heart [50]) for PTH action.

The downregulation of the mRNA of the PTH–PTHrP receptor in various organs in uremia is prevented by parathyroidectomy or by treatment with a calcium channel blocker. Because these latter procedures normalize the basal levels of $[Ca^{2+}]$i in CRF, one may suggest that the elevation of $[Ca^{2+}]$i in CRF plays a major role in the downregulation of the PTH–PTHrP receptor. Such an effect may be mediated by the interference of the high levels of $[Ca^{2+}]i$ with the molecular machinery of the cells. The chronic increase in $[Ca^{2+}]i$ may impair the transcription or processing and/or turnover of the mRNA of the receptor.

The available data are consistent with the proposition that the PTH-mediated rise in the basal levels of $[Ca^{2+}]i$ in CRF provides a negative feedback mechanism through which the mRNA of the PTH–PTHrP receptor is downregulated to protect the cells against continued increase in blood levels of PTH, which further augments the elevation in $[Ca^{2+}]i$ to reach a level that would result in cell death. However, this useful adaptive process is not without an adverse effect. The tradeoff may be a downregulation of other hormone receptors if their molecular machinery is affected in a similar manner by the elevated $[Ca^{2+}]i$ of CRF. Indeed, the mRNA of angiotensin II (AT_1) and of vasopressin (AV1a) are downregulated in CRF (51). Again, this downregulation of these two receptors is prevented by parathyroidectomy or by treatment with a calcium channel blocker. This potential generalized effect of the elevation in the basal levels $[Ca^{2+}]i$ in CRF may provide an explanation for the resistance to the action of many hormones commonly encountered in CRF. Indeed, the calcium signals induced by PTH, angiotensin II, vasopressin, or glucagon in hepatocytes of rats with CRF are reduced (51).

Role of Parathyroid Hormone-Mediated Elevation in $[Ca^{2+}]i$ in the Genesis of the Uremic Syndrome

Available data indicate that the elevation in the basal levels of $[Ca^{2+}]i$ in various cells in uremia plays a paramount role in the genesis of the manifestations of the uremic syndrome. First, the prevention of the rise in $[Ca^{2+}]i$ in animals with CRF by prior parathyroidectomy or by their treatment with verapamil from day 1 of CRF was associated with correction of the uremic derangements (52–70). Second, reduction of blood levels of PTH by subtotal parathyroidectomy or by the medical suppression of the parathyroid gland activity with 1,25-dihydroxyvitamin D_3 ($1,25(OH)_2D_3$) in humans was associated with improvement of the uremic abnormalities (71–82). Third, treatment of humans or animals with preexisting CRF with calcium channel blockers (verapamil or nifedipine) reversed the uremic manifestations (59,79, 83,84). Table 8.3 provides data on the relationship between PTH and organ dysfunction in animals with CRF, and Table 8.4 provides these data regarding humans with CRF. It should be mentioned that chronic excess of PTH may affect organ function in CRF through other mechanisms besides the elevation in basal levels of $[Ca^{2+}]i$.

CYTOSOLIC CALCIUM IN PHOSPHATE DEPLETION

Chronic phosphate depletion is associated with multiple organ dysfunction (85–141). (These derangements are listed in Table 8.5). This is not surprising because two critical disturbances occur during chronic and marked phosphate depletion. First, there is a decrease in 2,3-diphosphoglycerate in the red blood cells (91,92), and this change is associated with increased affinity for hemoglobin to oxygen (91,92), resulting in tissue hypoxia. Second, there is also a decrease in tissue content of ATP (88,90,97,98,111,113, 119,120,123) and, therefore, a decrease in the availability of energy-rich phosphate compounds that are essential for cell function.

The available data indicate that ATP of cells starts to fall several weeks after a significant decrease in their inorganic phosphorus content. ATP continues to decrease thereafter (111,123), suggesting that other cellular metabolic disturbance(s) may contribute to the decrease in ATP besides phosphorus deficiency.

It has been shown that a chronic increase in calcium burden of cells inhibits mitochondrial oxidation and hence ATP production (107,111,142,143). It is theoretically possible that phosphate depletion is associated with a rise in $[Ca^{2+}]i$, and such an increment contributes significantly to the decrease in ATP content of cells through an effect on mitochondrial oxidation and/or phosphorylation. Indeed, several studies have demonstrated that phosphate depletion is associated with a significant rise in basal levels of $[Ca^{2+}]i$ in brain synaptosomes (141), pancreatic islets (119,120), and PMNLs (97) (Fig. 8.8).

Calcium entry into cells may be increased in phosphate depletion because the latter affects the phospholipid metabolism of cells (89,112). Smogorzewski et al. (89) reported significant decrements in total phospholipid content and in the contents of phosphatidylinositol, phosphatidylserine, and phosphatidylethanolamine of brain synaptosomes (Fig. 8.9). These changes can render the cell membrane more permeable to calcium and lead to augmented entry of this ion into cells (145,146).

The initial fall of ATP secondary to phosphorus deficiency and/or secondary to increased calcium entry into cells may be followed by reduction in the activity of the calcium pumps, leading to reduced calcium extrusion out of the cells and consequently to a rise in basal levels of $[Ca^{2+}]i$. Also, alterations in phospholipid metabolism of cell membrane adversely affect the activity of Na^+-K^+ATPase (147) and, therefore, also contribute to reduced calcium extrusion out of the cell and to the rise in $[Ca^{2+}]i$. Indeed, studies in brain synaptosomes (88,145) and in pancreatic islets (119, 120) have shown that the V_{max} of Ca^{2+}ATPase and Na^+-K^+ATPase are reduced in phosphate depletion (Fig. 8.10).

Thus, the available data are consistent with the notion that calcium entry into cells is increased and calcium extrusion out of the cells is decreased in phosphate depletion, These derangements lead to a rise in $[Ca^{2+}]i$, an event that would inhibit mitochondrial oxidation and phosphorylation and hence reduce ATP production. Therefore, it seems that the fall in ATP content of cells in phosphate depletion

TABLE 8.3. UREMIC MANIFESTATIONS ATTRIBUTED TO PTH-MEDIATED RISE IN [Ca^{2+}]i IN ANIMALS WITH CHRONIC RENAL FAILURE

Organ	Derangement	Prevented or Reversed by: Total Parathyroidectomy	Prevented or Reversed by: Calcium Channel Blocker	Induced by PTH Administration in Normal Animals
Brain	Abnormal EEG	+		+
Brain synaptosomes	Decreased NE content	+	+	+
	Decreased NE release	+	+	+
	Decreased NE uptake	+	+	+
	Reduced V_{max} of tyrosine hydroxylase	+		
	Increased Km of monoamine oxidase	+		
	Reduced total phospholipid content, phosphoinositol phosphatidylserine, and phosphatidylethanolamine	+	+	+
	Increased Ach content and release	+	+	
	Reduced choline kinase activity	+	+	
	Decreased choline content	+	+	
	Increased choline uptake	−	−	
	Increased choline release	−	−	
Peripheral nerves	Prolonged motor nerve conduction velocity	+		+
Heart	Impaired mitochondrial oxidation	+	+	+
	Impaired energy shuttle[a]	−		+
	Impaired energy use[a]	−		+
	Impaired fatty acid oxidation	+	+	+
	Decreased cardiac output[a]	−		+
	Right ventricular hypertrophy	+		
Lungs	Impaired diffusion capacity	+		
	Increased mean pulmonary wedge pressure	+		
Pancreas	Impaired glucose-induced insulin secretion	+	+	+
	Reduced leucine-induced insulin secretion	+	+	
	Decreased potassium-induced insulin secretion	+	+	
Lipid metabolism	Triglyceridemia	+	+	
	Impaired fat tolerance	+	+	
	Reduced postheparine lipolytic activity	+	+	
	Decreased hepatic lipase activity	+	+	
Polymorphonuclear leukocytes	Impaired phagocytosis	+	+	
	Reduced oxygen consumption	+	+	
Erythrocytes	Shortened survival	+		
Testes	Reduced blood levels of testosterone	+		+
B cells	Impaired immunoglobulin production	+		

PTH, parathyroid hormone; EEG, electronecephalogram; NE, norepinephrine; Ach, acetylcholine.
[a]Total parathyroidectomy did not correct these abnormalities because normal amounts of PTH are required for the synthesis of creatinine phosphokinase.

TABLE 8.4. UREMIC MANIFESTATIONS ATTRIBUTED TO EXCESS PTH IN PATIENTS WITH CHRONIC RENAL FAILURE

		Improved or Normalized by		
Organ	Derangements	Parathyroidectomy	Suppression of Parathyroid Glands Activity by $1,25(OH)_2D_3$ or Vitamin D_3	Calcium Channel Blocker
Brain	Abnormal EEG	+	+	
Peripheral nerve	Prolonged motor nerve conduction velocity[a]			
Heart	Decreased cardiac index	+	+	
	Reduced left ventricular ejection fraction	+		
	Decreased percent fiber shortening	+	+	
Pancreas	Impaired insulin secretion	+	+	
Polymorphonuclear	Impaired phagocytosis			+
	Impaired glycogen metabolism		+	+
Itching		+		
Tissue necrosis		+		
Soft-tissue calcification		+	+	
Bone resorption		+	+	
Sexual function, impotence		+	+	

PTH, parathyroid hormone; EEG, electroencephalogram.
[a]A relationship between the derangement in motor nerve conduction velocity and blood levels of PTH was documented.

TABLE 8.5. ORGAN DYSFUNCTION AND METABOLIC DERANGEMENTS IN PHOSPHATE DEPLETION

Central nervous system (85–89)
Irritability, paresthesia, dysarthria, anisocoria, hyperreflexia, confusion, obtundation, convulsion, coma, abnormal norepinephrine metabolism of brain, derangements in phospholipid metabolism of brain synaptosomes, and ↓ ATP, and ↑ cytosolic calcium in brain synaptosomes.

Hematopoietic system
Red blood cells (90–95): ↓ ATP content; ↓ hexokinase activity; ↓ 2,3-diphosphoglycerate; ↑ oxygen affinity; ↑ rigidity; ↓ life span, spherocytosis, and hemolysis.
Leukocytes (96,97): ↓ chemotactic, phagocytic, and bactericidal activity and ATP content and elevated cytosolic calcium.
Platelets (98): ↓ ATP content, thrombocytopenia, shortened platelet survival, impaired clot retraction, megakaryocytosis of the marrow.

Hypofunction of parathyroid glands (99–101)

Skeletal abnormalities (102,103)
Bone pain, pseudofractures, rickets or osteomalacia, and bone resorption.

Muscular dysfunction (102,104–107)
Marked muscular weakness, rhabdomyolysis, ↑ blood creatine phosphokinase and aldolase levels, low transmembrane resting potential difference in muscle, and impaired bioenergetic processes.

Cardiovascular system (108–114)
↓ Myocardial stroke work
↓ Cardiac contractility
↑ Left ventricular end-diastolic pressure, congestive heart failure, impaired bioenergetic and phospholipid metabolism of heart
↓ ATP of heart and blood vessels and impaired pressor response to norepinephrine and angiotensin

Impaired pulmonary muscle performance (115)

Impaired carbohydrate tolerance (116–119)
Hyperglycemia, peripheral resistance to the action of insulin, impaired insulin secretion and abnormalities in cellular metabolism of pancreatic islets including ↓ ATP content and ↑ cytosolic calcium.

Disturbances in renal function and electrolyte metabolism (101,102,116,121–141)
Elevation in serum calcium, hypomagnesemia, metabolic acidosis, fall in GFR hypercalciuria, hypermagnesiuria, hypophosphaturia, blunted phosphaturic response to extracellular fluid volume expansion or PTH administration, decreased proximal sodium reabsorption without natriuresis, decreased Tm bicarbonate and bicarbonaturia, decreased Tm glucose, reduced titratable acid excretion, decreased renal content of inorganic phosphorus and ATP, decreased cellular hydrogen ion concentration, decreased renal gluconeogenesis, decreased urinary excretion of cyclic AMP, and stimulation of 25-hydroxycholecalciferol-1-α-hydroxylase and increased 1,25 $(OH)_2D$ production.

ATP, adenosine triphosphate; PTH, parathyroid hormone; AMP, adenosine monophosphate.
Modified from Massry SG. The clinical syndrome of phosphate depletion. *Adv Exp Med Biol* 1978;103:301–307, with permission.

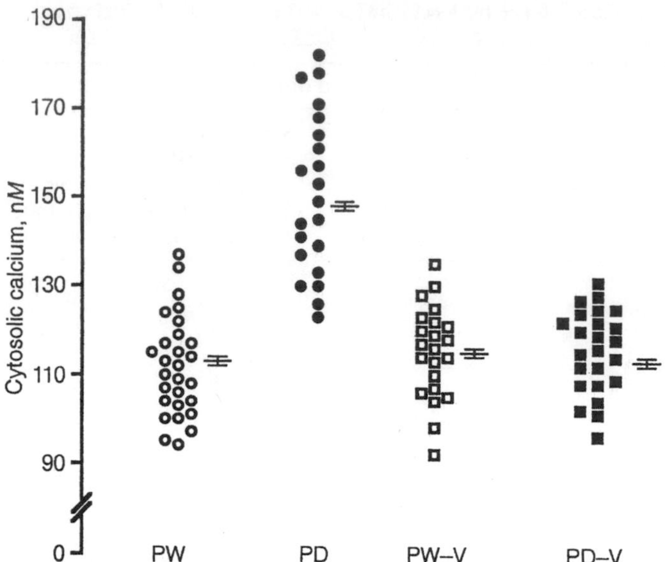

FIGURE 8.8. Cytosolic calcium in polymorphonuclear leukocytes of phosphate-depleted (*PD*), pair-weighed (*PW*), and PD and PW rats treated with verapamil (*V*). Each datum point represents one study and brackets denote mean ± 1 SE. (From Kiersztejn M, Chervu I, Smogorzewski M, et al. On the mechanism of impaired phagocytosis in phosphate depletion. *J Am Soc Nephrol* 1992;2: 1484–1489, with permission.)

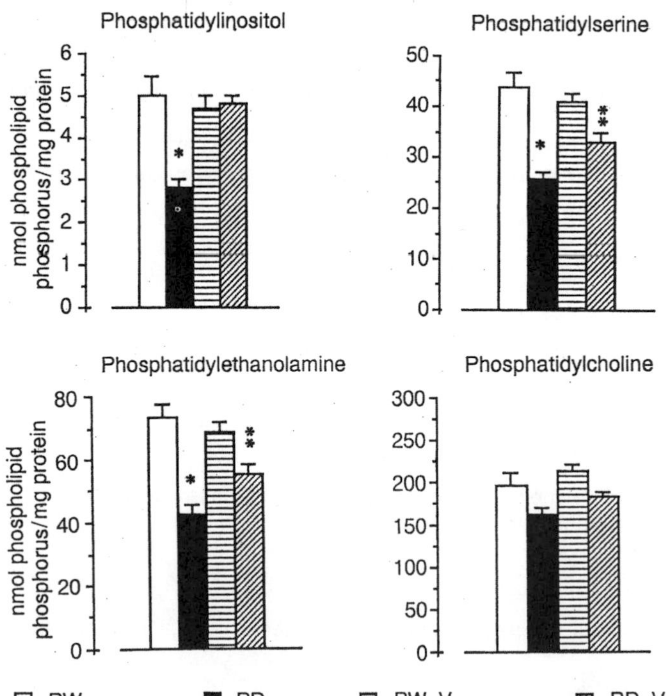

FIGURE 8.9. Various phospholipid contents of brain synaptosomes of phosphate-depleted (*PD*), pair-weighed (*PW*), and PD and PW rats treated with verapamil (*V*). Columns represent mean values, and brackets denote 1 SE. *$p < 0.01$ versus all groups; **$p < 0.01$ versus PW rats. (Based on data from Smogorzewski M, Islam A, Koureta P, et al. Reduced phospholipid content of brain synaptosomes in phosphate depletion. *Am J Physiol* 1991;261:742–747, with permission.)

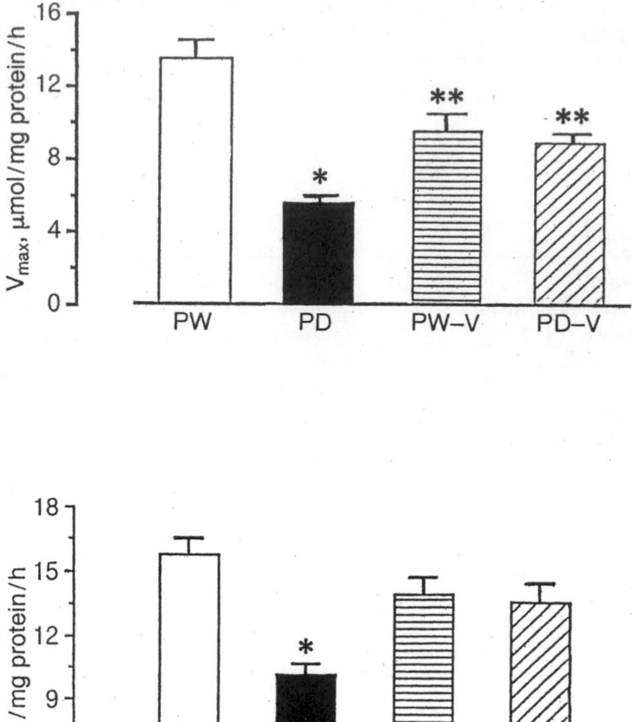

FIGURE 8.10. V_{max} of Ca^{2+}ATPase (*upper panel*) and Na^+-K^+-ATPase (*lower panel*) of pancreatic islets of phosphate-depleted (*PD*), pair-weighed (*PW*), and PD and PW rats treated with verapamil (*V*). Each column represents mean values, and brackets denote SE. *$p < 0.01$ versus all groups; **$p < 0.01$ versus PW rats. (From Fadda GZ, Hajjar SM, Zhou X-I, et al. Verapamil corrects abnormal metabolism of pancreatic islets and insulin secretion in phosphate depletion. *Endocrinology* 1992;130:193–202, with permission.)

is not only the result of the phosphorus deficiency but also to the increase in $[Ca^{2+}]i$. The proposed model for these events is depicted in Fig. 8.11.

If an increase in calcium entry occurs in phosphate depletion and if this plays an important role in the sequence of events described in Fig. 8.12, one should be able to ameliorate or prevent these cellular derangements by blocking calcium entry into the cells. Indeed, the treatment of phosphate-depleted rats with the calcium channel blocker verapamil improved or normalized both the metabolic profile and the function of many cells (88,89,97,119,120) (Figs. 8.8, 8.9, 8.10, 8.12, 8.13, and 8.14). Of special interest is the observation that despite chronic and marked phosphate depletion, cell ATP increased toward normal levels when the elevation in $[Ca^{2+}]i$ was prevented by verapamil (Fig. 8.12). This again points toward an important role for

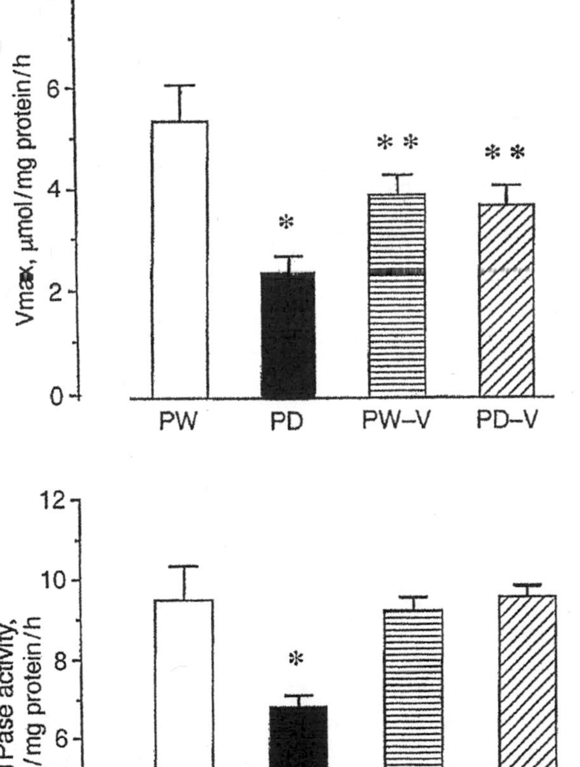

FIGURE 8.11. V_{max} of Ca^{2+}ATPase (*upper panel*) and Na^+-K^+-ATPase (*lower panel*) of brain synaptosomes of phosphate-depleted (*PD*), pair-weighed (*PW*), and PD and PW rats treated with verapamil (*V*). Each column represents mean values, and brackets denote SE. *$p < 0.01$ versus all groups; **$p < 0.01$ versus PW rats. (Based on data from Massry SG, Hajjar SM, Koureta P, et al. Phosphate depletion increases cytosolic calcium of brain synaptosomes. *Am J Physiol* 1991;260:F12–F18, with permission.)

the rise in $[Ca^{2+}]i$ in the genesis of the decrease in ATP content of cells in phosphate depletion.

The elevation in basal levels of $[Ca^{2+}]i$ in phosphate depletion could also adversely affect cell function. As stated earlier in this chapter, calcium serves as a second messenger in cell function, and in order for calcium to act as such, the rise in $[Ca^{2+}]i$ ($\Delta[Ca^{2+}]i$) and/or the ratio between ($\Delta[Ca^{2+}]i$)/basal $[Ca^{2+}]i$ induced by an agonist should be of appropriate magnitude. A smaller or a larger than normal $\Delta[Ca^{2+}]i$ and/or $\Delta[Ca^{2+}]i$/basal $[Ca^{2+}]i$ ratio may result in a defective cell response. Indeed, in phosphate depletion both of these parameters are abnormal in pancreatic islets in response to glucose (119,120) or potassium (148), in brain synaptosomes in response to potassium (88), and in PMNLs in response to FMLP (formylMet-Leu-Phe) (97). Prevention of the rise in the basal levels of $[Ca^{2+}]i$ by treatment of phosphate-depleted rats with verapamil was associated with normalization of the calcium signal and the ($\Delta[Ca^{2+}]i$)/basal $[Ca^{2+}]i$ in response to agonists (88,119, 120,148) and normalization of cell function. These observations indicate that phosphate depletion causes a rise in basal levels of $[Ca^{2+}]i$ and assign a critical role for this derangement in the genesis of the decrease in cell ATP and in the organ dysfunction in phosphate depletion.

CYTOSOLIC CALCIUM IN DIABETES MELLITUS

Diabetes mellitus is associated with complications affecting almost every organ, including vasculopathy, neuropathy, central nervous system dysfunction, retinopathy, cataracts, nephropathy, cardiomyopathy in the absence of appreciable coronary artery disease, atherosclerosis, and impaired function of PMNLs and B lymphocytes. The mechanisms responsible for this wide range of organ dysfunctions are not fully understood. Many factors may be involved, such as hyperglycemia, genetic predisposition, environment, hypertension, insulin deficiency (type I diabetes mellitus), and elevated blood levels of insulin (type II diabetes mellitus). Thus, dissection of the role of the entire spectrum of these factors in the genesis of diabetic complications is a very difficult and taxing endeavor.

Support for the "glucose hypothesis," implying an important role for hyperglycemia in the pathogenesis of diabetic complications, is growing. Epidemiologic studies (149), investigations with experimental diabetes (150,151), and the results of the Diabetes Control and Complications Trials (DCCT) (152) provide strong evidence that hyperglycemia is a major culprit in the genesis of diabetic complications. The availability of the assay of glycosylated hemoglobin (HbA_{1c}) (153), as a measure of glycemic control, has permitted better and more reliable epidemiologic studies exploring the relationship between hyperglycemia and diabetic complications. Data are now available supporting a relationship between hyperglycemia and retinopathy in both type I (154,155) and type II diabetes (156). In addition, Singer et al. (157) reported an association between prevalence of cardiovascular disease and HbA_{1c} levels. In addition, data from animal research showed that stringent control of hyperglycemia in animals with diabetes mellitus was associated with amelioration of the microvascular disease (150) or glomerulopathy (151). Similar observations were reported in humans with diabetes mellitus. Indeed, the DCCT clearly demonstrated that intensive therapy for the control of hyperglycemia in patients with type I diabetes was associated with significant reductions in retinopathy, neuropathy, and nephropathy (152). It stands to reason, therefore, that strict control of hyperglycemia is necessary

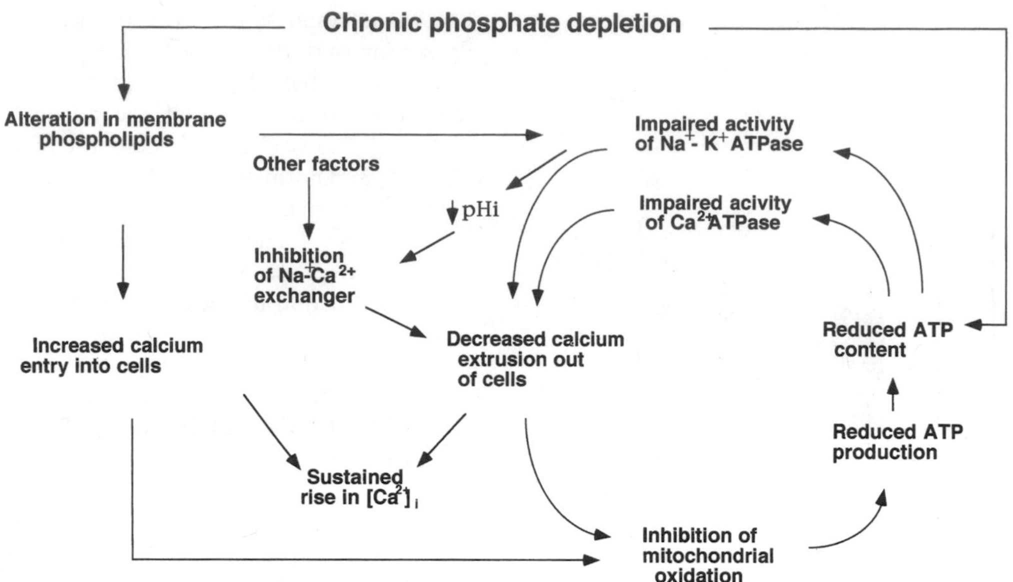

FIGURE 8.12. Schematic presentation of the processes that lead to derangements in the metabolic profile of the cell in phosphate depletion. $[Ca^{2+}]i$, cytosolic calcium; $[Na^{+}]i$, intracellular sodium.

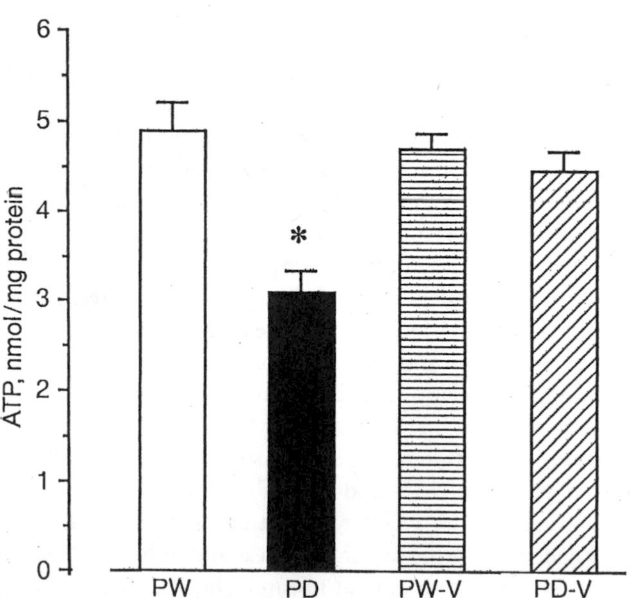

FIGURE 8.13. Adenosine triphosphate (ATP) content of pancreatic islets of phosphate-depleted (*PD*), pair-weighed (*PW*), and PD and PW rats treated with verapamil (*V*). Each column represents mean values, and brackets denote SE. *$p < 0.01$ versus all groups; **$p < 0.01$ versus PW rats. Verapamil treatment only partially, but significantly, corrected the reduction in ATP content of phosphate depletion. (From Fadda GZ, Hajjar SM, Zhou X-I, et al. Verapamil corrects abnormal metabolism of pancreatic islets and insulin secretion in phosphate depletion. *Endocrinology* 1992; 130:193–202, with permission.)

for the control of the diabetic complications. However, a very large segment of the population of patients with diabetes does not have good hyperglycemic control, and this is especially true for those with type II. In fact, in a large survey of a population of such patients in the Denver, Colorado area, the average fasting blood glucose was found to be about 200 mg/dL and their HbA_{1c} was 11.5% to 12.0%, independent of their treatment with insulin or oral hypoglycemic agents (158). It is apparent, therefore, that understanding the mechanisms through which hyperglycemia exerts its deleterious effects is critical for designing therapeutic approaches to ameliorate the complications of diabetes mellitus. Many issues need to be considered. These include, but are not limited to, four aspects that we mention because we believe that they provide the initial investigative steps in researching the deleterious effects of hyperglycemia.

1. How does hyperglycemia mediate its deleterious effects?
2. Are the mechanisms underlying the hyperglycemia-induced complications uniform and applicable to all organs? Are there differences in the response of various organs to hyperglycemia?
3. Are the pathways through which hyperglycemia exerts its deleterious effects preventable even if the hyperglycemia is not adequately controlled?
4. Are there medical therapeutic approaches to treat the complications in patients with poorly controlled diabetes mellitus?

Certain data are available regarding these issues. Two consequences of hyperglycemia have received a great deal of attention. First, the aldose reductase-sorbitol pathway, which is activated by hyperglycemia, leads to the accumula-

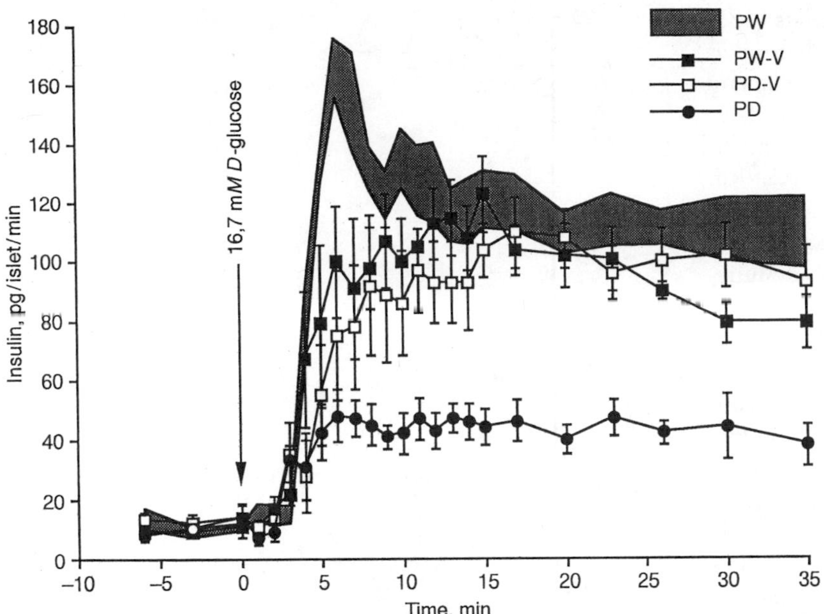

FIGURE 8.14. Dynamic data on glucose-insulin secretion by pancreatic islets from phosphate-depleted (*PD*), pair-weighed (*PW*), and PD and PW rats treated with verapamil (*V*). Shaded area represent mean ± 1 SE. Each datum point represents mean value, and brackets denote ± 1 SE. (From Fadda GZ, Hajjar SM, Zhou X-I, et al. Verapamil corrects abnormal metabolism of pancreatic islets and insulin secretion in phosphate depletion. *Endocrinology* 1992;130:193–202, with permission.)

tion of sorbitol in cells (159,160). The increase in sorbitol content may be harmful to cell function. Indeed, sorbitol accumulation is associated with an increased osmotic gradient and swelling of cells, reduced myoinositol content, and deranged energy metabolism (160–162). Available data show that sorbitol accumulation is harmful to the eye lens and may lead to cataracts, and it can damage the pericytes and nerve tissue and may contribute to neuropathy. These data have prompted the use of aldose reductase inhibitors in the management of the neuropathy of diabetes mellitus with encouraging results in animal models (163,164) but unconvincing outcomes in humans (165–167). It must be mentioned that the activation of aldose reductase occurs only in cells into which glucose can enter independently of insulin. Thus, the stimulation of this pathway may not occur uniformly in all cells of animals or humans with hyperglycemia. This may explain why sorbitol accumulation is implicated in the genesis of cataracts and neuropathy but not in other complications of diabetes mellitus. Thus, even if the use of aldose reductase inhibitors is helpful, their usefulness may be limited to only some diabetic complications.

The second consequence of hyperglycemia, which has received much attention and may play an important role in the genesis of the complications of diabetes, is the production of advanced glycosylation end products (AGEs) (168). The initial step of this process is the Maillard reaction (169), which involves the nonenzymatic glycosylation of amino acids by glucose, with the early products being the Schiff base and the Amadori adducts (170–172). The production and breakdown of these two compounds are fixed, and an equilibrium between them and a protein of sufficient life span is reached within hours or days; once this has happened, the amount of Amadori adducts bound to the protein does not change over time (173). These products are the precursors of AGEs that form slowly by rearrangement, oxidation, dehydration, and polymerization processes of the Amadori products (174). The latter may undergo oxidative cleavage, and the resulting products do not propagate advanced glycosylation (175,176). Therefore, the formation of these cleavage products may limit the progressive accumulation of AGEs. These compounds are attached irreversibly to proteins for the entire life span of the protein (173, 174), but their formation *in vivo* may be retarded by the action of reductase enzymes that reduce 3-deoxy-D-glucosone to less reactive 3-deoxy-D-fructose (175,176). Inhibition of reductase enzymes may lead to an increase in AGE accumulation. Furthermore, the net accumulation of AGE proteins in tissue matrix reflects a balance between glucose-accelerated accumulation and macrophage-mediated removal (174). Inhibition of macrophage activity would result in an increase in AGEs. Because AGEs are cleared by the kidney (177), renal failure is associated with high AGE levels (178,179). The circulating levels of AGEs and their tissue content are elevated in diabetes mellitus (173,174,178), and a large body of evidence suggests that the accumulation of AGEs in patients with diabetes plays an important role in the pathogenesis of many of the complications in these patients (173,174,178). Studies on the usefulness of AGE inhibitors by aminoguanidine in the management of diabetic complication are being investigated.

A third potential mechanism that may participate in the pathogenesis of diabetic complications that has received less attention is a derangement in the cellular homeostasis of calcium and elevation in the basal levels of $[Ca^{2+}]i$. Indeed, a review of the literature indicates that the basal level of

$[Ca^{2+}]i$ is elevated on erythrocytes (180), platelets (181, 182), and adipocytes (183,184) of patients with diabetes as well as in many cells of animals with experimental diabetes mellitus (185–188). This phenomenon led Levy et al. (189) to propose that many of the complications of diabetes mellitus are, at least in part, related to the elevation in $[Ca^{2+}]i$. This is a plausible proposition because other conditions in which the basal levels of $[Ca^{2+}]i$ are elevated, such as CRF and phosphate depletion, are associated with organ dysfunctions similar to those seen in diabetes mellitus. Demonstration of a relationship between the elevation in $[Ca^{2+}]i$ in diabetes mellitus and a specific cell dysfunction is limited. We have reported that the basal levels of $[Ca^{2+}]i$ of both PMNLs (190) (Fig. 8.15) and B lymphocytes (191) (Fig. 8.16) from patients with type II diabetes and poorly controlled hyperglycemia are elevated, and there were significant correlations between the $[Ca^{2+}]i$ of these cells and the degree of the hyperglycemia (Figs. 8.17 and 8.18). The elevation in $[Ca^{2+}]i$ was associated with impaired phagocytosis of PMNLs (190) and with impaired proliferation of B cells (191); normalization of blood glucose of these patients with the oral hypoglycemic agent, glyburide, was associated with reversal of the $[Ca^{2+}]i$ derangements in these cells and their abnormal functions. These observations suggested that hyperglycemia causes a rise in $[Ca^{2+}]i$ of these cells and the high $[Ca^{2+}]i$ interferes with their function.

The mechanisms responsible for the hyperglycemia-induced elevation in basal levels of $[Ca^{2+}]i$ are not well understood. Hyperglycemia may be associated with increased calcium influx into cells with a consequent acute rise in $[Ca^{2+}]i$. Indeed, certain studies have shown that a high glucose concentration induces an acute rise in $[Ca^{2+}]i$ of insulinoma cells (192), pancreatic islets (193), cultured rat tail artery vascular smooth muscle cells (194), PMNLs (195), and human red blood cells (196).

The pathways that mediate the acute rise in $[Ca^{2+}]i$ of cells exposed to a high glucose concentration are not fully elucidated. It has been reported that hyperglycemia may increase the activity (197) or the translocation of protein kinase C (198) or both (199). Activation of protein kinase C causes a rise in $[Ca^{2+}]i$ of many cells including thymocytes (36), pancreatic islets (200), hepatocytes (37), adipocytes (201), and renal proximal tubular cells (202). It is, therefore, possible that activation of protein kinase C by glucose participates in the glucose-induced rise in $[Ca^{2+}]i$ of PMNLs. In an effort to gain insight into the cellular pathways responsible for the glucose-induced acute rise in $[Ca^{2+}]i$, we carried out studies in PMNLs of rats exposed to high glucose concentrations (203) and found that hyperglycemia, through its osmotic effect and cell shrinkage, stim-

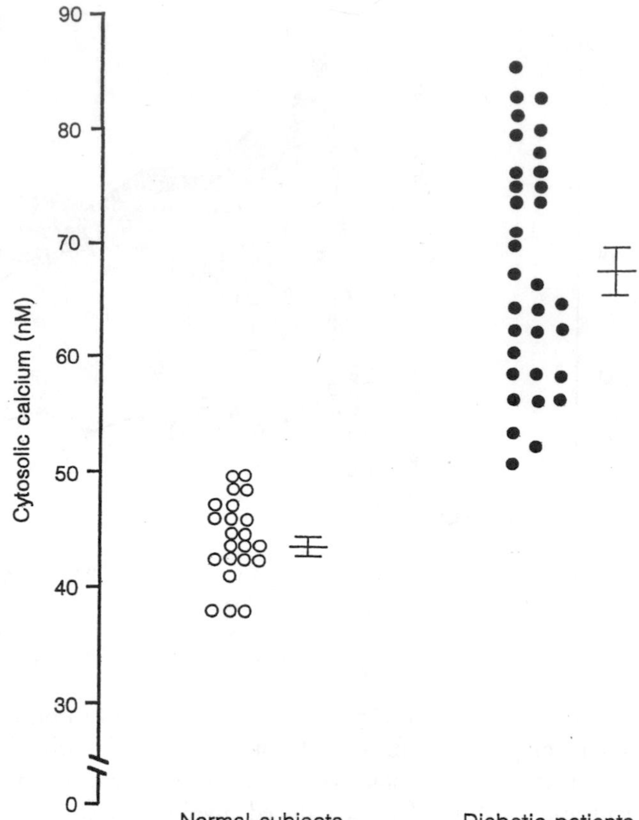

FIGURE 8.16. Basal levels of cytosolic calcium of polymorphonuclear leukocytes from normal subjects and patients with type II diabetes mellitus. Each point represents one subject, and the horizontal line denotes the mean (± 1 SE). (Modified from Alexiewicz JM, Kumar D, Smogorzewski M, et al. Polymorphonuclear leukocytes in non-insulin-dependent diabetes mellitus: Abnormalities in metabolism and function. *Ann Intern Med* 1995;123:919–924, with permission.)

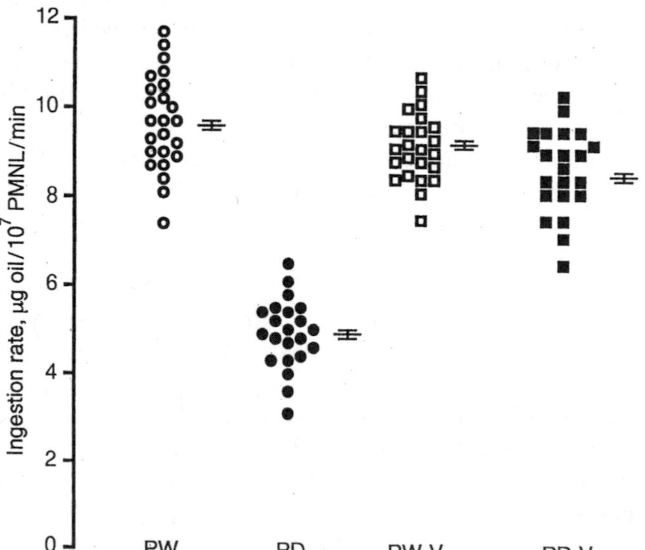

FIGURE 8.15. Ingestion of oil particles (phagocytosis) by polymorphonuclear leukocytes of phosphate-depleted (*PD*), pair-weighed (*PW*), and PD and PW rats treated with verapamil (*V*). Each datum point represents one study, and brackets denote ± 1 SE. (From Kiersztejn M, Chervu I, Smogorzewski M, et al. On the mechanism of impaired phagocytosis in phosphate depletion. *J Am Soc Nephrol* 1992;2:1484–1489, with permission.)

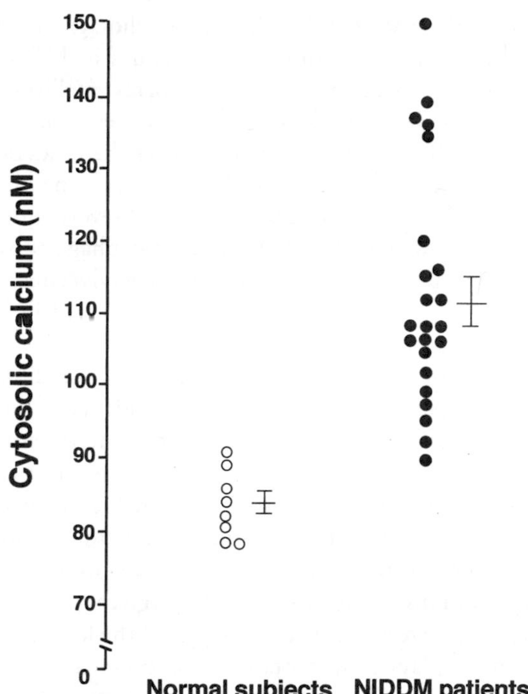

FIGURE 8.17. Basal levels of cytosolic calcium of B cells from normal subjects and patients with type II diabetes mellitus. Each point represents one subject, and the horizontal line denotes the mean (± 1 SE). (From Alexiewicz JM, Kumar D, Smogorzewski M, et al. Elevated cytosolic calcium and impaired proliferation of B lymphocytes in type II diabetes mellitus. *Am J Kidney Dis* 1997;(30)1:98–104, with permission.)

ulates a myriad of intracellular pathways including G proteins, the adenylate cyclase-cAMP protein kinase A system, and the phospholipase C pathway with consequent activation of protein kinase C. These cellular events activate calcium channels, which permit calcium influx into cells, and mobilize calcium from intracellular stores (Fig. 8.19). Indeed, the calcium channel blockers verapamil, nifedipine, or amlodipine markedly inhibited the magnitude of the glucose-induced rise in $[Ca^{2+}]i$. These effects of hyperglycemia are mimicked by equimolar concentrations of mannitol or choline chloride, demonstrating that the effects described earlier are not related to glucose *per se* but to its osmotic activity. Similar effects occurred in renal proximal tubular cells (204), cardiac myocytes (205), and hepatocytes (206).

As stated earlier in this chapter, an increase in calcium influx into cells by itself is not adequate to cause an increase in the basal levels of $[Ca^{2+}]i$ because cells are endowed with powerful mechanisms that directly $[Ca^{2+}$-ATPase, Na^{+}-Ca^{2+} exchanger) and indirectly (Na^{+}-K^{+}-ATPase) extrude calcium from cells. Therefore, for the basal levels of $[Ca^{2+}]i$ to increase, the function of these pumps must be impaired. Certain data indicate that Ca^{2+}-ATPase activity is reduced in sarcolemmal preparations of hearts from rats with streptozotocin-induced diabetes (207) and in erythrocytes of Zucker diabetic rats (208). Furthermore, Na^{+}-K^{+}-ATPase is reduced in the heart of rats with type II diabetes (186), in the sciatic nerve of rats with streptozotocin-induced diabetes (209), and in the platelets of patients with type II diabetes (210). In addition, Kuriyama et al. (211) found that vascular smooth muscle cells cultured in media containing high glucose had elevated levels of $[Ca^{2+}]i$ and reduced Na^{+}-K^{+}-ATPase activity. Finally, the Na^{+}-Ca^{2+} exchanger was found to be reduced in sarcolemmal preparations of heart from diabetic rats (186,207). It is not known, however, whether derangements in these pumps that may be associated with diabetes mellitus are present in other cells.

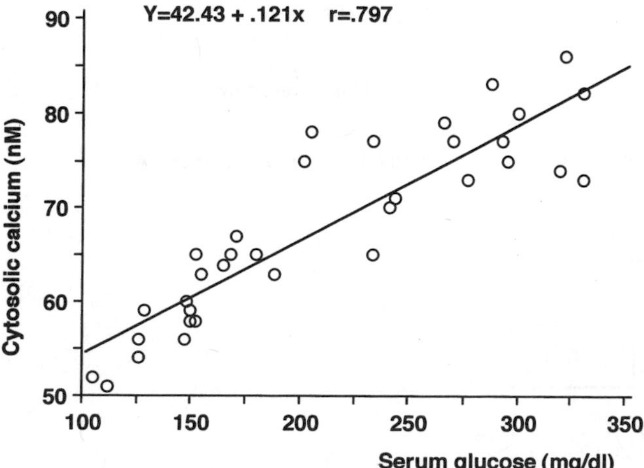

FIGURE 8.18. Relationship between cytosolic calcium of polymorphonuclear leukocytes and blood levels of glucose in 34 patients with type II diabetes mellitus. (From Alexiewicz JM, Kumar D, Smogorzewski M, et al. Polymorphonuclear leukocytes in non-insulin-dependent diabetes mellitus: Abnormalities in metabolism and function. *Ann Intern Med* 1995;123:919–924, with permission.)

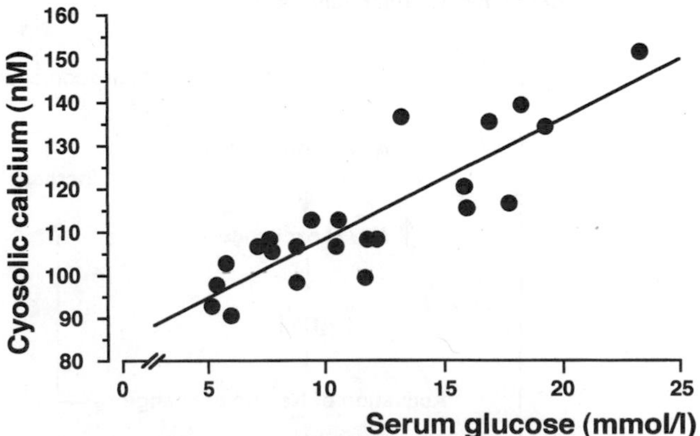

FIGURE 8.19. Relationship between cytosolic calcium of B cells and blood levels of glucose in 23 patients with type II diabetes mellitus. (From Alexiewicz JM, Kumar D, Smogorzewski M, et al. Elevated cytosolic calcium and impaired proliferation of B lymphocytes in type II diabetes mellitus. *Am J Kidney Dis* 1997;(30)1: 98–104, with permission.)

Thus, the limited available data permit the proposition that the initial event leading to the rise in the basal levels of [Ca^{2+}]i in diabetes is the hyperglycemia-induced calcium influx into cells. This is supported by the observation that the control of hyperglycemia is associated with normalization of the basal levels of [Ca^{2+}]i at least in two cell types (i.e., PMNLs [190] and B cells [191]). Chronic and sustained entry of calcium into cells that occurs with uncontrolled hyperglycemia may result in a decrease in cellular ATP content. Indeed, it has been found that sustained entry of calcium into cells in other settings is associated with inhibition of mitochondrial oxidation and phosphorylation and, hence, reduced ATP production (142,143) and a fall in ATP content. We reported that the ATP content of PMNLs of patients with type II diabetes is reduced, returning to normal after the control of hyperglycemia and normalization of PMNLs [Ca^{2+}]i (190). Because ATP is required for the normal function of Ca^{2+}-ATPase and Na^{+}-K^{+}-ATPase, a decrease in ATP content may be followed by a decrease in the activity of these enzymes. Understanding the mechanisms responsible for the elevation in the basal levels of [Ca^{2+}]i would permit the development of therapeutic approaches to prevent the rise in [Ca^{2+}]i, even if the hyperglycemia is uncontrolled.

If the initial event leading to the rise in the basal levels of [Ca^{2+}]i in diabetes mellitus is the hyperglycemia-induced increase in calcium influx, blocking this effect may prevent the rise in the basal levels of [Ca^{2+}]i, despite the hyperglycemia. Further, if the rise in the basal levels of [Ca^{2+}]i plays an important role in the genesis of the diabetic complications, preventing the rise in [Ca^{2+}]i may ameliorate or reverse cell dysfunction. We examined these issues in PMNLs of rats with streptozotocin-induced diabetes mellitus. We found that the basal levels of [Ca^{2+}]i in these cells are increased and phagocytosis is impaired after the induction of diabetes mellitus. Treatment of these rats with the calcium channel blocker amlodipine prevented and reversed the rise in [Ca^{2+}]i basal levels and the impaired phagocytosis of PMNLs despite sustained and marked hyperglycemia (212) (Fig. 8.20). It is of interest that Pierce et al. (213) found that treatment of rats with streptozotocin-induced diabetes with the calcium channel blockers verapamil or diltiazem markedly and significantly reduced the incidence of cataract and partially protected against the development of retinopathy despite sustained hyperglycemia. The lenses of the diabetic rats had a high calcium content, which correlated significantly with cataract formation. Verapamil treatment caused significant reduction in lenticular calcium. These *in vivo* observations again show that hyperglycemia is associated with an increased calcium content of the lens, that this derangement plays an important role in cataract formation, and that both abnormalities could be mitigated by treatment with calcium channel blockers (Figs. 8.21 and 8.22).

The mechanisms through which an elevation in the basal levels of [Ca^{2+}]i in diabetes mellitus adversely affect cell function are not known. An elevation in [Ca^{2+}]i in other conditions such as CRF or phosphate depletion is associated with (a) reduced cellular ATP content (119); (b) an inhibitory effect on many enzymes such as Ca^{2+}-ATPase (57, 120), Na^{+}-K^{+}-ATPase (57), synaptosomal tyrosine hy-

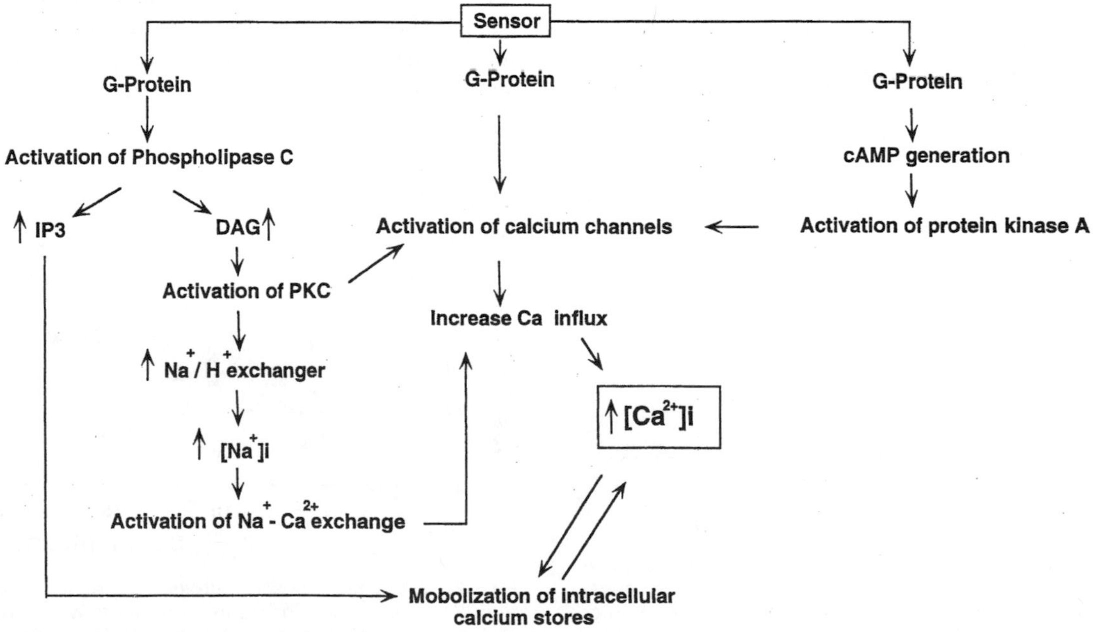

FIGURE 8.20. Schematic representation of the potential cellular events that lead to an elevation in cytosolic calcium ([Ca^{2+}]i) of polymorphonuclear leukocytes exposed to a high glucose concentration (30 mM) *in vitro.* IP3, inositol triphosphate; DAG, diacylglycerol; PKC, protein kinase C.

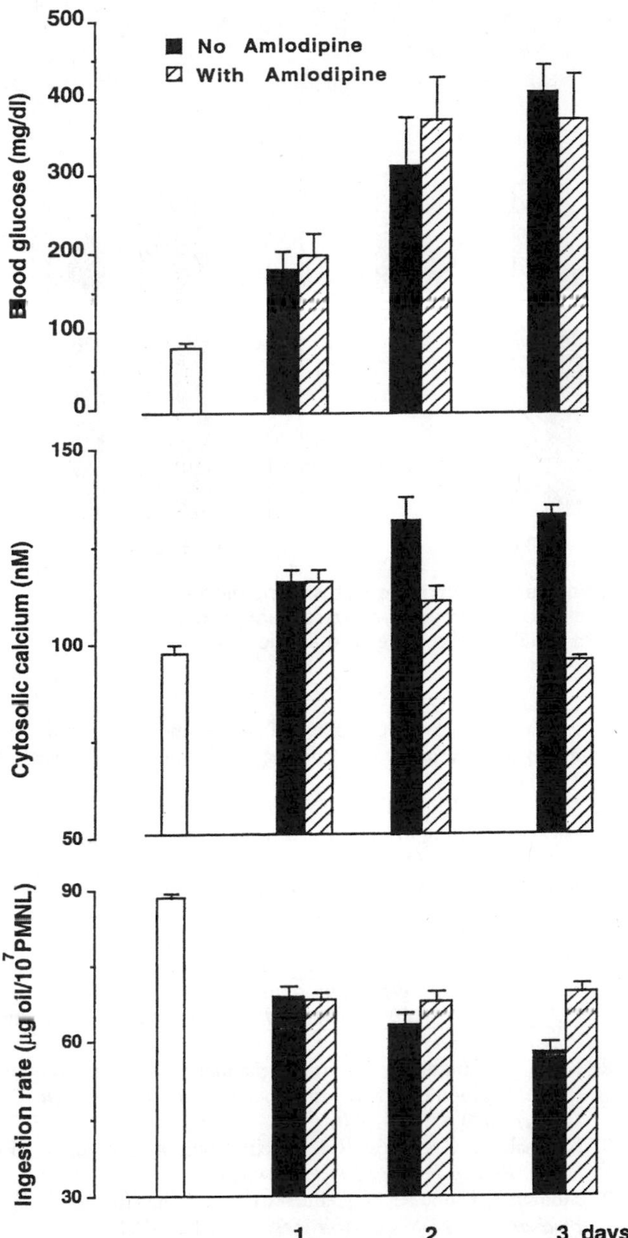

FIGURE 8.21. Blood glucose concentration, basal levels of $[Ca^{2+}]i$, and phagocytosis of polymorphonuclear leukocytes of rats with 1, 2, and 3 days of diabetes with and without treatment with amlodipine. Data from normal rats (□) also are shown. Each bar represents the mean (± 1 SE) of six to seven studies of diabetic rats and 21 studies of normal rats. (From Seyrek N, Marcinkowski W, Smogorzewski M, et al. Amlodipine prevents and reverses the elevation in $[Ca^{2+}]i$ and the impaired phagocytosis of PMNLs of diabetic rats. *Nephrol Dial Transplant* 1997;12:265–272, with permission.)

droxylase and monoamine oxidase (214), choline kinase (215), hepatic lipase (216), lipoprotein lipase (217,218), and pancreatic islets phosphofructokinase 1 (219); (c) an inhibitory effect on transport systems such as the Na^+-Ca^{2+} exchanger (42) and Na^+-H^+ antiport (57,220); (d) reduced phospholipid contents in brain synaptosomes (45, 89) and myocardium (112); and (e) alterations in the molecular machinery of the cells (49,50,221). Indeed, an elevation in the basal levels of $[Ca^{2+}]i$ in CRF or in phosphate depletion is associated with downregulation of the mRNA of many proteins. These include the mRNA of the PTH–PTHrP receptors of the kidney (49,221), heart (50), and liver (5,49); the mRNA of the angiotensin II and vasopressin receptors of the liver (50); and the mRNA of hepatic lipase (216). Normalization of $[Ca^{2+}]i$ of the various cells by treatment of animals with CRF or phosphate depletion with a calcium channel blocker normalized $[Ca^{2+}]i$ and significantly mitigated or completely reversed the downregulation of the mRNA of these proteins (49,50,221).

Similar effects of an elevation in basal levels of $[Ca^{2+}]i$ may occur in diabetes mellitus. We already have mentioned that reduced ATP content and impairment in the activity of Ca^{2+}-ATPase, Na^+-K^+-ATPase, and the Na^+-Ca^{2+} exchanger have been observed in diabetes mellitus. Some data are also available incriminating the rise in $[Ca^{2+}]i$ in alterations in the molecular machinery of cells. We examined the effect of streptozotocin-induced diabetes mellitus in rats on the $[Ca^{2+}]i$ of the renal proximal tubular cells and on the expression of mRNA for the PTH–PTHrP, vasopressin, and angiotensin receptors in these cells (222) and found that the levels of $[Ca^{2+}]i$ are elevated and the mRNAs for the hormone receptors are downregulated. Normalization of $[Ca^{2+}]i$ levels in these cells by treatment of the rats with amlodipine normalized the expression of the mRNAs of these receptors. Weiss et al. (223) also reported that diabetes mellitus in rats is associated with downregulation of the insulinlike growth factor-I (IGF-I) gene and upregulation of IGF-I receptor in rat kidneys. These observations again demonstrate an effect of diabetes on the molecular machinery of cells. These authors, however, did not measure kidney cell $[Ca^{2+}]i$, but concluded that these changes are related to the hyperglycemia. Studer and Ganas (224) found that the basal levels of $[Ca^{2+}]i$ of hepatocytes from diabetic rats are elevated and the vasopressin-, angiotensin-, and glucagon-induced rise in $[Ca^{2+}]i$ is reduced. They did not measure the mRNA or the proteins of these receptors, and it is possible that the reduced calcium signal induced by these hormones is the result of a reduction in their receptors. Mene et al. (225) found that the calcium signals induced by angiotensin II, prostaglandin F_2, and arginine vasopressin in mesangial cells cultured for 5 days in media containing 22 mM glucose are reduced significantly. This observation is consistent with alterations in the receptors of these agonists in the mesangial cells. Tanaka et al. (226) reported that cell surface ($^3H^+$)-bunazosin binding by cardiac myocytes from rats with streptozotocin-induced diabetes is markedly reduced. This binding reflects the number and/or affinity of the α-adrenoreceptors. The generation of IP3 after stimulation of the cardiac myocytes with noradrenaline also is reduced. Treatment of these animals with verapamil corrected these abnormalities despite persistent

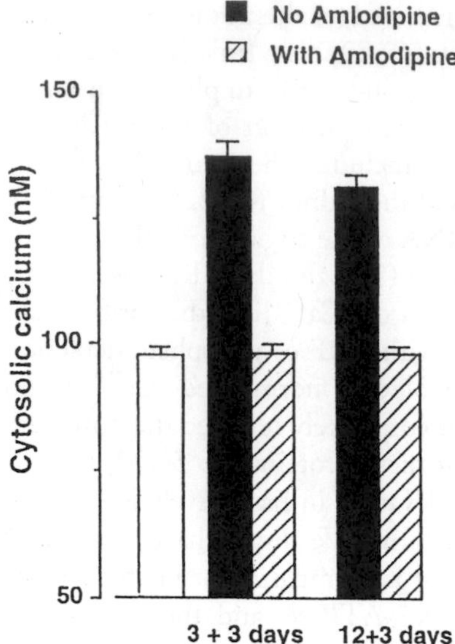

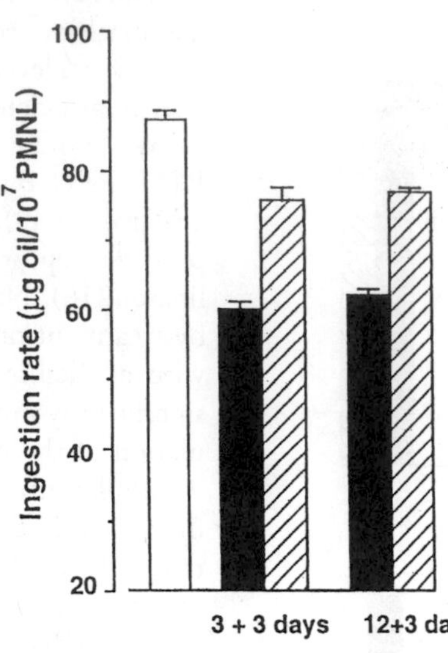

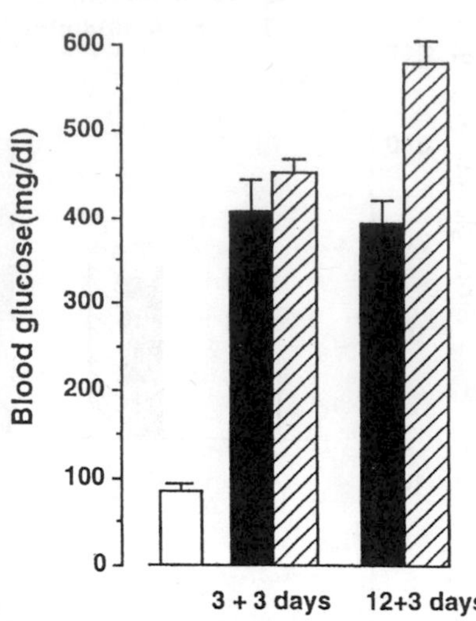

FIGURE 8.22. Basal levels of ([Ca^{2+}]i) of polymorphonuclear leukocytes, phagocytosis, and blood glucose levels in 21 normal rats (□) and in 3 to 12 day diabetic rats, which then were treated for 3 days with amlodipine. Each bar represents the mean (± 1 SE) of six studies of diabetic rats.

hyperglycemia. These data are consistent with adverse effects of diabetes on the molecular machinery and on cell signaling. Because verapamil corrected these derangements, it is reasonable to suggest that elevated levels of [Ca^{2+}]i of cardiac myocytes are responsible for these derangements.

It is apparent from this discussion that (a) derangements in cellular regulation of calcium are present in both type I and type II diabetes, (b) these abnormalities could adversely affect cell function through many pathways, and (c) a potential therapeutic approach may be available to combat these disturbances and their effects on cell function. Thus, the comprehensive study of the abnormalities in cellular calcium homeostasis in diabetes, an understanding of their mechanisms, and the evaluation of potential approaches for their prevention and/or management are of extreme clinical importance, especially for those patients with uncontrolled hyperglycemia. The data that would be generated by such studies may yield information enabling the formulation of new therapeutic approaches that may be useful in the treatment of many of the complications in patients with uncontrolled hyperglycemia.

REFERENCES

1. Rothinger JA, Iverson JG. Ruled by waves? Intracellular and extracellular calcium signaling. *Acta Physiol Scand* 2002;169: 203–219.
2. Alexiewicz JM, Smogorzewski M, Fadda GZ, et al. Impaired phagocytosis in dialysis patients: Studies on mechanisms. *Am J Nephrol* 1992;11:102–111.
3. Ahmed A, Krol E, Smogorzewski M, et al. Effect of amlodipine therapy on the monoclonal antibody 3G8-induced calcium signal in polymorphonuclear leukocytes of hemodialysis patients. *Am J Nephrol* 1999;19:505–508.
4. Fadda GZ, Massry SG. Impaired glucose-induced calcium signal in pancreatic islets in chronic renal failure. *Am J Nephrol* 1991;11:475–478.
5. Massry SG, Klin M, Ni Z, et al. Impaired agonist-induced calcium signaling in hepatocytes from chronic renal failure rats. *Kidney Int* 1995;48:1324–1331.
6. Koureta P, Smogorzewski M, Massry SG. Effect of potassium chloride on cytosolic calcium of brain synaptosomes of rats with chronic renal failure. *Miner Elect Metab* 1991;17:194–197.
7. Slupsky CM, Sykes BD. The structural basis of regulation by calcium-binding EF-hand proteins. In: Carafoli E, Klee C, eds. *Calcium as a cellular regulator.* New York: Oxford University Press, 1999:73–99.
8. Brini M, Carafoli E. Calcium signaling: a historical account, recent developments and future perspectives. *CMLS, Cell Mol Life Sci* 2000;57:354–370.
9. Kawasaki H, Kretsinger RH. Calcium-binding proteins I: EF-hands. *Protein Profile* 1994;1:342–391.
10. Mooren F, Kinne RKH. Cellular calcium in health and disease. *Biochemica et Biophysia Acta* 1998;1406:127–151.
11. Tsien RW, Wheeler DB. Voltage-gated calcium channels. In: Carafoli E, Klee C, eds. *Calcium as a cellular regulator.* New York: Oxford University Press, 1999:171–200.
12. Putney JW Jr. Receptor-regulated calcium entry. *Pharmacol Ther* 1990;48:427–434.
13. Tsien RW, Tsien RY. Calcium channels, stores and oscillations. *Ann Rev Cell Dev Biol* 1990;6:715–760.
14. Hume RI, Honig MG. Excitatory action of ATP on embryonic chick muscle. *J Neurosci* 1986;6:681–690.
15. Benham CD, Tsien RW. A novel receptor-operated Ca^{2+}-permeable channel activity by ATP in smooth muscle. *Nature* 1987;328:275–278.
16. Friel DD, Bean BP. Two ATP-activated conductances in bullfrog atrial cells. *J Gen Physiol* 1988;91:1–27.
17. Bean BP. ATP-activated channels in rat and bullfrog sensory neurons: concentration dependence and kinetics. *J Neurosci* 1990;10:1–10.
18. Alonso-Torre SR, Trautmann A. Calcium responses elicited by nucleotides in macrophages. Interaction between two receptor subtypes. *J Biol Chem* 1993;268:18640–18647.

19. Vincent P. Cationic channels sensitive to extracellular ATP in rat lacrimal cells. *J Physiol* (London) 1992;449:313–331.
20. Dolphin AC. Regulation of calcium channel activity by GTP binding proteins and second messengers. *Biochemica et Biophysia Acta* 1991;1091:68–80.
21. Berridge MJ. Capacitative calcium entry. *Biochem J* 1995;312: 1–11.
22. Berridge MJ. Inositol triphosphate and calcium signaling. *Nature* 1993;301:315–325.
23. Hoth M, Penner R. Depletion of intracellular calcium stores activates a calcium current in mast cells (comment). *Nature* 1992;355(6358):353–356.
24. Yang X-C, Sachs F. Block of stretch-activated ion channels in Xenopus oocytes by gadolinium and calcium ions. *Science* 1989; 243:1068–1071.
25. Carafoli E. The Ca^{2+}pump of the plasma membrane. *J Biol Chem* 1992;267:2115–2118.
26. Jarrett HW, Penniston JT. Partial purification of the [Ca^{2+} + Mg^{2+}] ATPase activator from human erythrocytes: its similarity to the activator of 3′-5′-cyclic nucleotide phosphodiesterase. *Biochem Biophys Res Commun* 1977;4:1210–1216.
27. Carafoli E. The calcium pumping ATPase of the plasma membrane. *Ann Rev Physiol* 1991;53:531–547.
28. Philipson KD. Sodium-calcium exchange. In: Carafoli E, Klee C, eds. *Calcium as a cellular regulator.* New York: Oxford University Press, 1999:279–294.
29. Berridge MJ. The endoplasmic reticulum: a multifunctional signaling organelle. *Cell Calcium* 2002;32:235–249.
30. McCormack JG, Denton RM. Calcium in the regulation of intramitochondrial enzymes. In: Carafoli E, Klee C, eds. *Calcium as a cellular regulator.* New York: Oxford University Press, 1999:520–554.
31. Pappenheimer AM, Wilens SL. Enlargement of the parathyroid gland in renal disease. *Am J Pathol* 1935;11:73.
32. Berson SA, Yalow RS. Parathyroid hormone in plasma in adenomatous hyperparathyroidism, uremia and bronchogenic carcinoma. *Science* 1966;154:907.
33. Arnaud CD. Hyperparathyroidism and renal failure. *Kidney Int* 1973;4:89–95.
34. Borle AB. Effect of purified parathyroid hormone on the calcium metabolism of monkey kidney cells. *Endocrinology* 1968; 6:1316–1322.
35. Massry SG, Smogorzewski M. The mechanisms responsible for the PTH-induced rise in cytosolic calcium in various cells are not uniform. *Miner Elect Metab* 1995;21:13–28.
36. Stojceva-Taneva O, Fadda GZ, Smogorzewski M, et al. Parathyroid hormone increases cytosolic calcium of thymocytes. *Nephron* 1993;64:592–599.
37. Klin M, Smogorzewski M, Khilnani H, et al. Mechanisms of PTH-induced rise in cytosolic calcium in adult rat hepatocytes. *Am J Physiol* 1994;267:G754–G763.
38. Urenia P, Kong X-F, Abu-Samra A-B, et al. Parathyroid hormone (PTH)/PTH-related peptide receptor messenger ribonucleic acids are widely distributed in rat tissue. *Endocrinology* 1993;133:617–623.
39. Tian J, Smogorzewski M, Kedes L, et al. Parathyroid hormone related protein receptor messenger RNA is present in many tissues besides the kidney. *Am J Nephrol* 1993;13:210–213.
40. Massry SG. Divalent ion metabolism and renal osteodystrophy. In: Massry SG, Glassock RJ, eds. *Textbook of nephrology*, 3rd ed. Baltimore: Williams and Wilkins, 1995:1441–1473.
41. Massry SG, Smogorzewski M. Mechanisms through which parathyroid hormone mediates its deleterious effects on organ function in uremia. *Semin Nephrol* 1994;14:219–231.
42. Zhang Y-B, Ni Z, Smogorzewski M, et al. Altered cytosolic calcium homeostasis in rat cardiac myocytes in CRF. *Kidney Int* 1994;45:1113–1119.
43. Hruska KA, Moskowitz D, Esbirt P, et al. Stimulation of inositol triphosphate and diacylglycerol production in renal tubular cells by parathyroid hormone. *J Clin Invest* 1987;79:230–239.
44. Brautbar N, Chakraborty J, Coates J, et al. Calcium, parathyroid hormone and phospholipid turnover of human red blood cells. *Miner Elect Metab* 1985;11:111–116.
45. Islam A, Smogorzewski M, Massry SG. Effect of chronic renal failure and parathyroid hormone on phospholipid content of brain synaptosomes. *Am J Physiol* 1989;256:F705–F710.
46. Carafoli E. Intracellular calcium homeostasis. *Ann Rev Biochem* 1987;56:395–433.
47. Levi E, Fadda GZ, Thanakitcharu P, et al. Chronology of cellular events leading to derangements in function of pancreatic islets in chronic renal failure. *J Am Soc Nephrol* 1992;3: 1139–1146.
48. Urena P, Kubrusky M, Mannstadt M, et al. The renal PTH/PTHrP receptor is down-regulated in rats with chronic renal failure. *Kidney Int* 1994;45:605–611.
49. Tian J, Smogorzewski M, Kedes L, et al. PTHPTHrP receptor is down-regulated in chronic renal failure. *Am J Nephrol* 1994; 14:41–46.
50. Smogorzewski M, Tian J, Massry SG. Down-regulation of PTH–PTHrP receptor of heart in CRF: role of [Ca^{2+}]i. *Kidney Int* 1995;47:1182–1186.
51. Massry SG, Klin M, Ni Z, et al. Impaired agonist-induced calcium signaling in hepatocytes from chronic renal failure rats. *Kidney Int* 1995;48:1324–1331.
52. Akmal M, Goldstein DA, Multani S, et al. Role of uremia, brain calcium, and parathyroid hormone on changes in electroencephalogram in chronic renal failure. *Am J Physiol* 1984;246: F575–F576.
53. Akmal M, Massry SG. Role of parathyroid hormone in the decreased motor nerve conduction velocity of chronic renal failure. *Proc Soc Exp Biol Med* 1990;195:202–207.
54. El-Balbessi S, Brautbar N, Anderson K, et al. Effect of chronic renal failure on heart: Role of secondary hyperparathyroidism. *Am J Nephrol* 1986;6:369–375.
55. Fadda GZ, Akmal M, Prendas H, et al. Insulin release from pancreatic islets: Effect of CRF and excess PTH. *Kidney Int* 1988;33:1066–1072.
56. Akmal M, Perkins S, Kasim SE, et al. Verapamil prevents chronic renal failure-induced abnormalities in lipid metabolism. *Am J Kidney Dis* 1993;22:158–163.
57. Fadda GZ, Hajjar SM, Perna AF, et al. On the mechanisms of impaired insulin secretion in chronic renal failure. *J Clin Invest* 1991;87:255–261.
58. Chervu I, Kiersztejn M, Alexiewicz JM, et al. Impaired phagocytosis in chronic renal failure is mediated by secondary hyperparathyroidism. *Kidney Int* 1992;41:1501–1505.
59. Kiersztejn M, Smogorzewski M, Thanakitcharu P, et al. Decreased O_2 consumption by polymorphonuclear leukocytes from humans and rats with CRF. Role of secondary hyperparathyroidism. *Kidney Int* 1992;42:602–609.
60. Islam A, Smogorzewski M, Massry SG. Effect of verapamil on CRF-induced abnormalities in phospholipid contents of brain synaptosomes. *Proc Soc Exp Biol Med* 1990;194:1620.
61. Smogorzewski M, Campese VM, Massry SG. Abnormal norepinephrine uptake and release in brain synaptosomes in chronic renal failure. *Kidney Int* 1989;36:458–465.
62. Smogorzewski M, Piskorska G, Borum PR, et al. Chronic renal failure, parathyroid hormone and fatty acids oxidation in skeletal muscle. *Kidney Int* 1988;31:555–560.
63. Perna AF, Smogorzewski M, Massry SG. Verapamil reverses

PTH- or CRF-induced abnormal fatty acid oxidation in muscle. *Kidney Int* 1988;34:774–778.
64. Smogorzewski M, Perna AF, Borum PR, et al. Fatty acid oxidation in the myocardium: Effects of parathyroid hormone and chronic renal failure. *Kidney Int* 1988;34:797–803.
65. Perna AF, Smogorzewski M, Massry SG. Effects of verapamil on the abnormalities in fatty acid oxidation of myocardium. *Kidney Int* 1989;36:453–457.
66. Smogorzewski M, Islam A, Minasian R, et al. Verapamil corrects abnormalities in norepinephrine metabolism of brain synaptosomes in CRF. *Am J Physiol* 1990;258:F1036–F1041.
67. Thanakitcharu P, Fadda GZ, Hajjar SM, et al. Verapamil prevents the metabolic and functional derangements in pancreatic islets in chronic renal failure rats. *Endocrinology* 1991;129: 1749–1754.
68. Fadda GZ, Akmal M, Soliman AR, et al. Correction of glucose intolerance and the impaired insulin release of chronic renal failure by verapamil. *Kidney Int* 1989;36:773–779.
69. Ni Z, Smogorzewski M, Massry SG. Derangements in acetylcholine metabolism in brain synaptosomes in chronic renal failure. *Kidney Int* 1993;44:630–637.
70. Akmal M, Kasim SE, Soliman AR, et al. Excess parathyroid hormone adversely affects lipid metabolism in chronic renal failure. *Kidney Int* 1990;37:854–858.
71. Cogan MG, Covey CM, Arieff AI, et al. Central nervous system manifestations of hyperparathyroidism. *Am J Med* 1978;65: 963–970.
72. Massry SG, Gordon A, Coburn JW, et al. Vascular calcification and peripheral necrosis in a renal transplant patient: Reversal of lesions following subtotal parathyroidectomy. *Am J Med* 1970;49:416–422.
73. Massry SG, Popovtzer MM, Coburn JW, et al. Pruritus as a manifestation of secondary hyperparathyroidism in uremia: Disappearance of itching following subtotal parathyroidectomy. *N Engl J Med* 1968;279:697–700.
74. Hampers CL, Katz AI, Wilson RE, et al. Disappearance of "uremic" itching after subtotal parathyroidectomy. *N Engl J Med* 1968;279:695–697.
75. Gipstein RH, Coburn JW, Adams DA, et al. Calciphylaxis in man. A syndrome of tissue necrosis and vascular calcification in 11 patients with chronic renal disease. *Arch Intern Med* 1976; 13:1273–1280.
76. Drueke T, Fleury I, Toure Y, et al. Effect of parathyroidectomy on left ventricular function in hemodialysis patients. *Lancet* 1980;1:112–114.
77. McGonigle RJS, Fowler MB, Timmis AB, et al. Uremic cardiomyopathy: Potential role of vitamin D and parathyroid hormone. *Nephron* 1989;36:94–100.
78. Goldstein DA, Feinstein EI, Chui LA, et al. The relationship between the abnormalities in electroencephalogram and blood levels of PTH in dialysis patients. *J Clin Endocrinol Metab* 1980; 51:130–134.
79. Haag-Weber M, Mai B, Horl WH. Normalization of enhanced neutrophil cytosolic calcium of hemodialysis patients with 1,25-dihydroxyvitamin D_3 and calcium channel blocker. *Am J Nephrol* 1993;13:467–472.
80. Mak RHK, Bettinelli A, Turner C, et al. The influence of hyperparathyroidism on glucose metabolism in uremia. *J Clin Endocrinol Metab* 1985;60:229–233.
81. Massry SG, Goldstein DA, Procci WR. Impotence in patients with uremia: A possible role for parathyroid hormone. *Nephron* 1977;19:305–310.
82. Malluche HH, Goldstein DA, Massry SG. Management of renal osteodystrophy with $1,25(OH)_2D_3$. II. Effects on histopathology of bone: Evidence for healing of osteomalacia. *Miner Elect Metab* 1979;2:48–55.
83. Thanakitcharu P, Fadda GZ, Hajjar SM, et al. Verapamil reverses glucose intolerance in pre-existing chronic renal failure: Studies on mechanisms. *Am J Nephrol* 1992;12:179–187.
84. Alexiewicz JM, Smogorzewski M, Akmal M, et al. Nifedipine reverses the abnormalities in $[Ca^{2+}]i$ and proliferation of B cells from dialysis patients. *Kidney Int* 1996;50:1249–1254.
85. Silvis SE, Paragas PV Jr. Fatal hyperalimentation syndrome. Animal studies. *J Lab Clin Med* 1971;78:918–930.
86. Silvis SE, Paragas PV Jr. Parasthesias, weakness, seizures and hypophosphatemia in patients receiving hyperalimentation. *Gastroenterology* 1972;62:513–517.
87. Bhaskaran D, Massry SG, Campese VM. Effect of hypophosphatemia on brain catecholamines content in the rat. *Miner Elect Metab* 1987;13:469–472.
88. Smogorzewski M, Islam A, Koureta P, et al. Abnormal norepinephrine metabolism in rat brain synaptosomes in phosphate depletion. *Am J Nephrol* 1993;13:43–52.
89. Smogorzewski M, Islam A, Koureta P, et al. Reduced phospholipid content of brain synaptosomes in phosphate depletion. *Am J Physiol* 1991;261:742–747.
90. Lichtman MA, Miller DR, Freeman RB. Erythrocyte adenosine triphosphate depletion during hypophosphatemia in a uremic subject. *N Engl J Med* 1969;280:240–244.
91. Lichtman MA, Miller DR, Cohen I, et al. Reduced red cell glycolysis, 2,3-diphosphoglycerate and adenosine triphosphate concentration, and increased hemoglobin-oxygen affinity caused by hypophosphatemia. *Ann Intern Med* 1971;74: 562–568.
92. Travis SF, Sugerman HJ, Rubergy RL, et al. Alterations of red cell glycolytic intermediates and oxygen transport as a consequence of hypophosphatemia in patients receiving intravenous hyperalimentation. *N Engl J Med* 1971;285:763–768.
93. Jacob ES, Amsden T. Acute hemolytic anemia with rigid red cell hypophosphatemia. *N Engl J Med* 1971;285:1446–1450.
94. Klock JC, Williams HE, Mentzer WC. Hemolytic anemia and somatic cell dysfunction in severe hypophosphatemia. *Arch Intern Med* 1974;134:360–364.
95. Territo MD, Tanaka KR. Hypophosphatemia in chronic alcoholism. *Arch Intern Med* 1974;134:445–447.
96. Craddock PR, Yawata Y, Van Santen L, et al. Acquired phagocyte dysfunction. A complication of the hypophosphatemia of parenteral hyperalimentation. *N Engl J Med* 1974:290: 1403–1407.
97. Kiersztejn M, Chervu I, Smogorzewski M, et al. On the mechanism of impaired phagocytosis in phosphate depletion. *J Am Soc Nephrol* 1992;2:1484–1489.
98. Yawata Y, Hebbel RP, Silvis S, et al. Blood cell abnormalities complicating the hypophosphatemia of hyperalimentation: Erythrocytes and platelet ATP deficiency associated with hemolytic anemia and bleeding in hyperalimented dog. *J Lab Clin Med* 1974;84:643–653.
99. Stoerk HC, Carnes WH. The relation of the dietary Ca:P ratio to serum Ca and to parathyroid volume. *J Nutr* 1945;29:43–50.
100. Slatopolsky E, Caglar S, Pennell JP, et al. On the pathogenesis of hyperparathyroidism in chronic experimental renal insufficiency in the dog. *J Clin Invest* 1971;50:492–499.
101. Dominguez JH, Fray RW, Leman J Jr. Dietary phosphate deprivation in women and men. Effects of mineral and acid balances, parathyroid hormone and the metabolism of 25-OH-vitamin D. *J Clin Endocrinol Metab* 1976;43:1056–1068.
102. Lutz M, Ney R, Bartter FC. Osteomalacia and debility resulting from phosphorus depletion. *Trans Assoc Am Physicians* 1964; 77:281–295.
103. Abrams DE, Silcott RB, Terry R, et al. Antacid induction of phosphate depletion syndrome in renal failure. *West J Med* 1974; 120:157–161.

104. Tuller MA. Myoglobinuria with or without drug usage. *JAMA* 1971;217:1868.
105. Knochel JP, Bilbrey CL, Fuller TJ, et al. The muscle cell in chronic alcoholism. The possible role of phosphate depletion in alcoholic myopathy. *Ann NY Acad Sci* 1975;252:274–291.
106. Fuller TJ, Carter NW, Barcenas C, et al. Reversible changes of the muscle cell in experimental phosphorus deficiency. *J Clin Invest* 1976;57:1019–1024.
107. Baczynski R, Massry SG, Maggott M, et al. Effect of parathyroid hormone on energy metabolism of skeletal muscle. *Kidney Int* 1985;28:722–727.
108. O'Connor LR, Wheeler WS, Bethune JE. Effect of hypophosphatemia on myocardial performance in man. *N Engl J Med* 1977;297:901–903.
109. Fuller RJ, Nichols WW, Brenner BJ, et al. Effects of phosphorus depletion on left ventricular energy generation. *Adv Exp Med Biol* 1978;103:395–400.
110. Darsee JR, Natter D. Reversible severe congestive heart failure in three cases of hypophosphatemia. *Ann Intern Med* 1978;89: 867–870.
111. Baczynski R, Massry SG, Kohan R, et al. Effect of parathyroid hormone on myocardial energy metabolism in the rat. *Kidney Int* 1985;27:718–725.
112. Brautbar N, Tabernero-Romo J, Coats J, et al. Impaired myocardial lipid metabolism in phosphate depletion. *Kidney Int* 1984;26:18–23.
113. Saglikes Y, Massry SG, Iseki K, et al. Effect of phosphate depletion on blood pressure and vascular reactivity to norepinephrine and angiotensin. *Am J Physiol* 1985;248:F93–F99.
114. Kreusser W, Schotz H, Rascher W, et al. Circulatory response to pressor agents in phosphorus depletion. *Adv Exp Med Biol* 1982;151:259–265.
115. Planas RF, McBrayer RH, Koen PA. Effect of hypophosphatemia on pulmonary muscle performance. *Adv Exp Med Biol* 1982;151:283–290.
116. Gold LW, Massry SG, Friedler RM. Effect of phosphate depletion on renal tubular reabsorption of glucose. *J Lab Clin Med* 1977;89:554–559.
117. Harter HR, Santiago JV, Rutherford WE, et al. The relative roles of calcium, phosphorus and parathyroid hormone on glucose- and tolbutamide-mediated insulin release. *J Clin Invest* 1976;58:359–367.
118. Simonson D, DeFronzo RA. Hypophosphatemia and glucose intolerance. *Adv Exp Med Biol* 1982;151:217–228.
119. Zhou X-J, Fadda GZ, Perna AF, et al. Phosphate depletion impairs insulin secretion by pancreatic islets. *Kidney Int* 1991; 39:120–128.
120. Fadda GZ, Hajjar SM, Zhou X-I, et al. Verapamil corrects abnormal metabolism of pancreatic islets and insulin secretion in phosphate depletion. *Endocrinology* 1992;130:193–202.
121. Freeman S, McLean FC. Experimental rickets. Blood and tissue changes in puppies receiving a diet very low in phosphorus, with and without vitamin D. *Arch Pathol* 1941;32:387–408.
122. Skikita M, Tsurnfuji S, Ito Y. Adaptation in renal phosphorus excretion under the influence of parathyroids: A study of ureterally catheterized rats. *Endocrinol Jpn* 1962;9:171.
123. Kreusser WJ, Kurokawa K, Aznar E, et al. Phosphate depletion: Effect of renal inorganic phosphorus and adenine nucleotides, urinary phosphate and calcium, and calcium balance. *Miner Elect Metab* 1978;1:30–42.
124. Cuisinier-Gleizes P, Thomasset M, Saioteny-Debove I, et al. Phosphorus deficiency, parathyroid hormone, and bone resorption in the growing rat. *Calcif Tiss Res* 1976;20:235–249.
125. Kreusser WI, Kurokawa K, Aznar E, et al. Effect of phosphate depletion on magnesium homeostasis. *J Clin Invest* 1978;61: 573–581.
126. Barzel US. Parathyroid hormone, blood phosphorus, and acid-base metabolism. *Lancet* 1971;i:1329–1331.
127. Gold LW, Massry SG, Arieff AI, et al. Renal bicarbonate wasting during phosphate depletion: A possible cause of altered acid-base homeostasis in hyperparathyroidism. *J Clin Invest* 1973; 52:2556–2562.
128. Massry SG, Kurokawa K, Arieff AI, et al. Metabolic acidosis of hyperparathyroidism. *Arch Intern Med* 1974;134:385–387.
129. Emmett M, Goldfarb S, Agus ZS, et al. The pathophysiology of acid-base changes in chronically phosphate-depleted rats: Bone kidney interaction. *J Clin Invest* 1977;59:291–298.
130. Coburn JW, Massry SG. Changes in serum and urinary calcium during phosphate depletion: Studies on mechanisms. *J Clin Invest* 1970;49:1073–1087.
131. Day HG, McCollum EV. Mineral metabolism, growth, and symptomatology of rats on a diet extremely deficient in phosphorus. *J Biol Chem*, 1939;130:269–283.
132. Young VR, Lofgreen GP, Luick JR. The effects of phosphorus depletion and of calcium and phosphorus intake on the endogenous excretion of these elements by sheep. *Br J Nutr* 1966;20: 795–805.
133. Steele TH, Engel JE, Tanaka Y, et al. On the phosphatemic action 1,25-dihydroxy vitamin D_3. *Am J Physiol* 1975;229: 489–495.
134. Steele TH, DeLuca HF. Influence of dietary phosphorus on renal phosphate reabsorption in the parathyroidectomized rats. *J Clin Invest* 1976;57:867–874.
135. Trohler V, Bonjour JP, Fleish J. Inorganic phosphate homeostasis: Renal adaptation to the dietary intake in intact and thyroparathyroidectomized rats. *J Clin Invest* 1976;57:264–273.
136. Beck N. Effect of dietary phosphorus (P) intake on renal actions of parathyroid hormone (PTH) and cyclic AMP (CaMP) (abstract). *Proc Am Soc Nephrol* 1976;9:1.
137. Goldfarb S, Wesby GR, Goldberg M, et al. Renal tubular effects of chronic phosphate depletion. *J Clin Invest* 1977;59:770–779.
138. Kreusser WJ, Descoeudres C, Oda Y, et al. Effects of phosphate depletion (PD) on renal gluconeogenesis (GNG) (abstract). *Proc Am Soc Nephrol* 1977;10:90A.
139. Tanaka Y, DeLuca HP. The control of 25-hydroxyvitamin D metabolism by inorganic phosphorus. *Arch Biochem Biophys* 1973;154:566–570.
140. Hughes MR, Brumbauch PF, Haussler MR, et al. Regulation of serum 1,25-dihydroxyvitamin D_3 by calcium and phosphate in the rat. *Science* 1975;190:578–580.
141. Massry SG. The clinical syndrome of phosphate depletion. *Adv Exp Med Biol* 1978;103:301–307.
142. Denton RM, McCormack JG. Ca^{2+} transport by mammalian mitochondria and its role in hormone action. *Am J Physiol* 1985; 249:E543–E554.
143. Trump BE, Berezsky IK. The role of ion deregulation in toxic cell injury. *Adv Modern Envir Toxicol* 1987;14:27–50.
144. Massry SG, Hajjar SM, Koureta P, et al. Phosphate depletion increases cytosolic calcium of brain synaptosomes. *Am J Physiol* 1991;260:F12–F18.
145. Deuticke B, Haest CWM. Lipid modulation of transport proteins in vertebral cell membranes. *Ann Rev Physiol* 1987;49: 221–235.
146. Yeagle DL. Lipid regulation of cell membrane structure and function. *FASEB J* 1989;3:1833–1842.
147. Sanderman M Jr. Regulation of membrane enzymes by lipids. *Biochem Biophys Acta* 1978;515:209–237.
148. Fadda GZ, Thanakitcharu P, Massry SG. Phosphate depletion reduces potassium-induced insulin secretion. *Proc Exp Biol Med* 1991;198:742–746.
149. Pirart I. Diabetes mellitus and its degenerative complications:

A prospective study of 4,400 patients observed between 1947 and 1973. *Diabetes Care* 1978;1:168–188.
150. Engerman R, Bloodworth SM Jr, Nelson S. Relationship of microvascular disease in diabetes to metabolic control. *Diabetes* 1977;26:760–769.
151. Cohen AJ, McGill PD, Rossetti RG, et al. Glomerulopathy in spontaneously diabetic rat: Impact of glycemic control. *Diabetes* 1987;36:944–951.
152. Diabetes Control and Complications Trial Research Group. The effect of intensive treatment of diabetes on the development and progression of long-term complications in insulin-dependent diabetes mellitus. *N Engl J Med* 1993;329:977–986.
153. Nathan DM, Singer DE, Hurxthal K, et al. The clinical information value of the glycosylated hemoglobin assay. *N Engl J Med* 1984;310:341–346.
154. Klein R, Klein BE, Moss SE, et al. The Wisconsin epidemiologic study of diabetic retinopathy. III: Prevalence and risk of diabetic retinopathy when age at diagnosis is 30 or more years. *Arch Ophthalmol* 1984;102:527–532.
155. Nathan DM, Singer DE, Godine JE, et al. Retinopathy in older type II diabetics: Association with glucose control. *Diabetes* 1985;35:797–801.
156. Klein R, Klein BE, Moss SE, et al. Glycosylated hemoglobin predicts the incidence and progression of diabetic retinopathy. *JAMA* 1988;260:2864–2871.
157. Singer DE, Nathan DM, Anderson KM, et al. Association of HbA_1C with prevalent cardiovascular disease in the original cohort of the Framingham Heart Study. *Diabetes* 1992;41: 202–208.
158. Estacio RO, Jeffers BW, Hiatt WR, et al. The effect of nisoldipine as compared with enalapril on cardiovascular outcomes in patients with non-insulin dependent diabetes and hypertension. *N Engl J Med* 1998;338:645–652.
159. Gabby KH, Merola LO, Field RA. Sorbitol pathway: Presence in nerve and cord with substrate accumulation in diabetes. *Science* 1966;151:209–210.
160. Gabby KH. The sorbitol pathway and the complications of diabetes. *N Engl J Med* 1973;288:831–836.
161. Greene DA, Lattimer SA, Sima AA. Sorbitol, phosphoinositides, and sodium-potassium ATPase in the pathogenesis of diabetic complications. *N Engl J Med* 1987;316:599–606.
162. Greene DH, Lattimer SA, Sima AA. Are disturbance of sorbitol, phosphoinositide, and Na^+-K^+-ATPase regulation involved in pathogenesis of diabetic neuropathy. *Diabetes* 1988;37: 688–693.
163. Beyer-Mears A, Cruz E. Reversal of diabetic cataract by sorbinil, an aldose reductase inhibitor. *Diabetes* 1985;4:15–21.
164. Engerman RL, Kern TS, Larson ME. Nerve conduction and aldose reductase inhibition during 5 years of diabetic of galactosaemia in dogs. *Diabetologia* 1994;37:141–144.
165. Fagius J, Brattberg A, Jameson S, et al. Limited benefit of treatment of diabetic polyneuropathy with an aldose reductase inhibitor: A 24-week controlled trial. *Diabetologia* 1985;28:323–329.
166. Krentz AJ, Monigsberger L, Ellis SH, et al. A 12 month randomized controlled study of the aldose reductase inhibitor ponalrestat in patients with chronic synaptosomes diabetic neuropathy. *Diabetic Med* 1992;9:413–418.
167. Sima AA, Prashar A, Nathaniel V, et al. Overt diabetic neuropathy: Repair of axo-glial dysfunction and axonal atrophy by aldose reductase inhibition and is a correlation to improvement in nerve conduction velocity. *Diabetic Med* 1993;10:115–121.
168. Brownlee M, Vlassara H, Cerami A. Nonenzymatic glycosylation and the pathogenesis of diabetic complications. *Ann Intern Med* 1984;101:527–537.
169. Maillard LC. Action des acides amines sur les sucres: Formation des melanoidines par voie methodique. *CR Acad Sci* 1912;154: 66–68.
170. Patton AR, Hill EG. Inactivation of nutrients by heating with glucose. *Science* 1941;107:68–69.
171. Mohammad A, Fraenkel-Conrat H, Olcott HS. The "browing" reaction of proteins with glucose. *Arch Biochem* 1949;24: 157–158.
172. Bunn HF, Haney DN, Gabbay KM, et al. Further identification of the nature and linkage of the carbohydrate hemoglobin Alc. *Biochem Biophys Res Commun* 1975;67:103–109.
173. Bucala R, Cerami A, Vlassara H. Advanced glycosylation end products in diabetic complications. *Diabetes Rev* 1995;3: 258–268.
174. Bucala R, Cerami A. Advanced glycosylation: Chemistry, biology, and implications for diabetes and aging. *Adv Pharmacol* 1993;23:1–34.
175. Ahmed MV, Thrope SR, Baynes JW. Identification of carboxymethyllysine as a degradation product or fructosyllysine in glycated protein. *J Biol Chem* 1986;261:4889–4894.
176. Ahmed MV, Dunn JA, Walla MD, et al. Oxidative degradation of glucose adducts to protein. *J Biol Chem* 1988;263: 8816–8821.
177. Gugliucci A, Bendayan M. Renal fate of circulating advanced glycated end products (AGE): Evidence for reabsorption and catabolism of ACE-peptides by renal proximal tubular cells. *Diabetologia* 1996;39:149–160.
178. Makita Z, Radoff S, Rayfield EJ, et al. Advanced glycosylation end products in patients with diabetic nephropathy. *N Engl J Med* 1991;325:836–842.
179. Makita Z, Bucala R, Rayfield EJ, et al. Diabetic-uremic serum advanced glycosylation end products are chemically reactive and resistant to dialysis therapy: Role in mortality of uremia. *Lancet* 1994;343:1519–1522.
180. Resnik LM, Gupta RK, Bhargava KK, et al. Cellular ions in hypertension diabetes and obesity: A nuclear magnetic resonance spectroscopic study. *Hypertension* 1991;17:951–957.
181. Tschöpe D, Rösen P, Gried FA. Increase in the cytosolic concentration of calcium in platelets of diabetic type II. *Thromb Res* 1991;62:421–428.
182. Pellegatta F, Folli F, Ronchi P, et al. Deranged platelet calcium homeostasis in poorly controlled IDDM patients. *Diabetes Care* 1993;16:178–183.
183. Segal S, Lloyd S, Sherman N, et al. Postprandial changes in cytosolic free calcium and glucose uptake in adipocytes in obesity and non-insulin-dependent diabetes mellitus. *Horm Res* 1990;34:39–44.
184. Draznin B, Sussman KE, Eckel RH, et al. Possible role of cytosolic free calcium concentrations in mediating insulin resistance of obesity and hyperinsulinemia. *J Clin Invest* 1988;28: 1848–1852.
185. Studer RK, Gansas L. Effect of diabetes on hormone-stimulated and basal hepatocyte calcium metabolism. *Endocrinology* 1989; 125:2421–2433.
186. Allo SN, Lincoln TM, Wilson GL, et al. Non-insulin-dependent diabetes induced defects in cardiac cellular calcium regulation. *Am J Physiol* 1991;260:C1165–C1171.
187. Schaffer SW. Cardiomyopathy associated with non-insulin-dependent diabetes. *Mol Cell Biochem* 1991;107:1–20.
188. Ohara T, Sussman KE, Draznin B. Effect of diabetes on cytosolic free Ca^{2+} and Na^+-K^+-ATPase in rat aorta. *Diabetes* 1991;40:1560–1563.
189. Levy J, Gavin JR III, Sowers JR. Diabetes mellitus: A disease of abnormal cellular calcium metabolism. *Am J Med* 1994;96: 260–273.
190. Alexiewicz JA, Kumar D, Smogorzewski M, et al. Polymorphonuclear leukocytes in non-insulin-dependent diabetes mellitus:

Abnormalities in metabolism and function. *Ann Intern Med* 1995;123:919–924.

191. Alexiewicz JM, Kumar D, Smogorzewski M, et al. Elevated cytosolic calcium and impaired proliferation of B lymphocytes in type II diabetes mellitus. *Am J Kidney Dis* 1997;(30)1: 98–104.
192. Hoenig M, Sharp GW. Glucose induces insulin release and a rise in cytosolic calcium concentration in a transplantable rat insulinoma. *Endocrinology* 1985;119:2502–2507.
193. Fadda GZ, Massry SG. Impaired glucose-induced calcium signal in pancreatic islets in chronic renal failure. *Am J Nephrol* 1991;11:475–478.
194. Barbagallo M, Shan I, Pang PKT, et al. Glucose-induced alterations of cytosolic free calcium in cultured rat tail artery vascular smooth muscle cells. *J Clin Invest* 1995;95:763–767.
195. Demerdash TM, Seyrek N, Smogorzewski M, et al. The pathways through which glucose induces a rise in $[Ca^{2+}]i$ of Polymorphonuclear leukocytes of rats. *Kidney Int* 1996;50: 2032–2040.
196. Resnick LM. Ionic basis of hypertension, insulin resistance, and related disorder: Mechanisms of syndrome X. *Am J Hypertens* 1993;5:296–301.
197. Draznin B, Leitner JW, Sussman KE, et al. Insulin and glucose modulate protein kinase C activity ín rats adipocytes. *Biochem Biophys Res Commun* 1988;156:570–575.
198. Lee TS, Saltsman KA, Ohashi H, et al. Activation of protein kinase C by elevation of glucose concentration: Proposal for a mechanism in the development of diabetic vascular complications. *Proc Natl Acad Sci U S A* 1989;86:5141–5145.
199. Sahai A, Fadda GZ, Massry SG. Parathyroid hormone activates protein kinase C of pancreatic islets. *Endocrinology* 1992;131: 1889–1894.
200. Fadda GZ, Thanakitcharu M, Smogorzewski M, et al. Parathyroid hormone raises cytosolic calcium in pancreatic islets: Study on mechanism. *Kidney Int* 1993;43:554–560.
201. Ni Z, Smogorzewski M, Massry SG. Effect of PTH on $[Ca^{2+}]i$ of rat adipocytes. *Endocrinology* 1994;135:1837–1844.
202. Tanaka H, Smogorzewski M, Koss M, et al. Pathways involved in PTH-induced rise in cytosolic Ca^{2+} concentration of rat renal proximal tubule. *Am J Physiol* 1995;268:F330–F337.
203. Demerdash TM, Seyrek N, Smogorzewski M, et al. Pathways through which glucose induces a rise in $[Ca^{2+}]i$ of polymorphonuclear leukocytes of rats. *Kidney Int* 1996;50:2032–2040.
204. Zhang YB, Smogorzewski M, Ni Z, et al. Elevation of cytosolic calcium of rat cardiac myocytes in phosphate depletion. *Kidney Int* 1996;49:251–254.
205. Aleksayan J, Smogorzewski M, Massry SG. High glucose concentration causes a rise in $[Ca^{2+}]i$ of hepatocytes of the rat: Studies on mechanism. *J Am Soc Neph* 1998;9:VA3204, abstract.
206. Symonian M, Smogorzewski M, Marcinkowski W, et al. Mechanisms through which high glucose concentration raises $[Ca^{2+}]i$ in renal proximal tubular cells. *Kidney Int* 1998;54:1206–1213.
207. Makino N, Dhalla KS, Elimban V, et al. Sarcolemmal Ca^{2+} transport in streptozotocin-induced diabetic cardiomyopathy in rats. *Am J Physiol* 1987;253:E202–E207.
208. Zemel MB, Sowers JR, Shehin S, Walsh MF, et al. Impaired calcium metabolism associated with hypertension in Zuker obese rats. *Metabolism* 1990;39:704–708.
209. Green DA, Lattimer SA. Impaired rat sciatic nerve sodium-potassium adenosine triphosphate in acute streptozotocin diabetes and its correction by dietary myoinositol supplementation. *J Clin Invest* 1983;72:1958–1963.
210. Mazzanti L, Rabini RA, Faloia E, et al. Altered cellular Ca^{2+} and Na^{+} transport in diabetes mellitus. *Diabetes* 1990;39: 850–854.
211. Kuriyama S, Tokudome C, Tomonari H, et al. Differential regulation of cation transport of vascular smooth muscle in a high glucose concentration milieu. *Diabetes Res Clin Pract* 1994; 29:77–84.
212. Seyrek N, Marcinkowski W, Smogorzewski M, et al. Amlodipine prevents and reverses the elevation in $[Ca^{2+}]i$ and the impaired phagocytosis of PMNLs of diabetic rats. *Nephrol Dial Transplant* 1997;12:265–272.
213. Pierce GN, Afzal N, Kroeger EA, et al. Cataract formation is prevented by administration of verapamil to diabetic rats. *Endocrinology* 1989;125:730–735.
214. Islam A, Smogorzewski M, Zayed A, et al. Effect of chronic renal failure with and without secondary hyperparathyroidism on the activities of synaptosomal tyrosine hydroxylase and monoamine oxidase. *Nephron* 1992;61:32–36.
215. Ni Z, Smogorzewski M, Massry SG. Derangements in acetylcholine metabolism in brain synaptosomes in chronic renal failure. *Kidney Int* 1993;44:630–637.
216. Klin M, Smogorzewski M, Ni Z, et al. Abnormalities in hepatic lipase in chronic renal failure: Role of excess parathyroid hormone. *J Clin Invest* 1996;97:2167–2173.
217. Akmal M, Perkins S, Kasim SE, et al. Verapamil prevents chronic renal failure-induced abnormalities in lipid metabolism. *Am J Kidney Dis* 1993;22:1158–1163.
218. Akmal M, Kasim SE, Soliman AR, et al. Excess parathyroid hormone adversely affects lipid metabolism in chronic renal failure. *Kidney Int* 1990;37:854–858.
219. Perna AF, Fadda GZ, Massry SG. Inhibition of phosphofructokinase activity in pancreatic islets in phosphate depletion. *Miner Elect Metab* 1991;17:8–11.
220. Michnowska M, Smogorzewski M, Massry SG. Impaired Na^{+}-H^{+}exchanger activity of hepatocytes in CRF. *J Am Soc Nephrol* 1997;8:929–934.
221. Marcinkowski W, Smogorzewski M, Zhang G, et al. Renal mRNA of PTH–PTHrP receptor, $[Ca^{2+}]i$ and phosphaturic response to PTH in phosphate depletion. *Miner Elect Metab* 1997;23:48–57.
222. Marcinkowski W, Zhang G, Smogorzewski M, et al. Elevation of $[Ca^{2+}]i$ of renal proximal tubular cells and downregulation of mRNA of PTH–PTHrP, Vla and AT_1 receptors in kidney of diabetic rats. *Kidney Int* 1997;51:1950–1955.
223. Weiss O, Anner H, Nephesh I, et al. Insulin-like growth factor-I (IGF-I) and IGF-I receptor gene expression in the kidney of the chronically hypoinsulinemic rat and hyperinsulinemic rat. *Metabolism* 1995;8:982–986.
224. Studer RK, Ganas L. Effect of diabetes on hormone stimulated and basal hepatocytes calcium metabolism. *Endocrinology* 1989; 125:2421–2433.
225. Mene P, Pugliese G, Pricci F, et al. High glucose inhibits cytosolic calcium signaling in cultured rat mesangial cells. *Kidney Int* 1993;43:585–591.
226. Tanaka Y, Kashiwage A, Saeki V, et al. Effects of verapamil on the cardiac alpha 1-adrenoreceptor signalling system in diabetic rats. *Eur J Pharmacol* 1993;244:105–109.

9

METABOLIC AND NUTRITIONAL RESPONSES TO ACIDEMIA

HAROLD A. FRANCH
WILLIAM E. MITCH

When considering what properties a uremic toxin must have, the ability to cause weight loss and muscle wasting are naturally at the top of the list. Our experience with patients tells us that the loss of lean body mass and the loss of bone mineral are hallmarks of uremia. Epidemiologic data suggest that markers associated with a poor nutritional status correlate strongly with outcomes among dialysis patients (1). Although metabolic acidosis is only one of many potential toxins that could cause the complications of uremia, it is the only toxin with a demonstrated ability to enhance catabolism, making it an attractive target for treatment (2).

Ironically, most of the catabolic response to acidemia is caused by chronic activation of the body's own mechanisms that buffer and excrete excess hydrogen ions (3). The body tolerates acute metabolic acidosis readily. For example, the blood pH falls below 7.2 during strenuous exercise without immediate adverse effects. In some ways acute acidosis helps the body during exercise or acute illness. Principally, increased tissue oxygen delivery that occurs via the Bohr effect (shifting oxygen from hemoglobin to tissues), vasodilation, and stimulation of the respiratory drive acts to aid tissue respiration and minimize lactic acidosis (4). Chronically, however, the body does not tolerate even small degrees of acidosis. The chronic buffering of acid by bone leads to a loss of bone mineral related to a multitude of hormonal changes (5). To increase net acid excretion, muscle protein is broken down to yield amino acids that are converted to glutamine. Glutamine, in turn, is delivered to the kidney where it forms the substrate for ammonium secretion (6). In this chapter, we will examine the catabolic effects of acid. We will first examine the effect on the endocrine system and then discuss the integrated effects on bone and muscle.

ENDOCRINE ABNORMALITIES

Much attention has been given to acid-induced changes in the function of endocrine organs, including the release of cortisol, insulin, thyroxin, insulinlike growth factor (IGF-1), aldosterone, and parathyroid hormone (PTH). In many cases, activation of endocrine responses enhances the ability of a normal kidney to excrete acid, but in chronic renal failure (CRF) the same responses can cause catabolism and contribute to uremic symptoms. In addition, other uremic toxins can interact with endocrine mediators; in many cases, direct-effects acidemia appears to have an additive effect with these endocrine responses.

Acidemia increases circulating adrenal cortical hormones (7). Adrenocorticotropin hormone (ACTH) levels increase after an infusion of inorganic acids to stimulate the production of both glucocorticoid and aldosterone (8). There also may be direct effect of a low pH on the adrenal gland to stimulate the release of aldosterone, a response that depends on an increase in intracellular calcium (9). Because both cortisol and aldosterone increase renal-acid excretion in subjects with normal renal function (10,11), the increase in ACTH can be seen as a homeostatic mechanism that acts to increase net acid excretion. Acidosis also appears to lower 11-β hydroxysteroid dehydrogenase activity in the aldosterone-sensitive cells in the kidney, and this prevents destruction of cortisol, allowing it to activate to the aldosterone receptor (12). It is interesting that acidosis is not the only cause of elevated glucocorticoid levels in uremia because adding bicarbonate to the diet to block the development of acidosis in rats with CRF does not normalize glucocorticoid production (13). This uremia-associated stimulation of glucocorticoid production is a crucial factor that induces abnormalities of calcium and protein metabolism (see later in this chapter) (14). In contrast, the role of aldosterone in uremic complications is not well established. Only two studies suggest direct involvement. A newer report indicates that spironalactone can help prevent mortality in patients with congestive heart failure and suggests that aldosterone might exacerbate some of the cardiovascular complications seen in kidney failure (15). Similar evidence of an effect of spironolactone blocking progression of CRF suggests that acid-induced increases in aldosterone may lead to renal damage (16).

Acidosis suppresses the clinical effect and cellular signaling stimulated by both insulin and IGF-1, but it does so in different ways. Acidosis does not alter islet-cell secretion of insulin, but it does induce resistance to insulin action in peripheral tissues; reversal of acidosis improves the sensitivity of glucose metabolism to insulin (17). In contrast, acidosis reduces growth hormone release from the pituitary, and this leads to lower levels of IGF-1 production.

The response to an infusion of physiologic concentrations of growth hormone may be very mildly impaired in acidosis, but larger concentrations completely reverse the effects of acidosis. Two factors appear to blunt the response to administered growth hormone: the density of IGF-1 receptors in muscle is lowered by acidemia and a defect in the signaling that results from the binding of IGF-1 (18–20). IGF-1 resistance in uremia does not improve with correction of acidosis, suggesting that separate mechanisms (possibly including corticosteroids) play a role (21,22). It has been shown that administration of super-physiologic doses of growth hormone reduces renal nitrogen loss (23). IGF-1 (like insulin) is a major determinant of amino acid release from the muscle, although part of the beneficial response on nitrogen balance may involve improvement in plasma cortisol or aldosterone (24). These studies point out how complex interactions occurring between the different endocrine mediators can work together to either exacerbate or relieve the effects of acidemia. Abnormalities in insulin and IGF-1 also play an important role in the growth suppression seen in children with acidosis (25).

Acidosis increases the sensitivity of the parathyroid gland to changes in ionized calcium and also stimulates the release of PTH (26). In normal adults, PTH long has been known to increase renal net acid secretion by inhibiting bicarbonate reclamation (27). In these subjects, acidosis decreases proximal tubular phosphate reabsorption, resulting in hypophosphatemia; this causes a secondary stimulation of 1,25 vitamin D production. Thus, in subjects with normal renal function, the resulting increase in the activation of vitamin D counteracts the direct effects of acidosis on the parathyroid, so that serum PTH concentrations usually are unchanged or even fall slightly with acidosis (28). In patients undergoing dialysis, acidosis has almost no effect on phosphate excretion or the production of 1,25 vitamin D levels because of the loss of kidney mass. Instead, acidosis increases PTH by a direct effect on the parathyroid glands (26,28, 29). It is important that correction of acidosis in patients undergoing hemodialysis who have secondary hyperparathyroidism improves the ability of an increase in plasma calcium to suppress the parathyroid gland's release of PTH (26).

Similar to kidney failure, acidosis lowers serum levels of the thyroid hormones, free T3 and T4; unlike kidney failure, however, it may raise reverse T3 slightly (30,31). Although resistance to the effects of TSH occurs within the thyroid gland, TSH remains within the normal range during acidosis. Although the clinical significance of the lower free T3 levels during acidosis is not apparent, it is postulated to limit the loss of muscle protein in uremia (32). In contrast to PTH, there is no evidence that low T3 has any effect on bone metabolism in uremia (33). Thus, the response of thyroid hormone to acidosis appears to be an exception to the overall paradigm of hormonal alterations contributing to acid-induced catabolism.

CALCIUM METABOLISM

Acids are buffered initially by the bicarbonate system followed by protein and bone buffering (Table 9.1). Bone will buffer acid directly because hydrogen ion exchanges with sodium and potassium in bone mineral. This exchange does not result in an equivalent loss of calcium for every hydrogen ion absorbed (34). Most acids interact with bone carbonates to release bound calcium (35). However, in respiratory acidosis, the high carbonate concentration in blood (derived from CO_2) prevents bone resorption by this mechanism. Secondly, metabolic acidosis stimulates bone-reabsorbing osteoclasts and at the same time suppresses the activity of the bone-stimulating osteoblasts (36). Acid acts to suppress the growth of osteoblasts and the formation of bone-matrix proteins at a transcriptional level (29). This direct effect of acidosis to demineralize bone appears to occur by different mechanisms than those induced by cortisol, PTH, or IGF-1. For example, parathyroidectomy does not block the effect of acidosis on bone; these effects of acidosis are additive to the response to PTH (29).

TABLE 9.1. CATABOLIC EFFECTS OF CHRONIC METABOLIC ACIDOSIS ON CALCIUM AND PROTEIN METABOLISM

1. Dissolution of bone
   a. Direct effect of acid on bone mineral content
   b. Increased osteoclast and decreased osteoblast activity
   c. Increased plasma glucocorticoids
   d. Increased serum parathyroid hormone (clinically apparent in uremia only)
   e. Decreased plasma insulinlike growth factor-1
2. Hypercalciuria and hyperphosphaturia leading to phosphate and calcium wasting
   a. Increased filtered load of calcium and phosphorous
   b. Decreased tubular reabsorption of calcium and phosphorous
3. Protein malnutrition and muscle wasting
   a. Activation of the ubiquitin-proteasome proteolytic system
      i. Decreased effect of pH
      ii. Increased plasma glucocorticoids
      iii. Insulin resistance in nonhepatic organs
   b. Activation of branched-chain ketoacid dehydrogenase
      i. Direct effect of pH
      ii. Increased plasma glucocorticoids
   c. Increased hepatic glutamine synthesis and renal glutamine extraction

In patients who have normal renal function, the effect of acidosis to mobilize calcium from bone increases renal calcium excretion. If there is a rise in serum calcium resulting from the mobilization of bone calcium, the amount of calcium filtered at the glomerulus increases, but the major effect of acidosis on urinary calcium is a direct inhibition of tubular calcium reabsorption that occurs independently of the level of filtered calcium (3). Thus, acidosis contributes directly to negative calcium balance by causing dissolution of bone and by increasing renal calcium loss. Together with the hypocitrituria that is induced by increased proximal tubular reabsorption of citrate (37) and the lower urine pH from acidosis, hypercalciuria contributes to an increased incidence of nephrolithiasis in acidotic patients (3,38).

Given these mechanisms and responses, it is not surprising that correction of acidosis has been shown to improve bone mineralization and histology in acidotic patients, including those treated by hemodialysis (39). Still, it has not been documented that reduced fracture rates or other outcomes are correlated with improved acid–base status in patients undergoing dialysis.

PROTEIN MALNUTRITION

Experimental studies have revealed detailed mechanisms of how excess acid accumulation causes loss of muscle mass. Metabolic acidosis acts not only through stimulation of glucocorticoids; it also stimulates renal ammonia excretion. The latter occurs when the kidney extracts glutamine from plasma to form ammonia and augment acid excretion. The mechanism by which acid directly stimulates glutamine production is accelerating muscle-protein degradation, leading to release of amino acids that are used to synthesize glutamine in the liver (7). Moreover, the oxidation of branched-chain amino acids (BCAA) rises in muscle to provide much of the nitrogen used in the hepatic synthesis of glutamine (40). The evidence for the latter response is that metabolic acidosis activates the rate-limiting enzyme for the irreversible decarboxylation of BCAA, branched-chain ketoacid dehydrogenase (BCKAD) in muscle, and this response accounts for BCAA degradation (40). Plasma levels of BCAA in uremic rats are low compared to pair-fed control rats and these low levels are linked to increased oxidation in muscle (41). The influence of acidosis in initiating and maintaining these processes was proved by adding $NaHCO_3$ to the diet to correct the metabolic acidosis of chronic uremia; both plasma levels of BCAA and rates of amino acid oxidation in muscle were restored to normal (41). We believe this response reflecting activation of BCKAD activity occurs in the muscle of acidotic patients as well. Studies of normal adults confirm that an acid diet results in a 25% stimulation of BCAA decarboxylation (42).

Acidosis has a similar effect to stimulate muscle-protein breakdown. In chronically uremic rats, muscle-protein degradation is high and correction of the acidosis of CRF reduces protein catabolism to normal levels, but impairment of protein synthesis persists after correction of acidosis (13, 43). Metabolic acidosis overrides the body's normal adaptive responses to a low-protein diet that includes a suppression of the oxidation of essential amino acids and the degradation of protein (44). In nondialysis patients, a switch to an isocaloric, low-protein diet decreased skeletal muscle and whole-body protein degradation, presumably because the low-protein diet reduced acidosis (45). Thus, evidence from experimental models and human studies demonstrate that metabolic acidosis accelerates irreversible oxidation of BCAA and degradation of skeletal muscle protein.

The mechanisms causing proteolysis involve direct and indirect responses. Regarding the direct effect, when the pH in the media of cultured myocytes is lowered, there is a slight decrease in protein synthesis plus an increase in protein degradation compatible with a direct effect of acidosis to change protein metabolism (46,47). In uremic rats, however, there also must be an indirect effect because the pH in muscle measured is normal *in vivo* in the resting state as well as during recovery from acidification (48). This suggests that other factors must act as signals to increase protein degradation. One of these factors is glucocorticoids because they are known to be released by acidosis and they directly induce catabolism (7,13). To test this in rats, we found that adrenalectomy blocks the effect that acidosis induced on protein and amino acid catabolism, but adding a physiologic amount of glucocorticoid restores the catabolic influence of acidosis *in vivo* (Fig. 9.1) (49). Both acidosis and glucocorticoid also are required to increase the activity of BCKAD and the ubiquitin–proteasome proteolytic system in muscle and cultured myocytes (47,50).

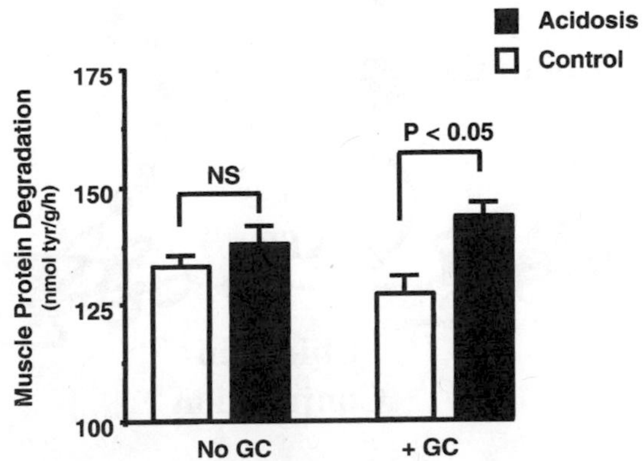

FIGURE 9.1. Acidosis requires glucocorticoids (GC) to stimulate muscle-protein breakdown, but glucocorticoids are not the only mediator. Protein degradation was measured in the muscles of adrenalectomized rats (no GC) and adrenalectomized rats given glucocorticoids (+ GC) with and without acidosis. The rate of protein breakdown is significantly higher in acidosis only when glucocorticoids are present. Because the amount of glucocorticoids given is the same with and without acidosis in the + GC rats, another factor must be increasing protein breakdown. (Modified from reference 49, with permission.)

METABOLIC ACIDOSIS STIMULATES THE UBIQUITIN–PROTEASOME PROTEOLYTIC PATHWAY

In all cells, including skeletal muscle, there are multiple proteolytic systems. These pathways include lysosomal proteolytic pathways (microautophagy, macroautophagy, and chaperone-mediated autophagy), the calcium-activated proteases in the cytoplasm, and adenosine triphosphate (ATP)-independent and ATP-dependent cytosolic pathways (51). The best described ATP-dependent cytosolic pathway is the ubiquitin–proteasome system (Fig. 9.2) (51). In the ubiquitin–proteasome pathway, proteins are targeted for degradation by ATP-dependent conjugation to ubiquitin, a small protein found in all cells. Protein–ubiquitin conjugates are degraded in another ATP-dependent process by the 26S proteasome, a large multicatalytic, multiple subunit proteolytic complex. The proteasome is found in the nucleus and cytoplasm of all cells (51).

Activation of the ATP-dependent ubiquitin–proteasome pathway in acidosis requires glucocorticoid; the increase in ATP-dependent proteolysis occurring in skeletal muscle of acidotic rats is abolished by adrenalectomy and restored by physiologic doses of glucocorticoid (7,52). It is interesting that the response to acidosis includes activation of gene transcription. The abundance of ubiquitin messenger RNA (mRNA) and mRNA-encoding subunits of the proteasome increases in muscle of acidotic rats with chronic uremia and acidosis (43). Newer studies show that the changes in mRNA require glucocorticoids and are the result of increased gene transcription (43,52).

The role of other hormonal abnormalities in mediating acid-induced protein degradation are more controversial. Insulin and IGF-1 suppress protein degradation in the body, and insulin resistance occurs with acidosis (21,53). Rats with insulin-dependent diabetes also exhibit increased muscle proteolysis via the ubiquitin–proteasome system, suggesting that reduced insulin activity could contribute to activation of this important pathway (54). However, diabetes induces other metabolic interactions that may not be present in acidosis, so the contribution of acidosis to insulin resistance in uremia and of insulin resistance to protein wasting in acidosis remains to be determined.

Whereas acidosis activates the ubiquitin–proteasome system in muscle leading to wasting, the response in the kidney is the opposite. Acidosis suppresses protein breakdown in the renal cortex and in suspensions of isolated tubules (55). The high ammonia concentrations present in acidosis suppress lysosomal proteolysis in renal tubular cells in culture, causing increased accumulation of proteins destroyed in lysosomes (56). This lysosomal pathway is known as chaperone-mediated autophagy (57). Because chaperone-mediated autophagy controls the half-life of many proteins important for growth, including glycolytic enzymes and the Pax-2 transcription factor, blocking this pathway could contribute to renal tubular hypertrophy and hyperplasia (58). Shechter et al. examined rats fed ammonium chloride *in vivo* and found that there is a decrease in lysosomal cathepsin activity

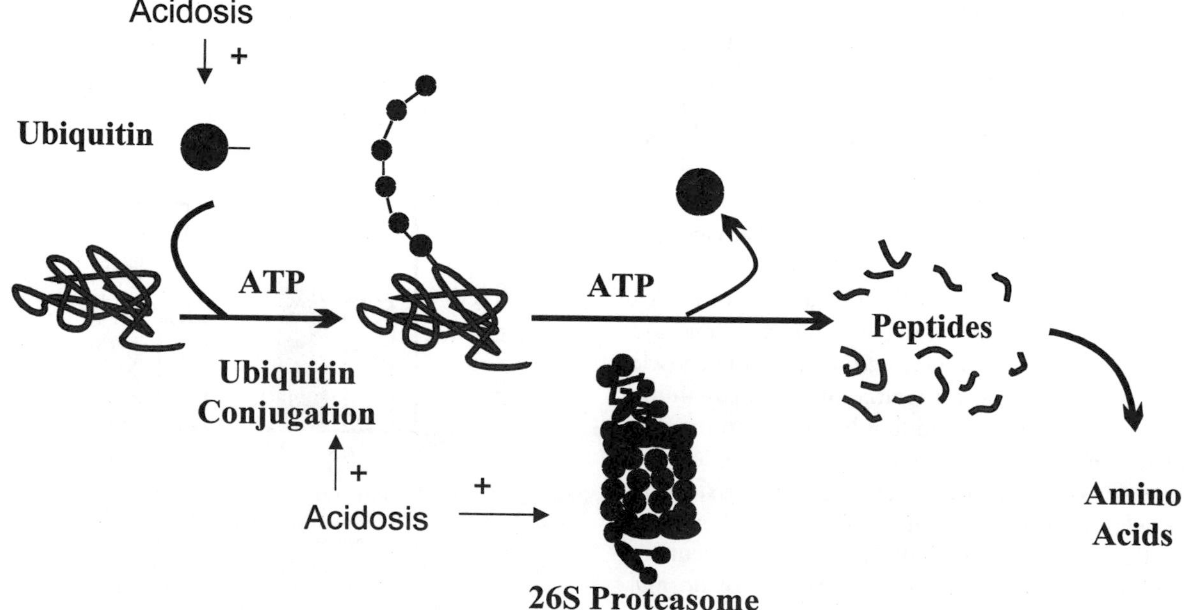

FIGURE 9.2. Acidosis stimulates the ubiquitin–proteasome system by effecting multiple steps. Proteins targeted for destruction are conjugated with ubiquitin, and the ubiquitin targets them to the proteasome where they are destroyed. Acidosis increases the amount of ubiquitin and proteasomes and also increases the conjugation of protein with ubiquitin.

in the renal cortex (55). Thus, the amino acids that are being lost by muscle are metabolized to ammonia, and the latter response provides a stimulus to cause growth of the kidney. The growth of the kidney is beneficial in that it increases the capacity for net acid secretion and increases the single nephron glomerular filtration rate (59). In kidney disease, these responses could be detrimental. For example, feeding rats acid diets worsens cyst formation in the kidney in rodent models of polycystic kidney disease (60). To date, there have been no human studies on the relation of acidosis to the progression of genetic or acquired cystic disease.

CLINICAL IMPLICATIONS FOR PROTEIN NUTRITION

How does metabolic acidosis affect nutritional status? It has long been felt that anorexia contributes to protein malnutrition in patients with metabolic acidosis, but it has been difficult to quantify the relative contribution of anorexia to protein malnutrition. However, there is evidence that excessive protein catabolism is the dominant mechanism for loss of lean body mass. First, in rats with CRF high-protein diets were associated with metabolic acidosis, stunted growth, and a lower efficiency of using dietary protein for growth (61). Secondly, in poorly growing infants with metabolic acidosis, nitrogen excretion does not correlate with protein intake, suggesting that their poor nitrogen balance is the result of increased catabolism rather than decreased diet (62). Thirdly, normal adults with experimentally induced metabolic acidosis eating a constant diet exhibit increased oxidation of the essential, branched-chain amino acids as well as protein degradation (42). Fourth, hemodialysis and patients with acidosis undergoing continuous ambulatory peritoneal dialysis exhibit excessive protein catabolism that can be suppressed when acidosis is corrected with dietary alkali supplements (63,64). Fifth, in patients undergoing hemodialysis there is a strong linear correlation between the degree of acidosis measured just before a dialysis treatment and the free valine concentration in a muscle biopsy (65), and treating dialysis patients with sodium bicarbonate was shown to raise the levels of branched-chain amino acids in muscle; this strategy will provide more essential amino acids that can be used in the synthesis of muscle protein (66). Besides taking supplements of sodium bicarbonate, patients undergoing dialysis will experience a reduction in the severity of acidosis when they are fed a low-protein diet. Either strategy is effective because both improve nitrogen balance and raise the plasma concentrations of the branched-chain amino acids (45,67).

Taken together, these clinical studies support the concept that correcting acidosis is a strategy that will improve protein metabolism in patients undergoing dialysis. However, there are significant factors to consider in the measurement of acid–base status in this population. Kirschbaum reported that the standard practice of using distant reference laboratories to measure bicarbonate levels led to falsely low values (68). Local laboratories also can give falsely low bicarbonate values when the sample is left open and carbon dioxide escapes (68). Consequently, decisionmaking should be based on the entire constellation of clinical data regardless of the location of the laboratory. Because most cross-sectional studies of the effects of acid–base status on nutritional parameters rely on a mixture of data from different laboratories, there is serious concern about the interpretation. For example, it is difficult to evaluate the observation that a single measurement of low predialysis bicarbonate may reflect the acid load from a higher protein intake in that particular interdialytic interval when the authors do not report the technique for measuring serum bicarbonate (69). Thus, one must take as much care in evaluating the acid–base status of patients in the literature as with one's own patients.

Finally, the similarity between the complications of chronic metabolic acidosis and those of aging suggest there is a link between acid homeostatic responses and osteoporosis and protein malnutrition in the geriatric population (2,3,70,71). The fall in the glomerular filtration rate that occurs with aging coupled with a diet that generates a large daily acid load as a result of the consumption of excess amino and nucleic acids in meat could lead to a chronic activation of mechanisms to buffer and excrete acid. This is especially true for poor people in Western countries, who typically consume inadequate amounts of organic bases from fruits and vegetables but are able to consume excessive protein. The metabolic responses just discussed will impair calcium and protein metabolism and also could result in plasma bicarbonate concentrations that are in the low-normal range (3). This has been called the "eubicarbonatemic" metabolic acidosis hypothesis because compensatory and buffering mechanisms keep the serum bicarbonate normal despite an ongoing acid-induced catabolic response. There are only limited clinical data supporting the eubicarbonatemic metabolic acidosis hypothesis, but elderly subjects who have normal serum bicarbonate levels develop improved calcium and nitrogen balance when they are given oral potassium bicarbonate supplements (70,71).

In summary, there is abundant evidence from experimental animals and cultured cells and from normal adults and patients with kidney disease that metabolic acidosis is a major factor causing abnormalities in calcium and protein metabolism (Table 9.1). Although interpretation of serum bicarbonate values is sometimes difficult, the treatment is straightforward and results in a gain of weight, bone density, and muscle mass (39,72). In short, the simple acts of restricting dietary protein (before the start of dialysis) or supplementing alkali (before or after the start of dialysis) can powerfully reduce the risk of major complications of uremia.

REFERENCES

1. Steinman TI. Serum albumin: its significance in patients with ESRD. *Semin Dial* 2000;13:404–408.

2. Franch HA, Mitch WE. Catabolism in uremia: the impact of metabolic acidosis. *J Am Soc Nephrol* 1998;9:S78–S81.
3. Alpern RJ, Sakhaee K. The clinical spectrum of chronic metabolic acidosis: Homoeostatic mechanisms produce significant morbidity. *Am J Kidney Dis* 1997;29:291–302.
4. Hsia CCW. Respiratory function of hemoglobin. *N Engl J Med* 1998;338:239–247.
5. Slatopolsky E, Caglar S, Pennell JP, et al. On the pathogenesis of hyperparathyroidism in chronic experimental renal insufficiency in the dog. *J Clin Invest* 1971;50:492–499.
6. Mitch WE, Price SR, May RC, et al. Metabolic consequences of uremia: Extending the concept of adaptive responses to protein metabolism. *Am J Kidney Dis* 1994;23:224–228.
7. May RC, Kelly RA, Mitch WE. Metabolic acidosis stimulates protein degradation in rat muscle by a glucocorticoid-dependent mechanism. *J Clin Invest* 1986;77:614–621.
8. Wood CE, Isa A. Intravenous acid infusion stimulates ACTH secretion in sheep. *Am J Physiol* 1991;260:E154–E161.
9. Kramer RE, Robinson TV, Schneider EG, et al. Direct modulation of basal and angiotensin II-stimulated aldosterone secretion by hydrogen ions. *J Endocrinol* 2000;166:183–194.
10. Wilcox CS, Cemerikic DA, Giebisch G. Differential effects of acute mineralo- and glucocorticosteroid administration on renal acid elimination. *Kidney Int* 1982;21:546–556.
11. Henger A, Tutt P, Riesen WF, et al. Acid-base and endocrine effects of aldosterone and angiotensin II inhibition in metabolic acidosis in human patients. *J Lab Clin Med* 2000;136:379–389.
12. Thompson A, Bailey MA, Michael AE, et al. Effects of changes in dietary intake of sodium and potassium and of metabolic acidosis on 11beta-hydroxysteroid dehydrogenase activities in rat kidney. *Exp Nephrol* 2000;8:44–51.
13. May RC, Kelly RA, Mitch WE. Mechanisms for defects in muscle protein metabolism in rats with chronic uremia: The influence of metabolic acidosis. *J Clin Invest* 1987;79:1099–1103.
14. Mitch WE, Wilcox CS. Disorders of body fluids, sodium and potassium in chronic renal failure. *Am J Med* 1982;72:536–550.
15. Pitt B, Zannad F, Remme WJ, et al. The effect of spironolactone on morbidity and mortality in patients with severe heart failure. Randomized Aldactone Evaluation Study Investigators. *N Engl J Med* 1999;341:709–717.
16. Greene EL, Kren S, Hostetter TH. Role of aldosterone in the remnant kidney model in the rat. *J Clin Invest* 1996;98: 1063–1068.
17. Mak RHK. Insulin resistance but IGF-1 sensitivity in chronic renal failure. *Am J Physiol* 1996;271:F114–F119.
18. Ding H, Gao X-L, Hirschberg R, et al. Impaired actions of insulin-like growth factor-1 on protein synthesis and degradation in skeletal muscle of rats with chronic renal failure: Evidence for a postreceptor defect. *J Clin Invest* 1996;97:1064–1075.
19. Ordonez FA, Santos F, Martinez V, et al. Resistance to growth hormone and insulin-like growth factor-I in acidotic rats. *Pediatr Nephrol* 2000;14:720–725.
20. Ding H, Qing DP, Kopple JD. IGF-1 resistance in chronic renal failure: current evidence and possible mechanisms. *Kidney Int Suppl* 1997;62:S45–S47.
21. Bereket A, Wilson TA, Kolasa AJ, et al. Regulation of the insulin-like growth factor system by acute acidosis. *Endocrinology* 1996; 137:2238–2245.
22. Brungger M, Hulter HN, Krapf R. Effect of chronic metabolic acidosis on the growth hormone/IGF-1 endocrine axis: New cause of growth hormone insensitivity in humans. *Kidney Int* 1997;51:216–221.
23. Mahlbacher K, Sicuro A, Gerber H, et al. Growth hormone corrects acidosis-induced renal nitrogen wasting and renal phosphate depletion and attenuates renal magnesium wasting in humans. *Metab Clin Exp* 1999;48:763–770.
24. Sicuro A, Mahlbacher K, Hulter HN, et al. Effect of growth hormone on renal and systemic acid-base homeostasis in humans. *Am J Physiol* 1998;274(4 Pt 2):F650–F657.
25. Hanna JD, Krieg RJ, Jr., Scheinman JI, et al. Effects of uremia on growth in children. *Semin Nephrol* 1996;16:230–241.
26. Graham KA, Reaich D, Channon SM, et al. Correction of acidosis in hemodialysis patients increases the sensitivity of the parathyroid glands to calcium. *J Am Soc Nephrol* 1997;8:627–631.
27. Arruda JA, Nascimento L, Westenfelder C, et al. Effect of parathyroid hormone on urinary acidification. *Am J Physiol* 1977; 232:F429–F433.
28. Krapf R, Vetsch R, Vetsch W, et al. Chronic metabolic acidosis increases the serum concentration of 1,25-dihydroxyvitamin D in humans by stimulating its production rate. *J Clin Invest* 1992; 90:2456–2463.
29. Bushinsky DA, Frick KK. The effects of acid on bone. *Curr Opin Nephrol Hypertens* 2000;9:369–379.
30. Brungger M, Hulter HN, Krapf R. Effect of chronic metabolic acidosis on thyroid hormone homeostasis in humans. *Am J Physiol* 1997;272:F648–F653.
31. Kaptein EM, Feinstein EI, Nicoloff JT, et al. Serum reverse triiodothyronine and thyroxine kinetics in patients with chronic renal failure. *J Clin Endocrinol Metab* 1983;57:181–189.
32. Lim VS, Tsalikian E, Flanigan MJ. Augmentation of protein degradation by L-triiodothyronine in uremia. *Metabolism* 1989; 38:1210–1215.
33. Kraut JA. Disturbances of acid-base balance and bone disease in end-stage renal disease. *Semin Dial* 2000;13:261–266.
34. Bushinsky DA, Chabala JM, Gavrilov KL, et al. Effects of in vivo metabolic acidosis on midcortical bone ion composition. *Am J Physiol* 1999;277:F813–F819.
35. Bushinsky DA. The contribution of acidosis to renal osteodystrophy. *Kidney Int* 1995;47:1816–1832.
36. Bushinsky DA. Bone disease in moderate renal failure: Cause, nature and prevention. *Annu Rev Med* 1997;48:167–176.
37. Melnick JZ, Srere PA, Elshourbagy NA, et al. Adenosine triphosphate citrate lyase mediates hypocitraturia in rats. *J Clin Invest* 1996;98:2381–2387.
38. Mitch WE, Walser M, Sapir DG. Nitrogen-sparing induced by leucine compared with that induced by its keto-analogue, alpha-ketoisocaproate, in fasting obese man. *J Clin Invest* 1981;67: 553–562.
39. Lefebvre A, de Vernejoul MC, Gueris J, et al. Optimal correction of acidosis changes progression of dialysis osteodystrophy. *Kidney Int* 1989;36:1112–1118.
40. May RC, Hara Y, Kelly RA, et al. Branched-chain amino acid metabolism in rat muscle: Abnormal regulation in acidosis. *Am J Physiol* 1987;252:E712–E718.
41. Hara Y, May RC, Kelly RA, et al. Acidosis, not azotemia, stimulates branched-chain amino acid catabolism in uremic rats. *Kidney Int* 1987;32:808–814.
42. Reaich D, Channon SM, Scrimgeour CM, et al. Ammonium chloride-induced acidosis increases protein breakdown and amino acid oxidation in humans. *Am J Physiol* 1992;263: E735–E739.
43. Bailey JL, Wang X, England BK, et al. The acidosis of chronic renal failure activates muscle proteolysis in rats by augmenting transcription of genes encoding proteins of the ATP-dependent, ubiquitin-proteasome pathway. *J Clin Invest* 1996; 97:1447–1453.
44. Price SR, Mitch WE. Metabolic acidosis and uremic toxicity: Protein and amino acid metabolism. *Semin Nephrol* 1994;14: 232–237.
45. Williams B, Hattersley J, Layward E, et al. Metabolic acidosis and skeletal muscle adaptation to low protein diets in chronic uremia. *Kidney Int* 1991;40:779–786.

46. England BK, Chastain J, Mitch WE. Extracellular acidification changes protein synthesis and degradation in BC3H-1 myocytes. *Am J Physiol* 1991;260:C277–C282.
47. Isozaki Y, Mitch WE, England BK, et al. Interaction between glucocorticoids and acidification results in stimulation of proteolysis and mRNAs of proteins encoding the ubiquitin-proteasome pathway in BC3H-1 myocytes. *Proc Natl Acad Sci U S A* 1996; 93:1967–1971.
48. Bailey JL, England BK, Long RC, et al. Experimental acidemia and muscle cell pH in chronic acidosis and renal failure. *Am J Physiol* 1995;269:C706–C712.
49. May RC, Bailey JL, Mitch WE, et al. Glucocorticoids and acidosis stimulate protein and amino acid catabolism in vivo. *Kidney Int* 1996;49:679–683.
50. Mitch WE, Medina R, Greiber S, et al. Metabolic acidosis stimulates muscle protein degradation by activating the ATP-dependent pathway involving ubiquitin and proteasomes. *J Clin Invest* 1994;93:2127–2133.
51. Mitch WE, Goldberg AL. Mechanisms of muscle wasting: The role of the ubiquitin-proteasome system. *N Engl J Med* 1996; 335:1897–1905.
52. Price SR, England BK, Bailey JL, et al. Acidosis and glucocorticoids concomitantly increase ubiquitin and proteasome subunit mRNAs in rat muscle. *Am J Physiol* 1994;267:C955–C960.
53. DeFronzo RA, Beckles AD. Glucose intolerance following chronic metabolic acidosis in man. *Am J Physiol* 1979;236: E328–E334.
54. Price SR, Bailey JL, Wang X, et al. Muscle wasting in insulinopenic rats results from activation of the ATP-dependent, ubiquitin-proteasome pathway by a mechanism including gene transcription. *J Clin Invest* 1996;98:1703–1708.
55. Shechter P, Shi JD, Rabkin R. Renal tubular cell protein breakdown in uninephrectomized and ammonium chloride-loaded rats. *J Am Soc Nephrol* 1994;5:1201–1207.
56. Franch HA, Curtis PV, Mitch WE. Mechanisms of renal tubular cell hypertrophy: Mitogen-induced suppression of proteolysis. *Am J Physiol* 1997;273:C843–C851.
57. Cuervo AM, Dice JF. Lysosomes, a meeting point of proteins, chaperones, and proteases. *J Mol Med* 1998;76:6–12.
58. Franch HA, Sooparb S, Du J, et al. A mechanism regulating proteolysis of specific proteins during renal tubular cell growth. *J Biol Chem* 2001;276:19126–19131.
59. Preisig PA, Franch HA. Renal epithelial cell hyperplasia and hypertrophy. *Semin Nephrol* 1995;15:327–340.
60. Torres VE, Mujwid DK, Wilson DM, et al. Renal cystic disease and ammoniagenesis in Han:SPRD rats. *J Am Soc Nephrol* 1994; 5:1193–1200.
61. Meireles CL, Price SR, Pereira AML, et al. Nutrition and chronic renal failure in rats: What is an optimal dietary protein? *J Am Soc Nephrol* 1999;10:2367–2373.
62. Kalhoff H, Manz F, Diekmann L, et al. Decreased growth rate of low-birth-weight infants with prolonged maximum renal acid stimulation. *Acta Ped* 1993;82:522–527.
63. Graham KA, Reaich D, Channon SM, et al. Correction of acidosis in hemodialysis decreases whole-body protein degradation. *J Am Soc Nephrol* 1997;8:632–637.
64. Graham KA, Reaich D, Channon SM, et al. Correction of acidosis in CAPD decreases whole body protein degradation. *Kidney Int* 1996;49:1396–1400.
65. Bergstrom J, Alvestrand A, Furst P. Plasma and muscle free amino acids in maintenance hemodialysis patients without protein malnutrition. *Kidney Int* 1990;38:108–114.
66. Lofberg E, Wernerman J, Anderstam B, et al. Correction of metabolic acidosis in dialysis patients increases branched-chain and total essential amino acid levels in muscle. *Clin Nephrol* 1997; 48:230–237.
67. Mochizuki T. The effect of metabolic acidosis on amino and keto acid metabolism in chronic renal failure. *Nippon Jinzo Gakkai Shi* 1991;33:213–224.
68. Kirschbaum B. Spurious metabolic acidosis in hemodialysis patients. *Am J Kidney Dis* 2000;35:1068–1071.
69. Uribarri J, Levin NW, Delmez J, et al. Association of acidosis and nutritional parameters in hemodialysis patients. *Am J Kidney Dis* 1999;34:493–499.
70. Sebastian A, Harris ST, Ottaway JH, et al. Improved mineral balance and skeletal metabolism in postmenopausal women treated with potassium bicarbonate. *N Engl J Med* 1994;330: 1776–1781.
71. Frassetto L, Morris RC, Sebastian A. Potassium bicarbonate reduces urinary nitrogen excretion in postmenopausal women. *J Clin Endocrinol Metab* 1997;82:254–259.
72. Stein A, Moorhouse J, Iles-Smith H, et al. Role of an improvement in acid-base status and nutrition in CAPD patients. *Kidney Int* 1997;52:1089–1095.

10

MANAGEMENT OF CARDIOVASCULAR RISK FACTORS IN RENAL FAILURE

M. SIVALINGHAM
ROBERT NICHOLAS FOLEY

Cardiovascular mortality rates in patients with end-stage renal disease (ESRD) are staggering. For example, 30-year-old patients being treated with dialysis therapy have the cardiovascular mortality rates of 80 year olds in the general population—the incidence of ischemic heart disease and cardiac failure are approximately 10% per annum for each condition (1). For coronary heart disease in the general population, a predicted rate probability of 20% per decade defines high risk, requiring earlier pharmacologic intervention for risk factors such as hypertension and hypercholesterolemia (2,3). Cardiac risk in renally impaired patients may be an order of magnitude higher than this arbitrary threshold. The degree to which shared risk factors (for renal and cardiovascular disease) contribute to this apparently deadly synergy is not known. It is likely that cardiovascular disease and renal disease accelerate each other's progression. It has been known for decades that cardiovascular disease worsens prognosis in patients with renal disease (4), and recent data suggest that even mild to moderate renal impairment worsens prognosis in patients at high cardiovascular risk (5).

It never has been demonstrated convincingly that uremia accelerates atherogenesis, although this is a highly prevalent concept. Left ventricular (LV) (1) enlargement and a stiff vascular tree are characteristic features of ESRD. Progressive renal impairment is a state of progressive hemodynamic stress, with profound demands on vascular and ventricular adaptive mechanisms. These compensatory mechanisms begin early in renal impairment and are likely to involve maladaptive trade-offs when the hemodynamic stresses/adaptation pathways are not interrupted. Animal models suggest that the nonredeemable costs of sustained hemodynamic stress include cardiac fibrosis and enhanced rates of apoptosis (6). Thus, the concept of overload cardiomyopathy is well described, even in subjects with normal coronary perfusion who begin life with intrinsically normal hearts (7). Abnormalities of ventricular structure and function are highly characteristic features and predictive of cardiac failure and death in ESRD. LV enlargement is present in more than one-third of patients with chronic renal insufficiency. The prevalence rises with declining renal function, increasing to 75% or more by the onset of ESRD (8,9). More recently, the enhanced arterial stiffness seen in patients with ESRD also has been shown to be highly predictive of death (10).

At the cellular level, several features are notable in animal models of uremia. These include hypertrophy of ventricular myocytes, cardiac fibrosis, poor capillary blood supply relative to LV muscle mass, a limited ability to adjust cardiac output to alterations in preload and afterload, limited supplies of high-energy phosphate metabolites in uremic myocytes, endothelial dysfunction, increased oxidative stress, and upregulation of procoagulation pathways (11).

HEMODYNAMIC STRESS

Anemia

Anemia and hypertension are modifiable hemodynamic stresses that consistently are associated with LV enlargement in observational studies (12,13). Anemia also has been shown to predict mortality and hospitalization in patients with ESRD (14,15). There is overwhelming evidence that partial correction of anemia, to at least 11 g/dL, leads to benefit in patients with renal impairment, principally in terms of quality of life, cognitive function, and partial regression of LV hypertrophy (16–21). Several newer studies have examined the question of full normalization of renal anemia. The studies reported to date have intervened late in the process by which sustained anemia may lead to end-stage overload cardiomyopathy. Numerous ongoing trials are examining the more preventive approaches of early intervention and anemia avoidance. In the United States Normal Hematocrit Trial, 1,233 patients with ischemic heart disease or cardiac failure undergoing hemodialysis were randomly assigned to hematocrit targets of 30% or 42%. The incidence of death or first nonfatal myocardial infarction was similar in both groups, but patients assigned to the higher target had more vascular access loss and a small but statistically significant decline in the adequacy of dialysis when compared to patients assigned to the lower hematocrit. On the positive side, the physical-function score on the quality-of-life questionnaire at 12 months was improved by higher hematocrit (22).

In the Canadian Normalization of Hemoglobin trial, 146 patients with either concentric LV hypertrophy or LV dilatation being treated with hemodialysis were randomly assigned to hemoglobin targets of 10 g/dL or 13.5 g/dL. In patients with concentric LV hypertrophy, the changes in LV mass index were similar in both target groups. The changes in cavity volume index were similar in both targets in the LV dilatation group. In the concentric LV hypertrophy group there was a correlation between the change in LV volume index and hemoglobin level achieved. Normalization of hemoglobin led to improved quality of life in terms of fatigue, depression, and relationships. The incidence of vascular access loss and death was similar in both target groups. More antihypertensives were needed to achieve similar blood pressure control, and a small but statistically significant reduction in dialysis adequacy was observed (23).

McMahon et al. performed a prospective, randomized, double-blinded crossover study in 14 patients undergoing hemodialysis; they were compared at rest and during a maximal incremental cycling exercise at a hemoglobin concentration of 10 g/dL and 14 g/dL following an initial baseline test. Peak work rate and VO_2 peak (oxygen consumption) were significantly high er at a hemoglobin of 14 g/dL than at 10 g/dL. Quality of life also was reported to be better at higher hemoglobin levels (24,25).

Newer evidence increasingly suggests that early intervention and a proactive approach to the treatment of renal anemia may achieve better cardiovascular outcomes than the traditional approach of late intervention that we have used to date. These hypotheses are being tested in several controlled clinical trials worldwide. While these trials are awaited, target levels of hemoglobin of 11 to 12 g/dL seem reasonable for most patients with renal impairment.

Blood Pressure

Rising blood pressure is a feature of early renal disease, its prevalence rising with declining renal function, to the extent that 90% of patients nearing end-stage renal failure have hypertension by conventional definitions (26). LV hypertrophy clearly is related to hypertension (27–30) and is associated with new ischemic heart disease, cardiac failure, and death in patients with ESRD (31). Hypertension and ischemic heart disease are both precursors of cardiac failure and LV dilatation—powerful predictors of early death in patients undergoing dialysis (32).

Hypertension may become refractory in patients with ESRD, despite multiple medications. This is often the result of subclinical salt and water overload, even in the absence of peripheral or pulmonary edema (33–35). This was underscored in a crossover trial comparing short daily and conventional (three times weekly) hemodialysis. Although weekly urea removal was similar with either strategy, blood pressure was dramatically better in the daily dialysis group, in whom antihypertensives were discontinued in most patients. This was accompanied by regression of LV hypertrophy, which very likely resulted from lowering of extracellular fluid volume (36).

Relatively few newer observational studies have associated hypertension and shorter survival in patients undergoing dialysis. In one dialysis population with very good blood pressure control as a result of long, slow dialysis, survival was better in those with a mean arterial pressure of below the median level of 98 mm Hg (37). In another study of patients who were hypertensive at commencement of regular dialysis, survival was better in those whose systolic blood pressure improved after initiation of dialysis therapy (38). These studies, however, are the exception, and most studies have shown an association between low blood pressure and increased mortality, or they have shown a "U"-shaped relationship, with both low and high blood pressure being associated with an increased relative risk of death (39–42). A plausible explanation for the findings is that the patient sample includes a considerable proportion of patients with established, or incipient, cardiac decompensation. Cardiac failure (as well as lower systolic and diastolic blood pressure levels) is known to be associated with a poor prognosis in patients undergoing dialysis (13).

Arterial rigidity is a hallmark of renal failure, and in many ways the cardiovascular system in uremia exhibits most features of premature senescence. A very interesting report from the Framingham Heart Study suggests that parameters such as systolic and diastolic blood pressure have less predictive power in subjects older than age 60 years. In older subjects, high pulse pressures are more highly predictive of adverse cardiovascular events (43). This type of analytic approach makes pathophysiologic sense, with an underlying premise that high stroke volumes lead to further vascular remodeling and exacerbate the problem of excessive arterial stiffness. If pulse pressure is indeed the culprit parameter, then analyses that use either systolic or diastolic blood pressure alone should have less predictive power for survival, and more predictive power should occur in analyses that include both systolic and diastolic blood pressure parameters simultaneously and in analyses that use pulse pressure alone. To date, almost all mortality analyses in patients with ESRD have used the former approach. A newer analysis from the United States Renal Data System showed all of these three characteristics, especially for postdialysis blood pressure levels, implicating high pulse pressure as a bad prognostic parameter. In addition, interdialytic weight gain above 5% of body weight was associated with shorter survival, whereas use of beta blockers was independently associated with longer survival.

The latter finding was highly noteworthy because beta blockers should have a greater impact on pulse pressure than other antihypertensive classes (44). Alternative explanations than analytic confounding are possible for the inverse association between blood pressure and mortality in dialysis populations. It is possible that low blood pressure impairs coronary perfusion, and, in the presence of a fixed stenosis, altered cardiac energetics, diastolic dysfunction, and decreased capillary density lead to myocardial ischemia. Clearly, only controlled trials in ESRD populations of blood pressure therapeutic strategies will resolve this troubling issue. However, the weight of evidence argues for aggressive treatment of hypertension because of evidence from observational and therapeutic studies in the general population and because such an approach slows the progression of chronic kidney diseases. Achieving euvolemia is a prerequisite for good blood pressure control in renal impairment. Because they repeatedly have been shown to slow the progression of chronic renal disorders (45–47), because of their salutary effect in cardiac failure (48,49), because they lengthen survival in populations at high cardiovascular risk (50), and because they appear to aid in regression of LV hypertrophy in patients undergoing dialysis (51,52), angiotensin converting enzyme (ACE) inhibitors are currently the antihypertensive of first choice in subjects with renal impairment. The choice of second-line agents is less clear-cut. However, because they prolong mortality in subjects with essential hypertension, reduce mortality in survivors of myocardial infarction, have safe antiarrhythmic effects, and improve outcome in cardiac failure, beta blockers probably are indicated most obviously. In practice, many authors feel that achievement of ideal blood pressure is of greater priority than the types of antihypertensives used.

MODIFIABLE GENERAL POPULATION RISK FACTORS

Hyperlipidemia

Table 10.1 shows selected targets for intervening in cardiovascular risk factors in patients with chronic kidney disease. Hyperlipidemia is common in patients with renal impairment. The most typical pattern consists of elevated triglycerides and low high-density lipoprotein (HDL) cholesterol but variable levels of low-density lipoprotein (LDL) cholesterol. In patients with chronic renal impairment and patients undergoing hemodialysis, LDL levels are low on average, whereas typical peritoneal dialysis and transplant recipients exhibit high LDL levels. Qualitative lipid abnormalities and high levels of lipoprotein(a), which are common in these populations, are not easily treatable pharmacologically and will not be discussed further in this chapter.

TABLE 10.1. THERAPEUTIC TARGETS

Blood pressure < 130/85, < 120/75 if proteinuria > 1 g/day, angiotensin-converting enzyme inhibitor as first-line agents unless contraindicated (2) [online]
Low-density lipoprotein cholesterol < 100 mg/dL (3)
Hemogobin 11–12 g/dL (75)
Initiate renal replacement therapy when glomerular filtration rate reaches 10.5 mL/min/1.73 m^2 (75)
Kt/V_{urea} of at least 1.2 (single-pool, variable volume, equivalent to urea reduction ratio of 65%) in patient undergoing hemodialysis (75)
For continuous ambulatory peritoneal dialysis, total Kt/V_{urea} of at least 2.0 per week and a total creatinine clearance of at least 60 L/wk/1.73 m^2 for high and high-average transporters, and 50 L/wk/1.73 m^2 in low and low-average transporters (75)
Nonsmoking
Glycosylated hemoglobin < 7% in patients with diabetes (76)

Several studies have shown that treatment of hypercholesterolemia with statins is safe and improves hard clinical outcomes in populations at high cardiovascular risk (53,54). There are no completed studies of lipid-lowering interventions on cardiovascular outcome in renal populations, although several are ongoing. Large-scale epidemiologic studies in patients undergoing hemodialysis have shown an inverse relationship between serum cholesterol and subsequent mortality, a situation that is eerily analogous to the blood pressure–mortality confusion discussed earlier in this chapter (55,56). This inverse association also may reflect reverse causation because chronic disease, chronic inflammation, and malnutrition all lower hepatic production of cholesterol and are very likely to be independent risk markers for death. General population guidelines suggest introduction of statin therapy to achieve LDL-cholesterol levels less than 100 mg/dL in subjects with coronary event rates above 20% per decade, diabetes, and overt vascular disease (2). Patients with renal impairment, with and without diabetes or vascular disease, have actual event rates far beyond this threshold value. Thus, while awaiting the results of pivotal trials, it seems reasonable to suggest this therapeutic target for patients with renal impairment, given the safety of statin therapy.

Hyperhomocystinemia

Homocysteine levels and renal function are inversely related (57). Correction of folic-acid deficiency reduces plasma homocysteine in patients with renal impairment. High doses of folic acid or methylated derivates can reduce homocysteine levels in subjects with renal failure, but full correction has not been shown convincingly. The evidence that hyperhomocystinemia is associated longitudinally with atherogenesis in patients with renal impairment is inconclusive. There is no evidence that lowering homocysteine levels reduces the risk of cardiovascular disease in the general population. Similarly, no randomized trials with hard outcomes have been performed in patients with renal disease. Thus, there is a strong rationale to monitor folate levels and to treat folate deficiency, but there is little evidence, yet, that supersupplementation confers benefit. It is also true, however, that such an approach is virtually risk free, which poses an interesting dilemma, given the huge cardiovascular risk and the difficulties in performing large randomized trials in patients with renal impairment.

Smoking, Glycemic Control in Patients with Diabetes, and Exercise

It is highly unlikely that several "sensible" cardiovascular risk factors will be supported by definitive, level 1 evidence in large populations with renal impairment. However, it seems illogical not to stress intervention regarding smoking, glycemic control in patients with diabetes, and adequate exercise in a population of patients at such pronounced cardiovascular risk.

THE UREMIC STATE

Inflammation, Endothelial Dysfunction, and Oxidative Stress

Several newer observational studies suggest that low-grade inflammation is common in patients with uremia, especially those with cardiovascular disease and malnutrition, and it may be one of the reasons for the strong association between hypoalbuminemia and cardiovascular events in renal impairment (58,59). In one study, vitamin E and C-reactive protein (CRP) levels were associated with ultrasound carotid intima-media thickness, whereas the presence of plaques was associated with older age, oxidized LDL levels, and small apo(a) isoform size (60). Serum levels of hyaluronan, an inflammatory marker, appear to be elevated in predialysis patients. Hyaluronan levels, which appear to be highest in subjects with malnutrition, inflammation, and cardiovascular disease, have been associated with short survival on dialysis (61). Similar observations were seen when soluble adhesion molecules were chosen as candidate cytokine (62).

It is difficult to tell whether these observations reflect causality or whether the associations are a result of cardiovascular disease. Both possibilities are plausible. The evidence that inflammation leads to cardiovascular disease is convincing in terms of biologic plausibility and observational epidemiology in nonuremic populations. For example, from a prospective cohort study of 14,916 initially healthy U.S. male physicians followed for 9 years, 140 cases developed symptomatic peripheral arterial disease. Of the 11 candidate biomarkers assessed at baseline, the total cholesterol HDL-C ratio and CRP were the strongest independent predictors of development of peripheral arterial disease (63). In another noteworthy study, CRP was measured at baseline and after 1 year in 5,742 participants in a 5-year randomized trial of lovastatin for the primary prevention of acute coronary events. Coronary events and baseline CRP were directly correlated. It is intriguing that lovastatin therapy reduced the CRP level by 14.8%. As expected, lovastatin reduced coronary event rates in the overall patient group. In subjects with total cholesterol to HDL cholesterol ratios higher than the median ratio, the benefit of lovastatin was largely independent of baseline CRP levels. Lovastatin was also beneficial, however, among those with lower total-HDL cholesterol ratios whose CRP levels fell in the upper 50% of the distribution. Lovastatin was of no benefit in subjects with lower levels of both parameters (64).

Several mechanisms have been proposed by which inflammation may promote atherogenesis (65). For example, increased expression of adhesion molecules on endothelial surfaces promotes the binding and activation of mononuclear cells and neutrophils. Downstream effects include increased oxidation of LDL. The acute-phase reaction includes the hepatic release of atherogenic proteins such as fibrinogen and lipoprotein(a) and proteins that reduce the function of HDL. For example, serum amyloid A protein displaces apolipoprotein A-1, reducing its ability to reduce oxidized LDL. In the presence of inflammatory cytokines, mononuclear cells can become lipid-rich macrophages. The overall pathobiology linking inflammation to atherosclerosis is not understood completely but is susceptible to intervention at several levels.

Renal impairment appears to be a state of endothelial dysfunction, with high levels of oxidative stress (66), features that clearly overlap with chronic activation of inflammatory systems. Oxidative stress is greater in patients undergoing hemodialysis with cardiovascular disease, suggesting a possible role for oxidative stress in the excess of cardiovascular disease. A noteworthy study examined the effect of high-dose vitamin E supplementation on cardiovascular outcomes in 196 patients undergoing hemodialysis with preexisting cardiovascular disease, randomly assigned to receive 800 IU/day of vitamin E or matching placebo for a median of 519 days. The primary endpoint was a composite variable consisting of fatal or nonfatal myocardial infarction, ischemic stroke, peripheral vascular disease, or unstable angina. Of patients, 16% assigned to vitamin E and 33% of those assigned to placebo had a primary endpoint ($p = 0.014$). The beneficial impact of vitamin E was most marked for myocardial infarction, with a threefold reduction in event rates compared to placebo (67). These data are even more noteworthy because they have not been matched in much larger trials of antioxidant therapies in nonrenal populations. They point to the potential of novel, nonclassical interventions and suggest different major pathophysiologic pathways in patients with renal disease. Clearly, these data need confirmation in larger groups of patients with renal disease to enhance their generalizability.

UREMIA AND ITS TREATMENT

There is considerable animal evidence that uremia is cardiotoxic. Induction of uremia leads to increased heart size, fibrosis, thickening of cardiac arterioles, and a reduction of capillary density. In these experimental studies, parathyroid hormone is a permissive factor, and some of the morphologic changes can be prevented with ACE inhibition, blockade of central sympathetic outflow, and endothelin antagonists. Immunohistochemical studies of signal transduction suggest accelerated rates of apoptosis—key information to suggest that morphologic adaptations induced by uremia are maladaptive (11,68). Functionally, the uremic environment leads to impaired cardiac function and inability to respond to perturbations in loading conditions in association with abnormal cardiac energetics and increased susceptibility to ischemic damage.

Disordered myocardial calcium use may be contributory (69). The best, although indirect, clinical evidence to date to suggest that uremia exerts an independent impact on cardiac morphology and function comes from renal transplantation series. LV hypertrophy, dilatation, and systolic dysfunction improve considerably after transplantation (70), the improvement continuing for several years after transplantation (71). This is in sharp contrast to the observations on dialysis therapy, in which progressive cardiac enlargement and decompensation is the norm. There have been few systematic studies to define threshold levels of dialysis time and toxin removal. However, "more" is likely to be better than "less."

Abnormalities of calcium–phosphate homeostasis are rife in renal impairment. Parathyroid hormone, which acts as a calcium ionophore, is a true uremic toxin at high levels, and experimental studies have shown deleterious effects on cardiac myocytes, as in all tissue types studied to date. Some studies have shown improvement in LV function and size after parathyroidectomy, whereas the inadequate hypertrophic response that typifies the dilated cardiomyopathy of renal impairment has been related to high parathyroid hormone levels in another study (72). Recently the role of calcium deposition, which has been contentious because it is difficult to determine whether it is an innocent bystander or a true pathogenic factor, has received more attention. High calcium x phosphate product has been associated independently with shorter survival in patients undergoing hemodialysis (73). In one study, 120 patients undergoing hemodialysis underwent B-mode ultrasonography of the common carotid artery, aorta, and femoral arteries to determine arterial distensibility, the elastic incremental modulus, and the presence of vascular calcifications. Arterial and aortic stiffness were significantly related to the degree of arterial calcification. The extent of arterial calcification, which is in part responsible for increased LV afterload, increased with age, duration of hemodialysis, the fibrinogen level, and the prescribed dose of calcium-based phosphate binders (74). If these results represent cause and effect, they suggest that randomized controlled trials are needed to test the hypotheses that phosphate-reduction strategies that minimize calcium load may improve cardiovascular outcomes in subjects with renal impairment.

CONCLUSION

The sheer number of cardiovascular risk factors that can, and possibly should, be addressed in patients with renal disease is intimidating. It is illogical to concentrate on one risk factor and ignore others given the enormous underlying risk. There has been a growing realization that clinical trials—many of them—are needed to rationalize therapy.

REFERENCES

1. Churchill DN, Taylor DW, Cook RI, et al. Canadian Hemodialysis Morbidity Study. *Am J Kidney Dis* 1992;19:214–234.
2. National Institutes of Health. National Heart, Lung, and Blood Institute. National Cholesterol Education Program. *Third report of the expert panel on detection, evaluation, and treatment of high blood cholesterol in adults* (Adult Treatment Panel III). Bethesda, MD: NIH, November 19, 2002, www.nhlbi.nih.gov/guidelines/cholesterol.
3. National Institutes of Health. National Heart, Lung, and Blood Institute. National High Blood Pressure Education Program. *The sixth report of the Joint National Committee on Prevention, Detection, Evaluation, and Treatment of High Blood Pressure.* NIH publication no. 98-4080. Bethesda, MD: NIH, November 1997, www.nhlbi.nih.gov/guidelines/hypertension.
4. Hutchinson TA, Thomas DC, MacGibbon B. Predicting survival in adults with end-stage renal disease: an age equivalence index. *Ann Intern Med* 1992;96:417–423.
5. Mann JF, Gerstein HC, Pogue J, et al. Renal insufficiency as a predictor of cardiovascular outcomes and the impact of ramipril: the HOPE randomized trial. *Ann Intern Med* 2001;134:629–636.
6. Hunter JJ, Chien KR. Signaling pathways for cardiac hypertrophy and failure. *N Engl J Med* 1999;341:1276–1283.
7. Katz AM. The cardiomyopathy of overload: an unnatural growth response in the hypertrophied heart. *Ann Intern Med* 1994;121:363–371.
8. Levin A, Thompson CR, Ethier J, et al. Left ventricular mass index increase in early renal disease: impact of decline in hemoglobin. *Am J Kidney Dis* 1999;34:125–134.
9. Foley RN, Parfrey PS, Harnett JD, et al. Clinical and echocardiographic disease in patients starting end-stage renal disease therapy. *Kidney Int* 1995;47:186–192.
10. Blacher J, Guerin AP, Pannier B, et al. Impact of aortic stiffness on survival in end-stage renal disease. *Circulation* 1999;99:2434–2439.
11. Middleton RI, Parfrey PS, Foley RN. Left ventricular hypertrophy in the renal patient. *J Am Soc Nephrol* 2001;12:1079–1084.
12. Foley RN, Parfrey PS, Hamett JD, et al. The impact of anemia on cardiomyopathy, morbidity, and mortality in end-stage renal disease. *Am J Kidney Dis* 1996;28:53–61.
13. Foley RN, Parfrey PS, Harnett JD, et al. Impact of hypertension on cardiomyopathy, morbidity and mortality in end-stage renal disease. *Kidney Int* 1996;49:1379–1385.

14. Ma JZ, Ebben J, Xia H, et al. Hematocrit level and associated mortality in hemodialysis patients. *J Am Soc Nephrol* 1999;10: 610–619.
15. Xia H, Ebben J, Ma JZ, Collins AJ. Hematocrit levels and hospitalization risks in hemodialysis patients. *J Am Soc Nephrol* 1999; 10:1309–1316.
16. Evans RW, Rader B, Manninen DL, et al. The quality of life of hemodialysis recipients treated with recombinant human erythropoietin. *JAMA* 1990;263:825–830.
17. Beusterien KM, Nissenson AR, Port FK, et al. The effects of recombinant human erythropoietin on functional health and well-being in chronic dialysis patients. *J Am Soc Nephrol* 1996; 7:763–773.
18. Marsh JT, Brown WS, Wolcott D, et al. rHuEPO treatment improves brain and cognitive function of anemic dialysis patients. *Kidney Int* 1991;39:155–163.
19. Canadian Erythropoietin Study Group. Association between recombinant human erythropoietin and quality of life and exercise capacity of patients receiving haemodialysis. *BMJ* 1990;300: 573–578.
20. London GM, Zins B, Pannier B, et al. Vascular changes in hemodialysis patients in response to recombinant human erythropoietin. *Kidney Int* 1989;36:878–882.
21. Sikole A, Polenakovic M, Spirovska V, et al. Analysis of heart morphology and function following erythropoietin treatment of anemic dialysis patients. *Artif Organs* 1993;17:977–984.
22. Besarab A, Kline Bolton W, Browne JK, et al. The effects of normal as compared with low hematocrit in patients with cardiac disease who are receiving hemodialysis and epoetin. *N Engl J Med* 1998;339:584–590.
23. Foley RN, Parfrey PS, Morgan J, et al. Effect of hemoglobin levels in hemodialysis patients with asymptomatic cardiomyopathy. *Kidney Int* 2000;58:1325–1335.
24. McMahon LP, McKenna MJ, Sangkabutra T, et al. Physical performance and associated electrolyte changes after haemoglobin normalization: a comparative study in haemodialysis patients. *Nephrol Dial Transplant* 1999;14:1182–1187.
25. McMahon LP, Mason K, Skinner SL, et al. Effects of haemoglobin normalization on quality of life and cardiovascular parameters in end-stage renal failure. *Nephrol Dial Transplant* 2000 Sep; 15(9):1425–1430.
26. Buckalew VM Jr, Berg RL, Wang SR, et al. Prevalence of hypertension in 1,795 subjects with chronic renal disease: the modification of diet in renal disease study baseline cohort. Modification of Diet in Renal Disease Study Group. *Am J Kidney Dis* 1996; 28:811–821.
27. Levin A, Singer J, Thompson CR, et al. Prevalent left ventricular hypertrophy in the predialysis population: identifying opportunities for intervention. *Am J Kidney Dis* 1996;27:347–354.
28. Foley RN, Parfrey PS, Harnett JD, et al. Impact of hypertension on cardiomyopathy, morbidity, and mortality in end-stage renal disease. *Kidney Int* 1996;49:1379–1385.
29. Savage T, Giles M, Tomson CV, et al. Gender differences in mediators of left ventricular hypertrophy in dialysis patients. *Clin Nephrol* 1998;49:107–112.
30. Tucker B, Fabbian F, Giles M, et al. Left ventricular hypertrophy and ambulatory blood pressure monitoring in chronic renal failure. *Nephrol Dial Transplant* 1997;12:724–728.
31. Parfrey PS, Foley RN, Harnett JD, et al. Outcome and risk factors for left ventricular disorders in chronic uraemia. *Nephrol Dial Transplant* 1996;11:1277–1285.
32. Harnett JD, Foley RN, Kent GM, et al. Congestive heart failure in dialysis patients: prevalence, incidence, prognosis and risk factors. *Kidney Int* 1995;47:884–890.
33. Rahman M, Dixit A, Donley V, et al. Factors associated with inadequate blood pressure control in hypertensive hemodialysis patients [see comments]. *Am J Kidney Dis* 1999;33:498–506.
34. Fishbane S, Natke E, Maesaka JK. Role of volume overload in dialysis-refractory hypertension. *Am J Kidney Dis* 1996;28: 257–261.
35. Scribner BH. Can antihypertensive medications control BP in haemodialysis patients: yes or no? *Nephrol Dial Transplant* 1999; 14:2599–2601.
36. Fagugli RM, Reboldi G, Quintaliani G, et al. Short daily hemodialysis: blood pressure control and left ventricular mass reductions in hypertensive hemodialysis patients. *Am J Kidney Dis* 2001;38: 371–376.
37. Charra B, Calemard E, Laurent G. Importance of treatment time and blood pressure control in achieving long-term survival on dialysis. *Am J Nephrol* 1997;16:35–44.
38. Fernandez JM, Carbonell ME, Mazzuchi N, et al. Simultaneous analysis of morbidity and mortality factors in chronic hemodialysis patients. *Kidney Int* 1992;41:1029–1034.
39. USRDS 1992 Annual Data Report. Comorbid conditions and correlations with mortality risk among 3,399 incident hemodialysis patients. *Am J Kidney Dis* 1992;20:32–38.
40. Iseki K, Miyasato F, Tokuyama K, et al. Low diastolic blood pressure, hypoalbuminemia, and risk hemodialysis patients. *Kidney Int* 1997;51:1212–1217.
41. Port FK, Hulbert-Shearon TE, Wolfe RA, et al. Predialysis blood pressure and mortality risk in national hemodialysis patients [see comments]. *Am J Kidney Dis* 1999;33:507–517.
42. Zager PG, Nikolic J, Brown RH, et al. ÒU curve association of blood pressure and mortality in hemodialysis patients. Medical Directors of Dialysis Clinic, Inc [published erratum appears in *Kidney Int* 1998 Oct;54(4):1417]. *Kidney Int* 1998;54:561–569.
43. Franklin SS, Larson MG, Khan SA, et al. Does the relation of blood pressure to coronary heart disease risk change with aging? The Framingham Heart Study. *Circulation* 2001;103: 1245–1249.
44. Foley RN, Herzog CA, Collins AJ. Pre and post-dialysis blood pressure patterns and mortality in dialysis patients. The USRDS Wave 3 & 4 Study. *J Am Soc Nephrol* 2001 (abstract).
45. Lewis EJ, Hunsicker LG, Bain RP, et al. The effect of angiotensin-converting-enzyme inhibition on diabetic nephropathy. The Collaborative Study Group. *N Engl J Med* 1993;329:1456–1462.
46. Maschio G, Alberti D, Janin G, et al. Effect of the angiotensin-converting-enzyme inhibitor benazepril on the progression of chronic renal insufficiency. The Angiotensin-Converting-Enzyme Inhibition in Progressive Renal Insufficiency Study Group. *N Engl J Med* 1996;334:939–945.
47. Ruggenenti P, Perna A, Gherardi G, et al. Renal function and requirement for dialysis in chronic nephropathy patients on long-term ramipril: REIN follow-up trial. Gruppo Italiano di Studi Epidemiologici in Nefrologia (GISEN). Ramipril Efficacy in Nephropathy. *Lancet* 1998;352:1252–1256.
48. Pfeffer MA, Braunwald E, Moye LA, et al. Effect of captopril on mortality and morbidity in patients with left ventricular dysfunction after myocardial infarction. Results of the survival and ventricular enlargement trial. The SAVE Investigators. *N Engl J Med* 1992;327:669–677.
49. Effect of enalapril on mortality and the development of heart failure in asymptomatic patients with reduced left ventricular ejection fractions. The SOLVD Investigators. *N Engl J Med* 1992; 327:685–691.
50. Vusuf S, Sleight P, Pogue J, et al. Effects of an angiotensin-converting-enzyme inhibitor, ramipril, on cardiovascular events in high-risk patients. The Heart Outcomes Prevention Evaluation Study Investigators. *N Engl J Med* 2000;342:145–153.
51. London GM, Pannier B, Guerin AP, et al. Cardiac hypertrophy, aortic compliance, peripheral resistance, and wave reflection in

end-stage renal disease. Comparative effects of ACE inhibition and calcium channel blockade. *Circulation* 1994;90:2786–2796.
52. Cannella G, Paoletti E, Barocci S, et al. Angiotensin-converting enzyme gene polymorphism and reversibility of uremic left ventricular hypertrophy following long-term antihypertensive therapy. *Kidney Int* 1998;54:618–626.
53. Grodos D, Tonglet R. Scandinavian simvastatin study (4S). *Lancet* 1994 Dec 24–31;344(8939–8940):1768.
54. Shepherd J, Cobbe SM, Ford I, et al. Prevention of coronary heart disease with pravastatin in men with hypercholesterolemia. West of Scotland Coronary Prevention Study Group. *N Engl J Med* 1995;333:1301–1307.
55. Lowrie EG, Lew NL. Death risk in hemodialysis patients: the predictive value of commonly measured variables and an evaluation of death rate differences between facilities. *Am J Kidney Dis* 1990;15:458–482.
56. Goldwasser P, Mittman N, Antignani A, et al. Predictors of mortality in hemodialysis patients. *J Am Soc Nephrol* 1993;3: 1613–1622.
57. Bostom AG, Culleton BF. Hyperhomocysteinemia in chronic renal disease. *J Am Soc Nephrol* 1999;10:891–900.
58. Yeun JY, Levine RA, Mantadilok V, et al. C-Reactive protein predicts all-cause and cardiovascular mortality in hemodialysis patients. *Am J Kidney Dis* 2000;35:469–476.
59. Foley RN, Parfrey PS, Hamett JD, et al. Hypoalbuminemia, cardiac morbidity, and mortality in end-stage renal disease. *J Am Soc Nephrol* 1996;7:728–736.
60. Stenvinkel P, Heimburger O, Paultre F, et al. Strong association between malnutrition, inflammation, and atherosclerosis in chronic renal failure. *Kidney Int* 1999;55(5):1899–1911.
61. Stenvinkel P, Heimburger O, Wang T, et al. High serum hyaluronan indicates poor survival in renal replacement therapy. *Am J Kidney Dis* 1999;34:1083–1088.
62. Stenvinkel P, Lindholm B, Heimburger M, et al. Elevated serum levels of soluble adhesion molecules predict death in pre-dialysis patients: association with malnutrition, inflammation, and cardiovascular disease. *Nephrol Dial Transplant* 2000;15:1624–1630.
63. Ridker PM, Stampfer MJ, Rifai N. Novel risk factors for systemic atherosclerosis: a comparison of C-reactive protein, fibrinogen, homocysteine, lipoprotein(a), and standard cholesterol screening as predictors of peripheral arterial disease. *JAMA* 2001;285: 2481–2485.
64. Ridker PM, Rifai N, Clearfield M, et al. Measurement of C-reactive protein for the targeting of statin therapy in the primary prevention of acute coronary events. *N Engl J Med* 2001;344: 1959–1965.
65. Kaysen GA. The microinflammatory state in uremia: causes and potential consequences. *J Am Soc Nephrol* 2001;12:1549–1557.
66. Handelman GJ, Walter MF, Adhikarla R, et al. Elevated plasma FZ-isoprostanes in patients on long-term hemodialysis. *Kidney Int* 2001;59:1960–1966.
67. Boaz M, Smetana S, Weinstein T, et al. Secondary prevention with antioxidants of cardiovascular disease in endstage renal disease (SPACE): randomised placebo-controlled trial. *Lancet* 2001; 356:1213–1218.
68. Amann K, Wiest G, Zimmer G, et al. Reduced capillary density in the myocardium of uremic rats—a stereological study. *Kidney Int* 1992;42:1079–1085.
69. Raine AE, Seymour AM, Roberts AF, et al. Impairment of cardiac function and energetics in experimental renal failure. *J Clin Invest* 1993;92:2934–2940.
70. Parfrey PS, Harnett JD, Foley RN, et al. Impact of renal transplantation on uremic cardiomyopathy. *Transplantation* 1995;60: 908–914.
71. Rigatto C, Foley RN, Kent GM, et al. Long-term changes in left ventricular hypertrophy after renal transplantation. *Transplantation* 2000;70:570–575.
72. London GM, Fabiani F, Marchais SJ, et al. Uremic cardiomyopathy: an inadequate left ventricular hypertrophy. *Kidney Int* 1987; 31:973–980.
73. Block GA, Hulbert-Shearon TE, Levin NW, et al. Association of serum phosphorus and calcium x phosphate product with mortality risk in chronic hemodialysis patients: a national study. *Am J Kidney Dis* 1998;31:607–617.
74. Guerin AP, London GM, Marchais SJ, et al. Arterial stiffening and vascular calcifications in end-stage renal disease. *Nephrol Dial Transplant* 2001;15:1014–1021.
75. National Kidney Foundation. Kidney Disease Outcomes Quality Initiative. www.kidney.org/professionals/doqi/guidelines.
76. Position statement: Standards of medical care for patients with diabetes mellitus. *Diabetes Care* 2001;24 (Suppl 1).

11

CAUSES OF PROTEIN-ENERGY MALNUTRITION IN CHRONIC RENAL FAILURE

RAJNISH MEHROTRA
JOEL D. KOPPLE

Many studies, both single and multicenter, from various parts of the world indicate that protein-energy malnutrition (PEM) is present in a significant proportion of nondialyzed patients with advanced chronic renal failure (CRF) and in those who have just commenced maintenance dialysis (MD) therapy (1–9). Similarly, surveys of patients undergoing MD suggest that, on average, about 40% of these patients have PEM (10–23). The evidence for nutritional decline in nondialyzed patients with CRF and patients undergoing MD includes low visceral protein concentrations (e.g., serum albumin, transferrin, prealbumin) (1,3,4,6–8,11,20) and serum cholesterol and total body nitrogen (13,14); a plasma and muscle amino acid profile consistent with PEM (24–27); low body mass index (4,6,20) and fat-free, edema-free mass (i.e., lean body mass) (2,4,6–8,20); decreased skeletal muscle circumference, diameter, or cross-sectional area (10,12,14, 18,23) and hand-grip muscle strength (7,28); and decreased subjective global assessment scores (1,4,7–9,15,16,21).

These findings are of particular importance because nutritional parameters at the time of initiation of dialysis are strong predictors of subsequent patient outcome (8,29–34) and the predictive value of PEM as a mortality risk factor in these patients persists for at least 5 years (35). Similarly, in prevalent patients undergoing MD, measures of PEM are associated with increased morbidity and mortality (1,8, 11,29–32,35–51). Hence, understanding the mechanisms that lead to malnutrition may be critical for improving the outcome of these patients.

ETIOLOGY OF PROTEIN-ENERGY MALNUTRITION IN PATIENTS UNDERGOING MAINTENANCE DIALYSIS

Patients with CRF constitute a highly heterogeneous group of individuals, and the etiology of PEM in these patients is clearly multifactorial. Potential causes are summarized in Table 11.1. In a given patient, varying combinations of these causes result in PEM, and the relative contribution of some or all of these factors varies widely between patients. We present an overview of the most important causes, except that of inflammation that leads to PEM in patients with CRF. Inflammation, most likely another important contributor to nutritional decline in individuals with CRF, is discussed in Chapter 13.

Low Nutrient Intake

Several lines of evidence suggest that a low nutrient intake is one of the most important causes for the development of PEM in patients with CRF and those undergoing MD.

Energy and Protein Requirements in Patients with Chronic Renal Failure and Patients Undergoing Maintenance Dialysis

The ideal study design to determine the protein and energy requirements for patients at various stages of renal failure would be to conduct a prospective, controlled trial in patients who are randomized to receive different levels of energy and protein intake and to study the effect of nutrient intake on nutritional status, morbidity, quality of life, and mortality. It is unlikely that such a trial will be conducted in the near future in the United States; hence, we are obliged to depend on such surrogate measures as metabolic-balance studies, body composition, and serum biochemical measures of nutritional status to determine the requirements. The rigorous methodology used in metabolic-balance studies permits an accurate estimation of protein and energy requirements; therefore they usually involve small numbers of patients studied at clinical research centers.

Energy and Protein Requirements for Nondialyzed Patients with Chronic Renal Failure

To maintain neutral energy balance, energy intake should equal energy expenditure. Several studies have demonstrated

TABLE 11.1. CAUSES OF PROTEIN-ENERGY MALNUTRITION IN PATIENTS WITH CHRONIC RENAL FAILURE

1. Inflammation
2. Low nutrient intake
   A. Anorexia induced by:
      i. Inadequate clearance of anorexigens
      ii. Impaired gastric emptying
      iii. Increased leptin levels
      iv. Comorbid illnesses
      v. Intraperitoneal instillation of dialysate
   B. Superimposed illnesses leading to:
      i. Altered gastrointestinal motility
      ii. Altered digestive or absorptive processes
3. Nutrient losses during dialysis
4. Metabolic acidemia
5. Comorbidity
6. Endocrine disorders of uremia
   A. Resistance to insulin
   B. Resistance to insulinlike growth factor-1 and growth hormone
   C. Hyperparathyroidism
   D. Hyperglucagonemia
   E. Hypotestosteronemia
7. Blood loss
   A. Occult gastrointestinal bleeding
   B. Venipuncture
   C. Sequestration in hemodialyzer

that the energy expenditure in nondialyzed patients with CRF is about the same as in healthy adults under a variety of conditions (Table 11.2) (52–54). Moreover, in most patients consuming about 0.60 g/kg/day, diets providing about 35 kcal/kg/d appear to be necessary to maintain neutral nitrogen balance (53). One study, however, concluded that nondialyzed patients with CRF and diabetes mellitus had higher resting energy expenditure than those without diabetes mellitus (55). If other investigators reproduce these findings, recommendations for energy intake may have to be tailored to the presence or absence of diabetes mellitus.

Similarly, amino acid turnover and nitrogen-balance studies in nondialyzed patients with CRF suggest that a diet providing 0.60 g/kg/day of predominantly high biologic value (HBV) protein will maintain neutral nitrogen balance, as long as an adequate energy supply (about 35 kcal/kg/d for those younger than 61 years old) is ensured (56–59). Long-term studies have demonstrated the nutritional safety of these low-protein diets; in all but one study, the energy intakes of patients exceeded 30 kcal/kg/d (57,60–63). In patients with nephrotic syndrome, a diet providing 0.8 g/kg/day of protein maintains nitrogen balance, as long as the dietary energy intake (DEI) is about 35 kcal/kg/d and urinary protein losses are roughly 5 g/day or less (64).

Energy and Protein Requirements for Patients Undergoing Maintenance Hemodialysis

Several studies have demonstrated that the energy expenditure in patients being treated with maintenance hemodialysis (MHD) is similar to that of healthy adults during a variety of activities (Table 11.2) (52,54,65); only one study demonstrated higher resting energy expenditure (by 7.3%) (66). The effect of the HD procedure remains uncertain because the two studies that addressed this issue came to conflicting conclusions (66,67). In the study by Ikizler et al., which demonstrated a 20% increase in energy expenditure

TABLE 11.2. ENERGY REQUIREMENTS OF PATIENTS WITH CHRONIC RENAL FAILURE

	Nondialyzed CRF	MHD	CPD
Energy expenditure studies			
Lying	Normal (52–54) Higher in diabetics (55)	Normal (52,54,65) 7.3% increase (66)	Normal (80)
Sitting	Normal (52)	Normal (52)	
Postprandial	Normal (52)	Normal (52)	
Exercise	Normal (52)	Normal (52)	
Dialysis procedure		No different from resting (67) 20% greater than resting (66)	Normal (80)

Nutritional Parameter	Energy Intake with Unchanging Parameter (kcal/kg desirable body weight)	
	Nondialyzed CRF (53)	MHD (68)
Energy intake and nutritional parameters		
Body weight (kg)	23.1	32.4
Nitrogen balance minus unmeasured losses (g/day)	34	38.5
Midarm circumference (cm)		34.1
Midarm muscle area (cm^2)		33
Body fat (%)		32

CRF, chronic renal failure; MHD, maintenance hemodialysis; CPD, chronic peritoneal dialysis.

during HD (66), patients had eaten shortly before the onset of the dialysis procedure and this increase in energy expenditure actually may reflect the specific dynamic action of food. The study by Olevitch et al. reported normal energy expenditure in patients undergoing MHD (67). Studies of nitrogen balances and a variety of anthropometric parameters have been used to determine the energy intake necessary to maintain a stable nutritional status in patients undergoing MHD who are consuming an average of 1.13 g/kg/day of protein (Table 11.2) (68). These analyses suggest that such an energy intake should be between 31.1 and 38.5 kcal/kg/d (Table 11.2).

To our knowledge, there are six published studies that have evaluated nitrogen balance to ascertain the DPI in patients undergoing MHD (Table 11.3) (68–73). In addition, several observational studies have demonstrated a relationship between DPI and morbidity and mortality (36–38, 74), whereas others were unable to demonstrate such a relationship (75,76).

Based on these studies, the National Kidney Foundation Kidney/Dialysis Outcome Quality Initiative (NKF-K/DOQI) suggests a DEI of 35 kcal/kg/d for patients undergoing MHD who are 60 years of age or younger and between 30 and 35 kcal/kg/d for patients older than 65 years of age, who tend to be sedentary (77). Furthermore, the NKF-K/DOQI workgroup suggests that using standard criteria for establishing dietary recommendations (78), a DPI of 1.2 g/kg/day is necessary to ensure neutral or positive nitrogen balance in most clinically stable patients undergoing MHD; at least 50% of the DPI should be HBV (77). There are currently no studies available to determine energy and protein requirements in patients undergoing MHD older than 60 years of age, and the recommendations for this age group are based on extrapolation from younger age groups and data obtained from normal older individuals.

Energy and Protein Requirements for Patients Undergoing Chronic Peritoneal Dialysis

Energy intake in patients undergoing peritoneal dialysis (PD) represents the sum of dietary intake and the quantity of glucose (dextrose) absorbed from the dialysate. At least three published studies have addressed the issue of energy requirements in chronic peritoneal dialysis (CPD) patients (79–81). The resting energy expenditure of patients undergoing CPD is similar to that of healthy, normal adults (80). Metabolic-balance studies in patients undergoing continuous ambulatory peritoneal dialysis (CAPD) eating their usual diets showed a strong correlation between total energy intake and nitrogen balance, irrespective of the duration for which the patients were on dialysis (79). In this investigation energy and protein intake were not varied independently of each other. Nonetheless, based primarily on the energy expenditure studies, the NKF-K/DOQI guidelines suggest a DEI of 35 kcal/kg/d for patients undergoing CPD 60 years of age or younger and between 30 and 35 kcal/kg/d for patients older than 60 years old (77). In a study published in 1998, Uribarri et al. demonstrated stable total body weight; edema-free, fat-free mass; and anthropometric parameters

TABLE 11.3. DIETARY PROTEIN REQUIREMENTS, AS DETERMINED BY NITROGEN BALANCE, IN PATIENTS UNDERGOING MAINTENANCE HEMODIALYSIS[a]

First Author and Year Published	n	Age Range (years)	Diabetics	Study Duration (days)	Dialysis Frequency	Energy Intake (kcal/kg/day)	Protein Intake (g/kg/day)	Mean Nitrogen Balance (g/day)
Ginn,'68 (69)	4	17–22	None	7–32	2x/week	50–55	0.4–1.48 HBV 0.14–0.95 LBV	Neutral/+ at 0.75 g/kg HBV protein Negative at 0.95 LBV protein
Kopple,'69 (70)	3		None	21–28	2x/week	35–45	0.75 (0.63 HBV) 1.25 (0.88 HBV)	Neutral Neutral
Borah,'78 (71)	5	35–65	None	7	3x/week	20.5–30.9	0.5 (37% HBV)	−1.98
Lim,'85 (72)[b]	6	20–59	None	9	3x/week	29.5 ± 1.5	0.87 ± 0.06	0.37 ± 1.0
Slomowitz,'89 (68)	6	24–64	None	21–23	3x/week	37.3 ± 2.1	1.13 ± 0.2	0.57 ± 0.42 (0/+ 4/6
Rao,'00 (73)[c]	15	18–55	None	7	3x/week	33 ± 6.5 32.8 ± 6.7	0.61 ± 0.1 1.06 ± 0.18	0.17 4.03

HBV, high biologic value; LBV, low biologic value.
[a]Nitrogen balances were not adjusted for unmeasured losses through the skin, hair and nail growth, and sweat and flatus.
[b]Energy intake was not constant from patient to patient.
[c]Great caution must be used in interpreting these data because subjects lived at home and all nitrogen output were estimated and not measured directly.

TABLE 11.4. DIETARY PROTEIN REQUIREMENTS, AS DETERMINED BY NITROGEN BALANCE, IN PATIENTS UNDERGOING CHRONIC PERITONEAL DIALYSIS

First Author and Year Published	n	Age Range (years)	Diabetics	Study Duration (days)	Dialysis Regimen	Protein Intake (g/kg/day)	Total Energy Intake (kcal/kg/day)	Nitrogen Balance (g/day)
Giordano, '80 (82)	8				CAPD	1.2		0/+ in 7/8
Blumenkrantz, '82 (83)	8[a]	27–59	None	14–33	CAPD	0.98 ± 0.03	41.3 ± 1.9	+0.35 ± 0.83
						1.44 ± 0.02	42.1 ± 1.2	+2.94 ± 0.54
Bergstrom, '93 (79)	12	27–62	None	6–11	CAPD	0.76–2.09	28–50	+ correlation with DPI
	9	27–62	None	6–11	CAPD	0.64–1.69	25–51	No correlation with DPI

CAPD, continuous ambulatory peritoneal dialysis; DPI, dietary protein intake.
[a]14 studies conducted in eight patients being treated with CAPD.

in 49 patients undergoing CPD on a total energy intake of about 29 kcal/kg/day and a DPI of about 1 g/kg/day over a 6-month period (81). However, the patients undergoing CPD were relatively obese for their height and if adjusted for the patients' overweight condition, the energy intake in these patients increased to the recommended levels.

To our knowledge, three sets of nitrogen-balance studies have been conducted in patients undergoing CPD (Table 11.4) (79,82,83). These studies indicate that a DPI of 1.1 g/kg/day or greater almost always is associated with neutral or positive nitrogen balance. Moreover, several studies have shown a relationship between DPI, as determined by the normalized protein equivalent of total nitrogen appearance, and the serum albumin and total body protein balance (79, 82,83) as well as mortality (1). Based on the currently available data and allowing 20% variability for individual differences as recommended by the Food and Nutrition Board of the U.S. National Academy of Sciences (78), the NKF-K/DOQI recommended a DPI of 1.2 to 1.3 g/kg/day for clinically stable patients undergoing CPD (77). There are currently no studies available for patients receiving automated peritoneal dialysis (APD). However, there is no reason to believe that their requirements will be materially different from those undergoing CAPD. Hence, until more specific data for patients undergoing APD are available, it would seem reasonable to make the same recommendations for dietary protein and energy intake for patients undergoing APD as for CAPD.

Spontaneous Protein and Energy Intake in Patients with Chronic Renal Failure

Some of the studies that have examined the spontaneous dietary energy and protein intake in patients with CRF are

TABLE 11.5. SPONTANEOUS DIETARY ENERGY AND PROTEIN INTAKE IN NONDIALYZED PATIENTS WITH CHRONIC RENAL FAILURE

First Author and Year Published	n	GFR Range (mL/min)	Dietary Energy Intake (kcal/kg/day)	Dietary Protein Intake (g/kg/day)
Williams '91 (215)	6	9–16[a]	38.3	1.2[b]
Walser '93 (237)	16	10–29[a]		0.82[c]
Mehrotra '97 (85)	45	4–53[d]		0.95[c]
Park '97 (3)	64	0–33		0.8
Pollock '97 (90)	766	84 ± 2[e]		0.98[c]
Chauveau '99 (63)	10	3–23[a]	27.8	0.78[b]
Aparcio '00 (238)	239	4–23[a]		0.85[b]
Kopple '00 (5)	1,785	12–82[a]		
Males			29.4	1.05[b]
Females			27.2	0.95[b]
Avesani '01 (55)				
Diabetics	24	43 ± 25[e]	23.4	0.89[b]
Nondiabetics	24	38 ± 18[e]	24.8	0.76[b]

GFR, glomerular fitration rate.
[a]Renal function determined by ^{51}Cr-EDTA or ^{99m}Tc-DTPA or iothalamte clearances.
[b]Dietary protein intake estimated by use of food diaries.
[c]Dietary protein intake estimated by urinary urea nitrogen excretion and urinary protein losses.
[d]Renal function determined by mean of urinary urea and creatinine clearances.
[e]Renal function estimated by 24-hour creatinine clearance.

TABLE 11.6. SPONTANEOUS DIETARY PROTEIN AND ENERGY INTAKE IN PATIENTS UNDERGOING MAINTENANCE HEMODIALYSIS AND CHRONIC PERITONEAL DIALYSIS

First Author and Year Published	n	Dietary Energy Intake (kcal/kg/day)	Dietary and Peritoneal Energy Intake	Dietary Protein Intake
Maintenance hemodialysis				
Pollock '90 (13)	11	29.8		1.09[a]
Rayner '91 (14)	52	74% of recommended		1.0[b]
Chauveau '96 (239)	50	30.1		1.2[b]
Dwyer '98 (19)	49	22.8		0.94[b]
Ge '98 (98)	75	28.1		1.0[b]
Sharma '99 (240)	106	29		0.93[a]
Lorenzo '01 (193)	207	24.7		1.0[b]
Chazot '01 (129)				
HD <10 yr	10	35.1		1.53[b]
HD >10 yr	10	31.0		1.19[b]
Chronic peritoneal dialysis				
Pollock '90 (13)	35	27.1		1.04[a]
Bergstrom '93 (79)	12	33.6	41.1	1.4[c]
Uribarri '98 (81)	48		28.8	61.7 (g/day)[d]
Caravaca '99 (131)	9		37.6	1.08[b]
Grzegorzewska '99 (241)	8	27.7	34.1	0.86[b]

HD, hemodialysis; DPI, dietary protein intake.
[a]DPI estimated using 24-hour recall.
[b]DPI estimated using food diaries.
[c]DPI estimated from dietary nitrogen intake.
[d]DPI estimated using urea kinetic modeling.

summarized in Tables 11.5 and 11.6, respectively. Declines in spontaneous dietary energy and protein intake are apparent in patients with CRF long before they reach end-stage renal disease and commence dialysis (5,84,85). Moreover, dialysis therapy is unable to eradicate anorexia in many patients (86). Hence, the mean intakes of both energy and protein in patients treated with MD are substantially lower than the reported nutritional needs of these patients; this deficit in the energy intake is greater than the decrement in protein intake. There is evidence that reduced energy intake may be more important than the lower protein intake in determining the nutritional status of patients undergoing MD. An insufficient energy intake, even in the face of adequate protein intake, can result in a negative nitrogen balance in patients with CRF (53,68,87). In the nitrogen-balance studies by Bergstrom et al. in patients undergoing CPD in which both energy and protein intake were varied (79), DEI correlated significantly with nitrogen balance in all studies, whereas the DPI correlated with nitrogen balance only in patients who recently had started dialysis. Finally, in the studies by Pollock et al., in both MHD and patients undergoing CPD, total body protein as measured by neutron-activation analysis correlated with estimated energy intake rather than with protein intake (47).

Low Nutrient Intake Is Important in Inducing Protein-Energy Malnutrition

Evidence of nutritional decline begins long before patients with progressive CRF develop end-stage renal disease. During the screening (baseline) phase of the Modification of Diet in Renal Disease (MDRD) study, a cross-sectional assessment of 1,785 clinically stable patients with moderate to advanced CRF (mean ± S.D. glomerular filtration rate, or GFR: 39.8 ± 21.1 mL/min/1/73 m^2) demonstrated a high prevalence of a decline in measures of nutritional status (5). Moreover, there was a direct association between various anthropometric and serum markers of nutritional status with GFR in this and another study (5,84). Several other cross-sectional studies have demonstrated a progressive decline in DEI and DPI with decreasing GFR (5,85,88–91); this observation has been confirmed in longitudinal studies as well (84,92). Because DPI and various nutritional markers covary with GFR and energy intakes are abnormally low even at modest declines in GFR, it has been postulated that low nutrient intake contributes to the nutritional decline observed during the predialysis phase; until recently, this hypothesis remained untested. In an analysis of the baseline phase of the MDRD study, the association of GFR with several of the anthropometric and biochemical and nutritional parameters either was attenuated or eliminated after controlling for protein and energy intakes (5).

Similar associations between measures of nutritional decline and dietary protein and energy intake have been demonstrated in patients treated with MD. Hence, in cross-sectional studies, the DPI has been shown to correlate with serum albumin (20,28,90,93–96) and prealbumin (20); plasma amino acids (24,28); subjective global assessment (16,97); body mass index (20,90,96); triceps skinfold thickness (96,98); percent body fat (96); fat-free, edema-free mass (20); total body nitrogen (13,99); and nitrogen balance (73,79,83). Furthermore, DEI has been correlated with body fat (24), nitrogen balance (68,79), plasma amino acids (68), and total body nitrogen (47). However, not all studies have been able to demonstrate a consistent relationship between estimates of DPI and several measures of nutritional decline. One of the cardinal reasons for this discrepancy is probably the fact that the DPI often is normalized to the current body weight; in severely malnourished individuals, this may result in an artifactually higher DPI. Indeed, several investigators now have demonstrated that malnourished individuals have a significantly lower DPI when the total daily protein intake is normalized to desirable body weight or fat-free, edema-free weight rather than actual body weight (18,28,100). Finally, interventions that result in an increased supply of energy and/or protein have been reported to result in an improvement in various nutritional parameters in patients undergoing MD (101–111).

Causes of Anorexia in Patients Undergoing Maintenance Dialysis

There are probably several causes for anorexia in patients being treated with MD. In this section, we present an overview of some of the key factors suspected to play a role. More recently, the potential contribution of inflammation to PEM, through its anorexigenic and catabolic effects, in patients undergoing MD has been investigated (see Chapter 13). The potential roles of comorbidity and inflammation in suppressing appetite are discussed in the following paragraphs.

Inadequate Solute Clearances

Anorexia is a cardinal uremic manifestation in patients with CRF, and this anorexia tends to improve over several days or weeks after initiation of MD (86). Based on these observations, it has been proposed that there are uremic toxins that accumulate during the progressive decline of renal function that are removed, to variable degrees, by dialysis. This hypothesis initially was tested in cross-sectional studies, and these analyses demonstrated a significant relationship between measures of small solute removal (Kt/V) and DPI (nPNA) in both nondialyzed patients with CRF and patients undergoing MD (9,79,85,91,99,112–116). This led to the assumption that there are small–molecular-weight uremic toxins that are responsible for anorexia in patients with CRF. It now is believed that part, but not all, of this relationship is the result of mathematic coupling (117,118) because both measures are derived from the terms used to calculate the rate of urinary nitrogen appearance and are normalized to the volume of distribution of urea. However, several investigators have demonstrated a relationship between the dose of urea removal and DPI, calculated from dietary records and interviews (79,117). The relationship is statistically significant, even when the dose of urea and creatinine removal is not normalized to body size (79,85, 116). Moreover, DEI also has been shown to correlate with small solute clearances in patients undergoing CPD (97).

There are four lines of evidence that suggest that an increase in solute clearances will lead to an increase in DPI. First, initiation of dialysis in uremic patients with CRF usually results in an increase in DPI; this effect has been demonstrated for patients undergoing treatment with either MHD (86,90) or CPD (33,90). Second, several longitudinal studies over the past few years lend support to the notion that an increase in solute clearances may result in an increase in dietary intake of nutrients. At least one randomized, controlled trial demonstrated that an increase in the dose of dialysis in patients undergoing MHD with a DPI of less than 1.0 g/kg/day resulted in an increase in DPI over the 3-month follow-up period (119). At least three uncontrolled studies have shown that there is an increase in dietary protein and/or energy intake with an increase in small solute clearances in patients undergoing CPD (97,120,121). More recently, a prospective, randomized trial confirmed the beneficial effect of an increase in dialytic clearances on the DPI in patients undergoing CPD (122). The only study that was unable to demonstrate a relationship between an increase in dialysis volumes and DPI in patients undergoing CPD did not achieve any increase in total clearances, which, in turn, were below the currently recommended minimum standards for adequacy of PD (123). Third, uncontrolled observations in small numbers of patients have shown that a new approach to dialysis therapy—daily treatment with nocturnal hemodialysis, which results in substantial increases in solute clearances—results in significant increases in dietary energy (124) and protein intake (124–126). Finally, nutritional status has been consistently and inversely correlated with the duration of MHD (127–129). The daily energy and protein intake has been demonstrated to be lower in those patients undergoing MHD who have been on dialysis for several years when compared to those who have commenced dialysis treatment only recently (129,130). The duration of dialysis may serve as a surrogate for the residual renal function because an inexorable decline occurs in glomerular filtration rate to zero or near zero over about 1 to 2 years in patients undergoing MHD and over 2 to 4 years in patients undergoing CPD. Hence, it is possible that the decline in nutrient intake is related to a loss of residual renal function. In patients undergoing CPD, a clear and consistent correlation has been demonstrated between dietary protein intake and small solute clearances from the native kidney (33,131,132).

Significant progress has been made in elucidating the nature of uremic toxins that result in anorexia in patients with uremia. Early observations suggested that for the same level of small solute clearances by dialysis, patients undergoing CPD had a higher DPI than patients undergoing MHD dialyzed with low-flux membranes (114). In one study in patients undergoing MHD dialyzed with high-flux membranes, the DPI for a given level of small solute clearance was demonstrated to be higher than in patients dialyzed with low-flux membranes (112). Because high-flux membranes remove more molecules of a higher molecular weight and because PD seems to have a higher weekly removal of the larger molecules than does hemodialysis, it was inferred that this improvement in DPI might be related to the removal, by dialysis, of substances of larger molecular weight—the so-called middle molecules. Recent experimental data suggest that middle-molecule fractions in the 1 to 5 kD range that can be isolated from both the dialyzer ultrafiltrate of plasma and from normal urine inhibit food intake in rats in a dose-dependent manner (133). It is likely that these middle-molecule fractions act in the splanchnic region and/or brain to inhibit food intake and that the effect is specific for ingestive behavior (134). However, a recent study was unable to demonstrate an increase in DPI with the presumptive increase in middle-molecule clearances by transferring patients undergoing MHD from a low-flux to a high-flux dialyzer (135).

Delayed Gastric Emptying

Gastroparesis is a well-known complication of diabetes mellitus and probably contributes to the low nutrient intake in this subgroup of patients. Gastroparesis also occurs not uncommonly in patients undergoing MD who do not have diabetes. Several studies have shown impairment in gastric motility in patients being treated with MHD and CPD using both radionuclide studies (136–140) and electric gastrography (EGG) (141,142). In a study using EGG, more than 50% of patients undergoing MHD and CPD who do not have diabetes demonstrated abnormal gastric emptying (142). However, it should be pointed out that not all investigators have demonstrated abnormalities in gastric emptying in patients undergoing MD (143,144). Nevertheless, it is possible that occult gastroparesis contributes to the pathogenesis of PEM in some patients undergoing MD who do not have diabetes; administration of prokinetic agents to hypoalbuminemic nondiabetic patients undergoing MHD with occult gastroparesis resulted in improvement in gastric emptying accompanied by an increase in serum albumin (145,146). The etiology of this gastroparesis remains unclear, and it has been postulated that derangements in the endocrine system of the gut may play a pathogenic role. In patients undergoing CPD, instillation of dialysate into the peritoneal cavity may contribute to abnormal gastric electrical activity (142) as well as the prolongation in gastric emptying time (147).

Increased Serum Leptin Levels

Leptin is a polypeptide that is encoded by the *ob* gene (148). In rodents, leptin acts on the hypothalamus to regulate food intake and energy expenditure (149–151); hence, it plays a key role in regulating body weight. The role of leptin in regulating body weight in humans is less clear. Several investigators have demonstrated elevated serum leptin levels in nondialyzed patients with CRF (152–156) and those undergoing MD (152,153,155,157–164). Thus, elevated leptin levels may play a role in determining the nutritional status of patients undergoing MD. Several cross-sectional studies have shown an inverse correlation between serum leptin levels and DPI (153,161); others have been unable to demonstrate a relationship between recent weight change or other nutritional measures and serum leptin levels (158). A more recent study has demonstrated a positive correlation between serum leptin levels and DPI in patients undergoing MHD (165). However, three recent longitudinal studies have reported that increased serum leptin levels are associated with weight loss in patients being treated with MHD (163) or CPD (152,164).

The etiology of hyperleptinemia in patients undergoing MD is most likely multifactorial. First, leptin is metabolized, at least in part, in the kidney and, hence, should accumulate in renal failure (159,166,167). This is believed to be the major cause for the accumulation of leptin in individuals with loss of renal function. Several investigators have demonstrated an inverse relationship between glomerular filtration rate and serum leptin levels (154,155). It should be noted that not all patients with CRF have elevated serum leptin levels (168,169). Second, insulin stimulates leptin synthesis (170,171), and the association of hyperinsulinemia with hyperleptinemia in patients with CRF may suggest a causal relationship (162,168,172). However, in a small study in nondialyzed patients with CRF, treatment with very–low-protein diets, supplemented with essential amino acids and ketoanalogues of amino acids, led to a reduction in hyperinsulinemia but had no effect on serum leptin levels (156). Moreover, renal transplantation is associated with a rapid decrease in serum leptin levels, although hyperinsulinemia persists (173,174). Third, such other hormones as growth hormone and insulinlike growth factor-I (IGF-I) can modify serum leptin levels (169). Fourth, there is evidence to suggest that intraperitoneal production of leptin may occur in patients undergoing CPD; its clinical relevance remains uncertain (175–177). Finally, activation of the acute-phase response may result in increased leptin levels; recent cross-sectional studies in patients undergoing CPD demonstrated a significant direct correlation between markers of inflammation and serum leptin levels (164,176). Other investigators have failed to demonstrate such a relationship (178,179). Moreover, a recent longitudinal study in patients undergoing MHD suggests that leptin behaves as a negative rather than a positive-acute phase reactant, adding greater complexity to the role of leptin in mediating the low nutrient intake in patients with CRF (180).

Intraperitoneal Instillation of Dialysate

Clinical experience suggests that patients undergoing CPD are more likely to report early satiety or feelings of fullness.

A study of eating behavior in patients undergoing CPD indicates that they have a lower food intake, as measured by the weight of the food ingested, than patients undergoing MHD, and this is associated with a constant feeling of fullness, a lower ranking of palatability of food, and a lower eating drive when compared to the predialysis state (181, 182). Impairment in gastric emptying, as discussed earlier, may contribute to this abnormality. The following two probable explanations have been offered to explain the suppression of appetite in patients undergoing CPD.

The abdominal distention produced either by intraperitoneal instillation of large volumes of dialysate or large ultrafiltration induced by the PD solutions, which are hyperosmolar, may have a direct inhibitory effect on appetite, independent of the absorption of nutrients, as has been demonstrated in a rabbit model of PD (183). If this hypothesis is true, the suppression of appetite should be uniform for all kinds of nutrients. In a PD model designed to study the ingestive behavior of rats, instillation of glucose-based dialysate resulted in a dose-dependent suppression of only carbohydrate intake, whereas the instillation of an amino acid–based dialysate resulted in a dose-dependent suppression of both carbohydrate and protein intake (184). This suggests that the inhibition of appetite caused by PD solutions seems to be specific for various nutritional constituents of the diet and is not simply an effect of hyperosmolality or large filling volumes. This observation is highly relevant because the PD solutions that are currently commercially available use glucose as an osmotic agent; up to 70% of the instilled glucose is absorbed, accounting for 20% to 30% of the total energy intake in patients undergoing CPD (185). Not withstanding these observations, there is no clear evidence that dietary energy or protein intake is lower in patients undergoing CPD than in patients undergoing MHD (Table 11.6).

Impact of Comorbidity on Nutritional Status

In the United States, patients undergoing MD have a high incidence and prevalence of comorbidity (186). More than 50% of the patients commencing MD are older than age 65 years, and almost one-half are diabetic (186). There is a high prevalence of cardiovascular disease at the time of initiating MD—almost one-third have a history of congestive heart failure and almost one-fourth have a history of ischemic heart disease (186). Moreover, this high prevalence of comorbidity generally is acknowledged to be an underestimate of the true burden of disease; a more rigorous review of a sample of the national cohort demonstrated a significantly higher prevalence of associated diseases than is reported in the National Registry (187). Each year, 10% to 15% of prevalent patients undergoing MD are diagnosed with atherosclerotic heart disease, congestive heart failure, peripheral vascular disease, and/or cerebrovascular disease (186). In 1999, patients undergoing MD in the United States were hospitalized an average of 1.5 times and spent a mean of 14 days per year in the hospital (186). It has been estimated that 80% of patients undergoing MHD admitted to hospital wards are in negative nitrogen balance (188). There is also a high incidence of complications resulting from the dialysis vascular access or peritoneal catheter in both MHD and patients undergoing CPD (i.e., infectious complications, vascular access thromboses), which may or may not require hospitalization but which add to the disease burden of these individuals. These comorbidities are responsible for a substantial proportion of the medicines prescribed to such patients treated with MD on an average day. During 1996 and 1997, the median number of medications consumed per day by patients undergoing MD ranged from 8 to 10 (189); 26% to 30% of all patients were prescribed proton pump inhibitors, and 13% were prescribed an agent that promotes gastrointestinal motility (189).

It is likely that the associated comorbidities, intercurrent illnesses, and medications consumed by patients undergoing MD contribute not only to the high prevalence of PEM but also to the association between malnutrition and the high morbidity and mortality in patients undergoing MD. The presence of comorbid illnesses has been shown to increase the mortality risk in patients undergoing CPD and MHD (190,191). An older age, the presence of diabetes mellitus, or the presence of cardiac disease are each associated with an increased risk of death in patients undergoing MD (186), each one of which is, in turn, associated with a higher prevalence or greater severity of PEM or a lower nutrient intake (9,28,40,47,192,193). It truly is the question of "which came first." On the one hand, in some epidemiologic analyses that adjust for the presence of comorbid illnesses, such measures of PEM as serum albumin lose their value as predictors of mortality in patients undergoing MD (190). On the other hand, the excess risk of death associated with diabetes mellitus is eliminated if the analyses are adjusted for predialysis serum albumin, creatinine, and urea (194). Such illnesses would be expected to reduce nutrient intake.

Associated illnesses might both increase morbidity and mortality and cause malnutrition by ways in which malnutrition makes little or no contribution to elevated mortality. Alternatively, a comorbid illness might cause an increase in morbidity and mortality in part by lowering nutrient intake or impairing intestinal absorption of nutrients. Associated illnesses also may result in the activation of the acute-phase response; one study has reported that elevated serum levels of acute-phase proteins are restricted to older patients undergoing MD (28), who in turn are likely to have greater comorbidities. Finally, inadequate nutrient intake as a result of anorexia (e.g., caused by chronic uremia) may predispose to many illnesses, thereby increasing morbidity and mortality.

Inflammation

There is increasing evidence demonstrating an association between cytokines and acute-phase proteins with various markers of nutritional decline, particularly with low serum albumin levels and greater morbidity and mortality of patients with chronic renal failure. Epidemiologic data indicate that inflammation may play an important role in the pathogenesis of PEM in a significant proportion of these patients. This issue is discussed in great detail in Chapter 13.

Endocrine Disorders in Uremia

A wide variety of hormonal derangements accompany the uremic state. It is likely that many of these derangements may promote PEM. In rat models of CRF, resistance to the actions of such anabolic hormones as insulin, growth hormone, and IGF-I consistently has been demonstrated (195,196); a postreceptor defect appears to underlie the insulin resistance seen in uremia and appears to be one of the causes of IGF-I resistance in CRF (197). Moreover, hyperparathyroidism, a common accompaniment of progressive renal failure, may decrease the ability of the pancreatic β cells to secrete insulin and also enhance gluconeogenesis and protein wasting (198).

In humans with CRF, evidence suggests that, although the insulin-induced inhibition of protein degradation is intact (199,200), the insulin-induced stimulation of protein synthesis may be impaired (200). Although the serum levels of growth hormone are increased in progressive renal failure, there is experimental evidence to suggest that uremia is associated with decreased hepatic growth hormone receptor and hepatic IGF-I messenger RNA expression (201,202). This may be explained by the finding in rats with CRF indicating that there is a postreceptor defect for the action of growth hormone in the liver of these animals. This defect may result in an attenuation of the anabolic response to growth hormone. Finally, there is clear evidence for resistance to the action of IGF-1 in humans undergoing MHD or CPD (203,204). (See Chapter 32.)

Moreover, uremia is associated with elevated serum concentrations of potentially catabolic hormones such as glucagon and parathyroid hormone (205,206). Furthermore, it has been suggested that vitamin D deficiency, commonly associated with progressive renal failure, may promote malnutrition. Indeed, a recent study has documented a direct correlation between serum 1,25 dihydroxycholecalciferol concentrations and serum albumin levels in nondialyzed patients with CRF (207). Finally, the thyroid hormone profile of patients with CRF is characterized by low serum concentrations of thyroxine and triiodothyronine (208). It has been suggested that this hormonal profile is a maladaptive response to a low energy intake.

Metabolic Acidemia

In animals with and without renal failure, acidemia enhances the decarboxylation of branched-chain amino acids and causes protein catabolism (209,210). These catabolic effects of acidosis in the skeletal muscle appear to be secondary to a transcriptional induction of the adenosine triphosphate–dependent cytosolic ubiquitin–proteasome proteolytic pathway (211,212). In humans, metabolic acidemia suppresses albumin synthesis, promotes negative nitrogen balance, and induces protein degradation (213,214). Furthermore, in nondialyzed patients with CRF, metabolic acidemia results in increased protein degradation and amino acid oxidation (215,216). Similar findings have been reported in individuals being treated with MD (217–219). Moreover, the intracellular concentration of branched-chain amino acids correlates directly with the serum bicarbonate concentration in patients undergoing MHD, and correction of the acidemia increases their concentrations of these amino acids in the muscle of these patients (220). However, cross-sectional and longitudinal studies in patients undergoing MD have demonstrated no relationship between serum bicarbonate and measures of visceral and somatic protein stores (221,222). On the contrary, a significant inverse relationship exists between the serum bicarbonate concentration and DPI (222), suggesting that the adverse nutritional effects of acidemia may be counterbalanced by an increased nutrient supply in these individuals or with better health associated with greater protein intake, thereby ameliorating or attenuating the nutritional consequences of metabolic acidemia.

The pathophysiologic role of metabolic acidemia is corroborated further by a decrease in protein degradation and an improvement in nitrogen balance in nondialyzed patients with CRF with the correction of metabolic acidemia, either by sodium bicarbonate supplementation or initiation of MHD (215,216,218,219,223). A study in 1988 reported an increase in serum albumin following the correction of metabolic acidemia in patients undergoing MHD (224). Improved weight gain and greater mid-arm circumference are reported in patients undergoing CPD who were given a higher concentration of alkali in the dialysate, which raised the serum bicarbonate concentration, in comparison to patients undergoing CPD treated with the usual alkali concentration (225).

Nutrient Losses in Dialysate

Each hemodialysis procedure results in the loss of about 6 to 12 g of amino acids (226–229) and 2 to 3 g of peptides (230); the magnitude of loss depends on the size and flux of the dialyzer, the blood and dialysate flow, the duration of the dialysis procedure, and whether the patient is postabsorptive or postprandial. However, the protein losses during a hemodialysis treatment are small. Until a few years ago, polysulfone dialyzers that were reprocessed with bleach and formaldehyde promoted large albumin losses (up to 14 g/hemodialysis treatment) as a result of increases in the dialysis membrane pore sizes (229,231). Since these reports, the manufacturing process of these dialyzers has been modified so that these dramatic changes in porosity no longer occur with reuse.

Patients undergoing CAPD lose 2 to 4 g of amino acids and 6 to 10 g of protein (4 to 6 g of albumin) per day (13,96,232–234). Additionally, the amino acid losses range between 1 to 3 g/d, and the magnitude of the losses of individual proteins correlates with their serum levels (234). To the authors' knowledge, peptide losses with CPD have not been studied. Peritoneal amino acid and protein losses with APD have not been well studied. The clinical relevance of these losses is unclear. It appears that these albumin losses result in an increase in the rate of albumin synthesis and a decrease in the catabolic rate in patients undergoing CPD, and this is associated with only a slight reduction in serum albumin levels when compared to patients undergoing MHD (235). However, these losses are exaggerated in patients with even mild episodes of peritonitis and can increase to dramatic levels if antibiotic therapy is delayed. During severe episodes of peritonitis, peritoneal protein losses may remain substantially elevated for several weeks despite appropriate antimicrobial therapy (233,236). Hence, it is likely that these nitrogen losses into the dialysate, although unlikely to induce PEM, contribute to PEM in a significant proportion of patients undergoing MD who have reduced nutrient intake or other disorders that promote PEM.

REFERENCES

1. Canada-USA Peritoneal Dialysis Study Group. Adequacy of dialysis and nutrition in continuous peritoneal dialysis: association with clinical outcomes. *J Am Soc Nephrol* 1996;7:198–207.
2. Woodrow G, Oldroyd B, Turney JH, et al. Whole body and regional body composition in patients with chronic renal failure. *Nephrol Dial Transplant* 1996;11:1613–1618.
3. Park JS, Jung HH, Yang WS, et al. Protein intake and the nutritional status in patients with pre-dialysis chronic renal failure on unrestricted diet. *Korean J Intern Med* 1997;12:115–121.
4. Stenvinkel P, Heimburger O, Paultre F, et al. Strong association between malnutrition, inflammation, and atherosclerosis in chronic renal failure. *Kidney Int* 1999;55:1899–1911.
5. Kopple JD, Greene T, Chumlea WC, et al. Relationship between nutritional status and the glomerular filtration rate: Results from the MDRD study. *Kidney Int* 2000;57:1688–1703.
6. Tan SH, Lee E, Tay ME, et al. Protein nutritional status of adult patients starting chronic ambulatory peritoneal dialysis. *Adv Perit Dial* 2000;16:291–296.
7. Heimburger O, Qureshi AR, Blaner WS, et al. Hand-grip muscle strength, lean body mass, and plasma proteins as markers of nutritional status in patients with chronic renal failure close to start of dialysis therapy. *Am J Kidney Dis* 2000;36:1213–1225.
8. Chung SH, Lindholm B, Lee HB. Influence of initial nutritional status on continuous ambulatory peritoneal dialysis patient survival. *Perit Dial Int* 2000;20:19–26.
9. Caravaca F, Arrobas M, Pizarro JL, et al. Uraemic symptoms, nutritional status and renal function in pre-dialysis end-stage renal failure patients. *Nephrol Dial Transplant* 2001;16:776–782.
10. Jacob V, Le Carpentier JE, Salzano S, et al. IGF-1, a marker of undernutrition in hemodialysis patients. *Am J Clin Nutr* 1990;52:39–44.
11. Lowrie EG, Lew N. Death risk in hemodialysis patients: the predictive value of commonly measured variables and an evaluation of death rate differences between facilities. *Am J Kidney Dis* 1990;15:458–482.
12. Nelson EE, Hong CD, Pesce AL, et al. Anthropometric norms for the dialysis population. *Am J Kidney Dis* 1990;16:32–37.
13. Pollock CA, Allen BJ, Warden RA, et al. Total body nitrogen by neutron activation analysis in maintenance dialysis patients. *Am J Kidney Dis* 1990;16:38–45.
14. Rayner HC, Stroud DB, Salamon KM, et al. Anthropometry underestimates body protein depletion in hemodialysis patients. *Nephron* 1991;59:33–34.
15. Young GA, Kopple JD, Lindholm B, et al. Nutritional assessment of continuous ambulatory peritoneal dialysis patients. *Am J Kidney Dis* 1991;17:462–471.
16. Cianciaruso B, Brunori G, Kopple JD, et al. Cross-sectional comparison of malnutrition in continuous ambulatory peritoneal dialysis and hemodialysis patients. *Am J Kidney Dis* 1995;26:475–486.
17. Palop L, Martinez JA. Cross-sectional assessment of nutritional and immune status in renal patients undergoing continuous ambulatory peritoneal dialysis. *Am J Clin Nutr* 1997;66:498S–503S.
18. Marcen R, Teruel JL, de la Cal MA, et al. The impact of malnutrition in morbidity and mortality in stable haemodialysis patients. Spanish Cooperative Study of Nutrition in Hemodialysis. *Nephrol Dial Transplant* 1997;12:2324–2331.
19. Dwyer JT, Cunniff PJ, Maroni BJ, et al. The hemodialysis (HEMO) pilot study: Nutrition program and participant characteristics at baseline. *J Renal Nutr* 1998;8:11–20.
20. Aparicio M, Cano N, Chauveau P, et al. Nutritional status of haemodialysis patients: a French national cooperative study. French Study Group for Nutrition in Dialysis. *Nephrol Dial Transplant* 1999;14:1679–1686.
21. Chung SH, Na MH, Lee SH, et al. Nutritional status of Korean peritoneal dialysis patients. *Perit Dial Int* 1999;19 (Suppl 2):S517–522.
22. Park YK, Kim JH, Kim KJ, et al. A cross-sectional study comparing the nutritional status of peritoneal dialysis and hemodialysis patients. *J Ren Nutr* 1999;9:149–156.
23. Williams AJ, McArley A. Body composition, treatment time, and outcome in hemodialysis. *J Ren Nutr* 1999;9:157–162.
24. Young GA, Swanepoel CR, Croft MR, et al. Anthropometery and plasma valine, amino acids and protein in the nutritional assessment of hemodialysis patients. *Kidney Int* 1982;21:492–499.
25. Wolfson M, Strong CJ, Minturn D, et al. Nutritional status and lymphocyte function in maintenance hemodialysis patients. *Am J Clin Nutr* 1984;39:547–555.
26. Bergstrom J, Alvestrand A, Furst P. Plasma and muscle free amino acids in maintenance hemodialysis patients without protein malnutrition. *Kidney Int* 1990;38:108–114.
27. Oksa H, Ahonen K, Pasternack A, et al. Malnutrition in hemodialysis patients. *Scand J Urol Nephrol* 1991;25:157–161.
28. Qureshi AR, Alvestrand A, Danielsson A, et al. Factors predicting malnutrition in hemodialysis patients: a cross-sectional study. *Kidney Int* 1998;53:773–782.
29. Churchill DN, Taylor DW, Cook RJ, et al. Canadian hemodialysis morbidity study. *Am J Kidney Dis* 1992;19:214–234.
30. Comorbid conditions and correlations with mortality among

3,399 incident hemodialysis patients. *Am J Kidney Dis* 1992;20:32–38.
31. Rocco MV, Jordan JR, Burkart JM. The efficacy number as a predictor of morbidity and mortality in peritoneal dialysis patients. *J Am Soc Nephrol* 1993;4:1184–1191.
32. Iseki K, Uehara H, Nishime K, et al. Impact of the initial levels of laboratory variables on survival in chronic dialysis patients. *Am J Kidney Dis* 1996;28:541–548.
33. McCusker FX, Teehan BP, Thorpe KE, et al. How much peritoneal dialysis is necessary for maintaining a good nutritional status? *Kidney Int Suppl* 1996;56:S56–S61.
34. Barrett BJ, Parfrey PS, Morgan J, et al. Prediction of early death in end-stage renal disease patients starting dialysis. *Am J Kidney Dis* 1997;29:214–222.
35. Leavey SF, Strawderman RL, Jones CA, et al. Simple nutritional indicators as independent predictors of mortality in hemodialysis patients. *Am J Kidney Dis* 1998;31:997–1006.
36. Degoulet P, Legrain M, Reach I, et al. Mortality risk factors in patients treated by chronic hemodialysis: Report of the Diaphane Collaborative Study. *Nephron* 1982;31:103–110.
37. Acchiardo SR, Moore LW, Latour PA. Malnutrition as the main factor in morbidity and mortality of hemodialysis patients. *Kidney Int Suppl* 1983;16:S199–203.
38. Parker TF, Laird NM, Lowrie EG. Comparison of the study groups in the National Cooperative Dialysis Study and a description of morbidity, mortality, and patient withdrawal. *Kidney Int Suppl* 1983;13:S42–49.
39. Teehan BP, Schleifer CR, Brown JM, et al. Urea kinetic analysis and clinical outcome in CAPD: a five-year longitudinal study. *Adv Perit Dial* 1990;6:181–185.
40. Blake PG, Flowerdew G, Blake R, et al. Serum albumin in patients on continuous ambulatory peritoneal dialysis—predictors and correlations with outcomes. *J Am Soc Nephrol* 1993;3:1501–1510.
41. Goldwasser P, Mittman N, Antignani A, et al. Predictors of mortality in hemodialysis patients. *J Am Soc Nephrol* 1993;3:1613–1622.
42. Iseki K, Kawazoe N, Fukiyama K. Serum albumin is a strong predictor of death in chronic dialysis patients. *Kidney Int* 1993;44:115–119.
43. Owen WF Jr, Lew NL, Liu Y, et al. The urea reduction ratio and serum albumin concentration as predictors of mortality in patients undergoing maintenance hemodialysis. *N Engl J Med* 1993;14:1001–1006.
44. Collins AJ, Ma JZ, Umen A, et al. Urea index (Kt/V) and other predictors of hemodialysis patient survival. *Am J Kidney Dis* 1994;23:272–282.
45. Avram MM, Mittman N, Bonomini L, et al. Markers for survival in dialysis: a seven-year prospective study. *Am J Kidney Dis* 1995;26:209–219.
46. Davies SJ, Russell L, Bryan J, et al. Comorbidity, urea kinetics, and appetite in continuous ambulatory peritoneal dialysis patients: their interrelationship and prediction of survival. *Am J Kidney Dis* 1995;26:353–361.
47. Pollock CA, Ibels LS, Ayass W, et al. Total body nitrogen as a prognostic marker in maintenance dialysis. *J Am Soc Nephrol* 1995;6:86–88.
48. Culp K, Flanigan M, Lowrie EG, et al. Modeling mortality risk in hemodialysis patients using laboratory values as time-dependent co-variates. *Am J Kidney Dis* 1996;28:741–746.
49. Mailloux LU, Napolitano B, Bellucci AG, et al. The impact of co-morbid risk factors at the start of dialysis upon the survival of ESRD patients. *ASAIO J* 1996;42:164–169.
50. Arora P, Strauss BJ, Bronvnicar D, et al. Total body nitrogen predicts long-term mortality in hemodialysis patients—a single center experience. *Nephrol Dial Transplant* 1998;13:1731–1736.
51. Perez RA, Blake PG, Spanner E, et al. High creatinine excretion ratio predicts a good outcome in peritoneal dialysis patients. *Am J Kidney Dis* 2000;36:362–367.
52. Monteon FJ, Laidlaw SA, Shaib JK, et al. Energy expenditure in patients with chronic renal failure. *Kidney Int* 1986;30:741–747.
53. Kopple JD, Monteon FJ, Shaib JK. Effect of energy intake on nitrogen metabolism in nondialyzed patients with chronic renal failure. *Kidney Int* 1986;29:734–742.
54. Schneeweiss B, Graninger W, Stockenhuber F, et al. Energy metabolism in acute and chronic renal failure. *Am J Clin Nutr* 1990;52:596–601.
55. Avesani CM, Cuppari L, Silva AC, et al. Resting energy expenditure in pre-dialysis diabetic patients. *Nephrol Dial Transplant* 2001;16:556–565.
56. Kopple JD, Coburn JW. Metabolic studies of low protein diets in uremia. I. Nitrogen and potassium. *Medicine* 1973;52:583–595.
57. Mitch WE, Abras E, Walser M. Long-term effects of a new ketoacid-amino acid supplement in patients with chronic renal failure. *Kidney Int* 1982;22:48–53.
58. Goodship TH, Mitch WE, Hoerr RA, et al. Adaptation to low-protein diets in renal failure: leucine turnover and nitrogen balance. *J Am Soc Nephrol* 1990;1:66–75.
59. Masud T, Young VR, Chapman T, et al. Adaptive responses to very low protein diets: the first comparison of ketoacids to essential amino acids. *Kidney Int* 1994;45:1182–1192.
60. Alvestrand A, Ahlberg M, Fürst P, et al. Clinical results of long-term treatment with a low protein diet and a new amino acid preparation in patients with chronic uremia. *Clin Nephrol* 1983;19:67–73.
61. Walser M. Does prolonged protein restriction preceding dialysis lead to protein malnutrition at the onset of dialysis? *Kidney Int* 1993;44:1139–1144.
62. Tom K, Young VR, Chapman T, et al. Long-term adaptive responses to dietary protein restriction in chronic renal failure. *Am J Physiol* 1995;268:E668–677.
63. Chauveau P, Barthe N, Rigalleau V, et al. Outcome of nutritional status and body composition of uremic patients on a very low protein diet. *Am J Kidney Dis* 1999;34:500–507.
64. Maroni BJ, Staffeld C, Young VR, et al. Mechanisms permitting nephrotic patients to achieve nitrogen equilibrium with a protein-restricted diet. *J Clin Invest* 1997;99:2479–2487.
65. Tabakian A, Juillard L, Laville M, et al. Effects of recombinant growth factors on energy expenditure in maintenance hemodialysis patients. *Miner Electr Metab* 1998;24:273–278.
66. Ikizler TA, Wingard RL, Sun M, et al. Increased energy expenditure in hemodialysis patients. *J Am Soc Nephrol* 1996;7:2646–2653.
67. Olevitch LR, Bowers BM, DeOreo PB. Measurement of resting energy expenditure via indirect calorimetery during adult hemodialysis treatment. *J Renal Nutr* 1994;4:192–197.
68. Slomowitz LA, Monteon FJ, Grosvenor M, et al. Effect of energy intake on nutritional status in maintenance hemodialysis patients. *Kidney Int* 1989;35:704–711.
69. Ginn HE, Frost A, Lacy WW. Nitrogen balance in hemodialysis patients. *Am J Clin Nutr* 1968;21:385–393.
70. Kopple JD, Shinaberger JH, Coburn JW, et al. Optimal dietary protein treatment during chronic hemodialysis. *Trans Am Soc Artif Int Org* 1969;15:302–308.
71. Borah MF, Schonfeld PY, Gotch FA, et al. Nitrogen balance during intermittent dialysis therapy of uremia. *Kidney Int* 1978;14:491–500.
72. Lim VS, Flanigan MJ, Zavala DC, et al. Protective adaptation

of low serum triiodothyronine in patients with chronic renal failure. *Kidney Int* 1985;28:541–549.
73. Rao M, Sharma M, Juneja R, et al. Calculated nitrogen balance in hemodialysis patients: influence of protein intake. *Kidney Int* 2000;58:336–345.
74. Harter HR. Review of significant findings from the National Cooperative Dialysis Study and recommendations. *Kidney Int Suppl* 1983;13:S107–112.
75. Movilli E, Filippini M, Brunori G, et al. Influence of protein catabolic rate on nutritional status, morbidity and mortality in elderly uraemic patients on chronic hemodialysis: a prospective 3-year follow-up study. *Nephrol Dial Transplant* 1995;10: 514–518.
76. Movilli E, Mombelloni S, Gaggiotti M, et al. Effect of age on protein catabolic rate, morbidity and mortality in ureamic patients with adequate dialysis. *Nephrol Dial Transplant* 1993; 8:735–739.
77. Clinical practice guidelines for nutrition in chronic renal failure. K/DOQI, National Kidney Foundation. *Am J Kidney Dis* 2000; 35 (6 Suppl 2):S1–S140.
78. Panel on Micronutrients, Subcommittees on Upper Reference Levels of Nutrients and of Interpretation and Use of Dietary Reference Intakes, and the Standing Committee on the Scientific Evaluation of Dietary Reference Intakes. *Dietary reference intakes for vitamin A, vitamin K, arsenic, boron, chromium, copper, iodine, iron, manganese, molybdenum, nickel, silicon, vanadium and zinc.* Washington, DC: National Academy Press, 2002:29–43.
79. Bergstrom J, Furst P, Alvestrand A, et al. Protein and energy intake, nitrogen balance and nitrogen losses in patients treated with continuous ambulatory peritoneal dialysis. *Kidney Int* 1993;44:1048–1057.
80. Harty J, Conway L, Keegan M, et al. Energy metabolism during CAPD: a controlled study. *Adv Perit Dial* 1995;11:229–233.
81. Uribarri J, Leibowitz J, Dimaano F. Caloric intake in a group of peritoneal dialysis patients. *Am J Kidney Dis* 1998;32: 1019–1022.
82. Giordano C, De Santo G, Pluvio M, et al. Protein requirements of patients on CAPD: a study of nitrogen balance. *Int J Artif Org* 1980;3:11–14.
83. Blumenkrantz MJ, Kopple JD, Moran JK, et al. Metabolic balance studies and dietary protein requirements in patients undergoing continuous ambulatory peritoneal dialysis. *Kidney Int* 1982;21:849–861.
84. Ikizler TA, Greene JH, Wingard RL, et al. Spontaneous dietary and protein intake during progression of chronic renal failure. *J Am Soc Nephrol* 1995;6:1386–1391.
85. Mehrotra R, Saran R, Moore HL, et al. Toward targets for initiation of chronic dialysis. *Perit Dial Int* 1997;17:497–508.
86. Mehrotra R, Berman N, Alistwani A, et al. Improvement of nutritional status after initiation of maintenance hemodialysis. *Am J Kidney Dis* 2002;40:133–142.
87. Sargent JA, Gotch FA, Borah M, et al. Urea kinetics: a guide to nutritional management of renal failure. *Am J Clin Nutr* 1978;31:1696–1702.
88. Kopple JD, Berg R, Houser H, et al. Nutritional status of patients with different levels of chronic renal insufficiency. Modification of Diet in Renal Disease (MDRD) Study Group. *Kidney Int Suppl* 1989;27:S184–194.
89. Coggins CH, Dwyer JT, Greene T, et al. Serum lipid changes associated with modified protein diets: results from the feasibility phase of the Modification of Diet in Renal Disease Study. *Am J Kidney Dis* 1994;23:514–523.
90. Pollock CA, Ibels LS, Zhu FY, et al. Protein intake in renal disease. *J Am Soc Nephrol* 1997;8:777–783.
91. Jansen MAM, Korevaar JC, Dekker FW, et al. Renal function and nutritional status at the start of dialysis treatment. *J Am Soc Nephrol* 2001;12:157–163.
92. Saran R, Moore H, Mehrotra R, et al. Longitudinal evaluation of renal Kt/V urea of 2.0 as a threshold for initiation of dialysis. *ASAIO J* 1998;44:M677–681.
93. Kaysen GA, Stevenson FT, Depner TA. Determinants of albumin concentration in hemodialysis patients. *Am J Kidney Dis* 1997;29:658–668.
94. Kaysen GA, Dubin JA, Muller HG, et al. The acute-phase response varies with time and predicts serum albumin levels in hemodialysis patients. *Kidney Int* 2000;58:346–352.
95. Kaysen GA, Chertow GM, Adhikarla R, et al. Inflammation and dietary protein intake exert competing effects on serum albumin and creatinine in hemodialysis patients. *Kidney Int* 2001;60:333–340.
96. Pollock CA, Ibels LS, Caterson RJ, et al. Continuous ambulatory peritoneal dialysis. Eight years of experience at a single center. *Medicine* 1989;68:293–308.
97. Davies SJ, Phillips L, Griffiths AM, et al. Analysis of the effects of increasing delivered dialysis treatment to malnourished peritoneal dialysis patients. *Kidney Int* 2000;57:1743–1754.
98. Ge YQ, Wu ZL, Xu YZ, et al. Study on nutritional status of maintenance hemodialysis patients. *Clin Nephrol* 1998;50: 309–314.
99. Fung L, Pollock CA, Caterson RJ, et al. Dialysis adequacy and nutrition determine prognosis in continuous ambulatory peritoneal dialysis patients. *J Am Soc Nephrol* 1996;7:737–744.
100. Kloppenburg WD, Stegman CA, de Jong PE, et al. Relating protein intake to nutritional status in hemodialysis patients: how to normalize the protein equivalent of total nitrogen appearance. *Nephrol Dial Transplant* 1999;14:2165–2172.
101. Heidland A, Kult J. Long-term effects of essential amino acids supplementation in patients on regular dialysis treatment. *Clin Nephrol* 1975;3:234–239.
102. Piraino AJ, Firpo JJ, Powers DV. Prolonged hyperalimentation in catabolic chronic dialysis therapy patients. *JPEN J Parenter Enteral Nutr* 1981;5:463–477.
103. Bruno M, Bagnis C, Marangella M, et al. CAPD with an amino acid dialysis solution: a long-term, cross-over study. *Kidney Int* 1989;35:1189–1194.
104. Allman MA, Stewart PM, Tiller DJ, et al. Energy supplementation and the nutritional status of hemodialysis patients. *Am J Clin Nutr* 1990;51:558–562.
105. Cano N, Labastie-Coeyrehourq J, Lacombe P, et al. Perdialytic parenteral nutrition with lipids and amino acids in malnourished hemodialysis patients. *Am J Clin Nutr* 1990;52:726–730.
106. Tietze IN, Pedersen EB. Effect of fish protein supplementation on amino-acid profile and nutritional status in haemodialysis patients. *Nephrol Dial Transplant* 1991;6:948–954.
107. Schulman G, Wingard RL, Hutchison RL, et al. The effects of recombinant human growth hormone and intradialytic parenteral nutrition in malnourished hemodialysis patients. *Am J Kidney Dis* 1993;21:527–534.
108. Kopple JD, Bernard D, Messana J, et al. Treatment of malnourished CAPD patients with an amino acid based dialysate. *Kidney Int* 1995;47:1148–1157.
109. Jones M, Hagen T, Algrim Boyle C, et al. Treatment of malnutrition with 1.1% amino acid peritoneal dialysis solution: results of a multicenter study. *Am J Kidney Dis* 1998;32:761–769.
110. Kuhlmann MK, Schmidt F, Köhler H. High protein/energy vs. standard protein/energy nutritional regimen in the treatment of malnourished hemodialysis patients. *Miner Electr Metab* 1999;25:306–310.
111. Eustace JA, Coresh J, Kutchey C, et al. Randomized double-blind trial of oral essential amino acids for dialysis-associated hypoalbuminemia. *Kidney Int* 2000;57:2527–2538.

112. Lindsay RM, Spanner E. A hypothesis: The protein catabolic rate is dependent upon the type and amount of treatment in dialyzed uremic subjects. *Am J Kidney Dis* 1989;13:382–389.
113. Lysaght MJ, Pollock CA, Hallet MD, et al. The relevance of urea kinetic modeling to CAPD. *ASAIO Trans* 1989;35:784–790.
114. Bergstrom J, Alvestrand A, Lindholm B, et al. Relationship between Kt/V and protein catabolic rate (PCR) is different in continuous peritoneal dialysis and hemodialysis patients. *J Am Soc Nephrol* 1991;2:358.
115. Goodship TH, Passlick-Deetjen J, Ward MK, et al. Adequacy of dialysis and nutritional status in CAPD. *Nephrol Dial Transplant* 1993;8:1366–1371.
116. Nolph KD, Moore HL, Prowant B, et al. Cross sectional assessment of weekly urea and creatinine clearances and indices of nutrition in continuous ambulatory peritoneal dialysis patients. *Perit Dial Int* 1993;13:178–183.
117. Harty J, Boulton H, Faragher B, et al. The influence of small solute clearance on dietary protein intake in continuous ambulatory peritoneal dialysis patients: a methodologic analysis based on cross-sectional and prospective studies. *Am J Kidney Dis* 1996;28:535–560.
118. Uehlinger DE. Another look at the relationship between protein intake and dialysis dose. *J Am Soc Nephrol* 1996;7:166–168.
119. Lindsay R, Spanner E, Heienheim P, et al. Which comes first, Kt/V or PCR—chicken or egg? *Kidney Int* 1992;42 (suppl 3): S32–S37.
120. Ginsberg N, Fishbane D, Lynn R. The effect of improved dialytic efficiencies on measures of appetite in peritoneal dialysis patients. *J Renal Nutr* 1996;6:217–221.
121. Malhotra D, Tzamaloukas AH, Murata GH, et al. Serum albumin in continuous ambulatory peritoneal dialysis: its predictors and relationship to urea clearance. *Kidney Int* 1996;50: 243–249.
122. Mak S-K, Wong P-N, Lo K-Y, et al. Randomized prospective study of the effect of increased dialytic dose on nutritional and clinical outcome in continuous ambulatory peritoneal dialysis patients. *Am J Kidney Dis* 2000;36:105–114.
123. Harty J, Boulton H, Venning M, et al. Impact of increasing dialysis volume on adequacy targets: a prospective study. *J Am Soc Nephrol* 1997;8:1304–1310.
124. O'Sullivan DA, McCarthy JT, Kumar R, et al. Improved biochemical variables, nutrient intake, and hormonal factors in slow nocturnal hemodialysis: a pilot study. *Mayo Clin Proc* 1998;73:1035–1045.
125. Pierratos A, Ouwendyk M, Francoeur R, et al. Nocturnal hemodialysis: three year experience. *J Am Soc Nephrol* 1998;9: 859–868.
126. McPhatter LL, Lockridge RS Jr, Albert J, et al. Nightly home hemodialysis: improvement in nutrition and quality of life. *Adv Renal Rep Ther* 1999;6:358–365.
127. Kopple JD, Henry DA, Roberts CE, et al. *Relationship between nutritional status of patients undergoing maintenance hemodialysis and duration of dialysis therapy*. Milan, Italy: Wichtig Editore, 1981.
128. Chertow GM, Johansen KL, Lew N, et al. Vintage, nutritional status, and survival in hemodialysis patients. *Kidney Int* 2000; 57:1176–1181.
129. Chazot C, Laurent G, Charra B, et al. Malnutrition in long-term haemodialysis survivors. *Nephrol Dial Transplant* 2001; 16:61–69.
130. Suda T, Hiroshige K, Ohta T, et al. The contribution of residual renal function to overall nutritional status in chronic haemodialysis patients. *Nephrol Dial Transplant* 2000;15:396–401.
131. Caravaca F, Arrobas M, Dominguez C. Influence of residual renal function on dietary protein and caloric intake in patients on incremental peritoneal dialysis. *Perit Dial Int* 1999;19: 350–356.
132. López-Menchero R, Miguel A, García-Ramón R, Pérez-Contreras J, et al. Importance of residual renal function in continuous ambulatory peritoneal dialysis: its influence on different parameters of renal replacement treatment. *Nephron* 1999;83: 219–225.
133. Anderstam B, Mamoun AH, Sodersten P, et al. Middle-sized molecule fractions isolated from uremic ultrafiltrate and normal urine inhibit ingestive behavior in the rat. *J Am Soc Nephrol* 1996;7:2453–2460.
134. Mamoun AH, Södersten P, Anderstam B, et al. Evidence of splanchnic-brain signaling in inhibition of ingestive behavior by middle molecules. *J Am Soc Nephrol* 1999;10:309–314.
135. Marcus RG, Cohl E, Uribarri J. Middle molecule clearance does not influence protein intake in hemodialysis patients. *Am J Kidney Dis* 1998;31:491–494.
136. Grodstein GP, Harrison A, Roberts C, et al. Impaired gastric emptying in hemodialysis patients. *Kidney Int* 1979;16:952 A (abstr).
137. Brown-Cartwright D, Smith HJ, Feldman M. Gastric emptying of an indigestible solid in patients with end-stage renal disease on continuous ambulatory peritoneal dialysis. *Gastroenterology* 1988;95:49–51.
138. Bird NJ, Streather CP, O'Doherty MJ, et al. Gastric emptying in patients with chronic renal failure on continuous ambulatory peritoneal dialysis. *Nephrol Dial Transplant* 1994;9:287–290.
139. Kao CH, Hsu YH, Wang SJ. Delayed gastric emptying in patients with chronic renal failure. *Nucl Med Commun* 1996;17: 164–167.
140. Van Vlem B, Schoonjans R, Vanholder R, et al. Delayed gastric emptying in dyspeptic chronic hemodialysis patients. *Am J Kidney Dis* 2000;36:962–968.
141. Ko CW, Chang CS, Wu MJ, et al. Transient impact of hemodialysis on gastric myoelectrical activity of uremic patients. *Dig Dis Sci* 1998;43:1159–1164.
142. Lee SW, Song JH, Kim GA, et al. Effect of dialysis modalities on gastric myoelectrical activity in end-stage renal disease patients. *Am J Kidney Dis* 2000;36:566–573.
143. Wright RA, Clemente R, Wathen R. Gastric emptying in patients with chronic renal failure receiving hemodialysis. *Arch Intern Med* 1984;144:495–496.
144. Soffer EE, Geva B, Helman C, et al. Gastric emptying in chronic renal failure patients on hemodialysis. *J Clin Gastroenterol* 1987; 9:651–653.
145. Ross EA, Koo LC. Improved nutrition after detection and treatment of occult gastroparesis in nondiabetic dialysis patients. *Am J Kidney Dis* 1998;31:62–66.
146. Silang R, Regalado M, Cheng TH, et al. Prokinetic agents increase plasma albumin in hypoalbuminemic chronic dialysis patients with delayed gastric emptying. *Am J Kidney Dis* 2001; 37:287–293.
147. Kim DJ, Kang W-H, Kim HY, et al. The effect of dialysate dwell on gastric emptying time in patients on continuous ambulatory peritoneal dialysis. *Perit Dial Int* 1999;19 (suppl 2):S176–S178.
148. Zhang Y, Proenca R, Maffei M, et al. Positional cloning of the mouse obese gene and its human homologue. *Nature* 1994;372: 425–432.
149. Campfield LA, Smith FJ, Guisez Y, et al. Recombinant mouse OB protein: evidence for a peripheral signal linking adiposity and central neural networks. *Science* 1995;269:546–549.
150. Halaas JL, Gajiwala KS, Maffei M, et al. Weight-reducing effects of the plasma protein encoded by the obese gene. *Science* 1995; 269:543–546.
151. Pelleymounter MA, Cullen MJ, Baker MB, et al. Effects of the

obese gene product on body weight regulation in ob/ob mice. *Science* 1995;269:540–543.
152. Heimburger O, Lonnqvist F, Danielsson A, et al. Serum immunoreactive leptin concentration and its relation to the body fat content in chronic renal failure. *J Am Soc Nephrol* 1997;8: 1423–1430.
153. Young GA, Woodrow G, Kendall S, et al. Increased plasma leptin/fat ratio in patients with chronic renal failure: a cause of malnutrition? *Nephrol Dial Transplant* 1997;12:2318–2323.
154. Nordfors L, Lönnqvist F, Heimbürger O, et al. Low leptin gene expression and hyperleptinemia in chronic renal failure. *Kidney Int* 1998;54:1267–1275.
155. Fontan MP, Rodriguez-Carmona A, Cordido F, et al. Hyperleptinemia in uremic patients undergoing conservative management, peritoneal dialysis, and hemodialysis: A comparative analysis. *Am J Kidney Dis* 1999;34:824–831.
156. de Precigout V, Chauveau P, Delclaux C, et al. No change of hyperleptinemia despite a decrease in insulin concentration in patients with chronic renal failure on a supplemented very low protein diet. *Am J Kidney Dis* 2000;36:1201–1206.
157. Howard JK, Lord GM, Clutterbuck EJ, et al. Plasma immunoreactive leptin concentration in end-stage renal disease. *Clin Sci (Lond)* 1997;93:119–126.
158. Merabet E, Dagogo-Jack S, Coyne DW, et al. Increased plasma leptin concentration in end-stage renal disease. *J Clin Endocrinol Metab* 1997;82:847–850.
159. Sharma K, Considine RV, Michael B, et al. Plasma leptin is partly cleared by the kidney and is elevated in hemodialysis patients. *Kidney Int* 1997;51:1980–1985.
160. Dagogo-Jack S, Ovalle F, Landt M, et al. Hyperleptinemia in patients with end-stage renal disease undergoing continuous ambulatory peritoneal dialysis. *Perit Dial Int* 1998;18:34–40.
161. Johansen KL, Mulligan K, Tai V, et al. Leptin, body composition, and indices of malnutrition in patients on dialysis. *J Am Soc Nephrol* 1998;9:1080–1084.
162. Nishizawa Y, Shoji T, Tanaka S, et al. Plasma leptin level and its relationship with body composition in hemodialysis patients. *Am J Kidney Dis* 1998;31:655–661.
163. Odamaki M, Furuya R, Yoneyama T, et al. Association of the serum leptin concentration with weight loss in chronic hemodialysis patients. *Am J Kidney Dis* 1999;33:361–368.
164. Stenvinkel P, Lindholm B, Lonnqvist F, et al. Increases in serum leptin levels during peritoneal dialysis are associated with inflammation and a decrease in lean body mass. *J Am Soc Nephrol* 2000;11:1303–1309.
165. Koo JR, Pak KY, Kim KH, et al. The relationship between plasma leptin and nutritional status in chronic hemodialysis patients. *J Korean Med Sci* 1999;14:546–551.
166. Meyer C, Robson D, Rackovsky N, et al. Role of the kidney in human leptin metabolism. *Am J Physiol* 1997;273:E903–907.
167. Jensen MD, Møller N, Nair KS, et al. Regional leptin kinetics in humans. *Am J Clin Nutr* 1999;69:18–21.
168. Stenvinkel P, Heimbürger O, Lönnqvist F. Serum leptin concentrations correlate to plasma insulin concentrations independent of body fat content in chronic renal failure. *Nephrol Dial Transplant* 1997;12:1321–1325.
169. Fouque D, Juillard L, Lasne Y, et al. Acute leptin regulation in end-stage renal failure: the role of growth hormone and IGF-1 (see comments). *Kidney Int* 1998;54:932–937.
170. Kolaczynski JW, Nyce MR, Considine RV, et al. Acute and chronic effects of insulin on leptin production in humans: Studies in vivo and in vitro. *Diabetes* 1996;45:699–701.
171. Malmstrom R, Taskinen MR, Karonen SL, et al. Insulin increases plasma leptin concentrations in normal subjects and patients with NIDDM. *Diabetologia* 1996;39:993–996.
172. Kagan A, Haran N, Leschinsky L, et al. Leptin in CAPD patients: serum concentrations and peritoneal loss. *Nephrol Dial Transplant* 1999;14:400–405.
173. Kokot F, Adamczak M, Wiecek A. Plasma leptin concentration in kidney transplant patients during the early post-transplant period. *Nephrol Dial Transplant* 1998;13:2276–2280.
174. Landt M, Brennan DC, Parvin CA, et al. Hyperleptinaemia of end-stage renal disease is corrected by renal transplantation. *Nephrol Dial Transplant* 1998;13:2271–2275.
175. Arkouche W, Juillard L, Delawari E, et al. Peritoneal clearance of leptin in continuous ambulatory peritoneal dialysis (see comments). *Am J Kidney Dis* 1999;34:839–844.
176. Heimbürger O, Wang T, Lönnqvist F, et al. Peritoneal clearance of leptin in CAPD patients: impact of local insulin administration. *Nephrol Dial Transplant* 1999;14:723–727.
177. Tsujimoto Y, Shoji T, Tabata T, et al. Leptin in peritoneal dialysate from continuous ambulatory peritoneal dialysis patients (see comments). *Am J Kidney Dis* 1999;34:832–838.
178. Landt M, Parvin CA, Dagogo-Jack S, et al. Leptin elimination in hyperleptinaemic peritoneal dialysis patients. *Nephrol Dial Transplant* 1999;14:732–737.
179. Parry RG, Johnson DW, Carey DG, et al. Serum leptin correlates with fat mass but not dietary energy intake in continuous ambulatory peritoneal dialysis patients. *Perit Dial Int* 1998;18: 569–575.
180. Don BR, Rosales LM, Levine NW, et al. Leptin is a negative acute phase protein in chronic hemodialysis patients. *Kidney Int* 2001;59:1114–1120.
181. Hylander B, Barkeling B, Rossner S. Eating behavior in continuous ambulatory peritoneal dialysis and hemodialysis patients. *Am J Kidney Dis* 1992;20:592–597.
182. Hylander B, Barkeling B, Rossner S. Changes in patients' eating behavior: in the uremic state, on continuous ambulatory peritoneal dialysis treatment, and after transplantation. *Am J Kidney Dis* 1997;29:691–698.
183. Balaskas EV, Rodela H, Oreopoulos DG. Effects of intraperitoneal infusion of dextrose and amino acids on the appetite of rabbits. *Perit Dial Int* 1993;13:S490–498.
184. Mamoun AH, Anderstam B, Sodersten P, et al. Influence of peritoneal dialysis solutions with glucose and amino acids on ingestive behavior in rats. *Kidney Int* 1996;49:1276–1282.
185. Grodstein GP, Blumenkratz MJ, Kopple JD, et al. Glucose absorption during continuous ambulatory peritoneal dialysis. *Kidney Int* 1981;19:564–567.
186. United States Renal Data System. U.S. Department of Public Health and Human Services, Public Health Service. Bethesda, MD: National Institutes of Health, 2001.
187. United States Renal Data System. U.S. Department of Public Health and Human Services, Public Health Service. Bethesda, MD: National Institutes of Health, 1999.
188. Ikizler TA, Greene JH, Yenicesu M, et al. Nitrogen balance in hospitalized chronic hemodialysis patients. *Kidney Int Suppl* 1996;57:S53–S56.
189. United States Renal Data System. U.S. Department of Public Health and Human Services, Public Health Service. Bethesda, MD: National Institutes of Health, 1998.
190. Keane WF, Collins AJ. Influence of co-morbidity on mortality and morbidity in patients treated with hemodialysis. *Am J Kidney Dis* 1994;24:1010–1018.
191. Struijk DG, Krediet RT, Koomen GC, et al. The effect of serum albumin at the start of continuous ambulatory peritoneal dialysis treatment on patient survival. *Perit Dial Int* 1994;14:121–126.
192. Leavey SF, Strawderman RL, Young EW, et al. Cross-sectional and longitudinal predictors of serum albumin in hemodialysis patients. *Kidney Int* 2000;58:2119–2128.
193. Lorenzo V, Martin M, Rufino M, et al. Protein intake, control of serum phosphorus, and relatively low levels of parathyroid

hormone in elderly hemodialysis patients. *Am J Kidney Dis* 2001;37:1260–1266.

194. Lowrie EG, Lew NL, Huang WH. Race and diabetes as death risk predictors in hemodialysis patients. *Kidney Int* 1992;42: S22–S31.
195. Krieg RJ Jr, Santos F, Chan JC. Growth hormone, insulin-like growth factor and the kidney. *Kidney Int* 1995;48:321–336.
196. Ding H, Gao XL, Hirschberg R, et al. Impaired actions of insulin-like growth factor 1 on protein Synthesis and degradation in skeletal muscle of rats with chronic renal failure. Evidence for a postreceptor defect. *J Clin Invest* 1996;97: 1064–1075.
197. DeFronzo RA, Alvestrand A, Smith D, et al. Insulin resistance in uremia. *J Clin Invest* 1996;67:563–568.
198. Mak RH, Bettinelli A, Turner C, et al. The influence of hyperparathyroidism on glucose metabolism in uremia. *J Clin Endocrinol Metab* 1985;60:229–233.
199. Reaich D, Graham KA, Channon SM, et al. Insulin-mediated changes in PD and glucose uptake after correction of acidosis in humans with CRF. *Am J Physiol* 1995;268:E121–126.
200. Castellino P, Solini A, Luzi L, et al. Glucose and amino acid metabolism in chronic renal failure: effect of insulin and amino acids. *Am J Physiol* 1992;262:F168–176.
201. Chan W, Valerie KC, Chan JC. Expression of insulin-like growth factor-1 in uremic rats: growth hormone resistance and nutritional intake. *Kidney Int* 1993;43:790–795.
202. Tönshoff B, Edén S, Weiser E, et al. Reduced hepatic growth hormone (GH) receptor gene expression and increased plasma GH binding protein in experimental uremia. *Kidney Int* 1994; 45:1085–1092.
203. DeFronzo RA, Tobin JD, Rowe JW, et al. Glucose intolerance in uremia: quantification of pancreatic beta cell sensitivity to glucose and tissue sensitivity to insulin. *J Clin Invest* 1978;62: 425–435.
204. Fouque D, Peng SC, Kopple JD. Impaired metabolic response to recombinant insulin-like growth factor-1 in dialysis patients. *Kidney Int* 1995;47:876–883.
205. Sherwin RS, Bastl C, Finkelstein FO, et al. Influence of uremia and hemodialysis on the turnover and metabolic effects of glucagon. *J Clin Invest* 1976;57:722–731.
206. Moxley MA, Bell NH, Wagle SR, et al. Parathyroid hormone stimulation of glucose and urea production in isolated liver cells. *Am J Physiol* 1974;227:1058–1061.
207. Yonemura K, Fujimoto T, Fujigaki Y, et al. Vitamin D deficiency is implicated in reduced serum albumin concentrations in patients with end-stage renal disease. *Am J Kidney Dis* 2000; 36:337–344.
208. Kaptein EM, Feinstein EI, Massry SG. Thyroid hormone metabolism in renal diseases. *Contrib Nephrol* 1982;33:122–135.
209. Hara Y, May RC, Kelly RA, et al. Acidosis, not azotemia, stimulates branched-chain, amino acid catabolism in uremic rats. *Kidney Int* 1987;32:808–814.
210. May RC, Hara Y, Kelly RA, et al. Branched-chain amino acid metabolism in rat muscle: abnormal regulation in acidosis. *Am J Physiol* 1987;252:E712–718.
211. Mitch WE, Medina R, Grieber S, et al. Metabolic acidosis stimulates muscle protein degradation by activating the adenosine triphosphate-dependent pathway involving ubiquitin and proteasomes. *J Clin Invest* 1994;93:2127–2133.
212. Bailey JL, Wang X, England BK, et al. The acidosis of chronic renal failure activates muscle proteolysis in rats by augmenting transcription of genes encoding proteins of the ATP-dependent ubiquitin-proteasome pathway. *J Clin Invest* 1996;97:1447–1453.
213. Reaich D, Channon SM, Scrimgeour CM, et al. Ammonium chloride-induced acidosis increases protein breakdown and amino acid oxidation in humans. *Am J Physiol* 1992;263: E735–739.
214. Ballmer PE, McNurlan MA, Hulter HN, et al. Chronic metabolic acidosis decreases albumin synthesis and induces negative nitrogen balance in humans. *J Clin Invest* 1995;95:39–45.
215. Williams B, Hattersley J, Layward E, et al. Metabolic acidosis and skeletal muscle adaptation to low protein diets in chronic uremia. *Kidney Int* 1991;40:779–786.
216. Reaich D, Channon SM, Scrimgeour CM, et al. Correction of acidosis in humans with CRF decreases protein degradation and amino acid oxidation. *Am J Physiol* 1993;265:E230–235.
217. Graham KA, Reaich D, Channon SM, et al. Correction of acidosis in CAPD decreases whole body protein degradation (published erratum appears in *Kidney Int* 1997 May;51(5):1662). *Kidney Int* 1996;49:1396–1400.
218. Graham KA, Reaich D, Channon SM, et al. Correction of acidosis in hemodialysis decreases whole-body protein degradation. *J Am Soc Nephrol* 1997;8:632–637.
219. Lim VS, Yarasheski KE, Flanigan MJ. The effect of uraemia, acidosis, and dialysis treatment on protein metabolism: a longitudinal leucine kinetic study. *Nephrol Dial Transplant* 1998;13: 1723–1730.
220. Löfberg E, Wernerman J, Anderstam B, et al. Correction of acidosis in dialysis patients increases branched-chain and total essential amino acid levels in muscle. *Clin Nephrol* 1997;48: 230–237.
221. Dumler F, Falla P, Butler R, et al. Impact of peritoneal dialysis modality and acidosis on nutritional status in peritoneal dialysis patients. *Adv Perit Dial* 1998;14:205–208.
222. Uribarri J, Levin NW, Delmez J, et al. Association of acidosis and nutritional parameters in hemodialysis patients. *Am J Kidney Dis* 1999;34:493–499.
223. Papadoyannakis NJ, Stefanidis CJ, McGeown M. The effect of the correction of metabolic acidosis on nitrogen and potassium balance of patients with chronic renal failure. *Am J Clin Nutr* 1984;40:623–627.
224. Movilli E, Zani R, Carli O, et al. Correction of metabolic acidosis increases serum albumin concentrations and decreases kinetically evaluated protein intake in haemodialysis patients: a prospective study. *Nephrol Dial Transplant* 1998;13:1719–1722.
225. Stein A, Moorhouse J, Iles-Smith H, et al. Role of an improvement in acid-base status and nutrition in CAPD patients. *Kidney Int* 1997;52:1089–1095.
226. Tepper T, van der Hem GK, Klip HG, et al. Loss of amino acids during hemodialysis: effect of oral essential amino acid supplementation. *Nephron* 1981;29:25–29.
227. Wolfson M, Jones MR, Kopple JD. Amino acid losses during hemodialysis with infusion of amino acids and glucose. *Kidney Int* 1982;21:500–506.
228. Gutierrez A, Bergström J, Alvestrand A. Hemodialysis-associated protein catabolism with and without glucose in the dialysis fluid. *Kidney Int* 1994;46:814–822.
229. Ikizler TA, Flakoll PJ, Parker RA, et al. Amino acid and albumin losses during hemodialysis. *Kidney Int* 1994;46:830–837.
230. Kopple JD, Swendseid ME, Shinaberger JH, et al. The free and bound amino acids removed by hemodialysis. *Trans Am Soc Artif Intern Organs* 1973;19:309–313.
231. Kaplan AA, Halley SE, Lapkin RA, et al. Dialysate protein losses with bleach processed polysulphone dialyzers. *Kidney Int* 1995; 47:573–578.
232. Katirtzoglou A, Oreopoulos DG, Husdan H, et al. Reappraisal of protein losses in patients undergoing continuous ambulatory peritoneal dialysis. *Nephron* 1980;26:230–233.
233. Blumenkrantz MJ, Gahl GM, Kopple JD, et al. Protein losses during peritoneal dialysis. *Kidney Int* 1981;19:593–602.

234. Kopple JD, Blumenkrantz MJ, Jones MR, et al. Plasma amino acid levels and amino acid losses during continuous ambulatory peritoneal dialysis. *Am J Clin Nutr* 1982;36:395–402.
235. Kaysen GA, Schoenfeld PY. Albumin homeostasis in patients undergoing continuous ambulatory peritoneal dialysis. *Kidney Int* 1984;25:107–114.
236. Bannister DK, Acchiardo SR, Moore LW, et al. Nutritional effects of peritonitis in continuous ambulatory peritoneal dialysis (CAPD) patients. *J Am Diet Assoc* 1987;87:53–56.
237. Walser M, Hill SB, Ward L, et al. A crossover comparison of progression of chronic renal failure: ketoacids versus amino acids. *Kidney Int* 1993;43:933–939.
238. Aparicio M, Chauveau P, De Précigout V, et al. Nutrition and outcome on renal replacement therapy of patients with chronic renal failure treated by a supplemented very low protein diet. *J Am Soc Nephrol* 2000;11:708–716.
239. Chauveau P, Naret C, Puget J, et al. Adequacy of haemodialysis and nutrition in maintenance haemodialysis patients: clinical evaluation of a new on-line urea monitor. *Nephrol Dial Transplant* 1996;11:1568–1573.
240. Sharma M, Rao M, Jacob S, et al. A dietary survey in Indian hemodialysis patients. *J Ren Nutr* 1999;9:21–25.
241. Grzegorzewska AE, Mariak I, Dobrowolska-Zachwieja A, et al. Effects of amino acid dialysis solution on the nutrition of continuous ambulatory peritoneal dialysis patients. *Perit Dial Int* 1999;19:462–470.

12

MALNUTRITION AS A RISK FACTOR OF MORBIDITY AND MORTALITY IN PATIENTS UNDERGOING MAINTENANCE DIALYSIS

KAMYAR KALANTAR-ZADEH
JOEL D. KOPPLE

In the United States, there are currently more than 250,000 individuals with end-stage renal disease (ESRD) who are dependent on maintenance hemodialysis (MHD) or chronic peritoneal dialysis (CPD) treatment for their survival (1). According to the estimates of the United States Renal Data System (USRDS), the number of patients undergoing maintenance dialysis (MD) will approach one-half million or even higher by the year 2010. These patients experience lower quality of life, greater morbidity, higher hospitalization rates, and increased mortality as compared to the general population (1,2). The annual mortality rate among patients undergoing MD in the United States continues to remain unacceptably high (i.e., approximately 20%) despite many recent improvements in dialysis treatment (1,3).

Many reports indicate that in patients undergoing MD there is a high prevalence of protein-energy malnutrition (PEM) (up to 40% or more) and a strong association between PEM and greater morbidity and mortality (4–8). Such prevalence rates for PEM are reported to be equally high among MHD and CPD patients. Evidence indicates that nutritional decline begins before ESRD develops, often even when the reduction in glomerular filtration rate is modest, and it is likely that a decrease in dietary protein and energy intake plays an important role (5,9,10).

In highly industrialized, affluent countries, PEM is an uncommon cause of poor outcome in the general population, whereas *over*nutrition is associated with a greater risk of cardiovascular disease and has an immense epidemiologic impact on the burden of this disease and on shortened survival. In contrast, in patients undergoing MD *under*nutrition is one of the most common risk factors for adverse cardiovascular events (5,9,11,12). The terms "reverse epidemiology" (9,12–14) or "risk factor paradox (or reversal)" (15) underscore this paradoxical observation. These terms indicate that certain markers that predict a low likelihood of cardiovascular events and an improved survival in the general population, such as decreased body mass index and lower serum cholesterol, become risk factors for increased cardiovascular morbidity and death in patients undergoing MD. Moreover, some indicators of overnutrition actually predict improved outcome in patients undergoing MD (11, 12) (Fig. 12.1).

Many recent studies suggest that patients undergoing MD with PEM and especially with hypoalbuminemia have an increased prevalence of markers of inflammation, which may be associated with a decreased quality of life, higher risk of cardiovascular events, and increased morbidity and mortality (16–19). The nature of the relationships between PEM and inflammation and the degree of the independent or joint contributions of these two conditions to adverse outcomes have not been established unequivocally (9,20). It also is commonly believed that some comorbid conditions in patients undergoing MD may contribute to the development of PEM (21–23). Moreover, the number of months or years on dialysis, also referred to as "vintage" (24), is reported to influence nutritional status and, hence, outcome in patients undergoing MD.

Although patients undergoing MD are at increased risk for malnutrition of protein, energy, certain vitamins, macrominerals and trace elements, this discussion will focus on PEM because this type of malnutrition is most associated with poor outcome. This chapter reviews pertinent outcomes, the association between measures of outcome and nutritional status, and the current thinking concerning the pathophysiology for the poor outcome that is associated with PEM in patients undergoing MD.

PERTINENT OUTCOMES IN PATIENTS UNDERGOING MAINTENANCE DIALYSIS

In recent years, there has been much growth in *outcome research* in patients with ESRD. The aim of much of this

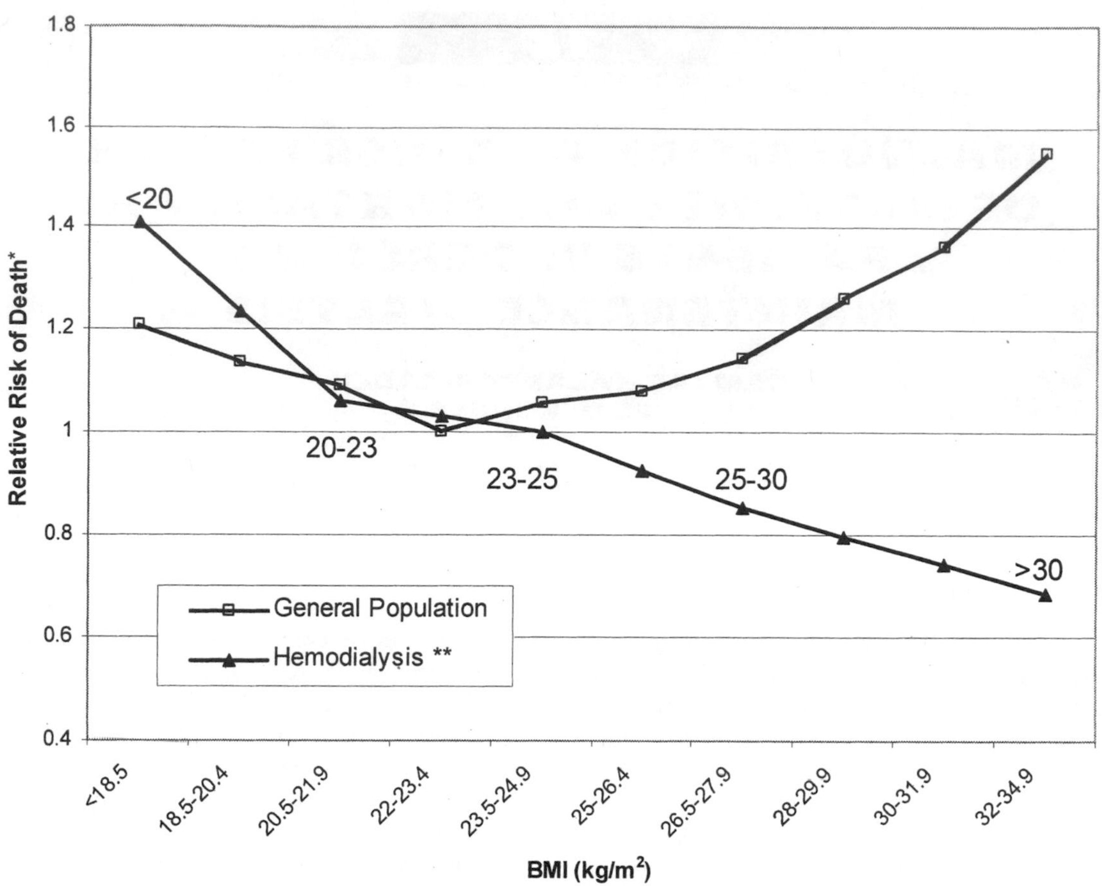

FIGURE 12.1. Reverse epidemiology of mortality risk factors in patients undergoing maintenance dialysis. Comparison between the effects of body mass index (BMI) on all-cause mortality in the general population (□) versus in the maintenance hemodialysis population (▲). *Note that each population has a different follow-up period: 14 years for the general population versus 4 years for hemodialysis patients. **BMI stratifications are different in two populations: X-axis is based on the original graph of the general population, and the original hemodialysis BMI subgroup ranges are printed additionally along the hemodialysis curve. (From Kalantar-Zadeh K, Block G, Humphreys M, et al. Reverse epidemiology of cardiovascular risk factor in maintenance dialysis patients. *Kidney Int* 2003;63(3):793–808, with permission.)

research has been to identify and define the scope and impact of modifiable and nonmodifiable risk factors in patients undergoing MD. These issues are of particular importance because these patients continue to consume a considerable portion of the Medicare budget, yet they have unacceptably poor outcome (3). Advances in statistical and epidemiologic methods, the availability of robust multivariate techniques that adjust for confounding and case-mix factors, and databases from large MD patient populations, including the USRDS (1) have contributed to the advances in this field. The data generated from these techniques and population-based studies suggest that both PEM and inflammation play important roles in poor outcome in patients undergoing MD.

Mortality

Mortality is the most definitive and objective outcome (25). The occurrence of death regardless of its etiology and type of surrounding circumstances (i.e., *all-cause mortality*) is usually used to evaluate death rate among patients undergoing MD (1). This, nevertheless, includes occasional rare deaths that may not be directly related to ESRD, such as homicide or motor-vehicle accidents. Despite such potential limitations, mortality remains the most objective and meaningful outcome in studies pertaining patients undergoing MD (25).

There is a high burden of cardiac disease and cardiovascular mortality in malnourished patients undergoing MD, accounting for more than 50% of deaths in these individuals (26,27). Hence, mortality of patients undergoing MD, currently about 20% per year in the United States, is not only much higher than that of the general population, but the proportion of deaths from cardiovascular diseases also may be much higher in this group (1,26,27).

Because of the heterogeneity of clinical and demographic characteristics of patients undergoing MD, *standardized mortality rates* (SMR) are used to remove the case-mix effects of gender, age, and race and the underlying causes of kidney disease such as diabetes mellitus (1,28). Some of the variability in the reported relationships between nutrition and inflammation and mortality may be the result of the statistical model used. For example, a mortality odds ratio based on logistic regression analysis does not control for the duration of time to death, whereas survival models such as Cox proportional hazard analysis do.

Hospitalization

The length and frequency of hospitalizations are linked closely to morbidity, and patients undergoing MD have a much higher rate of hospitalization as compared to the general population—on average 10 to 15 days per year for each patient treated with MD in the United States (1). Hospitalization rates are commonly used outcome measures (1,18). Hospitalization, however, is a less objective outcome measure when compared to mortality because the decision to admit, retain, or discharge a patient in the hospital can be affected by subjective and nonstandardized factors, such as regional insurance or health care policies (25). Moreover, many hospital admissions in both MHD and CPD patients are dialysis-access–related, which may or may not be a direct consequence of PEM or chronic inflammation. It, however, has been argued that patients undergoing MD with malnutrition-inflammation complex syndrome are more prone to develop access failure events (19).

In most outcome studies, the *hospitalization frequency* (e.g., total number of hospital admissions) and/or the total number of *hospitalization days* are calculated for a given period (e.g., within a 12-month period) (1). Simple or multivariate regression analyses can be used to evaluate the effect of measures of PEM on hospitalization rates and to estimate correlation coefficients (19,29). Alternatively, Poisson regression models can be used to estimate the hospitalization *rate ratios* and their 95% confidence intervals (CI) to study the effect of changes in nutritional measures on hospitalization (29). Moreover, for study subgroups or sample sizes with infrequent hospitalization, *time to first hospitalization* within a predetermined interval can be analyzed using survival-like models (30). The USRDS reports national ESRD hospitalization rates in this manner as *standardized hospitalization ratios* (SHR), similar to mortality rates (SMR). In calculating the SHR, the first hospitalization event for each individual per year is considered and the subsequent hospitalizations during this interval are ignored, which may be a limitation of SHR.

Quality of Life

Monitoring patient's functional status and the subjective sense of well-being, together known as quality of life (QOL) measurements, is of particular importance in patients with ESRD because the physical and emotional debility experienced by patients with PEM undergoing MD can be severe (31–33). The QOL measurements have become an important outcome measure and are relied on heavily as a key outcome not only by physicians and scientists but also by the U.S. Food and Drug Administration and other health policy authorities. Although QOL measures are subjective, studies repeatedly have shown that these measures are reproducible and reliable predictors of prospective mortality and hospitalizations in patients undergoing MD (18).

A number of instruments have been used to assess sense of well-being and functional and health status in rather broad categories, whereas some others have a more limited focus. Some of these tools have been validated and even modified for patients undergoing MD (18,33). The Karnofsky score is based on a simple questionnaire and assesses the functional status (34). The Short Form Health Survey with 36 questions (SF36) is one of the most commonly used instruments for QOL evaluation in patients undergoing MD (18,33). It is used both as a stand-alone measure of QOL and as a core component of several major assessment tools including the Kidney Disease Quality of Life (KDQOL™) survey instrument, which has been validated for patients undergoing MD (35). The Beck Depression Inventory (BDI) is another frequently used self-administered QOL questionnaire, which focuses on the presence or degree of depression among patients undergoing MD (36).

Other Pertinent Outcome Measures

The nature (infection, occlusion, stenosis) and frequency of dialysis access complications and the survival of different dialysis access modalities (fistula, graft, and tunneled catheter) may have some association with the nutritional and inflammatory processes in patients undergoing MD and, hence, can be analyzed as an outcome (37–39). The degree of refractoriness of anemia in patients undergoing MD is another suggested outcome (19,39,40). The ESRD-associated anemia is a multifactorial disorder that can be managed relatively successfully by recombinant erythropoietin (EPO) and iron therapy. The EPO and iron requirement to maintain the recommended hemoglobin concentration (11 to 12 g/L) may increase when inflammation and/or malnutrition is present (40–43). The ratio of the EPO dose to the hematocrit for each patient is referred to as the "EPO resistance index" (37). Changes over time in this index can be used as both a risk factor and an outcome measure. The EPO index is higher in patients undergoing MD with malnutrition (43), hepatitis-C virus infection (38), and high serum C-reactive protein (CRP) values (37,44).

ASSOCIATION OF MEASURES OF NUTRITION WITH OUTCOME

Many studies describe significant correlations between measures of PEM and such clinical outcomes as worsened QOL and increased rates of hospitalization and mortality in patients undergoing MD. As is discussed in this chapter and at greater length in Chapter 13, some indicators of PEM also may reflect the presence or the severity of inflammation (19,27,45,46). Measures of PEM in patients undergoing MD can be divided into four major categories, which are listed in Table 12.1 along with an indication of whether they predict hospitalization or mortality. The first category denotes measures of dietary protein and energy intake, which can be analyzed either directly (e.g., by means of diet records and questionnaires) or indirectly based on total nitrogen appearance. The second category includes methods to estimate body composition (e.g., based on body weight and size, caliper anthropometry, or energy-beam emission). Laboratory measures and composite-scoring systems based on nutritional markers comprise the third and fourth categories, respectively.

Each of these methods has both practical values and limitations. For example, serum albumin, transferrin, and prealbumin are negative acute-phase reactants and may reflect inflammation (46). The nutritional scoring systems also may reflect the severity of illness in patients undergoing MD (43). During acute catabolic states, the urea nitrogen appearance may increase transiently independent of food intake (47). Diet records are subject to wide within-person variability, and caliper anthropometrics are subject to errors due to interobserver and intraobserver variability (48). Finally, despite the abundance of nutritional methods and the

TABLE 12.1. ASSESSMENT TOOLS THAT HAVE BEEN USED TO EVALUATE PROTEIN-ENERGY MALNUTRITION (PEM) IN PATIENTS UNDERGOING MAINTENANCE DIALYSIS AS THEY RELATE TO OUTCOME

A. Nutritional Intake	**Mortality**	**Hospitalization**
A.1. Direct assessment: diet recalls, diaries with interview, and food-frequency questionnaires	(82)	(88)
A.2. Indirect assessment: based on urea nitrogen appearance: nPNA (nPCR)	(63,66,67)	(52,53,63–65)
B. Body Composition	**Mortality**	**Hospitalization**
B.1. Weight-based measures: BMI; weight-for-height; and edema-free, fat-free weight	(4,11,68,69,164)	(11,164)
B.2. Other anthropometrics: skinfold (trlceps, biceps, etc.) and arm-muscle circumference	(56,115)	No relevant publication detected
B.3. Total body elements: total body nitrogen and potassium	(165,166)	No relevant publication detected
B.4. Energy-beam methods: DEXA, BIA, NIR	(79)	(19,86)
C. Laboratory Values (serum levels)	**Mortality**	**Hospitalization**
C.1. Visceral proteins/negative acute-phase reactants:		
Albumin	(4,8,64,80–85,98,101, 167–171)	(19,64,85–88,168,169,172)
Prealbumin (transthyretin)	(95,170,173)	(86)
Transferrin	(85)	(85,86)
C.2. Lipids: cholesterol, other lipids, and lipoproteins	(68,98,101) (19)	(19)
C.3. Somatic proteins and nitrogen surrogates:		
Creatinine	(81,83,97,98,101,170)	(86)
SUN	(63,68,98,174)	(63,64)
C.4. Positive acute-phase reactants and cytokines:		
CRP	(104–106)	(86)
Others: IL, TNF-α, SAA, ferritin	(85,107,175)	(85)
C.5. Blood cell counts: total lymphocyte count	(80,81,87)	No relevant publication detected
D. Nutritional Scoring Systems	**Mortality**	**Hospitalization**
D.1. Conventional SGA and its derivatives (MIS, DMS, CANUSA, etc.)	(7,19,116)	(19,116)
D.2. Non-SGA composite scores: HD-PNI, others (Wolfson, Merkus, Merckman)	(56,118,176)	(118,176)

nPNA, normalized protein nitrogen appearance; nPCR, normalized protein catabolic rate; BMI, body mass index; DEXA, dual energy x-ray absorptiometry; BIA, bioelectrical impedance analysis; NIR, near infrared interactance; SUN, serum urea nitrogen; IGF-1, insulinlike growth factor 1; CRP, C-reactive protein; IL, interleukin (e.g., IL-1 and IL-6); TNF-α, tumor necrosis factor alpha; SAA, serum amyloid A; SGA, subjective global assessment of nutritional status; MIS, malnutrition inflammation score; DMS, dialysis malnutrition score; CANUSA, Canada–USA study-based modification of the SGA; HD-PNI, hemodialysis prognostic nutritional index.

[a]SUN/creatinine ratio was studied.

[b]Study included patients with chronic kidney disease (pre-end-stage renal disease).

many studies of nutritional status in patients undergoing MD, there is still no consensus as to what are the best measures of the nutritional status in these individuals. This problem is compounded because many of these measures have little or no association with each other (49). For example, an obese patient being treated with MD may have hypoalbuminemia, and decreased body fat may be seen in a patient who has normal serum albumin and transferrin.

Nutrient Intake and Outcome

Diet records (diaries) with or without interviews and food recalls examine the food intake over relatively short intervals of time (i.e., usually from 1 or 2 days to one a week). They are historically among the first and most commonly used tools to assess directly the intake of protein and energy and other nutrients in patients undergoing MD. However, they are subject to wide within-person variability because of their restricted time frame and patient unreliability (50,51). The National Cooperative Dialysis Study (NCDS) was one of the first large-scale studies that examined the diet intake in patients undergoing MD; 165 individuals were monitored with repeated 5-day food records (52–54). Somewhat earlier, Thunberg et al. (55) used 3-day dietary recalls to assess food intake in 58 patients being treated with MHD. Wolfson et al. (56) used dietary records and other nutritional measures to assess 30 clinically stable male dialysis veterans who were followed over an average of 43 months. By constructing a composite score based on such nutritional measures, the latter investigators showed that the death rate in the "malnourished" group was higher than among normally nourished patients undergoing MD (56).

Food frequency questionnaires (FFQ) comprise a set of questions about an individual's food intake history and often give multiple-choice options for the answers. Compared to diet records and recalls, the FFQ questions provide data for much more extended intervals (i.e., several weeks, months, or even years), but the data generated may be less accurate (57). The FFQ has been used extensively in epidemiologic studies to evaluate the food intake among diverse populations and is a valuable tool for large cohorts and case-control studies (58). The pattern and type of foods and nutrients can be assessed rather accurately; data concerning total food and nutrient intake tend to be less reliable. The use of FFQ in patients undergoing MD has been restricted to a few cross-sectional studies with small samples. Facchini et al. used Block's FFQ in 85 patients undergoing dialysis and concluded that patients with ESRD ingest an atherogenic diet (59). Kalantar-Zadeh et al. used Block's FFQ in 30 patients undergoing MHD and 30 nondialytic controls and found that the patients treated with MHD consumed abnormally low amounts of vitamin C, potassium, and fiber (57). Preliminary data of the authors of this chapter indicate that FFQ-based data concerning the quantity and type of nutrients ingested may be associated with outcome in patients undergoing dialysis (unpublished data).

The normalized protein equivalent of total nitrogen appearance (nPNA), also known as normalized protein catabolic rate (nPCR), is believed to reflect the daily protein intake in patients undergoing MD and is among the monthly reported laboratory measures in many dialysis centers in the United States. The nPNA, which may be confounded as a result of its mathematical coupling with Kt/V (60), has been shown in many studies (including the NCDS [52–54]) but not in all reports (60–62) to be a predictor of hospitalization (52,53,63–65) and mortality (63,66,67) in patients undergoing MD. Some studies have shown that nPCR is not associated with serum albumin but is still correlated with clinical outcome (64). Even among patients undergoing MD who have a reportedly adequate Kt/V (>1.20), there is a strong association between the nPNA and outcome with dialysis outcome (30). In this latter study, 122 patients undergoing MHD with a delivered Kt/V or more than 1.20 at the start of the study were followed for 12 months. Serum albumin and nPNA were the only variables with significant correlations with both mortality and three measures of hospitalization (i.e., hospitalization days, frequency of hospitalization, and time to first hospital admission) (30).

Body Composition and Outcome

The postdialysis (dry) weight, which usually is obtained after each hemodialysis treatment among patients undergoing MHD or after emptying the abdominal dwell in patients undergoing peritoneal dialysis, is an easy and reliable measure of nutritional status in patients undergoing MD and is a predictor of outcome (4,7,11,68,69) (Fig. 12.1). However, weight must be standardized by height or other confounding factors such as gender or race. Kopple et al. (70) reported a significant correlation between standardized body weight (i.e., weight-for-height) and survival in 12,965 patients undergoing MHD. The investigators showed that body weight-for-height was an independent predictor of higher mortality in those patients undergoing MHD who were in the lower 50th percentile for this measurement. In another study of 3,607 patients undergoing MHD (4), the body mass index (BMI) (i.e., weight in kg divided by height in meters squared) was shown to be a strong, independent predictor of mortality. BMI remained a death risk factor for up to 5 years after the date of measurement with a relative mortality rate of 0.67 for each BMI unit *increase*; these epidemiologic associations indicate the protective effect of increased weight on outcome in patients undergoing MD (4).

These and other similar findings demonstrating a deleterious effect of lower body weight on outcome in patients undergoing MD are consistent with the theory of "reverse epidemiology" in patients undergoing MD (9,15) (see earlier and Figure 12.1). Studies in normal individuals denote that, unlike in patients undergoing MD, an increased, and not a decreased, BMI or weight-for-height is correlated with higher mortality (58). Several recent studies based on large sample sizes have indicated the same reversed correlation between weight and outcome in MHD and CPD patients in the United States and Europe and Japan (12). Some studies in the general population describe a left-sided domination of the "J" or "U" curve effect, which slightly resembles the epidemiologic association observed in patients undergoing MD (Fig. 12.1) (12,71). The effect of weight on QOL also may be "J" or "U" shaped. Although many studies have shown that malnourished patients undergoing MD with decreased weight have a worse QOL, a study in 2001 showed that patients undergoing MHD with a higher BMI and body fat percentage had less favorable QOL scores as well (18). This suggests that despite the survival advantages of obese patients undergoing MD, their obesity may interfere with their sense of well-being or daily activities.

Caliper anthropometry is a simple method to estimate body composition based on measuring skinfolds and extremity muscle circumference. Compared to weight- and height-based measures, skinfold and muscle mass measurements are less precise and have wider coefficients of variation, even if the anthropometrist is meticulous and well trained (72). However, they remain among classic nutritional measures for large-scale epidemiologic studies of nutritional status. Chazot et al. (73) showed that in patients undergoing MHD for more than 20 years, the arm-muscle circumference and triceps skinfold thickness were lower as compared to age- and gender-matched patients undergoing MHD with less than 5 years of vintage. To the authors' knowledge, a direct association between caliper-based measures and dialysis outcome has not been reported. However, body composition measurements and composite-based scoring systems that are based on caliper anthropometry occasionally have been shown to correlate with morbidity and mortality in patients undergoing MD (see later in this chapter).

Energy-beam methods measure body composition by x-ray, electric current, or light emission and are the foundation of dual-energy x-ray absorptiometry (DEXA), bioelectrical impedance analysis (BIA), and near infrared interactance (NIR), respectively. The DEXA has been shown to have a high degree of precision and accuracy in most validation studies (74). Dumler et al. reported that multiple compartment measurement by DEXA provided the best current "gold standard" for body composition analysis in patients undergoing MD (75). A limitation of DEXA in patients undergoing MHD is its inability to differentiate between muscle mass with normal water content and excess water (74,75). DEXA should be performed as close as feasible following the completion of a dialysis session to avoid the effects of excess water loss or gain during or between the dialysis treatments. The same limitation pertains to BIA, a measurement that may vary widely as a result of fluctuations in total body water in patients undergoing MD (74–76). However, NIR measurements, although less precise, appear to be independent of water status (77,78). Among the energy-beam measurements of body composition, so far only the BIA has been shown to be associated with dialysis outcome. Chertow et al. (79) conducted a cohort study in 3,009 adult patients undergoing MHD from 101 outpatient dialysis units who were followed for up to 12 months. Patients with narrow (low) BIA phase angle experienced an increased relative risk (RR) of death. The RRs for a phase angle less than 4 degrees remained statistically significant after adjusting for age, gender, race, serum albumin and creatinine concentrations, and dialysis intensity (phase angle less than 3 degrees, RR 2.2, 95% CI 1.6 to 3.1; 3 to 4 degrees, RR 1.3, 95% CI 1.0 to 1.7, compared with patients with a phase angle of 4 degrees or greater). More prospective studies to examine the association of measurements of body composition and dialysis outcome currently are in progress.

Laboratory Measures and Outcome

Among visceral proteins, serum albumin is the most studied laboratory measure in outcome studies in patients undergoing MD. Many studies with valid methodologies and robust multivariate techniques show strong significant correlations between serum albumin concentration and mortality (4,8, 19,80–84), hospitalization (19,85–88), and QOL (18) in both MHD and CPD patients. The effect of serum albumin on survival has been shown to remain significant even up to 12 years of follow-up (89). The controversy exists, however, as to whether serum albumin is a *nutritional* measure. Many studies by Kaysen and others point out the role of serum albumin as a negative acute-phase reactant (16,90, 91). Struijk et al. (92) studied serum albumin in 61 patients treated with CPD who were followed for 2 years. Although serum albumin was associated with survival in univariate analysis, in a multivariate model that was controlled for age, hemoglobin, and presence of systemic diseases, serum albumin was no longer a statistically significant predictor of mortality. Serum albumin was lower in patients with systemic disease, highlighting the controversy regarding the use of serum albumin as a measure of nutrition, rather than as a nonspecific marker of comorbid conditions and/or inflammation (see also Chapters 13 and 15). At the least, PEM may reduce serum albumin concentrations to about 3.0 g/dL, if not lower, but very low serum albumin levels (e.g., 2.0 g/dL or less) appear to require the presence of inflammation, albumin losses (e.g., loss of albumin into the urine, gastrointestinal tract or through peritoneal dialysis), or liver failure (9).

Serum prealbumin and transferrin also have been used to measure nutritional status in patients undergoing MD (93). A theoretic advantage over serum albumin is their shorter half-lives—1.8 and 8 days, respectively (43). Hence, these two proteins are reported to be early predictors of changes in serum albumin and nutritional status (94). In a study of more than 1,600 patients undergoing MHD, serum prealbumin was inversely related to mortality, with a relative risk reduction of 6% per 1 mg/dL increase in prealbumin, even after adjusting for case mix, serum albumin, and other nutritional indicators (95). Prealbumin also is called transthyretin because it binds to (and carries) thyroid hormone and retinol-binding protein. Serum prealbumin is elevated in renal insufficiency probably because renal degradation of retinol-binding protein decreases when the kidney fails (95). Serum prealbumin concentrations associated with the lowest mortality risk in patients undergoing MD are about 30 mg/dL or greater. Because in individuals with renal insufficiency who do not have ESRD serum prealbumin may vary according to the degree of renal failure, this protein is probably not a good measure of nutritional status in the latter individuals (93).

Serum transferrin, as measured by total iron-binding capacity, may be a survival predictor in patients undergoing MHD (85). However, serum transferrin levels are affected by their iron stores (43). It also should be noted that, as with serum albumin, both serum transferrin and prealbumin are negative acute-phase reactants (96), and, hence, the same controversy involves the role of these latter proteins as indicators of nutritional status.

Serum creatinine reflects a somatic protein and particularly muscle-protein content; therefore it is also an indicator of the nutritional status in patients undergoing MD (81,83,97,98). There is a strong association between decreased serum creatinine concentrations and increased mortality in both MHD (98–100) and CPD patients (99,100). Paradoxically, in the general population, an *elevated* serum creatinine is a risk factor for adverse cardiovascular events and mortality—a phenomenon that can be regarded as yet another example of the "reverse epidemiology" (12) (see earlier in this chapter). Serum urea nitrogen (SUN), a rather imprecise indicator of protein intake and total nitrogen appearance, is also an indicator of outcome in patients undergoing MD (63,68,98). The major determinant of total nitrogen appearance is the urea nitrogen appearance. Urea is the major metabolite of protein and amino acid degradation. Thus the net rate of urea production correlates closely with net protein degradation (see Chapters 15 and 23). This relationship may be stronger in patients undergoing MD because they excrete little or no ammonia in the urine so a greater fraction of the nitrogen released from degraded protein and amino acids is converted to urea. Both serum creatinine and SUN can be affected by the dose of dialysis treatment and residual renal function, and epidemiology of these compounds should be adjusted for these factors.

Lower serum cholesterol is associated with poor outcome in patients undergoing MD (68,98,101,102). Iseki et al. reported a "U"-shaped correlation between serum cholesterol and poor outcome in patients undergoing MD in that not only low (less than 150 mg/dL) but also high serum cholesterol levels (greater than 220 mg/dl) are associated with increased mortality in Japanese patients undergoing MHD (Fig. 12.2) (102). However, in American patients undergoing MHD, hypocholesterolemia appears to have a more dominant effect on mortality than hypercholesterolemia (98). Such findings provide additional evidence for the "reverse epidemiology" theory described in patients undergoing MD, as compared to the general population in whom a lower serum cholesterol is a marker of improved survival (12,14). The effect of other lipid components, however, appears to be similar to that of general population; increased serum low-density lipoprotein or lipoprotein(a), for instance, are associated with a poor outcome in patients undergoing MD (14,103).

Many other laboratory measures that are considered to be markers of inflammation or cardiovascular disease may

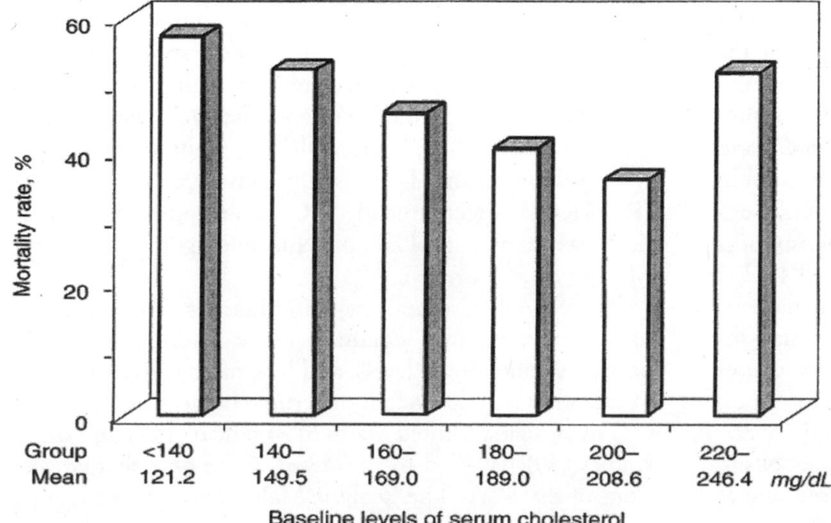

FIGURE 12.2. Relationship between mortality rate and subgroups of baseline levels of serum cholesterol. Cohort of chronic hemodialysis patients (n = 1,167) was followed prospectively for 10 years. (From Iseki K, Yamazato M, Tozawa M, et al. Hypocholesterolemia is a significant predictor of death in a cohort of chronic hemodialysis patients. *Kidney Int* 2002;61(5):1887–1893, with permission.)

be related indirectly to PEM. Serum CRP, interleukins (IL), and other positive acute-phase reactants and proinflammatory cytokines have been studied with regard to their possible associations with PEM and poor outcome in patients undergoing MD (104–106). Elevated CRP is reported to be more common in malnourished patients undergoing MD (20) and to be associated with erythropoietin resistance (37) and mortality (104). Catabolic cytokines, including tumor necrosis factor-alpha (TNF-α), IL-1β, and IL-6, are markers of inflammation in patients undergoing MD and are associated with increased risk of death (107,108). Abdullah et al. showed that TNF-α levels were higher in malnourished patients undergoing MD and have a negative correlation with their mid-arm muscle circumference (108). Bologa et al. reported that IL-6 was a strong predictor of dialysis mortality among patients undergoing MD as compared to other proinflammatory cytokines (109). Serum ferritin, another positive acute-phase reactant and an indicator of iron stores, correlates with the degree of malnutrition (43) and may predict hospitalization and mortality (85) as well as resistance to erythropoietin (37) in patients undergoing MHD. Serum levels of insulinlike growth factor-I (IGF-I) correlate with protein intake, estimated from the nPNA, in patients undergoing MHD (110). Some studies suggest a low level of correlation between hyperleptinemia and measures of PEM (111). A cross-sectional study of 117 patients undergoing MHD paradoxically found a lower plasma homocysteine level in patients with adverse cardiovascular events; this association may be related to the higher prevalence of PEM and hypoalbuminemia in this group of patients undergoing MHD (112). It may represent another example of the "reverse epidemiology."

Several serum electrolytes and solutes may be affected by nutritional intake. Serum potassium, calcium, phosphorus, bicarbonate, and the anion gap may not necessarily be affected by protein-energy nutritional status, but abnormal serum levels may occur in circumstances where low nutrient intake plays a role (98). Most of these measures also may be altered by nonnutritional factors, and clinical judgment is necessary to accurately evaluate the significance of the aberration. For example, serum phosphorus and calcium may vary based on the quality and quantity of the phosphorus binders. Patients with a low daily intake of protein and energy often have low intakes of phosphorus and potassium and consequently low serum values of these elements. Both very low and very high concentrations of serum phosphorus and potassium, according to some (98) but not all studies (113), are associated with poor outcome in patients undergoing MD. However, high-protein intake may increase the generation of acidic compounds with a consequent lowered serum bicarbonate and increased anion gap. Hence, a high-protein intake increases the likelihood of acidemia and a propensity for increased protein catabolism. High-protein diets also are associated with increased probability of survival, possibly because such patients have better nutritional status and/or because an increased appetite indicates greater health (114). Finally, although not a serum chemistry, total lymphocyte count (TLC) also has been used as an indicator of PEM (81). The Spanish Cooperative Study of Nutrition in Hemodialysis found that TLC and serum albumin were the only two nutritional measures that were associated with morbidity and mortality in patients undergoing MHD (87).

Nutritional Scoring Systems and Outcome

Because various nutritional measures may independently predict outcome and may assess different aspects of nutritional status, several researchers have tried to develop a composite nutritional score. Ideally, such a score would not only reflect the overall nutritional status of an MD patient but would predict outcome. Wolfson et al. (56) introduced a composite score based on body weight, mid-arm muscle circumference, and serum albumin and found that 70% of patients undergoing MHD were malnourished. Marckmann et al. (115) developed a nutritional scoring system based on serum transferrin, relative body weight, triceps skinfold, and mid-arm muscle circumference. They studied 16 patients treated with peritoneal dialysis and 32 patients undergoing MHD and reported that those patients with the worst initial composite score were more likely to die during a 24-month follow-up.

The subjective global assessment (SGA) of nutritional status was designed to evaluate surgical patients primarily with gastrointestinal diseases (43). It has been used in a number of epidemiologic studies and clinical trials in patients undergoing MD (43). In initial studies, the original techniques for assessing SGA were used. The techniques since have been modified to more effectively evaluate the nutritional status of patients with renal failure. SGA is discussed more extensively in Chapter 15. The SGA is significantly correlated with morbidity and mortality among patients undergoing MD (7,116). Some studies suggest that the SGA measures the degree of sickness as well as nutritional status (43). However, that is the point of this chapter—that PEM is predictive of and associated with comorbidity and death. The National Kidney Foundation (NKF) Kidney Disease and Dialysis Outcome Quality Initiative (K/DOQI) has recommended SGA as an appropriate nutritional assessment tool for patients undergoing CPD and MHD (49).

The SGA has several major limitations. These include its subjective features, semiquantitative grading restricted to only three nutritional levels, and lack of objective measures of nutrition such as weight or serum chemistries (49). CANUSA (Canada-United States of America) (117) and other studies (40) have led to improved, more quantitative versions of the SGA. The Dialysis Malnutrition Score is such an example (40). Because there are epidemiologic and causal associations between PEM and inflammation and measures of each of these conditions have outcome-predictive value, it is reasonable to consider developing a composite score that combines the measures of protein-energy nutritional status and inflammation. Such a score might give a more precise prediction of outcome. The Malnutrition-Inflammation Score (MIS) is based on the SGA, body mass index, and serum albumin and transferrin concentrations (19). In a study of 83 patients undergoing MHD, the MIS was strongly correlated with 12-month hospitalization rates and mortality (19).

The hemodialysis prognostic nutrition index (HD-PNI) has been proposed by Kelly et al. (118) and is based on serum creatinine and albumin concentrations and 6-month retrospective hospitalization data. The HD-PNI correlated with mortality and prospective hospitalization in a large group of patients undergoing MHD (118). Its major limitations include the need for a sophisticated linear mathematic equation and its dependence on historical hospitalization data to predict prospective hospitalization rates.

Nutritional Interventions and Outcome

Because PEM is a powerful predictor of death risk for patients undergoing MD and if PEM is treatable, it is possible that nutritional interventions may improve poor outcome in patients undergoing MD. Experience with nutritional support of sick or malnourished individuals may provide some insight as to the independent role of PEM on clinical outcome in patients undergoing MD. Ample evidence suggests that maintaining an adequate nutritional intake in patients with a number of acute or chronic catabolic illnesses may improve their nutritional status (119,120). In some of these studies, such improvement is associated with reduced morbidity and mortality and improved quality of life (121). However, evidence as to whether nutritional treatment may improve morbidity and mortality in patients undergoing MD is limited. There are no large-scale, randomized prospective interventional studies that have examined these questions. Among studies based on food intake, Kuhlmann et al. reported that prescription of 45 kcal/kg/d and 1.5 g protein/kg/d induced weight gain and improved serum albumin and other measures of nutritional status in malnourished patients undergoing MHD (122). Leon et al. reported that tailored nutritional intervention improved serum albumin levels in 52 patients undergoing MHD, and this effect was observed even among patients with high serum CRP levels (123). Several retrospective studies demonstrated a beneficial effect of intradialytic parenteral nutrition (IDPN) on clinical outcome (124–127), but a number of other studies of IDPN failed to show improvement in nutritional status or clinical outcome in patients undergoing MHD (128,129). However, many of these studies used small sample sizes, failed to restrict study subjects to those with PEM, did not control for concurrent food intake, did not define or adjust appropriately for comorbid conditions, performed nutritional interventions for only short periods, or had only a short period of follow-up. Until large-scale, prospective randomized interventional studies are conducted, it will be difficult to ascertain the potential benefits of increasing nutritional intake in malnourished patients undergoing MD (129).

A number of other techniques have been used for the prevention or treatment of PEM in patients undergoing MD. Routine methods include preventing PEM before the onset of dialysis therapy, dietary counseling, maintenance of an adequate dose of dialysis, avoidance of acidemia, and aggressive treatment of superimposed catabolic illness (6). More novel, nondietary interventions in addition to IDPN include an appetite stimulant, such as megestrol acetate (130), L-carnitine (73,131), and growth factors including recombinant human growth hormone (rhGH) (132), IGF-1 (133), and anabolic steroids (134). Iglesias et al. used rhGH in a small group of malnourished patients undergoing MD and found that patients gained weight and serum transferrin levels increased (135). Recombinant IGF-1 and nandrolone also have been used in the treatment of malnourished dialysis patients (132,133). Nonetheless, although these treatments have improved nutritional status, with the probable exceptions of the effect of L-carnitine administration on QOL, none of these treatments have yet been shown to improve QOL, morbidity, or mortality in patients undergoing MD. Nutritional interventions for patients undergoing MD are discussed in greater depth in Chapters 25, 26, 27, and 32.

Hypotheses Explaining the Link between Protein-Energy Malnutrition and Poor Outcome

Measures of nutritional status, both at the time of initiation of dialysis and during the course of maintenance dialysis therapy, are strong predictors of subsequent outcome (4, 40,98). The causes of PEM in patients undergoing MD are discussed in Chapter 11. In brief, these include: (a) low nutrient intake (e.g., from anorexia caused by uremic toxins or impaired gastric emptying; (b) clinically apparent comorbid illnesses; (c) inflammation without clinically apparent superimposed illness; (d) nutrient losses during dialysis; (e) endocrine disorders of uremia (e.g., resistance to insulin, growth hormone, and IGF-1); (f) acidemia; and (g) blood losses. Several theories have been proposed to explain the link between PEM and high morbidity and mortality, particularly from cardiovascular disease, in patients undergoing MD. These are discussed in the following section.

Suggested Pathophysiologies for Poor Outcome as a Consequence of Protein-Energy Malnutrition

According to a traditional theory, PEM is associated with increased morbidity and mortality because it impairs host resistance (136,137). There is evidence that certain nutrients may enhance the immune response (138,139). Arginine and glutamine are reported to be among such nutrients (140). Patients undergoing MD may be particularly susceptible to zinc (141,142), vitamin B6 (pyridoxine), vitamin C, and folic-acid deficiencies (143,144), most of which can induce alterations in host defense, such as diminished antibody response, polymorphonuclear leukocyte or lymphocyte dysfunction, and impaired wound healing. Preliminary data suggest that levocarnitine may protect against endotoxins and also suppress elaboration of TNF-α from monocytes (145). Because uremia itself and associated comorbid illnesses may compromise the immune system (146,147), it is possible that patients undergoing MD may be particularly susceptible to the immune-attenuating effects of PEM. Impaired host resistance, aggravated by PEM in these individuals, may predispose to inflammatory diseases, such as infections, which in turn may engender cardiovascular disease (see later in this chapter). Thus, PEM may be a cause as well as a risk factor for morbidity and mortality in patients undergoing MD. Indirect arguments also suggest that malnutrition might increase cardiac death as a consequence of decreased L-arginine availability and the ensuing diminished synthesis of nitric oxide (14).

Several independent studies have shown a relationship between inflammatory processes, most commonly indicated by elevated serum CRP concentrations, and risk of cardiovascular death among patients undergoing MD (17,148). Because inflammation may be associated with both anorexia and increased net protein catabolism (i.e., the difference between protein synthesis and protein degradation), inflammation may be the link between PEM and morbidity and mortality. Inflammation may induce endothelial cell damage and atherogenesis (see Chapter 13 and later in this chapter) (149).

Another theory is based on the character of food ingested by patients undergoing MD. According to this theory, patients with chronic kidney disease (CKD) without ESRD and patients undergoing MD may tend to consume an atherogenic diet (57,150). Because of difficulty in maintaining adequate energy intake on low-protein, low-potassium diets, patients may tend to rely more on high-fat food sources. Also, many patients with CKD have received extensive treatment with glucocorticoids, which may increase serum lipid levels. Moreover, two recent studies based on food-frequency questionnaires indicate that patients undergoing MHD take significantly lower amounts of potassium, dietary fiber, vitamin C, and some cardioprotective carotenoids (57,59). Such patients appear to have a lower intake of most nutrients including minerals and vitamins but a higher intake of cholesterol. Facchini et al. showed that of six dietary constituents associated with cardioprotective effects (folate, vitamin E, vitamin A-retinoids, total carotenoids, beta carotene, and vitamin C), all but vitamin E were significantly lower in the ESRD diet (59). These results were consistent with another report indicating that most patients with ESRD, like nondialyzed patients with CKD, are exposed to traditional restrictions in potassium intake, which may result in reduced fruit and vegetable intake, leaving meat and other high-fat foods as the main source of calories (57). This theory suggests that the atherogenic nature of the diet, and not a deficiency of protein and energy (i.e., the cause of PEM), is the cause of the poor outcome. Moreover, much attention has been drawn toward the role of excessive calcium intake, such as from ingestion of calcium-containing phosphorus binders, and high dietary and serum phosphorus in the development of coronary artery calcification and subsequent increased risk of cardiovascular events in patients undergoing MD (151). If vascular disease is promoted by high calcium and phosphorus intake, the connection to PEM is not clear.

Comorbid illnesses also may serve as a link between PEM and morbidity and mortality in patients undergoing MD. Patients undergoing MD who have the lowest serum albumin levels or body weights-for-height are more likely to have severe underlying diseases such as longstanding diabetes mellitus, chronic lung or heart failure, or peripheral vascular insufficiency (70). Hence, a statistically significant correlation between measures of PEM and morbidity and mortality does not indicate which of these variables is the cause of the other; our hypothesis is that each one contributes to the other. Even if PEM is not the primary cause, improving nutritional status may mitigate the high risk of adverse outcomes (see earlier in this chapter). Among patients undergoing MD with less severe comorbid condition, epidemiologic studies indicate that deficient nutrient intake and PEM are still independent causes of increased morbidity and mortality (9,152).

Is Inflammation the Missing Link?

Infection and/or inflammation may predispose patients undergoing MD to atherosclerosis as well as to anorexia, a net catabolic state, and hypoalbuminemia (16,46,91,149). It is suggested that the superimposed illnesses frequently encountered by patients undergoing MD contribute to the hypercatabolic state and the development of inflammatory conditions (47,153) (Fig. 12.3). Models to investigate the causes of inflammation (e.g., infection by *Chlamydia pneumoniae*) and their impact on atherosclerosis and coronary disease have been developed in nonuremic patients (154, 155). Recent studies indicate that many patients undergoing MD, especially those with hypoalbuminemia, are in an inflammatory state associated with elevated serum levels of positive acute-phase proteins (including CRP) and certain proinflammatory cytokines (such as IL-1 and IL-6 and TNF-α) and decreased serum negative acute-phase proteins (including albumin, transferrin, and prealbumin) (104, 149). Epidemiologic studies indicate that inflammation, as manifested by altered serum acute-phase proteins and cer-

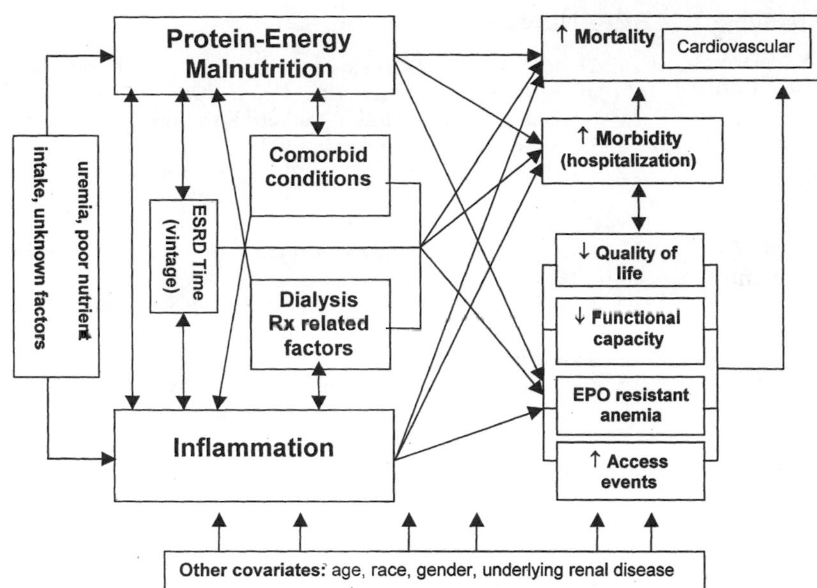

FIGURE 12.3. A hypothetical model of the complex interrelationships among the predictors (inflammation and malnutrition) and outcomes (quality of life, morbidity, and mortality).

tain proinflammatory cytokines, is another major risk factor for increased morbidity and mortality in patients undergoing MD (148). Thus, the acute-phase inflammatory process that is a normal host-defense mechanism, under some circumstances, might play a detrimental role in patients undergoing MD and contribute to the risk for cardiovascular events (104).

Indeed, several investigators suggest that PEM in patients undergoing MD is a consequence of chronic inflammatory processes (9,46,156) (see Chapter 13). According to this model, inflammation is associated with an increase in plasma and probably tissue levels of catabolic cytokines, which then promote PEM. TNF-α, for instance, not only promotes catabolic processes, engendering both protein degradation and suppression of protein synthesis (157), but also induces anorexia (158,159). Elevation of inflammatory proteins and catabolic cytokines occur in nondialyzed patients with advanced chronic renal insufficiency and in patients undergoing MD (160). Evidence suggests that albumin synthesis is suppressed when serum CRP is elevated (16). Morbid conditions that are associated temporally with PEM or chronic inflammation, along with the effect of dialysis vintage, may be major determinants of the low QOL and adverse outcomes in patients undergoing MD (6,9) (Fig. 12.3). Thus, chronic inflammation may be the missing link or factor that causally ties PEM to morbidity and mortality. It has been argued that PEM is a result rather than the cause of inflammation and, hence, that PEM may be a secondary marker itself and not a causal agent in its own right of poor outcome in patients undergoing MD (27,45, 149). The paradoxical relationship between protein-energy undernutrition and cardiovascular disease in patients undergoing MD, which appears to be causally connected through inflammation, has been referred to as the Malnutrition Inflammation Complex Syndrome (19,85) or Malnutrition Inflammation Atherosclerosis syndrome (27) to underscore the high prevalence of cardiovascular disease among malnourished patients undergoing MD with inflammation.

The extent to which PEM and inflammation may each be the cause of the other and the degree to which they can independently cause adverse outcomes in patients undergoing MD have not been defined clearly. The data that thus far connect PEM to inflammation are epidemiologic in nature, and there is a paucity of interventional studies that could more definitively evaluate the interrelationships between PEM, inflammation, and outcome in patients undergoing MD. Evidence suggests that PEM is not caused exclusively by chronic inflammatory processes and circulating proinflammatory cytokines in patients with ESRD. In patients undergoing MD, the association between serum albumin and CRP is not precise; and the reported correlation coefficients are usually less than 0.50 (16,45). Serum albumin and CRP are shown to be independent predictors of morbidity and mortality even after adjusting for each other (86,105). Moreover, serum albumin concentrations usually do not fluctuate on a month-to-month basis, whereas serum CRP appears to do so (46,161). In some but not all studies, serum albumin and other indicators of protein-energy nutritional status correlate with nPNA, an indicator of protein intake (20,161). A study performed by Owen et al. (162) based on 1,044 blood samples in a large number of patients undergoing MHD did not show any significant association between the odds ratio of death and CRP, and the patients' risk of mortality was thought to be influenced primarily through depletion of body proteins, not inflammation.

The fact that inflammatory cytokines may cause anorexia

does not indicate that a low protein-energy intake resulting from this anorexia may not have its own adverse effects. Indeed, the whole field of nutritional support is based on the tenet that acutely or chronically ill patients who either do not eat because they are anorexic or who are physically incapable of ingesting, digesting, or processing food may benefit from nutritional therapy (138). Evidence demonstrates that at least in some acute or chronic illnesses, the provision of adequate nutrition does improve hypoalbuminemia (123) and clinical outcome (121). Hence, inflammation or morbid events may be caused, in part, by inadequate nutritional intake, as has been shown for other illnesses associated with an inflammatory response. The positive association of measures of PEM with inflammation may result, in part, from the generation of cytokines in the setting of low protein and energy intake (9). These considerations, although not yet definitively proven, suggest that factors other than the catabolic consequences of inflammation also affect serum albumin and other nutritional measures and that nutrient intake is very likely such a factor. In summary, although in patients undergoing MD PEM may be associated with poor outcome because of the contribution of inflammation, existing data remain consistent with the possibility that nutrient intake may affect outcome independently.

Is Protein-Energy Malnutrition a Main Contributor to Poor Outcome in End-Stage Renal Disease?

The relationship between undernutrition and adverse outcome in patients undergoing MD is so strong that it practically reverses the association that is seen in the general population; thus, it is referred to as the "reverse epidemiology" theory. Although no uniform approach is available for rating the overall severity of PEM in patients undergoing MD, measures of food intake, laboratory measurements of nutritional status, body composition tools, and nutritional scoring systems are all predictors of outcome in these individuals. The pathophysiology of PEM as it relates to poor clinical outcome and the methods of treating PEM are not yet well understood. Although epidemiologic evidence suggests that inflammation is a cause of both PEM and the morbidity and mortality associated with PEM, much of this association could be the result of anorexia and poor nutrient intake engendered by inflammatory processes. There is strong evidence indicating that PEM may independently contribute to adverse outcomes and that nutritional therapy may be beneficial for patients undergoing MD with PEM. There is, however, a paucity of information concerning the effect of nutritional therapy on morbidity and mortality in patients undergoing MD. Large-scale, randomized, clinical trials of the effects of nutritional intake, nutritional status, and inflammation on clinical outcome would greatly help to better define the causal relationships between these factors in patients undergoing MD (163).

REFERENCES

1. United States Renal Data System 2003 annual data report. *Atlas of end-stage renal diseases in the United States*. Bethesda, MD: National Institute of Health, National Institute of Diabetes and Digestive and Kidney Diseases, 2003.
2. Nicolucci A, Procaccini DA. Why do we need outcomes research in end stage renal disease? *J Nephrol* 2000;13(6): 401–404.
3. Morbidity and mortality of dialysis. *NIH Consens Statement* 1993;11(2):1–33.
4. Leavey SF, Strawderman RL, Jones CA, et al. Simple nutritional indicators as independent predictors of mortality in hemodialysis patients. *Am J Kidney Dis* 1998;31(6):997–1006.
5. Mehrotra R, Kopple JD. Nutritional management of maintenance dialysis patients: why aren't we doing better? *Annu Rev Nutr* 2001;21:343–379.
6. Kopple JD. Nutritional status as a predictor of morbidity and mortality in maintenance dialysis patients. *Asaio J* 1997;43(3): 246–250.
7. Chung SH, Lindholm B, Lee HB. Influence of initial nutritional status on continuous ambulatory peritoneal dialysis patient survival. *Perit Dial Int* 2000;20(1):19–26.
8. Williams AJ, McArley A. Body composition, treatment time, and outcome in hemodialysis patients. *J Ren Nutr* 1999;9(3): 157–162.
9. Kalantar-Zadeh K, Kopple JD. Relative contribution of malnutrition and inflammation to clinical outcome in dialysis patients. *Am J Kidney Dis* 2001;38(6):1343–1350.
10. Kopple JD, Greene T, Chumlea WC, et al. Relationship between nutritional status and the glomerular filtration rate: results from the MDRD study. *Kidney Int* 2000;57(4): 1688–1703.
11. Fleischmann E, Teal N, Dudley J, et al. Influence of excess weight on mortality and hospital stay in 1346 hemodialysis patients. *Kidney Int* 1999;55(4):1560–1567.
12. Kalantar-Zadeh K, Block G, Humphreys M, et al. Reverse epidemiology of cardiovascular risk factors in maintenance dialysis patients. *Kidney Int* 2003;63(3):793–808.
13. Coresh J, Longenecker JC, Miller ER, et al. Epidemiology of cardiovascular risk factors in chronic renal disease. *J Am Soc Nephrol* 1998;9:S24–S30.
14. Ritz E. Why are lipids not predictive of cardiovascular death in the dialysis patient? *Miner Electrolyte Metab* 1996;22(1–3): 9–12.
15. Fleischmann EH, Bower JD, Salahudeen AK. Risk factor paradox in hemodialysis: better nutrition as a partial explanation. *Asaio J* 2001;47(1):74–81.
16. Kaysen GA, Stevenson FT, Depner TA. Determinants of albumin concentration in hemodialysis patients. *Am J Kidney Dis* 1997;29(5):658–668.
17. Kaysen GA. Inflammation nutritional state and outcome in end stage renal disease. *Miner Electrolyte Metab* 1999;25(4–6): 242–250.
18. Kalantar-Zadeh K, Kopple JD, Block G, et al. Association between SF36 quality of life measures and nutrition, hospitalization, and mortality in hemodialysis patients. *J Am Soc Nephrol* 2001;12(12):2797–2806.
19. Kalantar-Zadeh K, Kopple JD, Block G, et al. A malnutrition inflammation score is correlated with morbidity and mortality in hemodialysis patients. *Am J Kidney Dis* 2001;38(6): 1251–1263.
20. Kaysen GA, Chertow GM, Adhikarla R, et al. Inflammation and dietary protein intake exert competing effects on serum albumin and creatinine in hemodialysis patients. *Kidney Int* 2001;60(1):333–340.

21. Fried L, Bernardini J, Piraino B. Charlson comorbidity index as a predictor of outcomes in incident peritoneal dialysis patients. *Am J Kidney Dis* 2001;37(2):337–342.
22. Beddhu S, Bruns FJ, Saul M, et al. A simple comorbidity scale predicts clinical outcomes and costs in dialysis patients. *Am J Med* 2000;108(8):609–613.
23. Longenecker JC, Coresh J, Klag MJ, et al. Validation of comorbid conditions on the end-stage renal disease medical evidence report: the CHOICE study. Choices for Healthy Outcomes in Caring for ESRD. *J Am Soc Nephrol* 2000;11(3):520–529.
24. Chertow GM, Johansen KL, Lew N, et al. Vintage, nutritional status, and survival in hemodialysis patients. *Kidney Int* 2000; 57(3):1176–1181.
25. Vonesh E, Schaubel D, Hao W, et al. Statistical methods for comparing mortality among ESRD patients: Examples of regional/international variations. *Kidney Int* 2000;57:19–27.
26. Bergstrom J. Nutrition and mortality in hemodialysis. *J Am Soc Nephrol* 1995;6(5):1329–1341.
27. Stenvinkel P, Heimburger O, Lindholm B, et al. Are there two types of malnutrition in chronic renal failure? Evidence for relationships between malnutrition, inflammation and atherosclerosis (MIA syndrome). *Nephrol Dial Transplant* 2000;15(7): 953–960.
28. Wolfe RA, Gaylin DS, Port FK, et al. Using USRDS generated mortality tables to compare local ESRD mortality rates to national rates. *Kidney Int* 1992;42(4):991–996.
29. Sehgal AR, Dor A, Tsai AC. Morbidity and cost implications of inadequate hemodialysis. *Am J Kidney Dis* 2001;37(6): 1223–1231.
30. Kalantar-Zadeh K, Supasyndh O, Lehn RS, et al. Normalized protein nitrogen appearance is correlated with hospitalization and mortality in hemodialysis patients with Kt/V greater than 1.20. *J Ren Nutr* 2003;13(1):15–25.
31. Blake C, Codd MB, Cassidy A, et al. Physical function, employment and quality of life in end-stage renal disease. *J Nephrol* 2000;13(2):142–149.
32. Chen YC, Hung KY, Kao TW, et al. Relationship between dialysis adequacy and quality of life in long-term peritoneal dialysis patients. *Perit Dial Int* 2000;20(5):534–540.
33. Diaz-Buxo JA, Lowrie EG, Lew NL, et al. Quality-of-life evaluation using Short Form 36: comparison in hemodialysis and peritoneal dialysis patients. *Am J Kidney Dis* 2000;35(2): 293–300.
34. Jofre R, Lopez-Gomez JM, Moreno F, et al. Changes in quality of life after renal transplantation. *Am J Kidney Dis* 1998;32(1): 93–100.
35. Kutner NG, Zhang R, McClellan WM. Patient-reported quality of life early in dialysis treatment: effects associated with usual exercise activity. *Nephrol Nurs J* 2000;27(4):357–367; discussion 368, 424.
36. Daneker B, Kimmel PL, Ranich T, et al. Depression and marital dissatisfaction in patients with end-stage renal disease and in their spouses. *Am J Kidney Dis* 2001;38(4):839–846.
37. Gunnell J, Yeun JY, Depner TA, et al. Acute-phase response predicts erythropoietin resistance in hemodialysis and peritoneal dialysis patients. *Am J Kidney Dis* 1999;33(1):63–72.
38. Kalantar-Zadeh K, Rodriguez R, Kelly M, et al. Cuffed dialysis catheter and hepatitis C are associated with malnutrition in hemodialysis patients. *J Am Soc Neph* 1999;10:246A Suppl (abstract A1245).
39. Goicoechea M, Caramelo C, Rodriguez P, et al. Role of type of vascular access in erythropoietin and intravenous iron requirements in haemodialysis. *Nephrol Dial Transplant* 2001;16(11): 2188–2193.
40. Kalantar-Zadeh K, Kleiner M, Dunne E, et al. A modified quantitative subjective global assessment of nutrition for dialysis patients. *Nephrol Dial Transplant* 1999;14(7):1732–1738.
41. Kalantar-Zadeh K, Hoffken B, Wunsch H, et al. Diagnosis of iron deficiency anemia in renal failure patients during the post-erythropoietin era. *Am J Kidney Dis* 1995;26(2):292–299.
42. Madore F, Lowrie EG, Brugnara C, et al. Anemia in hemodialysis patients: variables affecting this outcome predictor. *J Am Soc Nephrol* 1997;8(12):1921–1929.
43. Kalantar-Zadeh K, Kleiner M, Dunne E, et al. Total iron-binding capacity-estimated transferrin correlates with the nutritional subjective global assessment in hemodialysis patients. *Am J Kidney Dis* 1998;31(2):263–272.
44. Barany P, Divino Filho JC, Bergstrom J. High C-reactive protein is a strong predictor of resistance to erythropoietin in hemodialysis patients. *Am J Kidney Dis* 1997;29(4):565–568.
45. Qureshi AR, Alvestrand A, Danielsson A, et al. Factors predicting malnutrition in hemodialysis patients: a cross-sectional study. *Kidney Int* 1998;53(3):773–782.
46. Kaysen GA. Malnutrition and the acute-phase reaction in dialysis patients—how to measure and how to distinguish. *Nephrol Dial Transplant* 2000;15(10):1521–1524.
47. Grodstein GP, Blumenkrantz MJ, Kopple JD. Nutritional and metabolic response to catabolic stress in uremia. *Am J Clin Nutr* 1980;33(7):1411–1416.
48. Dwyer JT, Cunniff PJ, Maroni BJ, et al. The hemodialysis pilot study: nutrition program and participant characteristics at baseline. The HEMO Study Group. *J Ren Nutr* 1998;8(1): 11–20.
49. National Kidney Foundation (NKF) Kidney Disease and Dialysis Outcome Initiative (K/DOQI). Clinical practice guidelines for nutrition in chronic renal failure. *Am J Kidney Dis* 2000;35(6, suppl 2).
50. Kopple JD, Shinaberger JH, Coburn JW, et al. Evaluating modified protein diets for uremia. *J Am Diet Assoc* 1969;54(6): 481–485.
51. Slomowitz LA, Monteon FJ, Grosvenor M, et al. Effect of energy intake on nutritional status in maintenance hemodialysis patients. *Kidney Int* 1989;35(2):704–711.
52. Lowrie EG, Laird NM, Parker TF, et al. Effect of the hemodialysis prescription of patient morbidity: report from the National Cooperative Dialysis Study. *N Engl J Med* 1981;305(20): 1176–1181.
53. Harter HR. Review of significant findings from the National Cooperative Dialysis Study and recommendations. *Kidney Int Suppl* 1983(13):S107–S112.
54. Schoenfeld PY, Henry RR, Laird NM, et al. Assessment of nutritional status of the National Cooperative Dialysis Study population. *Kidney Int Suppl* 1983(13):S80–S88.
55. Thunberg BJ, Swamy AP, Cestero RV. Cross-sectional and longitudinal nutritional measurements in maintenance hemodialysis patients. *Am J Clin Nutr* 1981;34(10):2005–2012.
56. Wolfson M, Strong CJ, Minturn D, et al. Nutritional status and lymphocyte function in maintenance hemodialysis patients. *Am J Clin Nutr* 1984;39(4):547–555.
57. Kalantar-Zadeh K, Kopple J, Deepak S, et al. Food intake characteristics of hemodialysis patients as obtained by food frequency questionnaire. *J Renal Nutrition* 2002;12(1):17–31.
58. Hu FB, Manson JE, Stampfer MJ, et al. Diet, lifestyle, and the risk of type 2 diabetes mellitus in women. *N Engl J Med* 2001; 345(11):790–797.
59. Facchini F, Schoenfeld P, Dixon B, et al. ESRD patients consume an atherogenic diet. *J Am Soc Neph* 1997;7:S133 (Abstract A1079).
60. Blake PG, Sombolos K, Abraham G, et al. Lack of correlation between urea kinetic indices and clinical outcomes in CAPD patients. *Kidney Int* 1991;39(4):700–706.

61. Herselman M, Moosa MR, Kotze TJ, et al. Protein-energy malnutrition as a risk factor for increased morbidity in long-term hemodialysis patients. *J Ren Nutr* 2000;10(1):7–15.
62. Maiorca R, Brunori G, Zubani R, et al. Predictive value of dialysis adequacy and nutritional indices for mortality and morbidity in CAPD and HD patients. A longitudinal study. *Nephrol Dial Transplant* 1995;10(12):2295–2305.
63. Acchiardo SR, Moore LW, Latour PA. Malnutrition as the main factor in morbidity and mortality of hemodialysis patients. *Kidney Int Suppl* 1983;16:S199–S203.
64. Teehan BP, Schleifer CR, Brown JM, et al. Urea kinetic analysis and clinical outcome on CAPD. A five year longitudinal study. *Adv Perit Dial* 1990;6:181–185.
65. Parker TF, Laird NM, Lowrie EG. Comparison of the study groups in the National Cooperative Dialysis Study and a description of morbidity, mortality, and patient withdrawal. *Kidney Int Suppl* 1983(13):S42–S49.
66. Genestier S, Hedelin G, Schaffer P, et al. Prognostic factors in CAPD patients: a retrospective study of a 10-year period. *Nephrol Dial Transplant* 1995;10(10):1905–1911.
67. Germain M, Harlow P, Mulhern J, et al. Low protein catabolic rate and serum albumin correlate with increased mortality and abdominal complications in peritoneal dialysis patients. *Adv Perit Dial* 1992;8:113–115.
68. Degoulet P, Legrain M, Reach I, et al. Mortality risk factors in patients treated by chronic hemodialysis. Report of the Diaphane collaborative study. *Nephron* 1982;31(2):103–110.
69. Wolfe RA, Ashby VB, Daugirdas JT, et al. Body size, dose of hemodialysis, and mortality. *Am J Kidney Dis* 2000;35(1):80–88.
70. Kopple JD, Zhu X, Lew NL, et al. Body weight-for-height relationships predict mortality in maintenance hemodialysis patients. *Kidney Int* 1999;56(3):1136–1148.
71. Lew EA, Garfinkel L. Variations in mortality by weight among 750,000 men and women. *J Chronic Dis* 1979;32(8):563–576.
72. Nelson EE, Hong CD, Pesce AL, et al. Anthropometric norms for the dialysis population. *Am J Kidney Dis* 1990;16(1):32–37.
73. Chazot C, Laurent G, Charra B, et al. Malnutrition in long-term haemodialysis survivors. *Nephrol Dial Transplant* 2001;16(1):61–69.
74. Woodrow G, Oldroyd B, Smith MA, et al. Measurement of body composition in chronic renal failure: comparison of skinfold anthropometry and bioelectrical impedance with dual energy X-ray absorptiometry. *Eur J Clin Nutr* 1996;50(5):295–301.
75. Dumler F. Use of bioelectric impedance analysis and dual-energy X-ray absorptiometry for monitoring the nutritional status of dialysis patients. *Asaio J* 1997;43(3):256–260.
76. Chertow GM, Lowrie EG, Wilmore DW, et al. Nutritional assessment with bioelectrical impedance analysis in maintenance hemodialysis patients. *J Am Soc Nephrol* 1995;6(1):75–81.
77. Kalantar-Zadeh K, Block G, Kelly MP, et al. Near infra-red interactance for longitudinal assessment of nutrition in dialysis patients. *J Ren Nutr* 2001;11(1):23–31.
78. Kalantar-Zadeh K, Dunne E, Nixon K, et al. Near infra-red interactance for nutritional assessment of dialysis patients. *Nephrol Dial Transplant* 1999;14(1):169–175.
79. Chertow G, Jacobs D, Lazarus J, et al. Phase angle predicts survival in hemodialysis patients. *J Renal Nutrition* 1997;7(4):204–207.
80. Carvounis CP, Manis T, Coritsidis G, et al. Total lymphocyte count: a promising prognostic index of mortality in patients on CAPD. *Perit Dial Int* 2000;20(1):33–38.
81. Owen WF, Lowrie EG. C-reactive protein as an outcome predictor for maintenance hemodialysis patients. *Kidney Int* 1998;54(2):627–636.
82. Maiorca R, Cancarini GC, Brunori G, et al. Comparison of long-term survival between hemodialysis and peritoneal dialysis. *Adv Perit Dial* 1996;12:79–88.
83. Avram MM, Fein PA, Bonomini L, et al. Predictors of survival in continuous ambulatory peritoneal dialysis patients: a five-year prospective study. *Perit Dial Int* 1996;16(Suppl 1):S190–S194.
84. Owen WF Jr, Lew NL, Liu Y, et al. The urea reduction ratio and serum albumin concentration as predictors of mortality in patients undergoing hemodialysis. *N Engl J Med* 1993;329(14):1001–1006.
85. Kalantar-Zadeh K, Don BR, Rodriguez RA, et al. Serum ferritin is a marker of morbidity and mortality in hemodialysis patients. *Am J Kidney Dis* 2001;37(3):564–572.
86. Ikizler TA, Wingard RL, Harvell J, et al. Association of morbidity with markers of nutrition and inflammation in chronic hemodialysis patients: a prospective study. *Kidney Int* 1999;55(5):1945–1951.
87. Marcen R, Teruel JL, de la Cal MA, et al. The impact of malnutrition in morbidity and mortality in stable haemodialysis patients. Spanish Cooperative Study of Nutrition in Hemodialysis. *Nephrol Dial Transplant* 1997;12(11):2324–2331.
88. Fung L, Pollock CA, Caterson RJ, et al. Dialysis adequacy and nutrition determine prognosis in continuous ambulatory peritoneal dialysis patients. *J Am Soc Nephrol* 1996;7(5):737–744.
89. Avram MM, Sreedhara R, Fein P, et al. Survival on hemodialysis and peritoneal dialysis over 12 years with emphasis on nutritional parameters. *Am J Kidney Dis* 2001;37(1 Suppl 2):S77–S80.
90. Kaysen GA, Yeun J, Depner T. Albumin synthesis, catabolism and distribution in dialysis patients. *Miner Electrolyte Metab* 1997;23(3–6):218–224.
91. Yeun JY, Kaysen GA. Factors influencing serum albumin in dialysis patients. *Am J Kidney Dis* 1998;32(6 Suppl 4):S118–S125.
92. Struijk DG, Krediet RT, Koomen GC, et al. The effect of serum albumin at the start of continuous ambulatory peritoneal dialysis treatment on patient survival. *Perit Dial Int* 1994;14(2):121–126.
93. Kopple JD, Mehrotra R, Suppasyndh O, et al. Observations with regard to the National Kidney Foundation K/DOQI clinical practice guidelines concerning serum transthyretin in chronic renal failure. *Clin Chem Lab Med* 2002;40(12):1308–1312.
94. Neyra NR, Hakim RM, Shyr Y, et al. Serum transferrin and serum prealbumin are early predictors of serum albumin in chronic hemodialysis patients. *J Ren Nutr* 2000;10(4):184–190.
95. Chertow GM, Ackert K, Lew NL, et al. Prealbumin is as important as albumin in the nutritional assessment of hemodialysis patients. *Kidney Int* 2000;58(6):2512–2517.
96. Kaysen GA. The microinflammatory state in uremia: causes and potential consequences. *J Am Soc Nephrol* 2001;12(7):1549–1557.
97. De Lima JJ, Vieira ML, Abensur H, et al. Baseline blood pressure and other variables influencing survival on haemodialysis of patients without overt cardiovascular disease. *Nephrol Dial Transplant* 2001;16(4):793–797.
98. Lowrie EG, Lew NL. Death risk in hemodialysis patients: the predictive value of commonly measured variables and an evaluation of death rate differences between facilities. *Am J Kidney Dis* 1990;15(5):458–482.
99. Avram MM, Mittman N, Bonomini L, et al. Markers for survival in dialysis: a seven-year prospective study. *Am J Kidney Dis* 1995;26(1):209–219.
100. Lowrie EG, Huang WH, Lew NL. Death risk predictors among peritoneal dialysis and hemodialysis patients: a preliminary comparison. *Am J Kidney Dis* 1995;26(1):220–228.

101. Gamba G, Mejia JL, Saldivar S, et al. Death risk in CAPD patients. The predictive value of the initial clinical and laboratory variables. *Nephron* 1993;65(1):23–27.
102. Iseki K, Yamazato M, Tozawa M, et al. Hypocholesterolemia is a significant predictor of death in a cohort of chronic hemodialysis patients. *Kidney Int* 2002;61(5):1887–1893.
103. Yang WS, Kim SB, Min WK, et al. Atherogenic lipid profile and lipoprotein(a) in relation to serum albumin in haemodialysis patients. *Nephrol Dial Transplant* 1995;10(9):1668–1671.
104. Yeun JY, Levine RA, Mantadilok V, et al. C-Reactive protein predicts all-cause and cardiovascular mortality in hemodialysis patients. *Am J Kidney Dis* 2000;35(3):469–476.
105. Iseki K, Tozawa M, Yoshi S, et al. Serum C-reactive protein (CRP) and risk of death in chronic dialysis patients. *Nephrol Dial Transplant* 1999;14(8):1956–1960.
106. Noh H, Lee SW, Kang SW, et al. Serum C-reactive protein: a predictor of mortality in continuous ambulatory peritoneal dialysis patients. *Perit Dial Int* 1998;18(4):387–394.
107. Stenvinkel P, Lindholm B, Heimburger M, et al. Elevated serum levels of soluble adhesion molecules predict death in pre-dialysis patients: association with malnutrition, inflammation, and cardiovascular disease. *Nephrol Dial Transplant* 2000;15(10):1624–1630.
108. Abdullah MS, Wild G, Jacob V, et al. Cytokines and the malnutrition of chronic renal failure. *Miner Electrolyte Metab* 1997;23(3–6):237–242.
109. Bologa RM, Levine DM, Parker TS, et al. Interleukin-6 predicts hypoalbuminemia, hypocholesterolemia, and mortality in hemodialysis patients. *Am J Kidney Dis* 1998;32(1):107–114.
110. Lindgren BF, Friis K, Ericsson F. Insulin-like growth factor I correlates with protein intake estimated from the normalized protein catabolic rate in hemodialysis patients. *Am J Nephrol* 2000;20(4):255–262.
111. Rodriguez-Carmona A, Perez Fontan M, et al. Hyperleptinemia is not correlated with markers of protein malnutrition in chronic renal failure. A cross-sectional study in predialysis, peritoneal dialysis and hemodialysis patients. *Nephron* 2000;86(3):274–280.
112. Wrone EM, Zehnder JL, Hornberger JM, et al. An MTHFR variant, homocysteine, and cardiovascular comorbidity in renal disease. *Kidney Int* 2001;60(3):1106–1113.
113. Greene SV, Falciglia G, Rademacher R. Relationship between serum phosphorus levels and various outcome measures in adult hemodialysis patients. *J Ren Nutr* 1998;8(2):77–82.
114. Dumler F, Falla P, Butler R, et al. Impact of dialysis modality and acidosis on nutritional status. *Asaio J* 1999;45(5):413–417.
115. Marckmann P. Nutritional status and mortality of patients in regular dialysis therapy. *J Intern Med* 1989;226(6):429–432.
116. Lawson JA, Lazarus R, Kelly JJ. Prevalence and prognostic significance of malnutrition in chronic renal insufficiency. *J Ren Nutr* 2001;11(1):16–22.
117. Adequacy of dialysis and nutrition in continuous peritoneal dialysis: association with clinical outcomes. Canada-USA (CANUSA) Peritoneal Dialysis Study Group. *J Am Soc Nephrol* 1996;7(2):198–207.
118. Beto JA, Bansal VK, Hart J, et al. Hemodialysis prognostic nutrition index as a predictor for morbidity and mortality in hemodialysis patients and its correlation to adequacy of dialysis. Council on Renal Nutrition National Research Question Collaborative Study Group. *J Ren Nutr* 1999;9(1):2–8.
119. Kopple JD. The nutrition management of the patient with acute renal failure. *JPEN J Parenter Enteral Nutr* 1996;20(1):3–12.
120. Mortelmans AK, Duym P, Vandenbroucke J, et al. Intradialytic parenteral nutrition in malnourished hemodialysis patients: a prospective long-term study. *JPEN J Parenter Enteral Nutr* 1999;23(2):90–95.
121. Koretz RL. Does nutritional intervention in protein-energy malnutrition improve morbidity or mortality? *J Ren Nutr* 1999;9(3):119–121.
122. Kuhlmann MK, Schmidt F, Kohler H. High protein/energy vs. standard protein/energy nutritional regimen in the treatment of malnourished hemodialysis patients. *Miner Electrolyte Metab* 1999;25(4–6):306–310.
123. Leon JB, Majerle AD, Soinski JA, et al. Can a nutrition intervention improve albumin levels among hemodialysis patients? A pilot study. *J Ren Nutr* 2001;11(1):9–15.
124. Foulks CJ. The effect of intradialytic parenteral nutrition on hospitalization rate and mortality in malnourished hemodialysis patients. *J Renal Nutr* 1994;4:5–10.
125. Chertow GM, Ling J, Lew NL, et al. The association of intradialytic parenteral nutrition administration with survival in hemodialysis patients. *Am J Kidney Dis* 1994;24(6):912–920.
126. Capelli JP, Kushner H, Camiscioli TC, et al. Effect of intradialytic parenteral nutrition on mortality rates in end-stage renal disease care. *Am J Kidney Dis* 1994;23(6):808–816.
127. Siskind MS, Lien YH. Effect of intradialytic parenteral nutrition on quality of life in hemodialysis patients. *Int J Artif Organs* 1993;16(8):599–603.
128. Pupim LB, Kent P, Hakim R. The potential of intradialytic parenteral nutrition: A review. *Miner Electrolyte Metab* 1999;25(4–6):317–323.
129. Foulks CJ. An evidence-based evaluation of intradialytic parenteral nutrition. *Am J Kidney Dis* 1999;33(1):186–192.
130. Boccanfuso JA, Hutton M, McAllister B. The effects of megestrol acetate on nutritional parameters in a dialysis population. *J Ren Nutr* 2000;10(1):36–43.
131. Semeniuk J, Shalansky KF, Taylor N, et al. Evaluation of the effect of intravenous l-carnitine on quality of life in chronic hemodialysis patients. *Clin Nephrol* 2000;54(6):470–477.
132. Johannsson G, Bengtsson BA, Ahlmen J. Double-blind, placebo-controlled study of growth hormone treatment in elderly patients undergoing chronic hemodialysis: anabolic effect and functional improvement. *Am J Kidney Dis* 1999;33(4):709–717.
133. Fouque D, Peng SC, Shamir E, et al. Recombinant human insulin-like growth factor-1 induces an anabolic response in malnourished CAPD patients. *Kidney Int* 2000;57(2):646–654.
134. Johnson CA. Use of androgens in patients with renal failure. *Semin Dial* 2000;13(1):36–39.
135. Iglesias P, Diez JJ, Fernandez-Reyes MJ, et al. Recombinant human growth hormone therapy in malnourished dialysis patients: a randomized controlled study. *Am J Kidney Dis* 1998;32(3):454–463.
136. Haag-Weber M, Horl WH. Altered cellular host defence in malnutrition and uremia. *Contrib Nephrol* 1992;98:105–111.
137. Haag-Weber M, Dumann H, Horl WH. Effect of malnutrition and uremia on impaired cellular host defence. *Miner Electrolyte Metab* 1992;18(2–5):174–185.
138. Souba WW. Nutritional support. *N Engl J Med* 1997;336(1):41–48.
139. Hulsewe KW, van Acker BA, von Meyenfeldt MF, et al. Nutritional depletion and dietary manipulation: effects on the immune response. *World J Surg* 1999;23(6):536–544.
140. Alexander JW. Immunoenhancement via enteral nutrition. *Arch Surg* 1993;128(11):1242–1245.
141. Kimmel PL, Phillips TM, Lew SQ, et al. Zinc modulates mononuclear cellular calcitriol metabolism in peritoneal dialysis patients. *Kidney Int* 1996;49(5):1407–1412.
142. Erten Y, Kayatas M, Sezer S, et al. Zinc deficiency: prevalence and causes in hemodialysis patients and effect on cellular immune response. *Transplant Proc* 1998;30(3):850–851.
143. Dobbelstein H, Korner WF, Mempel W, et al. Vitamin B6

deficiency in uremia and its implications for the depression of immune responses. *Kidney Int* 1974;5(3):233–239.
144. Casciato DA, McAdam LP, Kopple JD, et al. Immunologic abnormalities in hemodialysis patients: improvement after pyridoxine therapy. *Nephron* 1984;38(1):9–16.
145. De Simone C, Famularo G, Tzantzoglou S, et al. Carnitine depletion in peripheral blood mononuclear cells from patients with AIDS: effect of oral L-carnitine. *Aids* 1994;8(5):655–660.
146. Vanholder R, Dell'Aquila R, Jacobs V, et al. Depressed phagocytosis in hemodialyzed patients: in vivo and in vitro mechanisms. *Nephron* 1993;63(4):409–415.
147. Vanholder R, Van Loo A, Dhondt AM, et al. Influence of uraemia and haemodialysis on host defence and infection. *Nephrol Dial Transplant* 1996;11(4):593–598.
148. Bergstrom J, Lindholm B, Lacson E Jr, et al. What are the causes and consequences of the chronic inflammatory state in chronic dialysis patients? *Semin Dial* 2000;13(3):163–175.
149. Stenvinkel P. Inflammatory and atherosclerotic interactions in the depleted uremic patient. *Blood Purif* 2001;19(1):53–61.
150. Dolson GM. Do potassium deficient diets and K+ removal by dialysis contribute to the cardiovascular morbidity and mortality of patients with end stage renal disease? *Int J Artif Organs* 1997; 20(3):134–135.
151. Goodman WG, Goldin J, Kuizon BD, et al. Coronary-artery calcification in young adults with end-stage renal disease who are undergoing dialysis. *N Engl J Med* 2000;342(20):1478–1483.
152. Kopple JD. McCollum Award Lecture, 1996: protein-energy malnutrition in maintenance dialysis patients. *Am J Clin Nutr* 1997;65(5):1544–1557.
153. Keane WF, Collins AJ. Influence of co-morbidity on mortality and morbidity in patients treated with hemodialysis. *Am J Kidney Dis* 1994;24(6):1010–1018.
154. Becker AE, de Boer OJ, van Der Wal AC. The role of inflammation and infection in coronary artery disease. *Annu Rev Med* 2001;52:289–297.
155. Pieniazek P, Karczewska E, Stepien E, et al. Incidence of Chlamydia pneumoniae infection in patients with coronary artery disease subjected to angioplasty or bypass surgery. *Med Sci Monit* 2001;7(5):995–1001.
156. Bergstrom J, Lindholm B. Malnutrition, cardiac disease, and mortality: an integrated point of view. *Am J Kidney Dis* 1998; 32(5):834–841.
157. Flores EA, Bistrian BR, Pomposelli JJ, et al. Infusion of tumor necrosis factor/cachectin promotes muscle catabolism in the rat. A synergistic effect with interleukin 1. *J Clin Invest* 1989;83(5): 1614–1622.
158. McCarthy DO. Cytokines and the anorexia of infection: potential mechanisms and treatments. *Biol Res Nurs* 2000;1(4): 287–298.
159. McCarthy DO. Tumor necrosis factor alpha and interleukin-6 have differential effects on food intake and gastric emptying in fasted rats. *Res Nurs Health* 2000;23(3):222–228.
160. Witko-Sarsat V, Friedlander M, Nguyen Khoa T, et al. Advanced oxidation protein products as novel mediators of inflammation and monocyte activation in chronic renal failure. *J Immunol* 1998;161(5):2524–2532.
161. Kaysen GA, Dubin JA, Muller HG, et al. The acute-phase response varies with time and predicts serum albumin levels in hemodialysis patients. The HEMO Study Group. *Kidney Int* 2000;58(1):346–352.
162. Owen WF Jr, Chertow GM, Lazarus JM, et al. Dose of hemodialysis and survival: differences by race and sex. *JAMA* 1998; 280(20):1764–1768.
163. Hakim RM. Proposed clinical trials in the evaluation of intradialytic parenteral nutrition. *Am J Kidney Dis* 1999;33(1): 217–220.
164. Johnson DW, Herzig KA, Purdie DM, et al. Is obesity a favorable prognostic factor in peritoneal dialysis patients? *Perit Dial Int* 2000;20(6):715–721.
165. Arora P, Strauss BJ, Borovnicar D, et al. Total body nitrogen predicts long-term mortality in haemodialysis patients—a single-centre experience. *Nephrol Dial Transplant* 1998;13(7): 1731–1736.
166. Pollock CA, Ibels LS, Allen BJ, et al. Total body nitrogen as a prognostic marker in maintenance dialysis. *J Am Soc Nephrol* 1995;6(1):82–88.
167. Collins AJ, Ma JZ, Umen A, et al. Urea index and other predictors of hemodialysis patient survival. *Am J Kidney Dis* 1994; 23(2):272–282.
168. Churchill DN, Taylor DW, Cook RJ, et al. Canadian Hemodialysis Morbidity Study. *Am J Kidney Dis* 1992;19(3):214–234.
169. Blake PG, Flowerdew G, Blake RM, et al. Serum albumin in patients on continuous ambulatory peritoneal dialysis—predictors and correlations with outcomes. *J Am Soc Nephrol* 1993; 3(8):1501–1507.
170. Avram MM, Goldwasser P, Erroa M, et al. Predictors of survival in continuous ambulatory peritoneal dialysis patients: the importance of prealbumin and other nutritional and metabolic markers. *Am J Kidney Dis* 1994;23(1):91–98.
171. Spiegel DM, Breyer JA. Serum albumin: a predictor of long-term outcome in peritoneal dialysis patients. *Am J Kidney Dis* 1994;23(2):283–285.
172. Spiegel DM, Anderson M, Campbell U, et al. Serum albumin: a marker for morbidity in peritoneal dialysis patients. *Am J Kidney Dis* 1993;21(1):26–30.
173. Sreedhara R, Avram MM, Blanco M, et al. Prealbumin is the best nutritional predictor of survival in hemodialysis and peritoneal dialysis. *Am J Kidney Dis* 1996;28(6):937–942.
174. De Lima JJ, da Fonseca JA, Godoy AD. Baseline variables associated with early death and extended survival on dialysis. *Ren Fail* 1998;20(4):581–587.
175. Stenvinkel P, Heimburger O, Wang T, et al. High serum hyaluronan indicates poor survival in renal replacement therapy. *Am J Kidney Dis* 1999;34(6):1083–1088.
176. Merkus MP, Jager KJ, Dekker FW, et al. Predictors of poor outcome in chronic dialysis patients: The Netherlands Cooperative Study on the Adequacy of Dialysis. The NECOSAD Study Group. *Am J Kidney Dis* 2000;35(1):69–79.

13

ROLE OF INFLAMMATION IN MALNUTRITION AND ATHEROSCLEROSIS IN CHRONIC RENAL FAILURE

PETER STENVINKEL
JANE Y. YEUN

Cardiovascular disease (CVD) remains the main cause of morbidity and mortality in patients with chronic renal failure (CRF). The annual mortality rate from CVD is approximately 9%, which is 10- to 20-fold higher than that in the general population, even when adjusted for age, gender, race, and the presence of diabetes mellitus (1). This high cardiovascular mortality suggests that patients with CRF may be subjected to a process of accelerated atherogenesis (2). In fact, the death rate among patients with CRF with signs of inflammation, malnutrition, and atherosclerosis are comparable to that of many cancer patients with metastases (3). The causes of atherosclerotic CVD in patients with CRF are probably multifactorial. Factors proven to contribute to atherosclerosis in the general population, such as dyslipidemia, left-ventricular hypertrophy, diabetes mellitus, hypertension, and tobacco smoking, are prevalent in patients with CRF. Thus, intuitively, it appears reasonable to assume that these traditional risk factors also apply to patients with CRF. However, a recent study suggests that the burden of traditional risk factors may not be sufficient to account for the higher mortality and morbidity from CVD in CRF (4). Instead, nontraditional risk factors, such as oxidative stress and inflammation, also may contribute to the excessive CVD mortality (3,5). Over the last several years, inflammation has been found to play a key role in atherosclerosis in the general population (6) and also may be an important contributor to both malnutrition and increased cardiovascular morbidity and mortality in patients with CRF.

SERUM ALBUMIN IS VULNERABLE TO THE EFFECTS OF INFLAMMATION

A low serum albumin concentration is a powerful predictor of mortality in patients with CRF (7). Previously this finding was interpreted to indicate the presence of malnutrition, possibly arising from inadequate dialysis and the resultant anorexia. Unfortunately, measures to improve nutrition through oral and intradialytic parenteral supplementation have not been very effective in normalizing serum albumin levels (8), and it seems that patients undergoing dialysis cannot "feed themselves out" of morbidity and mortality. It must be emphasized that not only is the serum albumin concentration a function of decreased protein intake; it is influenced also by external losses of albumin and the presence of inflammation (9). Indeed, the synthetic rates of albumin and other serum proteins commonly used as markers of malnutrition, such as prealbumin and retinol-binding protein, are decreased during inflammation (10–13). Consequently, their use as nutritional markers in patients undergoing dialysis may be problematic. Instead, nutritional markers such as subjective global assessment (14) and anthropometry may be more accurate.

TWO TYPES OF MALNUTRITION IN PATIENTS WITH CHRONIC RENAL FAILURE

It is well established that a large proportion of patients with CRF considered to be malnourished, as determined by anthropometry and subjective global assessment, also have evidence for chronic inflammation and CVD (12,13). Thus, comorbidity and/or inflammation also may contribute to malnutrition in patients with CRF, as suggested by several lines of evidence. First, Kaizu et al. (15) demonstrated that circulating interleukin (IL)-6 levels adversely affected, at least in part, the nutritional status in patients being treated with maintenance hemodialysis (MHD). Moreover, IL-6 transgenic mice had a muscle-wasting syndrome that was completely blocked by treatment with an IL-6 receptor antibody (16). In healthy subjects subjected to semistarvation

(17) and in patients with anorexia nervosa (18), serum albumin levels declined only modestly. Even in adult marasmus (protein-calorie malnutrition without inflammation) cases, Bistrian et al. (19) showed that serum albumin levels are preserved. In fact, the only direct dietary cause for severe hypoalbuminemia is inadequate energy intake when the protein intake is severely limited (20). Indeed, low serum albumin levels discriminated poorly between well-nourished and malnourished patients with CRF, as identified by anthropometric and subjective global assessment, whereas they are closely associated with the presence of inflammation (14). Based on these findings we have proposed that patients with CRF may have at least two types of malnutrition (21). Type 1 malnutrition is associated with anorexia resulting from the uremic syndrome; the type 2 malnutrition is "cytokine-driven" and associated with significant comorbidity, inflammation, and increased protein catabolism and oxidative stress, as outlined in Table 13.1. Clinically it is obvious that both types often may coexist. Indeed, it is possible that protein-energy malnutrition, perhaps by predisposing to infection, also may predispose to inflammation.

MARKERS OF INFLAMMATION PREDICT CLINICAL OUTCOME IN CHRONIC RENAL FAILURE

Because both inflammation and inadequate nutritional intake may decrease the concentration of commonly used biochemical markers of malnutrition, much of the previously reported relationship between serum albumin and total and cardiovascular mortality in patients undergoing MHD (7) or chronic peritoneal dialysis (CPD) (22) may have been caused by an inflammatory process rather than poor nutritional intake. Indeed, since the first report by Bergström et al. (23) of an association between an elevated C-reactive protein (CRP) level and increased mortality, several groups have reported similar findings in both MHD (9,24,25) and CPD (26) patients. Available evidence suggests that CRP is a precise and objective index of inflammatory activity and that it accurately reflects the generation of proinflammatory cytokines, such as IL-1, IL-6, and tumor necrosis factor-α (TNF-α). Indeed, elevated serum levels of various proinflammatory cytokines also are associated with increased mortality in patients undergoing dialysis (27,28). The fact that an elevated CRP level is such a strong predictor of cardiovascular mortality (9,24) suggests that the association between inflammation and atherosclerosis is particularly strong in patients undergoing dialysis. Indeed, CRP independently predicts the number and the extent of atherosclerotic carotid plaques in patients undergoing dialysis (29). Even in patients with CRF not yet on dialysis a strong relationship between malnutrition, elevated CRP levels, and atherosclerosis exists (13). Moreover, serum hyaluronan, another inflammatory marker generated in response to proinflammatory cytokines, strongly predicts mortality in patients with CRF (30).

It is interesting that these findings in patients with CRF are mirrored by several publications evaluating the association between cardiovascular risk and CRP levels in patients without renal disease. Even small increases in the levels of proinflammatory cytokines such as IL-6 (31) or acute-phase proteins such as CRP (32) predicted CVD in otherwise healthy adults. A meta analysis by Danesh et al. (33) reported that the risk ratio for coronary heart disease was two times higher in subjects with elevated CRP. In addition, the risk of CVD seems to be markedly increased in other patient groups with a chronic inflammatory state. Notably, women with systemic lupus erythematosus were more than 50 times more likely to have a myocardial infarction than were women of similar age (34). Similarly, in a Finnish study patients with rheumatoid arthritis had increased mortality from CVD (35). Finally, recent evidence suggests that even young patients with the human immunodeficiency virus (HIV) patients had accelerated coronary atherosclerosis (36).

TABLE 13.1. PROPOSED FEATURES OF TYPE-1 AND TYPE-2 MALNUTRITION

	Type-1	Type-2
S-albumin	Normal/low	Low
Comorbidity	Uncommon	Common
Presence of inflammation	No	Yes
Food intake	Low	Low/normal
Resting energy expenditure	Normal	Elevated
Oxidative stress	Increased	Markedly increased
Protein catabolism	Decreased	Increased
Reversed by dialysis and nutritional support	Yes	No

INFLAMMATION AND ANEMIA

Anemia, which is associated with increased cardiovascular and all-cause mortality in patients with CRF (37), may be one of many links between inflammation, raised levels of proinflammatory cytokines, and poor outcome in patients with CRF. Indeed, Lowrie (38) postulated that anemia and malnutrition share the inflammatory response as a common cause. Several lines of evidence in animal studies suggest that elevated levels of proinflammatory cytokines may cause anemia. First, IL-1 and TNF-α have suppressive effects on erythropoiesis (39), which may be the main mechanism by which cytokines cause anemia. Proinflammatory cytokines also inhibit erythropoietin production (40) and induce intestinal bleeding (41). Thus, other cytokine-mediated mechanisms also may contribute to the anemia associated with inflammation. Finally, inflammation affects mucosal uptake and transfer of iron, thus reducing the absorption of oral iron and further contributing to the anemia (42). In human studies, Barany et al. (43) and Beguin et al. (44) found that patients undergoing MHD with an elevated CRP level or fibrinogen level, another marker for the acute-phase response, were less responsive to erythropoietin. Gunell et al. (45) further showed that both low serum albumin and high CRP levels predicted erythropoietin resistance in both MHD and CPD patients, lending additional support to the contention that the inflammatory response is responsible for both the low serum albumin and the anemia.

RELATIONSHIPS BETWEEN INFLAMMATION, MALNUTRITION, AND ATHEROSCLEROSIS

Although hypoalbuminemia (7,22) and inflammation (9, 24) are important predictors of mortality in patients undergoing dialysis, complications from malnutrition and inflammation are not the most common causes of mortality in this patient group (46). In fact, malnutrition accounts for less than 5% of deaths, whereas atherosclerotic CVD is by far the most common cause of mortality in the dialysis population (1). This apparent paradox may be explained by the strong interactions between atherosclerotic CVD and inflammatory and nutritional parameters in patients with CRF (13). Based on these findings we (21) have suggested the presence of a syndrome consisting of malnutrition, inflammation, and atherosclerosis (MIA syndrome), which is present in many patients starting dialysis treatment and is associated with a high mortality rate on dialysis (3). Indeed, inflammation is more common in malnourished patients (12), and Ikizler et al. (47) showed that the nutritional status and the inflammatory response are independent predictors of hospitalization in patients undergoing MHD. Moreover, the presence of malnutrition (48) and inflammation (24) is associated with a higher cardiovascular mortality rate in patients undergoing MHD, and nutritional and inflammatory markers are linked closely to cardiovascular disease in patients with CRF (*vide supra*). It is interesting that Wang et al. (49) demonstrated in patients undergoing CPD that cardiac valve calcification is associated with the presence of inflammation and malnutrition, independent of abnormal calcium-phosphate metabolism, suggesting that cardiac calcification also may be associated with the MIA syndrome. Taken together, there seems to be a vicious circle of malnutrition, inflammation, and atherosclerosis in patients with CRF, and elevated levels of proinflammatory cytokines appear to play a central role in this scenario (21).

CAUSES OF INFLAMMATION IN CHRONIC RENAL FAILURE

About 30% to 50% of predialysis (13), MHD (9,12,24,29, 50), and CPD (51) patients in various European and North American studies have serologic evidence of an activated inflammatory response (Table 13.2). Patients of Asian origin undergoing dialysis appear to have a lower prevalence of elevated CRP (25,26), and genetic factors, such as IL-6 promotor polymorphism (52), may contribute to the observed variations in the prevalence of inflammation. It should be emphasized that CRP measurements in most cross-sectional studies were made at a single time point, which may complicate interpretation because CRP is a *moving target.* In fact, in 2000 Kaysen et al. (53) showed that the acute-phase response is intermittent and varies significantly with time despite no change in dialyzer type or dialysis

TABLE 13.2. RECENT CLINICAL STUDIES THAT HAVE ASSESSED PREVALENCE OF ELEVATED CRP AMONG PATIENTS WITH CRF

Authors	Year	No.	CRP (mg/L)	Prevalence of Elevated CRP (%)
Europe and North America				
Zoccali et al. (29)	1998	112 HD	>5	65
Owen et al. (50)	1998	1,054 HD	>8	35
Qureshi et al. (12)	1998	128 HD	>10	53
Zimmermann et al. (24)	1999	280 HD	>8	46
Yeun et al. (9)	2000	91 HD	>5.2	51
Stenvinkel et al. (13)	1999	109 CRF	>10	32
Asia				
Iseki et al. (25)	1999	163 HD	>10	21
Noh et al. (26)	1998	106 PD	>8	14

CRP, C-reactive protein; HD, hemodialysis; CRF, chronic renal failure.

TABLE 13.3. POTENTIAL CAUSES OF INFLAMMATION IN CHRONIC RENAL FAILURE

Potential Cause in Predialysis Stage	Additional Causes in HD	Additional Causes in PD
Reduced renal clearance	Graft and fistula infection	Peritonitis
Cytokines	Bioincompatible HD-membrane	Peritoneal access infection
Ages		Bioincompatible dialysate
Genetic factors	Endotoxin exposure from contaminated dialysate	Endotoxin exposure from contaminated dialysate
Comorbidity		
Chronic heart failure	Backfiltration	
Atherosclerosis		
Occult persistent infections		
Chlamydia pneumoniae		
Tuberculosis		
Dental and/or gingival infections		

HD, hemodialysis; PD, peritoneal dialysis.

treatment. This observation by Kaysen et al. (53) together with the high prevalence of elevated CRP in prepatients undergoing dialysis (13) suggest that factors unrelated to dialysis therapy may be largely responsible for the elevated CRP levels in patients undergoing dialysis (Table 13.3). The responsible factors may be the presence of comorbidity or the renal failure itself.

DECREASED RENAL CLEARANCE OF CYTOKINES

Available evidence suggests an upregulation of proinflammatory cytokine activity in patients with CRF, and markedly elevated levels of cytokines have been found both before and after the start of dialysis treatments (27,54–56). The cause(s) of elevated serum levels of proinflammatory cytokines in CRF are not well understood. However, in some studies no difference in the serum levels of IL-1, IL-6, and TNF-α was observed between long-term and not-yet-dialyzed patients, suggesting that CRF may be a more important cause of elevated cytokine levels than the dialysis procedure (54,55). Indeed, the deterioration of renal function has been associated with a significant increase in serum cytokine levels (57), and a strong positive correlation between creatinine clearance and various cytokines and their soluble receptors has been demonstrated in nondialyzed patients with varying degrees of renal failure (58–60). Moreover, patients with CRF have a lower urinary IL-6 receptor excretion rate than controls (61), and Bolton et al. (56) found in a multiple regression analysis that creatinine was the sole determinant of IL-6 levels in a group of predialysis and dialysis patients. Finally, reduced renal function may affect both TNF (62) and IL-1 (63) clearance in nephrectomized rats, suggesting that proinflammatory cytokines actually could be regarded as uremic toxins. The importance of the kidney in cytokine handling further is underscored by Hession et al. (64) who demonstrated that the Tamm-Horsfall glycoprotein might regulate the activity of potent cytokines such as IL-1 and TNF. However, because the half-life of various cytokines is short and because local tissue degradation may be the most important way to inactivate cytokines, more research is needed to determine the relative importance of the kidney in cytokine clearance.

COMORBIDITY

Other non–dialysis-related causes of elevated CRP and cytokine levels in patients with CRF may include factors such as chronic heart failure (CHF) with edema (65) and the atherosclerotic process. By virtue of its acute-phase behavior, CRP may be a marker for severe and progressive atherosclerosis (66). However, because some patients with stable and unstable angina pectoris have normal levels of acute-phase proteins, increased CRP levels cannot be attributed solely to the presence and severity of atherosclerosis (67). The highly skewed distribution of CRP and IL-6, in predialysis and dialysis patients (Fig. 13.1) suggests that patient-specific processes—such as clotted access grafts with occult infections (68); percutaneous peritoneal dialysis catheter infections; and persistent *Chlamydia pneumoniae* (29,69,70), tuberculosis, and dental/gingival (71) infections—may play an important role in causing inflammation in patients with CRF.

ADVANCED GLYCATION END PRODUCTS

When aldehyde or ketone groups of carbohydrates react nonenzymatically with amino acids a variety of complex

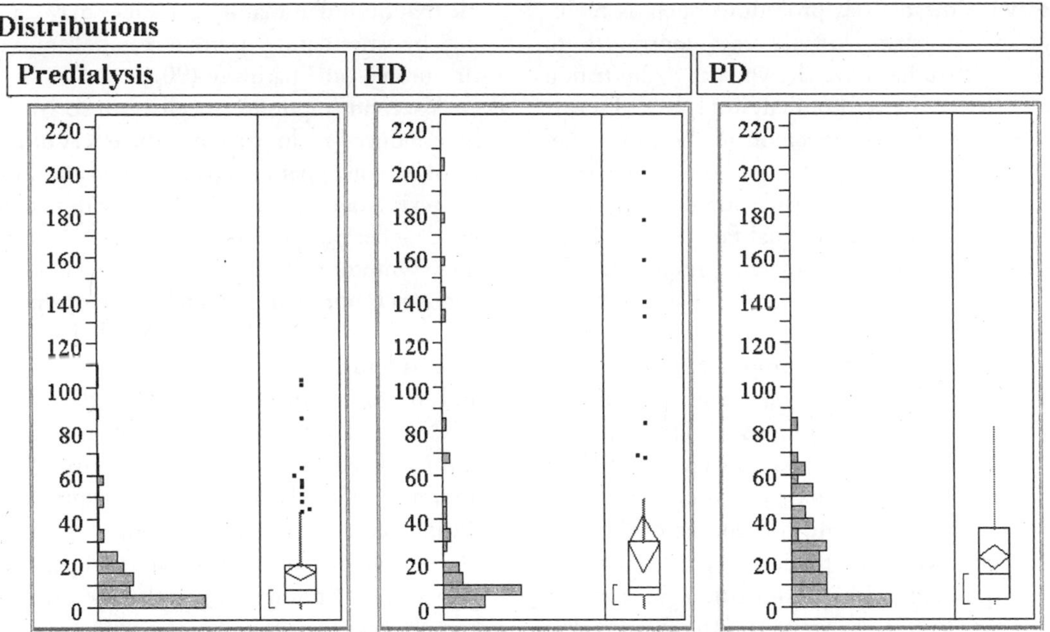

FIGURE 13.1. Distribution of C-reactive protein in 112 predialysis (median 8.2; range 0.2 to 102.0 mg/L), 54 maintenance hemodialysis (median 8.9; range 0.2 to 200.2 mg/L), and 51 chronic peritoneal dialysis patients (median 15.0; range 1.0 to 81.0 mg/L). Predialysis and maintenance hemodialysis patients were treated in Stockholm, Sweden, and the chronic peritoneal dialysis patients were treated in Sacramento, California, United States.

compounds called advanced glycation end products (AGEs) are formed. AGEs may promote atherosclerosis through binding to their endothelial receptors, with sequential expression of adhesion molecules and attraction of circulating monocytes to the vessel wall (72). In patients with rheumatoid arthritis, CRP levels correlate strongly with pentosidine, an AGE (73). Several *in vitro* studies show that AGEs induce cytokine production and trigger an inflammatory response (74–76). Thus, it is possible that the accumulation of AGEs in patients with CRF from decreased renal clearance may promote inflammation. As speculated by Schwedler et al. (77), monocyte stimulation by AGEs could be the initial signal of an important inflammatory cascade leading to CRP production.

THE DIALYSIS PROCEDURE

Some studies reported that increased levels of proinflammatory cytokines are found primarily in patients undergoing dialysis (78,79), suggesting that the dialysis procedure with extracorporeal circulation of blood also may contribute to inflammation (Table 13.3). Haubitz et al. (80) reported that CRP levels 24 hours after hemodialysis were significantly greater than predialysis values. Indeed, exposure of mononuclear cells to the hemodialysis membrane is a potential source for increased cytokine levels (81). Several hemodialysis-related factors have been proposed to contribute to the inflammatory response, including dialysis against bioincompatible membranes (61,82), the use of nonsterile dialysate (83), and the back-leak of dialysate (84) across the dialysis membrane. However, optimized hemodialysis therapy using ultrapure dialysate and biocompatible dialyzer membranes reduces CRP but does not normalize it, suggesting dialysis-related factors are not the main cause of inflammation in patients undergoing hemodialysis (85).

The PD process itself may contribute significantly to inflammation because of the use of bioincompatible PD solutions (86). Haubitz et al. (87) suggested that induction of the inflammatory activity is lower during PD as compared to hemodialysis, and Takahashi et al. (88) showed that PD treatment stimulates the production of IL-6 to a lesser extent than does hemodialysis. However, in our experience with European and North American patients, the prevalence of elevated CRP levels are similar in patients undergoing CPD or MHD (Fig. 13.1).

INFLAMMATION AS A CAUSE OF MALNUTRITION IN CHRONIC RENAL FAILURE

Protein-energy malnutrition and wasting are common phenomena among patients with CRF. Although various factors associated with the dialysis procedure, such as bioincompatibility and nutrient losses, may contribute to malnutrition, recent studies have shown that malnutrition is common even before the start of dialysis (13,89). Disturbances in protein and energy metabolism, hormonal derangements, and a spontaneous reduction in dietary energy and protein intake may be responsible for the decline in nutritional status with progressive renal failure (89). Little is known about the specific mechanism(s) responsible for the altered appetite and metabolism with renal disease, although a role for cytokines, such as TNF-α (also called cachectin), IL-1, and IL-6, has been proposed (90). In older patients without renal disease, cachexia is associated usually with higher-than-normal concentrations of TNF-α, IL-1, and IL-6 (91). The effects of cytokines may result from direct action on the gastrointestinal system or indirect effects on the central nervous system. Indeed, increased levels of proinflammatory cytokines predict hypoalbuminemia (28) and are associated with malnutrition in patients undergoing dialysis (15,92). Kaizu et al. (15) showed that the body-weight loss over 3 years was significantly higher and the serum albumin levels was significantly lower in patients undergoing dialysis with high IL-6 levels. These data suggest that chronic inflammation and elevated levels of proinflammatory cytokines may be one important cause of wasting in patients with CRF.

Proinflammatory cytokines may mediate malnutrition in CRF through several mechanisms (Table 13.4). One important mechanism is increased protein hydrolysis and increased muscle-protein breakdown. It has been shown that TNF-α activated the transcription factor nuclear factor kappa B (NF-κB) to suppress MyoD messenger RNA (mRNA) at the posttranscriptional level, thus disrupting skeletal muscle differentiation and repair of damaged muscle tissue (93). This may be one mechanism through which proinflammatory cytokines induce skeletal muscle decay. A decrease in muscle mass also may be caused by activation of the ubiquitin–proteasome proteolytic system, which accelerates degradation of muscle protein (94). Proinflammatory cytokines, such as TNF-α, increase ubiquitin gene expression in skeletal muscle (95). Consequently, it is possible that proinflammatory cytokines may cause muscle wasting by stimulating protein catabolism via the ubiquitin–proteosome pathway (90).

TABLE 13.4. EFFECTS BY WHICH PROINFLAMMATORY CYTOKINES MAY CAUSE MALNUTRITION

Affect skeletal muscle differentiation and mass
Activate nuclear factor kappa B (NF-κB) by suppressing MyoD (93)
Stimulate the ubiquitin-proteosome pathway (95)
Inhibit feeding
Suppress appetite (97–99)
Inhibit gastric emptying and intestinal motility (90)

A second important mechanism for the proposed cytokine-induced malnutrition is the effect of proinflammatory cytokines on appetite and eating behavior. PD patients with anorexia alone or in combination with nausea and vomiting have higher plasma levels of TNF-α than patients without these symptoms (96). The mechanism of cytokine-induced anorexia is not clear, although some studies have implicated leptin. Grunfeld et al. (97) found that administration of TNF-α and IL-1 increased leptin mRNA levels in hamsters and noted a strong inverse correlation between leptin mRNA level and subsequent food intake. Sarraf et al. (98) and Moshyedi et al. (99) reported similar findings in mice. Serum leptin levels (98) and leptin expression (99) increased during acute inflammation induced by the administration of multiple cytokines or by bacterial peritonitis. Taken together, these findings suggest that elevated leptin levels may be responsible for the anorexia observed during inflammatory conditions in animal models. However, a recent study in humans with CRF suggests that leptin levels may be suppressed during inflammation and actually may act as a negative acute-phase protein, much like albumin (100). It is obvious that more studies are needed, especially in humans, to test the hypothesis that cytokines mediate anorexia either through leptin or through direct effects on the hypothalamic nuclei. Finally, cytokines also may contribute to malnutrition by decreasing gastric motility and/or by modifying gastric-acid secretion (91).

CHRONIC HEART FAILURE

Chronic heart failure, a common feature of CRF (101), is associated with both malnutrition (cardiac cachexia) and increased levels of proinflammatory cytokines in the general population (102,103). Thus, it could be hypothesized that the proinflammatory cytokines, generated in response to factors such as reduced tissue perfusion and altered gut permeability and congestion, may play an important role in the loss of lean body mass in patients with CHF. Because changes in proinflammatory cytokines and acute-phase reactants in CHF are dynamic and increased levels occur mainly with decompensated heart failure, it is important to distinguish between compensated and decompensated CHF when studying the importance of acute-phase reactants or cytokines in the pathogenesis of CHF (104). Because cardiac cachexia is a strong independent risk factor for mortality in nonrenal patients with CHF (105), it seems not unlikely that CHF also may contribute to wasting, elevated levels of proinflammatory cytokines, and increased mortality in patients with CRF.

ATHEROGENIC POTENTIAL OF ACUTE-PHASE REACTANTS AND CYTOKINES

Although the association between CVD and inflammation is well documented in the dialysis patient population, it is unknown if the acute-phase response is merely an epiphenomenon reflecting established atherosclerotic disease or if the acute-phase reactants actually are involved in the initiation and/or progression of atherosclerosis (Table 13.5). Several lines of evidence suggest that CRP may contribute directly to atherogenesis. First, Torzewski et al. (106) demonstrated the presence of CRP deposits in the arterial wall of early atherosclerotic lesions. Second, CRP was shown to colocalize with complement in heart tissue during acute myocardial infarction, leading to the hypothesis that CRP may directly cause tissue damage (107). Third, CRP has been shown to induce adhesion molecule expression in the presence of serum, suggesting a direct proinflammatory effect on human endothelial cells (108). Other acute-phase reactants also may contribute to an accelerated atherosclerotic process. During inflammation serum amyloid A is incorporated into HDL and renders the normally protective HDL atherogenic (109). Several additional interactions between the inflammatory mediators and the various lipoprotein moieties and their metabolism result in altered lipoprotein structure and composition, providing another link between inflammation and accelerated atherosclerosis (110). Finally, other acute-phase reactants, such as lipoprotein(a) (111) and fibrinogen (112), also may have direct atherogenic and/or thrombogenic properties.

TABLE 13.5. SOME DIRECT AND INDIRECT EFFECTS BY WHICH PROINFLAMMATORY CYTOKINES AND ACUTE-PHASE REACTANTS MAY CAUSE ATHEROSCLEROSIS

Direct Effects	Indirect Effects
C-reactive protein	Endothelial dysfunction
Deposits in the arterial wall	Insulin resistance
Causes endothelial dysfunction	Increased oxidative stress
Serum amyloid A	Chronic persistent infections
Affects lipoprotein structure	
Lipoprotein(a)	
Promotes atherogenesis and thrombogenesis	
Fibrinogen	
Promotes atherogenesis and thrombogenesis	
Generates tumor necrosis factor-α	
Downregulates apolipoprotein(E) secretion	
Causes endothelial dysfunction	
Promotes vascular calcification	
Interleukin-6	
Deposits in the arterial wall	

Proinflammatory cytokines also may have direct atherogenic properties. TNF-α has been shown to downregulate apoprotein E (important in the metabolism of intermediate-density lipoprotein) secretion (113), promote *in vitro* calcification of vascular cells (114), and cause endothelial dysfunction (115). IL-6 also may have atherogenic properties because injections of recombinant IL-6 exacerbated early atherosclerosis in mice (116). Moreover, IL-6 may activate the endothelium to produce vasoconstrictor substances and may have procoagulant properties (52). Further support for the atherogenicity of IL-6 comes from studies showing that elevated IL-6 levels predicted myocardial infarction in healthy men (31) and predicted cardiovascular mortality in elderly patients followed for 5 years (117). Whether this atherogenic effect is the result of the subsequent generation of acute-phase reactants, to IL-6 itself, or to an as-yet-unidentified mechanism is not clear. Although acute-phase reactants and cytokines may promote atherogenesis directly, the association between chronic inflammation and CVD may, in part, be indirect. Chronic inflammation is associated with several features known to cause atherosclerosis, such as endothelial dysfunction, insulin resistance, and increased oxidative stress (118).

INFLAMMATION AND ENDOTHELIAL DYSFUNCTION

Normal endothelial function is important for maintaining cardiovascular homeostasis, and endothelial injury may result in lipid accumulation, smooth-muscle proliferation, and vasospasm. Endothelial dysfunction is a prominent feature in predialysis (119), CPD (120), and MHD (121) patients. Recent studies have shown strong associations between markers of inflammation such as CRP and TNF-α and endothelial dysfunction in patients with coronary heart disease (122,123) and following heart transplantation (124). Moreover, infusion of endotoxins or proinflammatory cytokines (115) or vaccination with *Salmonella typhi* (125) to induce an inflammatory state generated a selective impairment of endothelium-dependent relaxation. Finally, long-term exposure of vascular endothelium to IL-1β and TNF-α caused endothelial dysfunction, intimal thickening, and coronary vasospasm in pigs (126). Thus far, to the best of our knowledge, no prospective study has addressed whether chronic or intermittent inflammation generates endothelial dysfunction in patients with CRF. However, because various circulating markers of endothelial activation correlate with the markers of inflammation in patients with CRF (56,127), such a relationship is also likely to exist in this patient group. Indeed, a cross-sectional study demonstrated significant negative correlations between endothelium-dependent vasodilation and inflammatory markers, such as IL-6, TNF-α, and fibrinogen, in a group of predialysis patients and patients undergoing dialysis (56). Taken together, available data suggest that endothelial dysfunction from chronic inflammation may contribute to the observed cardiovascular risk in patients with CRF.

INFLAMMATION AND INSULIN RESISTANCE

Insulin resistance is a well-documented feature of CRF (128) and is associated with premature atherosclerosis. In nonrenal patient populations, elevated CRP levels are associated with several different features of the insulin resistance syndrome; these include increased body mass index (129–131), serum lipid levels (129,130), and fasting glucose levels (129). In 2000, Festa et al. (132) demonstrated that one-third of 1,008 patients without diabetes had impaired glucose tolerance and that there was a linear increase in CRP with increasing numbers of metabolic disorders. Consequently, chronic low-grade inflammation may be part of the insulin-resistance syndrome.

INFLAMMATION AND INCREASED OXIDATIVE STRESS

Oxidative stress results when there is excessive free radical production or low antioxidant levels. It has emerged as an important cofactor for the development of endothelial dysfunction and atherogenesis (133). Free radicals generate oxidized low-density lipoprotein (LDL), which damages the vascular wall and causes atherosclerotic lesions. Increased oxidative stress appears to be present in patients undergoing MHD as evidenced by the presence of various products of oxidation (134) and of autoantibodies to oxidatively modified LDL (135) in these patients. The loss of antioxidants, such as vitamins C, E, and serum albumin, and the decreased activity of reducing enzymes that occur in patients with CRF either from renal failure or as a consequence of dialysis treatment likely contribute to the oxidative stress (134).

In particular, malnourished patients undergoing dialysis have increased oxidative stress, which may contribute to the high prevalence of CVD seen in patients with CRF that are both malnourished and inflamed (136). Indeed, supplementation with vitamin E, 800 IU/day, reduced cardiovascular endpoints and myocardial infarction in patients undergoing dialysis (137). The cause(s) of increased oxidative stress in malnutrition are not well understood. However, in view of the documented strong relationship between malnutrition and inflammation, it is possible that a chronic inflammatory response may be the primary cause of increased oxidative stress in malnourished patients with CRF. Indeed, Memon et al. (138) demonstrated that LDL isolated from animals treated with bacterial lipopolysaccharide (LPS) was more susceptible to *ex vivo* oxidation with copper than LDL isolated from saline-treated animals. Thus, one could speculate that chronic inflammation causes increased oxidative stress. Two clinical studies suggest that this link may be operative in patients with CRF. First, Nguyen-Khoa et al. (139) suggested that the presence of inflammation and the duration of dialysis are the most important determinants of oxidative stress in patients treated with hemodialysis. Second, Handelman et al. (140) reported an association between F2-isoprostanes, an indicator of oxidative stress, and CRP levels in patients undergoing MHD, further supporting a link between inflammation and increased oxidative stress.

INFLAMMATION AND ANGIOGENESIS

Neovascularization and excessive angiogenesis are present in many chronic inflammatory disorders in humans (141) because proinflammatory mediators stimulate neutrophil-directed angiogenesis (142). The vascular endothelial growth factor (VEGF) may be the most potent proangiogenic cytokine and may play a central role in mediating new blood vessel formation (141). McCourt et al. (142) demonstrated that inflammatory stimuli, such as LPS and TNF-α, caused significant release of VEGF from neutrophils. It is interesting that increased angiogenesis is found in the failing peritoneal membrane during prolonged PD (143), a condition known to be associated with inflammation and poor outcome (144). Thus, inflammation and angiogenesis seem to be interrelated and closely involved in the pathophysiology of the failing peritoneal membrane. Moreover, Moulton et al. (145) suggested that neovascularization may promote growth of the atherosclerotic plaque and that antiangiogenic therapy may be an effective strategy to interrupt the development of atherosclerosis. These findings suggest that antiangiogenic treatment strategies have a potential future clinical application in managing patients with chronic inflammatory diseases.

Among other drugs with antiangiogenic potential, thalidomide appears promising because it prevents VEGF-induced neovascular growth (146) and selectively inhibits the production of TNF-α (147). In clinical trials, thalidomide reversed the wasting syndrome associated with other inflammatory disorders, such as HIV (148) and tuberculosis (149). Prospective clinical studies are needed to investigate whether thalidomide is safe and has beneficial effects on the cardiovascular and nutritional status and mortality rate in patients with CRF who have signs of wasting and inflammation.

TREATMENT STRATEGIES OF THE PATIENT WITH CHRONIC RENAL FAILURE AND INFLAMMATION

Although many patients with CRF are inflamed, little is known about how to manage chronic inflammation in these individuals. Some basic tenets are obvious and apply to all patients regardless of whether they are on dialysis. Occult infections when found should be treated with antibiotics. Optimal treatment of CHF and coronary heart disease is essential because these comorbidities may cause or contribute to inflammation. Research demonstrates that angiotensin converting enzyme (ACE) inhibitors may suppress the production of catabolic cytokines, such as TNF-α or IL1-β, both *in vitro* in human monocytes (150) and *in vivo* (151), in mice. Indeed, in patients with severe CHF, high-dose ACE-inhibitor treatment (40 mg/day) is associated with a significant decrease in IL-6 activity (152). In patients with CRF, it has been found that the use of ACE-inhibitors is associated with lower TNF-α and CRP levels (153). Whether the observed decrease in cytokine and acute-phase proteins levels is the result of a direct suppressive effect of ACE inhibitors on cytokine production or the result of an indirect effect from amelioration of CHF is not clear, but further clinical studies are indicated.

Aspirin is known to reduce both CRP and IL-6 levels in patients with angina pectoris (154). Moreover, the aspirin-induced reduction in the risk of myocardial infarction seems to be directly related to the level of CRP (32). Thus, aspirin may be a good choice for treating patients with CRF and inflammation. However, in view of the significant side effect of bleeding (155), generalized use of aspirin cannot be advocated in patients with CRF until the results of prospective randomized studies are available. In 2001, 3-hydroxy-3-methylglutaryl coenzyme A (HMG-CoA) reductase inhibitors were shown to reduce CRP levels by about 15%, independent of lipid-lowering effects (156). Thus, statins may be another treatment strategy to consider in the patient with CRF and inflammation. The ongoing AURORA (157) and 4D trials, when completed, may provide more information on the role of statins in patients undergoing dialysis.

Because available evidence suggests that the hemodialysis procedure itself may cause an inflammatory response and that using bioincompatible membrane (82,85) and ultrapure dialysate (158) reduces it, optimizing the hemodialysis treatment is important, especially in patients with inflammation undergoing MHD. Similarly, as new and more biocompatible PD solutions become available, they should be considered in patients undergoing CPD with signs of the MIA syndrome (159). In addition to being more biocompatible, amino acid–based PD solutions can correct protein malnutrition and replace amino acids lost during PD (160), which may decrease susceptibility to infections and also improve oxidative stress.

Chronic heart failure with fluid overload is a common feature in patients undergoing CPD or MHD (101). Niebauer et al. (65) demonstrated that fluid overload may be an important cause of inflammation in CHF and that control of volume status with diuretics decreases serum endotoxin levels. Thus, rigorous control of fluid overload in the patient undergoing dialysis might be another measure to prevent and treat the MIA syndrome. In this respect icodextrin-containing PD solutions may be beneficial because they allow sustained ultrafiltration with long dialysate dwell times. By analogy, long hemodialysis sessions to optimize volume control might reduce or prevent the acute-phase response in patients undergoing MHD.

Because oxidation products may mediate inflammation in patients with CRF (161) nutrients and/or antioxidants that modulate cytokine biology (162) are of particular interest. In nonrenal patients, vitamin E supplementation decreased CRP (163,164) and monocyte IL-6 levels (163). In patients undergoing MHD, vitamin E supplements reduced cardiovascular endpoints and myocardial infarction in a randomized placebo-controlled trial (137), and vitamin E–coated dialysis filters reduced oxidative stress (121,165). Unfortunately, neither study addressed the impact of vitamin E supplementation on inflammatory parameters in patients with CRF. Because inflammation, oxidative stress, and atherosclerosis are closely intertwined further studies are needed to investigate the ability of oral vitamin E–coated dialyzers to reduce inflammatory markers and improve outcome in patients undergoing MHD.

CONCLUSIONS

Chronic renal failure is characterized by an exceptional mortality rate, much of which results from CVD. Chronic inflammation, as evidenced by increased levels of proinflammatory cytokines and CRP, is a common feature in European and North American patients with CRF and may cause both malnutrition and atherosclerotic CVD through various pathogenetic mechanisms. The cause(s) of the inflammation are probably multifactorial. Although the acute-phase reaction may reflect simply the underlying CVD, it may also directly cause vascular injury. Available data suggest that proinflammatory cytokines may play a central role in the genesis of both inflammation-driven malnutrition and CVD. Suppression, or disruption, of the vicious cycle of malnutrition, inflammation, and atherosclerosis (MIA syndrome) may improve survival in patients undergoing dialysis. As yet, there is no recognized or proposed treatment for patients with CRF with noninfectious chronic inflammation. Future research should focus on elucidating the etiology of the inflammation and studying the long-term effects of various antiinflammatory treatment strategies on the nutritional and cardiovascular status and outcome in patients with CRF.

REFERENCES

1. Foley RN, Parfrey PS, Sarnak MJ. Clinical epidemiology of cardiovascular disease in chronic renal failure. *Am J Kidney Dis* 1998;32(Suppl 5):S112–S119.

2. Lindner A, Charra B, Sherrard DJ, et al. Accelerated atherosclerosis in prolonged maintenance haemodialysis. *N Engl J Med* 1974;290:697–701.
3. Stenvinkel P. Inflammatory and atherosclerotic interactions in the depleted uremic patient. *Blood Purif* 2001;19:53–61.
4. Cheung AK, Sarnak MJ, Yan G, et al. Atherosclerotic cardiovascular disease risks in chronic hemodialysis patients. *Kidney Int* 2000;58:353–362.
5. Sarnak MJ, Levey AS. Cardiovascular disease and chronic renal disease: a new paradigm. *Am J Kidney Dis* 2000;35:S117–S131.
6. Ross R. Atherosclerosis: an inflammatory disease. *N Engl J Med* 1999;340:115–126.
7. Lowrie EG, Lew NL. Death risk in hemodialysis patients: The predictive value of commonly measured variables and an evaluation of death rate differences between facilities. *Am J Kidney Dis* 1990;15:458–482.
8. Foulks CJ. An evidence-based evaluation of intradialytic parenteral nutrition. *Am J Kidney Dis* 1999;33:186–192.
9. Yeun JY, Levine RA, Mantadilok V, et al. C-reactive protein predicts all-cause and cardiovascular mortality in hemodialysis patients. *Am J Kidney Dis* 2000;35(3):469–476.
10. Kaysen GA, Rathore V, Shearer GC, et al. Mechanisms of hypoalbuminemia in hemodialysis patients. *Kidney Int* 1995;48: 510–516.
11. Kaysen GA, Stevenson FT, Depner TA. Determinants of albumin concentration in hemodialysis patients. *Am J Kidney Dis* 1997;29:658–668.
12. Qureshi AR, Alvestrand A, Danielsson A, et al. Factors influencing malnutrition in hemodialysis patients. A cross-sectional study. *Kidney Int* 1998;53:773–782.
13. Stenvinkel P, Heimbürger O, Paultre F, et al. Strong associations between malnutrition, inflammation and atherosclerosis in chronic renal failure. *Kidney Int* 1999;55:1899–1911.
14. Heimbürger O, Qureshi AR, Blaner WS, et al. Hand-grip muscle strength, lean body mass and plasma proteins as markers of nutritional status in patients with chronic renal failure close to start of dialysis therapy. *Am J Kidney Dis* 2000;36:1213–1225.
15. Kaizu Y, Kimura M, Yoneyama T, et al. Interleukin-6 may mediate malnutrition in chronic hemodialysis patients. *Am J Kidney Dis* 1998;31:93–100.
16. Tsujinaka T, Fujita J, Ebisuri C, et al. Interleukin-6 receptor antibody inhibits muscle atrophy and modulates proteolytic systems in interleukin-6 transgenic mice. *J Clin Invest* 1996;97: 244–249.
17. Keys A, Brozek J, Henschel A, et al. *The biology of human starvation.* Minneapolis: University of Minnesota Press, 1950.
18. Smith G, Robinsson PH, Fleck A. Serum albumin distribution in early treated anorexia nervosa. *Nutrition* 1996;12:677–684.
19. Bistrian B, Sherman M, Blackburn G, et al. Cellular immunity in adult marasmus. *Arch Intern Med* 1977;137:1408–1411.
20. Lunn P, Austin S. Dietary manipulation of plasma albumin concentrations. *J Nutr* 1983;113:1791–1801.
21. Stenvinkel P, Heimbürger O, Lindholm B, et al. Are there two types of malnutrition in chronic renal failure? Evidence for relationships between malnutrition, inflammation and atherosclerosis (MIA-syndrome). *Nephrol Dial Transpl* 2000;15: 953–960.
22. Avram MM, Fein PA, Bonomini L, et al. Predictors of survival in continuous ambulatory peritoneal dialysis patients: A five year prospective study. *Perit Dial Int* 1996;16(Suppl 1): S190–S194.
23. Bergström J, Heimbürger O, Lindholm B, et al. Elevated serum C-reactive protein is a strong predictor of increased mortality and low serum albumin in hemodialysis (HD) patients (abstract). *J Am Soc Nephrol* 1995;6:573.
24. Zimmermann J, Herrlinger S, Pruy A, et al. Inflammation enhances cardiovascular risk and mortality in hemodialysis patients. *Kidney Int* 1999;55:648–658.
25. Iseki K, Tozawa M, Yoshi S, et al. Serum C-reactive (CRP) and risk of death in chronic dialysis patients. *Nephrol Dial Transpl* 1999;14:1956–1960.
26. Noh H, Lee SW, Kang SW, et al. Serum C-reactive protein: a predictor of mortality in continuous ambulatory peritoneal dialysis patients. *Nephrol Dial Transpl* 1998;18:387–394.
27. Kimmel PL, Phillips TM, Simmens SJ, et al. Immunologic function and survival in hemodialysis patients. *Kidney Int* 1998;54: 236–244.
28. Bologa RM, Levine DM, Parker TS, et al. Interleukin-6 predicts hypoalbuminemia, hypocholesterolemia, and mortality in hemodialysis patients. *Am J Kidney Dis* 1998;32:107–114.
29. Zoccali C, Benedetto FA, Mallamaci F, et al. Inflammation is associated with carotid atherosclerosis in dialysis patients. *J Hypertens* 2000;18:1207–1213.
30. Stenvinkel P, Heimbürger O, Wang T, et al. High serum hyaluronan indicate poor survival in renal replacement therapy. *Am J Kidney Dis* 1999;34:1083–1088.
31. Ridker PM, Rifai N, Stampfer MJ, et al. Plasma concentration of interleukin-6 and the risk of future myocardial infarction among apparently healthy men. *Circulation* 2000;101: 1767–1772.
32. Ridker PM, Cushman M, Stampfer MJ, et al. Inflammation, aspirin and the risk of cardiovascular disease in apparently healthy men. *N Engl J Med* 1997;336:973–979.
33. Danesh J, Whincup P, Walker M, et al. Low grade inflammation and coronary heart disease: prospective study and updated meta-analyses. *BMJ* 2000;321:199–204.
34. Manzi S, Meilahn EN, Rairie JE, et al. Age-specific incidence rates of myocardial infarction and angina in women with systemic lupus erythematosus: comparison with Framingham study. *Am J Epidemiol* 1997;145:408–415.
35. Mutru O, Laakso M, Isomäki H, et al. Cardiovascular mortality in patients with rheumatoid arthritis. *Cardiology* 1989;76: 71–77.
36. Tabib A, Leroux C, Mornex JF, et al. Accelerated coronary atherosclerosis and arteriosclerosis in young human-immunodeficiency-virus-positive patients. *Coron Artery Dis* 2000;11: 41–46.
37. Murphy ST, Parfrey PS. The impact of anemia correction on cardiovascular disease in end-stage renal disease. *Semin Nephrol* 2000;20:350–355.
38. Lowrie EG. Acute-phase inflammatory process contributes to malnutrition, anemia, and possible other abnormalities in dialysis patients. *Am J Kidney Dis* 1998;32 (Suppl 4):S105–S112.
39. Macdougall IC. Role of uremic toxins in exacerbating anemia in renal failure. *Kidney Int* 2001;78:S67–S72.
40. Jelkmann W, Pagel H, Wolff M, et al. Monokines inhibiting erythropoietin production in human hepatoma cultures and in isolated perfused rat kidneys. *Life Sci* 1992;50:301–308.
41. Jongen-Lawrencic M, Peeters HRM, Rozemuller H, et al. IL-6 induced anaemia in rats: possible pathogenetic implications for anaemia observed in chronic inflammations. *Clin Exp Immunol* 1996;103:328–334.
42. Koistra M, Niemantsverdriet E, van ES A, et al. Iron absorption in erythropoietin-treated haemodialysis patients: effects of iron availability, inflammation and aluminum. *Nephrol Dial Transpl* 1998;13:82–88.
43. Barany P, Divino-Filho JC, Bergström J. High C-reactive protein is a strong predictor of resistance to erythropoietin in hemodialysis patients. *Am J Kidney Dis* 1997;29:565–568.

44. Beguin Y, Loo M, R'Zik S, et al. Early prediction of response to recombinant human erythropoietin in patients with the anemia of renal failure by serum transferrin receptor and fibrinogen. *Blood* 1993;82:2010–2016.
45. Gunell J, Yeun J, Depner TA, et al. Acute-phase response predicts erythropoietin resistance in hemodialysis and peritoneal dialysis patients. *Am J Kidney Dis* 1999;33:63–72.
46. United States Renal Data System. Excerpts from the USRDS 1999 annual data report. *Am J Kidney Dis* 1999;34(Suppl 1): S87–S89.
47. Ikizler TA, Wingard RL, Harvell J, et al. Association of morbidity with markers of nutrition and inflammation in chronic hemodialysis patients: A prospective study. *Kidney Int* 1999;55: 1945–1951.
48. Keane WF, Collins AJ. Influence of co-morbidity on mortality and morbidity of hemodialysis patients. *Am J Kidney Dis* 1994; 24:1010–1018.
49. Wang AYM, Woo J, Wang M, et al. Association of inflammation and malnutrition with cardiac valve calcification in continuous ambulatory peritoneal dialysis patients. *J Am Soc Nephrol* 2001;12:1927–1936.
50. Owen WF, Lowrie EG. C-reactive protein as an outcome predictor for maintenance hemodialysis patients. *Kidney Int* 1998; 54:627–636.
51. Yeun JY, Kaysen GA. Acute phase proteins and peritoneal dialysate albumin loss are the main determinants of serum albumin in peritoneal dialysis patients. *Am J Kidney Dis* 1997;30: 923–927.
52. Yudkin JS, Kumari M, Humphries SE, et al. Inflammation, obesity, stress and coronary heart disease: is interleukin-6 the link? *Atherosclerosis* 2000;148:209–214.
53. Kaysen GA, Dublin JA, Müller HG, et al. The acute-phase response varies with time and predicts serum albumin levels in hemodialysis patients. *Kidney Int* 2000;58:346–352.
54. Pereira BJG, Shapiro L, King AJ, et al. Plasma levels of IL-1β, TNF-α and their specific inhibitors in undialyzed chronic renal failure, CAPD and hemodialysis patients. *Kidney Int* 1994;45: 890–896.
55. Herbelin A, Urena P, Nguyen AT, et al. Elevated circulating levels of interleukin-6 in patients with chronic renal failure. *Kidney Int* 1991;39:954–960.
56. Bolton CH, Downs LG, Victory JGG, et al. Endothelial dysfunction in chronic renal failure: roles of lipoprotein oxidation and pro-inflammatory cytokines. *Nephrol Dial Transpl* 2001; 16:1189–1197.
57. Nakanishi I, Moutabarrik A, Okada N, et al. Interleukin-8 in chronic renal failure and dialysis patients. *Nephrol Dial Transpl* 1994;9:1435–1442.
58. Brockhaus M, Bar-Khayim Y, Gurwicz S, et al. Plasma tumour necrosis factor soluble receptors in chronic renal failure. *Kidney Int* 1992;42:663–667.
59. Descamps-Latscha B, Herbelin A, Nguyen AT, et al. Balance between IL-1β, TNF-α, and their specific inhibitors in chronic renal failure and maintenance dialysis. *J Immunol* 1995;154: 882–892.
60. van Riemsdijk-van Overbeeke IC, Baan CC, Hesse CJ, et al. TNF-α:mRNA, plasma protein levels and soluble receptors in patients with chronic hemodialysis, on CAPD and with end-stage renal failure. *Clin Nephrol* 2000;53:115–123.
61. Memoli B, Postiglione L, Cianciaruso B, et al. Role of different dialysis membranes in the release of interleukin-6 soluble receptor in uremic patients. *Kidney Int* 2000;58:417–424.
62. Bemelmans MH, Gouma DJ, Buurman WA. Influence of nephrectomy on tumor necrosis factor clearance in murine model. *J Immunol* 1993;150:2007–2017.
63. Poole S, Bird TA, Selkirk S, et al. Fate of injected interleukin 1 in rats: Sequestration and degradation in the kidney. *Cytokine* 1990;2:416–422.
64. Hession C, Decker JM, Sherblom AP, et al. Uromodulin (Tamm-Horsfall glycoprotein): a renal ligand for lymphokines. *Science* 1987;237:1479–1484.
65. Niebauer J, Volk HD, Kemp M, et al. Endotoxin and immune activation in chronic heart failure: a prospective cohort study. *Lancet* 1999;353:1838–1842.
66. Heinrich J, Schulte H, Schönfeld R, et al. Association of variables of coagulation, fibrinolysis and acute-phase with atherosclerosis in coronary and peripheral arteries and those arteries supplying the brain. *Thromb Haemost* 1995;73:374–378.
67. Liuzzo G, Biasucci LM, Gallimore JR, et al. Prognostic value of C-reactive protein and plasma amyloid A protein in severe unstable angina. *N Engl J Med* 1994;331:417–424.
68. Ayus JC, Sheikh-Hamad D. Silent infection in clotted hemodialysis access grafts. *J Am Soc Nephrol* 1998;9:1314–1321.
69. Stenvinkel P, Heimbürger O, Jogestrand T, et al. Does persistent infection with *Chlamydia pneumoniae* increase the risk of atherosclerosis in chronic renal failure? *Kidney Int* 1999;55: 2531–2532.
70. Haubitz M, Brunkhorst R. C-reactive protein and chronic *Chlamydia pneumonia* infection—long term predictors of cardiovascular disease survival in patients on peritoneal dialysis. *Nephrol Dial Transpl* 2001;16:809–815.
71. Spittle M, Craig R, Adhikarla R, et al. Relationship between antibodies to peridontal pathogens and C-reactive protein (CRP) levels in hemodialysis patients. *J Am Soc Nephrol* 2000; 11:299A.
72. Schmidt AM, Hori O, Chen JX, et al. Advanced glycation endproducts interacting with their endothelial receptor induce expression of vascular cell adhesion molecule (VCAM-1) in cultured human endothelial cells and in mice. A potential mechanism for the accelerated vasculopathy of diabetes. *J Clin Invest* 1995;96:1395–1403.
73. Miyata T, Ishiguro N, Yasuda Y, et al. Increased pentosidine, an advanced glycation end product, in plasma and synovial fluid from patients with rheumatoid arthritis and its relation with inflammatory markers. *Biochem Biophys Res Comm* 1998;244: 45–49.
74. Li JJ, Dickson D, Hof PR, et al. Receptors for advanced glycosylation end products in human brain: Role in brain homeostasis. *Molecular Med* 1998;4:46–60.
75. Morohoshi M, Fujisawa K, Uchimura I, et al. Glucose-dependent interleukin 6 and tumor necrosis production by human peripheral blood monocytes in vitro. *Diabetes* 1996;45: 954–959.
76. Vlassara H, Brownlee M, Manogue R, et al. Cachectin/TNF and IL1 induced by glucose-modified proteins: Role in normal tissue remodeling. *Science* 1988;240:1546–1548.
77. Schwedler S, Schinzel R, Vaith P, et al. Inflammation and advanced glycation end products in uremia: simple coexistence, potentiation or causal relationship? *Kidney Int* 2001;59 (Suppl 78):S32–S36.
78. Cavaillon JM, Poignet JL, Fitting C, et al. Serum interleukin-6 in long-term hemodialysed patients. *Nephron* 1992;60: 307–313.
79. Libetta C, De Nicola L, Rampino T, et al. Inflammatory effects of peritoneal dialysis: evidence of systemic monocyte activation. *Kidney Int* 1996;49:506–511.
80. Haubitz M, Schulze M, Koch KM. Increase of C-reactive pro-

tein serum values following haemodialysis. *Nephrol Dial Transpl* 1990;5:500–503.
81. Zaoui P, Hakim RM. The effects of the dialysis membrane on cytokine release. *J Am Soc Nephrol* 1994;4:1711–1718.
82. Schouten WEM, Grooteman MPC, et al. Effects of dialyser and dialysate on the acute phase response in clinical bicarbonate dialysis. *Nephrol Dial Transpl* 2000;15:379–384.
83. Tielemans C, Husson C, Schurmans T, et al. Effects of ultrapure and non-sterile dialysate on the inflammatory response during in vitro hemodialysis. *Kidney Int* 1996;49:236–243.
84. Panichi V, Migliori M, De Pietro S, et al. Plasma C-reactive protein in hemodialysis patients: a cross-sectional and longitudinal survey. *Blood Purif* 2000;18:30–36.
85. Schindler R, Boenisch O, Fischer C, et al. Effect of the hemodialysis membrane on the inflammatory reaction in vivo. *Clin Nephrol* 2000;53:452–459.
86. Zemel D, Krediet RT. Cytokine pattern in the effluent of continuous ambulatory peritoneal dialysis: relationship to peritoneal permeability. *Blood Purif* 1996;14:198–216.
87. Haubitz M, Brunkhorst R, Wrenger E, et al. Chronic induction of C-reactive protein by hemodialysis, but not by peritoneal dialysis therapy. *Perit Dial Int* 1996;16:158–162.
88. Takahashi T, Kubota M, Nakamura T, et al. Interleukin-6 gene expression in peripheral mononuclear cells from patients undergoing hemodialysis or continuous ambulatory peritoneal dialysis. *Ren Fail* 2000;22:345–354.
89. Kopple JD, Greene T, Chumlea WC, et al. Relationship between GFR and nutritional status: results from the MDRD study. *Kidney Int* 2000;57:1688–1703.
90. Plata-Salamán CR. Cytokines and anorexia: A brief overview. *Semin Oncol* 1998;25:64–72.
91. Yeh SS, Schuster MW. Geriatric cachexia: the role of cytokines. *Am J Clin Nutr* 1999;70:183–197.
92. King AJ, Kehayias JJ, Roubenoff R, et al. Cytokine production and nutritional status in hemodialysis patients. *Int J Artif Organs* 1998;21:4–11.
93. Guttridge DC, Mayo MW, Madrid LV, et al. NF-κB-induced loss of MyoD messenger RNA: Possible role in muscle decay and cachexia. *Cytokine* 2000;289:2363–2365.
94. Mitch WE, Du J, Bailey JL, et al. Mechanisms causing muscle proteolysis in uremia: the influence of insulin and cytokines. *Miner Elect Metab* 1999;25:216–219.
95. García-Martínez C, Llovera M, Agell N, et al. Ubiquitin gene expression in skeletal muscle is increased by tumor necrosis factor-α. *Biochem Biophys Res Comm* 1994;201:682–686.
96. Aguilera A, Codoceo R, Selgas R, et al. Anorexigen (TNF-alpha, cholecystokinin) and orexigen (neuropeptide Y) plasma levels in peritoneal dialysis (PD) patients. Their relationship with nutritional parameters. *Nephrol Dial Transpl* 1998;13:1476–1483.
97. Grunfeld C, Zhao C, Fuller J, et al. Endotoxin and cytokines induce expression of leptin, the ob gene product in hamsters. A role for leptin in the anorexia of infection. *J Clin Invest* 1996; 97:2152–2157.
98. Sarraf P, Frederich RC, Turner EM, et al. Multiple cytokines and acute inflammation raise mouse leptin levels: potential role in inflammatory anorexia. *J Exp Med* 1997;185:171–175.
99. Moshyedi AK, Josephs MD, Abdalla EK, et al. Increased leptin expression in mice with bacterial peritonitis is partially regulated by tumor necrosis factor alpha. *Infect Immun* 1998;66: 1800–1802.
100. Don BR, Rosales LM, Levine NW, et al. Leptin is a negative acute phase protein in chronic hemodialysis patients. *Kidney Int* 2001;59:1114–1120.
101. Parfrey PS, Foley RN, Harnett JD, et al. Outcome and risk factors for left ventricular disorders in chronic uremia. *Nephrol Dial Transpl* 1996;11:1277–1285
102. Levine B, Kalman J, Mayer L, et al. Elevated circulating levels of tumor necrosis factor in severe chronic heart failure. *N Engl J Med* 1990;323:236–241.
103. Munger MA, Johnsson B, Amber IJ, et al. Circulating concentrations of proinflammatory cytokines in mild or moderate heart failure secondary to ischemic or idiopathic dilated cardiomyopathy. *Am J Cardiol* 1996;77:723–727.
104. Sato Y, Takatsu Y, Kataoka K, et al. Serial circulating concentrations of C-reactive protein, interleukin (IL)-4, and IL-6 in patients with acute left heart decompensation. *Clin Cardiol* 1999; 22:811–813.
105. Anker SD, Ponikowski P, Varney S, et al. Wasting as independent risk factor for mortality in chronic heart failure. *Lancet* 1997;349:1050–1053.
106. Torzewski J, Torzewski M, Bowyer DE, et al. C-reactive protein frequently colocalizes with the terminal complement complex in the intima of early atherosclerotic lesions of human coronary arteries. *Arterioscler Tromb Vasc Biol* 1998;18:1386–1392.
107. Lagrand WK, Niessen HWM, Wolbink G-J, et al. C-reactive protein colocalizes with complement in human hearts during acute myocardial infarction. *Circulation* 1997;95:97–103.
108. Pasceri V, Willerson JT, Yeh ET. Direct proinflammatory effect of C-reactive protein on human endothelial cells. *Circulation* 2000;102:2165–2168.
109. Van Lenten BJ, Hama SY, de Beer FC, et al. Anti-inflammatory HDL becomes pro-inflammatory during the acute phase response. Loss of protective effect of HDL against LDL oxidation in aortic wall cell cocultures. *J Clin Invest* 1995;96:2758–2767.
110. Khovidhunkit W, Memon RA, Feingold KR, et al. Infection and inflammation-induced proatherogenic changes of lipoproteins. *J Infect Dis* 2000;181(Suppl 3):S462–S472.
111. Sandkamp M, Funke H, Schulte H, et al. Lipoprotein(a) is an independent risk factor for myocardial infarction at a young age. *Clin Chem* 1990;36:20–23.
112. Smith EB, Thompson WD. Fibrin as a factor in atherogenesis. *Thromb Res* 1994;73:1–19.
113. Zuckerman SH, O'Neal L. Endotoxin and GM-CSF-mediated down-regulation of macrophage apo E secretion is inhibited by a TNF-specific monoclonal antibody. *J Leukoc Biol* 1994;55: 743–748.
114. Tintut Y, Patel J, Parhami F, et al. Tumor necrosis factor-α promotes in vitro calcification of vascular cells via the cAMP pathway. *Circulation* 2000;102:2636–2642.
115. Bhagat K, Vallance P. Inflammatory cytokines impair endothelium-dependent dilatation in human veins in vivo. *Circulation* 1997;96:3042–3047.
116. Huber SA, Sakkinen P, Conze D, et al. Interleukin-6 exacerbates early atherosclerosis in mice. *Arterioscler Thromb Vasc Biol* 1999; 19:2364–2367.
117. Harris TB, Ferrucci L, Tracy RP, et al. Association of elevated interleukin-6 and C-reactive protein levels with mortality in the elderly. *Am J Med* 1999;106:506–512.
118. Stenvinkel P. Malnutrition and chronic inflammation as risk factors for cardiovascular disease in chronic renal failure. *Blood Purif* 2001;19:143–151.
119. Annuk M, Lind L, Linde T, et al. Impaired endothelium-dependent vasodilation in renal failure in humans. *Nephrol Dial Transpl* 2001;16:302–306.
120. van Guldener C, Janssen MJ, Lambert J, et al. Endothelium-dependent vasodilation is impaired in peritoneal dialysis patients. *Nephrol Dial Transpl* 1998;13:1782–1786.
121. Miyazaki H, Matsuoka H, Itabe H, et al. Hemodialysis impairs endothelial function via oxidative stress. Effects of vitamin E-coated dialyzer. *Circulation* 2000;101:1002–1006.
122. Fichtscherer S, Rosenberger G, Walter DH, et al. Elevated C-reactive protein levels and impaired endothelial vasoreactivity

in patients with coronary heart disease. *Circulation* 2000;102: 1000–1006.
123. Sinisalo J, Paronen J, Mattila KJ, et al. Relation of inflammation to vascular function in patients with coronary heart disease. *Atherosclerosis* 2000;149:403–411.
124. Holm T, Aaukrust P, Andersen AK, et al. Peripheral endothelial dysfunction in heart transplant recipients: possible role of proinflammatory cytokines. *Clin Transpl* 2000;14:218–225.
125. Hingorani AD, Cross J, Kharbanda RK, et al. Acute systemic inflammation impairs endothelium-dependent dilation in humans. *Circulation* 2000;102:994–999.
126. Shimokawa K, Ito A, Fukumoto Y, Kadokami T, et al. Chronic treatment with interleukin-1 beta induces coronary intimal lesions and vasospastic responses in pigs in vivo: The role of platelet derived growth factor. *J Clin Invest* 1996;97:769–776.
127. Stenvinkel P, Lindholm B, Heimbürger M, et al. Elevated serum levels of soluble adhesion molecules predicts death in predialysis patients: Association with malnutrition, inflammation and cardiovascular disease. *Nephrol Dial Transpl* 2000;15:1624–1630.
128. DeFronzo RA, Alvestrand A, Smith D, et al. Insulin resistance in uremia. *J Clin Invest* 1981;67:563–568.
129. Mendall MA, Patel P, Ballam L, et al. C reactive protein and its relation to cardiovascular risk factors: a population based cross sectional study. *BMJ* 1996;312:1061–1065.
130. Yudkin JS, Stehouwer CD, Emeis JJ, et al. C-reactive protein in healthy subjects: associations with obesity, insulin resistance, and endothelial dysfunction: a potential role for cytokines originating from adipose tissue. *Arterioscler Thromb Vasc Biol* 1999; 19:972–978.
131. Visser M, Bouter LM, McQuillan GM, et al. Elevated C-reactive protein levels in overweight and obese adults. *JAMA* 1999; 282:2131–2135.
132. Festa A, D'Agostino R, Howard G, et al. Chronic subclinical inflammation as part of the insulin resistance syndrome. *Circulation* 2000;102:42–47.
133. Halliwell B. The role of oxygen radicals in human disease with particular reference to the vascular system. *Haemostasis* 1993; 23(Suppl 1):118–126.
134. Yeun JY, Kaysen GA. C-reactive protein, oxidative stress, homocysteine, and troponin as inflammatory and metabolic predictors of atherosclerosis in ESRD. *Curr Opin Nephrol Hypertens* 2000;9:621–630.
135. Maggi E, Bellazzi R, Gazo A, et al. Autoantibodies against oxidatively-modified LDL in uremic patients undergoing dialysis. *Kidney Int* 1994;46:869–876.
136. Stenvinkel P, Holmberg I, Heimbürger O, et al. A study of plasmalogen as an index of oxidative stress in patients with chronic renal failure. Evidence of increased oxidative stress in malnourished patients. *Nephrol Dial Transpl* 1998;13: 2594–2600.
137. Boaz M, Smetana S, Weinstein T, et al. Secondary prevention with antioxidants of cardiovascular disease in endstage renal disease (SPACE): randomised placebo-controlled trial. *Lancet* 2000;356:1213–1218.
138. Memon RA, Staprans I, Noor M, et al. Infection and inflammation induce LDL oxidation in vivo. *Arterioscler Thromb Vasc Biol* 2000;20:1536–1542.
139. Nguyen-Khoa T, Massy ZA, De Bandt JP, et al. Oxidative stress and haemodialysis: role of inflammation and duration of dialysis treatment. *Nephrol Dial Transpl* 2001;16:335–340.
140. Handelman GJ, Walter MF, Adhikarla R, et al. Elevated plasma F2-isoprostanes in patients on long-term hemodialysis. *Kidney Int* 2001;59:1960–1966.
141. Griffioen AW, Molema G. Angiogenesis: Potentials for pharmacological intervention in the treatment of cancer, cardiovascular disease, and chronic inflammation. *Pharm Rev* 2000;52: 237–268.
142. McCourt M, Wang JH, Sookhai S, et al. Proinflammatory mediators stimulate neurophil-directed angiogenesis. *Arch Surg* 1999;134:1331–1332.
143. Combet S, Miyata T, Moulin P, et al. Vascular proliferation and enhanced expression of endothelial nitric oxide synthase in human peritoneum exposed to long-term peritoneal dialysis. *J Am Soc Nephrol* 2000;11:717–728.
144. Chung SH, Heimbürger O, Stenvinkel P, et al. Association between residual renal function, inflammation, and patient survival in new peritoneal dialysis patients. *Nephrol Dial Transplant* 2003;18(3):590–597.
145. Moulton KS, Heller E, Konerding MA, et al. Angiogenesis inhibitors endostatin or TNP-470 reduce intimal neovascularization and plaque growth in apolipoprotein E-deficient mice. *Circulation* 1999;99:1726–1732.
146. Kruse FE, Joussen AM, Rohrschneider K, et al. Thalidomide inhibits corneal angiogenesis induced by vascular endothelial growth factor. *Graefes Arch Clin Exp Ophthalmol* 1998;236: 461–466.
147. Corral LG, Haslett PA, Muller GW, et al. Differential cytokine modulation and T cell activation by two distinct classes of thalidomide analogues that are potent inhibitors of TNF-alpha. *J Immunol* 1999;163:380–386.
148. Reyes-Terán G, Sierra-Madero JG, Martínez del Cerro V, et al. Effects of thalidomide on HIV-associated wasting syndrome: a randomized, double blind, placebo-controlled clinical study. *AIDS* 1996;10:1501–1507.
149. Tramontana JM, Utaipat U, Molloy A, et al. Thalidomide treatment reduces tumour necrosis factor-α production and enhances weight gain in patients with pulmonary tuberculosis. *Molecular Med* 1995;1:384–397.
150. Schindler R, Dinarello CA, Koch KM. Angiotensin-converting enzyme inhibitors suppress synthesis of tumor necrosis factor and interleukin 1 by human peripheral blood mononuclear cells. *Cytokine* 1995;7:526–533.
151. Fukuzawa M, Satoh J, Sagara M, et al. Angiotensin-converting enzyme inhibitors suppress production of tumor necrosis factor-alpha in vitro and in vivo. *Immunopharmacology* 1997;36: 49–55.
152. Gullestad L, Aukrust P, Ueland T, et al. Effect of high- versus low-dose angiotensin converting enzyme inhibition on cytokine levels in chronic heart failure. *J Am Coll Cardiol* 1999;34: 2061–2067.
153. Stenvinkel P, Andersson P, Wang T, et al. Do ACE-inhibitors suppress tumor necrosis factor-α production in advanced chronic renal failure? *J Intern Med* 1999;246:503–507.
154. Ikonomidis I, Andreotti F, Economou E, et al. Increased proinflammatory cytokines in patients with chronic stable angina and their reduction by aspirin. *Circulation* 1999;100:793–798.
155. Livio M, Benigni A, Vigano G, et al. Moderate doses of aspirin and risk of bleeding in renal failure. *Lancet* 1986;1:414–416.
156. Ridker PM, Rifai N, Lowenthal SP. Rapid reduction in C-reactive protein with cerivastatin among 785 patients with primary hypercholesterolemia. *Circulation* 2001;103:1191–1193.
157. Fellström BC, Holdaas H, Jardine AG. Why do we need a statin trial in hemodialysis patients? *Kidney Int* 2003;84:204–206.
158. Sitter T, Bergner A, Schiffl H. Dialysate related cytokine induction and response to recombinant human erythropoietin in haemodialysis patients. *Nephrol Dial Transpl* 2000;15: 1207–1211.
159. Chung SH, Stenvinkel P, Bergström J, et al. Biocompatibility of new peritoneal dialysis solutions: What can we hope to achieve? *Perit Dial Int* 2000;20:S57–S67.

160. Kopple JD, Bernard D, Messana J, et al. Treatment of malnourished CAPD patients with an amino acid based dialysate. *Kidney Int* 1995;47:1148–1157.
161. Witko-Sarsat V, Friedlander M, Khoa TN, et al. Advanced oxidation protein products as novel mediators of inflammation and monocyte activation in chronic renal failure. *J Immunol* 1998;161:2524–2532.
162. Grimble RF. Nutritional modulation of cytokine biology. *Nutrition* 1998;14:634–640.
163. Devaraj S, Jialal I. Alpha tocopherol supplementation decreases serum C-reactive protein and monocyte interleukin-6 levels in normal volunteers and type-2 diabetic patients. *Free Radic Biol Med* 2000;29:790–792.
164. Uppritchard JE, Sutherland WHF, Mann JI. Effect of supplementation with tomato juice, vitamin E, and vitamin C on LDL oxidation and products of inflammatory activity in type 2 diabetes. *Diabetes Care* 2000;23:733–738.
165. Satoh M, Yamasaki Y, Nagake Y, et al. Oxidative stress is reduced by the long-term use of vitamin E-coated dialysis filters. *Kidney Int* 2001;59:1943–1950.

14

EFFECT OF MALNUTRITION AND CHANGES IN PROTEIN INTAKE ON RENAL FUNCTION

SAULO KLAHR

Protein intake is an important modulator of renal hemodynamics (1,2). A sustained change from a low- to a high-protein diet increases renal blood flow and glomerular filtration rate (GFR) by 30% to 60% in several species (3–6). Acute administration of protein also increases renal blood flow and GFR by similar amounts for several hours after ingestion of a protein load (7–10). Changes in renal hemodynamics are not observed after ingestion of carbohydrates or fats, suggesting that this effect is unique to protein intake (3). Administration of individual amino acids by stomach tube (11) or as an intravenous infusion (12,13) mimics the response to protein feeding with respect to renal blood flow and GFR. Protein intake increases single-nephron GFR and renal plasma flow per nephron.

Several mechanisms, which may not be mutually exclusive, have been proposed to explain the increase in renal blood flow and GFR observed after a protein meal or during chronic protein administration. First, humoral factors, either circulating or local, are released in response to elevation in plasma amino acid levels and subsequently stimulate renal vasodilation.

Increased protein intake stimulates the secretion of growth hormone, glucagon, dopamine, eicosanoids, and renin. A role for amino acids as metabolic substrates in causing these changes has been suggested, and intrinsic renal mechanisms including tubuloglomerular feedback and tubular transport mechanisms may be involved.

CIRCULATING FACTORS

Growth Hormone and Glucagon

Both growth hormone and glucagon have been implicated in the renal vasodilation that follows a protein load (14–16). Indeed, both hormones, when infused intravenously, increased renal blood flow and GFR (14,17,18). However, the role of growth hormone in this phenomenon is questionable because renal blood flow and GFR increase after a meat meal (8) or during amino acid infusion (19) before plasma growth hormone levels rise. Also, renal plasma flow and GFR may rise in the absence of increased levels of plasma growth hormone (20). In addition, patients deficient in growth hormone exhibit renal vasodilation after an amino acid infusion (19,21). Glucagon release may play a role in the increase in renal blood flow and GFR after a protein meal. Protein meals and amino acid administration stimulate the release of glucagon. However, carbohydrate meals, which do not affect renal hemodynamics, do not increase plasma glucagon (6). Administration of branched-chain amino acids does not cause renal vasodilation and does not increase glucagon release (22,23). Also, GFR and effective renal plasma flow increase in parallel with the changes in plasma glucagon after a meat meal in children with type I diabetes (24). Furthermore, infusion of glucagon in humans to achieve plasma levels comparable to those obtained during arginine infusion also increases GFR and renal plasma flow (25). However, there are also contradictory results that do not support a role of glucagon in the renal vasodilation that occurs after a protein meal (26,27). Other studies (5, 28,29) suggest that an increase in plasma glucagon is not needed for protein or amino acid–stimulated renal vasodilation and hyperfiltration. It is possible that a combination of increased amino acids and increased glucagon is necessary for the hemodynamic effects to occur.

Glucagon increases sodium excretion. However, this action of the peptide may be indirect because infusion of glucagon into the renal artery does not produce natriuresis. Glucagon increases circulating cyclic adenosine monophosphate (cAMP), which may decrease tubular sodium absorption.

Renin-Angiotensin System

The renin-angiotensin system may mediate protein or amino acid–induced renal vasodilation and increases in GFR. This effect of protein on the renin-angiotensin system may be more important during long-term changes in protein intake rather than with the acute administration of a protein load. Most studies indicate that plasma renin activity and angiotensin II concentration do not increase during the acute infusion of amino acids or following a meat meal (20,30,31). Several investigators have examined the effects of ACE inhibitors on the renal hemodynamic responses to protein feeding or amino acid infusion. Woods et al. (30) found that infusion of captopril to conscious dogs did not modify the increase in renal plasma flow and GFR observed after a meat meal. The same was the case in humans (32). However, with long-term increases in dietary protein, the synthesis and release of renin is augmented (33). Renal renin messenger RNA (mRNA) was higher in rats fed a high-protein diet (50% protein) than in rats fed a standard rat chow (24% protein). A lower protein intake (6% protein) decreased the activity of renal renin mRNA in rats (33). Rosenberg et al. (10) also examined the effects of dietary protein on GFR, renin activity, and excretion of eicosanoids in humans with glomerular disease. The high-protein diet was accompanied by higher plasma renin activity and an increased excretion of prostaglandin E_2 (PGE_2) and 6-keto $PGE_1\alpha$ in the urine. These changes were observed in patients with a wide spectrum of severity of disease and in the absence of changes in weight, mean arterial pressure, or serum protein levels. The finding of increased eicosanoid excretion in patients ingesting high-protein diets suggests that augmented eicosanoid synthesis may mediate the increased release of renin in such patients.

Dopamine

Because dopamine increases renal plasma flow and GFR, as well as solute excretion, intrarenal dopamine was suggested as the mediator of several of the renal effects of protein or amino acid administration (34). A protein load increased dopamine levels in plasma (when carbidopa, a dopamine decarboxylase inhibitor, was present) and caused natriuresis and increased osmolal clearance (34). Without carbidopa, plasma dopamine did not increase, but dopamine excretion promptly increased.

Atrial Peptides

The administration of atrial peptide (ANP) increases GFR, but it probably does not mediate the renal hemodynamic changes observed after a meat meal or amino acid loading because (a) sodium intake and markers of plasma volume suggest no greater stimulus toward atrial peptide secretion after the meat meal, and (b) atrial peptide administration in animals increases GFR to a greater extent than renal plasma flow (35), a pattern somewhat different from that observed after a meat meal. Several studies have reported no increase in atrial peptide after a meat meal in humans (36,37). In another study, atrial peptide was found to be constant or only slightly elevated in plasma after a meat meal despite a significant increase in creatinine clearance (38). Thus, atrial peptide does not appear to play a major role in mediating the changes in renal blood flow and GFR that occur after a protein meal.

Infusion of ANP leads to variable but short-lived effects on renal blood flow. The renal vasodilation observed during ANP infusion is most likely an autoregulatory adjustment compensatory for the fall in blood pressure.

LOCAL FACTORS

Eicosanoids

Protein intake conditions the synthesis of eicosanoid in isolated glomeruli from rats (39,40). Glomeruli obtained from rats fed a high-protein diet produced significantly greater amounts of PGE_2, 6-keto $PGE_1\alpha$, and thromboxane A_2 under basal conditions than glomeruli obtained from rats fed a low-protein diet. To investigate the potential role of the renin-angiotensin system in the protein-induced modulation of glomerular eicosanoid production, rats ingesting either a high- or low-protein diet were randomized to groups receiving an ACE inhibitor (enalapril) or no therapy. Enalapril attenuated the protein-induced augmentation in glomerular eicosanoid production. This effect occurred only when enalapril was administered *in vivo*. The active metabolite enalaprilate did not alter PGE_2 production by isolated glomeruli when added *in vitro*. Thus, dietary protein modulates glomerular eicosanoid synthesis in the rat, and this effect seems to be mediated by the renin-angiotensin system. Yanagisawa et al. (40) also found that addition of angiotensin II to isolated glomeruli *in vitro* increased the synthesis of eicosanoids. The increment was greater in glomeruli obtained from rats fed a high-protein diet than in glomeruli from rats fed a low-protein diet. To examine the potential mechanisms by which changes in protein intake may modify eicosanoid synthesis, we determined the activities of phospholipase A_2 and phospholipase C (40).

There was a significant increase in phosphatidyl ethanolamine-specific phospholipase A_2 activity in glomeruli from rats fed a high-protein diet when compared with glomeruli from rats fed a low-protein diet. In contrast, phosphatidyl-specific phospholipase A_2 activity was decreased significantly in glomeruli from rats fed a high-protein diet. No significant changes in phosphatidyl inositol biphosphate (PIP_2) and phospholipase C activities were detected between glomeruli of the two dietary groups. The content and activity of cyclooxygenase was significantly greater in glomeruli from rats fed a high-protein diet than in glomeruli from rats fed a low-protein diet. These rat studies indicate that the greater synthesis of eicosanoids in glomeruli isolated from rats fed a high-protein diet may be mediated by increases in the amount and activity of cyclooxygenase coupled with enhanced activity of phosphoethanolamine-specific phospholipase A_2. The greater release of arachidonic acid, as a result of enhanced activity of phosphoethanolamine-specific phospholipase A_2 and the increased activity of cyclooxygenase, would result in increased eicosanoid synthesis. In rats fed a high-protein diet, inhibition of the synthesis of angiotensin II using an ACE inhibitor prevented the increases in the activities of phospholipase A_2 and cyclooxygenase observed in untreated rats. This observation suggests that increased protein intake augments renin-angiotensin production. The increased activity of angiotensin II, in turn, conditions the production of eicosanoids. Dietary protein intake also modulated glomerular eicosanoid production in three models of experimental renal disease in the rat: streptozotocin-induced diabetes mellitus, Heymann nephritis, and partial renal ablation (41,42). Vasodilatory eicosanoids (PGE_2, prostacyclin) may account for the increase in renal plasma flow and GFR observed after protein administration.

Nitric Oxide

Besides eicosanoids, another locally acting humoral factor that may participate in the vasodilation of amino acid administration is nitric oxide. Several laboratories have demonstrated that inhibitors of L-arginine metabolism and other inhibitors of nitric oxide synthesis prevent or at least blunt amino acid–stimulated renal vasodilation and the increase in GFR in rats and dogs (43–46). Arginine is not responsible for the vasodilation of amino acid mixtures because infusion of amino acid mixtures without arginine produces vasodilation. Consequently, nitric oxide does not account for the vasodilatory role of other amino acids. Agmatine, an active metabolite of arginine metabolism, is also a vasodilatory compound (47).

ROLE OF SPECIFIC AMINO ACIDS

Whether specific amino acids increase GFR directly or through some mediator is also unknown. Glycine can increase GFR when infused intravenously in dogs (48). An infusion of mixed amino acids has a similar effect in rats (49). Brezis et al. (50) examined the functional effects of different amino acid mixtures in the isolated perfused rat kidney. Addition of either an amino acid mixture or 2 mM glutamine to the glucose-containing perfusate markedly decreased renal vascular resistance. Oxygen consumption increased, which suggested metabolism of amino acids by tubular cells. Amino acid–induced vasodilation was blocked by antimycin or rotenone, inhibitors of mitochondrial respiration, or when the kidney was perfused with α-aminoisobutyrate or other nonmetabolizable amino acids. The conclusion reached was that enhanced renal metabolism accounted for the decrease in vascular resistance.

INTRINSIC RENAL MECHANISMS

The third potential factor involved in mediating protein or amino acid–stimulated renal vasodilation is the action of intrinsic renal mechanisms including tubuloglomerular feedback and tubular transport. Tubuloglomerular balance has been examined in rats with subtotal nephrectomy fed isocaloric diets containing 6% or 40% casein for 10 days prior to study. Rats fed the 40% casein diet required a greater tubular flow rate to initiate a decrease in single-nephron GFR. A 40% to 50% decreased sensitivity of the tubuloglomerular feedback mechanism was observed, which led to the conclusion that a high-protein diet causes a failure of the normal mechanisms controlling GFR (51). The mechanism may be related to changes in angiotensin production or vascular response to its action or to increased reabsorption of sodium and chloride by the thick ascending limb of the loop of Henle. The increased reabsorption of sodium chloride may be the result of marked hypertrophy of the thick ascending limb of Henle observed in rats fed a high-protein diet (52).

In summary, the mechanisms underlying the variable increase in GFR in response to an acute protein load (1,2) are not well characterized. The increase in GFR may be conditioned by the previous level of dietary protein intake, protein source, volume status, renal disease that may be present, activity of the renin-angiotensin system, and production of renal eicosanoids. In contrast to the variable and transient response of GFR to short-term protein loads, more long-term changes in protein intake apparently affect the level of GFR in a more sustained fashion. How this change in GFR relates to the progression of renal insufficiency has not been defined.

EFFECTS OF MALNUTRITION OR PROTEIN DEPRIVATION ON RENAL FUNCTION

A decreased protein intake has been shown to decrease GFR and renal plasma flow in normal subjects. Normal subjects fed a calorie-deficient diet, regardless of the percentage of calories derived from fat, protein, or carbohydrates, demonstrate a reduction in creatinine clearance (53). Also, normal subjects with decreased intake of protein as compared to the same subjects during the ingestion of a "normal" protein demonstrated a fall in inulin clearance and paraaminohippurate (PAH) clearance, surrogate measures of GFR, and effective renal plasma flow (4). Prolonged deprivation of calories and protein intake in the diet may result in calorie-protein malnutrition. Studies carried out in developing countries have shown that both children and adults with calorie-protein malnutrition sustain changes in renal function as a consequence of the dietary deprivation (54). Children with calorie-protein malnutrition demonstrated reductions in GFR and renal plasma flow (55). Values ranged

TABLE 14.1. GLOMERULAR FILTRATION RATE AND RENAL PLASMA FLOW IN MALNOURISHED SUBJECTS

	Malnourished				Repleted or Normal			
Investigator	No. of Subjects	C_{IN}	C_{PAH} (mL/min)	FF	No. of Subjects	C_{IN}	C_{PAH} (mL/min)	FF
Alleyne (6)	8 children	47.1	249.4	0.21	14 children	92.4	321.2	0.29
	7 children[a]	42.9	184.0	0.27				
Arroyave et al. (13)	9 children	13.7	—	—	9 children	33.9	—	—
					17 normal children	45.0		
Gordillo et al. (8)	10 children	23.0	108.4		25 normal children	64.0	294	0.23
Klahr (14,15)	10 adults	64.1	325.8	0.20	10 adults	88.3	381.1	0.24
McCance (17)	11 adults	119.4	—			—		
	11 adults	100.9	—			—		
Mollison (16)	2 adults[a]	53,70	230,383[b]			—		
	2 adults	124,141	340,710[b]			—		

C_{IN}, clearance of insulin; C_{PAH}, clearance of P-aminohippurate; FF, filtration fraction.
[a]Edema was present in these subjects at the time of study. Mean values are given in mL/min. The data for adults are corrected for 1.73 m^2. The data of Arroyave and Gordillo are expressed per (m^2). The data of Alleyne are corrected for height (m^3).
[b]Diodone clearances.
From Klahr S, Alleyne GAO. Effect of chronic protein-calorie malnutrition on the kidney. Editorial. *Kidney Int* 1973;3:129–141, with permission.

from 13 to 50 mL/min/1.73 m^2 for GFR and from 110 to 150 mL/min/1.73 m^2 for renal plasma flow. Filtration fraction, the ratio of GFR to renal plasma flow, was reduced. These changes in renal hemodynamics were not influenced by the presence or absence of edema. Following repletion and refeeding with protein, similar increases in GFR and renal plasma flow were observed in children with or without edema. Several studies also have revealed decreases in GFR and renal plasma flow in adults with calorie-protein malnutrition as assessed by the clearance of inulin and PAH. Such decreases could be reversed toward normal by protein repletion (54). Table 14.1 summarizes data on the clearances of inulin (GFR) and PAH and filtration fraction in children and adults before and after protein repletion.

LEVELS OF PLASMA CREATININE AND SERUM UREA NITROGEN IN PATIENTS WITH PROTEIN-ENERGY MALNUTRITION

A decrease in GFR usually is associated with increased plasma levels of creatinine and urea nitrogen. When production of urea or creatinine is decreased, however, moderate to severe impairment of renal function may not result in increased plasma levels of either of these two compounds. Patients with moderate to severe protein energy malnutrition usually present with low or normal plasma levels of creatinine and urea nitrogen despite marked reductions in GFR (56). Because the excretion of both creatinine and urea in the urine is markedly reduced in patients with calorie-protein malnutrition, it may be concluded that production of both of these substances is diminished in subjects with malnutrition. The decrease in creatinine production is probably the result of a marked decrease in muscle mass. The low levels of urea presumably result from decreased protein intake, slower tissue-protein breakdown, and/or possibly urea reutilization (57). During protein repletion, both SUN (serum urea nitrogen) and plasma creatinine increase despite an increase in GFR (56). The increase in the levels of SUN and creatinine presumably reflects increased entry of both end products of the metabolism of protein and creatine into body fluids; hence, during the period of protein repletion, urea and creatinine production exceeds their excretion. It has been noted that urea levels may rise above normal in children recovering from malnutrition. This rise simply may reflect the high-protein diets that usually are fed to such children. Besides affecting renal hemodynamics, energy-protein malnutrition results in changes in acid-base balance, the kidney's concentrating ability, and the kidney's ability to excrete sodium loads.

CONCENTRATION AND DILUTION OF THE URINE IN PATIENTS WITH PROTEIN-ENERGY MALNUTRITION

Polyuria and nocturia are frequent complaints of patients with malnutrition. The capacity to concentrate the urine in patients with calorie-protein malnutrition is diminished. However, the ability to excrete a minimally dilute urine is not reduced. Klahr et al. (58) studied the ability of patients with chronic calorie-protein malnutrition to dilute and concentrate their urine. After 14 hours of fluid deprivation, urine osmolality never exceeded 600 mOsm/kg water in 11 malnourished subjects. Protein repletion resulted in a progressive increase in urine osmolality in each patient after 14 hours of fluid deprivation (Fig. 14.1). Values for solute-free water reabsorption (TcH_2O) also were depressed in

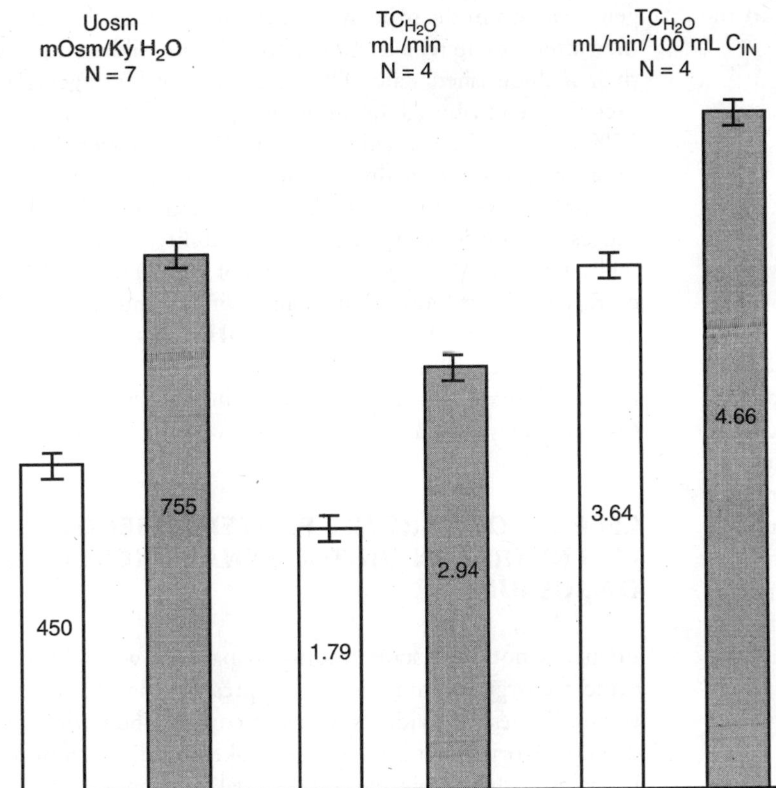

FIGURE 14.1. Urine osmolality (U_{osm}) and negative free water clearance (Tc_{H_2O}) in patients with chronic calorie-protein malnutrition before (*open bars*) and after (*striped bars*) protein repletion. (From Klahr S, Alleyne GAO. Effect of chronic protein-calorie malnutrition on the kidney. Editorial. *Kidney Int* 1973; 3:129–141, with permission.)

malnourished individuals given mannitol and vasopressin. However, the ability of malnourished individuals to produce a diluted urine was intact. During water loading, urine osmolality in seven adults with malnutrition averaged 57 mOsm/kg body water, a figure comparable to that observed in normal subjects. Values for free water clearance corrected per deciliter of GFR averaged 15.8 mL, a figure similar to that reported in healthy individuals.

The defect in concentrating the urine in malnourished subjects probably results from a decrease in osmolality in the renal medulla, most likely as a consequence of low levels of urea in this area of the kidney (58). The concentrating defect resolves slowly during protein repletion, presumably as a result of a markedly positive nitrogen balance in the initial weeks of protein repletion. During this period, urea excretion in the urine does not rise considerably for several weeks after the increase in dietary protein intake is initiated. Thus, rapid restoration of the renal medullary gradient for urea would not be expected. However, the oral administration of urea results in a rapid increase in the ability to concentrate the urine after 14 hours of fluid deprivation in malnourished subjects (58). The marked improvement in the concentrating ability of several malnourished subjects during protein repletion and the dramatic change observed during the administration of urea suggests that an anatomic alteration does not account for the concentrating defect. Rather, a functional disorder seems likely. Impaired resorption of sodium in the ascending segment of the loop of Henle may explain the concentrating defect; however, the finding of a normal capacity to dilute the urine would argue against such a postulate. Most likely, a marked decrease in urea, as an osmolal particle in the renal medulla effective in promoting the reabsorption of water from the cortical and medullary collecting ducts, accounts for the concentrating defect in patients with protein-energy malnutrition. An excellent correlation was found during protein repletion in patients with malnutrition between the values for urine osmolality and the concomitant 24-hour nitrogen excretion in the urine. These results support the suggestion that decreased urea concentration in the renal medulla accounts for the renal-concentrating defect of patients with chronic protein malnutrition.

Pennell et al. (59) examined by micropuncture techniques the effects of urea infusion on the urine-concentrating mechanisms of protein-depleted rats. These studies showed that the enhanced urinary osmolality of protein-depleted rats infused with urea was attended by (a) increased papillary hypertonicity, (b) increased urea concentration in all papillary structures, and (c) increased water removal from the descending limb. Crawford et al. (60) showed that in rats fed a low-protein diet and given injections of long-acting vasopressin, the administration of urea further reduced urine volume and increased urine-concentrating ability. From the preceding data, it is possible to ascribe the polyuria and the renal-concentrating defect observed in malnourished subjects to decreased urea concentration in the renal medulla.

ACID EXCRETION AND ACID-BASE BALANCE IN PATIENTS WITH CALORIE-PROTEIN MALNUTRITION

Adults with chronic calorie-protein malnutrition have normal blood pH and serum bicarbonate levels (61). However, the total excretion of net acid as measured by the sum of urine ammonium plus titratable acid minus urine bicarbonate is markedly decreased in patients with calorie-protein malnutrition. The finding of reduced acid excretion despite normal blood pH and bicarbonate levels suggests that endogenous acid production is reduced in malnutrition (61). The generation of hydrogen ions from metabolism usually is related to protein degradation. In normal subjects consuming daily a diet of constant composition, the rate of metabolic hydrogen ion production will be constant and the quantity of hydrogen excreted in the urine will equal the rate of hydrogen ion production. In patients with severe malnutrition, hydrogen ion production is decreased. When subjects with malnutrition are given protein, they retain nitrogen, and even in severely malnourished children there is a marked positive balance after protein administration. Thus, fewer amino acids are catabolized. Also, patients with malnutrition exhibit reduced protein turnover in muscle. In addition, there is a decrease in the activities of amino acid–activated enzymes of liver and a decrease in urea cycle enzymes; thus, amino acids from muscle are incorporated preferentially into protein and there is less wasteful degradation. Little is known about organic acid excretion in malnutrition. Uric acid excretion varies widely, and it would be expected that with severe potassium deficiency the renal excretion of organic acids may be altered. The net effect of all these adaptations is a reduction in the metabolic production of acid. Renal acid excretion increases during protein repletion without a change in the serum levels of bicarbonate or changes in blood pH (61). Administration of ammonium chloride leads to a greater degree of metabolic acidosis in malnourished patients than in the same subjects after a period of protein repletion. Klahr et al. found that although basal excretion of ammonia was lower in malnourished subjects, the increment after ammonium-chloride administration was approximately the same before and after protein repletion; however, the increment in titratable acid was four times greater in the protein-repleted state than in the malnourished state (61). This increment is related to the greater availability of phosphate in the urine, a consequence of increased dietary protein, which is a major source of dietary phosphorus during the period of repletion compared to the period of profound malnutrition, when excretion of phosphorus was less than 200 mg per day. A similar pattern of acid excretion has been observed in children. Total hydrogen excretion in the urine was greater in malnourished children after protein repletion than in the same children during their malnourished state. The percentage of hydrogen-ion excretion contributed by ammonium was approximately 75% in the malnourished state and 58% in recovered children. In adults with malnutrition the urine can be acidified to a pH as low as 4.5 during ammonium-chloride loading, suggesting no defect in the kidney's ability to produce a hydrogen gradient in distal segments of the nephron. However, it has been found that infants with malnutrition and gastroenteritis can lower their urine pH to a greater extent when they are well nourished than when they are malnourished. Therefore, an impairment in their ability to acidify the urine may be present in children with malnutrition.

EFFECTS OF CHRONIC PROTEIN-ENERGY MALNUTRITION ON THE RENAL EXCRETION OF SODIUM

Edema is not a constant finding in patients with chronic protein-energy malnutrition. The presence or absence of edema in these individuals seems to correlate best with the dietary history of salt intake. The intake of sodium chloride in malnourished subjects is quite variable. Among children with kwashiorkor, moderate to severe edema usually is present (62). Edema usually is present in the lower extremities, hands, and face (63). Edema-forming states are characterized by the renal retention of salt and water. Thus, in the edema-forming syndromes, the rate of excretion of sodium and water by the kidney is lower than the concurrent rate of acquisition. Common to all edema-forming states is the apparent need for expansion of effective extracellular fluid volume. Sodium-balance studies in nonedematous malnourished patients have shown that these subjects could conserve sodium adequately when fed a diet containing 10 mEq of salt daily. By contrast, when fed a diet containing 170 mEq of sodium, these patients demonstrated a mean positive sodium balance of 420 mEq and a weight gain of 2.8 kg after 5 days of such a diet. After protein repletion, the same individuals fed an identical diet demonstrated a mean positive sodium balance of only 150 mEq and a weight gain of 1.2 kg. The results of these balance studies suggest that subjects with protein malnutrition have impaired excretion of sodium loads (64). The capacity to excrete an equivalent sodium load improves after protein repletion.

The effects of acute administration of sodium chloride also have been studied in patients with chronic protein malnutrition before and after protein repletion. These malnourished subjects had a mean GFR of 41 mL/min, which increased to 45 mL/min during extracellular volume expansion. Basal excretion of sodium in the urine averaged 20.6 μEq/min and increased to 46 μEq/min after volume expansion. Fractional sodium excretion increased from

0.5% to 0.8% with expansion. When the same individuals were studied after protein repletion, basal GFR averaged 77 mL/min and increased to 87 mL/min after administration of saline. Absolute sodium excretion increased from 112 to 1,170 μEq/min, and fractional sodium excretion increased from 1.1% to 11% before and after saline expansion, respectively. Thus, the rapid intravenous administration of isotonic saline results in an almost negligible increase in fractional sodium excretion in the malnourished state. When the same studies were repeated after protein repletion, a pronounced increase in fractional sodium excretion was observed. Similar observations have been made in children with malnutrition. A smaller percentage of the saline load is excreted by children who are malnourished than by children who are protein-replete. The mechanisms of sodium retention in malnutrition are not clear, but systemic as well as intrinsic renal factors seem to have a role (Fig. 14.2). Decreased protein intake leads to hypoalbuminemia. It is controversial whether plasma volume is decreased in malnourished subjects; however, available evidence indicates that cardiac output is diminished (65). A decrease in cardiac output, in turn, will tend to decrease arterial pressure, leading to a fall in peritubular hydrostatic pressure and increased tubular reabsorption of salt and water. In addition, renal blood flow and GFR are diminished greatly in malnourished subjects, leading to a decrease in the filtered load of salt and water. Simultaneously, there is increased renin-angiotensin production (55) and presumably elevated levels of circulating aldosterone, which in turn will increase the tubular reabsorption of salt and water. The combination of a decreased filtered load of salt and water plus increased tubular reabsorption leads to net sodium retention and edema formation.

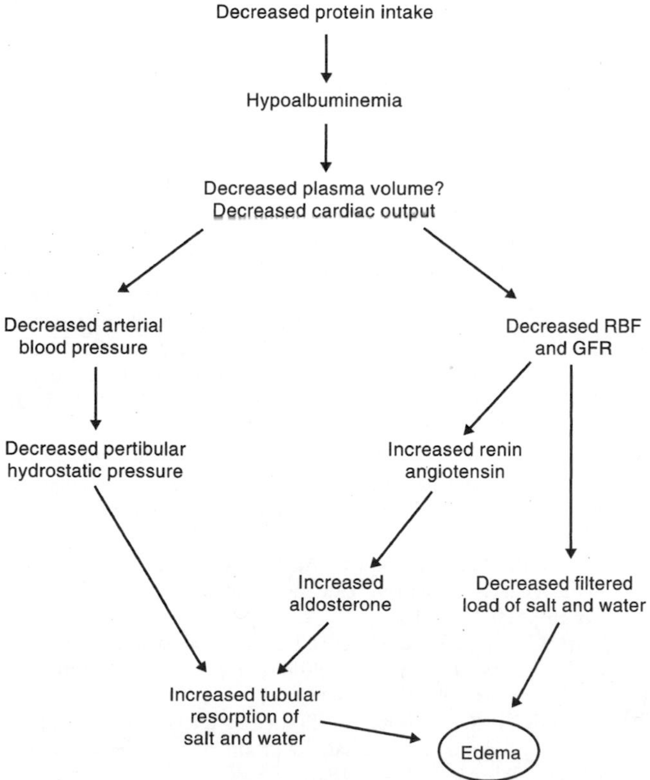

FIGURE 14.2. Possible mechanisms responsible for the development of edema in patients with chronic calorie-protein malnutrition. RBF, renal blood flow; GFR, glomerular filtration rate. (From Klahr S, Alleyne GAO. Effect of chronic protein-calorie malnutrition on the kidney. Editorial. *Kidney Int* 1973;3:129–141, with permission.)

MALNUTRITION IN ADVANCED RENAL DISEASE

Patients with advanced chronic renal disease often manifest signs of wasting and malnutrition. Most studies that have evaluated the nutritional status of patients with chronic renal failure have reported some degree of malnutrition in this population. The prevalence of malnutrition has been estimated to range from approximately 20% to 60% in different studies. A number of studies have documented the increased morbidity and mortality in patients with renal failure suffering from malnutrition (66–68).

SUMMARY

The effects of chronic calorie-protein malnutrition on renal function are summarized in Table 14.2. The decrease in GFR and the increased reabsorption of solutes observed in malnourished individuals would tend to minimize the loss of nutrients in the urine. In addition, the fall in the filtered load of sodium would decrease the metabolic requirements for sodium reabsorption in the kidney and hence lower the basal metabolic requirement in patients with chronic protein-energy malnutrition.

TABLE 14.2. EFFECTS OF CHRONIC CALORIE-PROTEIN MALNUTRITION ON RENAL FUNCTION

1. Decreased renal plasma flow and glomerular filtration rate
2. Impaired concentrating ability (polyuria) with normal diluting capacity
3. Impaired ability to excrete acid loads
   a. Normal ability to decrease urine pH
   b. Markedly decreased titratable acid excretion because of substantial reduction in phosphate excretion in urine
4. Impaired ability to excrete salt load

From Klahr S, Davis T. Changes in renal function with chronic calorie-protein malnutrition. In: Mitch WE, Klahr S, eds. *Nutrition and the kidney.* Boston: Little, Brown, 1988:59–79, with permission.

ACKNOWLEDGMENTS

The author gratefully acknowledges the assistance of Monica Waller in the preparation of this chapter.

REFERENCES

1. Klahr S. Effects of protein intake on the progression of renal disease. *Annu Rev Nutr* 1989;9:87–108.
2. Woods LL. Mechanisms of renal hemodynamic regulation in response to protein feeding. *Kidney Int* 1993;44:659–675.
3. Shannon JA, Jolliffe N, Smith HW. The excretion of urine in the dog. IV. The effect of maintenance diet, feeding, etc., upon the quantity of glomerular filtrate. *Am J Physiol* 1932;101: 625–638.
4. Pullman TN, Alving AS, Dern RJ, et al. The influence of dietary protein intake on specific renal functions in normal man. *J Lab Clin Med* 1954;44:320–332.
5. Schoolwerth AC, Sandler RS, Hoffman P, et al. Effects of nephron reduction and dietary protein content on renal ammoniagenesis in the rat. *Kidney Int* 1975;7:397–404.
6. Ando A, Kawata T, Hara Y, et al. Effects of dietary protein intake on renal function in humans. *Kidney Int* 1989;27:S64–S67.
7. O'Connor WJ, Summerill RA. The effect of a meal of meat on glomerular filtration rate in dogs at normal urine flows. *J Physiol* 1976;256:81–91.
8. Bergstrom J, Ahlberg M, Alvestrand A. Influence of protein intake on renal hemodynamics and plasma hormone concentrations in normal subjects. *Acta Med Scand* 1985;217:189–196.
9. Bosch JP, Lew S, Glabman S, et al. Renal hemodynamic changes in humans. Response to protein loading in normal and diseased kidneys. *Am J Med* 1986;81:809–815.
10. Rosenberg ME, Swanson JE, Thomas BL, et al. Glomerular and hormonal responses to dietary protein intake in human renal disease. *Am J Physiol* 1987;253:F1083–F1090.
11. Lee KE, Summerill RA. Glomerular filtration rate following administration of individual amino acids in conscious dogs. *Q J Exp Physiol* 1982;67:459–465.
12. Woods LL, Mizelle HL, Montani J-P, et al. Mechanisms controlling renal hemodynamics and electrolyte excretion during amino acids. *Am J Physiol* 1986;251:F303–F312.
13. Stummvoll HK, Luger A, Prager R. Effect of amino acid infusion on glomerular filtration rate. *N Engl J Med* 1983;308:159–160.
14. Premen AJ, Hall JE, Smith MJ Jr. Postprandial regulation of renal hemodynamics: Role of pancreatic glucagon. *Am J Physiol* 1985;248:F656–F662.
15. Brouhard BH, Lagrone LF, Richards GE, et al. Somatostatin limits rise in glomerular filtration rate after a protein meal. *J Pediatr* 1987;110:729–734.
16. Castellino P, Coda B, DeFronzo RA. Effect of amino acid infusion on renal hemodynamics in humans. *Am J Physiol* 1986;251: F132–F140.
17. Haffner D, Zacharewicz S, Mehls O, et al. The acute effect of growth hormone on GFR is obliterated in chronic renal failure. *Clin Nephrol* 1989;32:266–269.
18. White HL, Heinbecker P, Rolf D. Enhancing effects of growth hormone on renal function. *Am J Physiol* 1949;157:47–51.
19. Hirschberg R, Kopple JD. Role of growth hormone in the amino acid-induced acute rise in renal function in man. *Kidney Int* 1987; 32:382–387.
20. Wada L, Don BR, Schambelan M. Hormonal mediators of amino acid-induced glomerular hyperfiltration in humans. *Am J Physiol* 1991;260:F787–F792.
21. Ruilope L, Rodicio J, Miranda B, et al. Renal effects of amino acid infusions in patients with panhypopituitarism. *Hypertension* 1988;11:557–559.
22. Claris-Appiani A, Assael BM, Tirelli AS, et al. Lack of glomerular hemodynamic stimulation after infusion of branched-chain amino acids. *Kidney Int* 1988;33:91–94.
23. Castellino P, Levin R, Shohat J, et al. Effect of specific amino acid groups on renal hemodynamics in humans. *Am J Physiol* 1990;258:F992–F997.
24. Castellino P, De Santo NG, Capasso G, et al. Low protein alimentation normalizes renal haemodynamic response to acute protein ingestion in type I diabetic children. *Eur J Clin Invest* 1989;19:78–83.
25. Hirschberg RR, Zipser RD, Slomowitz LA, et al. Glucagon and prostaglandins are mediators of amino acid-induced rise in renal hemodynamics. *Kidney Int* 1988;33:1147–1155.
26. Friedlander G, Blanchet-Benque F, Nitenberg A, et al. Glucagon secretion is essential for amino acid-induced hyperfiltration in man. *Nephrol Dial Transplant* 1990;5:110–117.
27. Premen AJ. Importance of the liver during glucagon-mediated increases in canine renal hemodynamics. *Am J Physiol* 1985;249: F319–F322.
28. Smoyer WE, Brouhard BH, Rassin DK, et al. Enhanced GFR response to oral versus intravenous arginine administration in normal adults. *J Lab Clin Med* 1991;118:166–175.
29. De Santo NG, Anastasio P, Loguercio C, et al. Glucagon-independent renal hyperaemia and hyperfiltration after an oral protein load in Child A liver cirrhosis. *Eur J Clin Invest* 1992;22:31–37.
30. Woods LL. Mechanisms of renal vasodilation after protein feeding: role of the renin-angiotensin system. *Am J Physiol* 1993;264: R601–R609.
31. Ruilope LM, Rodicio J, Garcia Robles R, et al. Influence of a low sodium diet on the renal response to amino acid infusions in humans. *Kidney Int* 1987;31:992–999.
32. Slomowitz LA, Hirschberg R, Kopple JD. Captopril augments the renal response to an amino acid infusion in diabetic adults. *Am J Physiol* 1988;255:F755–F762.
33. Rosenberg ME, Chmielewski D, Hostetter TH. Effect of dietary protein on rat renin and angiotensinogen gene expression. *J Clin Invest* 1990;85:1144–1149.
34. Williams M, Young JB, Rosa RM, et al. Effect of protein ingestion on urinary dopamine excretion. Evidence for the functional importance of renal decarboxylation of circulating 3,4-dihydroxyphenylalanine in man. *J Clin Invest* 1986;78:1687–1693.
35. Maack T, Marion DN, Camargo MJ, et al. Effects of auriculin (Atrial Natriuretic Factor) on blood pressure, renal function and the renin-aldosterone system in dogs. *Am J Med* 1984;77: 1069–1075.
36. Cavatorta A, Buzio C, Pucci F, et al. Effects of antihypertensive drugs on glomerular function in normotensive and hypertensive subjects: Hormonal aspects. *J Hypertens* 1991;9(Suppl 6): S218–S219.
37. Moulin B, Dhib M, Coquerel A, et al. Atrial natriuretic peptide in the renal response to an acute protein load. *Int J Clin Pharmacol Res* 1990;10:211–216.
38. Tam SC, Tang LS, Lai CK, et al. Role of atrial natriuretic peptide in the increase in glomerular filtration rate induced by a protein meal. *Clin Sci* 1990;78:481–485.
39. Don BR, Blake S, Hutchison FN, et al. Dietary protein intake modulates glomerular eicosanoid production in the rat. *Am J Physiol* 1989;256:F711–F718.
40. Yanagisawa H, Morrissey J, Yates J, et al. Protein increases glomerular eicosanoid production and activity of related enzymes. *Kidney Int* 1992;41:1000–1007.
41. Stahl RA, Kudelka S, Helmchen U. High protein intake stimulates prostaglandin formation in remnant kidneys. *Am J Physiol* 1987;252:F1083–F1094.

42. Schambelan M, Blake S, Sraer J, et al. Increased prostaglandin production by glomeruli isolated from rats with streptozotocin-induced diabetes mellitus. *J Clin Invest* 1985;75:404–412.
43. De Nicola L, Blantz RC, Gabbai FB. Nitric oxide and angiotensin IT. Glomerular and tubular interaction in the rat. *J Clin Invest* 1992;89:1248–1256.
44. King AJ, Troy JL, Anderson S, et al. Nitric oxide: A potential mediator of amino acid-induced renal hyperemia and hyperfiltration. *J Am Soc Nephrol* 1991;1:1271–1277.
45. Murakami M, Suzuki H, Ichihara A, et al. Effects of Larginine on systemic and renal haemodynamics in conscious dogs. *Clin Sci* 1991;81:727–732.
46. Tolins JP, Raij L. Effects of amino acid infusion on renal hemodynamics. Role of endothelium-derived relaxing factor. *Hypertension* 1991;17:1045–1051.
47. Morrissey J, Klahr S. Effects of agmatine, an active metabolite of arginine metabolism, on the kidney. *Nephrol Dial Transplant* 1996;11:1217–1219.
48. Pitts RF. The effects of infusing glycine and of varying the dietary protein intake on renal hemodynamics of the dog. *Am J Physiol* 1944;142:355–365.
49. Meyer TW, Ichikawa I, Katz R, et al. The renal hemodynamic response to amino acid infusion in the rat. *Trans Assoc Am Physicians* 1983;96:76–83.
50. Brezis M, Silva P, Epstein FH. Amino acids induce renal vasodilatation in isolated perfused kidneys: Coupling to oxidative metabolism. *Am J Physiol* 1984;247:H999–H1004.
51. Seney FD, Wright FS. Dietary protein suppresses feedback control of glomerular filtration in rats. *J Clin Invest* 1985;75: 558–568.
52. Bankir L, Bouby N, Trin-Trang-Tan MM. Vasopressin dependent kidney hypertrophy: role of urinary concentration in protein-induced hypertrophy and in progression of chronic renal failure. *Am J Kidney Dis* 1991;17:661–665.
53. Sargent FIT, Johnson RE. The effect of diet on renal function in healthy men. *Am J Clin Nutr* 1956;4:466–481.
54. Klahr S, Alleyne GAO. Effects of chronic protein-calorie malnutrition on the kidney. *Kidney Int* 1973;3:129–141.
55. Alleyne GAO. The effect of severe protein-calorie malnutrition on the renal function of Jamaican children. *Pediatrics* 1967;39: 400–411.
56. Klahr S, Tripathy K. Evaluation of renal function in malnutrition. *Arch Intern Med* 1966;118:322–325.
57. Tripathy K, Klahr S, Lotero H. Utilization of exogenous urea nitrogen in malnourished adults. *Metabolism* 1970;19:253–262.
58. Klahr S, Tripathy K, Garcia FT, et al. On the nature of renal concentrating defect in malnutrition. *Am J Med* 1967;43:84–96.
59. Pennell JP, Sanjana V, Frey NR, et al. The effect of urea infusion on the urinary concentrating mechanism in protein depleted rats. *J Clin Invest* 1975;55:399–409.
60. Crawford JB, Doyle AP, Probst JH. Service of urea in renal water conservation. *Am J Physiol* 1959;196:545–548.
61. Klahr S, Tripathy K, Lotero H. Renal regulation of acid-base balance in malnourished man. *Am J Med* 1970;48:325–331.
62. Waterlow JC, Scrimshaw NS. The concept of kwashiorkor from a public health point of view. *Bull World Health Organ* 1957; 16:458–464.
63. Trowell HG, Davies JNP, Dean RFA. *Kwashiorkor.* London: Arnold, 1954.
64. Klahr S, Davis TA. Changes in renal function with chronic protein-calorie malnutrition In: Mitch WE, Klahr S, eds. *Nutrition and the kidney.* Boston: Little, Brown, 1988:59–79.
65. Alleyne GAO. Cardiac function in severely malnourished Jamaican children. *Clin Sci* 1966;30:553–562.
66. Qureshi AR, Alvestrand A, Danielsson A, et al. Factors predicting malnutrition in hemodialysis patients: a cross-sectional study. *Kidney Int* 1998;53:773–782.
67. Stenvinkel P, Heimburger O, Paultre F, et al. Strong association between malnutrition, inflammation, and atherosclerosis in chronic renal failure. *Kidney Int* 1999;55:1899–1911.
68. Ikizler TA, Hakim RM. Nutrition in end-stage renal disease. *Kidney Int* 1996;50:343–357.

15

ASSESSMENT OF PROTEIN-ENERGY NUTRITIONAL STATUS

LARA PUPIM
CATHI JACKSON MARTIN
T. ALP IKIZLER

Assessment and monitoring of protein and energy nutritional status are crucial to prevent, diagnose, and treat protein-energy malnutrition (PEM), a condition highly prevalent and strongly correlated with increased morbidity and mortality in multiple patient populations, including patients with renal failure (1–14) (see Chapters 10 and 11). Protein and energy nutritional status refers to the quantitative and qualitative status of protein in nonmuscle (visceral) and muscle (somatic) components, in addition to the energy-balance status (15). Assessment of protein and energy nutritional status is a broad and complex topic that involves indirect measures of visceral protein concentrations, somatic protein stores, and energy expenditure and requirements and precise measurements of protein and energy homeostasis (16). PEM can be defined as a state where net nutrient intake (i.e., intake corrected for losses) is lower than nutrient requirements, ultimately leading to various metabolic abnormalities, decreased tissue function, and loss of body mass (15,17). Further, PEM is a condition associated and interrelated with many diseases, such that it can be secondary to or causative of an underlying disease. Therefore, a clinically meaningful assessment of protein and energy nutritional status should be not only able to assess the risk of morbidity and mortality resulting from PEM, but also simultaneously able to distinguish the causes and consequences of both PEM and the underlying diseases. A meaningful method also should determine whether there is a possibility of benefit from nutritional interventions (17).

Assessment of protein and energy nutritional status usually requires multiple different measurements (18). There is no definitive single method to assess nutritional status and responses to nutritional intervention that can be considered as a "gold standard," and a number of the proposed methods currently are being used concomitantly (Fig. 15.1). In this chapter, we will describe these various types of methods to assess protein and energy nutritional status. Our aim is to expand and update data on the readily available indirect methods to assess protein stores and energy balance and to discuss more precise techniques to estimate protein and energy homeostasis. Special considerations of specific methods related to renal failure will be addressed as appropriate.

ASSESSMENT OF PROTEIN STORES

To have a healthy life, an adult must be able to maintain neutral nitrogen balance. Nitrogen balance can be defined as the difference between the intake and loss of nitrogen. A positive or negative protein balance is used to determine the adequacy of protein intake of the patient. Nitrogen balance is dependent on two components: protein anabolism and protein catabolism. Protein anabolism is highly dependent on dietary nutrient intake. Neutral nitrogen balance can be achieved with a dietary protein intake (DPI) as low as 0.6 g/kg/day in normal subjects, when energy intake is adequate (19–23). However, if protein and energy requirements are not met from the diet, compensatory mechanisms are activated to maintain neutral nitrogen balance (24,25). These mechanisms include a reduction in protein breakdown and amino acid oxidation, ultimately leading to more efficient utilization of nutrients (25). Still, it should be noted that these compensatory responses are limited to some extent, and there is a minimum requirement for DPI. If the protein requirements are not met, a state of protein catabolism ensues and is reflected as a worsening in protein nutritional status. In most cases, direct and precise measures of nitrogen balance are not readily available, and indirect measures of protein stores are necessary. The most commonly used measures are visceral protein concentrations and somatic protein stores.

Visceral Protein Concentrations

Visceral protein concentrations refer to biochemical markers used to identify protein deficiency. These markers are circulating proteins that estimate the size of the visceral protein

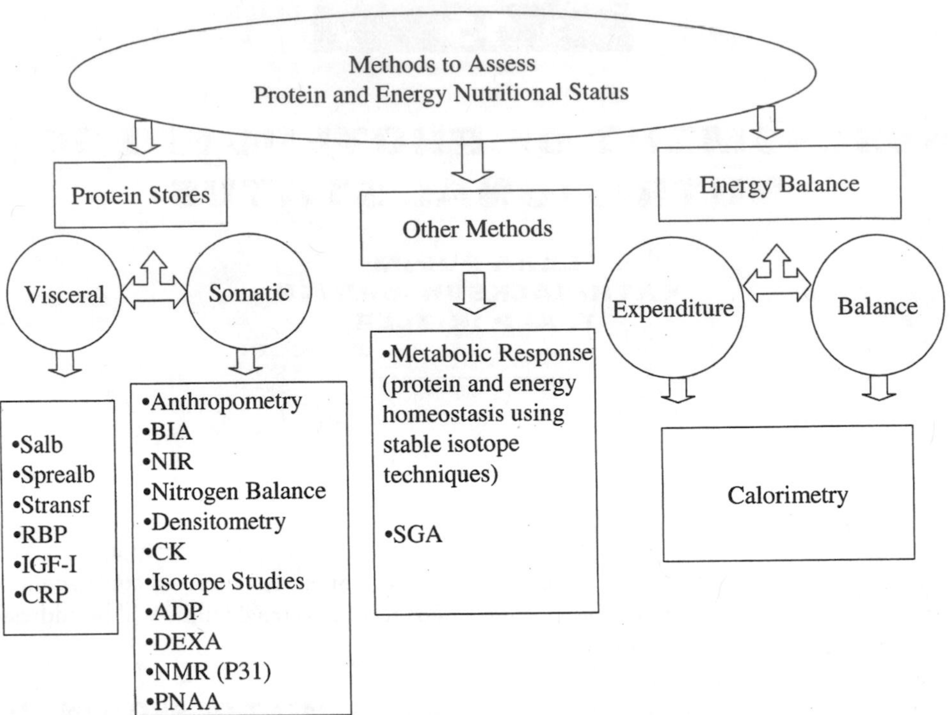

FIGURE 15.1. Salb, serum albumin; Sprealb, serum prealbumin; Stransf, serum transferrin; RBP, retinol-binding protein; IGF-I, insulinlike growth factor-1; CRP, C-reactive protein; BIA, bioelectrical impedance analysis; NIR, near infrared reactance; CK, creatine kinetics; DEXA, dual energy x-ray absorptiometry; ADP, air-displacement plethysmography; NMR, nuclear magnetic resonance; PNNA, prompt neutron activation analysis; SGA, subjective global assessment.

pool in the body (15). Almost all circulating visceral proteins have certain physiologic roles as carriers or binders or are actively involved in vital functions, such as the immune system. The most readily available and commonly used laboratory tests for visceral protein concentrations are depicted in Table 15.1. These include serum albumin, serum prealbumin (transthyretin), and serum transferrin. Other less available markers are serum retinol-binding protein, insulin-like growth factor-1 (IGF-I), pseudocholinesterase, and ribonuclease. Finally, certain positive acute-phase reactants (APRs) have been proposed as "nutritionally-related" markers because an increase in their concentrations usually is associated with a decrease in most of the visceral protein concentrations. These APRs include C-reactive protein (CRP), ceruloplasmin, complement components, fibrinogen, plasminogen-activator inhibitor-1, antiproteases, serum amyloid A, and fibronectin.

Serum Albumin

Serum albumin is a convenient, readily available laboratory test and by far the most extensively studied serum protein. Several studies have shown a strong correlation between low levels of serum albumin and increased risk of morbidity and mortality in many patient populations (26–30). It has been suggested that serum albumin is a marker of overall health status rather than a nutritional marker, an appropriate distinction when one understands its complex physiology. The concentration of serum albumin is the net result of its synthesis, breakdown, volume of distribution, and exchange between intravascular and extravascular spaces, as well as losses (31,32). Albumin is a highly water-soluble protein, located mainly in the extracellular space, with a total body pool of approximately 300 g (3.5 to 5.3 g/kg) in a normal average-weighted (70 kg) man. Approximately two-thirds of this pool is in the extravascular space, and the ratio of intravascular to extravascular albumin concentration varies in different tissues. Albumin is synthesized in the liver and secreted into the bloodstream, where it is equilibrated rapidly and has a half-life of approximately 20 days. Equilibration between intravascular and extravascular albumin pools is slower than within the intravascular space, varying from 7 to 10 days, depending on the tissue.

Inadequate DPI is characterized by a decrease in the rate of albumin synthesis (33), which in the short term may have little impact on serum albumin levels because albumin has a low turnover rate and large pool size. Serum albumin concentrations actually may increase during short-term fasting because of contraction of the intravascular space. Similarly, in the long term, low protein intake and decreased protein synthesis may be compensated by decreased albumin breakdown and also a shift from the extravascular to

TABLE 15.1. DIFFERENT METHODS TO ASSESS PROTEIN CONCENTRATIONS IN PATIENTS WITH RENAL FAILURE

Methods	Advantages	Disadvantages	Clinical Application
Serum albumin	Readily available Inexpensive Excellent outcome predictor	Long half-life (late marker) Influenced by extracellular volume Influenced by inflammatory response	Diagnosis and/or screening Longitudinal evaluation[a] Clinical and research
Serum prealbumin	Readily available Inexpensive Excellent outcome predictor Short half-life (can detect early changes) Low influence of extracellular volume	Influenced by level of renal function Influenced by inflammatory response	Diagnosis and/or screening Longitudinal evaluation[a] Clinical and research
Serum transferrin	Readily available Inexpensive Short half-life (can detect early changes) Low influence of extracellular volume	Influenced by iron stores Influenced by inflammatory response Not validated in large-scale studies	Diagnosis and/or screening Longitudinal evaluation[a] Clinical and research
Retinol-binding protein	Short half-life (can detect early changes)	Limited availability Expensive Influenced by level of renal function Influenced by inflammatory response Decreased in hyperthyroidism Decreased in vitamin A deficiency	Diagnosis and/or screening Longitudinal evaluation[a] Research
Serum IGF-I	Good association with other proteins Short half-life (can detect early changes)	Limited availability Expensive Acutely affected by dietary intake Not validated in large-scale studies	Diagnosis and/or screening Longitudinal evaluation[a] Research

IGF-I; insulinlike growth factor-1.
[a]Repeated measurements in the same patient allow detection of more subtle changes to guide nutritional interventions.

the intravascular space, maintaining serum albumin concentrations. Indeed, studies have shown that long-term protein and energy restriction in healthy subjects and patients with anorexia nervosa leads to significant decrease in body weight but little change in serum albumin concentration (17). However, because the exchange between intravascular and extravascular albumin pools is so large, small variations in this exchange can cause significant alterations in serum albumin levels over time in certain conditions where low DPI is maintained.

In addition to decreased DPI, hypoalbuminemia can be secondary to certain underlying conditions and diseases, such as hepatic and inflammatory disorders, which cause a decrease in albumin synthesis and increase in albumin breakdown (34–38). Serum albumin levels below 3.0 g/dL are usually the result of some cause other than solely low nutrient intake. Inflammatory processes may increase transcapillary losses of albumin (39). It is interesting that serum albumin levels fail to increase in patients with cancer after 21 days of intensive nutritional therapy (40) and in nursing home patients after enteral feeding (29), suggesting that the underlying inflammatory stress present in some disease conditions may perpetuate the hypoalbuminemia despite adequate protein and energy intake. Decreased albumin synthesis from liver failure as well as albumin losses by the gastrointestinal tract; by certain renal diseases; or from tissue injuries such as wounds, burns, and peritonitis also can lead to hypoalbuminemia.

Serum albumin is an important nutritional marker in patients with renal disease. Many studies have shown the predictive power of serum albumin for clinical outcomes, especially in the end-stage renal disease (ESRD) population. Levels below 2.5 g/dL (normal range 3.5 to 5.5 g/dL) have been associated with a risk of death 20 times higher compared to a reference level of 4.0 to 4.5 g/dL in patients undergoing hemodialysis, and levels of 3.5 to 4.0 g/dL (considered to be within the normal range) were associated with doubling the risk of death (30). Serum albumin levels also have been shown to decrease in renal disease as a result of inflammatory response and hypervolemia, both of which are highly prevalent in this patient population (41–43). Although longitudinal studies evaluating the validity of serum albumin as a nutritional marker in the presence of inflammation and altered volume status are limited, available data suggest that serum albumin levels are indeed directly related to nutrition, and serum albumin is a useful nutritional marker even in the presence of inflammation in patients with ESRD (43,44).

Serum Prealbumin

Serum prealbumin is the carrier protein for retinol-binding protein and thyroxin. It has some advantages for nutritional assessment as compared to serum albumin because it is less abundant than serum albumin in the body and its half-life is 2 to 3 days, making serum prealbumin a more sensitive test to detect subtle changes in visceral protein stores (45–47). Other advantages of serum prealbumin include the fact that it can be measured easily; it is less affected by liver disease than other serum proteins; and it has a high ratio of essential to nonessential amino acids, making it a distinct marker for protein synthesis (48,49). In addition, serum prealbumin concentration is not affected by hydration status (50). Low nutrient intake decreases serum prealbumin levels, which can be restored by refeeding (51), characteristics of a useful tool to monitor nutritional supplementation (45). Similar to serum albumin, serum prealbumin has been reported to be a reliable outcome predictor in many patient populations, including patients with renal failure (47,52–55). Limitations of its use as a marker to monitor nutritional status and intervention include the possible increase of serum prealbumin in patients with acute alcohol intoxication (56), during prednisone therapy, and while using progestational agents (57). Serum prealbumin levels may be decreased during zinc deficiency (58) and infections (59,60) as well as in response to cytokine and hormone infusions (61, 62), suggesting the same profile as serum albumin with regard to inflammatory response.

Serum prealbumin tends to increase as renal function decreases, and it may not be a reliable tool to assess protein stores in patients with progressive renal disease. However, in patients with ESRD, in whom renal function is relatively stable and essentially has disappeared, serum prealbumin may be a useful tool and a level below 29 mg/dL has been recommended to indicate PEM (14). Of note, this value is within the normal range (i.e., 10 to 40 mg/dL) for populations with normal renal function.

Serum Transferrin

The primary function of serum transferrin is to transport iron in the plasma. It has a half-life of 8 to 10 days and a small body pool, making it sensitive to nutritional changes (46,63,64). It can be measured directly by radioimmunoassay or turbidimetric reading or estimated by measurements of the total iron-binding capacity (TIBC) [serum transferrin = (0.8 × TIBC) − 43]. The normal range is between 250 and 300 mg/dL. Low levels of serum transferrin (<200 mg/dL) have been associated with poor clinical outcome in malnourished children and other hospitalized patient populations (65,66). Improvements in serum transferrin levels also have been observed with nutritional supplementation (67).

In patients with renal failure, assessment of serum transferrin as a marker of protein stores is problematic (68). Specifically, iron metabolism is altered in renal failure, which can significantly affect serum transferrin concentrations. In addition, routine iron loading in patients with ESRD; losses as a result of the nephrotic syndrome and gastrointestinal diseases; and, as with all the visceral proteins, any condition associated with inflammatory response or liver failure will affect serum transferrin concentrations (69,70). Therefore, serum transferrin is not a recommended tool for monitoring nutritional status in patients with ESRD. This is consistent with the National Kidney Foundation Kidney/Dialysis Outcome Quality Initiative Clinical Practice Guidelines (71).

Retinol-Binding Protein

Retinol-binding protein transports retinol and is linked with serum prealbumin at a constant molar ratio. The half-life of retinol-binding protein is about 10 hours, and, as with serum prealbumin, it has a small body pool and is a more specific marker of subtle changes in protein stores. Similar to serum albumin and serum prealbumin, retinol-binding protein levels decrease during inflammatory states. In addition, retinol-binding protein levels decrease in hyperthyroidism and vitamin A deficiency. In the renal failure population, the use of retinol-binding protein as a nutritional marker is more complicated than serum prealbumin because it is metabolized in the proximal tubular cells, making the serum levels and the half-life of retinol-binding proteins dependent on the level of renal function (72).

Insulin-like Growth Factor-I

IGF-I is a growth factor structurally related to insulin and is produced and released primarily by the liver, mainly in response to growth hormone. It has the benefit of a short half-life (2 to 6 hours) and being 95% bound to its specific binding-proteins concentrations, with very small changes in the daily serum concentrations (73). IGF-I levels decrease during fasting and increase with refeeding. Therefore, IGF-I concentrations have been used to assess nutritional status in different patient populations (74–77). Serum IGF-I concentrations may be affected by liver disease, in addition to its dependence on the binding and release from the binding proteins and growth hormone levels (73).

Limited studies in patients with ESRD suggest that IGF-I correlates more closely with markers of somatic protein stores, compared to serum albumin and serum transferrin (77), and longitudinal changes in IGF-I concentrations in patients undergoing maintenance hemodialysis are associated with changes in other nutritional parameters and can predict these changes, especially serum albumin (78,79). Nonetheless, the fact that serum IGF-I levels also reflect recent nutrient intake may limit its usefulness as an indicator of body composition.

C-Reactive Protein

CRP is a positive APR that correlates negatively with visceral protein concentrations. During inflammatory processes there is release of cytokines, which mediate an increase in hepatic synthesis of APRs, such as CRP, and suppression of the synthesis of negative-phase reactants, such as serum albumin (80). CRP is not a direct nutritional marker, but it is important to understand its role in the overall assessment of nutritional status. For example, in the face of low serum albumin or prealbumin levels (negative APR), it is important to evaluate for potential nonnutritional sources of protein depletion. If CRP levels are simultaneously high, sources of infection and/or inflammation should be investigated and if possible, resolved, along with nutritional supplementation as appropriate.

In renal failure, levels of serum CRP have been strongly and negatively correlated with concentrations of serum albumin, and patients with hypoalbuminemia have significantly higher values of CRP compared to patients with normal serum albumin undergoing hemodialysis (42,81,82). CRP also has been shown to be a strong predictor of death in patients undergoing hemodialysis (81,83).

Somatic Protein Stores

Assessment of somatic protein stores is an essential component of the evaluation of nutritional status (84). Evaluation of somatic protein stores involves determining body composition by measuring the individual compartments of water, fat, bone, muscle, and visceral organs (85). The techniques described in the subsequent sections of this chapter will discuss the various compartment models in detail and compare the benefits and drawbacks with a special emphasis on renal patients. When evaluating these techniques, the effects of aging, level of fitness, disease processes, and feasibility of the tests also should be considered (86).

Muscle mass comprises the majority of somatic protein stores and will be the focus of this discussion. Generally, somatic protein stores are preserved at the expense of other body fuels, such as fat, until severe catabolic illnesses occur, ultimately leading to PEM. There are many techniques available to determine body composition including anthropometry, bioelectrical impedance (BIA), dual energy x-ray absorptiometry (DEXA), prompt neutron activation analysis (PNAA), and hydrodensitometry. Table 15.2 illustrates several techniques, with their advantages, disadvantages, and clinical applications.

Anthropometry

Anthropometric measurements have been used for decades and include height and weight, calculated body mass index

TABLE 15.2. DIFFERENT METHODS FOR SOMATIC PROTEIN STORES AND BODY COMPOSITION ASSESSMENT ACCORDING TO COMPARTMENT MODELS

Methods	Advantages	Disadvantages	Clinical Application
Two-compartment			
Anthropometry	Easy, fast, and safe	High interobserver variability (anthropometry)	Diagnosis and/or screening
BIA[a]	Bedside	Dependent on operator skills	Longitudinal evaluation[a]
NIR*	Noninvasive	Influenced by extracellular volume	Clinical and research
Densitometry	Inexpensive	*Regression equations derived from healthy subjects	
	*Low interobserver and intraobserver variability		
Three-compartment			
Creatinine kinetics (CK)	Easy and safe (CK)	*Relatively invasive	Diagnosis and/or screening
Isotope dilution*	Inexpensive (CK)	*Time-consuming (CK)	Longitudinal evaluation[a]
TBK*	Not influenced heavily by extracellular volume	*Moderately expensive	Clinical and research
DEXA**	Accurate	*Requires specialized oral or intravenous formula	*Research only
		**Minimal radiation exposure	
Four-compartment			
ADP	Easy, fast, and safe	Expensive	Diagnosis and/or screening
PNAA*	Noninvasive	Not readily available	Longitudinal evaluation[a]
	Small influence of extracellular volume	*Minimal radiation exposure	Research
	Accommodates most body types	Requires time-consuming analysis	
	Accurate		
Five-compartment			
NMR	Very accurate	Very expensive	Diagnose and/or screening
	Ability to delineate organ size and body-fat distribution	Not readily available	Research
		Requires specialized personnel	
		Validity in abnormal water balance is not well established	

BIA, bioelectrical impedance analysis; NIR, near infrared interactance; TBK, total body potassium; DEXA, dual-energy x-ray absorptiometry; ADP, air displacement plethysmography; PNAA, prompt neutron activation analysis; NMR, nuclear magnetic resonance spectroscopy.
[a]Repeated measurements in the same patient allow detection of subtle changes to guide nutritional interventions.

(BMI), skinfold thickness (TSF), biceps and subscapular skinfolds, mid-arm circumference (MAC), and calculated mid-arm muscle circumference (MAMC) diameter or area (87). A detailed description of these techniques can be found elsewhere (88). This technique is a two-compartment model that involves measuring skinfolds and circumferences at standardized sites, usually on the right side of the body. Measurements are repeated three times, averaged, and compared to percentiles of the normal population. The most commonly used standards are those reported by Jelliffe (89, 90), based on European male military personnel and low-income American women, and those reported by Frisancho, which are based on white males and females who participated in the United States Health and Nutrition and Evaluation Survey (NHANES) (91,92). There is poor correlation between these two standards in classifying patients, and most clinicians prefer the Frisancho calculations as being the most accurate for the U.S. population. In fact, 20% to 30% of healthy control subjects would be considered malnourished based on these standards. These measurements can quantify indirectly the major compositional determinants of body weight and are well suited for identifying levels of lean (fat-free) body mass and total body fat in healthy individuals (93,94). Because almost half of the body's fat mass is found in the subcutaneous layer, these measurements can provide a reasonably accurate index of total body fat. They have the advantages of being inexpensive and easy to perform at the bedside, and there are well-established norms for comparison of healthy populations based on the NHANES III survey data. However, it has been suggested that they have limitations for specific patient populations, such as those with ESRD, because of the severely limited database and lack of correction for hydration status or effects of chronic illness (17).

Among various anthropometric measurements, BMI measurements tend to overestimate body fat and are not sensitive for detecting small changes in body composition (95–97). In addition, the calculation used to determine BMI {BM (kg) / ht^2 (m^2)} may not apply to people outside the norm. BMI is convenient and inexpensive to measure, and it does correlate strongly with mortality in patients undergoing maintenance hemodialysis (Chapter 12).

The techniques for measuring MAMC, MAC, and TSF are subjective and dependent on the technique of the clinician (87). There has been a reported difference of as much as 10% even when measures were repeated by the same clinician, and this is likely to be greater when more than one clinician is involved (98). In addition, anthropometry is not valid in patients with large shifts in body water as is frequently seen in renal failure and liver disease. Another shortcoming is the poor correlation reported between visceral protein stores and upper-arm measurements. In general, anthropometry is insensitive for detecting subtle changes in body composition compared to other methods. However, anthropometric measurements can be useful when tracked serially on a patient and when used in conjunction with other nutritional indices.

With regard to patients with renal failure, there are several important implications. Specifically, the patient undergoing maintenance hemodialysis should be assessed on the side opposite to the vascular access. In addition, caution should be used when comparing their measurements to the established norms because the measurements may vary along with alterations in fluid status. These measurements are perhaps among the least reliable for accuracy in patients with renal failure. Attempts have been made to establish standards for the dialysis population (99). However, the validity of these has been questioned because of the small sample size of the subjects and variability of results between clinicians (17).

Bioelectrical Impedance Analysis

BIA is a technique that has proved to be safe, generally accepted by patients, and easy to use (100,101). BIA is used for determining fluid management and increasingly for evaluating nutritional assessment. BIA is based on a two-compartment model that determines total body water (TBW) and soft tissue (i.e., fat mass [FM] and fat-free mass [FFM]) (102). It is based on the principle that the impedance of a cylindric conductor is related to its length, cross-sectional area, and applied signal frequency. Impedance is the vector sum of resistance and reactance. Figure 15.2 illustrates the detailed configuration of bioelectrical impedance. Mammalian tissues conduct an electrical current in proportion to their water and electrolyte content. Lean body tissues, which contain body fluids and electrolytes, have highly conductive, low resistance electrical pathways. Skin, bone, and fat, however, are very poor conductors and offer high resistance (103). Reactance is defined as the opposition to the flow of electrical current as a result of the electrical capacitance such as that found in the cell membrane wall. Because of this, cell membranes are the only component that offers reactance to electrical currents. The resistance and reactance components are aligned in both parallel and series orientations in the human body (104). Resistance is defined as the extracellular and intracellular fluid content, whereas the reactance is based on the cell-membrane content. In FFM, these fluid compartments are parallel components separated by cell membranes; therefore, parallel models are more accurate for determining their impedance.

BIA usually is measured by attaching two electrodes on the arm at the mid-wrist and the middle finger and two electrodes on the same side leg at the mid-ankle and foot just below the second and third toe. The electrodes are connected to a small machine that emits a tiny imperceptible current and measures the resistance and reactance. The entire process can be performed at the bedside and takes less than 5 minutes. BIA can be assessed through single frequency or multifrequency. The single-frequency BIA is

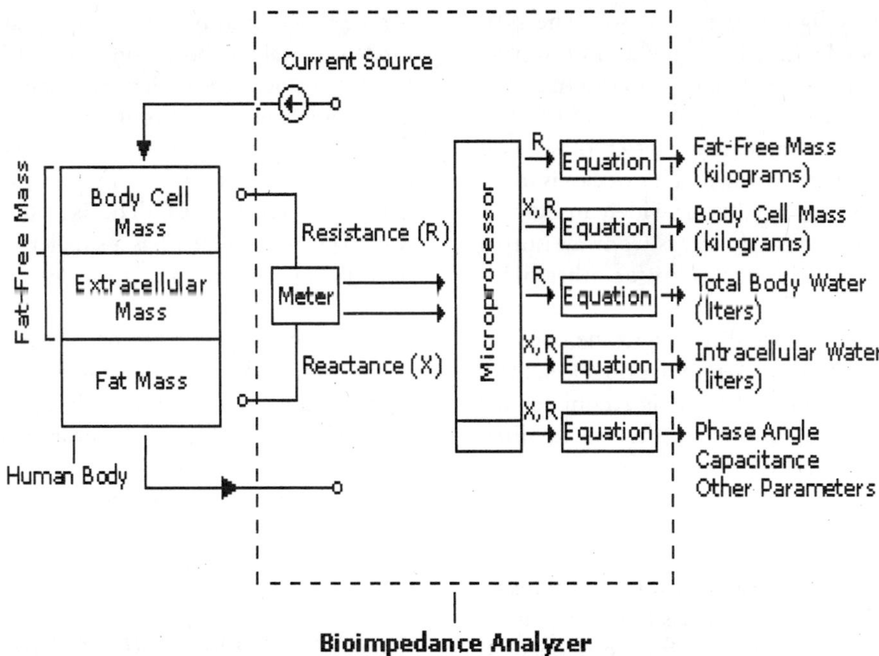

FIGURE 15.2. Schematic diagram of technical considerations for BIA. (From Biodynamics Corporation, Seattle, WA, USA, with permission.)

performed at 50 KHz and assumes a penetration of 50% to 60% intracellular space, whereas multifrequency BIA measures extracellular water with the lower frequency and TBW at a higher frequency of 500 MHz to 1 to 2 KHz (105). There is disparity regarding the accuracy between the two methods. Although arms and legs account for only 35% of total body volume, 85% of total body resistance is represented (106–108). Reactance, thought by some to represent cell integrity and nutritional health because cell walls and membranes possess electrical capacitance, has not been investigated as widely as resistance. Phase angle is a calculation derived from BIA that originally was used as a tool to diagnose metabolic disorders. Phase angle is defined as the arc tangent of the reactance to resistance ratio multiplied by 180 degrees and reflects the relative contribution of reactance to overall impedance. It has been found to positively correlate with total body protein and muscle mass as well as muscle strength (103). The two compartments that are defined by BIA are extracellular mass (ECM), which is primarily fluid and fat mass, and body cell mass (BCM), which is the metabolically active portion of the body (109). The ratio of ECM to BCM is a known sensitive marker of PEM; phase angle appears to reflect its prognostic significance. Consequently, a change in the ECM:BCM ratio is associated with a change in the phase angle. A phase angle of less than 4 degrees is associated with a significant increase in the risk of death in patients undergoing maintenance hemodialysis, whereas a phase angle of less than 3 degrees is related to a threefold increase in mortality (110). Conversely, high phase angles appear to be consistent with large quantities of intact cell membranes of skeletal muscle and body cell mass. Although phase angle may not be reliable in certain populations in detecting depletion of edema-free lean body mass, it may be superior in its ability to identify patients with clinically relevant PEM and poor prognosis (101,111).

There are some important limitations to accuracy of BIA in body composition analysis of patients with renal failure. Because patients with renal failure exhibit abnormal fluid balance, this can result in inaccurate estimations of lean body mass and fat mass (112). Therefore, for accurate results, BIA should be conducted when the patient is in an edema-free or near edema-free state, such as following hemodialysis. BIA should be assessed on the nonaccess side in patients undergoing maintenance hemodialysis. In patients being treated with peritoneal dialysis, BIA should be performed with the peritoneal cavity empty. In addition, the software packages that provide the calculations compare results to normal healthy individuals rather than to specific disease populations. However, there are recently published standards based on the maintenance hemodialysis population that are now available for comparison (113).

Near Infrared Interactance

Near infrared interactance (NIR) is based on light absorption and reflection using a near infrared light emission and is a noninvasive, simple, and rapid method of assessing the percentage of body fat. The device is commercially available and portable. The main body of the instrument is connected via a light cable to a tiny light-emitting sensor. The NIR sensor window is equipped with a light shield prior to placing it on the mid-upper arm to ensure that no external light interferes with the estimation of percent body fat (114). NIR measurements are obtained in a matter of seconds while the device is on the patient's arm. This device is moderately expensive and has been used most widely in Europe. Drawbacks of NIR include possible errors from measuring only one site (upper arm), the possibility of other light-source contamination in measurement, and unproven validity of the predictive equations used to determine body fat when applied to the hemodialysis population (114,115). For patients undergoing hemodialysis it is recommended that NIR be performed 10 to 20 minutes after the termination of dialysis on the nonaccess arm.

Densitometry

Densitometry provides a two-compartment model, measuring FM and FFM. It is based on the assumption that fat has a constant of 0.9 kg/L and the fat-free component is 1.1 kg/L. It measures body mass and volume and calculates body density by using Siri's equation for Caucasian populations [% fat $= 4.95/(D-4.5) \times 100$] and Shuttle's equation for African Americans [% fat $= 4.374/(D-3.928) \times 100$]. The "gold standard" of densitometry is underwater weighing (100,124). However, the process requires a special facility and can take anywhere from 30 to 45 minutes. In addition, the method may be uncomfortable for the subject because it requires them to be underwater for several seconds and is associated with technical difficulty for obese, elderly, or debilitated subjects when getting into or out of the apparatus.

Creatinine Kinetics

Creatinine kinetics is based on the principle that creatinine production is proportional to FFM and that in the steady state creatinine production is equal to the sum of creatinine excretion and metabolic degradation (116). This technique has correlated well with other methods of body composition analysis (117). However, the procedure requires the subject to collect his urine for a 24-hour period and, preferably, to keep the collection on ice, which may make this method less acceptable to the patient. There are only limited studies using creatinine kinetics in practice. Also, intake of meat (skeletal muscle, myocardium) may contribute up to 30% of urine creatinine excretion in normal adults and must be taken into consideration when calculating creatinine kinetics. Therefore, the reliability of this technique is not well established.

Diluted Isotope Studies

Isotope dilution generally is considered a more accurate method than multifrequency BIA for determining body FM from TBW. It can be used in three- and four-compartment models to evaluate body composition (118). This procedure involves using labeled elements that either are ingested orally or administered through intravenous routes and measuring their presence in saliva, plasma, and urine. The most commonly used isotopic compound for measuring TBW is deuterium oxide (D_2O). This is followed by doubly labeled water ($H_2{}^{18}O$), which has a smaller isotopic exchange with nonaqueous compounds, making it the preferred isotope. However, its cost is prohibitive for widespread use (96,119). Tritium-labeled water has been used previously but is less common now because of concerns over radioactivity. Advantages of isotope dilution techniques include the accuracy of TBW comparable to densitometry and moderate cost. Further, results are less likely to be compromised by errors of technique (120). However, these studies are somewhat invasive, requiring blood collection and the consumption of the tracers, and the analysis is time-consuming (96).

Air-Displacement Plethysmography

Air-displacement plethysmography (ADP) has become available for the measurement of body composition. ADP requires placing the subject in an egg-shaped, airtight, fiberglass chamber and uses pressure-volume relationships and body weight to derive TBW (121,122). In this technique, TBW is measured by determining the volume of air equal to the air displaced by the subjects' body when the subject sits inside the chamber. The subject's body volume is calculated indirectly by subtracting the volume of air remaining inside the chamber when the subject is inside from the volume of air in the chamber when it is empty.

ADP offers several advantages over other more established methods including the fact that it can accommodate a variety of body sizes; provides a rapid (6 to 10 minutes), safe, and comfortable measurement process; and is completely automated and noninvasive (123,124). However, the instrument is expensive, requires frequent calibration and establishment of isothermal conditions for each test, and is dependent on a highly trained technician. There are significant gender differences with ADP; ADP underestimates FM in males and slightly overestimates FM in females (124, 125). In addition, because it is a relatively new technique, the validity, reliability, and practicality of ADP in various populations, including patients with ESRD, has not yet been well defined.

Dual Energy X-Ray Absorptiometry

DEXA initially was used for the detection of osteoporosis by measuring bone density. Today, DEXA is also a leading "high-tech" method for measuring body composition (103). Unlike BIA, DEXA gives a direct measure of body composition based on a three-compartment model: FM, FFM, and bone density (126). DEXA is one of the most accurate determinations of body composition that is available at this time and has a precision error of 0.5% to 3.0% and an accuracy error of 3.0% to 9.0% (120,127). With this technique, body composition is calculated by ascertaining the amount of radiation attenuated by the bone or soft tissue while low- and high-energy radiograph beams (70 kVp and 140 kVp, respectively) are transmitted to a subject (103,128). This technique requires the subject to lie down on the examination surface as a scanning arm performs a series of transverse movements at 1-cm intervals while emitting photons at the two-energy levels indicated earlier. The soft-tissue mass reduces photon flux much less than bone mineral density, and differential absorption of the photons is measured and processed by the DEXA software to estimate bone mineral density, FM, and FFM (128). Each study can be performed in 6 to 15 minutes with minimal radiation exposure (<5 mrem) and minor discomfort to the patient. Because of the minimal radiation exposure, serial measurements can be obtained safely (87).

DEXA offers many advantages including the fact that it is suitable for virtually all ages and body sizes. It is easy to obtain, has excellent precision, and also can provide regional body composition. In addition, it has been shown to be quite sensitive for the detection of small changes in body composition, which makes it a very useful tool. However, it also has several limitations, including cost, which is a major factor. The DEXA instrument itself can cost more than $100,000, and there is also the expense of trained personnel to operate it. It is not a portable device; patients must come to a center for evaluation. Hence, there is a much bigger time commitment for the patient. Thus, patient acceptance of this examination may be less than other methods. As with most other methods, hydration status of the patient must be considered for each evaluation—an important consideration for patients with renal disease (104). Although the DEXA technology continues to improve, the accuracy of this technique for individuals who do not have stable fluid balance, such as the ESRD population, is not yet well defined (120,121).

Prompt Neutron Activation Analysis

The four-compartment method of PNAA has been available for 20 years and is considered to be the most accurate technique available for determining body protein stores. PNAA involves irradiating the subject with neutrons and measuring the gamma rays that are emitted by the individual during the procedure (129). This method offers quantitative assessment of nutritionally relevant components of body composition including total body nitrogen, which remains the most direct measure of total body protein, and total body potassium (130,131). Although this technique is considered to give the most accurate assessment of total body protein, the prohibitive cost and limited availability of the instrument and facility make this method impractical for the general population. Indeed, there are fewer than 10 facilities in the world that offer this technology. The radiation exposure to the subjects, approximately 0.2 mSv, is equivalent to the average chest x-ray (132), which can be a significant detriment and limits the feasibility of making serial measurements on patients. There are few studies using PNAA to assess nutritional status in patients with renal failure. However, it has been demonstrated that this method is much more sensitive than other techniques for detecting nitrogen depletion in these patients. Total body nitrogen correlated significantly with DPI, calculated from the urea nitrogen appearance as well as total energy intake, and is inversely associated with increased mortality (132).

Nuclear Magnetic Resonance Spectroscopy

Nuclear magnetic resonance spectroscopy, particularly using P-31, can provide unique and quantitative data that are not available from routine laboratory tests and is the method of choice for examining muscle wasting (133). This technique uses a five-compartment model that offers the ability to delineate organ size and structure, body-fat distribution, total body water, and muscle size without exposing the patient to radiation. In addition, it is very sensitive for detecting inflammatory processes in the muscle. The major drawback with this technique is cost, which is prohibitive for general clinical use (119). There are no studies in patients with renal disease in the current literature using this technique to assess body composition.

Subjective Global Assessment

Subjective global assessment (SGA) is a simple assessment method that draws on the experience of a clinician to make an overall assessment of nutritional status in a standardized way. It is based on a seven-point scale and is comprised of a medical history and a physical examination (Table 15.3). The medical history includes an anthropometric component involving present weight and height and comparing them to weight and height from the past 2 weeks as well as the previous 6 months. A score is assigned on a scale from 1 to 7 based on the amount of weight lost or gained compared to previous measurements. Disease states and comorbidities also are considered to take into account metabolic stress and nutritional requirements. In addition, gastrointestinal symptoms are evaluated based on the frequency and duration of symptoms such as diarrhea, anorexia, nausea, and vomiting. Finally, the patient is evaluated on functional capacity, which involves assessing how much difficulty the patient has carrying out normal activities of daily living. The physical assessment involves a hands-on examination of the patient by the practitioner. Loss of subcutaneous fat stores and muscle wasting are evaluated by observation and palpation. In addition, edema is evaluated in patients with an albumin of less than 2.8 gm/dL, and ascites

TABLE 15.3. DIFFERENT COMPONENTS OF SUBJECTIVE GLOBAL ASSESSMENT

Medical History		Physical Examination		
Component	**Outcomes**	**Component**	**Sites**	**Outcomes**
Weight history	Changes in dry weight—rate and pattern of loss >5–10%	Subcutaneous fat stores	Biceps, triceps, fat pads under eyes	Declining circumference, hollow under eyes
Diet intake review	Comparison to usual intake—degree and duration	Muscle wasting	Temple, quadriceps, deltoid, clavicle and shoulder, ribs, knee, calf, interosseous muscle, ribs, scapula	Prominent bone structure, flat or hollow areas
Gastrointestinal symptoms	Frequency and severity of symptoms that last more than 2 weeks	Edema	Extremities and facial features	Swelling when at dry weight
Functional status	Assess changes from baseline related to nutrition	Ascites (HD only)	Abdomen	Swelling in abdominal area after treatment
Acute stresses	Increased metabolic demands			

HD, hemodialysis.
Classification of ratings:
1 or 2 Severe malnutrition
3, 4, or 5 Moderate malnutrition
6 or 7 Mild to normal nutrition

may be assessed in patients undergoing maintenance dialysis (134). When this has been completed, an overall SGA rating is assigned to the patient, ranging from a rating of 1 or 2 for severe malnutrition indicating significant physical signs in most categories, 3 to 5 for mild to moderate malnutrition indicating no clear indication of normal status or severe malnutrition, and a 6 or 7 for very mild malnutrition to well-nourished (114,135).

The use of SGA mainly has been limited to patients with cancer, gastrointestinal surgical disorders, and renal failure rather than healthy populations. The direct relationship of SGA to various components of nutritional status has not been determined (136), and the reliability and validity remain somewhat controversial. Indeed, the very nature of this assessment is a subjective evaluation and scores can vary from practitioner to practitioner, although reliability between trained observers is good (134). The accuracy, reproducibility, and consistency of the SGA should be improved by using initial standard training, specific procedures, and an ongoing review of the procedures and results. It is important to point out that SGA does not replace formal nutrition assessment methods, but it can be used as a screening tool in conjunction with others to determine the aggressiveness of nutritional intervention and prioritize patient care. Research has shown that SGA is not a sensitive test or reliable predictor of the degree of PEM, although it can differentiate severely malnourished patients from those with normal nutrition (136,137). Overall SGA scores have been shown to correlate fairly strongly with outcomes in multiple studies, including those conducted in patients undergoing maintenance hemodialysis (135,137).

ASSESSMENT OF PROTEIN AND ENERGY HOMEOSTASIS

As previously mentioned, one should assess biomarkers that directly predict clinically important outcomes whenever possible (Table 15.4). When not possible, many surrogate markers are accepted for each disease or condition to be evaluated. Further, a meaningful biomarker should not only predict important clinical outcomes but also measure metabolic response to nutritional interventions. The nutritional markers discussed so far can accomplish these goals to some extent. However, they are limited in terms of precision and may not detect subtle changes in protein and energy stores, either quantitatively or qualitatively. In addition, the concentrations of visceral proteins and the somatic protein stores do not represent measures of metabolic abnormalities. The assessment of metabolic abnormalities, such as the bal-

TABLE 15.4. PROPOSED CHARACTERISTICS OF AN IDEAL NUTRITIONAL MARKER

✓ Readily available
✓ Inexpensive
✓ Short half-life
✓ Good outcome predictor
✓ Good association with other nutritional markers
✓ Distinguishes protein and energy malnutrition from underlying diseases
✓ Measures metabolic responses to nutritional interventions
✓ Low influence of extracellular volume
✓ Low influence of inflammatory status

ance between protein synthesis and breakdown as well as energy intake and expenditure, can be a precise way to detect metabolic changes and/or metabolic responses to interventions. This type of assessment has low variability and high sensitivity and specificity and is able to detect subtle and narrow changes. Further, the metabolic responses can be assessed in very short periods (hours), allowing the study of each patient as his own control, and therefore decreasing interpatient and intrapatient variability. In this respect, measurements of nitrogen balance and/or protein homeostasis using stable isotope–tracer techniques are potential approaches to accomplish these goals. These techniques comprise all these characteristics and with minimal risk to the patient. Further, metabolic studies of protein, carbohydrate, and lipids using stable isotopes, in addition to assessment of energy expenditure, are complex techniques that provide information on the link between nutrition, substrate metabolism, and substrate oxidation.

Nitrogen Balance

Nitrogen balance can be described as a measure of the net change in total body protein. This is based on the assumption that, except in azotemic individuals, almost all nitrogen in the body is found in protein. Protein contains approximately 16% nitrogen by weight, so 1 gram of nitrogen represents 6.25 grams of protein (138). Accordingly, classical nitrogen-balance techniques are a powerful, sensitive, and usually accurate tool for assessing the nutritional and metabolic response to changes in nutritional status. A major factor responsible for the precision and sensitivity of this technique is the precise control of the activities, diet, and environment of an individual during the studies (139).

Normal, healthy adults are in neutral balance with a nitrogen balance that is equal to about +0.5 g/d (to account for unmeasured nitrogen losses from sweat; skin desquamation; hair and nail growth; respiration; flatus; and, if present, sputum and salivary losses and menstruation). During neutral nitrogen balance, whole-body protein synthesis is equal to whole-body protein degradation (140). If nitrogen balance is positive, the subject is in a net anabolic state, whereas if the nitrogen balance is negative, the subject is in a net catabolic state such as from starvation or inadequate protein intake. This is an excellent tool for determining the amount of protein that is required for a subject to maintain a neutral or positive nitrogen balance depending on the individual's nutritional goals. However, it is not a tool that can be used in routine clinical practice, and specially equipped centers are required to conduct nitrogen-balance studies. Measurement of nitrogen balance requires meticulous detail, and a period of equilibration of 10 to 14 days is usually necessary before the effects of nutritional intervention can be assessed. After nitrogen equilibration is attained, it generally is necessary to measure nitrogen balance over a period of 5 to 10 days (141–143).

Despite the apparent advantages, there are important limitations inherent to the classical nitrogen-balance technique. Most of the measurements errors, such as losses of food on cooking and losses of feces and urine on toilet paper or in collection containers, lead to falsely positive balances. Further, the facilities necessary to carry out these studies are not widely available for general clinical use and are very expensive and the studies are time consuming. A less expensive but less precise estimate of nitrogen balance can be made by measuring urinary urea nitrogen and dietary nitrogen intake during the same 24-hour period. The information then is put into the following calculation for determining nitrogen balance:

$$\text{DPI (g)}/6.25 - \{\text{UUN} + (0.031 \times \text{weight})\} = \text{nitrogen balance}$$

where 0.031 is a constant used to estimate nonurea nitrogen losses (138). There are serious limitations to the accuracy of these latter techniques including overestimating intake and underestimating output, which can lead to falsely positive balances. The calculated results can be considered to provide only crude estimates of nitrogen balance (139).

For patients with renal failure, nitrogen balance must be adjusted for changes in the body nitrogen pool (i.e., the urea volume of distribution) by measuring the serum urea nitrogen daily. Using linear regression, the change in the urea pool then can be estimated and used to calculate nitrogen balance. An alternative approach for measuring nitrogen output has been designed for patients with ESRD using the calculation of the normalized protein nitrogen appearance (nPNA or nPCR) or urea nitrogen appearance (UNA) to estimate nitrogen output as long as the patient is edema-free and in a metabolically steady state. As indicated, nPNA and UNA are less precise measures of total nitrogen output as compared to the direct measurement of nitrogen in dialysate, urine, and feces. Total nitrogen output, estimated from the UNA or nPNA, then can be compared to DPI to provide a rough estimate of nitrogen balance.

Assessment of Protein Homeostasis

Although nitrogen balance is an excellent tool for determining protein requirements, it does not take into account the turnover of protein in the body, an event much greater than DPI (144). The balance between the protein breakdown and synthesis is the determinant of the net nitrogen balance. Protein balance is then a condition where protein synthesis and protein breakdown are equal or not significantly different, a condition in which edema-free lean body mass is supposed to be stable. A positive net balance of protein homeostasis reflects increased protein synthesis, decreased breakdown, or both. Contrarily, a negative net balance reflects decreased synthesis, increased breakdown, or both. Protein homeostasis can be measured most readily at the whole-body level and at the skeletal muscle level. An effective method for assessing protein homeostasis and also total protein synthesis and breakdown is the use of primed continuous infusion of isotopic tracers, such as leucine, valine, and lysine for the whole-body component and phenylalanine for the skeletal muscle component.

^{13}C-leucine is a common stable isotopic tracer used for metabolic studies at the whole-body level. The rate of appearance of endogenous leucine is an estimate of whole-body protein breakdown and can be calculated by dividing the labeled leucine (^{13}C-leucine) infusion rate by the plasma ^{13}C-ketoisocaproate (KIC) enrichment (145). It normally is expressed as mg/kg/min or, ideally, as mg/kg of fat-free, edema-free mass/min and should be corrected for any infused or lost amino acids during the study hours. The method also requires determination of breath $^{13}CO_2$ production, which can be calculated by multiplying the total carbon dioxide production (VCO_2) by the breath $^{13}CO_2$ enrichment. The rate of whole-body leucine oxidation can be calculated by dividing breath $^{13}CO_2$ production by 0.8 (correction factor for the retention of $^{13}CO_2$ in the bicarbonate pool) and by the plasma KIC enrichment (145). The nonoxidative leucine disappearance rate is an estimate of whole-body protein synthesis, and it can be determined indirectly by subtracting leucine oxidation from the corrected total leucine rate of disappearance. Therefore, determination of rates of whole-body protein breakdown and protein synthesis, using labeled leucine as a tracer, are complex but precise methods derived from the endogenous rate of leucine appearance, leucine oxidation rate, and the nonoxidative leucine rate of disappearance, respectively, assuming that 7.8% of whole-body protein is comprised of leucine (146).

Similar calculations are used to assess protein turnover in skeletal muscle. However, the plasma enrichment of labeled phenylalanine [(ring-$^2H_5$)-phenylalanine] is measured instead of leucine, valine, or lysine. This is because phenylalanine is not synthesized *de novo* or metabolized by skeletal muscle. Therefore, the rate of appearance of unlabeled phenylalanine reflects muscle-protein breakdown, and the rate of disappearance of labeled phenylalanine estimates muscle-protein synthesis (147). The measurements are adjusted for blood or plasma flow through the muscle, and data generally are expressed as μg/100 mL of blood or plasma flow/min (148).

In addition to measuring whole-body and skeletal muscle turnover, stable isotopes can be used to measure the fractional synthetic rate of individual proteins, such as albumin and transferrin. The detailed techniques are beyond the scope of this chapter and can be found elsewhere (145,148). Finally, skeletal muscle biopsies have been used in both *in vitro* (149) and *in vivo* studies in animals and human subjects to investigate protein synthesis and breakdown or amino acid kinetics (150–152). Although technically complex, it provides a means of measuring the transport rates of natural amino acids rather than inferring from the kinetics of its analogues, which may be different from one another. These techniques enable analysis of transmembrane transport of amino acids, the intracellular concentrations of many amino acids and their metabolites, the rates of protein breakdown and synthesis, the intramuscular *de novo* synthesis of amino acids, and concentrations of many other intracellular compounds in muscle (151,152).

Studies in patients with renal failure have shown the utility and validity of stable-isotope techniques as precise tools for evaluating metabolic responses to nutritional interventions, as well as the metabolic responses to the hemodialysis procedure. Several investigators have studied the metabolic effects of hemodialysis on whole-body and skeletal muscle turnover and energy metabolism (153–156). These techniques have been applied to measure the metabolic response to intradialytic parenteral nutrition in patients undergoing maintenance hemodialysis (157). Indeed, the technique has been shown to be feasible and reliable for these research purposes. In addition, it has been applied successfully to estimate fractional synthetic rates of body proteins in patients undergoing maintenance hemodialysis (158).

Despite the multiple advantages related to the use of stable-isotope kinetic studies, these techniques also have certain inherent errors and limitations. There is considerable variability of protein synthesis and degradation throughout the day as well as problems associated with isotope intracellular reentry throughout the studies. In general, it is difficult to perform long-term continuous isotope studies and a minimum of 3 to 4 weeks is required between studies in a certain individual. There is also significant cost associated with these studies. Therefore, the superiority of these techniques over classical nitrogen-balance studies for measuring protein balance is not conclusively justified, although stable isotope studies have other unique strengths.

Assessment of Energy Homeostasis

Energy balance is a major requirement for human cell function and is determined by energy intake and energy expenditure. Energy intake is derived from dietary carbohydrates, lipids, and proteins. These substrates are metabolized and converted into chemical energy (in the form of adenosine phosphate, or ATP, and other energy metabolites) and used for growth and maintenance of body tissues (159). If nutrient intake is inadequate to meet energy requirements, the result will be loss of body weight and gradual decrease in carbohydrate and lipid stores (160). Body protein stores also may be metabolized under these circumstances to generate the required energy, causing major metabolic alterations, such as acidosis, ketosis, loss of nitrogen, and dehydration.

Common terminology in energy balance includes total energy expenditure and its components: basal metabolic rate, resting energy expenditure (REE), physical activity, energy requirement, and the thermic effect of food. The REE, also known as resting metabolic rate, is the metabolism of the body at rest, reflected as the heat production of the body when in a state of complete mental and physical rest and in the postabsorptive state (i.e., after a 12-hour of fast) (161). Nutrient intake, exercise performance, sleep, changes in the external temperature, and disease states or external manipulations (e.g., hemodialysis) may change heat production and therefore the REE. The REE reflects the energy requirements to maintain and conduct normal metabolic activity of muscle, brain, liver, kidney, and other cells (159). The thermic effect of food refers to the increase in energy expenditure above the REE that occurs after a meal. It is a consequence of the extra energy released as a result of digestion, absorption, and metabolism of nutrients. Energy expenditure of physical activity is the energy required to perform body motion. In sedentary individuals, REE is the largest component of energy expenditure, encompassing about 65% to 80% of total daily energy expenditure. To prevent body wasting (fat and/or lean masses), the energy intake must be equal to the total expenditure during the same period (159,161). The World Health Organization has defined energy requirement as "the level of energy intake from food that will balance energy expenditure when the individual has a body size and composition, and level of physical activity, consistent with long term good health; and that will allow for the maintenance of economically necessary and sociably desirable physical activity. In children, pregnant or lactating women the energy requirement includes the energy needs associated with the deposition of tissues or the secretion of milk at rates consistent with good health" (162).

In summary, energy balance is neutral when the number of calories absorbed equals the amount of energy expended for body processes and activities with no weight change. When available energy exceeds the capacity of the body to expend it, a positive energy balance exists, causing weight gain with excess energy stored in the body primarily as adipose tissue. Adipose tissue will be maintained, will increase, or will become depleted, depending on the energy balance over time. When energy intake is not adequate for the requirement, a negative energy balance will occur, using adipose stores and other potential fuels (carbohydrates and proteins) and causing weight loss.

As with protein assessment, it is important to define the energy abnormalities in specific populations before assessing the energy balance. With regards to patients with renal failure, earlier studies concluded that energy requirement was similar between chronic renal failure and healthy subjects, both before and after initiation of renal replacement therapy (163–165). However, recent studies suggest that the REE is higher in patients with diabetes and chronic renal failure (166) and coronary heart disease, especially after adjusting for fat-free mass (167,168). Further, several studies have shown that REE increases during the hemodialysis procedure in the postabsorptive state (154,157,167). Overall, an energy intake of approximately 35 kcal/kg/day usually maintains visceral and somatic protein stores and nitrogen balance in CRF and maintenance dialysis patients, including patients with CRF fed a low-protein diet (71). It is important to keep in mind that because energy intake is prescribed based on weight, and in virtue of all the fluid/body weight variability found in patients with renal failure, desirable rather than actual body weight should be used. Another important point is that although their energy requirements are the same as for the healthy population, patients with CRF often ingest less than 35 kcal/kg/day, especially as glomerular filtration rate decreases below 25 mL/min, mainly from anorexia (169). This is important because appropriate energy intake is necessary for adequate utilization of protein, which is particularly important when low-protein diets are prescribed. Also, the level of energy requirement is increased during concurrent illnesses, particularly those requiring hospitalization.

Resting energy expenditure may be assessed by using standard equations and by indirect and direct measurements. The simplest method to estimate REE (kcal/day) is the calculation by the Harris-Benedict equation:

$$\text{Men: REE} = 66 + (13.7 \times \text{weight}) + (5 \times \text{height}) - (6.8 \times \text{age})$$

$$\text{Women: REE} = 655.1 + (9.6 \times \text{weight}) + (1.8 \times \text{height}) - (4.7 \times \text{age})$$

where weight is expressed in kg, height in cm, and age in years.

Although there is a general consensus that direct measures are always more precise than indirect ones, this may not be the case for energy assessment, where the term "indirect" refers to the assessment of energy expenditure generally performed by measuring oxygen consumption (VO_2) and carbon dioxide production (VCO_2), and "direct" in this context means measuring the direct heat transfer (170). Measurements of REE by indirect calorimetry, in general, are well correlated with direct calorimetry values and, in addition, provide an appreciation of substrate oxidation associated with heat production. Direct calorimetry measures the heat production directly, but it is much more difficult to perform and gives no information concerning the substrates used to generate the heat. Nonetheless, direct calorimetry traditionally is considered the gold standard for measurements of energy expenditure. However, indirect calorimetry is not only more convenient but it is particularly suitable if nutritional assessment is desirable (161,171). Because energy balance grossly equals energy intake minus energy expenditure and indirect calorimetry usually is measured for short periods with the subjects in the postabsorptive state, measurement of energy balance is mainly the measurement of energy output and is almost invariably performed by indirect calorimetry (172). Estimates are available so that short periods of assessment may be used to estimate 24-hour REE (172).

The most precise technique to indirectly measure calorimetry is the whole-room indirect calorimetry (metabolic chamber) (172). These are small rooms usually furnished with a bed and/or chair, toilet facilities, and telephone to allow the patient to be able to stay inside it comfortably enough for an adequate period of measurement. The metabolic chamber is designed to monitor patients for several days at a time. The metabolic rate is calculated based on the measurement of VO_2 and VCO_2, using standard estimation equations to return values of REE. Briefly, the chamber is ventilated with fresh air, and the airflow is measured continuously (outflow). The inflow-outflow difference in O_2 levels and the outflow-inflow difference in CO_2 concentrations are measured continuously. In steady-state conditions, airflow is set to maintain a concentration of CO_2 of less than 0.5% in the chamber. The subject's oxygen consumption then is calculated by the formula: $VO_2 = (VO_2 \text{ in-}VO_2 \text{ out}) + \Delta VO_2/\Delta t$, where ($VO_2$ in-VO_2 out) represents the difference between the flow rates of O_2 at the inlet and outlet of the chamber, and $\Delta VO_2/\Delta t$ represents the change in the O_2 content during the time Δt. The respiratory quotient (RQ) can be determined dividing VCO_2 by VO_2. There are some correction equations for differences between rates of VCO_2 and VO_2 because VCO_2 is usually smaller than VO_2. Special formulas for these corrections are out of the scope of this chapter and can be found elsewhere (172).

Another method of indirect calorimetry is to use the metabolic cart, which involves placing a plastic mask or ventilated hood to the patient's face to prevent the escape of expired air from the system. The air is drawn through the system and integrated into an O_2 and CO_2 analyzer attached to a computer for data analysis and storage, including all the parameters measured by the chamber (i.e., VO_2, VCO_2, metabolic rate, and RQ) (172). The metabolic carts are used widely in clinical practice and for research purposes. The accuracy of such carts has been proved inferior to whole-room indirect calorimetric chamber (173) because of some inherent technical limitations. For example, patients sometimes react adversely to a mask, mouthpiece, or ventilated hood and become agitated, with involuntarily hyperventilation, generating inappropriate high rates of VO_2 and VCO_2. A small percentage of subjects also experience a training effect, with resting EE decreasing significantly with repeated studies (173). Finally, some masks do not fit securely around the mouths and noses of malnourished patients, resulting in a leak of respiratory gases; also, these systems are not comfortable or practical to use for long periods (173). These limitations should be taken into account in clinical practice and in most of the research protocols because a metabolic cart is the most commonly used indirect calorimetry technique and a metabolic chamber is only available in very limited number of centers.

As previously discussed, total energy expenditure is composed of REE, the thermal effect of food, and physical activity, assuming an ideal situation of a postabsorptive state. Total energy expenditure can be precisely and directly measured by doubly labeled water—a safe and noninvasive technique, yet not of widespread use. It is done by oral ingestion or intravenous injection of two stable isotopes of water (i.e., $H_2{}^{18}O$ and ^2H_2O) in bolus. The disappearance of ^2H_2O is similar to water flux alone, but $H_2{}^{18}O$ is also lost in carbon dioxide (CO_2). The difference in the balance rates of these two tracers is a direct function of VCO_2 and can be used to calculate oxidation of carbohydrate, lipids, and protein (amino acids).

In summary, there are many different methods available for assessing protein and energy nutritional status. Some are easy to perform, readily available, and inexpensive, whereas others are sophisticated, not available in many centers, and either expensive or have an unfavorable cost-benefit ratio. A monthly nutritional screening can be performed easily at nearly any clinic or hospital by measuring serum albumin, serum prealbumin, serum transferrin, and bioimpedance values. However, if the goal is to precisely and longitudinally follow changes in body composition, one may want to use anthropometry, DEXA, and even more sophisticated methods, if available. For all methods, repeated measures and technical standardization are extremely important to reduce variability of results. Finally, complex and precise methods to assess protein-energy metabolism (i.e., stable isotope–tracer techniques), although not of widespread availability, are the methods of choice to measure acute changes or responses to metabolic interventions, minimizing variability and errors, making them the method of choice for research purposes. Regardless of the method, it is important to keep in mind that none is perfect and definitive, and the results should be analyzed in the clinical context of each individual patient.

REFERENCES

1. Allison SP. Malnutrition, disease, and outcome. *Nutrition* 2000; 16:590–593.
2. Bistrian BR, Blackburn GL, Vitale J, et al. Prevalence of malnutrition in general medical patients. *JAMA* 1976;235: 1567–1570.
3. Hill GL, Blackett RL, Pickford I, et al. Malnutrition in surgical patients. An unrecognised problem. *Lancet* 1977;1:689–692.
4. Sharma R, Florea VG, Bolger AP, et al. Wasting as an independent predictor of mortality in patients with cystic fibrosis. *Thorax* 2001;56:746–750.
5. Campos AC, Matias JE, Coelho JC. Nutritional aspects of liver transplantation. *Curr Opin Clin Nutr Metab Care* 2002;5: 297–307.
6. Ollenschlager G. [Nutritional deficiency during aggressive treatment of tumors]. *Fortschr Med* 1991;109:533–534.
7. Nitenberg G. Nutritional support in sepsis: still skeptical? *Curr Opin Crit Care* 2000;6:253–266.
8. Angus DC, Linde-Zwirble WT, Lidicker J, et al. Epidemiology of severe sepsis in the United States: analysis of incidence, out-

come, and associated costs of care. *Crit Care Med* 2001;29: 1303–1310.

9. Guarnieri G, Faccini L, Lipartiti T, et al. Simple methods for nutritional assessment in hemodialyzed patients. *Am J Clin Nutr* 1980;33:1598–1607.
10. Young GA, Swanepoel CR, Croft MR, et al. Anthropometry and plasma valine, amino acids, and proteins in the nutritional assessment of hemodialysis patients. *Kidney Int* 1982;21: 492–499.
11. Schoenfeld PY, Henry RR, Laird NM, et al. Assessment of nutritional status of the national cooperative dialysis study population. *Kidney Int* 1983;23:80–88.
12. Wolfson M, Strong CJ, Minturn RD, et al. Nutritional status and lymphocyte function in maintenance hemodialysis patients. *Am J Clin Nutr* 1984;37:547–555.
13. Cianciaruso B, Brunori G, Kopple JD, et al. Cross-sectional comparison of malnutrition in continuous ambulatory peritoneal dialysis and hemodialysis patients. *Am J Kidney Dis* 1995; 26:475–486.
14. Hakim RM, Levin N. Malnutrition in hemodialysis patients. *Am J Kidney Dis* 1993;21:125–137.
15. Sardesai VM. Fundamentals of nutrition. In: Sardesai VM, ed. *Introduction to clinical nutrition.* New York: Marcel Dekker, 1998:1–13.
16. Sardesai VM. Nutritional assessment. In: Sardesai VM, ed. *Introduction to clinical nutrition.* New York: Marcel Dekker, 1998: 295-307.
17. Jeejeebhoy KN. Nutritional assessment. *Nutrition* 2000;16: 585–590.
18. Identifying patients at risk: ADA's definitions for nutrition screening and nutrition assessment. Council on Practice (COP) Quality Management Committee. *J Am Diet Assoc* 1994;94: 838–839.
19. Requirements EaP. Report of a Joint FAO/WHO Ad Hoc Expert Committee. Technical Report Series, 1973;522.
20. Borah MF, Schoenfeld PY, Gotch FA, et al. Nitrogen balance during intermittent dialysis therapy of uremia. *Kidney Int* 1978; 14:491–500.
21. Ginn HE, Frost A, Lacy WW. Nitrogen balance in hemodialysis patients. *Am J Clin Nutr* 1968;21:385–393.
22. Kopple JD, Shinaberger JH, Coburn JW, et al. Optimal dietary protein treatment during chronic hemodialysis. *Trans Am Soc Artif Int Organs* 1969;15:302–308.
23. Lim VS, Flanigan MJ, Zavala DC, et al. Protective adaptation of low serum triiodothyronine in patients with chronic renal failure. *Kidney Int* 1985;28:541–549.
24. Motil KJ, Matthews DE, Bier DM, et al. Whole-body leucine and lysine metabolism: response to dietary protein intake in young men. *Am J Physiol* 1981;240:E712–721.
25. Price SR, Mitch WE. Metabolic acidosis and uremic toxicity: protein and amino acid metabolism. *Semin Nephrol* 1994;14: 232–237.
26. Anderson CF, Wochos DN. The utility of serum albumin values in the nutritional assessment of hospitalized patients. *Mayo Clin Proc* 1982;57:181–184.
27. Reinhardt GF, Myscofski JW, Wilkens DB, et al. Incidence and mortality of hypoalbuminemic patients in hospitalized veterans. *JPEN J Parenter Enteral Nutr* 1980;4:357–359.
28. Apelgren KN, Rombeau JL, Twomey PL, et al. Comparison of nutritional indices and outcome in critically ill patients. *Crit Care Med* 1982;10:305–307.
29. Kaw M, Sekas G. Long-term follow-up of consequences of percutaneous endoscopic gastrostomy (PEG) tubes in nursing home patients. *Dig Dis Sci* 1994;39:738–743.
30. Lowrie EG, Lew NL. Death risk in hemodialysis patients: The predictive value of commonly measured variables and an evaluation of death rate differences between facilities. *Am J Kidney Dis* 1990;15:458–482.
31. Jeejeebhoy KN. Nutritional assessment. *Gastroenterol Clin North Am* 1998;27:347–369.
32. Klein S. The myth of serum albumin as a measure of nutritional status. *Gastroenterology* 1990;99:1845–1846.
33. Kirsch R, Frith L, Black E, et al. Regulation of albumin synthesis and catabolism by alteration of dietary protein. *Nature* 1968; 217:578–579.
34. Kashihara T, Fujimori E, Oki A, et al. Protein-losing enteropathy and pancreatic involvement in a case of connective tissue disease. *Gastroenterol Jpn* 1992;27:246–251.
35. Chiu NT, Lee BF, Hwang SJ, et al. Protein-losing enteropathy: diagnosis with (99m)Tc-labeled human serum albumin scintigraphy. *Radiology* 2001;219:86–90.
36. Kaysen GA, Rathore V, Shearer GC, et al. Mechanisms of hypoalbuminemia in hemodialysis patients. *Kidney Int* 1995;48: 510–516.
37. Cueto Manzano AM. [Hypoalbuminemia in dialysis. Is it a marker for malnutrition or inflammation?]. *Rev Invest Clin* 2001;53:152–258.
38. Moshage HJ, Janssen JA, Franssen JH, et al. Study of the molecular mechanism of decreased liver synthesis of albumin in inflammation. *J Clin Invest* 1987;79:1635–1641.
39. Fleck A, Raines G, Hawker F, et al. Increased vascular permeability: a major cause of hypoalbuminaemia in disease and injury. *Lancet* 1985;1:781–784.
40. Gray GE, Meguid MM. Can total parenteral nutrition reverse hypoalbuminemia in oncology patients? *Nutrition* 1990;6: 225–228.
41. Kaysen GA, Dubin JA, Muller HG, et al. Relationships among inflammation nutrition and physiologic mechanisms establishing albumin levels in hemodialysis patients. *Kidney Int* 2002; 61:2240–2249.
42. Kaysen GA. The microinflammatory state in uremia: causes and potential consequences. *J Am Soc Nephrol* 2001;12:1549–1557.
43. Kaysen GA, Chertow GM, Adhikarla R, et al. Inflammation and dietary protein intake exert competing effects on serum albumin and creatinine in hemodialysis patients. *Kidney Int* 2001;60:333–340.
44. Ikizler TA, Wingard RL, Harvell J, et al. Association of morbidity with markers of nutrition and inflammation in chronic hemodialysis patients: a prospective study. *Kidney Int* 1999;55: 1945–1951.
45. Beck FK, Rosenthal TC. Prealbumin: a marker for nutritional evaluation. *Am Fam Physician* 2002;65:1575–1578.
46. Neyra NR, Hakim RM, Shyr Y, et al. Serum transferrin and serum prealbumin are early predictors of serum albumin in chronic hemodialysis patients. *J Ren Nutr* 2000;10:184–190.
47. Chertow GM, Ackert K, Lew NL, et al. Prealbumin is as important as albumin in the nutritional assessment of hemodialysis patients. *Kidney Int* 2000;58:2512–2517.
48. Spiekerman AM. Nutritional assessment (protein nutriture). *Anal Chem* 1995;67:429R–436R.
49. Spiekerman AM. Proteins used in nutritional assessment. *Clin Lab Med* 1993;13:353–369.
50. Mears E. Outcomes of continuous process improvement of a nutritional care program incorporating serum prealbumin measurements. *Nutrition* 1996;12:479–484.
51. Measurement of visceral protein status in assessing protein and energy malnutrition: standard of care. Prealbumin in Nutritional Care Consensus Group. *Nutrition* 1995;11:169–171.
52. Ingenbleek Y, DeVisscher M, DeNayer P. Measurement of prealbumin as index of protein-calorie malnutrition. *Lancet* 1972; 2:106–108.
53. Ingenbleek Y, Van Den Schrieck HG, De Nayer P, et al. Albu-

min, transferrin and the thyroxine-binding prealbumin/retinol-binding protein (TBPA-RBP) complex in assessment of malnutrition. *Clin Chim Acta* 1975;63:61–67.
54. Mittman N, Avram MM, Oo KK, et al. Serum prealbumin predicts survival in hemodialysis and peritoneal dialysis: 10 years of prospective observation. *Am J Kidney Dis* 2001;38:1358–1364.
55. Duggan A, Huffman FG. Validation of serum transthyretin (prealbumin) as a nutritional parameter in hemodialysis patients. *J Ren Nutr* 1998;8:142–149.
56. Staley MJ. Fructosamine and protein concentrations in serum. *Clin Chem* 1987;33:2326–2327.
57. Oppenheimer JH, Werner SC. Effect of prednisone on thyroxine-binding proteins. *J Clin Endocrinol Metab* 1966;26:715–721.
58. Le Moullac B, Gouache P, Bleiberg-Daniel F. Regulation of hepatic transthyretin messenger RNA levels during moderate protein and food restriction in rats. *J Nutr* 1992;122:864–870.
59. Winkler MF, Gerrior SA, Pomp A, et al. Use of retinol-binding protein and prealbumin as indicators of the response to nutrition therapy. *J Am Diet Assoc* 1989;89:684–687.
60. Hedlund JU, Hansson LO, Ortqvist AB. Hypoalbuminemia in hospitalized patients with community-acquired pneumonia. *Arch Intern Med* 1995;155:1438–1442.
61. Nieken J, Mulder NH, Buter J, et al. Recombinant human interleukin-6 induces a rapid and reversible anemia in cancer patients. *Blood* 1995;86:900–905.
62. O'Riordain MG, Ross JA, Fearon KC, et al. Insulin and counterregulatory hormones influence acute-phase protein production in human hepatocytes. *Am J Physiol* 1995;269:E323–330.
63. Huebers HA, Finch CA. The physiology of transferrin and transferrin receptors. *Physiol Rev* 1987;67:520–582.
64. Fletcher JP, Little JM, Guest PK. A comparison of serum transferrin and serum albumin as nutritional parameters. *J Parenter Enteral Nutr* 1987;11:144.
65. Briassoulis G, Zavras N, Hatzis T. Malnutrition, nutritional indices, and early enteral feeding in critically ill children. *Nutrition* 2001;17:548–557.
66. Han PD, Burke A, Baldassano RN, et al. Nutrition and inflammatory bowel disease. *Gastroenterol Clin North Am* 1999;28:423–443, ix.
67. Taylor SJ, Fettes SB, Jewkes C, et al. Prospective, randomized, controlled trial to determine the effect of early enhanced enteral nutrition on clinical outcome in mechanically ventilated patients suffering head injury. *Crit Care Med* 1999;27:2525–2531.
68. Qureshi AR, Alvestrand A, Danielsson A, et al. Factors predicting malnutrition in hemodialysis patients: a cross-sectional study. *Kidney Int* 1998;53:773–782.
69. Barany P, Peterson E, Ahlberg M, et al. Nutritional assessment in anemic hemodialysis patients treated with recombinant human erythropoietin. *Clin Nephrol* 1991;35:270–279.
70. Roza AM, Tuitt D, Shizgal HM. Transferrin: A poor measure of nutritional status. *J Parenter Enteral Nutr* 1984;8:523.
71. Clinical practice guidelines for nutrition in chronic renal failure. K/DOQI, National Kidney Foundation. *Am J Kidney Dis* 2000;35:S1–S140.
72. Cano N, Di Costanzo-Dufetel J, Calaf R, et al. Prealbumin-retinol-binding-protein-retinol complex in hemodialysis patients. *Am J Clin Nutr* 1988;47:664–667.
73. Kiess W, Kessler U, Schmitt S, et al. Growth hormone and insulin-like growth factor 1: Basic aspects. In: Flyvbjerg A, Orskov H, Alberti KG, eds. *Growth hormone and insulin-like growth factor 1*. New York: Wiley, 1993:1–21.
74. Raynaud-Simon A, Perin L, Meaume S, et al. IGF-I, IGF-I-binding proteins and GH-binding protein in malnourished elderly patients with inflammation receiving refeeding therapy. *Eur J Endocrinol* 2002;146:657–665.
75. Thissen JP, Ketelslegers JM, Underwood LE. Nutritional regulation of the insulin-like growth factors. *Endocr Rev* 1994;15:80–101.
76. Van den Berghe GH. Acute and prolonged critical illness are two distinct neuroendocrine paradigms. *Verh K Acad Geneeskd Belg* 1998;60:487–518; discussion 518–520.
77. Jacob V, Carpentier JEL, Salzano S, et al. IGF-1, a marker of undernutrition in hemodialysis patients. *Am J Clin Nutr* 1990;52:39–44.
78. Kagan A, Altman Y, Zadik Z, et al. Insulin-like growth factor-I in patients on CAPD and hemodialysis: relationship to body weight and albumin level. *Adv Perit Dial* 1995;11:234–238.
79. Parker III TF, Wingard RL, Husni L, et al. Effect of the membrane biocompatibility on nutritional parameters in chronic hemodialysis patients. *Kidney Int* 1996;49:551–556.
80. Gabay C, Kushner I. Acute-phase proteins and other systemic responses to inflammation. *N Engl J Med* 1999;340:448–454.
81. Owen WF, Lowrie EG. C-reactive protein as an outcome predictor for maintenance hemodialysis patients. *Kidney Int* 1998;54:627–636.
82. Harrison NA, Masterton RG, Bateman JM, et al. C-reactive protein in acute renal failure. *Nephrol Dial Transplant* 1989;4:864–869.
83. Panichi V, Migliori M, De Pietro S, et al. C reactive protein in patients with chronic renal diseases. *Ren Fail* 2001;23:551–562.
84. Locatelli F, Fouque D, Heimburger O, et al. Nutritional status in dialysis patients: a European consensus. *Nephrol Dial Transplant* 2002;17:563–572.
85. Ikizler TA, Hakim RM. Nutrition in end-stage renal disease. *Kidney Int* 1996;50:343–357.
86. Stenvinkel P, Barany P, Chung SH, et al. A comparative analysis of nutritional parameters as predictors of outcome in male and female ESRD patients. *Nephrol Dial Transplant* 2002;17:1266–1274.
87. Wang J, Thornton JC, Kolesnik S, et al. Anthropometry in body composition. An overview. *Ann N Y Acad Sci* 2000;904:317–326.
88. Chumlea WC, Guo SS, Vellas B. Assessment of protein-calorie nutrition. In: Kopple JD, Massry SG, eds. *Nutritional management of renal disease*. Baltimore, MD: Lippincott Williams & Wilkins, 1997:203–228.
89. Jelliffe DB, Jelliffe EF. An evaluation of upper arm measurements used in nutritional assessment. *Am J Clin Nutr* 1980;33:2058–2059.
90. Gurney JM, Jelliffe DB. Arm anthropometry in nutritional assessment: nomogram for rapid calculation of muscle circumference and cross-sectional muscle and fat areas. *Am J Clin Nutr* 1973;26:912–915.
91. Harries AD, Jones LA, Heatley RV, et al. Assessment of nutritional status by anthropometry: a comparison of different standards of reference. *Hum Nutr Clin Nutr* 1983;37:227–231.
92. Frisancho AR. Nutritional anthropometry. *J Am Diet Assoc* 1988;88:553–555.
93. de Onis M, Habicht JP. Anthropometric reference data for international use: recommendations from a World Health Organization Expert Committee. *Am J Clin Nutr* 1996;64:650–658.
94. Vansant G, Van Gaal L, De Leeuw I. Assessment of body composition by skinfold anthropometry and bioelectrical impedance technique: a comparative study. *JPEN J Parenter Enteral Nutr* 1994;18:427–429.
95. Ravasco P, Camilo ME, Gouveia-Oliveira A, et al. A critical approach to nutritional assessment in critically ill patients. *Clin Nutr* 2002;21:73–77.
96. Yao M, Roberts SB, Ma G, et al. Field Methods for Body

Composition Assessment are Valid in Healthy Chinese Adults. *Am Soc Nutr Sci* 2002:310–317.

97. Mei Z, Grummer-Strawn LM, Pietrobelli A, et al. Validity of body mass index compared with other body-composition screening indexes for the assessment of body fatness in children and adolescents. *Am J Clin Nutr* 2002;75:978–985.
98. Pollock ML, Jackson AS. Research progress in validation of clinical methods of assessing body composition. *Med Sci Sports Exerc* 1984;16:606–615.
99. Nelson EE, Hong CD, Pesce AL, et al. Anthropometric norms for the dialysis population. *Am J Kidney Dis* 1990;16:32–37.
100. Pupim LB, Kent P, Ikizler TA. Bioelectrical impedance analysis in dialysis patients. *Miner Electrolyte Metab* 1999;25:400–406.
101. Dumler F, Kilates C. Use of bioelectrical impedance techniques for monitoring nutritional status in patients on maintenance dialysis. *J Ren Nutr* 2000;10:116–124.
102. Evans EM, Arngrimsson SA, Cureton KJ. Body composition estimates from multicomponent models using BIA to determine body water. *Med Sci Sports Exerc* 2001;33:839–842.
103. Chertow GM. Estimates of body composition as intermediate outcome variables: are DEXA and BIA ready for prime time? *J Ren Nutr* 1999;9:138–141.
104. Dumler F. Use of bioelectric impedance analysis and dual-energy X-ray absorptiometry for monitoring the nutritional status of dialysis patients. *Asaio J* 1997;43:256–260.
105. Khaled MA, Kabir I, Goran MI, et al. Bioelectrical impedance measurements at various frequencies to estimate human body compositions. *Indian J Exp Biol* 1997;35:159–161.
106. Biggs J, Cha K, Horch K. Electrical resistivity of the upper arm and leg yields good estimates of whole body fat. *Physiol Meas* 2001;22:365–376.
107. Di Iorio BR, Terracciano V, Bellizzi V. Bioelectrical impedance measurement: errors and artifacts. *J Ren Nutr* 1999;9:192–197.
108. Wotton MJ, Thomas BJ, Cornish BH, et al. Comparison of whole body and segmental bioimpedance methodologies for estimating total body water. *Ann N Y Acad Sci* 2000;904: 181–186.
109. Kotler DP, Rosenbaum K, Allison DB, et al. Validation of bioimpedance analysis as a measure of change in body cell mass as estimated by whole-body counting of potassium in adults. *J Parenter Enteral Nutr* 1999;23:345–349.
110. Chertow GM, Jacobs DO, Lazarus JM, et al. Phase angle predicts survival in hemodialysis patients. *J Renal Nutr* 1997;7: 204–207.
111. Piccoli A, Fanos V, Peruzzi L, et al. Reference values of the bioelectrical impedance vector in neonates in the first week after birth. *Nutrition* 2002;18:383–387.
112. Woodrow G, Oldroyd B, Turney JH, et al. Measurement of total body water by bioelectrical impedance in chronic renal failure. *Eur J Clin Nutr* 1996;50:676–681.
113. Chertow GM, Lazarus JM, Lew NL, et al. Bioimpedance norms for the hemodialysis population. *Kidney Int* 1997;52: 1617–1621.
114. Elia M. Assessment of nutritional status and body composition. In: Rombeau JL, Rolandelli RH, eds. *Clinical nutrition: enteral and tube feeding*, 3rd ed. Philadelphia: W.B. Saunders, 1997: 155–173.
115. Kalantar-Zadeh K, Dunne E, Nixon K, et al. Near infra-red interactance for nutritional assessment of dialysis patients. *Nephrol Dial Transplant* 1999;14:169–175.
116. Keshaviah PR, Nolph KD, Moore HL, et al. Lean body mass estimation by creatinine kinetics. *J Am Soc Nephrol* 1994;4: 1475–1485.
117. Bhatla B, Moore H, Emerson P, et al. Lean body mass estimation by creatinine kinetics, bioimpedance, and dual energy x-ray absorptiometry in patients on continuous ambulatory peritoneal dialysis. *Asaio J* 1995;41:M442–M446.
118. Fuller NJ, Jebb SA, Laskey MA, et al. Four-component model for the assessment of body composition in humans: comparison with alternative methods, and evaluation of the density and hydration of fat-free mass. *Clin Sci (Lond)* 1992;82:687–693.
119. Forbes GB. Body composition. In: Ziegler EE, Filer LJ Jr, eds. *Present knowledge in nutrition*, 7th ed. Washington, DC: International Life Sciences Institutes Press, 1996:7–12.
120. Fogelholm M, van Marken Lichtenbelt W. Comparison of body composition methods: a literature analysis. *Eur J Clin Nutr* 1997;51:495–503.
121. Kyle UG, Genton L, Pichard C. Body composition: what's new? *Curr Opin Clin Nutr Metab Care* 2002;5:427–433.
122. Dempster P, Aitkens S. A new air displacement method for the determination of human body composition. *Med Sci Sports Exerc* 1995;27:1692–1697.
123. Fields DA, Goran MI, McCrory MA. Body-composition assessment via air-displacement plethysmography in adults and children: a review. *Am J Clin Nutr* 2002;75:453–467.
124. Levenhagen DK, Borel MJ, Welch DC, et al. A comparison of air displacement plethysmography with three other techniques to determine body fat in healthy adults. *JPEN J Parenter Enteral Nutr* 1999;23:293–299.
125. Biaggi RR, Vollman MW, Nies MA, et al. Comparison of air-displacement plethysmography with hydrostatic weighing and bioelectrical impedance analysis for the assessment of body composition in healthy adults. *Am J Clin Nutr* 1999;69:898–903.
126. Curtin F, Morabia A, Pichard C, et al. Body mass index compared to dual-energy x-ray absorptiometry: evidence for a spectrum bias. *J Clin Epidemiol* 1997;50:837–843.
127. Abrahamsen B, Hansen TB, Hogsberg IM, et al. Impact of hemodialysis on dual X-ray absorptiometry, bioelectrical impedance measurements, and anthropometry. *Am J Clin Nutr* 1996; 63:80–86.
128. Panotopoulos G, Ruiz JC, Guy-Grand B, et al. Dual x-ray absorptiometry, bioelectrical impedance, and near infrared interactance in obese women. *Med Sci Sports Exerc* 2001;33: 665–670.
129. Cohn SH, Brennan BL, Yasumura S, et al. Evaluation of body composition and nitrogen content of renal patients on chronic dialysis as determined by total body neutron activation. *Am J Clin Nutr* 1983;38:52–58.
130. Stall S, DeVita MV, Ginsberg NS, et al. Body composition assessed by neutron activation analysis in dialysis patients. *Ann N Y Acad Sci* 2000;904:558–563.
131. Morgan WD. Of mermaids and mountains. Three decades of prompt activation in vivo. *Ann N Y Acad Sci* 2000;904: 128–133.
132. Pollock CA, Ibels LS, Allen BJ, et al. Total body nitrogen as a prognostic marker in maintenance dialysis. *J Am Soc Nephrol* 1995;6:82–88.
133. Park JH, Olsen NJ. Utility of magnetic resonance imaging in the evaluation of patients with inflammatory myopathies. *Curr Rheumatol Rep* 2001;3:334–345.
134. Detsky AS, Baker JP, Mendelson RA, et al. Evaluating the accuracy of nutritional assessment techniques applied to hospitalized patients: methodology and comparisons. *JPEN J Parenter Enteral Nutr* 1984;8:153–159.
135. McCann L. Using subjective global assessment to identify malnutrition in the ESRD patient. *Nephrol News Issues* 1999;13: 18–19.
136. Cooper BA, Bartlett LH, Aslani A, et al. Validity of subjective global assessment as a nutritional marker in end-stage renal disease. *Am J Kidney Dis* 2002;40:126–132.
137. Duerksen DR, Yeo TA, Siemens JL, et al. The validity and

reproducibility of clinical assessment of nutritional status in the elderly. *Nutrition* 2000;16:740–744.
138. Goldstein DJ. Assessment of nutritional status in renal diseases. In: Mitch WE, Klahr S, eds. *Handbook of nutrition and the kidney*, 3rd ed. Philadelphia: Lippincott-Raven, 1998:46–86.
139. Kopple JD. Uses and limitations of the balance technique. *JPEN J Parenter Enteral Nutr* 1987;11:79S–85S.
140. Rao M, Sharma M, Juneja R, et al. Calculated nitrogen balance in hemodialysis patients: influence of protein intake. *Kidney Int* 2000;58:336–345.
141. Reifenstein EC, Albright F, Wells SL. The accumulation, interpretation, and presentation of data pertaining to metabolic balances, notably those of calcium, phosphorus, and nitrogen. *J Clin Endocrinol Metab* 1945;5:367–395.
142. Kopple JD, Coburn JW. Metabolic studies of low protein diets in uremia. I. Nitrogen and potassium. *Medicine (Baltimore)* 1973;52:583–595.
143. Calloway DH. Nitrogen balance of men with marginal intakes of protein and energy. *J Nutr* 1975;105:914–923.
144. Garlick PJ, Clugston GA, Swick RW, et al. Diurnal variations in protein metabolism in man. *Proc Nutr Soc* 1978;37:33A.
145. Wolfe RR. *Radioactive and stable isotope tracers in biomedicine: principles and practice of kinetic analysis.* New York: Wiley-Liss, 1992:283–316.
146. Garlick PJ, McNurlan MA, McHardy KC, et al. Rates of nutrient utilization in man measured by combined respiratory gas analysis and stable isotopic labeling: effect of food intake. *Hum Nutr Clin Nutr* 1987;41:177–191.
147. Barrett EJ, Revkin JH, Young LH, et al. An isotopic method for measurement of muscle protein synthesis and degradation in vivo. *Biochem J* 1987;245:223–228.
148. Gelfand RA, Barrett EJ. Effect of physiologic hyperinsulinemia on skeletal muscle protein synthesis and breakdown in man. *J Clin Invest* 1987;80:1–6.
149. Christensen HN. Role of amino acid transport and countertransport in nutrition and metabolism. *Physiol Rev* 1990;70: 43–77.
150. Shotwell MA, Kilberg MS, Oxender DL. The regulation of neutral amino acid transport in mammalian cells. *Biochim Biophys Acta* 1983;737:267–284.
151. Biolo G, Zhang XJ, Wolfe RR. Role of membrane transport in interorgan amino acid flow between muscle and small intestine. *Metabolism* 1995;44:719–724.
152. Biolo G, Fleming RY, Maggi SP, et al. Transmembrane transport and intracellular kinetics of amino acids in human skeletal muscle. *Am J Physiol* 1995;268:E75–E84.
153. Lim VS, Bier DM, Flanigan MJ, et al. The effect of hemodialysis on protein metabolism: a leucine kinetic study. *J Clin Invest* 1993;91:2429–2436.
154. Ikizler TA, Pupim LB, Brouillette JR, et al. Hemodialysis stimulates muscle and whole body protein loss and alters substrate oxidation. *Am J Physiol Endocrinol Metab* 2002;282:E107-16.
155. Goodship TH, Mitch WE, Hoerr RA, et al. Adaptation to low-protein diets in renal failure: leucine turnover and nitrogen balance. *J Am Soc Nephrol* 1990;1:66–75.
156. Goodship TH, Lloyd S, Clague MB, et al. Whole body leucine turnover and nutritional status in continuous ambulatory peritoneal dialysis. *Clin Sci (Lond)* 1987;73:463–469.
157. Pupim LB, Flakoll PJ, Brouillette JR, et al. Intradialytic parenteral nutrition improves protein and energy homeostasis in chronic hemodialysis patients. *J Clin Invest* 2002;110:483–492.
158. Caglar K, Peng Y, Pupim LB, et al. Inflammatory signals associated with hemodialysis. *Kidney Int* 2002;62:1408–1416.
159. Sardesai VM. Requirements for energy, carbohydrates, fat, and proteins. In: Sardesai VM, ed. *Introduction to clinical nutrition.* New York: Marcel Dekker, 1998:1–13.
160. Woo R, Daniels-Kush R, Horton ES. Regulation of energy balance. *Annu Rev Nutr* 1985;5:411–433.
161. Bursztein S, Elwyn DH, Asakanazi J, et al. *Energy metabolism, indirect calorimetry, and nutrition.* Baltimore: Lippincott Williams & Wilkins, 1989.
162. Consultation FWUE. Energy and protein requirements. Geneva: World Health Organization, 1985.
163. Monteon FJ, Laidlaw SA, Shaib JK, et al. Energy expenditure in patients with chronic renal failure. *Kidney Int* 1986;30: 741–747.
164. Schneeweiss B, Graninger W, Stokenhuber F, et al. Energy metabolism in acute and chronic renal failure. *Am J Clin Nutr* 1990;52:596–601.
165. Olevitch LR, Bowers BM, DeOreo PB. Measurement of resting energy expenditure via indirect calorimetry among adult hemodialysis patients. *J Renal Nutr* 1994;4:192–197.
166. Avesani CM, Cuppari L, Silva AC, et al. Resting energy expenditure in pre-dialysis diabetic patients. *Nephrol Dial Transplant* 2001;16:556–565.
167. Ikizler TA, Wingard RL, Sun M, et al. Increased energy expenditure in hemodialysis patients. *J Am Soc Nephrol* 1996;7: 2646–2653.
168. Neyra RN, Chen KY, Sun M, et al. Increased resting energy expenditure in patients with end-stage renal disease. *J Parenter Enteral Nutr* 2003;27:36–42.
169. Levey AS, Greene T, Beck GJ, et al. Dietary protein restriction and the progression of chronic renal disease: what have all of the results of the MDRD study shown? Modification of Diet in Renal Disease Study group. *J Am Soc Nephrol* 1999;10: 2426–2439.
170. Simonson DC, DeFronzo RA. Indirect calorimetry: methodological and interpretative problems. *Am J Physiol* 1990;258: E399–E412.
171. Ferrannini E, Elia M, Ravussin E, et al. Indirect calorimetry: theory and practice. In: Kinney JM, Tucker HN, eds. *Energy metabolism.* New York: Raven Press, 1992:1–113.
172. Jequier E, Acheson K, Schutz Y. Assessment of energy expenditure and fuel utilization in man. *Annu Rev Nutr* 1987;7: 187–208.
173. Leff ML, Hill JO, Yates AA, et al. Resting metabolic rate: measurement reliability. *JPEN J Parenter Enteral Nutr* 1987;11: 354–359.

16

INFLUENCE OF DIETARY PROTEIN INTAKE ON THE PROGRESSION OF CHRONIC RENAL INSUFFICIENCY

DENIS FOUQUE

For many decades, it has been recommended that patients with renal disease modify their nutrient intakes. Depending on the disease, these modifications generally are focused on salt, protein, potassium, calcium, phosphorus, alkaline derivatives, oxalates, citrates, products that engender uric acid, and water or fluid. In this chapter, we will focus on the experimental and clinical effects of protein intake on renal function in patients with a chronic reduction in glomerular filtration rate (GFR) who do not have end-stage renal disease, or ESRD (i.e., individuals with chronic renal insufficiency). We will address the potential benefits and risks of limiting the patient's protein intake to an optimal level and address how to monitor the actual intake of these diets. In addition, the clinical evidence that justifies such dietary interventions in patients with chronic renal insufficiency will be discussed.

ASSESSING THE PROGRESSION OF CHRONIC RENAL INSUFFICIENCY

One of the main questions that arises when investigators want to study nephroprotection is how progression of renal disease should be monitored. Experimental studies frequently present histologic data such as glomerular sclerosis, tubular atrophy, and interstitial fibrosis in response to diet interventions. However, such data are not available in humans because ethical reasons prevent the performance of serial kidney biopsies during dietary interventions. Because renal failure is the ultimate consequence of progressive renal disease, renal function and its impairment usually are considered key outcome measures in experimental and clinical trials. However, one of the main limitations of this approach is that renal function is directly affected by nutritional intake independently of injury to renal tissue. Thus, interpretation of traditional markers of renal function could be flawed by nutritional interventions. To illustrate this point, Levey et al. have summarized the renal function decrease during the Modification of Diet in Renal Disease (MDRD) study using different estimates of GFR in groups of people usual-protein–intake diets and low-protein–intake diets (Fig. 16.1) (1). If we accept the ^{125}I-iothalamate renal clearance as the gold standard for GFR measurement, it is easy to note that other traditional renal function markers are not as accurate measures of GFR and can lead to misinterpretation. Although it is not the aim of this chapter to present detailed information on how to monitor renal function in experimental and clinical studies, some brief comments related to nutritional influences may be warranted.

Serum creatinine has been used extensively to monitor renal function and to assess renal insufficiency in clinical trials (2). It is now well established that serum creatinine or its derivatives are not accurate indicators of renal function (3). Serum creatinine is largely produced by the catabolism of muscle creatine; 1.7% of the entire muscle creatine pool is converted to creatinine daily. This conversion rate does not appear to be extremely constant because the daily variability in this conversion rate in healthy volunteers has been reported to range from 6% to 26% (4). Serum creatinine also is affected by creatine and creatinine intake from ingested meat (5). Indeed, investigators reported that serum creatinine increased by as much as 50% from normal values within 2 to 4 hours after a meal containing 225 g of boiled beef (5). The half-life to achieve a new steady state in creatinine excretion following a change in creatine intake is 41 days (6). Thus, any change in creatine intake (e.g., in intake of animal skeletal muscle) will necessitate a minimum of three half-lives to reach a new plateau (e.g., 4 months after the start of the new diet and before any valid estimation of renal function from creatinine could be done). In addition, any change in the diet that leads to a variation of muscle mass will modify the creatine pool and creatinine production (7). For instance, intensive physical exercise leading to hypertrophy of skeletal muscle will induce an increase in serum creatinine independent of renal function change.

Serum creatinine also may vary independently of renal

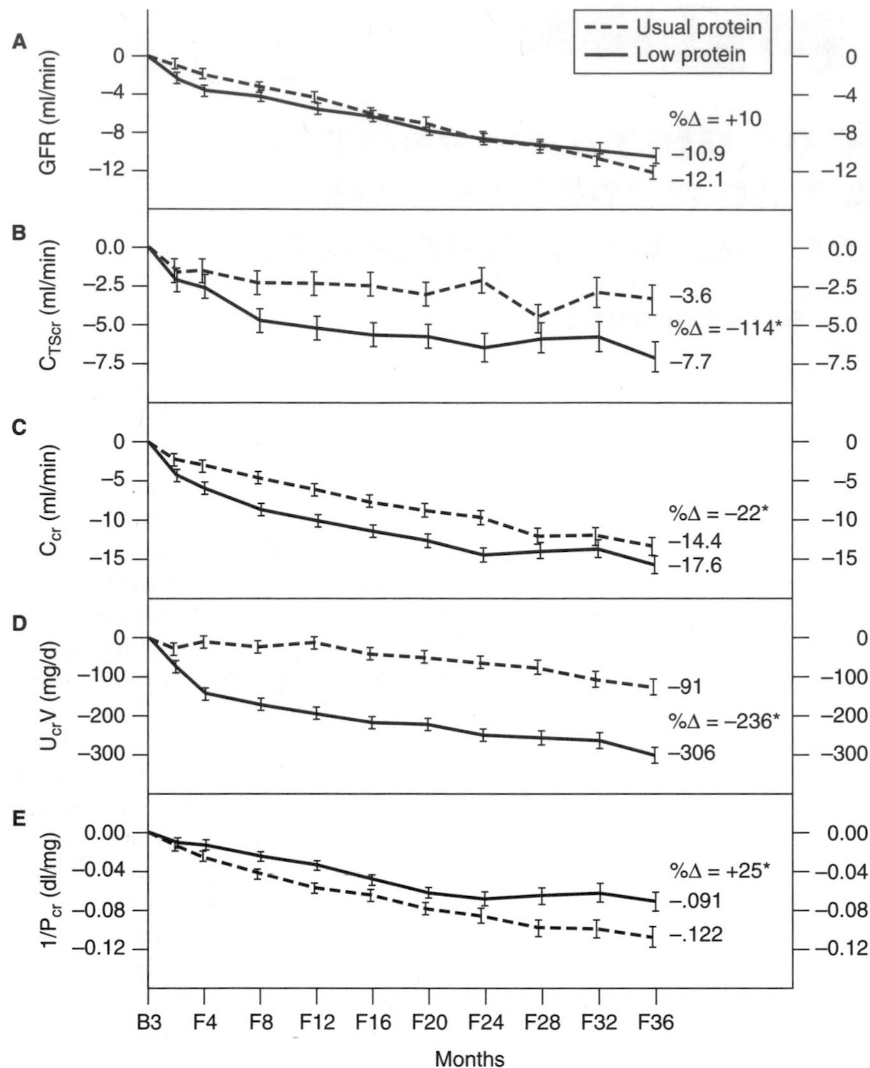

FIGURE 16.1. The rates of decline in renal function as measured by different techniques in Study A of the Modification of Diet in Renal Disease Study. *Dashed lines*, usual protein intake; *solid lines*, low-protein diet. **A:** ^{125}I-iothalamate plasma clearance; **B:** Tubular secretion of creatinine; **C:** Creatinine clearance; **D:** Creatinine excretion rate; **E:** Reciprocal serum creatinine. (From Modification of Diet in Renal Disease Study Group. Effects of diet and antihypertensive therapy on creatinine clearance and serum creatinine concentration in the modification of diet in renal disease study. *J Am Soc Nephrol* 1996;7:556–565, with permission.)

function and food intake for additional reasons. First, there is an intervariability between measurement techniques among different clinical laboratories that can exceed 30 to 40 μmol/L for the same sample. Second, the level of serum creatinine depends on the tubular secretion of creatinine, which has a great variability, particularly in the range of 40 to 80 mL/min of GFR (8). In addition, the tubular secretion of creatinine is impaired by many medications such as trimethoprim, cimetidine, salicylate, or probenecid. These drugs generally will block the tubular secretion of creatinine, increasing serum creatinine without a change in GFR. Creatinine also is metabolized by extrarenal routes, mostly degraded by intestinal microorganisms, and this extrarenal clearance may vary as renal failure progresses (9).

Because it has been shown that in most renal diseases there is a linear loss of renal function over time in more than 80% of patients, the inverse of serum creatinine (1/Screat), which also decreases linearly with time, has been used as a surrogate for estimating renal function. Unfortunately, all of the limitations that exist using the serum creatinine as an indication of GFR also pertain to the reciprocal of the serum creatinine, thus rendering this marker unsuitable for assessing diet impact on renal function.

Creatinine clearance, serially measured, has been proposed as an indicator of renal function loss. Creatinine clearance is not an ideal method for assessing glomerular filtration because it exceeds the GFR by 10 to 15 mL/min (in healthy adults) as a result of active tubular secretion. As renal function deteriorates further, the tubular secretion increases disproportionately and can overestimate renal function by 80% to 100% in cases of severe renal insufficiency (8,10). The correlation between the creatinine clearance and true GFR is weak and improves after administering cimetidine (800 or 1,200 mg), which blocks the tubular part of creatinine clearance, 1 to 2 hours before commencing the urine collection (10–12). In the pilot phase of the MDRD study, the mean correlation coefficient for the rate of change in creatinine clearance (24-hour urine collection) versus GFR (^{125}I-iothalamate clearance) was only 0.56 and 0.50 in studies A and B, respectively (13). Another important nonspecific cause of inaccurate estimation of renal function by the creatinine clearance is an incomplete urine collection. This inaccuracy tends to improve when short-period repeated urine collections are done over a 3- to 4-hour period (11, 14). Thus, to assess the effects of a given intervention on renal function in a clinical trial, creatinine clearance can be used under the following conditions: the range of renal function of patients should be wide, the treatment does not affect the tubular secretion of creatinine, and the clearance is measured during short periods (11,14). Whether cimetidine-treated creatinine clearance should be performed in diet intervention studies has not yet been validated but perhaps should be considered when true GFR measurements cannot be used.

A number of formulas have been derived from creatinine and various parameters such as age, gender, and weight (Equation 1) (15,16). These formulas appear convenient to use, can be computed directly from simple software or pocket organizers, and have broad applicability for the general treatment of renal disease. In 1999 Levey et al. reanalyzed the data obtained through the MDRD study and proposed a formula (Equation 2) (17) based on serum creatinine, serum urea, serum albumin, age, gender, and ethnicity, which seems more accurate than creatinine clearance or the Cockcroft–Gault equation (Equation 1) (15).

$$\text{Equation 1 (15): CCr} = [(140 - \text{age}) \times \text{Weight}] / (\text{Pcreat} \times 72) \text{ for men}$$

$$\text{CCr} = [(140 - \text{age}) \times \text{Weight}] / (\text{Pcreat} \times 85) \text{ for women}$$

Where CCr is creatinine clearance in mL/min, Pcreat is serum creatinine in mg/dL, and age is in years and weight is in kg (15).

$$\text{Equation 2 (17): GFR} = 170 \times [\text{Pcreat}]^{-0.999} \times [\text{Age}]^{-0.176} \times [0.762 \text{ if patient is female}] \times [1.180 \text{ if patient is black}] \times [\text{SUN}]^{-0.170} \times [\text{Alb}]^{0.318}$$

Where GFR is the glomerular filtration rate in mL/min/1.73 m^2, Pcreat is serum creatinine in mg/dL, SUN is serum urea nitrogen in mg/dL, and Alb is serum albumin in g/dL. Age is in years (17).

Although simple formulas can predict GFR with acceptable precision for routine use (Cockcroft–Gault formula overestimates GFR by only 16%—for example, 7 mL/min/1.73 m^2 [17]), for research purposes, more precise techniques should be used.

GFR is considered to be the gold standard for estimating renal function and for assessing the progression of renal disease (3). However, the GFR measurement is difficult to perform, is expensive, and presents some limitations. Traditional markers such as inulin have been challenged by radiotracers such as ^{125}I-iothalamate, ^{99m}Tc-DTPA, or ^{51}Cr-EDTA (ethylene-diamine-tetra-acetic acid). Measurements can be done after a single injection, either subcutaneously or intravenously, and include plasma and/or urine samples over 3 to 4 hours. Usually, when urine samples are needed, bladder catheterization is not necessary but may be required in cases of bladder dysfunction such as in diabetes or neurologic disease. To avoid prerenal azotemia, it generally is recommended to ensure a minimal urine output by ingesting a water load before the test. This has been challenged by Anastasio et al., who actually reported a decrease in GFR after patients received a large oral water load (4 mL/kg body weight every 30 min) during a 3-hour GFR measurement (18).

Finally, another more pragmatic approach has been proposed to assess the efficacy of a treatment in renal failure. The "renal death" was defined as the number of patients starting dialysis during a study (2,19). Because death from renal failure origin cannot be excluded formally, we have included the number of deaths within the "renal death" definition, as well as the number of renal transplantation before the start of dialysis if it happened during the study.

PROTEIN INTAKE AND CHRONIC RENAL INSUFFICIENCY: EXPERIMENTAL DATA

There is ample evidence, dating from the 1920s, that elevated protein intake or amino acid infusion alter renal hemodynamics and impair renal function and tissue in normal animals or experimental renal insufficiency (20–25). (For detailed reviews see references 26 through 28.) In many of these experiments, it is somewhat difficult to identify clearly the specific role of protein because sodium, energy, fluid, and phosphorus intakes obviously varied and were not always controlled. In addition, in case of severe experimental nephropathy, high-protein intake may have elicited superimposed uremic toxicity and mortality not directly related to further damage to renal function or injury to the kidney, thus adding confounding elements (21). We will review here the experimental data on the renal effects of a reduced protein intake.

The hemodynamic effects of dietary protein have been attributed to a number of mechanisms that increase GFR, induce and/or increase proteinuria, and eventually lead to glomerulosclerosis and renal insufficiency. Candidates for these mechanisms include hormones (glucagon, insulin, insulinlike growth factor-1 [IGF-1], and angiotensin II), cytokines (prostaglandins), and kinins (29–33). Intrarenal regulation of sodium transport also may be involved through the proximal sodium/amino acid cotransporter; activity of this transporter is enhanced in response to an increased filtered amino acid load, thus stimulating the tubuloglomerular feedback and increasing the GFR (34).

Protein restriction ablates most of the hemodynamic changes observed after renal ablation or 5/6 nephrectomy. Micropuncture studies provide direct evidence that the increase in single-*Nephron* GFR after renal mass reduction is responsible for the accelerated glomerular injury (35). Reducing protein intake decreases GFR in normal animals and blunts the renal hemodynamic changes induced by extensive renal ablation (i.e., increased glomerular pressure and flow). Subsequent studies in rats with less severe renal ablation showed that a low-protein intake also lowers hyperfiltration and retards the onset of proteinuria and glomerular fibrosis (23,36,37). In addition to these experimental data, low-protein intakes also increased survival in these animals with reduced renal function (21).

A reduced animal-protein intake (usually a diet containing 6% protein) allows control of glomerular hypertension by inducing afferent arteriolar vasoconstriction, which in turn decreases the glomerular plasma flow and reduces proteinuria (35). Protein restriction decreases the percentage of glomerular sclerosis and proteinuria. Indeed, Hostetter et al. reported that at 4 and 8 months after the onset of renal insufficiency created by a 5/6 nephrectomy, glomerulosclerosis was attenuated by 50% in animals receiving a 6% protein diet and proteinuria was lowered to 25% of that in rats receiving a 40% protein diet (23). Of importance, these benefits were observed at different levels of renal impairment (Fig. 16.2).

Micropuncture studies in 5/6 nephrectomized rats showed that a reduction in protein intake from 20% to 6% led to a reduction in single-*Nephron* GFR and normalized intraglomerular capillary pressure (25). Of interest, proteinuria in the 6% protein diet group was reduced to one-fifth of proteinuria observed in the 20% protein diet group. Both groups of rats were hypertensive, and there was no discussion on what the effects of a low-protein diet (LPD) would have been if the rats were normotensive (25). Thus, whereas a low dietary protein intake (DPI) shortly commenced after the onset of renal ablation seems to mainly blunt the increase in glomerular capillary pressure, delayed use of an LPD will reduce glomerular capillary pressure without lowering renal hyperperfusion or hyperfiltration (25,38). These data support the deleterious impact of glomerular hypertension and the protective role of a low-protein intake on the remnant renal function in experimental renal insufficiency.

Protein intake and protein trafficking through the kidney are associated with hypermetabolism (39) and oxidant stress (40). Oxygen consumption and ammonia production decreased by about 50% when rats were fed a 12% instead

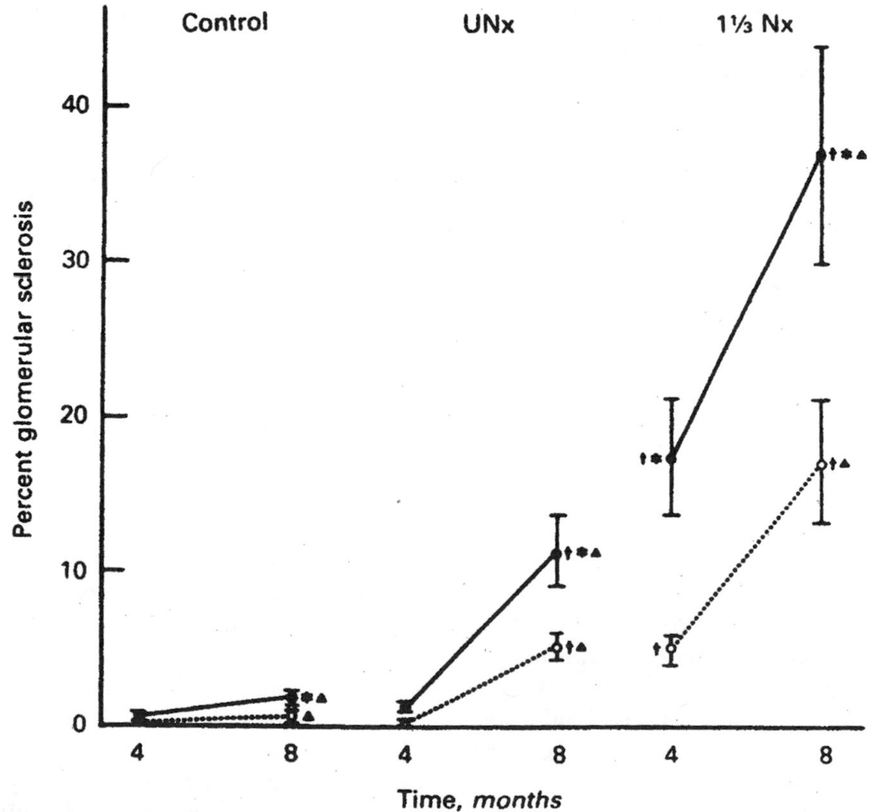

FIGURE 16.2. Percentage of sclerosed glomeruli in rats with two different levels of experimental renal insufficiency as compared with a control group of rats. *Open circles*, low protein intake; *closed circles*, high protein intake. (From Hostetter TH. Chronic effects of dietary protein in the rat with intact and reduced renal mass. *Kidney Int* 1986;30:509–517, with permission.)

of a 40% protein diet (40). This fact is explained primarily by a decrease in net sodium reabsorption (41). In another study, hypoxic injury of the thick ascending limb was mitigated by reducing the protein content of the diet (42). Additional metabolic data obtained through ^{31}P-NMR (phosphorus-nuclear magnetic resonance) spectroscopy also show that protein restriction reduces intracellular inorganic phosphate and pH, consistent with a decrease in oxygen consumption (43). This decrease in oxygen demand secondary to a reduction in protein diet from 30% to 6% may be responsible for reduced kidney production of glutathione and malondialdehyde (41,43).

The effect of the type of protein may deserve some comment. Based on the observation that vegetarians have lower GFR than omnivores (44,45), Williams et al. tested two different sources of protein derived from either animal or vegetable origin, casein or soya, in stable rats with chronic renal failure (CRF) (46). Both regular (24%) and moderately low (12%) protein intakes of each of those two protein sources were studied. After 3 months of dietary feeding, glomerulosclerosis and tubular dilation were found to be always greater in the casein-fed versus the soya-fed groups. Proteinuria was greatest with the 24% (99 ± 34(sd) mg/d) and 12% (64 ± 18) casein diet, lower in the 24% soya group (30 ± 5), and lowest in the 12% (35 ± 7) soya groups. There was no difference in the severity of the proteinuria or histologic lesions in the 24% versus the 12% soya groups (46). Although these results are convincing, it should be noted that, because of the different digestibility of protein, it is possible that vegetable proteins were less absorbed than the animal proteins by about 10%, thus reducing the true protein load with the former diet. It is interesting to note that particular amino acids may elicit specific renal hemodynamic effects. A diet enriched with L-arginine, the precursor of nitric oxide (NO), has been shown to reduce glomerular hypertension and glomerulosclerosis in 5/6 nephrectomized rats (47). Because NO is a potent vasodilation factor, locally enhanced NO production may be involved in these hemodynamic changes. L-arginine also stimulates growth hormone secretion, which also may cause renal vasodilation through release of IGF-1 and, consequently, NO.

Another interesting hypothesis was developed by Tapp et al. Because in most studies of protein reduction it is the whole food intake that is reduced, these authors studied the effects of energy restriction as compared with protein restriction (48). Five groups of 5/6 nephrectomized rats were fed a control diet, a 40% reduction in overall food, a 40% energy-reduced diet, a 40% protein-reduced diet, or a 40% salt-reduced diet. After 21 weeks of diet, histologic findings clearly showed protected kidneys in the low–energy-alone group, which disclosed less glomerulosclerosis as well as less interstitial inflammation, as compared with all other groups. Of interest, proteinuria was lowest in this calorie-restricted group (48). The discrepant finding of an absence of beneficial effects of the protein-reduced diet might be explained by a too modest reduction in protein intake as compared to the control diet. In a subsequent paper, these investigators reported that 2 weeks after 5/6 nephrectomy, the kidney IGF-1 content and the severity of inflammatory lesions were reduced with calorie restriction (49). Altogether, these results suggest that IGF-1 expression could be involved in the tubulointerstitial inflammatory response and controlled by a low energy intake. Of interest is the fact that proteinuria also was reduced by the low-calorie diet (49).

In a strain of mice (kd/kd) developing an autoimmune interstitial nephritis, Fernandes et al. showed that an LPD alone did not reduce mice mortality as compared with a combined protein and calorie restriction, which induced the largest survival in animals (50). However, the suppression of immune disease may be a more important cause of reduced mortality than any alteration in kidney metabolism or physiology in this experiment. Because in patients reducing energy intake to a level that may induce malnutrition is not considered appropriate or justifiable, the relevance of these energy intake–reducing studies to clinical medical care may be quite limited.

Studies have addressed the potential role of endothelin (ET) as a cause of puromycin-induced glomerulosclerosis. In addition, ET-1 gene expression has been reported to be elevated in other renal mass reduction experiments. Nakamura et al. reported that a 6% protein diet, as compared with a 22% protein diet, was able to reverse proteinuria and increase ET-receptor messenger RNA (mRNA), ET-1 mRNA, and protein in puromycin-induced glomerulosclerosis (51). Whether this improvement occurs through a reduction in factors that stimulate ET release (e.g., transforming growth factor-β [TGF-β] and tumor necrosis factor-α) has not been proved directly in this experiment but represents a possibility (52).

More recent studies have addressed the potential renal antifibrotic effect of an LPD. Nakayama et al. reported that in adriamycin-treated rats, expression of fibronectin and TGF-β in the kidney was reduced dramatically when animals received a 6% protein diet as compared with their littermates receiving a regular 20% protein diet (53). In addition, these investigators showed a posttranscriptional reduction in fibronectin synthesis after short-term (2 weeks) treatment with an LPD, whereas there was no difference in fibronectin gene expression. These interesting observations bear similarities to the effects of energy and protein intakes on the transcriptional and posttranscriptional regulation of IGF-1 synthesis in liver cells (54,55).

TGF-β, a potent profibrotic agent, has been reported to be decreased by intervention with LPDs. Peters et al. documented two sets of findings in this regard. First, L-arginine supplement augmented the propensity of an LPD (6%) to reduce the glomerular expression of TGF-β, fibronectin, and plasmin activator inhibitor 1 (PAI-1) in a model of immune glomerulonephritis (56), independent of NO metabolism. Second, whereas maximal angiotensin II (AII) blockade by very high doses of either angiotensin converting enzyme (ACE) or AII antagonists resulted in only a 45% decrease in TGF-β gene expression and protein production, the addition of an LPD to other well-established nephroprotective treatments resulted in a further 20% reduction in TGF-β expression and production, and this was associated with a similar decrease in fibronectin and PAI-1 (57). It should be emphasized that in both experiments, the control of profibrotic mediators was associated with a concomitant decrease in proteinuria. These findings provide good evidence that an LPD possesses its own therapeutic actions, independent from ACEI or AII antagonists, on renal scarring. Whether these antifibrotic properties will persist in chronic renal disease is unknown but certainly deserves further research.

It should be emphasized that the effects of an LPD in reducing proteinuria may affect tubular atrophy and apoptosis (58). Indeed, there is a toxic role of serum albumin on tubular cells in culture (59,60). Recently, two sets of experiments have highlighted the role of protein delivery to the tubule in increasing interstitial fibrosis (61) and tubule cell apoptosis (62). Indeed, the dramatic increase in proteinuria following intraperitoneal bovine serum albumin is associated with a profound tubular apoptotic reaction. Thus, because most experiments have shown that reducing protein intake is associated with a reduction in proteinuria (63), it is possible but not proven that a low-protein intake also reduces renal apoptosis.

In summary, there is a large set of evidence from experimental research indicating that high protein loads are hazardous to the kidney and that a large number of the physiopathologic changes that occur secondary to reduced functioning renal mass or renal insufficiency are corrected or, at most, improved by diets low in protein. However, these experiments use the extreme ends of dietary protein content to identify these histologic and hemodynamic changes. For example, Neugarten et al. reported that the renal injury and proteinuria of puromycin-treated rats improved with a diet providing 4% protein, as compared with a group of rats receiving a 50% protein diet (64). How do these extremely different protein diets compare with clinical studies? How would humans respond to LPDs? What is the evidence for the nutritional safety of LPDs? Could it be possible to adhere to such diets for long periods? How would one monitor compliance? These questions will be addressed in the following section.

PROTEIN INTAKE AND CHRONIC RENAL INSUFFICIENCY: CLINICAL STUDIES

Protein Requirements in Normal Individuals

In the United States, the daily average protein intake is about 90 to 110 g in adult men and 65 to 70 g in adult women (U.S. Department of Agriculture, 1983); in most European countries it is 1.3 g/kg. Protein intake tends to diminish by 15% by the age of 70 (28,65). In women, the mean protein intake is 30% to 50% lower than in men for the same age (66) and is in accord with their 40% lower muscle mass as compared with men (67). Thus, based on the Food and Agriculture Organization of the United Nations recommendations, most adults in occidental countries have protein intakes far above the recommended allowance, which currently is 0.75 g/kg/day (68). Furthermore, it should be emphasized that the 0.75 g/kg body weight value is defined as the safety level, including two standard deviations above the average requirement obtained through individual metabolic balances, thus guaranteeing that at least 97.5% of subjects will attain neutral or positive nitrogen balance (68). Fortunately, as a result of the gaussian distribution of protein requirements, many normal individuals will be in neutral protein balance with a lower level of protein intake. This fact partly may explain why in patients undergoing maintenance dialysis some individuals present with normalized protein equivalent of total nitrogen appearance (nPNA) lower than recommended and show little or no signs of protein malnutrition.

In patients with CRF, from the perspective of the nutritional needs to maintain healthy body composition, there is no need to increase or decrease these recommended dietary protein levels. Indeed, in stable adult patients, most nitrogen-balance and protein-turnover studies have confirmed these data (see later in this chapter). In addition, it should be noted that during the progression of renal insufficiency, spontaneous alterations in nutrient intake frequently occur, generally in the form of a reduction in energy and protein intake (69–71). Indeed, in a 2001 National Health and Nutrition Examination Survey survey, it was reported that in patients with an estimated GFR between 30 and 60 mL/min, spontaneous energy and protein intakes were 23.3 $\pm$ 0.7(SEM) kcal/kg/day and 0.91 $\pm$ 0.03 g protein/kg/day, and in patients with a GFR less than 30 mL/min the values were 20.9 $\pm$ 1.0 kcal/kg/day and 0.86 $\pm$ 0.03 g protein/kg/day (72). These findings are of particular clinical importance because when there is a deficient energy intake, the body cannot adjust as readily to a reduction in protein intake. Thus, in the absence of a dietary control and care plan, patients with chronic renal disease will do worse nutritionally than if they were enrolled in a diet of optimal moderately low protein and adequate energy intake (71,72).

Metabolic Effects of Low-Protein Diets in Humans

Effects of the Nature of Protein

Kontessis et al. examined the effects of protein of different sources on glomerular dynamics in 17 healthy volunteers (73). Although diets were not heavily restricted (intakes averaged about 1 g/kg body weight [BW]/day), a decrease in GFR (−10%), in urinary albumin excretion (−50%), and immunoglobulin G (IgG) clearance (−35%) was observed after 3 weeks of ingesting a vegetable protein as compared to a regular animal protein diet (73). In another study of similar design, these investigators measured GFR in nine diabetic patients without severe renal involvement (74). Again, there was a 15% and 40% decrease in GFR and in microalbuminuria, respectively, with the vegetable protein as compared with the animal protein diet. Interestingly, a marked decrease (−20%) in serum IGF-1, a strong GFR regulatory hormone, also was observed with the vegetarian protein diet, thus suggesting that protein intake might regulate renal hemodynamics, at least in part, through IGF-1 levels.

In 12 proteinuric patients with CRF, Rosenberg et al. examined, in a random crossover design, the effects of a marked reduction in protein intake from 2 to 0.55 g protein/kg/day for 11 days (75). There was a 35% decrease in proteinuria from 7.0 ± 3 to 4.7 ± 2 g/day and an improved glomerular permselectivity as determined by dextran clearances and from a disproportionate reduction in IgG as compared to albumin clearance; whereas there was no change in GFR and renal plasma flow (75), a net decrease in plasma renin activity and plasma aldosterone also was noted during the low-protein period, confirming experimental data.

Metabolic Adaptation to a Reduction in Protein Intake

Figure 16.3 shows the metabolic adaptation that occurs when an *ad libitum* protein diet (1.1 g/kg/day) is changed to a more limited protein intake (0.7 g/kg/day) in 12 patients with moderate chronic renal insufficiency without the nephrotic syndrome (76). Using a whole-body amino acid tracer (i.e., ^{13}C-leucine), the investigators reported a net decrease in leucine oxidation, which is considered to reflect the excess amino acid catabolism; these findings suggest a normal adaptation in protein metabolism, similar to that reported in healthy volunteers (77). There was no change in patients' body weight, serum albumin, or IGF-1 after the 3 months of this reduced protein intake, confirming the safety of this level of protein intake (0.7 g/kg/day) in CRF (76). Other studies have reported similar findings in patients with CRF undergoing different types of diet intervention but mostly with shorter studies. Goodship et al. studied six patients with moderate CRF during a short-term (1 week) regular (1 g protein/kg/d) or reduced (0.6 g protein/kg/d) protein intake and with energy intakes of 32.5 kcal/kg/day (78). Fasting leucine oxidation did not change significantly with the low-protein intake, whereas postprandial leucine oxidation decreased by about 25% ($p < 0.05$). As in nephrotic patients without CRF (79), these data show that patients with mild renal insufficiency can adapt their protein metabolism during acute or chronic reductions in protein intake by reducing amino acid oxidation during both the postprandial and the fasting state.

More restricted protein intakes have been shown to reduce amino acid oxidation by a greater magnitude. Masud et al. reported in six predialysis patients that a diet providing 0.35

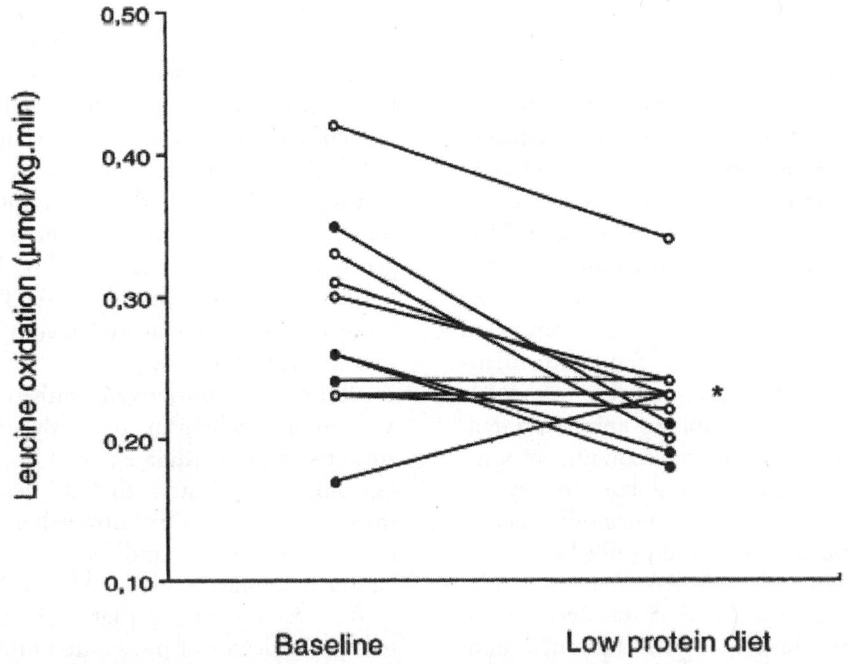

FIGURE 16.3. Total body leucine oxidation, a marker of protein metabolism, before and after ingestion of a low-protein diet (LPD) for 3 months in 12 patients with moderate chronic renal failure (1.1 g protein/kg/day in baseline versus 0.7 g/kg/day in LPD). The data demonstrate an adequate adaptation to a reduced protein intake (*$p < 0.05$ from baseline). (From Bernhard J, Beaufrere B, Laville M, et al. Adaptive response to a low-protein diet in predialysis chronic renal failure patients. *J Am Soc Nephrol* 2001;12:1249–1254, with permission.)

g protein/kg/day supplemented with either ketoacids or essential amino acids for 25 days maintained neutral nitrogen balance and body composition (80). These diets were associated with very low leucine oxidation rates, which were not different whether patients were supplemented with ketoanalogues or essential amino acids (80). In a long-term follow-up of these patients (16 months), the fasting leucine oxidation rate remained at the low level of 10.0 ± 2.2 μmol/kg/h (81). In response to a lower protein intake, these values for amino acid oxidation appear to be more reduced than was observed in studies with less restricted protein intakes (76, 78), suggesting a potential "functional reserve" for protein sparing in patients with CRF.

Maroni et al. studied patients presenting with heavy proteinuria (e.g., greater than 6 g/day) and moderate CRF (GFR: about 50 mL/min/1.73 m^2). Using leucine-turnover and nitrogen-balance techniques, they showed that a reduction from 1.85 to 1.00 g protein/kg/day in the patients induced adaptive protein-conserving mechanisms that were similar to those of healthy volunteers and that the patients sustained positive nitrogen balance (82). These results have been confirmed by Giordano et al., who showed that in seven patients with heavy proteinuria who underwent a reduction in protein intake from 1.20 to 0.66 g/kg/day for 1 month, their endogenous leucine flux decreased by 8% ($p < 0.05$), hepatic albumin synthesis decreased from 18.2 to 14.9 g/1.73 m^2 ($p < 0.03$), and serum albumin rose from 2.88 to 3.06 g/dL ($p < 0.03$) (79).

Other Metabolic Consequences of Reduced Protein Intakes

A reduction in protein intake induces a number of changes in the intake of many foods, and this may modify intakes of many dietary nutrients. It is of particular importance to ensure that the patient will not simply reduce intakes of all nutrients in addition to protein. A number of studies reported a dramatic decrease in energy intake when an LPD was prescribed (83,84). This finding has been used by critics to advise against such dietary interventions. Because these pitfalls are now well identified, LPDs can be administered safely under the adequate supervision of trained dietitians (85). Another consequence of reducing protein in the diet is the increase in the ratio of vegetable to animal protein. This may lead to a reduction in the total amount of saturated fat and cholesterol ingested. A reduction of protein intake from 1.11 to 0.71 g/kg/day in 12 normolipemic patients with mild CRF improved the lipid profile by increasing the Apo A1 lipoprotein and the Apo A1/B ratio, despite an increase in dietary carbohydrates that was necessary to maintain a sufficient energy intake (86). In addition, alcohol consumption (perhaps most beneficially from red wine origin) may be recommended in modest amounts (e.g., one drink per day) because of the numerous epidemiologic studies in the general population that indicate cardiovascular benefits from a regular intake of small quantities of alcoholic beverages (87,88).

Abnormal insulin sensitivity and insulin resistance can be improved by an LPD. When eight patients with advanced CRF (GFR: 13.2 ± 2.8(SEM) mL/min/1.73 m^2) were prescribed a very–low-protein intake supplemented by ketoanalogues of amino acids for 3 months, they showed an improvement in fasting serum glucose from 5.0 ± 0.1 to 4.7 ± 0.1 mmol/L ($p < 0.05$), a decrease in fasting plasma insulin from 82.4 ± 20.7 to 48.8 ± 8.0 pmol/L ($p < 0.05$), and a decrease in endogenous glucose production by 66% for comparable plasma insulin levels. These data indicate an improved sensibility to insulin (89).

Effects on Proteinuria

Because proteinuria clearly has been identified as an independent risk factor for progression of renal failure, it is relevant to examine the specific effects of LPDs on proteinuria. As discussed earlier, experimental studies almost unanimously report a reduction in proteinuria when animals are placed on an LPD. In humans, the acute 35% reduction in proteinuria observed by Rosenberg et al. (75) was confirmed during dietary therapy by Aparicio et al. (63). These investigators reported a decrease in proteinuria from 3.2 ± 1.2 to 1.8 ± 1.1 g/day ($p < 0.01$) in 15 patients with advanced chronic renal insufficiency after 6 months of a very–low-protein intake (0.3 g/kg/day) supplemented with ketoacids, whereas serum albumin increased concomitantly from 36.5 ± 4.0 to 40.8 ± 3.2 ($p < 0.01$) (Fig. 16.4) (63).

When Giordano et al. (79) changed from a 1.2 g protein/kg/day to a 0.66 g protein/kg/day protein diet in seven patients with the nephrotic syndrome, proteinuria decreased by 38%, and there was a linear relationship between the reduction in proteinuria and the achieved reduction in protein intake, as has been noted previously by Kaysen (90). It was proposed that a decrease in proteinuria is a stimulus for a reduction in albumin synthesis. Furthermore, fibrinogen synthesis rate also decreased by 30% with LPDs, from 4.6 to 3.0 g/1.73 m^2/day ($p < 0.03$); these synthesis rates, however, still were increased as compared with healthy volunteers (1.93 g/1.73 m^2/day) (79). The similar reductions in albumin and fibrinogen syntheses may be triggered by a common mechanism, presently unknown, but which is advantageously modulated by a low-protein intake. Thus, not only do patients with CRF generally adapt to LPDs; there also seems to be further benefits of such LPDs by reducing proteinuria and its consequent metabolic disturbances in nephrotic states.

It is well established that ACE inhibitors can markedly reduce the degree of proteinuria in most renal diseases. Of interest is the additional antiproteinuric effect of an LPD in combination with ACE inhibitors. This observation first was described by Ruilope et al. in a short-term study involving 17 patients with mild CRF (91). Enalapril, 20 mg/day,

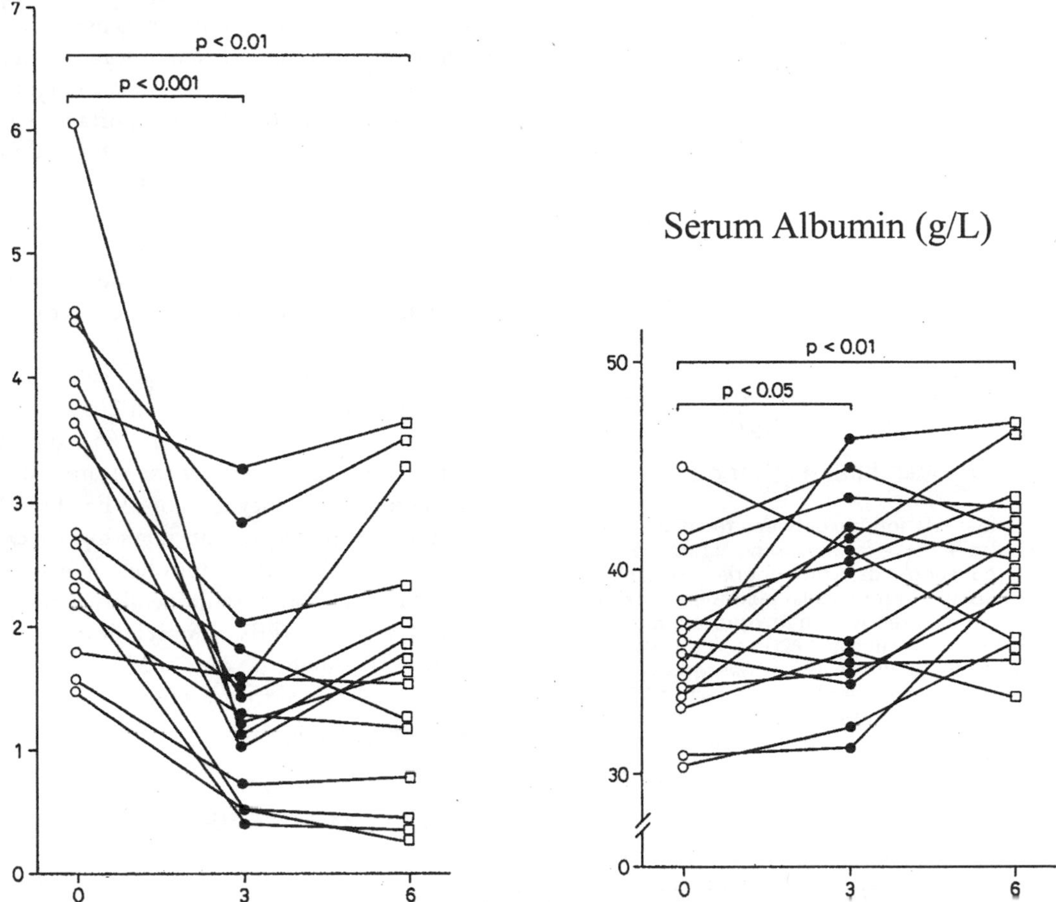

FIGURE 16.4. The decrease in proteinuria (*left panel,* g/day) and the increase in serum albumin (*right panel,* g/L) during 3 and 6 months of treatment with a very–low-protein diet (0.3 g/kg/day) in 15 patients with advanced chronic renal failure. (From Thomas ME, Brunskill NJ, Harris KPG, et al. Proteinuria induces tubular cell turnover: a potential mechanism for tubular atrophy. *Kidney Int* 1999;55:890–898, with permission.)

reduced proteinuria by about 20%; a 25% reduction in protein intake from 1 g/kg/day (estimated from urinary urea output) decreased proteinuria by 30%. However, the combination of both interventions induced a 55% decrease in proteinuria; this latter reduction in proteinuria was significantly greater than each separate intervention (91). These findings were confirmed by Gansevoort et al. (92), who studied in a crossover design 14 patients with modest renal impairment and nephrotic-range proteinuria. Enalapril, 10 mg/day, induced a reduction of proteinuria by 35%, whereas a 50% reduction in protein intake decreased proteinuria by 20%. Again, there was an additional effect of both treatments, with a 55% to 60% decrease in proteinuria by enalapril and low-protein intake. Furthermore, as shown in Fig. 16.5, there was a linear relation between the reduction in both protein intake and proteinuria (92).

The question of whether LPDs are safe has been a subject of some controversy (93) and has been examined by estimating the nutritional status and survival of patients who received reduced protein intakes for years. Chauveau et al. (94) reported regional body composition measured by dual-energy x-ray absorptiometry (DEXA) and nutritional status in 10 patients receiving a very–low-protein diet (LPD) (0.3 g protein/kg/day supplemented with amino acids and ketoanalogues) for 1 year. There was no change in anthropometric measures and serum biochemistry during the 1-year follow-up (94). DEXA analyses revealed a decrease in lean body mass during the first 3 months following the reduction in protein intake that was not fully corrected to baseline at 1 year (baseline: 46.2 kg; 1 year: 45.1 kg). Body fat mass increased slightly at three months and one year (baseline: 20.1 kg; 1 year: 21.4 kg, $p < 0.01$). It is interesting that

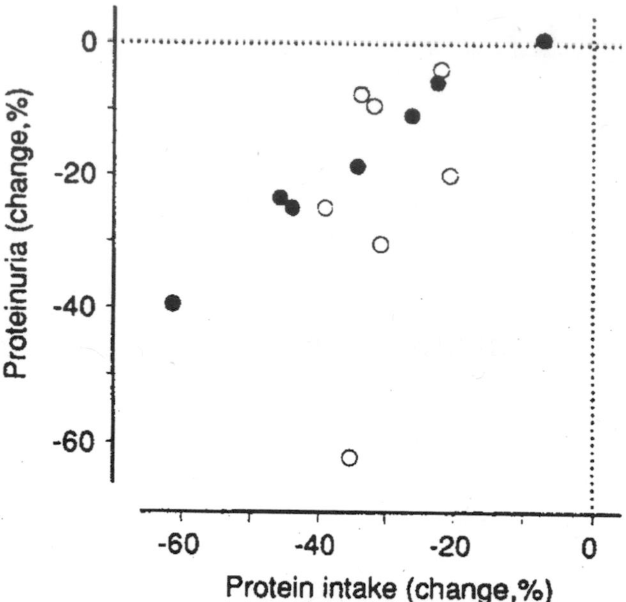

FIGURE 16.5. The linear relationship between the degree of reduction in dietary protein intake from baseline (1.0 to 1.5 g protein/kg/day) and the reduction in daily proteinuria in 14 nephrotic patients with normal to mild chronic renal failure ($r = 0.58$, $p < 0.05$). *Closed circles*, patients receiving a low-protein diet (LPD) only; *open circles*, patients receiving an LPD in addition to angiotensin converting enzyme inhibitors. (From Gansevoort RT, de Zeeuw D, de Jong PE. Additive antiproteinuric effect of ACE inhibition and a low-protein diet in human renal disease. *Nephrol Dial Transplant* 1995;10:497–504, with permission.)

there seemed to be a redistribution of lean body mass in favor of an increase in lean truncal mass that was sustained during the 1 year of follow-up (94). It should be mentioned that during this trial, energy intake was 27.8 ± 7.6 at baseline, 31.0 ± 8.1 at 3 months, and 29.8 ± 8.8 kcal/kg/day at 1 year. Thus, the alterations observed after 3 months of a very–low-protein intake spontaneously improved over time, became of no clinical importance after 1 year of follow-up, and occurred in association with the benefits observed with regard to improved insulin resistance and bone metabolism and reduction in uremic symptoms (94). Long-term low-protein interventions also have been reported to be safe by other investigators (95–98). In the MDRD study, body weight and composition were assessed every 3 months during the 2.2-year mean follow-up period (98). The actual reductions in protein intake were less than expected (actual versus prescribed: 0.71 versus 0.58 and 1.11 versus 1.3 g/kg BW/day, respectively, in Study A; 0.48 versus 0.28 and 0.72 versus 0.58 g/kg BW/day, respectively, in Study B). Furthermore, energy intake was low despite intensive counseling (range: 22.5 to 26.7 kcal/kg/day among different subgroups). Despite these values, overall clinical and biologic surveys, as well as endpoint recording, did not show evidence for protein–energy malnutrition during a follow-up period of 2 to 3 years (98). Figure 16.6 shows that serum albumin levels increased slightly in all groups from baseline, but this increase was greater in the LPD group as compared with the control group in Study A (Figure 16.6, top, solid line). The decrease in serum transferrin during the study is somewhat difficult to interpret because iron stores and the presence of inflammation were not monitored. Finally, although statistically significant, these changes in body composition may not be of clinical importance (−2 to 0 kg for body weight and −0.5 to +0.5% for body fat mass over 3 years). They underscore the importance for the physician to ensure that there is adequate nutritional monitoring and, where indicated, nutritional intervention in these patients (Table 16.1). It is important to note that no patient had to withdraw from the MDRD study because of impaired nutritional status.

What is the long-term consequence of LPDs on survival after dialysis therapy is started? In 2000 Aparicio et al. reported encouraging outcomes in 165 patients undergoing maintenance dialysis who were treated with very–low-protein diets before they developed ESRD (99). Walser et al. demonstrated that patients ingesting a very–low-protein diet who were followed carefully before they commenced dialysis treatments could postpone dialysis for many months, even with very low GFRs, before clinical symptoms occurred (100,101). It should be cautioned, however, that patients were not randomized to assess the effects of the LPDs in any of these foregoing studies.

LONG-TERM LOW-PROTEIN DIET CLINICAL TRIALS

For many years, it has been proposed that patients with advanced renal failure should reduce their protein intake to decrease uremic symptoms. In the mid-1970s, because a number of experimental studies reported beneficial effects of low-protein intakes on renal function, it was proposed to test this hypothesis in humans. Before analyzing in detail these studies, some general remarks should be made. First, as discussed earlier, most animal research studies were performed using extremely high or low levels of dietary protein (e.g., unphysiologic or very large differences in dietary protein content between groups) to identify mechanisms and explain therapeutic effects. Second, in many experiments, substantial numbers of animals died without analysis of the potential role of the diet in these deaths. Only data from the survivors were analyzed—a fact that would not apply to human research. Third, most laboratory research is short term and is carried out in animals that do not have other chronic diseases; this stands in contrast to the case in many patients with chronic renal disease. Thus, the effects of LPDs in patients with chronic renal insufficiency may differ from the results of experimental studies. Indeed, as compared with experimental research, there are specific caveats to clinical research, such as the variability of outcome, the

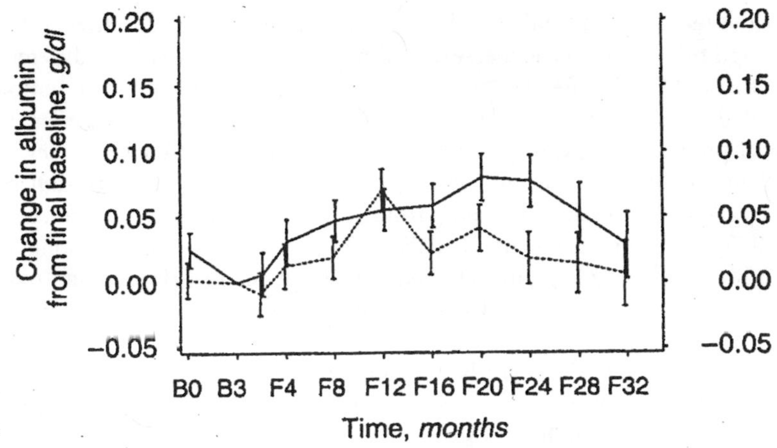

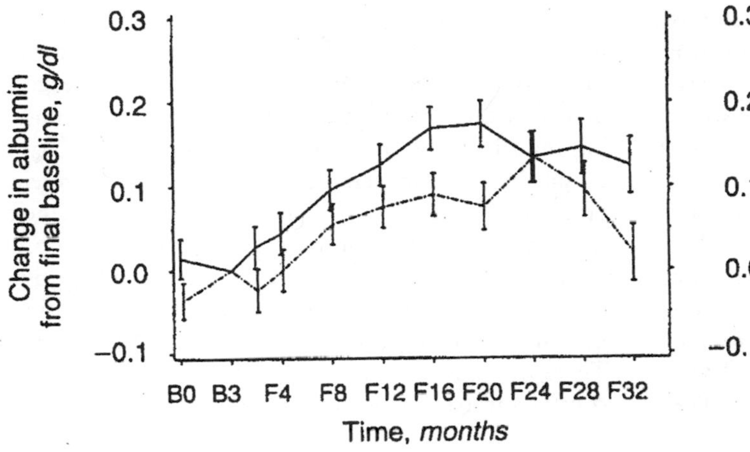

FIGURE 16.6. Mean changes in serum albumin from the end of baseline in Study A (*top*) and Study B (*bottom*) patients during the course of the Modification of Diet in Renal Disease Study. (From Kopple JD, Levey AS, Greene T, et al. Effect of dietary protein restriction on nutritional status in the Modification of Diet in Renal Disease Study. *Kidney Int* 1997;52: 778–791, with permission.)

issue of treatment compliance and medication effects, and (eventually) the phenotype of the population studied. These factors are one of the reasons why such large numbers of patients are required to test a single hypothesis in a clinical trial.

More than 50 trials have assessed the effects of LPDs in humans with renal disease. These studies have been reviewed by Fouque et al. (19). However, in many of these trials, the methodologic quality was judged to be poor based on uncontrolled design, nonrandom allocation of diets, or the use of retrospective analyses. Furthermore, many of these reports, undertaken in the early 1970s, did not use an adequate marker of renal function to assess the effect of the diet intervention, particularly because the serum creatinine or its derivatives (creatinine clearance, 1/serum creatinine) are influenced strongly by the primary intervention (e.g., reducing protein intake; see earlier). Because contradictory results often were reported, we will review only the largest trials of high methodologic quality (i.e., those large prospective, controlled trials with a random allocation of diet intervention).

The study of Rosman et al. reported the effects of two different levels of protein restriction in 247 patients followed for 2 to 4 years (102,103). Protein intake was reduced to 0.6 g/kg/day in patients with a GFR between 60 and 30 mL/min and to 0.4 g/kg/day in those with a GFR between 30 and 10 mL/min (103). Both of the control groups for these two LPD groups were allowed a free protein intake diet. Based on the 1/serum creatinine slope over time, it

TABLE 16.1. ESTIMATION OF DIETARY PROTEIN INTAKE IN A STABLE NONCATABOLIC 70-KG ADULT PATIENT INGESTING A 0.6-G PROTEIN/KG/DAY DIET, BASED ON A DAILY URINARY NITROGEN APPEARANCE

UNA = 4.8 g/day
DPI = 7.25 UNA + 10.9 = 45.7 g/day
DPI/kg = 45.7/70 = 0.65 g/kg

Compliance to the diet (e.g., an upper actual protein intake no greater than 20% over prescribed intake) is considered acceptable if this patient has a UNA no greater than 5.5 g/day.

UNA, urinary nitrogen appearance; DPI, dietary protein intake.
From Kopple JD, Gao XL, Qing DP. Dietary protein, urea nitrogen appearance and total nitrogen appearance in chronic renal failure and CAPD patients. *Kidney Int* 1997;52:486–494, with permission.

was concluded that not all patients benefited from the restricted diet: only males appeared to respond with significant slowing, and patients with polycystic kidney disease did not reduce their GFR decline with a restricted diet. Measurements of urinary urea excretion indicated that protein intake only decreased to 30% to 35% lower than the unrestricted diets, which ranged from 0.90 to 0.95 g/kg/day in the moderately impaired group and from 0.70 to 0.80 g/kg/day in the more advanced CRF group. Whereas no difference in survival was observed in the group with mild CRF, in the group with more advanced CRF there was a marked improvement in survival in the patients treated with protein restriction after 4 years of follow-up (percent survival off-dialysis, 60% versus 30%, $p < 0.025$) (103). The authors concluded that such dietary intervention would be more beneficial in some subgroups of patients whose CRF rapidly progresses, such as males, and patients with glomerulonephritis. They also noted that compliance was very good after a short period of training and was sustained over time and that protein restriction did not cause malnutrition (103).

The second large-scale randomized study was performed in Australia and published in 1989 (96). Ihle et al. studied 72 patients with advanced renal failure for 18 months. Patients were randomized to receive either a control diet or a diet providing 0.4 g protein/kg/day (LPD). The actual protein intakes, estimated from urinary urea output, was approximately 0.8 and 0.6 g/kg/day, respectively. GFR was measured every 6 months by ^{51}Cr-EDTA clearances. The GFR decreased only in the control group (15 to 6 mL/min over 18 months, $p < 0.01$), whereas no decrease occurred in the LPD group. The number of patients who started dialysis during the trial was significantly greater in the control group ($p < 0.05$). Body composition varied somewhat, with a significant loss of body weight only in the LPD group, whereas there was no change in other anthropometric measures or in serum albumin in either group. There was no dietary analysis of intakes, so that an insufficient energy intake could not be ruled out to explain the loss of weight with the LPD. The authors concluded that there was a beneficial effect of this moderately reduced protein intake ($p < 0.01$) (96).

Two years later, Williams et al. published the effects of three different nutritional interventions in 95 patients with advanced renal insufficiency (97). After a 6-month run-in period, patients were randomized to receive, for about 18 months, a 0.6 g protein/kg/day and 800 mg phosphate intake, a diet providing 1,000 mg phosphate/day plus phosphate binders and without specific protein restriction, or a protein- and phosphate-unrestricted diet. Dietary compliance was estimated by urinary urea output and dietary recalls and averaged 0.7, 1.02, and 1.14 g protein/kg/day and 815, 1,000, and 1,400 mg phosphorus/day, respectively. Slight weight losses were observed in the protein- and phosphorus-restricted groups (-1.3 and -1.65 kg BW for the LPD and low-phosphate group, respectively). Other anthropometric measures did not change. There was no difference in the decrease in creatinine clearance over time among any of the three groups. However, as discussed earlier, the creatinine clearance is of questionable accuracy as a measure of GFR, and thus no conclusion on renal protection can be drawn reliably from this study (97). Death or the commencement of dialysis therapy did not differ among the three groups (18 individuals on the low-protein and phosphate diet, 18 on the low-phosphate diet, and 16 in the control group).

The Northern Italian Cooperative Study Group, in 1991, reported the results of a large randomized controlled study in 456 patients with a GFR lower than 60 mL/min, who were followed for 2 years (104). Patients either received a control protein intake of 1 g/kg/day or a low-protein intake providing 0.6 g/kg/day; both diets provided an energy intake of at least 30 kcal/kg/day. The main outcome criterion was the renal survival defined as the commencement of dialysis therapy or the doubling of serum creatinine during the trial. DPI was serially monitored by urinary urea output in a random sample of patients. Actual protein intakes were, however, only slightly different because the control group ate 0.90 g protein/kg/day and the low-protein group ingested 0.78 g/kg/day, and there was a large overlap between individuals from the two groups (underlining the necessity for intensive dietary counseling and monitoring). There was only a borderline significant difference between control and restricted protein groups with slightly less patients in the latter group reaching a renal endpoint ($p = 0.059$).

A randomized trial in France, reported in 1999 by Malvy et al., examined the effects of more severe protein restriction (0.3 g protein/kg/day) supplemented with ketoanalogues (Ketosteril®, 0.17 g/kg BW/day) versus 0.65 g protein/kg/day in 50 patients with severe renal insufficiency (creatinine clearance lower than 20 mL/min) (95). Patients were followed until dialysis or until the creatinine clearance decreased under 5 mL/min/1.73 m^2. Kaplan-Meier survival analysis did not show differences in renal survival between the two diets, but the modest size of the study or the reduced protein intake of the control group may explain this result. There was a loss of 2.7 kg BW in the very–low-protein diet over 3 years that was derived equally from losses of fat and lean body mass. No weight loss or body composition change was observed in the groups prescribed the 0.65 g protein/kg diet. Serum calcium was maintained better in the very low supplemented diet as a result of the calcium salt content of the ketoanalogue supplement. This study does not clearly identify the respective effect of each intervention (i.e., a low [0.65 g protein/kg/day] versus a very low supplemented protein intake [0.3 g protein/kg/day]) because all patients had a baseline protein intake of 1.0 g protein/kg/day before starting the study and because no unrestricted protein group was studied for comparison (95). For those patients presenting with a severe renal failure at inclusion (GFR of about 15 mL/min/1.73 m^2), the "half-life" for renal death was 9 months in the 0.65 g protein/kg/day as compared to 21 months in the most restricted diet (0.3 g protein/kg/day), which still represents a clinical difference for the patients.

The MDRD study is the largest clinical study yet performed to test the effects of low-protein intake and strict blood pressure control on the progression of renal disease in more than 800 patients (1,13,69,105–118). Two groups of patients were studied, one with moderate renal dysfunction (Study A, GFR: 25 to 55 mL/min/1.73 m^2) and the second with a more advanced renal dysfunction (Study B, GFR: 13 to 24 mL/min/1.73 m^2). The patients were randomized to receive 1 g protein/kg/day or more versus 0.6 g/kg/day and to reach a mean blood pressure of 105 or 92 mmHg in group A and 0.6 g protein/kg/day versus 0.3 g/kg/day plus a ketoacid supplement and comparable blood pressure goals in group B. The primary objective was the effect of both interventions, in a latin square design and intention-to-treat analysis, on the progression of renal failure. This was estimated by the changes in ^{125}I-iothalamate clearance measured every 4 months over more than 2 years. The mean patient follow-up was 2.2 years (108). Actual protein intakes were 1.11 ± 0.19 versus 0.73 ± 0.15 g protein/kg/day in group A (n = 585) and 0.69 ± 0.12 versus 0.46 ± 0.15 g protein/kg/day in group B (n = 255). The overall results appeared somewhat disappointing at first glance. There was no difference between the groups with regard to the decline in GFR in Study A. In Study B, there was a borderline significantly greater rate of decline in GFR in the group prescribed the 0.6 g protein/kg/day diet versus the ketoacid-supplemented diet (p = 0.07).

These raw results require several comments. First, as shown in Fig. 16.7, during the first 4 months of diet intervention in Study A, there was a sharp initial decrease in GFR in the group with the more restricted protein intake (mean DPI, 0.73 g/kg/day). This was followed by a slower linear decrease than occurred with the larger protein intake (mean DPI, 1.11 g/kg/day). This initial 4-month decrease in GFR with the lower DPI now is considered to be the result of the well-described reduction in glomerular hemodynamics that follow protein restriction (28). Arguably, in retrospect, there should have been a run-in period that included the first several weeks of dietary protein treatment before the key GFR outcome data began to be collected. If this had been done, then the follow-up period of the study (e.g., from 4 months after the start until 3 years), the slope of GFR decrease, which was significantly lower in the more restricted protein group (Fig. 16.7, p = 0.009) (118), would have indicated a beneficial effect of dietary protein restriction in reducing the rate of decrease in GFR. Second, unexpectedly, the actual rate of progression of renal failure was lower than expected when the study was designed (i.e., in Study A, the reduction in GFR was 3.8 versus 6 mL/min/year) (105). This had a major negative impact on the ability of this study to demonstrate statistical differences. An

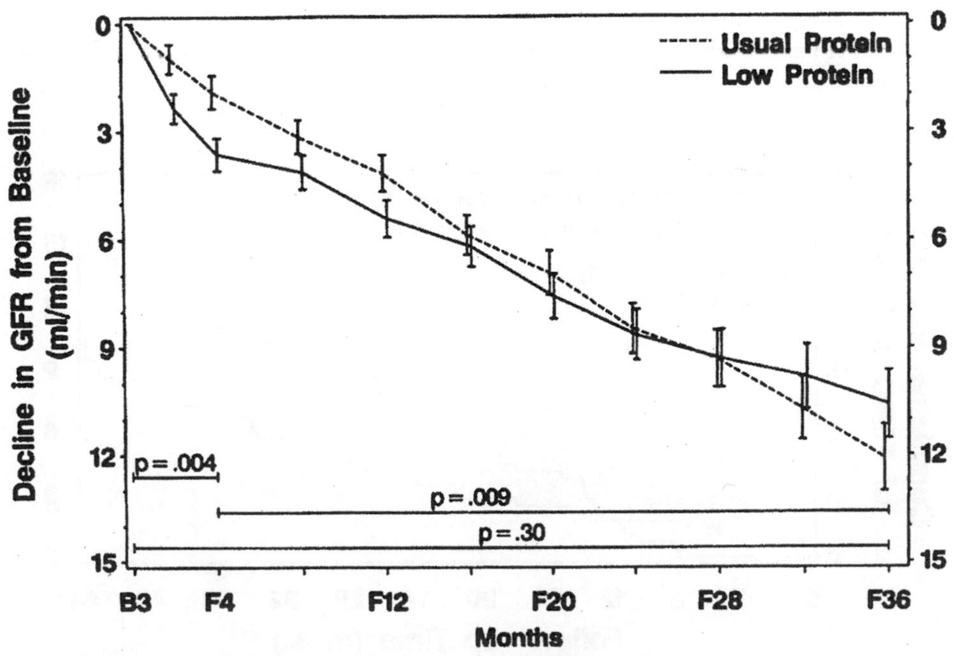

FIGURE 16.7. The glomerular filtration rate decline during the course of the Modification of Diet in Renal Disease Study (Study A) with separate analyses including and not including the first 4-month adaptation period. (From Levey AS, Greene T, Beck GJ, et al. Dietary protein restriction and the progression of chronic renal disease: what have all the results of the MDRD study shown? *J Am Soc Nephrol* 1999;10:2426–2439, with permission.)

additional 3-month period of follow-up would have been necessary to correct for this reduction in GFR decline. Thus, it is tempting to classify this large clinical trial as inconclusive rather than negative. In addition, when patients were followed in an open fashion after the end of the study and up to 44 months of diet, the difference in cumulative incidence of ESRD or death reached borderline significance in the patients who were assigned to the lower protein diet ($p = 0.056$, Fig. 16.8). It should be remembered that in the large Diabetes Complications and Control Trial for strict blood glucose control and its effects of renal impairment, no effect was detected at 2 years, and the suppressive effect of strict glucose control on the development of microalbuminuria or proteinuria was observed only after 4 years of treatment (119).

Although not definitive, correlational analyses may give further insights into the efficacy of dietary intervention, particularly when a flawed design, such as an observation period of inadequate duration, hampers interpretation of the main outcome measure. First, when patients were analyzed with regard to their actual protein intake, as estimated through either diet interviews and diaries or urea nitrogen appearance, and independently of the group to which they were randomized, a strong relation was found between the magnitude of protein intake and the GFR slope ($p = 0.011$) or renal death (e.g., risk of death or ESRD) ($p = 0.001$) (118). Indeed, for Study B, a regression model estimated that for every reduction in 0.2 g protein/kg/day, there was a 1.15 mL/min/year reduction in GFR decline and a 49% reduction in the incidence of renal death (118). There was no additional effect of ketoanalogue supplements on retardation of progression of renal failure. This finding contradicts a previous observation made in the MDRD Feasibility Study in which a trend for a protective effect ($p = 0.06$) of ketoacids was observed (116). These latter authors suggested that the different ketoanalogue composition used in the MDRD Study B, and particularly the greater tryptophan content, may account for the lack of effectiveness of the ketoacids in the MDRD study (116,120).

A comparable analysis in Study A showed a more moderate impact of protein restriction with a 0.32 mL/min/year slower GFR decline per each 0.2 g protein/kg/day reduction ($p = 0.075$). Thus, these secondary analyses of the MDRD study support a moderate beneficial effect of reduced protein intakes in patients with CRF; these effects were related, in a gradient fashion, to a reduction in the protein intake rather than to a well-identified degree of protein restriction that was necessary to slow progression. There was no apparent effect of either protein intake or blood pressure control in patients with polycystic kidney disease. Because these individuals constituted 25% of the total patients in the MDRD study, this fact also contributed to the ambiguous results (110).

LEVEL OF EVIDENCE IN CLINICAL TRIALS

Metaanalysis is a comprehensive method aimed at searching, selecting, and analyzing appropriately designed clinical trials to increase the number of patients or observations and improve the power of statistical analysis (e.g., by reducing the confidence interval) (2,121,122). To date, metaanalyses are considered to be second in validity of the evidence it provides, immediately behind the evidence provided by large randomized trials (considered to be level one) and equal to small randomized trials (123). Three metaanalyses have

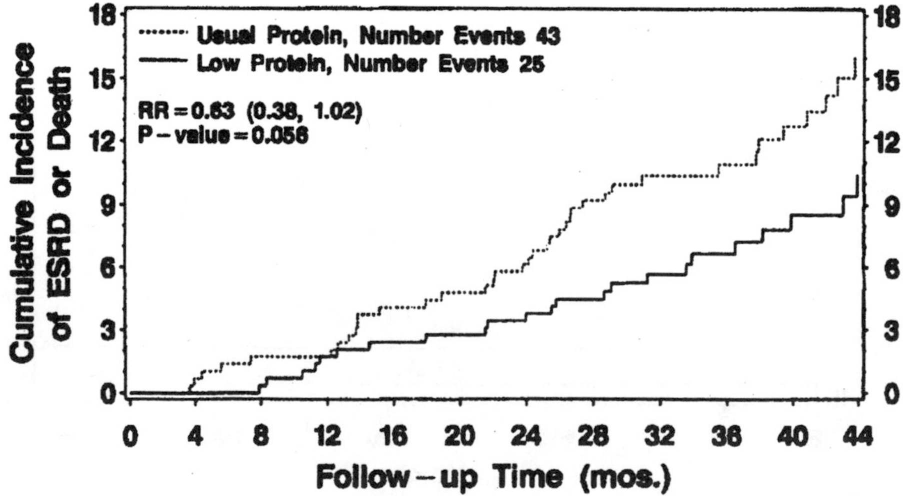

FIGURE 16.8. Occurrence of renal failure or death in Study A of the Modification of Diet in Renal Disease Study, including a 10-month additional follow-up after completion of the study (p = 0.056 between the two levels of protein intake). (From Levey AS, Greene T, Beck GJ, et al. Dietary protein restriction and the progression of chronic renal disease: what have all the results of the MDRD study shown? *J Am Soc Nephrol* 1999;10:2426–2439, with permission.)

been performed on LPDs (2,124,125), of which the first has been updated (19). These reports have searched the literature by different ways to ensure the most exhaustive collection of trials, including international databases in non-English languages. The most rigorous criterion for selecting or rejecting papers for analysis include consideration of randomized controlled trials only, because it generally is believed that nonrandomized controlled trials are more likely to give biased results than their randomized counterparts (125).

Based on this background, we have identified seven randomized controlled trials suitable for analysis among 50 clinical trials assessing the effects of LPDs for the treatment of patients with chronic renal insufficiency (19). Because, as seen earlier, most of these trials did not use an adequate marker of renal failure progression, we decided to define the renal death (e.g., death or the need to start dialysis during the study) as the primary outcome. This criterion was obtained easily by analysis of published papers or by direct contact with investigators in both the control and the restricted dietary protein groups of patients (Fig. 16.9). Gender and the nature of renal disease were distributed equally in control and more restricted groups; thus, those avoiding well-identified independent causes for more rapid progression of renal disease would not influence the results (19). The results are depicted in Fig. 16.9. Individual odds ratios are shown on the top of Fig. 16.9, and the pooled results are on the bottom line. Overall, there were 753 patients in the more restricted protein intake groups and 741 individuals in the higher protein intakes. One hundred and one renal deaths were found in the LPD group versus 141 in the control group, giving an odds ratio for low protein versus control of 0.61, with a 95% confidence interval of 0.46 to 0.83 ($p = 0.006$; Fig. 16.9). This indicates that LPDs may result in a 39% reduction for death or the need to start dialysis therapy as compared with larger or unlimited protein intakes. Pedrini et al. confirmed those findings in six trials, including the MDRD study (124). These authors reported an additional analysis for diabetic nephropathy, using different outcome measures: renal function or albuminuria. Of note is the fact that the average renal function of these patients with diabetes was less reduced, with a mean GFR of 77 mL/min, and the latter trials were of smaller size (n = 8 to 35). The overall results of this latter metaanalysis were also in favor of the LPD, with an odds ratio of 0.56 (CI: 0.40 to 0.77, $p < 0.001$). However, the patients' sample size was 108, a very small number rarely used in the metaanalytic process. Further larger-scale studies in patients with diabetic nephropathy appear necessary to confirm these results.

In a comparable attempt to examine the impact of LPDs on loss of GFR, Kasiske et al. summarized a total of 24 controlled clinical trials, of which 13 were randomized (125). The main outcome was the loss of GFR over time (mL/min/year) in groups receiving or not receiving an LPD. A total of 2,248 patients were collected, from which 1,919 were enrolled in randomized studies. GFR loss was lower by 0.53 mL/min/year (95% CI, 0.08 to 0.98) in the more protein restricted group ($p < 0.05$).

The number needed to treat (NNT) is a recently developed methodologic tool used to compare the efficacy of a given treatment in different studies (126). It theoretically represents the number of patients that must be treated by a given intervention to avoid one extra death per year. From the present metaanalysis data, NNT conferred by a low-protein intervention can be estimated to be comprised between four and 56 depending on the study. This is quite a narrow range and favorably compares with the well-accepted

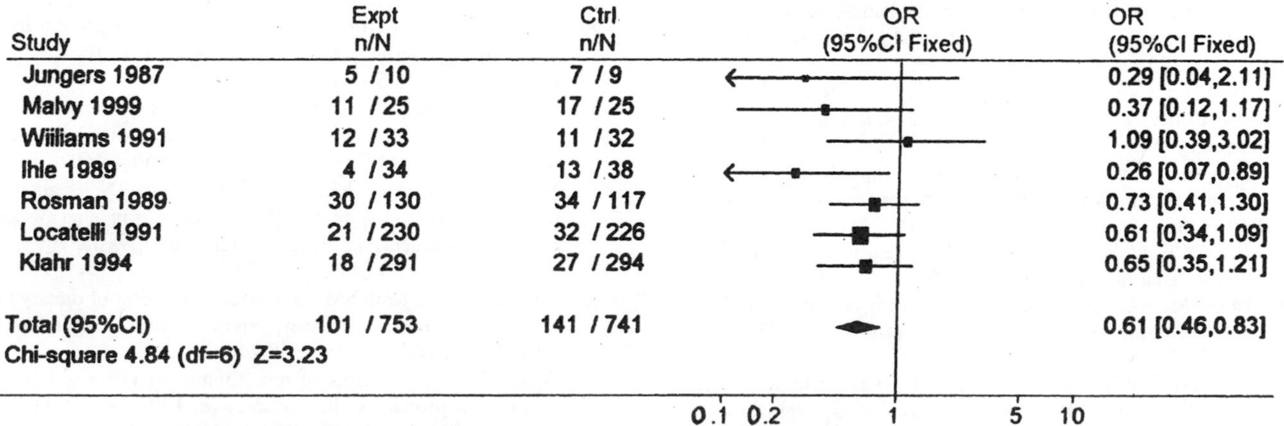

Study | Expt n/N | Ctrl n/N | OR (95%CI Fixed) | OR (95%CI Fixed)
Jungers 1987 | 5 / 10 | 7 / 9 | 0.29 [0.04,2.11]
Malvy 1999 | 11 / 25 | 17 / 25 | 0.37 [0.12,1.17]
Williams 1991 | 12 / 33 | 11 / 32 | 1.09 [0.39,3.02]
Ihle 1989 | 4 / 34 | 13 / 38 | 0.26 [0.07,0.89]
Rosman 1989 | 30 / 130 | 34 / 117 | 0.73 [0.41,1.30]
Locatelli 1991 | 21 / 230 | 32 / 226 | 0.61 [0.34,1.09]
Klahr 1994 | 18 / 291 | 27 / 294 | 0.65 [0.35,1.21]
Total (95%CI) | 101 / 753 | 141 / 741 | 0.61 [0.46,0.83]
Chi-square 4.84 (df=6) Z=3.23
0.1 0.2 1 5 10

FIGURE 16.9. Reduction in the odds of renal death in seven prospective randomized studies of protein restriction in patients with chronic renal insufficiency. A square denotes the odds ratio (treatment/control) for each trial, and the diamond indicates the overall results of the seven trials combined. Horizontal lines represent 95% confidence intervals (CI). Overall "common" odds ratio = 0.61 (95% CI: 0.46, 0.83), $p = 0.006$. (From Fouque D, Wang PH, Laville M, et al. Low protein diets delay end-stage renal disease in non-diabetic adults with chronic renal failure. *Nephrol Dial Transplant* 2000;15:1986–1992, with permission.)

mortality reduction obtained by statins in the 4S (Scandinavian Simvastatin Survival Study) trial (NNT = 30) and WOSCOPS (West of Scotland Coronary Prevention Study) (NNT = 111) (127). This analysis gives further support to the thesis that dietary protein restriction is an effective therapeutic intervention.

CONCLUSION

Many experimental studies provide evidence for the beneficial effects of low-protein intakes. These benefits include reduction in uremic toxicity; healthier nutritional status, particularly if energy intake is well maintained; slowing of the loss of renal function; and delay in the need for renal replacement therapy. Such LPDs, of course, do not prevent the loss of renal function in patients with chronic progressive renal disease. Thus, in patients with CRF, it may be of value to prescribe a reduction in DPI.

REFERENCES

1. Modification of Diet in Renal Disease Study Group. Effects of diet and antihypertensive therapy on creatinine clearance and serum creatinine concentration in the modification of diet in renal disease study. *J Am Soc Nephrol* 1996;7:556–565.
2. Fouque D, Laville M, Boissel JP, et al. Controlled low protein diets in chronic renal insufficiency: meta-analysis. *BMJ* 1992; 304:216–220.
3. Levey AS. Measurement of renal function in chronic renal disease. *Kidney Int* 1990;38:167–184.
4. Edwards OM, Bayliss RIS, Mullen S. Urinary creatinine excretion as an index of the completeness of 24-hour urine collections. *Lancet* 1969;2:1165.
5. Mayersohn M, Conrad KA, Achari R. The influence of a cooked meat meal on creatinine plasma concentration and creatinine clearance. *Br J Clin Pharmacol* 1983;15:227–230.
6. Mitch WE, Walser M. A proposed mechanism for reduced creatinine excretion in severe chronic renal failure. *Nephron* 1978; 21:248–253.
7. Crim MC, Calloway DH, Margen S. Creatine metabolism in men: urinary creatine and creatinine excretions with creatine feeding. *J Nutr* 1975;105:428–438.
8. Shemesh O, Golbetz H, Kriss JP, et al. Limitations of creatinine as a marker in glomerulopathic patients. *Kidney Int* 1985;28: 830–838.
9. Mitch WE, Collier VU, Walser M. Creatinine metabolism in chronic renal failure. *Clin Sci* 1980;58:327–335.
10. Walser M. Assessing renal function from creatinine measurements in adults with chronic renal failure. *Am J Kidney Dis* 1998;32:23–31.
11. Zaltzman JS, Whiteside C, Cattran DC, et al. Accurate measurement of impaired glomerular filtration using single-dose oral cimetidine. *Am J Kidney Dis* 1996;27:504–511.
12. Kemperman FA, Silberbusch J, Slaats EH, et al. Estimation of the glomerular filtration rate in NIDDM patients from plasma creatinine concentration after cimetidine administration. *Diabetes Care* 1998;21:216–220.
13. Modification of Diet in Renal Disease Study Group. The modification of diet in renal disease study (MDRD): Design, methods and results from the feasibility study. *Am J Kidney Dis* 1992; 20:18–33.
14. Levey AS. Assessing the effectiveness of therapy to prevent the progression of renal disease. *Am J Kidney Dis* 1993;22:207–214.
15. Cockcroft DW, Gault MH. Prediction of creatinine clearance from serum creatinine. *Nephron* 1976;16:31–41.
16. Walser M, Drew HH, Guldan JL. Prediction of glomerular filtration rate from serum creatinine concentration in advanced chronic renal failure. *Kidney Int* 1993;44:1145–1148.
17. Levey AS, Bosch JP, Lewis JB, et al. A more accurate method to estimate glomerular filtration rate from serum creatinine: a new prediction equation. Modification of Diet in Renal Disease Study Group. *Ann Intern Med* 1999;130:461–470.
18. Anastasio P, Cirillo M, Spitali L, et al. Level of hydration and renal function in healthy humans. *Kidney Int* 2001;60: 748–756.
19. Fouque D, Wang PH, Laville M, et al. Low protein diets delay end-stage renal disease in non-diabetic adults with chronic renal failure. *Nephrol Dial Transplant* 2000;15:1986–1992.
20. Farr LE, Smadel JE. The effects of dietary protein on the course of nephrotoxic nephritis in rats. *J Exp Med* 1939;70:615–627.
21. Kleinknecht C, Salusky IB, Broyer M, et al. Effects of various protein diets on growth, renal function, and survival of uremic rats. *Kidney Int* 1979;15:534–541.
22. Brenner BM. Nephron adaptation to renal injury or ablation. *Am J Physiol* 1985;249:F324–F337.
23. Hostetter TH. Chronic effects of dietary protein in the rat with intact and reduced renal mass. *Kidney Int* 1986;30:509–517.
24. Mauer SM, Steffes MW, Azar S, et al. Effects of dietary protein content in streptozotocin-diabetic rats. *Kidney Int* 1989;35: 48–59.
25. Nath KA, Krens SM, Hostetter TH. Dietary protein restriction in established renal injury in the rat. *J Clin Invest* 1986; 1199–1205.
26. Premen AJ. Potential mechanisms mediating postprandial hyperemia and hyperfiltration. *Faseb J* 1988;2:131–137.
27. Diamond JR. Effects of dietary interventions on glomerular pathophysiology. *Am J Physiol* 1990;258:F1–F8.
28. King AC, Levey AS. Dietary protein and renal function. *J Am Soc Nephrol* 1993;3:1723–1737.
29. Hirschberg R, Kopple JD. Response of insulin-like growth factor-1 and renal hemodynamics to a high- and low-protein diet in the rat. *J Am Soc Nephrol* 1991;1:1034–1039.
30. Don BR, Blake S, Hutchison FN, et al. Dietary protein intake modulates glomerular eicosanoid production in the rat. *Am J Physiol* 1989;256:F711–F717.
31. Jaffa AA, Vio CP, Silva RH, et al. Evidence for renal kinins as mediators of amino acid-induced hyperperfusion and hyperfiltration in the rat. *J Clin Invest* 1992;89:1460–1469.
32. Martinez-Maldonado M, Benabe JE, Wilcox JN, et al. Renal renin, angiotensinogen, and ANGI-converting enzyme gene expression: influence of dietary protein. *Am J Physiol* 1993;264: F981–F992.
33. Rosenberg ME, Kren SM, Hostetter TH. Effect of dietary protein on rat renin-angiotensin system in subtotally nephrectomized rats. *Kidney Int* 1990;38:240–248.
34. Woods LL. Mechanisms of renal hemodynamic regulation in response to protein feeding. *Kidney Int* 1993;44:659–666.
35. Hostetter TH, Olson HG, Rennke HG, et al. Hyperfiltration in remnant nephrons: a potentially adverse response to renal ablation. *Am J Physiol* 1981;241:F85–F93.
36. El Nahas AM, Paraskevakou H, Zoob S, et al. Effect of dietary protein restriction on the development of renal failure after subtotal nephrectomy in rats. *Clin Sci* 1983;65:399–406.
37. Kenner CH, Evan AP, Blomgren P, et al. Effect of protein intake

on renal function and structure in partially nephrectomized rats. *Kidney Int* 1985;27:739–750.

38. Meyer TW, Anderson S, Rennke HG, et al. Reversing glomerular hypertension stabilizes established glomerular injury. *Kidney Int* 1987;31:752–759.
39. Bankir L, Kriz W. Adaptation of the kidney to protein intake and to urine concentrating activity: similar consequences in health and CRF. *Kidney Int* 1995;47:7–24.
40. Harris DC, Tay C. Altered metabolism in the ex vivo remnant kidney. II. Effects of metabolic inhibitors and dietary protein. *Nephron* 1993;64:417–423.
41. Nath KA, Croatt AJ, Hostetter TH. Oxygen consumption and oxidant stress in surviving nephrons. *Am J Physiol* 1990;258: F1354–F1361.
42. Brezis M, Rosen SN, Epstein FH. The pathophysiological implications of medullary hypoxia. *Am J Kidney Dis* 1989;13: 253–259.
43. Jarusiripipat C, Shapiro JI, Chan L, et al. Reduction of remnant *Nephron* hypermetabolism by protein restriction. *Am J Kidney Dis* 1991;28:367–372.
44. Margetts BM, Beilin LJ, Vandongen R, et al. Vegetarian diet in mild hypertension: a randomised controlled trial. *BMJ* 1986; 293:1468–1471.
45. Wiseman MJ, Hunt R, Goodwin A, et al. Dietary composition and renal function in healthy subjects. *Nephron* 1987;46:37–42.
46. Williams AJ, Baker F, Walls J. Effect of varying quantity and quality of dietary protein intake in experimental renal disease in rats. *Nephron* 1987;46:83–90.
47. Katoh T, Takahashi K, Klahr S, et al. Dietary supplementation with L-arginine ameliorates glomerular hypertension in rats with subtotal nephrectomy. *J Am Soc Nephrol* 1994;4:1690–1694.
48. Tapp DC, Wortham WG, Addison JF, et al. Food restriction retards body growth and prevents end-stage renal pathology in remnant kidneys of rats regardless of protein intake. *Lab Invest* 1989;60:184–191.
49. Kobayaschi K, Venkatachalam MA. Differential effects of calorie restriction on glomeruli and tubules of the remnant kidney. *Kidney Int* 1992;42:710–717.
50. Fernandes G, Yunis EJ, Miranda M, et al. Nutritional inhibition of genetically determined renal disease and autoimmunity with prolongation of life in kd/kd mice. *Proc Natl Acad Sci USA* 1978;75:2888–2892.
51. Nakamura T, Fukui M, Ebihara I, et al. Effects of a low-protein diet on glomerular endothelin family gene expression in experimental focal glomerular sclerosis. *Clin Science* 1995;88:29–37.
52. Nakamura T, Ebihara I, Fukui M, et al. Altered glomerular steady-state levels of tumor necrosis factor-alpha mRNA during nephrotic and sclerotic phases of puromycin aminonucleoside nephrosis in rats. *Clin Science* 1993;84:349–356.
53. Nakayama M, Okuda S, Tamaki K, et al. Short- or long-term effects of a low-protein diet on fibronectin and transforming growth factor-beta synthesis in adriamycin-induced nephropathy. *J Lab Clin Med* 1996;127:29–39.
54. Straus DS, Takamoto CD. Effect of fasting on insulin-like growth factor-1 (IGF-1) and growth hormone receptor mRNA levels and IGF-1 gene transcription in rat liver. *Mol Endocrinol* 1991;4:91–100.
55. Straus DS. Nutritional regulation of hormones and growth factors that control mammalian growth. *Faseb J* 1994;8:6–12.
56. Peters H, Border WA, Noble NA. Tandem antifibrotic actions of L-arginine supplementation and low protein diet during the repair phase of experimental glomerulonephritis. *Kidney Int* 2000;57:992–1001.
57. Peters H, Border WA, Noble NA. Angiotensin II blockade and low-protein diet produce additive therapeutic effects in experimental glomerulonephritis. *Kidney Int* 2000;57:1493–1501.
58. Walls J. Relationship between proteinuria and progressive renal disease. *Am J Kidney Dis* 2001;37:S13–S16.
59. Dixon R, Brunskill NJ. Activation of mitogenic pathways by albumin in kidney proximal tubule epithelial cells: implications for the pathophysiology of proteinuric states. *J Am Soc Nephrol* 1999;10:1487–1497.
60. Erkan E, DeLeon M, Devarajan P. Albumin overload induces apoptosis in LLC-PK(1) cells. *Am J Physiol* 2001;280: F1107–F1114.
61. Wang SA, LaPage J, Hirschberg R. Role of glomerular ultrafiltration of growth factors in progressive interstitial fibrosis in diabetic nephropathy. *Kidney Int* 2000;57:1002–1014.
62. Thomas ME, Brunskill NJ, Harris KPG, et al. Proteinuria induces tubular cell turnover: a potential mechanism for tubular atrophy. *Kidney Int* 1999;55:890–898.
63. Aparicio M, Bouchet JL, Gin H, et al. Effect of a low-protein diet on urinary albumin excretion in uremic patients. *Nephron* 1988;50:288–291.
64. Neugarten J, Feiner HD, Schacht RG, et al. Amelioration of experimental glomerulonephritis by dietary protein restriction. *Kidney Int* 1983;24:595–601.
65. Subcommittee on the Tenth Edition of the Recommended Dietary Allowances, Food and Nutrition Board, Commission on Life Sciences, National Research Council. *Recommended Dietary Allowances*, 10th ed. Washington, DC: National Academies Press, 1989.
66. Munro HN, McGandy RB, Hartz SC, et al. Protein nutriture of a group of free-living elderly. *Am J Clin Nutr* 1987;46:586–592.
67. Cohn SH, Vartsky D, Yasumura S, et al. Compartmental body composition based on total body nitrogen, potassium and calcium. *Am J Physiol* 1980;239:E524–E530.
68. FAO/WHO/UNU. *Energy and protein requirements.* Geneva: World Health Organization, 1985;724:1–206.
69. Kopple JD, Greene T, Chumlea WC, et al. Relationship between nutritional status and GFR: results from the MDRD study. *Kidney Int* 2000;57:1688–1703.
70. Ikizler TA, Greene JH, Wingard RL, et al. Spontaneous dietary protein intake during progression of chronic renal failure. *J Am Soc Nephrol* 1995;6:1386–1391.
71. Pollock CA, Ibels LS, Zhu FY, et al. Protein intake in renal disease. *J Am Soc Nephrol* 1997;8:777–783.
72. Garg AX, Blake PG, Clark WF, et al. Association between renal insufficiency and malnutrition in older adults: Results from the NHANES III. *Kidney Int* 2001;60:1867–1874.
73. Kontessis P, Jones S, Dodds R, et al. Renal, metabolic and hormonal responses to ingestion of animal and vegetable proteins. *Kidney Int* 1990;38:136–144.
74. Kontessis P, Bossinakou I, Sarika L, et al. Renal, metabolic and hormonal responses to protein of different origin in normotensive, nonproteinuric type 1 diabetic patients. *Diabetes Care* 1995;18:1233–1240.
75. Rosenberg ME, Swanson JE, Thomas BL, et al. Glomerular and hormonal responses to dietary protein intake in human renal disease. *Am J Physiol* 1987;253:F1083–F1090.
76. Bernhard J, Beaufrere B, Laville M, et al. Adaptive response to a low protein diet in predialysis chronic renal failure patients. *J Am Soc Nephrol* 2001;12:1249–1254.
77. Quevedo MR, Price GM, Halliday D, et al. Nitrogen homoeostasis in man: diurnal changes in nitrogen excretion, leucine oxidation and whole body leucine kinetics during a reduction from a high to a moderate protein intake. *Clin Sci* 1994;86:185–193.
78. Goodship TJ, Mitch WE, Hoerr RA, et al. Adaptation to low protein diets in renal failure: Leucine turnover and nitrogen balance. *J Am Soc Nephrol* 1990;1:66–75.
79. Giordano M, DeFeo P, Lucidi P, et al. Effects of dietary protein

restriction on fibrinogen and albumin metabolism in nephrotic patients. *Kidney Int* 2001;60:235–242.

80. Masud T, Young VR, Chapman T, et al. Adaptive responses to very low protein diets: the first comparison of ketoacids to essential amino acids. *Kidney Int* 1994;45:1182–1192.
81. Tom K, Young VR, Chapman T, et al. Long-term adaptive responses to dietary protein restriction in chronic renal failure. *Am J Physiol* 1995;268:E668–E677.
82. Maroni BJ, Staffeld C, Young VR, et al. Mechanisms permitting nephrotic patients to achieve nitrogen equilibrium with a protein-restricted diet. *J Clin Invest* 1997;99:2479–2487.
83. Kopple JD, Berg R, Houser H, et al. Nutritional status of patients with different levels of chronic renal insufficiency. *Kidney Int* 1989;27:S184–S194.
84. Fouque D, Joly MO, Laville M, et al. Increase of serum insulin-like growth factor I (IGF 1) during chronic renal failure is reduced by low-protein diet. *Miner Electrolyte Metab* 1992;18: 276–279.
85. Clinical practice guidelines for nutrition in chronic renal failure. K/DOQI, National Kidney Foundation. *Am J Kidney Dis* 2000; 35:S1–S140.
86. Bernard S, Fouque D, Laville M, et al. Effects of low-protein diet supplemented with ketoacids on plasma lipids in adult chronic renal failure. *Miner Electrolyte Metab* 1996;22: 143–146.
87. Renaud SC, Gueguen R, Siest G, et al. Wine, beer, and mortality in middle-aged men from eastern France. *Arch Intern Med* 1999;159:1865–1870.
88. Gronbaek M, Becker U, Johansen D, et al. Type of alcohol consumed and mortality from all causes, coronary heart disease, and cancer. *Ann Intern Med* 2000;133:411–419.
89. Rigalleau V, Blanchetier V, Combe C, et al. A low-protein diet improves insulin sensitivity of endogenous glucose production in predialytic uremic patients. *Am J Clin Nutr* 1997;65: 1512–1516.
90. Kaysen GA, Gambertoglio J, Jimenez I, et al. Effects on dietary protein intake on albumin homeostasis in nephrotic patients. *Kidney Int* 1986;29:572–577.
91. Ruilope LM, Casal MC, Praga M, et al. Additive antiproteinuric effect of converting enzyme inhibition and a low protein intake. *J Am Soc Nephrol* 1992;3:1307–1311.
92. Gansevoort RT, de Zeeuw D, de Jong PE. Additive antiproteinuric effect of ACE inhibition and a low-protein diet in human renal disease. *Nephrol Dial Transplant* 1995;10:497–504.
93. Aparicio M, Chauveau P, Combe C. Are supplemented low-protein diets nutritionally safe? *Am J Kidney Dis* 2001;37: S71–S76.
94. Chauveau P, Barthe N, Rigalleau V, et al. Outcome of nutritional status and body composition of uremic patients on a very low protein diet. *Am J Kidney Dis* 1999;34:500–507.
95. Malvy D, Maingourd C, Pengloan J, et al. Effects of severe protein restriction with ketonanalogues in advanced renal failure. *J Am Coll Nutr* 1999;18:481–486.
96. Ihle B, Becker G, Withworth JA, et al. The effect of protein restriction on the progression of renal insufficiency. *N Engl J Med* 1989;321:1773–1777.
97. Williams PS, Stevens ME, Fass G, et al. Failure of dietary protein and phosphate restriction to retard the rate of progression of chronic renal failure: a prospective, randomized, controlled trial. *Q J Med* 1991;81:837–855.
98. Kopple JD, Levey AS, Greene T, et al. Effect of dietary protein restriction on nutritional status in the Modification of Diet in Renal Disease Study. *Kidney Int* 1997;52:778–791.
99. Aparicio M, Chauveau P, DePrecigout V, et al. Nutrition and outcome on renal replacement therapy of patients with chronic renal failure treated by a supplemented very low protein diet. *J Am Soc Nephrol* 2000;11:708–716.
100. Coresh J, Walser M, Hill S. Survival on dialysis among chronic renal failure patients treated with a supplemented low-protein diet before dialysis. *J Am Soc Nephrol* 1995;6:1379–1385.
101. Walser M, Hill S. Can renal replacement be deferred by a supplemented very-low protein diet? *J Am Soc Nephrol* 1999;10: 110–116.
102. Rosman JB, Ter Wee PM, Meijer S, et al. Prospective randomised trial of early dietary protein restriction in chronic renal failure. *Lancet* 1984;2:1291–1296.
103. Rosman JB, Langer K, Brandl M, et al. Protein-restricted diets in chronic renal failure: a four-year follow-up shows limited indications. *Kidney Int* 1989;27:S96–S102.
104. Locatelli F, Alberti D, Graziani G, et al. Prospective, randomised, multicentre trial of effect of protein restriction on progression of chronic renal insufficiency. *Lancet* 1991;337: 1299–1304.
105. Beck GJ, Berg RL, Coggins CH, et al. Design and statistical issues of the Modification of Diet in Renal Disease trial. *Control Clin Trial* 1991;12:566–586.
106. Greene T, Bourgoignie JJ, Habwe V, et al. Baseline characteristics in the Modification of Diet in Renal Disease study. *J Am Soc Nephrol* 1993;4:1221–1236.
107. Laidlaw SA, Berg RL, Kopple JD, et al. Patterns of fasting plasma amino acid levels in chronic renal insufficiency: Results from the feasibility phase of the Modification of Diet in Renal Disease study. *Am J Kidney Dis* 1994;23:504–513.
108. Klahr S, Levey AS, Beck GJ, et al. The effects of dietary protein restriction and blood-pressure control on the progression of chronic renal disease. Modification of Diet in Renal Disease Study Group. *N Engl J Med* 1994;330:877–884.
109. Peterson JC, Adler S, Burkart J, et al. Blood pressure control, proteinuria, and the progression of renal disease. *Ann Int Med* 1995;123:754–762.
110. Klahr S, Breyer JA, Beck GJ, et al. Dietary protein restriction, blood pressure control, and the progression of polycystic kidney disease. *J Am Soc Nephrol* 1995;5:2037–2047.
111. Klahr S. Role of dietary protein and blood pressure in the progression of renal disease. *Kidney Int* 1996;49:1783–1786.
112. Modification of Diet in Renal Disease Study Group. Short-term effects of protein intake, blood pressure, and antihypertensive therapy on glomerular filtration rate in the modification of diet in renal disease study. *J Am Soc Nephrol* 1996;7:2097–2109.
113. Levey AS, Adler S, Caggiula AW, et al. Effects of dietary protein restriction on the progression of advanced renal disease in the Modification of Diet in Renal Disease study. *Am J Kidney Dis* 1996;27:652–663.
114. Klahr S. Primary and secondary results of the Modification of Diet in Renal Disease study. *Miner Electrolyte Metab* 1996;22: 138–142.
115. Rocco MV, Gassman J, Wang SR, et al. Cross-sectional study of quality of life and symptoms in chronic renal disease patients: the modification of diet in renal disease study. *Am J Kidney Dis* 1997;29:888–896.
116. Teschan P, Beck GJ, Dwyer J, et al. Effect of a ketoacid-aminoacid-supplemented very low protein diet on the progression of advanced renal disease: a reanalysis of the MDRD feasibility study. *Clin Nephrol* 1998;50:273–283.
117. Hunsicker L, Adler S, Caggiula AW, et al. Predictors of the progression of renal disease in the Modification of Diet in Renal Disease study. *Kidney Int* 1997;51:1908–1919.
118. Levey AS, Greene T, Beck GJ, et al. Dietary protein restriction and the progression of chronic renal disease: what have all the

results of the MDRD study shown? *J Am Soc Nephrol* 1999; 10:2426–2439.

119. The effect of intensive treatment of diabetes on the development and progression of long-term complications in insulin-dependent diabetes mellitus. The Diabetes Control and Complications Trial. *N Engl J Med* 1993;1994:1194–1199.
120. Mitch WE, Walser M, Steinman T, et al. The effects of keto acid-amino acid supplement to a restricted diet on the progression of chronic renal failure. *N Engl J Med* 1984;311:623–629.
121. Abbe KA, Detsky AS, O'Rourke E. Meta-analysis in clinical research. *Ann Intern Med* 1987;107:224–233.
122. Sacks HS, Berrier J, Reitman D, et al. Meta-analyses of randomized controlled trials. *N Engl J Med* 1987;316:450–455.
123. Sackett DL. Rules of evidence and clinical recommendations on the use of antithrombotic agents. *Chest* 1989;95:S2–S4.
124. Pedrini MT, Levey AS, Lau J, et al. The effect of dietary protein restriction on the progression of diabetic and nondiabetic renal diseases: a meta-analysis. *Ann Intern Med* 1996;124:627–632.
125. Kasiske BL, Lakatua JD, Ma JZ, et al. A meta-analysis of the effects of dietary protein restriction on the rate of decline in renal function. *Am J Kidney Dis* 1998;31:954–961.
126. Altman DG, Andersen PK. Calculating the number needed to treat for trials where the outcome is a time to event. *BMJ* 1999; 319:1492–1495.
127. Skolbekken JA. Communicating the risk reduction achieved by cholesterol reducing drugs. *BMJ* 1998;316:1956–1958.

17

CALCIUM, PHOSPHORUS, AND VITAMIN D METABOLISM IN RENAL DISEASES AND CHRONIC RENAL FAILURE

SHARON M. MOE

In people with healthy kidneys, normal serum levels of phosphorus and calcium are maintained through the interaction of two hormones: parathyroid hormone (PTH) and 1,25(OH)2D (calcitriol), the active metabolite of vitamin D_3. These two hormones act on three target organs: bone, kidney, and intestine. The kidneys play a critical role in the regulation of normal serum calcium and phosphorus levels; thus, derangements occur quickly in patients with renal failure. Unfortunately, these are an important cause of morbidity and mortality in patients undergoing dialysis.

NORMAL PHYSIOLOGY

Normal Calcium Balance

Serum calcium levels are tightly controlled within a narrow range, usually 8.5 to 10.5 mg/dL (2.1 to 2.6 mmol/L). Intake of calcium by adults in the United States varies between 400 and 1,600 mg/day, with the median dietary intake being approximately 575 mg/day for women and 825 mg/day for men (1). Of the total dietary intake, only about 25% to 45% is absorbed (2). Fractional calcium absorption can increase with ingestion of a low-calcium diet or with administration of vitamin D compounds (3). The primary site for calcium excretion is the kidney. There is also an obligatory secretion of approximately 130 mg of calcium from the intestines per day (4). In normal individuals, the net calcium balance varies with age. Children and young adults are usually in a slightly positive net calcium balance; beyond age 25 to 35, when bones stop growing, the calcium balance tends to become negative or at least neutral (4). Normal individuals have protection against calcium overload by virtue of their ability to reduce intestinal absorption of calcium and increase renal excretion of calcium in response to excessive calcium intake. However, as renal function diminishes, the kidneys lose their ability to protect against calcium overload by increasing renal excretion of calcium.

The serum calcium level is a poor reflection of overall total body calcium because serum levels are only 0.1% to 0.2% of extracellular calcium, which in turn is only 1% of total body calcium. The remainder of total body calcium is stored in bone. The extracellular calcium is composed of the physiologically active ionized calcium (40% to 50% of total), as well as calcium bound to albumin and globulins (40%) and calcium bound to anions such as phosphate and citrate (10%). In individuals with normal homeostatic mechanisms, interactions of PTH and vitamin-D metabolites at target organs maintain the serum ionized calcium level within the normal range to ensure proper cellular function.

Normal Phosphorus Balance

Serum phosphorus levels normally are maintained within a narrow range, typically 2.5 to 4.5 mg/dL (0.8 to 1.5 mmol/L). Approximately 1,000 to 1,800 mg of phosphorus is ingested daily in the average Western diet (5,6). Of this amount, about 30% is excreted through the gastrointestinal tract and 70% is excreted by the kidneys (7). The dietary sources of phosphorus include all meats, dairy products, and many cereals and grains, thus making dietary restriction nearly impossible. The amount of phosphorus excreted by the kidneys is determined by the balance between ultrafiltration and reabsorption. As renal function and the ultrafiltration rate decline, serum phosphorus levels are maintained through a compensatory decrease in the rate of renal tubular reabsorption of phosphorus, mediated in part by elevation in the serum PTH (7). This adaptation allows for maintenance of normal serum phosphorus levels until the glomerular filtration rate (GFR) falls below 20 to 25 mL/min, at which point elevation in the serum PTH level cannot further increase phosphorus excretion and hyperphosphatemia develops (7–9). Thus, normal serum phosphorus levels are maintained well into advanced stages of renal failure but as a consequence of worsening secondary hyperparathyroidism.

Parathyroid Hormone

The primary function of PTH is to maintain calcium homeostasis by (a) increasing bone mineral dissolution, thus releasing calcium and phosphorus, (b) increasing renal reabsorption of calcium and excretion of phosphorus, and (c) enhancing the gastrointestinal absorption of both calcium and phosphorus indirectly through its effects on the synthesis of 1,25(OH)2D to increase serum calcium (Fig. 17.1). In healthy subjects, this increase in serum PTH level in response to hypocalcemia effectively restores serum calcium levels and maintains serum phosphorus levels. The kidneys are of key importance in this normal homeostatic response; thus, patients with renal failure may not be able to appropriately correct changes in serum-ionized calcium.

PTH is cleaved to an 84 amino acid protein in the parathyroid gland, where it is stored in secretory granules for release. Once released, the circulating 1-84 amino acid protein has a half-life of 2 to 4 minutes. It then is cleaved into N-terminal, C-terminal, and midregion fragments of PTH, which are metabolized in the liver and kidney (10,11). PTH secretion occurs in response to hypocalcemia, hyperphosphatemia, and 1,25(OH)2D deficiency. The extracellular concentration of ionized calcium is the most important determinant of minute-to-minute secretion of PTH from stored secretory granules in response to hypocalcemia. The secretion of PTH in response to low levels of ionized calcium is a sigmoidal relationship, as depicted in Fig. 17.2 (12), frequently referred to as the calcium-PTH curve. The rapid response, within seconds, of changes in ionized calcium concentration has long been hypothesized to be the result of a calcium-sensing receptor (CaR). This CaR now has been sequenced and cloned and is a member of the G-protein receptor superfamily, with a seven-membrane–spanning domain (13). Inactivating mutations have been associated with neonatal severe hyperparathyroidism and benign familial hypocalciuric hypercalcemia (14). These patients have asymptomatic elevations of serum calcium in the presence of nonsuppressed PTH, representing a true shift to the right of this curve. Activating mutations have been found in patients with autosomal dominant hypocalcemia (15). The CaR also has been localized to the thyroid C cells and the kidney, predominantly in the thick ascending limb where it controls renal excretion of calcium in response to changes in serum calcium (16,17).

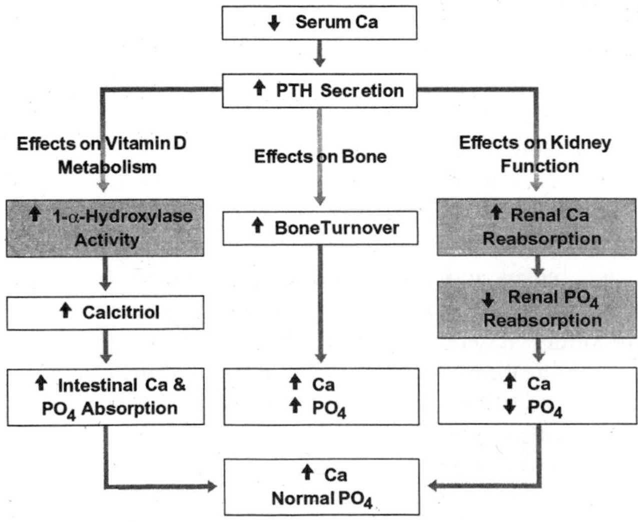

FIGURE 17.1. Interrelationship of calcium and phosphorus metabolism. Normal homeostatic response to decreased serum calcium. Note: Items in gray boxes are directly affected by decreased renal function.

PTH secretion also is regulated by vitamin D. 1,25(OH)2D decreases PTH synthesis by binding to the vitamin-D response element on the PTH gene as detailed later. 1,25(OH)2D also regulates the expression of the elevated vitamin-D receptor (VDR) itself and regulates parathyroid cell proliferation (18). In addition, elevated serum phosphorus also regulates proliferation of PTH cells and stimulates PTH secretion (19). The mechanism of this appears to be mediated via post-translational binding proteins (20,21), and downregulation of the CaR (22). This latter finding has important implications in patients with renal failure.

Early studies indicated that the calcium-PTH curve was shifted to the right in renal failure, creating an altered set point, defined as the calcium concentration that results in 50% maximal PTH secretion (23,24). The extrapolation of these data to clinical practice was that patients with renal failure required supraphysiologic serum levels of calcium to suppress PTH. However, several studies failed to confirm these findings (25). In rats fed a high phosphorus diet, the messenger RNA and protein expression of the CaR is downregulated in PTH glands (22). In parathyroid glands removed from patients with severe secondary hyperparathyroidism, there was altered sensitivity to calcium (a shift to the right of the curve) when glands were incubated in the presence of phosphorus (26). A 1998 study of patients undergoing dialysis demonstrated that an infusion of phosphorus shifts the calcium-PTH curve to the right (27). These studies indicate that phosphorus may regulate the CaR. Thus, it is possible that some of the earlier discrepancy in the literature regarding possible alterations of the set point in renal failure may have been the result of differences in serum phosphorus levels in the various studies (28), although methodologic differences also can explain some of this discrepancy (25). This interrelationship of calcium, phosphorus, and calcitriol in regulating PTH synthesis is complex, and nearly impossible to fully evaluate in humans,

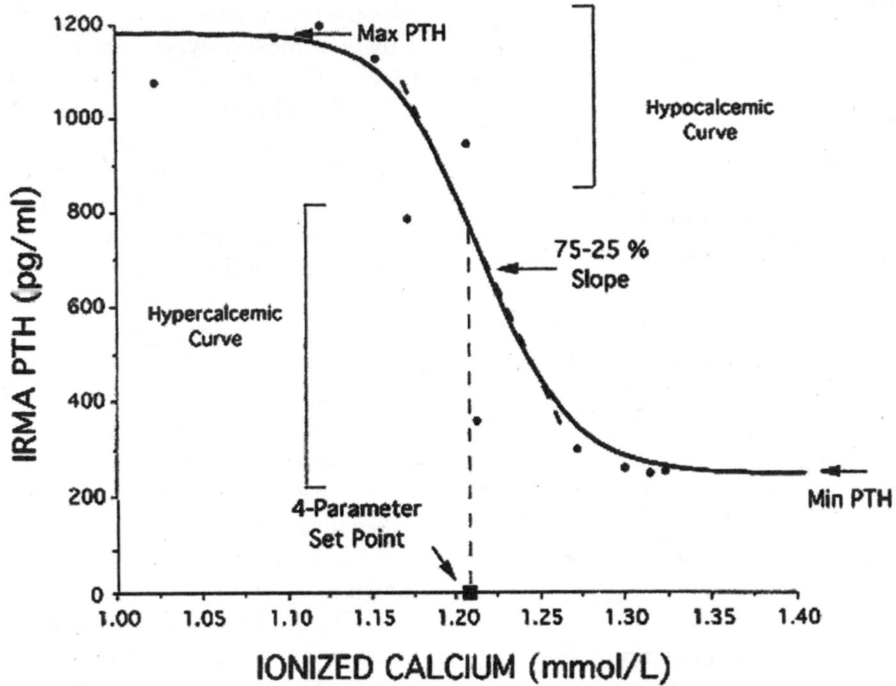

FIGURE 17.2. Plot of parathyroid hormone (PTH) (pg/mL) versus ionized calcium (iCa; mmol/L) from a representative patient undergoing hemodialysis. Data (•) obtained during successive dialyses against low calcium dialysate (hypocalcemic curve) and high calcium dialysate (hypercalcemic curve) were fitted using the four-parameter model (*solid line*). Fitted maximal (max) PTH and minimal (min) PTH are indicated. The four-parameter set point (*solid square*) is the iCa corresponding to a PTH midway between max and min PTH. The 75% to 25% nonnormalized slope (*dashed line*) also is shown. (From Ouseph R, Leiser JD, Moe SM. Calcitriol and the parathyroid hormone-ionized calcium curve: a comparison of methodologic approaches. *J Am Soc Nephrol* 1996;7: 497–505, with permission.)

because changes in one lead to rapid changes in the other parameters. However, based on these studies, it appears that calcium is more important in stimulating PTH release, whereas calcitriol is more important in inhibiting PTH release. The presence of hyperphosphatemia impairs both of these homeostatic mechanisms.

PTH binds to the PTH receptor, which is a member of the G-protein–linked seven-membrane–spanning receptor family (29). PTH receptors are located ubiquitously in the body, although most abundantly in kidney and bone. PTH-induced signaling predominately affects mineral metabolism; however, there are many extraskeletal manifestations of PTH excess. These include encephalopathy, anemia, extraskeletal calcification, peripheral neuropathy, cardiac dysfunction, hyperlipidemia, and impotence (30–33). After binding, PTH stimulates intracellular signaling by both cAMP (cyclic adenosine monophosphate) and IP_3/DAG (triphosphate diacylglycerol) pathways (34). PTH-related peptide, or PTHrp, is only homologous to PTH in the first 13 amino acids, but that minimal homology allows PTHrp to activate the PTH receptor (35). PTHrp is critical in developmental biology because the knockout mice die at birth (36). However, serum levels of PTHrp in the adult are low in normal individuals but can be elevated with ectopic production of PTHrp from certain tumors leading to humoral hypercalcemia of malignancy through traditional PTH-stimulated mineral metabolism pathways (37). In contrast, in healthy individuals PTHrp is expressed locally in multiple tissues including epithelia, mesenchymal tissue, endocrine glands, and the central nervous system. Thus, in contrast to PTH, which is synthesized to act systemically, PTHrp is synthesized locally for roles in cell biology (38). The importance of PTHrp in normal biology is only beginning to become unraveled.

The measurement of PTH is not easy, and there has been a progression of increasingly sensitive assays developed over the past few years. The major difficulty in accurately measuring PTH is the presence of circulating fragments, particularly in the presence of renal failure (10,11). Initial measurements of PTH using C-terminal assays were inaccurate in patients with renal disease because of impaired renal excretion, and thus retention, in renal failure. The development of the N-terminal assay brought hope of a more accurate reflection of end-organ effects of PTH, but it also detected inactive metabolites. The current standard of care is to use a two-site antibody "intact" assay, which is capable of detecting the intact PTH molecule by binding an antibody to the N-terminus and another to the C-terminus

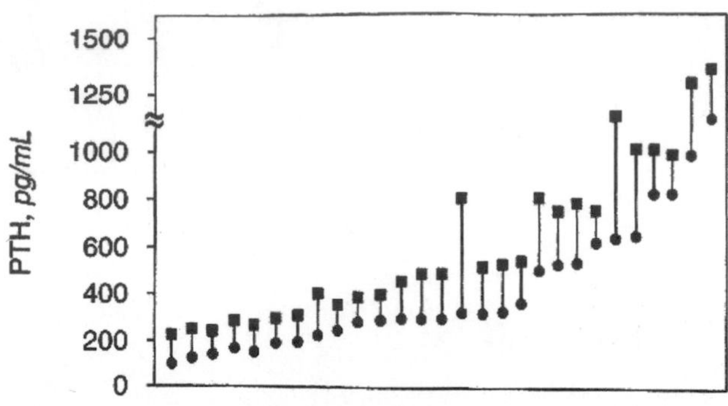

FIGURE 17.3. Comparison of the 1-84 amino acid and 7-84 amino acid parathyroid hormone (PTH) assays. Serum samples from uremic patients undergoing dialysis were analyzed by both PTH assays. The squares represent the "intact" PTH assay, and the circles represent the 1-84 amino acid "whole" PTH assay. The results of the intact assay were uniformly higher than the results with the whole assay. (From Slatopolsky E, Finch J, Clay P, et al. A novel mechanism for skeletal resistance in uremia. *Kidney Int* 2000;58: 753–761, with permission.)

(39). This intact assay is more discriminatory than N- or C-terminal assays in patients with renal failure (40); however, it does not correlate well with underlying bone histology (41,42). Recent data indicate that in renal failure, there is also accumulation of a 7-84 amino acid fragment, which is detected by the intact assay (43). In rats that have undergone parathyroidectomy, the injection of a truly whole 1-84 amino acid PTH was able to induce bone resorption, whereas the 7-84 amino acid fragment was antagonistic (44). In patients, the measurement of the intact PTH led to results that were always greater than the whole (1-84 amino acid only) assay, regardless of whether the patients had low or high PTH levels (Fig. 17.3) (44,45). These findings partially may explain the apparent end-organ resistance of PTH in patients being treated with dialysis (46), although there is also evidence for downregulation of PTH receptors in bone in uremia (40,47). At this time, it is unknown if the new whole PTH assay or the ratio of the 1-84 amino acid to 7-84 amino acid (active/antagonist) PTH levels more accurately reflect underlying bone histology than the intact assay.

Vitamin D

Although vitamin D_3 is metabolically inactive, it is metabolized in the liver to 25(OH)D and then converted in the kidney via the 1-α-hydroxylase enzyme to 1,25(OH)2D, which has a number of important effects (48). Its most important function is exerted on the small intestine, where it regulates the intestinal absorption of calcium and, to a lesser degree, phosphorus (49). Apart from its effect on calcium and phosphorus levels, 1,25(OH)2D also directly suppresses PTH synthesis, as described earlier (50), and may be important for normal bone turnover by enhancing formation of osteoclasts (51). Enhanced secretion of PTH in response to low levels of calcium increases 1-α-hydroxylase activity in the kidney, thereby raising serum 1,25(OH)2D levels. This resulting rise in serum calcium and 1,25(OH)2D feeds back on the parathyroid gland, decreasing PTH secretion, thus completing the typical endocrine feedback loop. PTH does not directly inhibit its own synthesis, which is one reason why PTH levels increase in the presence of renal failure where 1,25(OH)2D is no longer synthesized in sufficient amounts. The 1-α-hydroxylase enzyme in the kidney is also the site of regulation of 1,25(OH)2D synthesis by numerous factors, including PTH, low calcium, low phosphorus, estrogen, prolactin, growth hormone, and 1,25(OH)2D itself (52). Thus, there is 1,25(OH)2D deficiency in essentially all patients with renal disease, with an inability to respond appropriately to normal physiologic stimuli. In addition, many patients undergoing dialysis are also deficient in the precursor vitamin D_3 as a result of inadequate dietary intake and lack of sunlight.

1,25(OH)2D mediates its cellular function via both genomic and nongenomic mechanisms. 1,25(OH)2D circulates in the bloodstream with vitamin-D binding protein. The free form of 1,25(OH)2D enters the target cell where it interacts with its nuclear VDR. This complex then combines with the retinoic acid X receptor to form a heterodimer, which, in turn interacts with the vitamin-D response element (VDRE) on the target gene (Fig. 17.4). The findings of VDRE on multiple genes, and VDR in multiple

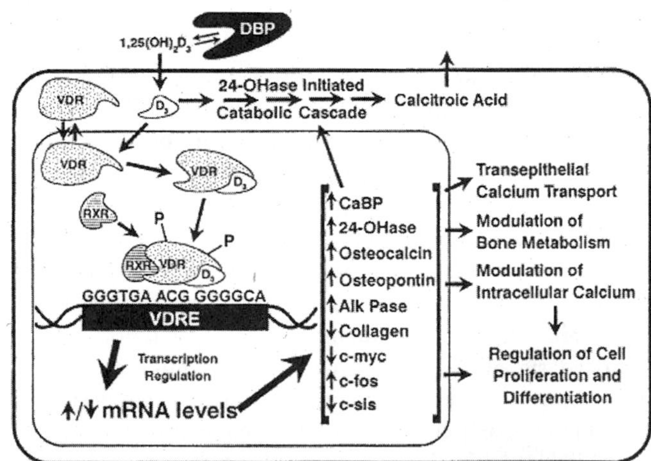

FIGURE 17.4. Proposed mechanism of action of $1,25(OH)_2D$ in target cells. The free form of vitamin D, $1,25(OH)_2D$, enters the target cell and interacts with its nuclear vitamin D receptor (VDR), which is phosphorylated (P). The $1,25(OH)_2D$-VDR complex combines with the retinoic acid X receptor (RXR) to form a heterodimer, which, in turn, interacts with the vitamin D-responsive element (VDRE), causing an enhancement or inhibition of transcription of vitamin D responsive genes such as osteocalcin. (From Holick MF. Vitamin D: photobiology, metabolism, mechanism of action, and clinical applications. In: Favus MJ, ed. *Primer on the metabolic bone diseases and disorders of mineral metabolism*, 4th ed. Philadelphia: Lippincott Williams and Wilkins, 1999:94, with permission.)

organ systems points to the wide spread systemic effects of vitamin D (53–55). In particular, it appears important in cell differentiation and proliferation, which has led to its therapeutic use in cancer and skin disorders (53,56). In addition to these nongenomic effects, 1,25(OH)2D facilitates the uptake of calcium by enhancing the production of the calcium-transport protein calbindin (9 kd in intestine and 28 kd in kidney) (57,58). Lastly, 1,25(OH)2D activates voltage-dependent calcium channels with increased intracellular calcium (59). To target 1,25(OH)2D to more specific cellular functions, the structure has been altered to produce several "designer" vitamin-D analogues that are in clinical use today. The vitamin-D analogues for use in renal failure are designed to maximize the effects on the PTH gland and minimize the effects on the intestine. Some of these vitamin-D analogues may be less hypercalcemic and may be useful in patients with renal failure, as described later.

Target Organs

Detailed descriptions of the cellular mechanisms of the target organs involved in calcium and phosphorus homeostasis are beyond the scope of this review, but a brief summary is included.

Intestinal Transport

The majority of calcium is absorbed in the duodenum and cecum, although absorption occurs throughout the intestinal tract. Calcium absorption is via a saturable active transport and an unsaturable passive transport. In addition, there is a low level of obligatory calcium secretion that occurs in the jejunum. The active calcium transport occurs in the intestinal brush border through calcium channels, down an electrochemical gradient. The process is facilitated by calbindin 9 kd, which ferries the calcium through the cell. The calcium then is extruded into the blood by a Ca/Mg/ATPase (adenosine triphosphatase), and a Na/Ca exchanger. Some calcium also is transported via paracellular pathways. 1,25(OH)2D enhances calcium uptake by the insertion of calcium channels, increasing the production of calbindin, enhancing the Ca/Mg/ATPase, and possibly enhancing paracellular pathways. Factors that increase intestinal calcium absorption predominately are mediated via 1,25(OH)2D, although low-calcium diet can directly affect absorption (60–63).

The absorption of phosphorus occurs throughout the small and large intestines but is maximal in the small intestine. The absorption occurs across the brush border, mediated by the Na/Pi exchanger. The energy for this is, in part, mediated by the Na gradient induced by the Na/K/ATPase exchanger. The ability of the intestines to acutely adapt to a low-phosphorus diet is the result of activation of stored Na/Pi cotransporters in the terminal web near the brush border. In addition, low-phosphorus diet induces the synthesis of 1,25(OH)2D, which enhances Na/Pi cotransport. There is also a concentration-dependent paracellular pathway (63,64).

Renal Transport

Compared to the intestine, the renal tubule reabsorbs 40-fold more calcium per day (8,000 mg versus 200 mg). The bulk of the reabsorption occurs in the proximal tubule (about 50% to 60%), but hormonal regulation predominates in the later renal segments. In the proximal tubule, calcium absorption parallels that of salt and water, and thus is likely passive, through paracellular pathways via convection (solvent drag) and electrochemical gradients. However, in the pars recta, approximately two-thirds of transport may be active. The predominance of convective mechanisms is why volume depletion can induce hypercalcemia. Approximately 20% of calcium is reabsorbed in the thick-ascending limb, of which about two-thirds is paracellular and the remaining is transcellular. The paracellular transport is mediated through a gradient established by the Na/K/2Cl exchanger and subsequent recycling of potassium. Inhibitors of the Na/K/2Cl exchanger, the loop diuretics, can inhibit the uptake of calcium in this segment and are useful for the treatment of hypercalcemia. The CaR is located predominately in the thick-ascending limb on the basolateral surface. Elevations in serum calcium levels turn on the CaR, which, through cell signaling pathways, inhibits transcellular transport of calcium. In so doing, the transport of NaCl in the thick-ascending limb is decreased, leading to decreased countercurrent multiplication. In addition, activation of the CaR appears to inhibit antidiuretic hormone's ability to insert aquaporin channels in the collecting duct, decreasing the ability to reabsorb water (16,65). These two phenomena may explain the polyuria observed with hypercalcemia, creating a vicious cycle of volume depletion and worsened hypercalcemia. Transport of calcium in the distal convoluted tubule and connecting tubule consists of apical entry of calcium through insertion of voltage-operated, dihydropyridine-sensitive calcium channels, which recently have been cloned (59,66). Transport through the basolateral membrane is via Ca-ATPase and Ca/Na exchangers. Alterations in normal sodium transport induced by either amiloride or thiazide diuretics can increase calcium reabsorption distally and are useful therapies for hypercalciuric nephrolithiasis.

Phosphorus is filtered freely at the glomerulus, and in normal situations the tubules reabsorb 80% to 90% of the filtered phosphorus. The vast majority of the reabsorption occurs in the proximal tubule via the Na/Pi cotransporter in a mechanism that parallels intestinal transport. Acute adaptation to low phosphorus diet occurs because of insertion of stored Na/Pi cotransporters, whereas chronic adaptation is the result of synthesis of new transporters (67). The ability of the tubules to absorb phosphorus becomes saturable at serum phosphorus levels of more than 6 mg/dL, the

Tm-Phosph. Phosphorus also is reabsorbed distally, although the mechanism is less clear (68).

The regulation of calcium and phosphorus transport in the kidneys is predominately through changes in the concentration of the ions themselves, through activity mediated by parathyroid hormone, and to a lesser extent by 1,25(OH)2D. PTH enhances calcium reabsorption through enhanced GFR, insertion of calcium channels in the thick-ascending limb, and probably through stimulation of the Na/Ca and Ca/ATPase exchangers in the distal tubule. PTH enhances phosphorus excretion primarily in the proximal tubule via changes in intracellular signaling that affect the Na/Pi exchanger. 1,25(OH)2D is also active in the kidney because the VDR is located through the nephron. However, the precise role is less clear than the effects of PTH. 1,25(OH)2D enhances the production of calbindin 28 kd, thus facilitating calcium reabsorption in distal segments (69). 1,25(OH)2D also inhibits the reabsorption of phosphorus in the proximal tubule. Although the mechanism of action of 1,25(OH)2D is not completely clear, it appears to be additive to the effects of PTH in that the excretion of calcium in the urine for any given serum level of calcium is markedly greater in the presence of both PTH and 1,25(OH)2D than either hormone alone (70).

Bone

The majority of the total body stores of calcium and phosphorus are located in bone. Trabecular (cancellous) bone is located predominately in the epiphyses of the long bones, which is 15% to 25% calcified, and serves a metabolic function with a relatively short turnover rate of ^{45}Ca (calcium). In contrast, cortical (compact) bone is in the shafts of long bones and is 80% to 90% calcified. This bone serves primarily a protective and mechanical function and has a calcium turnover rate of months. Bone consists predominately (90%) of highly organized cross-linked fibers of type I collagen; the remainder consists of proteoglycans and "noncollagen" proteins such as osteopontin, osteocalcin, osteonectin, and alkaline phosphatase. Hydroxyapatite—$Ca_{10}(PO_4)_6(OH)_2$—is the major bone salt.

The cellular components of bone are of utmost importance and consist of cartilage cells, which are key to bone development; osteoblasts, which are the bone-forming cells; and osteoclasts, which are the bone-resorbing cells. Osteoblasts are derived from progenitor mesenchymal cells located in the bone marrow. They then are induced to become osteoprogenitor cells, then endosteal or periosteal progenitor cells, then mature osteoblasts. The control of this differentiation pathway is the result of bone morphogenic proteins and the transcription factor Cbfa1 (core binding factor 1) early and other hormones and cytokines later. Once bone formation is complete, osteoblasts may become quiescent cells trapped within the mineralized bone in the form of osteocytes. The osteocytes are interconnected through a series of cannaliculi. Although these cells previously were thought to be of little importance, it is now clear that they serve to transmit the initial signaling involved with mechanical loading (71).

Osteoclasts are derived from hematopoietic precursor cells that differentiate and somehow are "signaled" to arrive at a certain place in the bone. Once there, they fuse to form the multinucleated cells known as osteoclasts, which become highly polarized, reabsorbing bone through the release of degradative enzymes. They move along a resorption surface via changes in the cytoskeleton. PTH, cytokines, and 1,25(OH)2D are all important in inducing the fusion of the committed osteoclast precursors. Once resorption is complete, estrogens, bisphosphonates, and cytokines can induce, and PTH can inhibit, apoptosis (72,73). Numerous hormones and cytokines have been evaluated, mostly *in vitro*, for their role in controlling osteoclast function.

The control of bone remodeling is highly complex but appears to occur in very distinct phases: (a) osteoclast resorption, (b) reversal, (c) preosteoblast migration and differentiation, (d) osteoblast matrix (osteoid or unmineralized bone) formation, (e) mineralization, and (f) quiescent stage. At any one time, less than 15% to 20% of the bone surface is undergoing remodeling, and this process in a single bone-remodeling unit can take 3 to 6 months. How a certain piece of bone is chosen to undergo a remodeling cycle and how the osteoclasts and osteoblasts signal each other is not completely clear.

Recently, the discovery of the osteoprotegerin (OPG) and RANK (receptor activator of nuclear-factor kB) system has shed new light on the control of osteoclast function and the long observed coupling of osteoblasts and osteoclasts. RANK is located on osteoclasts, and the OPG-ligand (OPG-L) is on osteoblasts. Osteoblasts also synthesize the protein OPG, which can bind to OPG ligand on osteoblasts and inhibit the subsequent binding of OPG-L to RANK on osteoclasts, thus inhibiting bone resorption. Alternatively, if OPG production is decreased, the OPG-L can bind with RANK on osteoclasts and induce osteoclastic bone resorption (Fig. 17.5). This fascinating control system is regulated by nearly every cytokine and hormone thought important in bone remodeling, including PTH, 1,25(OH)2D, estrogen, glucocorticoids, interleukins, prostaglandins, and members of the transforming growth factor-β superfamily of cytokines (74–76). OPG has been successful in preventing bone resorption in animal models of osteoporosis and tumor-induced bone resorption (77,78). Not surprisingly, OPG is being tested as a therapeutic agent for osteoporosis, and initial studies appear promising (79). It is interesting that abnormalities in the OPG/RANK have been found in renal failure (80), although the effect on bone remodeling is not yet clear.

The clinical assessment of bone remodeling is best done with a bone biopsy of the trabecular bone, usually at the iliac crest. The patient is given a tetracycline derivative ap-

NEED LESS BONE?

In the absence of OPG, OPG-L is available to bind to RANK, stimulating osteoclast mediated bone resorption

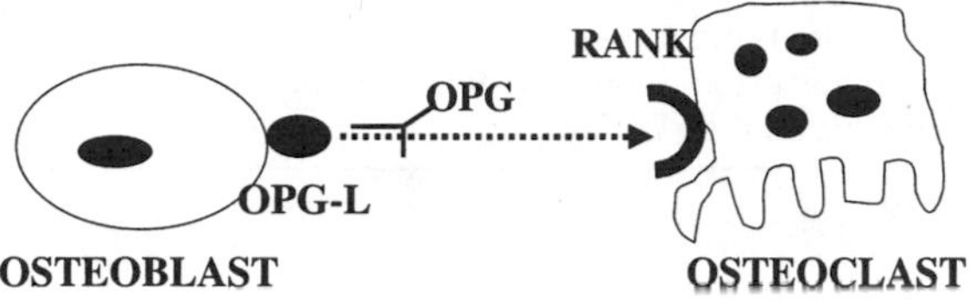

NEED MORE BONE?

OPG binds to OPG-L, interfering with binding of OPG-L to RANK, preventing osteoclast bone resorption

FIGURE 17.5. Role of osteoprotegerin in the regulation of osteoclast-mediated bone resorption. See text for details.

proximately 1 month before the bone biopsy and a different tetracycline derivative 3 to 5 days before the biopsy. Tetracycline binds to hydroxyapatite and emits fluorescence, thereby serving as a label of the bone. A core of predominately trabecular bone is taken, embedded in a plastic material, and sectioned. The use of this plastic material is why only some laboratories are equipped to process bone biopsies. Typical pathology labs normally decalcify tissue and paraffin embed, which will destroy the very architecture that is necessary to differentiate metabolic disorders.

The sections then can be visualized with special stains and under fluorescent microscopy to determine the amount of bone between the two tetracycline labels or that formed in the time interval between the two labels. This dynamic parameter assessed on bone biopsy is the basis for assessing bone turnover, which is key in discerning types of renal osteodystrophy, as detailed later in this chapter. In addition to dynamic indices, bone biopsies can be analyzed by histomorphometry for many static parameters. The nomenclature for these assessments has been standardized (81). Clinically, bone biopsies are most useful for differentiating types of renal osteodystrophy, as well as other undiagnosed metabolic disorders. However, with the advent of several new markers of bone turnover, the use of bone biopsy has been reserved primarily for the diagnosis of renal osteodystrophy and for research purposes (82). For renal osteodystrophy the most important parameters are fibrosis and osteoid (unmineralized bone) area as a percent of total bone area. These two static parameters, together with the dynamic bone turnover assessed by bone formation rate or activation frequency, can distinguish the various forms of renal osteodystrophy (Table 17.1). The histologic features will be described in more detail later.

ABNORMALITIES IN RENAL FAILURE: SECONDARY HYPERPARATHYROIDISM

As detailed earlier, the kidney plays an integral role in the maintenance of normal calcium and phosphorus homeostasis and bone health. As a result, severe abnormalities can occur in the presence of renal failure. As renal disease advances, the reduced mass of functioning renal tissue is unable to excrete the normal dietary intake of phosphorus. Early on, the serum level of phosphorus is maintained via stimulation of PTH release, leading to the development of secondary hyperparathyroidism, the "trade-off" hypothesis (7). Phosphorus retention further limits calcitriol production by inhibiting the activity of 1-α-hydroxylase, which converts 25(OH)-vitamin D_3 into active 1,25(OH)2D (calcitriol). The decreased 1,25(OH)2D leads directly to further increases in PTH release, as well as decreased calcium and phosphorus absorption from the gastrointestinal tract. The impaired calcium absorption leads to relative decreases in serum-ionized calcium, further augmenting secondary hyperparathyroidism. Over time, the parathyroid glands become less sensitive to the feedback suppression of calcium and calcitriol, causing continual secretion of PTH and secondary hyperparathyroidism (83). Continual stimulation of PTH secretion has been shown to induce irreversible hyperplasia of the parathyroid glands in uremic rats (84) through a number of abnormalities of gene and growth-factor expression (18). The continued elevated levels of PTH lead to increased bone remodeling and eventually oste-

TABLE 17.1. HISTOLOGIC CLASSIFICATION OF RENAL OSTEODYSTROPHY

Lesion	Area of Fibrosis (% of tissue area)	Area of Osteoid (% of total bone area)	Bone Formation Rate ($\mu m^2/mm^2$ tissue area day)
Mild	<0.5	<15	>108
Osteitis fibrosa	>0.5	<15	X[a]
Mixed	>0.5	>15	X[a]
Osteomalacia	<0.5	>15	X[a]
Adynamic	<0.5	<15	<108
Normal range	0	1–7	108–500

From Sherrard DJ, Hercz G, Pei Y, et al. The spectrum of bone disease in end-stage renal failure—an evolving disorder. *Kidney Int* 1993;43:436–442, with permission.
[a]X is not a diagnostic criterion.

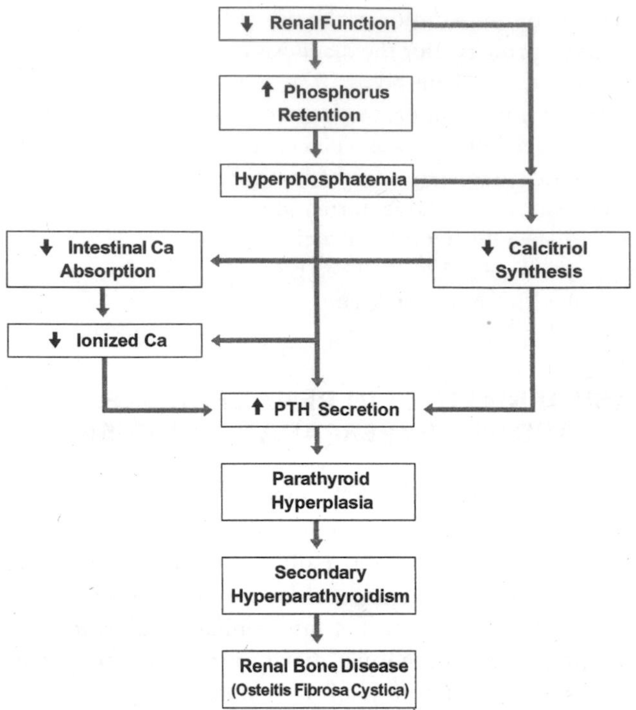

FIGURE 17.6. Succession of events in advanced renal disease leading to osteitis fibrosa cystica.

itis fibrosa cystica (Fig. 17.6). The latter bone pathology is characterized by excessive remodeling with increased osteoclast and osteoblast cell number and activity.

As indicated in Fig. 17.6, hyperphosphatemia has been shown to be one of the most important factors in the pathogenesis of secondary hyperparathyroidism. Although early studies suggested a hyperphosphatemia-induced decline in serum calcitriol, leading to low serum calcium, as the initial stimulus for enhanced PTH secretion (85), more recent evidence suggests that elevated serum phosphorus levels promote PTH secretion directly, independent of changes in serum calcium or calcitriol. Phosphorus restriction in dogs with renal failure (86) and in patients with chronic renal failure (87) have been shown to decrease PTH secretion directly, independently of changes in serum calcium or calcitriol. In uremic rats, phosphorus directly stimulates hyperparathyroidism and parathyroid gland hyperplasia (84). Moreover, high phosphorus levels have been shown to directly stimulate PTH secretion in intact rat parathyroid glands *in vitro* (86,88). In addition, in the presence of increased phosphorus load, the PTH–calcium curve probably is shifted to the right, creating resistance at the level of the PTH gland (28). Thus, there is now substantial evidence to support that phosphorus, calcium, and 1,25(OH)2D all act directly, and independently, to regulate PTH secretion.

RENAL OSTEODYSTROPHY

The term "renal osteodystrophy" encompasses all types of metabolic bone disease found in patients undergoing dialysis (Table 17.2). As detailed earlier, bone is a dynamic tissue and is remodeled constantly. Bone turnover is tightly regulated by numerous hormones and cytokines, of which PTH is of key importance. The prevalence of different forms of renal osteodystrophy has changed over the past decade. Whereas osteitis fibrosa cystica previously had been the predominant lesion, the prevalence of adynamic bone disease has increased (Table 17.3). These changes may reflect the numerous changes in the dialysis population, the dialysis regimen, and supportive care that have occurred during this period (82).

TABLE 17.2. CLASSIFICATION OF RENAL OSTEODYSTROPHY

High-turnover bone disease
Osteitis fibrosa cystica due to secondary hyperparathyroidism
Mixed uremic lesion
Low-turnover bone disease
Osteomalacia (aluminum or nonaluminum)
Adynamic/aplastic bone disease

In situations where PTH is elevated, bone turns over with excessive rapidity, replacing lamellar bone with structurally inferior woven bone. In addition, both osteoblastic bone formation and osteoclastic bone resorption are accelerated and fibrosis eventually develops, a pathology referred to as osteitis fibrosa cystica (Fig. 17.7A). In contrast, in low-turnover bone disease the pathology can be either osteomalacia, where there is increased osteoid (unmineralized bone), or adynamic bone where there is a paucity of cells (Fig. 17.7B). Mixed uremic osteodystrophy has components of both high turnover and increased osteoid. The histomorphometric features of the different forms of renal osteodystrophy are shown in Table 17.1.

Low-turnover bone disease usually is observed in the presence of normal to low levels of PTH. In osteomalacia, aluminum is deposited at the mineralization front, blocking mineralization. This leads to an accumulation of osteoid, or unmineralized bone, and is the hallmark of osteomalacia.

TABLE 17.3. CHANGING PATTERN OF RENAL OSTEODYSTROPHY IN PATIENTS UNDERGOING DIALYSIS

	Percentage of Patients			
			1993 (82)	
	1972 (237)	1986 (90)	HD	CAPD
Osteitis fibrosa cystica	22	68	38	9
Mild OF	45	0	13	21
Mixed uremic lesion	9	0	11	4
Osteomalacia	24	25	2	6
Adynamic bone disease	0	7	36	61

HD, hemodialysis; CAPD, continuous ambulatory peritoneal dialysis; OF, osteitis fibrosa.

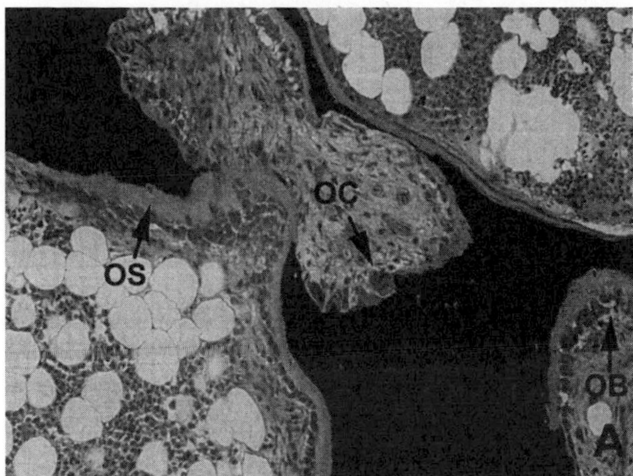

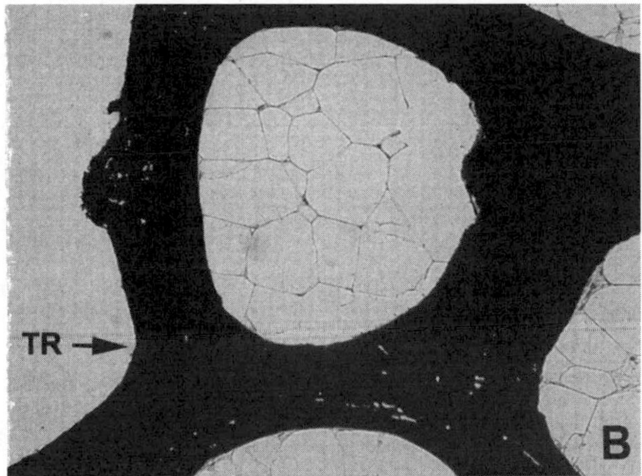

FIGURE 17.7. Histologic features of hyperparathyroid and adynamic bone disease. **(A):** Severe osteitis fibrosa cystica in a bone biopsy from a patient with severe secondary hyperparathyroidism (serum intact parathyroid hormone, or PTH, of 1,600 pg/mL). Stained with MacNeal's stain. The black area represents mineralized bone; the light gray area is unmineralized bone or osteoid (OS). The marrow space demonstrates severe fibrosis. There also is increased bone formation with activated osteoblasts (OB) and increased bone resorption with activated osteoclasts (OC). Tetracycline labeling (not shown) revealed an increased rate of bone formation. **(B):** Adynamic bone disease in a bone biopsy from a patient undergoing peritoneal dialysis with hypercalcemia and low serum PTH. The biopsy reveals only mineralized trabecular bone (TR) with a marked absence of cells and osteoid. Aluminum staining was negative.

Aluminum can induce many extraskeletal abnormalities as well, which are detailed later in this chapter. In contrast, adynamic (often called aplastic) bone disease is characterized by normal amounts of osteoid, an absence of tissue fibrosis, decreased numbers of osteoblasts and osteoclasts, and low rates of bone formation (82). The etiology of adynamic bone disease is unknown, but risk factors include age, oversuppression of PTH with vitamin D and calcium-containing phosphate binders, diabetes, and possibly calcium overload (82,89–91). In addition, there is evidence for altered osteoblast response to PTH as a result of downregulation of the PTH receptor in renal failure (92), which further contributes to the paucity of cells observed in adynamic bone disease. The predominance of adynamic bone disease in patients undergoing peritoneal dialysis may reflect the relative constant positive calcium balance in these patients, with resultant suppression of PTH compared to patients undergoing hemodialysis, although other factors are also likely.

Diagnosis of Renal Osteodystrophy

Studies evaluating the ability of the serum concentration of intact PTH to predict both low- and high-turnover bone disease have been disappointing. In general, the risk of high-turnover bone disease increases with the concentration of PTH (Fig. 17.8) (41,42). However, the ability to reliably predict the presence of high-turnover bone disease is poor until intact PTH levels of 450 to 500 pg/mL are reached. Levels of intact PTH under 100 pg/mL are fairly reliable for the prediction of low-turnover bone disease (41), but again, they are not perfect. These studies that correlate intact PTH with bone histology were done before the widespread use of vitamin D derivatives and may not be applicable in the current treatment environment. However, a study of patients undergoing peritoneal dialysis published in 2000 confirmed these findings (93). Thus, in general, levels of intact PTH below 100 to 150 pg/mL are indicative of low-turnover bone, whereas levels of intact PTH greater than 450 to 500 pg/mL are indicative of high-turnover bone on biopsy. Levels in between those two cutoff levels are not predictive of underlying bone histology, creating a clinical challenge for nephrologists. Studies in patients with chronic kidney disease not yet undergoing dialysis indicate that similar levels of PTH predict high-turnover bone disease (94–97), but these studies are small. It is possible that the new "whole" PTH assay (44,45) will be more predictive of bone histology, but this remains to be demonstrated.

Obviously, it is not practical to have all patients undergo a bone biopsy. Thus, we must use clinical judgment, PTH hormone levels, and various other bone markers. Initially, there was great hope for the new bone markers such as osteocalcin and bone alkaline phosphatase to be predictive of underlying bone histology. Unfortunately, these specialized tests offer little additive value to our usual measurement of calcium, phosphorus, PTH, and total alkaline phosphatase (98). Thus, we must look at multiple variables (Table 17.4). In contrast to the hypophosphatemia and hypercalcemia observed in primary hyperparathyroidism, patients with secondary hyperparathyroidism tend to be hyperphosphatemic (which leads to increased PTH). The serum level of calcium is variable and depends on the overall calcium balance, type of phosphate binder, vitamin D therapy, and calcium dialysate concentration. However, in advanced

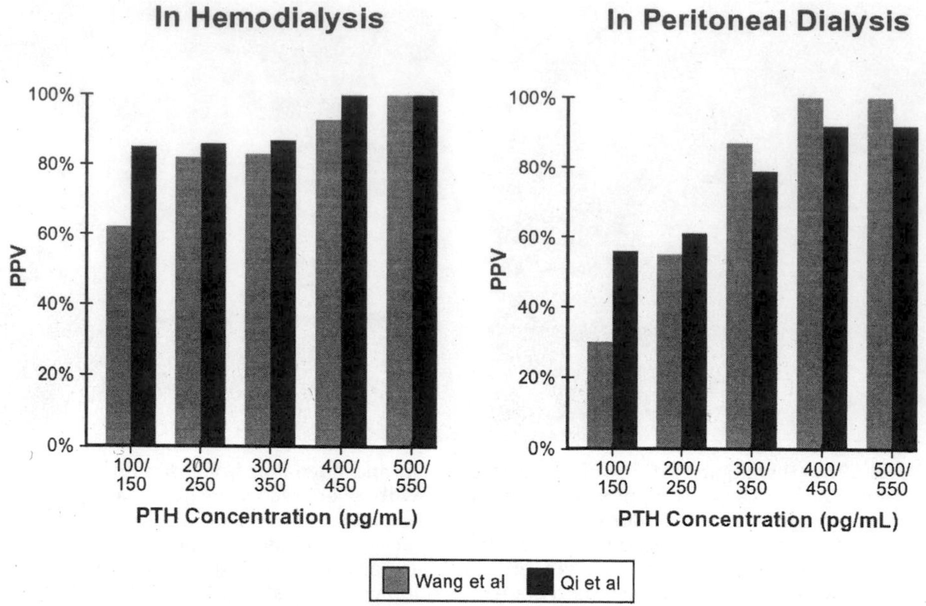

FIGURE 17.8. Positive predictive value (PPV) of serum PTH concentration in detecting high-turnover bone disease by bone biopsy in hemodialysis and peritoneal dialysis patients. (From Wang M, Hercz G, Sherrard DJ, et al. Relationship between intact 1-84 parathyroid hormone and bone histomorphometric parameters in dialysis patients without aluminum toxicity. *Am J Kidney Dis* 1995;26:836–844, with permission, and Qi Q, Monier-Faugere MC, Geng Z, et al. Predictive value of serum parathyroid hormone levels for bone turnover in patients on chronic maintenance dialysis. *Am J Kidney Dis* 1995;26:622–631, with permission.)

cases of secondary hyperparathyroidism, patients are both hypercalcemic and hyperphosphatemic, in part because of efflux from bone. It is also important to look at the trend of PTH values with time. Clearly, if the PTH concentration is above 150 pg/mL by intact assay and consistently rising, then the patient almost certainly has high-turnover bone. In contrast, patients with low-turnover bone are often hypercalcemic, in part because of the inability of low-turnover bone to buffer an acute calcium load (89). Bone biopsy is the only way to definitively differentiate if low-turnover bone is the result of adynamic bone or aluminum-induced osteomalacia, although deferoxamine-stimulation tests and random serum aluminum levels occasionally can be helpful, as discussed later.

General Treatment Strategies for Secondary Hyperparathyroidism

The treatment of secondary hyperparathyroidism should begin early in the course of renal failure. As detailed earlier, the ability to excrete a phosphorus load begins to decrease when the GFR approaches 30 to 40 mL/min. The serum

TABLE 17.4. FEATURES OF HIGH-TURNOVER AND LOW-TURNOVER RENAL OSTEODYSTROPHY

	High Turnover	Low Turnover
PTH	Increased	Decreased
Alkaline phosphatase	Increased	Normal
Bone alkaline phosphatase	Increased	Normal or decreased
Osteocalcin	Increased	Normal
Calcium	Variable	Can be increased
Phosphorus	Increased	Normal or increased
DFO stimulation test	Normal	Normal (adynamic) Elevated delta (aluminum OM)
Skeletal radiographs	Resorption, sclerosis	Normal
Symptoms	Usually asymptomatic unless very severe disease	Asymptomatic (adynamic) Symptomatic (aluminum OM)

PTH, parathyroid hormone; DFO; deferoxamine; OM, osteomalacia.

level thus is maintained at a normal level but only because of compensatory increases in serum levels of PTH. Thus, the mainstay of therapy at this level of GFR should be dietary phosphate restriction and consideration of the use of phosphate binders. Treatment with vitamin D compounds probably also should begin at GFR levels less than 30 mL/min. This is more controversial because of an early study demonstrating worsening renal failure with therapy (99). However, other studies have failed to demonstrate this (100,101). If vitamin D analogues are started, close monitoring of serum calcium, phosphorus, and creatinine is indicated. Treatment probably should begin at levels of intact PTH of 80 to 100 pg/mL, with the concept of preventing hyperparathyroidism. Based on animal data, the key to the successful treatment of secondary hyperparathyroidism is to prevent the development of hyperplasia because once that stage is reached, regression is unlikely (102). Unfortunately, recent bone biopsy studies indicate that nearly half of all patients beginning renal replacement therapy have significant secondary hyperparathyroidism (97). Thus, more aggressive and frequent monitoring of serum PTH, phosphorus restriction, and use of vitamin D is indicated in the predialysis patient population and will be recommended in the National Kidney Foundation Kidney/Dialysis Outcome Quality Initiative (NKF-K/DOQI) on Bone and Mineral Metabolism. However, there are no long-term studies of patients treated with this regimen prior to the initiation of dialysis.

For patients undergoing dialysis, the treatment strategies for secondary hyperparathyroidism are threefold: (a) phosphate restriction and use of phosphate binders, (b) normalizing serum calcium, and (c) use of vitamin D analogues. The current strategy is to monitor serum PTH levels quarterly, although more frequent monitoring is indicated, and reimbursed, in cases of more severe hyperparathyroidism or when therapy is adjusted. As detailed earlier, the target PTH is probably around 150–300 pg/mL by the intact assay.

Control of Phosphorus

Successful clinical management of phosphorus consists of several core components: a low phosphorus diet, adequate dialysis, and safe and effective phosphate-binding therapy. The efficacy of each of these components depends on patient compliance—the key for improving phosphorus control.

Phosphorus is contained in almost all foods. Unfortunately, foods high in phosphorus are generally also high in protein, and thus restricting the phosphorus intake means an intake of dietary protein lower than that required for proper nutrition. NKF-K/DOQI dietary guidelines for patients undergoing maintenance hemodialysis include a daily intake of 1.2 grams of protein per kilogram body weight (103). Protein requirements are even higher in patients receiving continuous ambulatory peritoneal dialysis (CAPD) than in patients undergoing hemodialysis because of the efflux of proteins into the dialysate (49,104). As a result, it is challenging to balance dietary phosphate restriction against the need for adequate protein intake, especially with malnutrition present in up to 50% of patients undergoing dialysis (105). Indeed, most well-nourished patients undergoing dialysis are in positive phosphorus balance. Roughly 60% to 70% of consumed phosphate is absorbed, so about 4,000 to 5,000 mg of phosphorus per week enters the extracellular fluid. Therefore, dietary phosphorus restriction alone, although an important component of effective phosphorus management, is not sufficient to control serum phosphorus levels in most patients undergoing dialysis. Table 17.5 lists some suggested alternatives to common foods that are high in phosphorus.

With the limitations of dietary phosphorus restriction, dialysis plays an important role in removing excess phosphorus from the patient's blood, eliminating about 2,700 to 3,000 mg phosphorus per week (106). However, a significant amount of the total body phosphorus is found in the intracellular compartment. Thus, the amount of phosphorus that can be removed during dialysis is limited. Kinetic studies indicate that phosphorus is cleared more efficiently in the first half of a hemodialysis treatment, when serum levels are highest (107). This correlation partly accounts for the rapid fall in serum phosphorus during the first 1 to 2 hours of treatment, followed by a plateau during which serum phosphorus levels remain between 1.9 and 3.4 mg/dL. The rate of phosphorus removal significantly decreases in the second half of treatment and generally is followed by a rebound in serum phosphorus levels in the first 3 to 4 hours following dialysis treatment (108,109). Nocturnal hemodialysis and other slow continuous methods offer a hope for the future because patients using these methods often require phosphorus repletion (110).

Phosphate Binders

Because of the limitations associated with dietary phosphorus restriction and the phosphorus removal with dialysis, dietary phosphate binders are required in nearly all patients undergoing dialysis. Unfortunately, no binder is perfect; the best binder is one the patient will take consistently. Thus, a trial of multiple binder regimens often is required. The dose of phosphate binder should be titrated to dietary intake of phosphorus for both the initial starting dose and subsequent dose adjustments.

Aluminum hydroxide is extremely efficient as a phosphate binder and, consequently, was the primary phosphate binder used from the time of its introduction in 1941 until the mid-1980s. Subsequently, it has been recognized that aluminum is absorbed from the gastrointestinal tract, and accumulation of even small amounts of aluminum in the body can cause toxic side effects such as aluminum bone disease (osteomalacia), dementia, myopathy, and anemia (49,111,112). It now is recognized that all patients undergo-

TABLE 17.5. PHOSPHORUS FOOD GUIDE

High-Phosphorus Food	Suggested Alternative
1 cup yogurt (353 mg)	1 cup sorbet (19 mg)
1/2 cup or 2.5 oz nuts, all kinds (315 mg)	1 cup unsalted popcorn or 1 oz pretzels (24 mg)
1 cup milk (236 mg)	1 cup nondairy creamer (frozen Coffee Rich, Morningstar, Dallas, TX) (132 mg)
1/2 cup macaroni and cheese (220 mg)	1/2 cup pasta noodles with margarine, garlic, and basil (150 mg)
1 oz chocolate (200 mg)	1 oz jelly beans, hard candy, gum drops, marshmallows (1 mg)
1 oz cheese, most kinds (150 mg)	1 oz cream cheese or Neufchatel cheese (34 mg)
1/2 cup bran cereal (143 mg)	1/2 cup cornflakes, rice cereals, or corn cereals (19 mg)
1/2 cup dried beans or peas (143 mg)	1/2 cup green beans or wax beans (19 mg)
1/2 cup custard (142 mg)	1/2 cup custard made with nondairy creamer (frozen Coffee Rich) (110 mg)
2 tbsp peanut butter (118 mg)	2 tbsp jam, jelly, or honey (2 mg)
2 slices of pizza (246 mg)	1 slice of pizza and 1 cup lettuce with Italian dressing (149 mg)
1/2 cup pudding (91 mg)	1/2 cup pudding made with nondairy creamer (frozen Coffee Rich) (33 mg)
1/2 cup oatmeal (88 mg)	1/2 cup cream of wheat or grits (16 mg)
1/2 cup brown rice (81 mg)	1/2 cup white rice (12 mg)
1/2 cup ice cream or ice milk (70 mg)	1/2 cup sherbet (38 mg) or 1 cup sorbet (19 mg)
12 oz cola (44 mg)	12 oz lemon-lime soda, ginger ale, grape soda, or root beer (0 mg)

ing dialysis receiving aluminum-containing binders are at risk for development of aluminum bone disease and other symptoms of aluminum intoxication, although patients with diabetes (113) and children (114) are at particularly high risk. Thus, aluminum-containing binders should be administered only when all other resources to control phosphorus have been exhausted.

Of the available calcium-containing binders, both calcium carbonate and calcium acetate have proven efficacy compared to placebo (115,116). In addition, calcium-containing phosphate binders have been shown to effectively lower phosphorus levels and help prevent the development of secondary hyperparathyroidism (49). Initial studies using sensitive balance studies demonstrated less calcium absorption from calcium acetate compared to calcium carbonate on a gram per gram basis (117,118). However, subsequent studies have not demonstrated consistently that calcium acetate can lead to less hypercalcemic episodes (119). Over the last 10 years, these two calcium-containing phosphate binders have become the mainstay of therapy, with choice depending primarily on patient preference. Other calcium supplements that have been used as phosphate binders include calcium ketoamino acids (120), calcium ketovaline (121), and calcium citrate. However, calcium citrate should be avoided because citrate can increase intestinal absorption of aluminum (122). The main side effects of calcium-containing phosphate binders are constipation, inability to swallow the tablets because of their size, altered taste, and increased calcium load. The latter will be discussed later.

A new noncalcemic, nonaluminum/metal-phosphate binder—sevelamer—received U.S. Food and Drug Administration approval in 1998. This binder is effective in controlling serum phosphorus (123,124) and leads to equivalent phosphate control but less hypercalcemia than does calcium acetate (125). In addition, this phosphate binder can be used together with calcium-containing phosphate binders and may allow the use of more vitamin D (126). This phosphate binder is also unique in that it lowers total cholesterol levels, principally by lowering low-density lipoprotein (LDL) levels (125,126). Recently, this phosphate binder was compared to calcium-containing phosphate binders in a randomized controlled year-long study. All binders showed excellent phosphate binder efficacy and relatively similar Ca X P products. However, sevelamer led to less hypercalcemia and less oversuppression of PTH. In addition, as detailed later, calcium-containing phosphate binders, but not sevelamer, led to progressive cardiac calcification by electron-beam computed tomography (EBCT) (Chertow et al., presented at the 2001 European Dialysis Transplant Association Annual Meeting; see reference 155). The main side effect of sevelamer is gastrointestinal distress, such as bloating, flatulence, and occasionally diarrhea. Unfortunately, sevelamer is much more expensive than the other phosphate binders and generally not affordable for patients in the United States without prescription drug coverage.

Other phosphate binders that are available include magnesium carbonate, usually in combination with calcium acetate. Magnesium carbonate is an effective phosphate binder. However, the dialysate magnesium concentration should be lowered in patients taking oral magnesium (127), which is not practical given that most dialysis units use premixed dialysis baths. Furthermore, no long-term studies have been done. This is of particular concern given that serum magnesium levels are a poor reflection of total body magnesium. Lanthanum carbonate, a heavy metal, has been effective in animal studies (128) and in patients undergoing dialysis in a preliminary report (129), but it is not yet approved. Most recent on the horizon are ferric compounds (130–132), which appear effective in limited studies. The breadth of choices of phosphate binders and the number of agents in development indicate that these medications continue to be the Achilles heel of patients undergoing dialysis with large numbers of pills required to control serum phosphorus. The number of pills required and the gastrointestinal side effects often lead to patient noncompliance. However, the physician and dietitian should be aggressive in finding a regimen agreeable to the patient. Frequent snacking without phosphate binders and taking calcium-based binders with oral iron supplements, which limit effectiveness, also can lead to hyperphosphatemia and can be adjusted easily. Lastly, some of the serum phosphorus derives from bone such that patients with high-bone turnover as a result of severe hyperparathyroidism may have hyperphosphatemia despite compliance with phosphate binders.

Therapy with Vitamin D Analogues

Berl et al. first demonstrated that orally administered 1,25(OH)2D, but not vitamin D_3, suppressed PTH in patients with renal failure (133), confirming that hydroxylation of the sterol at the level of the kidney is required for its actions on PTH. The intravenous formulation was introduced in 1984 by Slatopolsky et al., who found excellent suppression of PTH in patients undergoing hemodialysis who were given high dose (4 mcg) intravenous calcitriol thrice weekly (23). Andress et al. subsequently demonstrated improvement in bone histology with intravenous therapy (134). Unfortunately, this therapy, although quite effective, led to uniform elevations in serum calcium. Sprague and Moe subsequently demonstrated that in patients with mild to moderate hyperparathyroidism, low doses (0.5 to 1 mcg) given intravenously thrice weekly were effective in suppressing PTH with time, and led to only a minimal increase in serum calcium levels (135).

Based on these and many other studies, intravenous pulse calcitriol was felt to be the optimal therapy to allow direct bioavailability to the parathyroid gland and bypass some of the intestinal absorption of calcium and phosphorus. However, in Japan, where intravenous medications are not paid for as they are in the United States, oral pulse calcitriol proved equally efficacious to intravenous calcitriol (136). Subsequent studies also have demonstrated that oral and intravenous calcitriol are equally efficacious with a similar incidence of hypercalcemia and hyperphosphatemia, at least in patients with mild to moderate secondary hyperparathyroidism (137,138). This was followed by our study of patients undergoing peritoneal dialysis (139) and that of Herrmann of patients undergoing hemodialysis (140) demonstrating that daily and pulse therapy of calcitriol, when given in equivalent weekly doses, were also equally efficacious in suppressing PTH. Thus, these studies demonstrate that calcitriol is effective for the treatment of secondary hyperparathyroidism regardless of its route of administration. However, most of these studies treated only mild to moderate hyperparathyroidism. The VDR is downregulated in the PTH glands in advanced hyperparathyroid disease, based on examination of tissue removed during parathyroidectomy (141). In these patients, very high doses may indeed be required. In addition, none of these regimens completely remove the problematic side effect of increased intestinal calcium and phosphorus absorption, leading to the aggressive development of analogues with increased potency at the PTH gland.

Three "less calcemic" analogues are commercially available: 19-nor-1,25(OH)2D (paricalcitol) and 1α(OH)D2 (doxercalciferol) in the United States, and 22-oxa-1,25(OH)2D (OCT) in Japan. All of these analogues appear effective in suppressing hyperparathyroidism in patients with end-stage renal disease (ESRD) (100,142–146). Paricalcitol appears superior to calcitriol in terms of its hypercalcemic and hyperphosphatemic effects in comparison studies in rats (147), but no direct comparison studies in humans have been published. Similarly, there are no comparative trials of doxercalciferol or OCT to calcitriol. The lack of comparative trials makes blanket endorsement of preferential use of any of these analogues over calcitriol premature. Unfortunately, demonstrating this in a randomized comparative trial is difficult, given that the concomitant use of different phosphate binders may alter serum calcium and phosphorus levels independent of the effects of the vitamin D analogues. Doxercalciferol is also available orally, and a direct comparison study of the oral and intravenous formulations indicate that the oral agent may lead to more hypercalcemia than the intravenous formulation (100). At least in the United States, economics appears to drive the preferred analogue used in most dialysis units. Vitamin D also has other extraskeletal effects and is particularly important in cell cycle, leading to its use for the treatment of psoriasis and malignancies. Unfortunately, in the absence of functioning kidneys, the adverse effects of hypercalcemia outweigh any improvement in immune function (148).

Despite aggressive use of calcitriol and other vitamin D analogues, a significant number of patients remain refractory to therapy, either because of hyperphosphatemia and/or hypercalcemia leading to an elevated calcium X phosphorus product (Ca X P), or advanced hyperplasia of the parathyroid glands, rendering the secretion of PTH insuppressible. In these patients surgical parathyroidectomy offers the only current solution to the ill effects of hyperparathyroidism. Katoh et al. have suggested using PTH gland imaging to determine who will and will not respond to calcitriol therapy by detecting enlarged parathyroid glands (149), but this has not become widely accepted and requires a skilled ultrasonography. The surgical technique used for parathyroidectomy is not as important as the skills of the surgeon. The patient who undergoes a parathyroidectomy gets immediate relief of musculoskeletal discomfort and a rapid fall in both serum calcium and phosphorus as a result of the "hungry bone" syndrome. The potential adverse effects of the surgery are primarily recurrent laryngeal nerve damage in addition to the usual anesthetic risks. There has been a tendency to avoid this procedure, but in my opinion, we probably underuse it. Prior to the parathyroidectomy, a bone biopsy should be done to rule out coexistent aluminum bone disease in anyone with significant aluminum exposure. The problem is that the amount of "significant" exposure is unique for each patient, leading some experts to argue that a biopsy should be done in all cases preoperatively (150).

Calcimimetics

New to the horizon are the calcimimetics, pharmaceutical agents that increase the sensitivity of the calcium-sensing receptor in the parathyroid gland, leading to suppression of PTH release by "mimicking" hypercalcemia. The first-generation agents were shown to be very effective in suppressing PTH in animal models of renal failure and in improving bone histology (151,152). The initial trial in humans was encouraging (153); however, the agent had poor bioavailability and difficult pharmacokinetics. This led to the second-generation agent. In the initial studies, this agent proved quite effective in suppressing PTH but with some hypocalcemia (154). The larger, phase II trial had dramatic results: effective suppression of PTH by 26% over 18 weeks and lowering of both calcium and phosphorus, leading to a reduction in the Ca X P product of 17% (155). If subsequent long-term studies confirm these findings, this would be the first PTH-suppressive agent to also lower the Ca X P product. Given the recent studies demonstrating the need to lower the product well beneath previously accepted levels (see later in this chapter), calcimimetics may become an important therapeutic option for secondary hyperparathyroidism.

LOW-TURNOVER BONE DISEASE

Aluminum-Induced Osteomalacia

As detailed earlier, low-turnover bone disease in patients undergoing dialysis is generally the result of aluminum-induced osteomalacia or adynamic bone. In aluminum-induced osteomalacia, aluminum deposits at the mineralization front, leading to impaired mineralization and subsequent accumulation of unmineralized bone, or osteoid. The potential toxicity of aluminum initially was recognized by Alfrey et al., who identified a fatal neurologic syndrome in patients undergoing dialysis consisting of dyspraxia, seizures, and electroencephalogram abnormalities in association with high brain aluminum levels on autopsy (156,157). The source of aluminum in these severe cases was felt to be elevated concentrations in dialysate water. Subsequently, aluminum-containing phosphate binders also were identified as a source (158–160). The additional symptoms of fractures, myopathy, and microcytic anemia were described several years after the initial reports of the neurologic syndrome (160,161). In the more recent Toronto bone biopsy study, where unselected patients at three dialysis units underwent bone biopsies and noninvasive tests (n = 259), 69 patients had aluminum bone disease defined as greater than 25% surface aluminum staining. In this series, aluminum bone disease was the most common bone histologic disorder associated with proximal myopathy, pathologic fractures, unexplained bone pain, microcytic anemia, and hypercalcemia (162). The ingestion of aluminum-containing phosphate binders, sucralfate, and some over-the-counter antacids also can lead to aluminum accumulation (163). Children, diabetics, and individuals taking citrate are at increased risk of developing the disease (114,122,164).

The diagnosis of aluminum-induced bone disease can be difficult because aluminum toxicity is the result of tissue burden, not serum levels. Milliner et al. first described the deferoxamine stimulation test, where serum aluminum levels are induced to rise, by administering the chelator deferoxamine. An increment in plasma aluminum concentration of 200 μg/L was the threshold for best specificity (93%) but poor sensitivity (43%) (165). Pei et al. later found that the specificity of the deferoxamine stimulation test improved in patients with low levels of intact PTH (<200 pg/mL). However, the sensitivity of the test remains poor at 48% to 66% (162). Serum aluminum levels are also not predictive, with poor sensitivity and specificity (166). Thus, bone biopsy remains the gold standard. Treatment of aluminum bone disease is with deferoxamine, 1 g/week posthemodialysis or intraperitoneally. The duration of therapy must be individualized but is usually 6 months to 1 year. The treatment is beneficial, with a dramatic improvement in musculoskeletal symptoms (112) and bone histology (167) in nearly all patients. Unfortunately, the treatment is not without adverse effects including hearing loss, retinal damage, and infection with mucormycosis. The latter is nearly always fatal (168). These adverse effects were much more common when patients were treated with deferoxamine each dialysis treatment, as opposed to the current standard therapy of once-weekly administration. Fortunately, this disease is now uncommon, at least in the United

States, where aluminum-containing phosphate binders rarely are used.

Adynamic Bone Disease

In contrast to aluminum-induced osteomalacia where there is abnormal bone mineralization, in adynamic bone disease there is a paucity of cells with resultant low bone turnover. In addition, in contrast to osteomalacia in adynamic bone, there is no increase in osteoid or unmineralized bone. The lack of bone-cell activity led to the initial description of the disease as "aplastic" bone disease. Early studies felt the disease was still the result of aluminum, but it later was identified in the absence of positive staining for aluminum (40, 169). As shown earlier, the disease is increasing in prevalence and is particularly common in patients undergoing peritoneal dialysis (82,170). Various risk factors have been identified: diabetes, treatment with peritoneal dialysis, older age, high calcium dialysate, and white race (91,171–174). In addition, some of the low PTH is secondary to oversuppression with calcitriol (175) or with calcium load because changing to a low calcium dialysate (176) or sevelamer, a non–calcium-containing phosphate binder (177), can increase the PTH. Patients with adynamic bone disease are often asymptomatic, however, they are at increased risk of hypercalcemia as a result of the inability of bone to buffer an acute calcium load (89). The relative lack of symptoms usually can help differentiate aluminum-induced bone disease, which is often symptomatic, from adynamic bone disease. Theoretically, the lack of cells in adynamic bone disease may impair the ability of bone to repair microfractures and predispose to fractures. Indeed, low levels of PTH have been identified as risk factors for fracture (178, 179), which are particularly common in patients with ESRD (179,180). However, these studies did not examine bone histology. Clearly, longitudinal studies of patients with biopsy-proven adynamic bone disease are needed.

What Is the Optimal Phosphorus, Calcium, and Calcium X Phosphorus Product?

In the past, a Ca X P product of 70 mg^2/dL^2 was considered the threshold above which calcitriol should be withheld, thereby reducing the ability to use vitamin D therapy. This was felt to be the level above which metastatic calcification occurred. Unfortunately, this level of 70 was based on theoretic, *in vitro* data and extrapolations from case reports (181–183). In addition, this number originated when the process by which calcium and phosphorus deposited into tissues in the form of hydroxyapatite was felt to be purely the result of physicochemical interactions and supersaturation. However, there is now clear evidence in nondialysis patients that the process of vascular calcification is cell mediated with production of bone matrix proteins by vascular smooth-muscle cells (184–188). The production of these "bone" matrix proteins in calcification of the arterioles of skin (calciphylaxis) and in calcification in the inferior epigastric artery of patients undergoing dialysis also has been demonstrated (189,190). Thus, vascular calcification is clearly a cell-mediated process. *In vitro* work has demonstrated that vascular smooth-muscle cells can mineralize in the presence of elevated phosphorus concentrations (191), similar to the mechanisms for phosphorus-induced bone mineralization. The *in vitro* concentrations required to induce mineralization in vascular cells are well within the range of serum phosphorus observed in the majority of patients undergoing dialysis.

Epidemiologic studies have demonstrated that the serum phosphorus and the calcium X phosphorus product are associated with poor outcomes. Lowrie and Lew found that serum phosphorus levels greater than 7.0 mg/dL were associated with increased mortality (192), and Block et al. found that serum phosphorus levels greater than 6.5 mg/dL were associated with increased mortality (193). The latter study also demonstrated that a calcium X phosphorus product greater than 73 mg^2/dL^2 was associated with increased mortality, principally as a result of the effects of phosphorus (193). These studies were from data sets from more than 10 years ago, during the widespread use of aluminum-containing phosphate binders, and before aggressive use of vitamin D metabolites for the treatment of secondary hyperparathyroidism. However, the association of elevated serum phosphorus and mortality was confirmed by Chertow et al., who found an 88% higher relative risk of death for patients undergoing hemodialysis with serum phosphorus levels of more than 9 mg/dL compared to patients with phosphorus levels in the reference range of 5 to 6 mg/dL (194). He also found that the relative risk of death correlated directly to serum calcium levels, increasing 47% as the calcium level rises from 9 to 9.5 mg/dL to more than 11 mg/dL (194). Elevated serum phosphorus also is associated with poor outcomes in European studies (195). These studies suggest that to prevent mortality, the phosphorus should be less than 6.5 to 7.0 mg/dL, and the calcium should be less than 11 mg/dL. These values are for mortality—what about morbidity?

As discussed in the section on physiology, serum levels of calcium and phosphorus in patients undergoing dialysis may not accurately reflect total body balance because the normal homeostatic control mechanisms are impaired. As noted by Hsu et al., we probably have been overemphasizing serum levels and underemphasizing balance. We are successful in removing some phosphorus with dialysis (106) but clearly not enough to keep up with dietary intake, even with the use of phosphate binders, resulting in positive phosphorus balance. Nearly all patients are in positive calcium balance as well, regardless of the serum level of calcium. Patients have a net positive calcium influx during hemodialysis, even with the use of "low" (2.5 meq/L) calcium dialysate solution, thus adding to the total body calcium load (196). Patients undergoing CAPD experience an average net positive calcium balance of +122 mg/day to +198 mg/day depending on the amount of protein in the diet. Assuming both hemodialysis and peritoneal dialysis patients consume only 800 mg/day of dietary calcium, the calculated daily calcium balance for adult (ages 18 to 30) patients undergoing dialysis would exceed the average normal calcium threshold balance of 114 mg/day (2,196). Furthermore, patients receiving dialysis may be expected to absorb approximately 20% to 30% of the calcium ingested from calcium-containing phosphate binders (49,117,118). This additional calcium, combined with the calcium influx from the dialysate, results in positive calcium balance, as illustrated in Fig. 17.9. In normal individuals, this excessive calcium and phosphorus load is excreted in the urine; however, patients undergoing dialysis are effectively a "closed box," with retention of both calcium and phosphorus. The result, especially with calcium-containing phosphate binders, is that nearly all patients are in positive calcium balance. In individuals without renal failure, once linear bone growth stops around age 25 to 30 years, nature provides for neutral calcium balance (197). Thus, when we consider the age of our patients and the abnormal bone remodeling in renal failure, patients are clearly calcium and phosphorus overloaded.

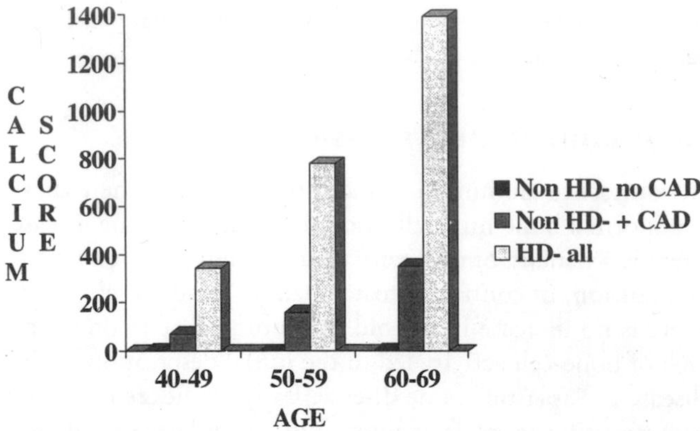

FIGURE 17.10. Median coronary artery calcification score in patients undergoing dialysis by electron-beam CT scan (EBCT). Fifty-seven patients undergoing hemodialysis (HD) were imaged by EBCT, and their calcification scores were determined. The results were compared to age-matched nondialysis patients with angiographically proven coronary artery disease (non-HD + CAD) and without angiographically proven coronary artery disease (non-HD − no CAD). The results demonstrate that patients undergoing dialysis have twofold to fivefold more coronary artery calcification than patients with proven coronary artery disease. (From Braun J, Oldendorf M, Moshage W, et al. Electron beam computed tomography in the evaluation of cardiac calcification in chronic dialysis patients. *Am J Kidney Dis* 1996;27:394–401, with permission.)

What evidence is there to support adverse outcomes with positive calcium and phosphorus balance and/or serum levels? In addition to the mortality data mentioned earlier, there is growing evidence for an adverse effect of mineral metabolism on the vascular system. This phenomenon has become easier to document with the advances in imaging in the recent decade, including EBCT scan and duplex ultrasonography. These techniques are much more reproducible than the older method of observing progression of vascular calcification on plain radiographs. EBCT allows rapid imaging of the heart in diastole, such that calcification in the coronary arteries can be distinguished and quantified easily. Braun et al. found in 1996 that patients undergoing hemodialysis had markedly increased coronary artery calcification compared to age- and sex-matched nonrenal failure individuals with angiographically proven coronary artery disease (Fig. 17.10). Furthermore, valvular calcification was present in 50% of patients, and the coronary artery calcification increased in all 57 patients over the course of 1 to 2 years (198). Goodman et al. found that this calcification

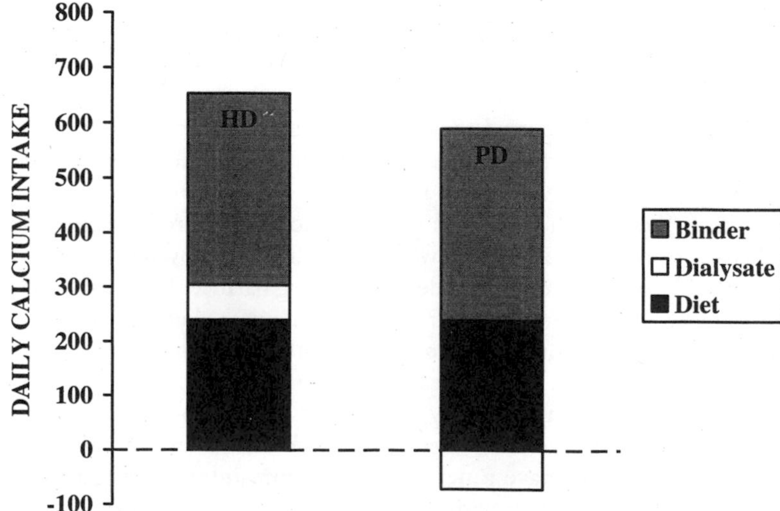

FIGURE 17.9. Daily calcium intake in patients undergoing dialysis with calcium-containing phosphate binders in hemodialysis (HD) and peritoneal dialysis (PD) patients. Patients undergoing dialysis ingest approximately 500 to 800 mg of calcium in their diet per day. If one conservatively assumes 20% to 40% absorption (2), approximately 300 mg per day of elemental calcium is absorbed. The dialysate with a 2.5-mEq bath leads to a minor influx of calcium in patients undergoing hemodialysis and a minor efflux in patients undergoing peritoneal dialysis (106,196). The remainder of the calcium ingested is from calcium-containing phosphate binders. Assuming the patient takes three tablets of calcium acetate with each of three meals (1.5 grams of elemental calcium) and absorbs 350 mg (117), the patient will be in net positive calcium balance of 600 to 700 mg per day.

also affected children and young adults undergoing dialysis. They demonstrated that the patients with increased coronary artery calcification were on dialysis for a longer time, had an elevated Ca X P product (65 + 10.6 versus 56.4 + 12.7 mg^2/dL^2, $p = 0.04$), increased intake of calcium-containing phosphate binder (6,456 + 4,278 versus 3,325 + 1,490 mg/day, $p = 0.02$), experienced a trend toward higher phosphorus levels (6.9 + 0.3 versus 6.3 + 1.2 mg/dL, $p = 0.06$), and had no difference in the serum calcium levels (203). Kimura et al. found an elevated Ca X P product of more than $60^2/dL^2$ on more than 25% of measurements correlated with severity of aortic calcification by abdominal CT (199). Marchais et al. found that patients with hyperphosphatemia of more than 6.2 mg/dL had higher diastolic and mean blood pressure and increased cardiac index caused by increased stroke index and heart rate. They also found increased carotid artery tensile stress in the patients who were hyperphosphatemic (200). This same group subsequently found increased arterial calcification was associated with increased intake of calcium-containing phosphate binders (201). In vascular calcification of the small arterioles of the skin (calciphylaxis), Ahmed et al. found elevated phosphorus and Ca X P product to be a risk factor in a case control study (189). This was confirmed by Mazhar et al., who found that the risk of calciphylaxis increased 3.51-fold for each mg/dL increase in serum phosphorus levels (202). Thus, there is mounting evidence that disturbances of mineral metabolism in renal failure contributes to the excessive cardiovascular disease observed in patients undergoing dialysis.

Although the molecular mechanisms responsible for vascular calcification in chronic renal failure are not yet fully elucidated, recent studies indicate that the process is similar to bone formation and involves bone-associated proteins and imbalances in calcium homeostasis (177,203). Recent morphologic analysis of coronary atherosclerotic lesions in patients with ESRD revealed that coronary plaques are more heavily calcified than in nonuremic control patients and the vessels are characterized by increased medial layer thickness with calcification (204). Extensive calcium content of atherosclerotic plaques and of the medial layer of arteries in patients with renal failure may contribute to the high rates of cardiovascular morbidity and mortality in these patients. Thus, techniques such as EBCT or spiral CT, may be particularly useful to detect both atherosclerotic plaque and medial-layer calcification. However, to date there are no studies using either technique demonstrating predictive value for future cardiac events or mortality in patients undergoing dialysis. However, an elevated calcium content in the coronary arteries does correlate with a history of coronary artery disease, peripheral vascular disease, and cerebrovascular disease in patients undergoing dialysis (205). The results of the recent randomized controlled trial comparing the phosphate binder sevelamer to calcium-containing phosphate binders using EBCT as one of the endpoints confirmed the role of calcium load. In the 80% of patients who had calcification at baseline, patients treated with sevelamer had a 6% (nonsignificant) increase in progression of coronary artery calcification, whereas patients treated with calcium-containing binders had a 25% (significant) increase in their median coronary artery calcification scores. This occurred despite excellent and equivalent phosphorus control (<5.5 mg/dL) and Ca X P product in both groups. Thus, the differences are most likely the result of the excess calcium load with the calcium-containing phosphate binders, although decreased levels of LDL cholesterol with sevelamer also may contribute (155). Whether this translates to improved outcomes remains to be determined.

Based on treatment approaches that were commonly used during the last decade, 60% of patients undergoing dialysis have serum phosphorus levels above 5.5 mg/dL (the usual upper limit of normal) and 40% of patients undergoing dialysis have a Ca X P product of more than 60 mg^2/dL^2 (193,206). It now appears that we may have been "accepting the unacceptable" (206). Previously accepted Ca X P product levels now are known to be associated with significant extraskeletal calcification and mortality. Excess total body calcium load, even in the presence of normal serum calcium and phosphorus levels, also may contribute to coronary calcification. Thus, we need to strive for lower values in our patients (206), which will be reflected in the target goals for the new bone and mineral NKF-K/DOQI: serum phosphorus levels at 3.5 to 5.5 mg/dL, Ca X P product below 55 mg^2/dL^2, and serum intact PTH levels near 150 to 300 pg/mL. Our ability to achieve these goals has improved dramatically with the advent of effective noncalcemic phosphate binders and less calcemic vitamin D analogues. The potential addition of calcimimetics to our regimen also will make these once formidable goals truly achievable.

Renal Transplant Bone Disease

Ideally, all of these complications of calcium and phosphorus imbalance and renal osteodystrophy would be cured with renal transplantation. Unfortunately, in many cases, renal transplantation returns individuals to chronic kidney disease and not normal renal function. In these patients, only partial improvement is observed. However, in the vast majority of cases aluminum-staining resolves, as does secondary hyperparathyroidism, although this can take longer. There are also unique bone and mineral metabolism disorders in the transplant recipient: hypophosphatemia and avascular necrosis. The etiology of the former is multifactorial and the subject of an excellent recent review (207). Avascular necrosis continues to plague transplant recipients, with little advancement of our understanding of the disease or effective therapies (208–210). Core decompression and joint replacement surgery remain the best treatment options (211).

There are limited studies evaluating bone histology in recipients of renal transplants. However, there appears to be a persistent mineralization defect (212). In some studies bone turnover normalized (212), but in others there is low turnover with histology consistent with adynamic bone disease (213). However, longitudinal studies are lacking. There does appear to be a consistent decrease in bone mineral densitometry, although more recent studies (214–216) have not found the dramatic decrease initially described (212). There is a corresponding increased fracture risk, although this risk is less than that observed with other solid organ transplants (217–221). The use of corticosteroids is the major determinant of low bone mass because these agents impair calcium absorption from the gastrointestinal tract and inhibit bone cell recruitment and function (222).

The diagnosis of corticosteroid induced osteoporosis (CIO) is best done with dual X-ray absorptiometry (DEXA) of the hips and spine for assessment of changes in trabecular bone. Osteoporosis, regardless of its etiology, is defined as a *t* score less than 2.5 standard deviations from the norm, which is a young adult mean. The rationale for use of this comparison group is that it is measuring current bone mass to peak bone mass. Furthermore, this value is the threshold below which there is increased fracture risk (223). This threshold value was confirmed in 2000 for corticosteroid-induced osteoporosis (224). The treatment for corticosteroid-induced osteoporosis is similar to that for other forms of osteoporosis: antiresorptive agents (osteoclast inhibitors) such as bisphosphonates, calcitonin, and estrogen in deficient women. There is substantial evidence from controlled trials in nontransplant, corticosteroid-induced osteoporosis that these agents, particularly bisphosphonates, are effective in preventing steroid-induced osteoporosis (225–227). However, there is only minimal controlled data on treatments with bisphosphonates available in renal transplantation (215,228). Theoretically, if there is adynamic bone in renal transplant patients, then bisphosphonates could worsen the disease by inhibiting the already defective bone-cell function. However, studies have not clearly demonstrated this. Thus, although there is concern about potential long-term consequences, the data to date support the use of antiresorptive therapies to prevent corticosteroid-induced osteoporosis. This last point deserves further emphasis: they are only effective in preventing bone loss and must be administered during the large dose of steroids given in the first 6 months posttransplant. Given the lack of longitudinal data and the long half-life of bisphosphonates (>15 to 20 years), only 6 months to 1 year of therapy should be given. The role of cyclosporin in this disease is somewhat controversial (219). However, recent studies in patients with kidney transplant showed a beneficial effect in corticosteroid-induced osteoporosis (229).

Ideally, there would be anabolic agents that actually build bone through stimulation of osteoblasts. Fluoride was the initial drug in this class, but longitudinal studies did not demonstrate benefit (230). PTH, when given subcutaneously in low, intermittent doses, is actually anabolic and a newly available treatment for osteoporosis (231) and corticosteroid-induced osteoporosis (232–234). This therapy has not been given to patients with renal impairment. New to the horizon is OPG as detailed earlier in this chapter, which appears promising in Phase I trials (79). This agent is particularly exciting for corticosteroid osteoporosis because the protein is known to be downregulated by corticosteroids *in vitro* (75,76). Thus, although the future is promising, we lack conclusive data on the optimal treatment at this time. That said, it is likely that patients will benefit from treatment with bisphosphonate or nasal spray calcitonin during the first 6 months of transplant when the greatest dose of steroids are given. This is also true for patients who are receiving corticosteroids for nontransplant purposes, such as treatment of glomerulonephritis.

Osteoporosis in Patients Undergoing Dialysis

The aging general population has brought great understanding and more aggressive treatments for osteoporosis. Given that the average age of patients undergoing dialysis is increasing, it is not surprising that many of these patients also suffer from osteoporosis. Osteoporosis is defined as a decrease in bone mass and is best quantified by DEXA. This test can detect only the overall density—not how the bone is arranged. In contrast to osteoporosis, renal osteodystrophy is a disorder of bone remodeling with resultant abnormal "arrangement" or histology. Renal osteodystrophy is best diagnosed by bone biopsy and can occur in the setting of decreased or increased overall bone mass. Thus, both osteoporosis and renal osteodystrophy can occur together in patients with ESRD. The appreciation of the potential impact of osteoporosis in patients undergoing dialysis has been through the work of Coco and Rush and Alem et al., demonstrating a substantial increase in the relative risk (fourfold to 18-fold) of hip fracture in patients undergoing dialysis compared to matched nondialysis patients (179, 180). In the latter study, a hip fracture in a patient undergoing dialysis was associated with a doubling of the mortality observed in hip fractures in nondialysis patients; in males the mortality increased from 36% to 61%, and in females it increased from 21% to 42% (179). The risk factors leading to hip fracture are multifactorial: age, female sex, white race, duration of dialysis, low PTH levels, and presence of peripheral vascular disease (179,235). However, none of these studies examined bone histology to determine the true impact of renal osteodystrophy. Indeed, it is not surprising that we see increased risk of hip fractures in patients undergoing dialysis when one considers all the risk factors. Both men and women frequently are hypogonadal ("renopause"); there is a J-shaped relationship with fractures and PTH in renal osteodystrophy (178,179), and the deposition

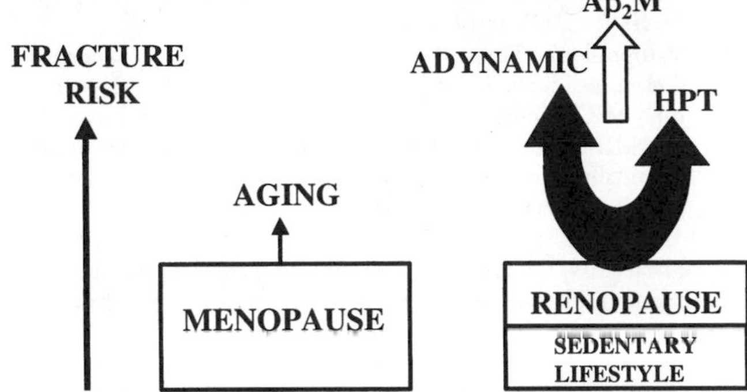

FIGURE 17.11. Fracture risk in end-stage renal disease. Patients undergoing dialysis have an increased risk of fracture compared to age-matched members of the general population as a result of multiple factors. These include a sedentary lifestyle, hypogonadism or "renopause," the J-shaped relationship of bone remodeling or turnover known as renal osteodystrophy, and the presence of β-2-microglobulin amyloidosis.

of β-2-microglobulin amyloid further increases fracture risk (236) (Fig. 17.11). The multifactorial cause of the problem increases the complexity of the therapeutic approach, and there are no studies to help guide therapy. Again, this is an important area for future research.

CONCLUSION

Multiple abnormalities of bone and mineral metabolism are observed in patients with renal failure. Our understanding of the cellular biology of parathyroid hormone and vitamin D in the last decade have led to new therapies that allow more aggressive treatment of renal osteodystrophy with less toxicity. This latter point is particularly important with the data of the role of abnormal mineral metabolism accumulating in cardiovascular disease, the leading cause of death in patients undergoing dialysis. Although significant progress has been made in our understanding of these disease states, there is much more knowledge to be gained.

ACKNOWLEDGMENTS

This chapter is dedicated to John and Michelle Moe for their unending support and patience. The author would like to thank Ms. Anni Hine for her expert administrative support in the preparation of this chapter.

REFERENCES

1. Walden O. The relationship of dietary and supplemental calcium intake to bone loss and osteoporosis. *J Am Diet Assoc* 1989; 89:397–400.
2. Coburn JW, Hartenbower DL, Massry SG. Intestinal absorption of calcium and the effect of renal insufficiency. *Kidney Int* 1973;4:96–104.
3. Favus MJ. Intestinal absorption of calcium, magnesium, and phosphorus. In: Coe FL, Favus MJ, eds. *Disorders of bone and mineral metabolism.* New York: Raven Press, Ltd., 1993:57–81.
4. Heaney R, Skillman T. Secretion and excretion of calcium by the human gastrointestinal tract. *J Lab Clin Med* 1964;64: 29–41.
5. Nordin BE. *Absorption of calcium, phosphorus and magnesium.* New York: Churchill Livingstone, 1976.
6. Delmez JA. Avoiding renal osteodystrophy in peritoneal dialysis patients. *Semin Dial* 1995;8:373–377.
7. Slatopolsky E, Bricker NS. The role of phosphorus restriction in the prevention of secondary hyperparathyroidism in chronic renal disease. *Kidney Int* 1973;4:141–145.
8. Slatopolsky E, Robson AM, Elkan I, et al. Control of phosphate excretion in uremic man. *J Clin Invest* 1968;47:1865–1874.
9. Brenner BM. *Disturbances of renal function.* New York: McGraw-Hill, 1994.
10. Martin KJ, Hruska KA, Lewis J, et al. The renal handling of parathyroid hormone. Role of peritubular uptake and glomerular filtration. *J Clin Invest* 1977;60:808–814.
11. Segre GV, Perkins AS, Witters LA, et al. Metabolism of parathyroid hormone by isolated rat Kupffer cells and hepatocytes. *J Clin Invest* 1981;67:449–457.
12. Brown EM. Four-parameter model of the sigmoidal relationship between parathyroid hormone release and extracellular calcium concentration in normal and abnormal parathyroid tissue. *J Clin Endocrinol Metab* 1983;56:572–581.
13. Brown EM, Gamba G, Riccardi D, et al. Cloning and characterization of an extracellular Ca(2+)-sensing receptor from bovine parathyroid. *Nature* 1993;366:575–580.
14. Pollak MR, Brown EM, Chou YH, et al. Mutations in the human Ca(2+)-sensing receptor gene cause familial hypocalciuric hypercalcemia and neonatal severe hyperparathyroidism. *Cell* 1993;75:1297–1303.
15. Pollak MR, Brown EM, Estep HL, et al. Autosomal dominant hypocalcaemia caused by a Ca(2+)-sensing receptor gene mutation. *Nat Genet* 1994;8:303–307.
16. Hebert SC. Extracellular calcium-sensing receptor: implications for calcium and magnesium handling in the kidney. *Kidney Int* 1996;50:2129–2139.
17. Brown EM, Pollak M, Hebert SC. Sensing of extracellular Ca2+ by parathyroid and kidney cells: cloning and characterization of an extracellular Ca(2+)-sensing receptor. *Am J Kidney Dis* 1995;25:506–513.
18. Drueke TB. Cell biology of parathyroid gland hyperplasia in chronic renal failure. *J Am Soc Nephrol* 2000;11:1141–1152.
19. Naveh-Many T, Rahamimov R, Livni N, et al. Parathyroid cell proliferation in normal and chronic renal failure rats. The effects of calcium, phosphate, and vitamin D. *J Clin Invest* 1995;96: 1786–1793.
20. Moallem E, Kilav R, Silver J, et al. RNA-Protein binding and post-transcriptional regulation of parathyroid hormone gene expression by calcium and phosphate. *J Biol Chem* 1998;273: 5253–5259.
21. Yalcindag C, Silver J, Naveh-Many T. Mechanism of increased parathyroid hormone mRNA in experimental uremia: roles of protein RNA binding and RNA degradation. *J Am Soc Nephrol* 1999;10:2562–2568.
22. Brown AJ, Ritter CS, Finch JL, et al. Decreased calcium-sensing receptor expression in hyperplastic parathyroid glands of uremic rats: role of dietary phosphate. *Kidney Int* 1999;55:1284–1292.
23. Slatopolsky E, Weerts C, Thielan J, et al. Marked suppression of secondary hyperparathyroidism by intravenous administra-

tion of 1,25-dihydroxy-cholecalciferol in uremic patients. *J Clin Invest* 1984;74:2136–2143.
24. Delmez JA, Tindira C, Grooms P, et al. Parathyroid hormone suppression by intravenous 1,25-dihydroxyvitamin D. A role for increased sensitivity to calcium. *J Clin Invest* 1989;83: 1349–1355.
25. Ouseph R, Leiser JD, Moe SM. Calcitriol and the parathyroid hormone-ionized calcium curve: a comparison of methodologic approaches. *J Am Soc Nephrol* 1996;7:497–505.
26. Almaden Y, Hernandez A, Torregrosa V, et al. High phosphate level directly stimulates parathyroid hormone secretion and synthesis by human parathyroid tissue in vitro. *J Am Soc Nephrol* 1998;9:1845–1852.
27. de Francisco AL, Cobo MA, Setien MA, et al. Effect of serum phosphate on parathyroid hormone secretion during hemodialysis. *Kidney Int* 1998;54:2140–2145.
28. Felsenfeld AJ, Rodriguez M. Phosphorus, regulation of plasma calcium, and secondary hyperparathyroidism: a hypothesis to integrate a historical and modern perspective. *J Am Soc Nephrol* 1999;10:878–890.
29. Juppner H, Abou-Samra AB, Freeman M, et al. A G protein-linked receptor for parathyroid hormone and parathyroid hormone-related peptide. *Science* 1991;254:1024–1026.
30. Massry SG. Neurotoxicity of parathyroid hormone in uremia. *Kidney Int Suppl* 1985;17:S5–11.
31. Slatopolsky E, Martin K, Hruska K. Parathyroid hormone metabolism and its potential as a uremic toxin. *Am J Physiol* 1980; 239:F1–12.
32. Potts JT Jr. Non-traditional actions of parathyroid hormone: an overview. *Miner Electrolyte Metab* 1995;21:9–12.
33. Feinfeld D. The role of parathyroid hormone as a uremic toxin: current concepts. *Semin Dial* 1992;5:48–53.
34. Abou-Samra AB, Juppner H, Force T, et al. Expression cloning of a common receptor for parathyroid hormone and parathyroid hormone-related peptide from rat osteoblast-like cells: a single receptor stimulates intracellular accumulation of both cAMP and inositol trisphosphates and increases intracellular free calcium. *Proc Natl Acad Sci U S A* 1992;89:2732–2736.
35. Segre GV. *Receptors for parathyroid hormone and parathyroid hormone-related protein.* New York: Academic Press, 1996.
36. Karaplis AC, Luz A, Glowacki J, et al. Lethal skeletal dysplasia from targeted disruption of the parathyroid hormone-related peptide gene. *Genes Dev* 1994;8:277–289.
37. Suva LJ, Winslow GA, Wettenhall RE, et al. A parathyroid hormone-related protein implicated in malignant hypercalcemia: cloning and expression. *Science* 1987;237:893–896.
38. Strewler GJ. The physiology of parathyroid hormone-related protein. *N Engl J Med* 2000;342:177–185.
39. Endres DB, Villanueva R, Sharp CF Jr, et al. Measurement of parathyroid hormone. *Endocrinol Metab Clin North Am* 1989; 18:611–629.
40. Cohen-Solal ME, Sebert JL, Boudailliez B. Comparison of intact, midregion, and carboxy-terminal assays of parathyroid hormone for the diagnosis of bone disease in hemodialyzed patients. *J Clin Endocrinol Metab* 1991;73:516–524.
41. Wang M, Hercz G, Sherrard DJ, et al. Relationship between intact 1-84 parathyroid hormone and bone histomorphometric parameters in dialysis patients without aluminum toxicity. *Am J Kidney Dis* 1995;26:836–844.
42. Qi Q, Monier-Faugere MC, Geng Z, et al. Predictive value of serum parathyroid hormone levels for bone turnover in patients on chronic maintenance dialysis. *Am J Kidney Dis* 1995;26: 622–631.
43. Gao P, Scheibel S, D'Amour P, et al. Development of a novel immunoradiometric assay exclusively for biologically active whole parathyroid hormone 1-84: implications for improvement of accurate assessment of parathyroid function. *J Bone Miner Res* 2001;16:605–614.
44. Slatopolsky E, Finch J, Clay P, et al. A novel mechanism for skeletal resistance in uremia. *Kidney Int* 2000;58:753–761.
45. John MR, Goodman WG, Gao P, et al. A novel immunoradiometric assay detects full-length human PTH but not amino-terminally truncated fragments: implications for PTH measurements in renal failure. *J Clin Endocrinol Metab* 1999;84: 4287–4290.
46. Massry SG, Coburn JW, Lee DB, et al. Skeletal resistance to parathyroid hormone in renal failure. Studies in 105 human subjects. *Ann Intern Med* 1973;78:357–364.
47. Urena P, Ferreira A, Kung VT, et al. Serum pyridinoline as a specific marker of collagen breakdown and bone metabolism in hemodialysis patients. *J Bone Miner Res* 1995;10:932–939.
48. Brickman AS, Coburn JW, Massry SG, et al. 1,25 Dihydroxy-vitamin D3 in normal man and patients with renal failure. *Ann Intern Med* 1974;80:161–168.
49. Delmez JA, Slatopolsky E. Hyperphosphatemia: its consequences and treatment in patients with chronic renal disease. *Am J Kidney Dis* 1992;19:303–317.
50. Silver J, Naveh-Many T, Mayer H, et al. Regulation by vitamin D metabolites of parathyroid hormone gene transcription in vivo in the rat. *J Clin Invest* 1986;78:1296–1301.
51. Roodman GD, Ibbotson KJ, MacDonald BR, et al. 1,25-Dihydroxyvitamin D3 causes formation of multinucleated cells with several osteoclast characteristics in cultures of primate marrow. *Proc Natl Acad Sci U S A* 1985;82:8213–8217.
52. Holick MF, Krane SM, Potts JT Jr. *Calcium, phosphorus, and bone metabolism: calcium-regulating hormones.* New York: McGraw-Hill, 1994.
53. Holick MF. *Vitamin D: photobiology, metabolism, mechanism of action, and clinical applications*, 4th ed. Philadelphia: Lippincott Williams & Wilkins, 1999.
54. Milde P, Merke J, Ritz E, et al. Immunohistochemical detection of 1,25-dihydroxyvitamin D3 receptors and estrogen receptors by monoclonal antibodies: comparison of four immunoperoxidase methods. *J Histochem Cytochem* 1989;37:1609–1617.
55. Berger U, Wilson P, McClelland RA, et al. Immunocytochemical detection of 1,25-dihydroxyvitamin D receptors in normal human tissues. *J Clin Endocrinol Metab* 1988;67:607–613.
56. Rice JS, Haverty T. Vitamin D and immune function in uremia. *Semin Dial* 1990;3:237–239.
57. Reichel H, Koeffler HP, Norman AW. The role of the vitamin D endocrine system in health and disease (see comments). *N Engl J Med* 1989;320:980–991.
58. Levitan IB. It is calmodulin after all! Mediator of the calcium modulation of multiple ion channels. *Neuron* 1999;22: 645–648.
59. Hoenderop JG, van der Kemp AW, Hartog A, et al. Molecular identification of the apical Ca2+ channel in 1, 25-dihydroxyvitamin D3-responsive epithelia. *J Biol Chem* 1999;274: 8375–8378.
60. Favus MJ. Factors that influence absorption and secretion of calcium in the small intestine and colon. *Am J Physiol* 1985; 248:G147–157.
61. Sheikh MS, Ramirez A, Emmett M, et al. Role of vitamin D-dependent and vitamin D-independent mechanisms in absorption of food calcium. *J Clin Invest* 1988;81:126–132.
62. Hurwitz S. Homeostatic control of plasma calcium concentration. *Crit Rev Biochem Mol Biol* 1996;31:41–100.
63. Lemann J Jr, Favus MJ. The intestinal absorption of calcium, magnesium, and phosphate. In: Favus MJ, ed. *Primer on the metabolic bone diseases and disorders of mineral metabolism*, 4th ed. Philadelphia: Lippincott Williams & Wilkins, 1999:63–67.

64. Murer H, Forster I, Hilfiker H, et al. Cellular/molecular control of renal Na/Pi-cotransport. *Kidney Int Suppl* 1998;65:S2–10.
65. Baum MA, Harris HW. Recent insights into the coordinate regulation of body water and divalent mineral ion metabolism. *Am J Med Sci* 1998;316:321–328.
66. Hoenderop JG, Muller D, Van Der Kemp AW, et al. Calcitriol controls the epithelial calcium channel in kidney. *J Am Soc Nephrol* 2001;12:1342–1349.
67. Lotscher M, Kaissling B, Biber J, et al. Role of microtubules in the rapid regulation of renal phosphate transport in response to acute alterations in dietary phosphate content. *J Clin Invest* 1997;99:1302–1312.
68. Friedlander G. Regulation of renal phosphate handling: recent findings. *Curr Opin Nephrol Hypertens* 1996;5:316–320.
69. Henry HL, Norman AW. Vitamin D: metabolism and biological actions. *Annu Rev Nutr* 1984;4:493–520.
70. Kurokawa K. Calcium-regulating hormones and the kidney (clinical conference). *Kidney Int* 1987;32:760–771.
71. Turner CH, Chandran A, Pidaparti RM. The anisotropy of osteonal bone and its ultrastructural implications. *Bone* 1995; 17:85–89.
72. Bonn D. Crumbling bones yield to molecular biology. *Lancet* 1999;353:1596.
73. Blair HC. How the osteoclast degrades bone. *Bioessays* 1998; 20:837–846.
74. Hofbauer LC, Khosla S, Dunstan CR, et al. The roles of osteoprotegerin and osteoprotegerin ligand in the paracrine regulation of bone resorption. *J Bone Miner Res* 2000;15:2–12.
75. Lories RJ, Luyten FP. Osteoprotegerin and osteoprotegerin-ligand balance: a new paradigm in bone metabolism providing new therapeutic targets. *Clin Rheumatol* 2001;20:3–9.
76. Sasaki N, Kusano E, Ando Y, et al. Glucocorticoid decreases circulating osteoprotegerin (OPG): possible mechanism for glucocorticoid induced osteoporosis. *Nephrol Dial Transplant* 2001;16:479–482.
77. Simonet WS, Lacey DL, Dunstan CR, et al. Osteoprotegerin: a novel secreted protein involved in the regulation of bone density. *Cell* 1997;89:309–319.
78. Akatsu T, Murakami T, Ono K, et al. Osteoclastogenesis inhibitory factor exhibits hypocalcemic effects in normal mice and in hypercalcemic nude mice carrying tumors associated with humoral hypercalcemia of malignancy. *Bone* 1998;23:495–498.
79. Bekker PJ, Holloway D, Nakanishi A, et al. The effect of a single dose of osteoprotegerin in postmenopausal women. *J Bone Miner Res* 2001;16:348–360.
80. Kazama JJ, Shigematsu T, Tsuda E, et al. Increased circulating osteoprotegerin/osteoclastogenesis inhibitory factor (OPG/OCIF) in patients with chronic renal failure. *J Am Soc Nephrol* 1999;10.
81. Parfitt AM, Drezner MK, Glorieux FH, et al. Bone histomorphometry: standardization of nomenclature, symbols, and units. Report of the ASBMR Histomorphometry Nomenclature Committee. *J Bone Miner Res* 1987;2:595–610.
82. Sherrard DJ, Hercz G, Pei Y, et al. The spectrum of bone disease in end-stage renal failure—an evolving disorder. *Kidney Int* 1993;43:436–442.
83. Feinfeld DA, Sherwood LM. Parathyroid hormone and 1,25(OH)2D3 in chronic renal failure. *Kidney Int* 1988;33: 1049–1058.
84. Slatopolsky E, Finch J, Denda M, et al. Phosphorus restriction prevents parathyroid gland growth. High phosphorus directly stimulates PTH secretion in vitro. *J Clin Invest* 1996;97: 2534–2540.
85. Portale AA, Halloran BP, Morris RC Jr. Physiologic regulation of the serum concentration of 1,25-dihydroxyvitamin D by phosphorus in normal men. *J Clin Invest* 1989;83:1494–1499.
86. Lopez-Hilker S, Dusso AS, Rapp NS, et al. Phosphorus restriction reverses hyperparathyroidism in uremia independent of changes in calcium and calcitriol. *Am J Physiol* 1990;259: F432–437.
87. Combe C, Aparicio M. Phosphorus and protein restriction and parathyroid function in chronic renal failure. *Kidney Int* 1994; 46:1381–1386.
88. Silver J, Moallem E, Kilav R, et al. New insights into the regulation of parathyroid hormone synthesis and secretion in chronic renal failure. *Nephrol Dial Transplant* 1996;11 Suppl 3:2–5.
89. Kurz P, Monier-Faugere MC, Bognar B, et al. Evidence for abnormal calcium homeostasis in patients with adynamic bone disease. *Kidney Int* 1994;46:855–861.
90. Llach F, Felsenfeld AJ, Coleman MD, et al. The natural course of dialysis osteomalacia. *Kidney Int Suppl* 1986;18:S74–79.
91. Couttenye MM, D'Haese PC, Deng JT, et al. High prevalence of adynamic bone disease diagnosed by biochemical markers in a wide sample of the European CAPD population. *Nephrol Dial Transplant* 1997;12:2144–2150.
92. Picton ML, Moore PR, Mawer EB, et al. Down-regulation of human osteoblast PTH/PTHrP receptor mRNA in end-stage renal failure. *Kidney Int* 2000;58:1440–1449.
93. Carmen Sanchez M, Auxiliadora Bajo M, Selgas R, et al. Parathormone secretion in peritoneal dialysis patients with adynamic bone disease. *Am J Kidney Dis* 2000;36:953–961.
94. Malluche HH, Ritz E, Lange HP, et al. Bone histology in incipient and advanced renal failure. *Kidney Int* 1976;9:355–362.
95. Hutchison AJ, Whitehouse RW, Boulton HF, et al. Correlation of bone histology with parathyroid hormone, vitamin D3, and radiology in end-stage renal disease. *Kidney Int* 1993;44: 1071–1077.
96. Torres A, Lorenzo V, Hernandez D, et al. Bone disease in predialysis, hemodialysis, and CAPD patients: evidence of a better bone response to PTH. *Kidney Int* 1995;47:1434–1442.
97. Bervoets RJ, Behets GJ, Spasovski G, et al. The spectrum of renal osteodystrophy (ROD) in end-stage renal failure patients not yet in dialysis (ESRD). *J Am Soc Nephrol* 2000;11:F615 (PS).
98. Urena P, De Vernejoul MC. Circulating biochemical markers of bone remodeling in uremic patients. *Kidney Int* 1999;55: 2141–2156.
99. Christiansen C, Rodbro P, Christensen MS, et al. Deterioration of renal function during treatment of chronic renal failure with 1,25-dihydroxycholecalciferol. *Lancet* 1978;2:700–703.
100. Maung HM, Elangovan L, Frazao JM, et al. Efficacy and side effects of intermittent intravenous and oral doxercalciferol (1alpha-hydroxyvitamin D(2)) in dialysis patients with secondary hyperparathyroidism: a sequential comparison. *Am J Kidney Dis* 2001;37:532–543.
101. Baker LR, Abrams L, Roe CJ, et al. 1,25(OH)2D3 administration in moderate renal failure: a prospective double-blind trial. *Kidney Int* 1989;35:661–669.
102. Slatopolsky E, Brown A, Dusso A. Role of phosphorus in the pathogenesis of secondary hyperparathyroidism. *Am J Kidney Dis* 2001;37:S54–57.
103. Kopple JD. National kidney foundation K/DOQI clinical practice guidelines for nutrition in chronic renal failure. *Am J Kidney Dis* 2001;37:S66–70.
104. Blumenkrantz MJ, Kopple JD, Moran JK, et al. Metabolic balance studies and dietary protein requirements in patients undergoing continuous ambulatory peritoneal dialysis. *Kidney Int* 1982;21:849–861.
105. Pastan S, Bailey J. Dialysis therapy. *N Engl J Med* 1998;338: 1428–1437.
106. Hsu SH, Zhao J, Ellman CF, et al. Calcium and phosphorus

fluxes during hemodialysis with low calcium dialysate. *Am J Kidney Dis* 1991;18:217–224.
107. Zucchelli P, Santoro A. Inorganic phosphate removal during different dialytic procedures. *Int J Artif Organs* 1987;10: 173–178.
108. Haas T, Hillion D, Dongradi G. Phosphate kinetics in dialysis patients. *Nephrol Dial Transplant* 1991;6:108–113.
109. Winchester JF, Rotellar C, Goggins M, et al. Calcium and phosphate balance in dialysis patients. *Kidney Int Suppl* 1993;41: S174–178.
110. Mucsi I, Hercz G, Uldall R, et al. Control of serum phosphate without any phosphate binders in patients treated with nocturnal hemodialysis. *Kidney Int* 1998;53:1399–1404.
111. Kates DM. Control of hyperphosphatemia in renal failure: role of aluminum. *Semin Dial* 1996;9:310–315.
112. Nebeker HG, Coburn JW. Aluminum and renal osteodystrophy. *Ann Rev Med* 1986;37:79–95.
113. Andress DL, Endres DB, Ott SM, et al. Parathyroid hormone in aluminum bone disease: a comparison of parathyroid hormone assays. *Kidney Int Suppl* 1986;18:S87–90.
114. Andreoli SP, Bergstein JM, Sherrard DJ. Aluminum intoxication from aluminum-containing phosphate binders in children with azotemia not undergoing dialysis. *N Engl J Med* 1984;310: 1079–1084.
115. Slatopolsky E, Weerts C, Lopez-Hilker S, et al. Calcium carbonate as a phosphate binder in patients with chronic renal failure undergoing dialysis. *N Engl J Med* 1986;315:157–161.
116. Emmett M, Sirmon MD, Kirkpatrick WG, et al. Calcium acetate control of serum phosphorus in hemodialysis patients. *Am J Kidney Dis* 1991;17:544–550.
117. Sheikh MS, Maguire JA, Emmett M, et al. Reduction of dietary phosphorus absorption by phosphorus binders. A theoretical, in vitro, and in vivo study. *J Clin Invest* 1989;83:66–73.
118. Mai ML, Emmett M, Sheikh MS, et al. Calcium acetate, an effective phosphorus binder in patients with renal failure. *Kidney Int* 1989;36:690–695.
119. d'Almeida Filho EJ, da Cruz EA, Hoette M, et al. Calcium acetate versus calcium carbonate in the control of hyperphosphatemia in hemodialysis patients. *Sao Paulo Med J* 2000;118: 179–184.
120. Macia M, Coronel F, Navarro JF, et al. Calcium salts of ketoamino acids, a phosphate binder alternative for patients on CAPD. *Clin Nephrol* 1997;48:181–184.
121. Schaefer K, von Herrath D, Erley CM, et al. Calcium ketovaline as new therapy for uremic hyperphosphatemia. *Miner Electrolyte Metab* 1990;16:362–364.
122. Nolan CR, Califano JR, Butzin CA. Influence of calcium acetate or calcium citrate on intestinal aluminum absorption. *Kidney Int* 1990;38:937–941.
123. Chertow GM, Burke SK, Lazarus JM, et al. Poly (allylamine hydrochloride) (RenaGel): a noncalcemic phosphate binder for the treatment of hyperphosphatemia in chronic renal failure. *Am J Kidney Dis* 1997;29:66–71.
124. Slatopolsky EA, Burke SK, Dillon MA. RenaGel, a nonabsorbed calcium- and aluminum-free phosphate binder, lowers serum phosphorus and parathyroid hormone. The RenaGel Study Group. *Kidney Int* 1999;55:299–307.
125. Bleyer AJ, Burke SK, Dillon M, et al. A comparison of the calcium-free phosphate binder sevelamer hydrochloride with calcium acetate in the treatment of hyperphosphatemia in hemodialysis patients. *Am J Kidney Dis* 1999;33:694–701.
126. Chertow GM, Dillon M, Burke SK, et al. A randomized trial of sevelamer hydrochloride (RenaGel) with and without supplemental calcium. Strategies for the control of hyperphosphatemia and hyperparathyroidism in hemodialysis patients. *Clin Nephrol* 1999;51:18–26.
127. Delmez JA, Kelber J, Norword KY, et al. Magnesium carbonate as a phosphorus binder: a prospective, controlled, crossover study. *Kidney Int* 1996;49:163–167.
128. Graff L, Burnel D. A possible non-aluminum oral phosphate binder? A comparative study on dietary phosphorus absorption. *Res Commun Mol Pathol Pharmacol* 1995;89:373–388.
129. Dewberry K, Fox J, Stewart J, et al. Lanthanum carbonate: A novel non-calcium containing phosphate binder. *J Am Soc Nephrol* 1997;8:A2610.
130. Hsu CH, Patel SR, Young EW. New phosphate binding agents: ferric compounds. *J Am Soc Nephrol* 1999;10:1274–1280.
131. Hergesell O, Ritz E. Stabilized polynuclear iron hydroxide is an efficient oral phosphate binder in uraemic patients. *Nephrol Dial Transplant* 1999;14:863–867.
132. Chang JM, Hwang SJ, Tsai JC, et al. Effect of ferric polymaltose complex as a phosphate binder in haemodialysis patients (letter). *Nephrol Dial Transplant* 1999;14:1045–1047.
133. Berl T, Berns AS, Hufer WE, et al. 1,25 dihydroxycholecalciferol effects in chronic dialysis. A double-blind controlled study. *Ann Intern Med* 1978;88:774–780.
134. Andress DL, Norris KC, Coburn JW, et al. Intravenous calcitriol in the treatment of refractory osteitis fibrosa of chronic renal failure (see comments). *N Engl J Med* 1989;321:274–279.
135. Sprague SM, Moe SM. Safety and efficacy of long-term treatment of secondary hyperparathyroidism by low-dose intravenous calcitriol. *Am J Kidney Dis* 1992;19:532–539.
136. Tsukamoto Y, Nomura M, Takahashi Y, et al. The 'oral 1,25-dihydroxyvitamin D3 pulse therapy' in hemodialysis patients with severe secondary hyperparathyroidism. *Nephron* 1991;57: 23–28.
137. Quarles LD, Yohay DA, Carroll BA, et al. Prospective trial of pulse oral versus intravenous calcitriol treatment of hyperparathyroidism in ESRD. *Kidney Int* 1994;45:1710–1721.
138. Levine BS, Song M. Pharmacokinetics and efficacy of pulse oral versus intravenous calcitriol in hemodialysis patients. *J Am Soc Nephrol* 1996;7:488–496.
139. Moe SM, Kraus MA, Gassensmith CM, et al. Safety and efficacy of pulse and daily calcitriol in patients on CAPD: a randomized trial. *Nephrol Dial Transplant* 1998;13:1234–1241.
140. Herrmann P, Ritz E, Schmidt-Gayk H, et al. Comparison of intermittent and continuous oral administration of calcitriol in dialysis patients: a randomized prospective trial. *Nephron* 1994; 67:48–53.
141. Drueke TB. Parathyroid gland hyperplasia in uremia. *Kidney Int* 2001;59:1182–1183.
142. Martin KJ, Gonzalez EA, Gellens M, et al. 19-Nor-1-alpha-25-dihydroxyvitamin D2 (Paricalcitol) safely and effectively reduces the levels of intact parathyroid hormone in patients on hemodialysis. *J Am Soc Nephrol* 1998;9:1427–1432.
143. Frazao JM, Chesney RW, Coburn JW. Intermittent oral 1alpha-hydroxyvitamin D2 is effective and safe for the suppression of secondary hyperparathyroidism in haemodialysis patients. 1alphaD2 Study Group. *Nephrol Dial Transplant* 1998;13 Suppl 3:68–72.
144. Frazao JM, Elangovan L, Maung HM, et al. Intermittent doxercalciferol (1alpha-hydroxyvitamin D(2)) therapy for secondary hyperparathyroidism. *Am J Kidney Dis* 2000;36:550–561.
145. Tan AU Jr, Levine BS, Mazess RB, et al. Effective suppression of parathyroid hormone by 1 alpha-hydroxy-vitamin D2 in hemodialysis patients with moderate to severe secondary hyperparathyroidism. *Kidney Int* 1997;51:317–323.
146. Akiba T, Marumo F, Owada A, et al. Controlled trial of falecalcitriol versus alfacalcidol in suppression of parathyroid hormone in hemodialysis patients with secondary hyperparathyroidism. *Am J Kidney Dis* 1998;32:238–246.

147. Slatopolsky E, Finch J, Ritter C, et al. A new analog of calcitriol, 19-nor-1,25-(OH)2D2, suppresses parathyroid hormone secretion in uremic rats in the absence of hypercalcemia. *Am J Kidney Dis* 1995;26:852–860.
148. Moe SM, Zekonis M, Harezlak J, et al. A placebo-controlled trial to evaluate immunomodulatory effects of paricalcitol. *Am J Kidney Dis* 2001;38(4):792–802.
149. Katoh N, Nakayama M, Shigematsu T, et al. Presence of sonographically detectable parathyroid glands can predict resistance to oral pulsed-dose calcitriol treatment of secondary hyperparathyroidism. *Am J Kidney Dis* 2000;35:465–468.
150. Malluche H. Renal bone disease 1982 to 1994: continued need for bone biopsies. *Mediguide to Nephrology* 1995;3:1–8.
151. Wada M, Nagano N, Furuya Y, et al. Calcimimetic NPS R-568 prevents parathyroid hyperplasia in rats with severe secondary hyperparathyroidism. *Kidney Int* 2000;57:50–58.
152. Chin J, Miller SC, Wada M, et al. Activation of the calcium receptor by a calcimimetic compound halts the progression of secondary hyperparathyroidism in uremic rats. *J Am Soc Nephrol* 2000;11:903–911.
153. Antonsen JE, Sherrard DJ, Andress DL. A calcimimetic agent acutely suppresses parathyroid hormone levels in patients with chronic renal failure. Rapid communication. *Kidney Int* 1998; 53:223–227.
154. Goodman WG, Frazao JM, Goodkin DA, et al. A calcimimetic agent lowers plasma parathyroid hormone levels in patients with secondary hyperparathyroidism. *Kidney Int* 2000;58:436–445.
155. Chertow GM, Burke SK, Raggi P. Sevelamer attenuates the progression of coronary and aortic calcification in hemodialysis patients. *Kidney Int* 2002;62(1):245–252.
156. Alfrey AC, Mishell JM, Burks J, et al. Syndrome of dyspraxia and multifocal seizures associated with chronic hemodialysis. *Trans Am Soc Artif Intern Organs* 1972;18:257–261.
157. Alfrey AC, LeGendre GR, Kaehny WD. The dialysis encephalopathy syndrome. Possible aluminum intoxication. *N Engl J Med* 1976;294:184–188.
158. Platts MM, Anastassiades E. Dialysis encephalopathy: precipitating factors and improvement in prognosis. *Clin Nephrol* 1981;15:223–228.
159. Platts MM, Goode GC, Hislop JS. Composition of the domestic water supply and the incidence of fractures and encephalopathy in patients on home dialysis. *BMJ* 1977;2:657–660.
160. Alfrey AC. Aluminum intoxication (editorial). *N Engl J Med* 1984;310:1113–1115.
161. Parkinson IS, Ward MK, Feest TG, et al. Fracturing dialysis osteodystrophy and dialysis encephalopathy. An epidemiological survey. *Lancet* 1979;1:406–409.
162. Pei Y, Hercz G, Greenwood C, et al. Non-invasive prediction of aluminum bone disease in hemo- and peritoneal dialysis patients. *Kidney Int* 1992;41:1374–1382.
163. Burgess E, Muruve D, Audette R. Aluminum absorption and excretion following sucralfate therapy in chronic renal insufficiency. *Am J Med* 1992;92:471–475.
164. Andress DL, Kopp JB, Maloney NA, et al. Early deposition of aluminum in bone in diabetic patients on hemodialysis. *N Engl J Med* 1987;316:292–296.
165. Milliner DS, Nebeker HG, Ott SM, et al. Use of the deferoxamine infusion test in the diagnosis of aluminum-related osteodystrophy. *Ann Intern Med* 1984;101:775–779.
166. Kausz AT, Antonsen JE, Hercz G, et al. Screening plasma aluminum levels in relation to aluminum bone disease among asymptomatic dialysis patients. *Am J Kidney Dis* 1999;34:688–693.
167. Andress DL, Nebeker HG, Ott SM, et al. Bone histologic response to deferoxamine in aluminum-related bone disease. *Kidney Int* 1987;31:1344–1350.
168. Boelaert JR, Fenves AZ, Coburn JW. Deferoxamine therapy and mucormycosis in dialysis patients: report of an international registry. *Am J Kidney Dis* 1991;18:660–667.
169. Moriniere P, Cohen-Solal M, Belbrik S, et al. Disappearance of aluminic bone disease in a long term asymptomatic dialysis population restricting A1(OH)3 intake: emergence of an idiopathic adynamic bone disease not related to aluminum. *Nephron* 1989;53:93–101.
170. Hutchison AJ, Whitehouse RW, Freemont AJ, et al. Histological, radiological, and biochemical features of the adynamic bone lesion in continuous ambulatory peritoneal dialysis patients. *Am J Nephrol* 1994;14:19–29.
171. Malluche HH, Monier-Faugere MC. Risk of adynamic bone disease in dialyzed patients. *Kidney Int Suppl* 1992;38:S62–67.
172. Hernandez D, Concepcion MT, Lorenzo V, et al. Adynamic bone disease with negative aluminium staining in predialysis patients: prevalence and evolution after maintenance dialysis. *Nephrol Dial Transplant* 1994;9:517–523.
173. Couttenye MM, D'Haese PC, Van Hoof VO, et al. Low serum levels of alkaline phosphatase of bone origin: a good marker of adynamic bone disease in haemodialysis patients. *Nephrol Dial Transplant* 1996;11:1065–1072.
174. Gupta A, Kallenbach LR, Zasuwa G, et al. Race is a major determinant of secondary hyperparathyroidism in uremic patients. *J Am Soc Nephrol* 2000;11:330–334.
175. Goodman WG, Ramirez JA, Belin TR, et al. Development of adynamic bone in patients with secondary hyperparathyroidism after intermittent calcitriol therapy. *Kidney Int* 1994;46: 1160–1166.
176. Montenegro J, Saracho R, Gonzalez O, et al. Reversibility of parathyroid gland suppression in CAPD patients with low i-PTH levels. *Clin Nephrol* 1997;48:359–363.
177. Moe SM, Peterson JM, Murphy CL, et al. Sevelamer HCl improves parathyroid hormone (PTH) and bone function in peritoneal dialysis (PD) patients with probable low turnover bone disease (*submitted*).
178. Atsumi K, Kushida K, Yamazaki K, et al. Risk factors for vertebral fractures in renal osteodystrophy. *Am J Kidney Dis* 1999; 33:287–293.
179. Coco M, Rush H. Increased incidence of hip fractures in dialysis patients with low serum parathyroid hormone. *Am J Kidney Dis* 2000;36:1115–1121.
180. Alem AM, Sherrard DJ, Gillen DL, et al. Increased risk of hip fracture among patients with end-stage renal disease. *Kidney Int* 2000;58:396–399.
181. Shear M, Kramer B. Composition of bone. III. Physicochemical mechanism. *J Biol Chem* 1928;79:125–145.
182. Nordin B. Primary and secondary hyperparathyroidism. *Adv Intern Med* 1957;9:81–105.
183. Parfitt AM. Soft-tissue calcification in uremia. *Arch Intern Med* 1969;124:544–556.
184. Bostrom K, Watson KE, Horn S, et al. Bone morphogenetic protein expression in human atherosclerotic lesions. *J Clin Invest* 1993;91:1800–1809.
185. Fitzpatrick LA, Severson A, Edwards WD, et al. Diffuse calcification in human coronary arteries. Association of osteopontin with atherosclerosis. *J Clin Invest* 1994;94:1597–1604.
186. Shanahan CM, Cary NR, Metcalfe JC, et al. High expression of genes for calcification-regulating proteins in human atherosclerotic plaques. *J Clin Invest* 1994;93:2393–2402.
187. Shanahan CM, Cary NR, Salisbury JR, et al. Medial localization of mineralization-regulating proteins in association with Monckeberg's sclerosis: evidence for smooth muscle cell-mediated vascular calcification. *Circulation* 1999;100:2168–2176.
188. Proudfoot D, Shanahan CM, Weissberg PL. Vascular calcification: new insights into an old problem (editorial; comment). *J Pathol* 1998;185:1–3.

189. Ahmed S, O'Neill KD, Hood AF, et al. Calciphylaxis is associated with hyperphosphatemia and increased osteopontin expression by vascular smooth muscle cells. *Am J Kidney Dis* 2001; 37:1267–1276.
190. Moe SM, O'Neill KD, Duan D, et al. Medial artery calcification in ESRD patients is associated with deposition of bone matrix proteins. *Kidney Int* 2002;61(2):638–647.
191. Jono S, McKee MD, Murry CE, et al. Phosphate regulation of vascular smooth muscle cell calcification. *Circ Res* 2000;87: E10–17.
192. Lowrie EG, Lew NL. Death risk in hemodialysis patients: the predictive value of commonly measured variables and an evaluation of death rate differences between facilities. *Am J Kidney Dis* 1990;15:458–482.
193. Block GA, Hulbert-Shearon TE, Levin NW, et al. Association of serum phosphorus and calcium x phosphate product with mortality risk in chronic hemodialysis patients: a national study. *Am J Kidney Dis* 1998;31:607–617.
194. Chertow GM, Lowrie EG, Lew NL. Mineral metabolism and mortality in dialysis. *J Am Soc Nephrol* 2000;11:Abstract A2958.
195. Ansell BM, Feest T, Taylor H. Serum phosphate and dialysis mortality in 1998: a multi-centre study from the UK. *Nephrol Dial Transplant* 2000;A182.
196. Hsu CH. Are we mismanaging calcium and phosphate metabolism in renal failure? *Am J Kidney Dis* 1997;29:641–649.
197. Heaney RP, Saville PD, Recker RR. Calcium absorption as a function of calcium intake. *J Lab Clin Med* 1975;85:881–890.
198. Braun J, Oldendorf M, Moshage W, et al. Electron beam computed tomography in the evaluation of cardiac calcification in chronic dialysis patients. *Am J Kidney Dis* 1996;27:394–401.
199. Kimura K, Saika Y, Otani H, et al. Factors associated with calcification of the abdominal aorta in hemodialysis patients. *Kidney Int Suppl* 1999;71:S238–241.
200. Marchais SJ, Metivier F, Guerin AP, et al. Association of hyperphosphataemia with haemodynamic disturbances in end-stage renal disease. *Nephrol Dial Transplant* 1999;14:2178–2183.
201. Guerin AP, London GM, Marchais SJ, et al. Arterial stiffening and vascular calcifications in end-stage renal disease. *Nephrol Dial Transplant* 2000;15:1014–1021.
202. Mazhar AR, Johnson RJ, Gillen D, et al. Risk factors and mortality associated with calciphylaxis in end-stage renal disease. *Kidney Int* 2001;60:324–332.
203. Goodman WG, Goldin J, Kuizon BD, et al. Coronary-artery calcification in young adults with end-stage renal disease who are undergoing dialysis. *N Engl J Med* 2000;342:1478–1483.
204. Schwarz U, Buzello M, Ritz E, et al. Morphology of coronary atherosclerotic lesions in patients with end-stage renal failure. *Nephrol Dial Transplant* 2000;15:218–223.
205. Raggi P, Boulay A, Chasan-Taber S, et al. Cardiac calcification in adult hemodialysis patients. A link between end-stage renal disease and cardiovascular disease? *J Am Coll Cardiol* 2002; 39(4):695–701.
206. Block GA, Port FK. Re-evaluation of risks associated with hyperphosphatemia and hyperparathyroidism in dialysis patients: recommendations for a change in management. *Am J Kidney Dis* 2000;35:1226–1237.
207. Levi M. Post-transplant hypophosphatemia. *Kidney Int* 2001; 59:2377–2387.
208. Usher BW Jr, Friedman RJ. Steroid-induced osteonecrosis of the humeral head. *Orthopedics* 1995;18:47–51.
209. Coombs RR, Thomas RW. Avascular necrosis of the hip. *Br J Hosp Med* 1994;51:275–280.
210. Mankin HJ. Nontraumatic necrosis of bone (osteonecrosis). *N Engl J Med* 1992;326:1473–1479.
211. Smith SW, Fehring TK, Griffin WL, et al. Core decompression of the osteonecrotic femoral head. *J Bone Joint Surg Am* 1995; 77:674–680.
212. Julian BA, Laskow DA, Dubovsky J, et al. Rapid loss of vertebral mineral density after renal transplantation. *N Engl J Med* 1991; 325:544–550.
213. Monier-Faugere MC, Mawad H, Qi Q, et al. High prevalence of low bone turnover and occurrence of osteomalacia after kidney transplantation. *J Am Soc Nephrol* 2000;11:1093–1099.
214. Kosch M, Hausberg M, Link T, et al. Measurement of skeletal status after renal transplantation by quantitative ultrasound. *Clin Nephrol* 2000;54:15–21.
215. Fan SL, Almond MK, Ball E, et al. Pamidronate therapy as prevention of bone loss following renal transplantation1 (see comments). *Kidney Int* 2000;57:684–690.
216. Lindberg JS, Moe SM. Osteoporosis in end-state renal disease. *Semin Nephrol* 1999;19:115–122.
217. Grotz WH, Mundinger FA, Gugel B, et al. Bone mineral density after kidney transplantation. A cross-sectional study in 190 graft recipients up to 20 years after transplantation. *Transplantation* 1995;59:982–986.
218. Grotz WH, Mundinger FA, Gugel B, et al. Bone fracture and osteodensitometry with dual energy X-ray absorptiometry in kidney transplant recipients. *Transplantation* 1994;58: 912–915.
219. Epstein S, Shane E, Bilezikian JP. Organ transplantation and osteoporosis. *Curr Opin Rheumatol* 1995;7:255–261.
220. Rodino MA, Shane E. Osteoporosis after organ transplantation. *Am J Med* 1998;104:459–469.
221. Shane E, Rivas M, McMahon DJ, et al. Bone loss and turnover after cardiac transplantation. *J Clin Endocrinol Metab* 1997;82: 1497–1506.
222. Moe SM. The treatment of steroid-induced bone loss in transplantation. *Curr Opin Nephrol Hypertens* 1997;6:544–549.
223. Hui SL, Slemenda CW, Johnston CC Jr. Age and bone mass as predictors of fracture in a prospective study. *J Clin Invest* 1988;81:1804–1809.
224. Selby PL, Halsey JP, Adams KR, et al. Corticosteroids do not alter the threshold for vertebral fracture. *J Bone Miner Res* 2000; 15:952–956.
225. Eastell R, Reid DM, Compston J, et al. A UK Consensus Group on management of glucocorticoid-induced osteoporosis: an update. *J Intern Med* 1998;244:271–292.
226. Adachi JD, Bensen WG, Bell MJ, et al. Salmon calcitonin nasal spray in the prevention of corticosteroid-induced osteoporosis. *Br J Rheumatol* 1997;36:255–259.
227. Adachi JD, Bensen WG, Brown J, et al. Intermittent etidronate therapy to prevent corticosteroid-induced osteoporosis (see comments). *N Engl J Med* 1997;337:382–387.
228. Geng Z, Monier-Faugere MC, Bauss F, et al. Short-term administration of the bisphosphonate ibandronate increases bone volume and prevents hyperparathyroid bone changes in mild experimental renal failure. *Clin Nephrol* 2000;54:45–53.
229. Westeel FP, Mazouz H, Ezaitouni F, et al. Cyclosporine bone remodeling effect prevents steroid osteopenia after kidney transplantation. *Kidney Int* 2000;58:1788–1796.
230. Riggs BL, Hodgson SF, O'Fallon WM, et al. Effect of fluoride treatment on the fracture rate in postmenopausal women with osteoporosis (see comments). *N Engl J Med* 1990;322:802–809.
231. Reeve J. PTH: a future role in the management of osteoporosis? (editorial). *J Bone Miner Res* 1996;11:440–445.
232. Lane N, Thompson J, Modin G, et al. Parathyroid hormone treatment of women with glucocorticoid-induced osteoporosis dramatically increases bone turnover. ASBMR 19th Annual Meeting 1997.
233. Lane NE, Thompson JM, Modin G, et al. Can parathyroid hormone treatment reverse steroid osteoporosis: preliminary re-

sults of biochemical markers and bone density. ASBMR 1996 T620.
234. Lane NE, Sanchez S, Modin GW, et al. Bone mass continues to increase at the hip after parathyroid hormone treatment is discontinued in glucocorticoid-induced osteoporosis: results of a randomized controlled clinical trial. *J Bone Miner Res* 2000; 15:944–951.
235. Stehman-Breen CO, Sherrard DJ, Alem AM, et al. Risk factors for hip fracture among patients with end-stage renal disease. *Kidney Int* 2000;58:2200–2205.
236. Hardy P, Benoit J, Donneaud B, et al. (Pathological fractures of the femoral neck in hemodialyzed patients. Apropos of 26 cases). *Rev Chir Orthop Reparatrice Appar Mot* 1994;80: 702–710.
237. Sherrard D, Baylink D, Wergedal J. Bone disease in uremia. *Trans Am Soc Artif Intern Organs* 1972;18:412–415.

18

NUTRITIONAL MANAGEMENT OF WATER, SODIUM, POTASSIUM, CHLORIDE, AND MAGNESIUM IN RENAL DISEASE AND RENAL FAILURE

MICHAEL E. FALKENHAIN
JUDITH A. HARTMAN
LEE HEBERT

The kidney plays the central role in regulating water and electrolyte balance. It does so by adjusting the excretion of these molecules in response to changes in intake. Thus, it should come as no surprise that, when the kidney is diseased, electrolyte and water balance can be abnormal. What is surprising is how well the impaired kidney is able to maintain water and electrolyte balance until virtually all kidney function has been lost. In this chapter we discuss water, sodium, chloride, potassium, and magnesium homeostasis and then show how the normal condition is perturbed by renal insufficiency. We provide specific guidelines for the dietary management of water, sodium, chloride, potassium, and magnesium in renal insufficiency. Chloride will be considered together with sodium because nearly all dietary chloride intake is the result of sodium chloride (NaCl or salt) intake (1).

SODIUM AND CHLORIDE

Sodium and the Control of Extracellular Fluid Volume

Sodium is the most abundant extracellular cation. Because sodium is actively excluded from cells and cell membranes generally are freely permeable to water, the amount of sodium in the extracellular space critically determines extracellular fluid volume (ECFV). Figure 18.1 shows that the intravascular fluid volume is a component of the ECFV and, in health, comprises approximately one-fourth of the ECFV. In many pathologic states the intravascular and interstitial fluid volume change in parallel; however, some disease states alter the distribution of fluid within the ECFV (Fig. 18.2). The highest priority in ECFV volume control is to maintain the intravascular volume at an optimum level (2). Thus, it follows that the goal in dietary management of sodium is to reestablish or help maintain an optimal intravascular volume.

A constellation of findings, when taken together, provides the clinician with an assessment of the intravascular volume. An overview of the diagnostic approach to assessing volume status is shown in Table 18.1. In the present context volume depletion is defined as a condition in which the patient will be benefited by increasing intravascular volume. Volume expansion is defined as a condition in which the patient will be benefited by decreasing intravascular volume.

Regulation of Sodium Balance in Health

There are several organ systems that "sense" the effective circulating volume (volume status): heart (3,4), arterial baroreceptors (5), liver (6), brain (7), and kidney (8). However, it is the kidney alone that is the effector organ in sodium homeostasis.

The normal kidney is able to maintain adequate volume status over a wide range of dietary sodium intake. For example, in healthy adults in the United States the average sodium intake is 170 mEq/day. In areas of Japan it can approach 300 mEq/day. It is less than 30 mEq/day in the New Guinea Highlands (9).

Although the kidney is remarkable in its ability to defend volume status over a wide range of sodium intake, the defense is not perfect. As shown in Fig. 18.3A, when NaCl intake is decreased abruptly from 150 mEq/day to 10 mEq/day in a normal individual, urine sodium gradually decreases over the next 4 days until sodium balance is achieved (i.e., urine sodium excretion approximates dietary sodium intake) (9,10). Before this steady state was reached, sodium output exceeded intake and a net loss of about 150 mEq

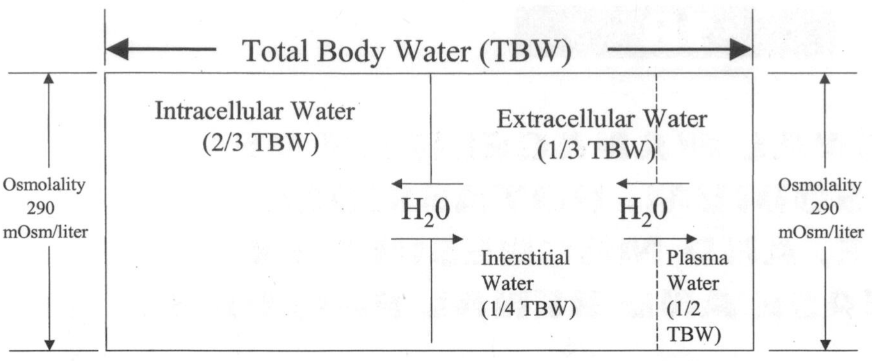

FIGURE 18.1. The nominal distribution and osmolality of body water. The short horizontal arrows indicate the presence of free diffusion of water among the body water compartments.

of sodium occurred. Because normal homeostasis requires that serum sodium concentration remain constant, a decrease in ECFV volume will occur (11). This is shown in Fig. 18.3A by the approximate 1-kg weight loss after the reduction in sodium intake. Concern has been raised that a persistently low sodium intake, through the reduction of intravascular volume and stimulation of angiotensin II, may accelerate tissue fibrosis and enhance cardiac mortality (12, 13). The potential detrimental effect of stimulating the renin angiotensin system is only a theoretic concern at this time (12). An extremely low-salt diet leading to a chronically low ECFV might render the individual more vulnerable to hypotension if rapid fluid and electrolyte loss occur, as in gastroenteritis.

Figure 18.3B shows that acutely increasing NaCl intake gradually increases urinary sodium excretion over the next 4 days until a new steady state is reached (9,10). During this period, a net gain of sodium occurs and is accompanied by water retention (approximately 1 kg) sufficient to maintain ECFV isotonicity. This traditional view was challenged in 2000 with the new concept of sodium storage (11). In this model, when NaCl intake is increased form baseline the intravascular volume will increase without a concomitant increase in ECFV or body weight (11). The clinical implica-

TABLE 18.1. CLINICAL AND LABORATORY ASSESSMENT OF VOLUME STATUS

Finding	Comment
Findings consistent with volume depletion	
Weight loss exceeding 0.25 kg/day	Weight loss exceeding this rate is usually the result of fluid and electrolyte deficits, not caloric deficits.
Blood pressure less than usual and/or orthostatic fall in blood pressure	A fall in systolic blood pressure by greater than 20 mmHg when changing from a supine to standing position with a rise in pulse rate suggests intravascular volume depletion. Autonomic neuropathy or alpha blockers can cause orthostatic hypotension in the absence of volume depletion; in this situation pulse rate does not rise.
Decreased skin turgor, cool or mottled extremities, collapsed peripheral veins	Elderly patients with arterial insufficiency can manifest these findings in the absence of volume depletion.
Elevated serum creatinine associated with a urine/plasma osmolality ratio >1.5 mEq/L and/or urine Na concentration < 20 mEq/L	These findings also can be seen in severe congestive heart failure or hepatic failure, in the absence of volume depletion.
Findings consistent with the absence of volume depletion and/or the presence of volume expansion	
Finding	**Comment**
Weight gain exceeding 0.25 kg/day	Weight gains exceeding this rate usually indicate fluid weight gains.
Onset of hypertension or worsening of previous hypertension	Those with salt-sensitive hypertension (e.g., African Americans, elderly) are particularly susceptible to hypertension with sodium and water retention.
Left ventricular failure (orthopnea, paroxysmal nocturnal dyspnea, rales at lung bases, audible third heart sound)	Patients with left ventricular failure are volume expanded (they will benefit from measures to decrease intravascular volume) regardless of other finding relating to volume status.
Peripheral edema, ascites, pleural effusions	These findings also can be the result of venous or lymphatic obstruction or severe hypoalbuminemia in the absence of volume expansion.

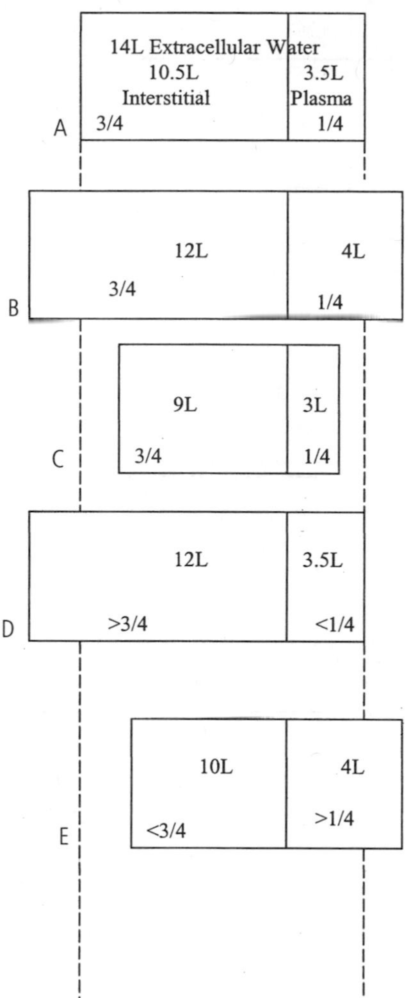

FIGURE 18.2. In a normal 70-kg person extracellular water (ECW) consists of 14 L of fluid divided between the intersitial (10.5 L) and intravascular (3.5 L) spaces (**A**). Illustrations B through E show various pathologic states can alter the amount and distributions of ECW. **A:** Distribution of ECW. Normal intersitial volume is three-fourths of ECW. Intravascular water (mainly plasma) is one-fourth of ECW. **B:** Interstitial and intravascular volume increase in parallel as occurs in: congestive heart failure; high salt intake; normal salt intake in ESRD. **C:** Interstitial and intravascular volume decrease in parallel as occurs in: gastrointestinal losses (vomiting and diarrhea); renal losses (diuretics, salt wasting); skin losses (sweating, burns). **D:** Interstitial volume increase but intravascular volume decreases or remains the same: calcium channel blocker therapy; hypoalbuminemia (liver disease, nephrotic syndrome, malnutrition). **E:** Intravascular volume increases but interstitial volume decreases or remains unchanged: rapid infusion of blood or colloid; head out water immersion.

tions of this model have yet to be elicited (14). Irrespective of this debate, in patients with "salt-sensitive" hypertension the increase in intravascular volume can result in an increase in blood pressure to abnormal levels (15). The determents of "salt sensitivity" are unknown, although renal insufficiency (15), older age (16), African-American race (16), and possibly being heterozygote for the adducin gene (17) appear to correlate. The human-adducin 460Trp allele may be a hypertension-favoring allele because it may affect blood pressure by increasing renal tubular reabsorption through the activation of Na-K-ATPase (sodium-potassium-adenosine triphosphatase). Whether a persistent increase in sodium intake is harmful to the general population is a matter of debate (18). The recently published dietary approaches to stop hypertension (DASH) diet in conjunction with sodium restriction added to the body of literature supporting salt reduction as a way to enhance blood pressure control. Patients provided a diet high in fruits, vegetables, and low-fat dairy products (DASH diet) had a significant reduction in blood pressure (19). When patients on the DASH diet where randomized to different amounts of sodium intake, patients on a lower sodium diet had a significant further reduction in blood pressure (20). It remains the recommendation of the National Heart, Lung, and Blood Institute that sodium intake be restricted in health (21). The Joint National Committee on Hypertension continues to recommend salt restriction in all patients with hypertension (22).

Regulation of Sodium Balance in Renal Diseases

The ability of patients with renal insufficiency to excrete a normal sodium intake usually remains intact until the glomerular filtration rate (GFR) falls to less than 15 mL/min (serum creatinine approximately 3 mg/dL) (23,24). Below a GFR of 15 mL/min, the kidneys often are unable to increase fractional excretion of sodium sufficiently to maintain satisfactory sodium balance on an average adult salt intake (120 to 170 mEq/day) (25). Thus, salt intake must be reduced in such patients to avoid an increase in intravascular volume (26). At a GFR of less than 50 mL/min but greater than 15 mL/min, mild to moderate renal sodium wasting occurs in many patients whose renal disease is not complicated by the nephrotic syndrome or other sodium-retaining state (27). That is, at this level of GFR, the patients usually lose the ability to reduce sodium excretion to less than 30 mEq/day (27). Thus, in such patients, acutely reducing dietary salt intake to less than 30 mEq/day can result in negative sodium and water balance. It is interesting that the ability to substantially reduce urine sodium excretion may be maintained in renal disease if dietary sodium is lowered gradually rather than abruptly (28).

Renal sodium wasting is accentuated if sodium is ingested as $NaHCO_3$ (sodium hydrogen carbonate) rather than NaCl. This was demonstrated when patients with various forms of renal insufficiency were fed a diet in which the source of sodium was 100 mEq/day of NaCl or 100 mEq/day of $NaHCO_3$. During NaCl feeding, patients maintained satisfactory sodium balance. However, during $NaHCO_3$ feeding, progressive negative sodium balances developed (29). The mechanism of this effect is thought to be a decreased capacity of renal tubular cells to reabsorb

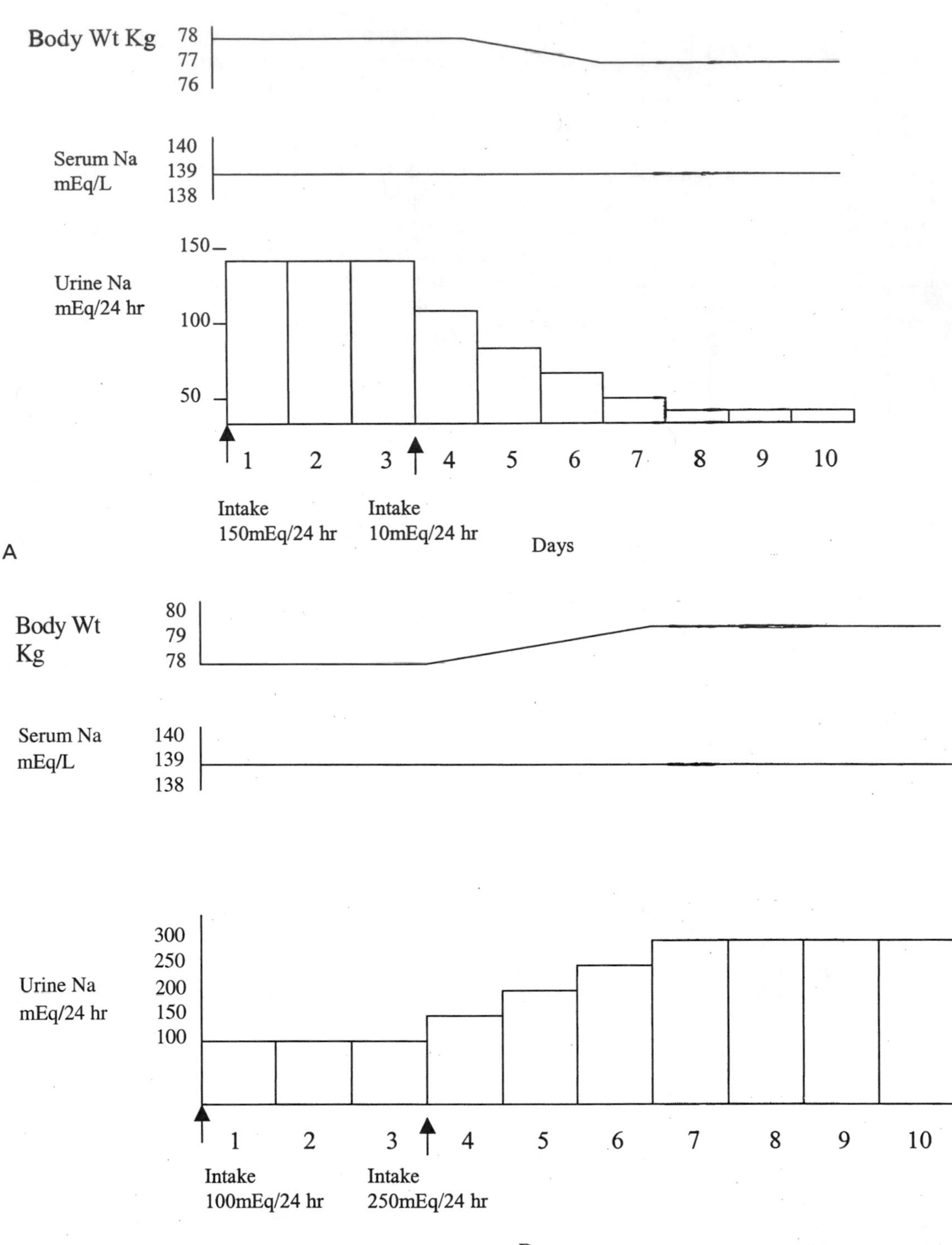

FIGURE 18.3. Change in body weight (Wt), serum sodium, and urine sodium. **A:** Dietary sodium intake is decreased to 10 mEq/day after a steady-state intake of 150 mEq/day. **B:** Dietary sodium intake increased to 250 mEq/day after steady-state intake of 100 mEq/day. (From Simpson FO. Sodium intake, body sodium, and sodium excretion. *Lancet* 1988;2:25–28, with permission.)

sodium unless it is accompanied by a highly reabsorbable anion such as chloride (30).

Effect of Calcium Channel Blocker Use on the Dietary Sodium Management

Unlike other classes of antihypertensive agents, the antihypertensive effects of calcium channel blockers may not be increased by salt restriction (31). This apparently occurs because calcium channel blockers promote natriuresis (32). Paradoxically, calcium channel blocker therapy often is associated with lower-extremity edema. Apparently, calcium channel blockers induce sufficient arteriolar vasodilatation of peripheral vessels to cause increased transmission of arterial hydrostatic pressure to tissue capillaries. This results in expansion of the interstitial volume. Lower-extremity edema also is seen with the use of other vasodilators such as minoxidil or hydralazine. The edema is usually a benign condition. Dietary salt restriction and diuretics can reduce the edema. However, vigorous salt restriction and diuresis are not recommended because it can result in reducing intravascular volume to less than normal.

Dietary NaCl Therapy in Patients with Renal Disease

The goal of NaCl therapy is to achieve optimum intravascular volume. Assessment of volume status is discussed in Table 18.1 and Fig. 18.2. Approximate levels of salt intake according to type and stage of renal disease are discussed in Table 18.2.

TABLE 18.2. RECOMMENDED DIETARY SODIUM INTAKE ACCORDING TO TYPE OR STAGE OF RENAL DISEASE

Increased need for dietary NaCl (generally >120 mM/day)
Medullary cystic disease
Fanconi's syndrome
Kidney–pancreas transplant with drainage of pancreatic secretions into the bladder
Renal insufficiency of any cause associated with excessive extra renal salt losses (e.g., diarrhea, excess sweating)
Hypercalcemia-associated renal impairment (the excess dietary sodium is needed to promote renal calcium excretion)
Polyuric recovery phase from acute renal injury, such as postobstructive or acute tubular necrosis

Usual need for dietary NaCl (generally 90 to 120 mM/day)
Renal disease that is not complicated by hypertension, edema, congestive heart failure, ascites, or pleural effusion

Decreased need for dietary NaCl (generally less than 100 mM/day)
Renal insufficiency complicated by hypertension, edema, congestive heart failure, ascites, or pleural effusion
Oliguric end-stage renal disease associated with normal volume status

TABLE 18.3. CONVERSION TABLE FOR DIETARY NaCl PRESCRIPTIONS (DAILY INTAKE) FOR ADULTS[a]

	Level of Salt Intake			
	Low	Recommended[b]	Average	High
Na				
g	2.0	2.3	3.9	4.6
mM	88	100	170	200
NaCl				
g	5.1	5.8	9.9	11.6
mM	88	100	170	200

[a]Molecular weights: Na 23, Cl 35.5.
[b]Approximately 1 to 1.3 mM/kg ideal body weight/day.

Dietary prescriptions for salt intake usually are written in milligrams or grams of sodium. Confusion can result when it is necessary to adjust dietary salt intake for increased losses of sodium in body fluids (usually measured in mEq/L). This problem is compounded if dietary NaCl intake is supplemented with NaCl tablets (usually formulated as 1-g NaCl tablets). It is unfortunate that tradition maintains this confusing situation. It would be easier if the dietary sodium prescription were provided in milliequivalents of sodium (or mmol/L of NaCl) rather than in milligrams or grams of sodium. To aid the clinician, Table 18.3 is a conversion table for the dietary sodium prescription.

High-Salt Diet

High salt intakes can be achieved consistently by using food with high salt contents (Table 18.4). NaCl tablets are also useful to increase NaCl intake. Compressed NaCl tablets, rather than enteric-coated tablets, are recommended because of more predictable absorption of the compressed tablet. Some patients dislike NaCl tablets because in doses greater than 6 gm daily nausea or a disagreeable salty aftertaste develops. The least effective means to substantially increase salt intake is to instruct the patient to simply add salt to the surface of food. Generally, the amount of salt actually added is small because the food becomes unpalatable if large amounts of surface salt are added. Increased dietary salt is more palatable if the salt is mixed with the food during preparation.

Low-Salt Diet

Low salt intakes consistently can be achieved with proper dietary counseling; the use of low-salt foods (Table 18.4), salt substitutes; and other flavor enhancers; and the judicious use of surface salt. Surface salt is much more efficiently tasted than is salt that is mixed with food. This is the reason that a serving of potato chips, which contains about 3 to 4 mEq of NaCl, tastes much "saltier" than a serving of bread, which contains about 5 to 8 mEq NaCl.

TABLE 18.4. SALT CONTENT OF VARIOUS FOODS

High (greater than 8 mEq per serving)	Low (less than 2 mEq per serving)
Dairy	
Processed American cheese	Nondairy creamer
Cottage cheese	Half and half cream
Buttermilk	
Meats/fish	
Processed meats	Lean beef
Bacon, sausage	Lean chicken
Canned meats	Fresh fish
Pickled herring	
Smoked salmon	
Breads and pastas	
Bread crumbs	Rice
Pita bread	Wheat germ
Bread stuffing	Cream of wheat
Cereals	Melba toast
Corn Flakes	Spaghetti
All Bran	
Waffles	
English muffins	
Legumes, fruits, and miscellaneous	
Coconut	Legumes
Refried beans	Tofu
Canned vegetables	Raw fruit
Canned soups	Raw carrots
Pickles	Lettuce
Corn chips, pretzels	Baked potato
Canned tomato products	Alcohol
Barbecue sauce	Soda
Canned gravy	Chocolate
Soy sauce	

From Mitch WE, Klahr S. Composition of common foods. In: Mitch WE, Klahr S, eds. *Nutrition and the kidney*. Boston: Little, Brown 1988:331, with permission.

Low-salt diets can be adhered to if processed foods are kept to a minimum and salt is avoided in cooking. To enhance the flavor of foods cooked without salt, flavor enhancers such as pepper, paprika, curry, thyme, and oregano can be used. Salt substitutes, which consist mostly of KCl, also can be used if potassium intake does not need to be reduced. Compared to flavor enhancers, salt substitutes have the advantage of tasting "saltier."

$NaHCO_3$ Therapy

Many patients with chronic renal disease require $NaHCO_3$ (or equivalent, such as NaCitrate) to treat the metabolic acidosis of renal failure. Usually $NaHCO_3$ can be administered in amounts sufficient to treat the metabolic acidosis without fear of inducing important sodium retention because, as discussed earlier, $NaHCO_3$therapy generally is not associated with sodium retention.

WATER

Water Metabolism in Health

By weight, the average human is 70% water—two-thirds in the intracellular space and one-third in the extracellular space (Fig. 18.1). Unlike sodium, in which excretion in health is adjusted to control blood volume, water excretion is adjusted to control blood osmolality. The normal kidney has the ability to conserve water (increase urinary osmolality as high as 1,200 mOsm/L) or excrete water (reduce urine osmolality to less than 50 mOsm/L) (33).

In health, daily metabolism and intake of nutrients produces about 600 mOsm that requires renal excretion. This "solute load" largely consists of urea produced from metabolism of protein and ingested Na, K, and their anions. If the urine is concentrated maximally (1,200 mOsm/L) the 600 mOsm can be excreted in 0.5 L of urine. Conversely, in states of maximum water intake, this same 600 mOsm can be excreted in about 12 L of urine (50 mOsm/L). This 12 L of urine can be viewed as consisting of 2 L of isotonic urine and 10 L of solute-free urine. The latter represents net water excretion.

The urinary volume in which the daily osmolar load is excreted depends on antidiuretic hormone (ADH). In the absence of ADH the collecting duct becomes impermeable to water, resulting in excretion of the dilute tubular fluid that is formed in the loop of Henle (34). Osmolality is the primary regulator of ADH release (35,36). However, there are nonosmotic stimuli for ADH release as well. These include nausea (37), hypoxia (38), insulin (39), norepinephrine (40), angiotensin II (41), and severe volume depletion (42). In health, water balance is achieved by adjusting renal excretion of water to compensate for variations in water intake and nonrenal water losses. The components of normal daily water balance in the adult are shown in Table 18.5.

Water Metabolism in Renal Insufficiency

Impaired ability to concentrate and dilute the urine occurs in all forms of renal disease, but it occurs earlier and more severely in primary tubulointerstitial renal diseases compared to primary glomerular diseases. However, in either form of renal disease, when the GFR falls to less than 20 mL/min, the maximum urine concentration barely exceeds plasma osmolality (300 mOsm/L) and the minimum urine osmolality can be reduced only to approximately 200 mOsm/L (24). Thus, in advanced renal insufficiency an osmolar load of 600 mOsm/day obligates a urine output of about 2 L/day. As a consequence, urine output is usually larger than normal in advanced renal insufficiency. It is only when end-stage renal disease (ESRD) is reached that urine

TABLE 18.5. COMPONENTS OF NORMAL DAILY WATER BALANCE IN THE ADULT

Water intake

Source of Water	Water Volume (mL/day)
Ingested as fluid	Variable,[a] usually 1,000–2,000
Ingested as solid food	Usually 800–1,000
Water production from oxidative metabolism	Usually 200–300
Total:	2,000–3,300

Water output

Routes of Water Loss	Water Volume (mL/day)
Urine	Variable,[b] usually 1,000–1,800
Sweat	Negligible, except in hot environment, when several thousand mL can be lost
Stool	100
Evaporation[c]	
Skin	450
Respiratory tract	450
Total:	2,000–3,300

[a]The amount of water ingested depends on cultural influences as well as serum osmolality.
[b]Depends on that need to achieve water balance.
[c]These are pure water losses. The losses are influenced by humidity and body temperature.

TABLE 18.6. GUIDELINE FOR DAILY WATER INTAKE IN ADULT PATIENTS WITH RENAL INSUFFICIENCY

Patients with impaired kidney function but not ESRD

Measured fluid intake (not including water in solid foods) of 2,000 ± 500 mL/24 hours is appropriate.

Higher water intake is required if the following conditions are present:

- "Salt-wasting" renal disease
- Nephrogenic diabetes insipidus
- Fever (increase fluid intake by 50 mL/day for each 1°F of fever)
- Hyperventilation (doubling the respiratory rate increases insensible losses from respiratory tract by about 200 mL/day)
- Increased sweating (the electrolyte content of sweat is not altered by renal failure)

Patients with oliguric acute renal failure or ESRD

Total daily fluid intake (including solid food) should approximate:
600 mL[a] + urine output + extrarenal water losses[b]

The above formula should be strictly adhered to in patients vulnerable to fluid overload (hypertension, congestive heart failure, etc.) or in those with hyponatremia.

More liberal intake is appropriate in patients not vulnerable to serious adverse effects of fluid overload. In these patients it is acceptable to permit up to 3-kg weight gains between hemodialysis treatments.

ESRD, end-stage renal disease.
[a]600 mL/day is the difference between daily insensible water losses (900 mL) and daily water production from metabolism of carbohydrates and fat (300 mL).
[b]Diarrhea, nasogastric suction, etc.

volume falls below normal in the face of a normal intake of water.

Because the patient with advanced renal insufficiency can neither conserve nor excrete water normally, the patient is vulnerable to hyponatremic volume expansion with a high water intake and hypernatremic volume contraction with a low water intake. Fortunately these problems rarely are encountered in ambulatory patients with renal failure because the thirst mechanism, which is not impaired in renal failure (43), usually dictates an appropriate water intake. However, in patients not in control of their fluid intake such as hospitalized patients, patients with diabetes in whom high serum glucose stimulates thirst (42), or patients with congestive heart failure in whom high angiotensin II levels stimulate thirst (44), water intake may exceed the impaired kidney's ability to excrete the free water load. In such patients, water intake must be controlled properly to avoid serious perturbations of water balance. Table 18.6 provides guidelines for water intake in patients with impaired kidney function.

Excessive Fluid Weight Gain in Patients with End-Stage Renal Disease Maintained on Dialysis

It is not uncommon for some patients with ESRD to gain 4 to 6 kg in fluid weight between hemodialysis treatments or during several days of continuous ambulatory peritoneal dialysis (CAPD) therapy. Many develop adverse effects of fluid overload such as hypertension or congestive heart failure. Often these patients are counseled to "drink less fluid." However, it is unlikely that the primary mechanism of the large fluid weight gains is excess water intake. If water intake were primarily responsible, such patients would develop frank hyponatremia (e.g., a 10% to 15% decrease in serum sodium concentration). In fact, these patients are usually normonatremic (unpublished observation). This suggests that the primary mechanism for the fluid weight gain is excess salt intake, which then drives excess water intake. Thus, the key to managing these patients is to reduce their salt intake. If their salt intake is controlled, their water intake (and fluid weight gains) will be controlled.

POTASSIUM

Normal Potassium Metabolism

Potassium is the most abundant intracellular cation. Only 2% of total body potassium is present in the extracellular space. Although the extracellular potassium concentration

TABLE 18.7. MAJOR CONSEQUENCES OF ABNORMAL PLASMA POTASSIUM CONCENTRATION

Hyperkalemia
Mild (serum potassium 5.5 to 6.5 mEq/L)[a]
 EKG: peaked T-wave, prolonged PR interval
 Symptoms: often none
Moderate to severe (serum potassium > 6.5 mEq/L)[a]
 EKG: loss of P wave, prolonged QRS interval, intraventricular conduction abnormalities progressing to bradycardia, sine wave complexes
 Symptoms: can be asymptomatic, muscle weakness and/or stiffness, especially leg muscles progressing to total paralysis of skeletal muscles

Hypokalemia
Mild (serum potassium 3.0 to 3.5 mEq/L)[a]
 EKG: prolonged QT interval; premature ventricular contractions, particularly in patients receiving digitalis and/or those with heart disease
 Symptoms: often none, except those attributable to arrhythmia
Moderate to severe (serum potassium <3.0 mEq/L)
 EKG: same as mild hypokalemia but tendency to ventricular tachycardia may be greater
 Symptoms: muscle weakness that can be severe, muscle cramping

EKG, electrocardiogram.
[a]The levels of serum potassium that provide serious signs and symptoms vary considerably among patients. Changes in serum potassium that come about gradually are usually better tolerated than those that occur acutely.

does not reflect total body potassium stores, measurement of serum potassium is useful because disturbances of serum potassium are clinically relevant (Table 18.7). In health the distribution of potassium between the intracellular and extracellular space is influenced primarily by insulin (45,46), catecholamines (47,48), acid–base status (49), and serum osmolality (50,51). Approximately 80% to 95% of the daily potassium intake is excreted in the urine, and 5% to 20% is excreted in the stool (52). The urinary excretion of a potassium load is not abrupt; rather, it occurs over 24 to 48 hours. To prevent life-threatening hyperkalemia, much of an administered or ingested potassium load is shifted into the intracellular space. Thus, potassium homeostasis is best considered in two categories: factors regulating potassium shift into cells and factors regulating renal excretion of potassium.

Extrarenal Potassium Handling in Health and in Renal Insufficiency

Insulin promotes the shift of potassium into the intracellular compartment in health and in renal insufficiency (45,46, 53–55). In the absence of insulin, infusion of a hypertonic solution such as glucose can induce hyperkalemia. The increase in potassium is secondary to the increase in plasma osmolality. Hyperkalemia from a rapid increase in serum osmolality also has been documented in patients with renal insufficiency as a result of administration of hypertonic saline or radiocontrast agents (50,51,56).

Catecholamines such as epinephrine cause a transient increase in extracellular fluid potassium followed by a sustained reduction in extracellular fluid potassium. The transient hyperkalemic response is mediated by the α-receptors, and the hypokalemic response is mediated by the β_2 receptors (48,57–59). Catecholamine-induced cellular potassium uptake can be impaired in renal failure and may explain the enhanced hyperkalemic response to α-adrenergic stimulation in renal failure (58,60). Despite this, patients with hyperkalemia and ESRD experience a decrease in serum potassium levels with β-agonist therapy (48,61).

Acidemia from inorganic acids, such as the infusion of HCl or NH_4Cl, results in hyperkalemia (49). However, metabolic acidosis that is the result of accumulation of organic acids, such as lactic acid or ketoacids, does not result in important transcellular shifts of potassium (62). Controversy exists regarding the effect of the metabolic acidosis of renal failure on transcellular potassium shifts (63,59).

Parathyroid hormone (PTH), through its ability to increase cytosolic calcium, interferes with the cellular uptake of potassium in renal disease and may play a role in the extrarenal handling of potassium in ESRD (64–66). Fasting in the patient with ESRD promotes hyperkalemia. This paradox is thought to result from insulinopenia and diminished response to catecholamines (57,60).

There is conflicting evidence about aldosterone's role in extrarenal potassium handling (55,57,67,68). In healthy individuals aldosterone's role in extrarenal potassium handling is minimal (69). In individuals who are anephric, disposal of an acute potassium load is impaired by an aldosterone receptor antagonist and is improved by an aldosterone agonist (70). There are also reports of impaired potassium handling in patients with renal insufficiency receiving heparin and angiotensin converting enzyme (ACE) inhibitors (71).

Renal Handling of Potassium in Health and in Renal Insufficiency

Plasma potassium is filtered freely at the glomerulus and then is reabsorbed extensively (90% to 95%) in the proximal nephron and loop of Henle. Potassium excretion is accomplished by distal tubular secretion. The renal tubular secretion of potassium is an energy-requiring process. Thus, disruption of tubular function by renal disease results in renal retention of potassium. This is in contrast to the renal handling of sodium in which damage to the kidney usually results in renal sodium wasting as a result of decreased sodium reabsorption.

In the distal-collecting duct potassium can be reabsorbed or secreted. Aldosterone is the primary factor influencing renal potassium handling (72). Increasing levels of aldosterone enhance potassium excretion by increasing the number of Na-K-ATPase pumps and sodium and potassium channels (73).

Renal potassium excretion is linked to distal nephron sodium absorption. Thus, increasing delivery of sodium to the distal tubule tends to increase urinary potassium excretion. Consequently, conditions such as high-salt diet, thiazide or loop diuretic therapy, Bartter's syndrome, and other acute or chronic salt-wasting renal diseases tend to cause hypokalemia. By contrast, low-salt diet or conditions that decrease distal delivery of sodium, such as congestive heart failure, tend to cause hyperkalemia. Positively charged ions such as trimethoprim and amiloride cause hyperkalemia by interfering with potassium excretion through blocking luminal sodium channels in the distal nephron (74). Spironolactone causes hyperkalemia by competitively inhibiting the action of aldosterone at its receptor. Chronic heparin therapy can inhibit aldosterone secretion (75,76).

Renal potassium excretion is maintained as GFR falls by increasing fractional excretion of potassium. At GFR above 15 mL/min (serum creatinine approximately 3.0 mg/dL), hyperkalemia rarely occurs unless aldosterone secretion or function is impaired. When the GFR falls below 15 mL/min, extrarenal handling of potassium, including increased gastrointestinal excretion, becomes more important in dissipating an acute potassium load (77).

When evaluating an elevated serum potassium level in the patient with renal impairment, many factors in addition to diet can play a role. As outlined earlier, fasting state, level of insulin, acid–base status, β-blocker therapy, serum PTH level, and heparin therapy can affect the plasma potassium level. Blood transfusion can be an important source of potassium because transfused blood can contain between 5 and 50 mEq/L of plasma potassium, depending on storage time of the blood (78).

Pseudohyperkalemia can result from lysis of erythrocytes if the venipuncture technique is flawed or if abnormally elevated levels of erythrocytes, platelets, or leukocytes are present (79–81). These cells release intracellular potassium when the blood is allowed to clot before obtaining serum. Collecting blood in heparin and using a syringe rather than a vacuum tube to collect the blood usually can avoid these causes of pseudohyperkalemia.

Dietary Management of Potassium

Most patients with renal insufficiency do not require aggressive dietary potassium restriction. That is, on a normal potassium intake (1 to 1.3 mEq/kg of ideal body weight/day) serum potassium will be maintained within the normal range. However, there are certain circumstances that may substantially limit renal potassium excretion in renal disease, making it necessary to reduce dietary potassium intake. There also are some conditions in patients with renal disease that may increase excretion of potassium, making it necessary to increase dietary potassium intake (Table 18.8).

TABLE 18.8. GUIDELINES FOR DIETARY POTASSIUM INTAKE IN ADULTS WITH RENAL INSUFFICIENCY

Condition usually requiring reduced potassium intake (50–60 mEq/day)
Mechanism: decreased aldosterone
Hyporenin-hypoaldosteronism
Beta blocker therapy
Chronic heparin therapy
Angiotensin converting enzyme inhibitor therapy
Angiotensin II receptor blockade
Mechanism: decreased sodium delivery to Na/K exchange site in distal tubule
Low NaCl intake
End-stage renal disease
Cyclosporine or tacralimus therapy
Conditions usually requiring an increase in potassium intake (100–120 mEq/day)
Type 1 or Type 2 renal tubular acidosis
Diuretic therapy
High-salt diets
$NaHCO_3$ therapy
Mineralocorticoid therapy (e.g., fludrocortisone, hydrocortisone)
Diuretic phase during recovery from acute tubular necrosis or obstructive uropathy
Bartter's or Gittleman's syndrome

Each gram of dietary protein generally contains about 1 mEq of potassium. Thus, it is difficult to design a diet that has a low potassium intake without also having a low protein intake. Fortunately, many patients with progressive renal disease are maintained on a reduced protein intake (e.g., 0.7 to 0.8 g/kg ideal body weight/day). Thus, potassium intake automatically is limited. If needed, potassium intake can be increased by increasing intake of nonprotein high-potassium food (Table 18.9).

MAGNESIUM

Total body magnesium is distributed primarily in bone and the intracellular fluid compartment, with only 1% of total body magnesium found in the ECFV. In health, approximately 40% of dietary magnesium is absorbed by the gastrointestinal tract; the remainder is excreted in the stool (82). Of plasma magnesium, 80% is filtered at the glomerulus, with all but 3% to 5% reabsorbed. Of the filtered load, 60% of magnesium is reabsorbed by the thick-ascending loop of Henle, 20% to 30% in the proximal tubule, and 5% in the distal tubule (34). In the face of low dietary magnesium intake, gastrointestinal absorption can increase to 70% and urinary excretion can be reduced to 0.5% of the filtered load. High dietary magnesium intake results in a reduction of gastrointestinal absorption to 20% and an increase in the fractional excretion of filtered magnesium.

TABLE 18.9. POTASSIUM CONTENT OF FOOD

Foods high in potassium (greater than 6.5 mEq per serving)
Imitation sour cream
Milk
Yogurt
Ice cream
Ground beef
Liver
Steak
Ham
Turkey
Flounder
Haddock
Tuna
Wheat germ
English muffins
Legumes[a]
Fruit[a]
Raw vegetables[a]
Potatoes[a]
Foods low in potassium (less than 2.5 mEq per serving)
Mozzarella and Swiss cheese
Parmesan cheese
Cream
Eggs
Shrimp
Breads
Rice
Spaghetti
Egg noodles
Raw grapes
Raw lemons
Alfalfa sprouts
Lettuce
Cucumber
Onion

[a]Foods that are high in potassium but low in protein.
From Mitch WE, Klahr S. Composition of common foods. In: Mitch WE, Kalhr S, eds. *Nutrition and the kidney.* Boston: Little, Brown, 1988:331, with permission.

Magnesium deficiency can result from dietary, gastrointestinal, or renal causes. In evaluating patients with hypomagnesemia, a 24-hour urinary magnesium content of greater than 0.5 mmol is abnormal and reflects renal magnesium wasting (32). With gastrointestinal losses of magnesium, urinary magnesium is reduced to 0.5 mmol per 24 hours or less. Low serum magnesium can interfere with the release of PTH and result in concomitant hypocalcemia (83). Hypomagnesemia also can result in tetany, muscle weakness, seizures, and supraventricular and ventricular arrhythmias (82).

TABLE 18.10. CONDITIONS ASSOCIATED WITH THE RENAL WASTING OF MAGNESIUM

Diuretics
Cisplatin-induced nephrotoxicity
Aminoglycoside-induced nephrotoxicity
Cyclosporine
Amphotericin B
Recovery phase of acute tubular necrosis
Acute alcohol intake
Hyperaldosteronism
Bartter's syndrome
Familial hypercalcemia
Hyperparathyroidism

TABLE 18.11. MANGESIUM CONTENT OF VARIOUS FOODS

High (greater than 20 mg per serving)
Meats
Green vegetables
Legumes
Dairy products
Low (less than 5 mg per serving)
Alcohol
Processed foods
Fat

Negative magnesium balance from decreased dietary intake is rare, except in the case of alcoholism. Alcoholics usually have a diet deficient in magnesium, and alcohol may promote renal magnesium wasting (84). Table 18.10 lists the causes of urinary magnesium wasting.

High serum magnesium levels occur almost exclusively in the face of renal insufficiency. At a GFR of less than 15 mL/min, the fractional excretion of magnesium may not increase sufficiently to prevent positive magnesium balance from occurring. This is especially true if dietary magnesium is supplemented with magnesium-containing antacids or cathartics (83). Mild increases in plasma magnesium are well tolerated, but at levels greater than 4 mEq/L loss of deep tendon reflexes, respiratory paralysis, and heart block may occur (83).

Dialysate for both hemodialysis and peritoneal dialysis contains magnesium concentrations that are below serum concentrations to help combat positive magnesium balance (83). Despite this, most patients undergoing dialysis have an increase in total body magnesium (85). The positive magnesium balance in patients with ESRD may contribute to renal osteodystrophy (86). Dietary magnesium manipulation usually is not addressed in ESRD unless the patient develops hypermagnesemia. On a diet containing the standard recommended daily allowance of magnesium (300 mg) serum magnesium levels usually will be maintained within normal limits. Table 18.11 lists the magnesium content of various food products.

REFERENCES

1. Whitescarver SA, Ott CE, Jackson BA, et al. Salt-sensitive hypertension: contribution of chloride. *Science* 1984;223(4643): 1430–1432.
2. Schrier RW. Pathogenesis of sodium and water retention in high-output and low-output cardiac failure, nephrotic syndrome, cirrhosis, and pregnancy (1). *N Engl J Med* 1988;319(16): 1065–1072.

3. Wennergren G, Henriksson BA, Weiss LG, et al. Effects of stimulation of nonmedullated cardiac afferents on renal water and sodium excretion. *Acta Physiol Scand* 1976;97(2):261–263.
4. de Bold AJ, Borenstein HB, Veress AT, et al. A rapid and potent natriuretic response to intravenous injection of atrial myocardial extract in rats. *Life Sci* 1981;28(1):89–94.
5. Epstein F. Effects of arteriovenous fistula on renal hemodynamics and electrolyte excretion. *J Clin Invest* 1953;32:233.
6. McCartney S, Cramb G. Effects of a high-salt diet on hepatic atrial natriuretic peptide receptor expression in Dahl salt-resistant and salt-sensitive rats. *J Hypertens* 1993;11(3):253–262.
7. Sumners C, Tang W, Paulding W, et al. Peptide receptors in astroglia: focus on angiotensin II and atrial natriuretic peptide. *Glia* 1994;11(2):110–116.
8. Fitzgibbons JP, Gennari FJ, Garfinkel HB, et al. Dependence of saline-induced natriuresis upon exposure of the kidney to the physical effects of extracellular fluid volume expansion. *J Clin Invest* 1974;54(6):1428–1436.
9. Simpson FO. Sodium intake, body sodium, and sodium excretion. *Lancet* 1988;2(8601):25–29.
10. Strauss MB. Surfeit and deficit of sodium. *Arch Intern Med* 1958; 102:527–537.
11. Heer M, Baisch F, Kropp J, et al. High dietary sodium chloride consumption may not induce body fluid retention in humans. *Am J Physiol Renal Physiol* 2000;278(4):F585–595.
12. Kurtzman NA. Should man live by low-salt bread alone? *Am J Kidney Dis* 2001;37(3):636–637.
13. Weinberger M, Fineberg N, Fineberg S, et al. Salt sensitivity, pulse pressure and death in normal and hypertensive humans. *Hypertension* 2001;37(2):429–432.
14. Humphreys MH. Salt intake and body fluid volumes: have we learned all there is to know? *Am J Kidney Dis* 2001;37(3): 648–652.
15. Murray RH, Luft FC, Bloch R, et al. Blood pressure responses to extremes of sodium intake in normal man. *Proc Soc Exp Biol Med* 1978;159(3):432–436.
16. Campase V. Salt sensitivity in hypertension. Renal and cardiovascular implications. *Hypertension* 1994;23:531.
17. Tripodi G, Valtorta F, Torielli L, et al. Hypertension-associated point mutations in the adducin alpha and beta subunits affect actin cytoskeleton and ion transport. *J Clin Invest* 1996;97(12): 2815–2822.
18. Taubes G. The (political) science of salt. *Science* 1998;281(5379): 898–901, 903–907.
19. Appel LJ, Moore TJ, Obarzanek E, et al. A clinical trial of the effects of dietary patterns on blood pressure. DASH Collaborative Research Group. *N Engl J Med* 1997;336(16):1117–1124.
20. Sacks FM, Svetkey LP, Vollmer WM, et al. Effects on blood pressure of reduced dietary sodium and the Dietary Approaches to Stop Hypertension (DASH) diet. DASH-Sodium Collaborative Research Group. *N Engl J Med* 2001;344(1):3–10.
21. US Department of Agriculture, US Department of Health and Human Services. Nutrition and your health: dietary guidelines for Americans, 4th ed. Home and Garden Bulletin No. 232; 1995.
22. Chobanian AV, Bakris GL, Black HR, et al. The seventh report of the joint national committee on prevention, detection, evalution, and treatment of high blood pressure: the JNC of report. *JAMA* 2003;289:2560–2571.
23. Bricker NS, Fine LG, Kaplan M, et al. "Magnification phenomenon" in chronic renal disease. *N Engl J Med* 1978;299(23): 1287–1293.
24. Fine L, Kurtz I, Woolf A, et al. Pathophysiology and nephron adaptation in chronic renal failure. In: Schrier RW, Gottschalk C, eds. *Diseases of the kidney.* Boston: Little, Brown, 1993: 1993–2703.
25. Kahn T, Mohammad G, Stein RM. Alterations in renal tubular sodium and water reabsorption in chronic renal disease in man. *Kidney Int* 1972;2(3):164–174.
26. Brod J, Bahlmann J, Cachovan M, et al. Development of hypertension in renal disease. *Clin Sci (Lond)* 1983;64(2):141–152.
27. Coleman A, Arias M, Carter N, et al. The mechanism of salt wastage in chronic renal disease. *Clin Invest* 1966;45:1116–1125.
28. Danovitch GM, Bourgoignie J, Bricker NS. Reversibility of the "salt-losing" tendency of chronic renal failure. *N Engl J Med* 1977;296(1):14–19.
29. Husted FC, Nolph KD, Maher JF. $NaHCO_3$ and NaCl tolerance in chronic renal failure. *J Clin Invest* 1975;56(2):414–419.
30. Reeves B, Te A. Tubular sodium transport. In: Schrier RW, Gottschalk CW, eds. *Diseases of the kidney.* Boston: Little, Brown, 1993:139.
31. Nicholson JP, Resnick LM, Laragh JH. The antihypertensive effect of verapamil at extremes of dietary sodium intake. *Ann Intern Med* 1987;107(3):329–334.
32. Krishna GG, Riley LJ Jr, Deuter G, et al. Natriuretic effect of calcium-channel blockers in hypertensives. *Am J Kidney Dis* 1991; 18(5):566–572.
33. Robertson G, Berl T. Pathophysiology of water metabolism. In: Brenner B, Rector F, eds. *The kidney.* Philadelphia: WB Saunders, 1991:677.
34. Teitelbaum I, Berl T, Kleeman C. The physiology of renal concentrating and diluting mechanisms. In: Maxwell M, Kleeman C, Narins RG, eds. *Clinical disorders of fluid and electrolyte metabolism.* St. Louis: McGraw-Hill, 1987:79.
35. Robertson GL. Thirst and vasopressin function in normal and disordered states of water balance. *J Lab Clin Med* 1983;101(3): 351–371.
36. Verney E. The antidiuretic hormone and the factors which determine its release. *Proc R Soc London* 1947;135:25.
37. Robertson GL. The regulation of vasopressin function in health and disease. *Recent Prog Horm Res* 1976;33:333–385.
38. Anderson RJ, Pluss RG, Berns AS, et al. Mechanism of effect of hypoxia on renal water excretion. *J Clin Invest* 1978;62(4): 769–777.
39. Baylis PH, Zerbe RL, Robertson GL. Arginine vasopressin response to insulin-induced hypoglycemia in man. *J Clin Endocrinol Metab* 1981;53(5):935–940.
40. Fisher DA. Norepinephrine inhibition of vasopressin antidiuresis. *J Clin Invest* 1968;47(3):540–547.
41. Keil LC, Summy-Long J, Severs WB. Release of vasopressin by angiotensin II. *Endocrinology* 1975;96(4):1063–1065.
42. Zerbe R, Robertson G. Osmotic and nonosmotic regulation of thirst and vasopressin secretion. In: Maxwell M, Kleeman C, Narins R, eds. *Clinical disorders of fluid and electrolyte metabolism.* New York: McGraw-Hill, 1987:61.
43. Argent NB, Burrell LM, Goodship TH, et al. Osmoregulation of thirst and vasopressin release in severe chronic renal failure. *Kidney Int* 1991;39(2):295–300.
44. Ramsay DJ, Rolls BJ, Wood RJ. The relationship between elevated water intake and oedema associated with congestive cardiac failure in the dog. *J Physiol* 1975;244(2):303–312.
45. DeFronzo RA, Sherwin RS, Dillingham M, et al. Influence of basal insulin and glucagon secretion on potassium and sodium metabolism. Studies with somatostatin in normal dogs and in normal and diabetic human beings. *J Clin Invest* 1978;61(2): 472–479.
46. DeFronzo RA, Felig P, Ferrannini E, et al. Effect of graded doses of insulin on splanchnic and peripheral potassium metabolism in man. *Am J Physiol* 1980;238(5):E421–427.
47. Brown M, Brown D, Murphy MB. Hypokalemia from beta2-receptor stimulation by circulating epinephrine. *N Engl J Med* 1983;309:1414–1419.
48. Castellino P, Bia MJ, DeFronzo RA. Adrenergic modulation of

potassium metabolism in uremia. *Kidney Int* 1990;37(2): 793–798.

49. Adler S, Fraley DS. Potassium and intracellular pH. *Kidney Int* 1977;11(6):433–442.
50. Conte G, Dal Canton A, Imperatore P, et al. Acute increase in plasma osmolality as a cause of hyperkalemia in patients with renal failure. *Kidney Int* 1990;38(2):301–307.
51. Moreno M, Murphy C, Goldsmith C. Increase in serum potassium resulting from the administration of hypertonic mannitol and other solutions. *J Lab Clin Med* 1969;73(2):291–298.
52. Rabelink TJ, Koomans HA, Hene RJ, et al. Early and late adjustment to potassium loading in humans. *Kidney Int* 1990;38(5): 942–947.
53. Alvestrand A, Wahren J, Smith D, et al. Insulin-mediated potassium uptake is normal in uremic and healthy subjects. *Am J Physiol* 1984;246(2 Pt 1):E174–180.
54. Silvia P, Brown R, Epstein F. Adaptation to potassium. *Kidney Int* 1977;11:466–475.
55. Brown RS. Extrarenal potassium homeostasis. *Kidney Int* 1986; 30(1):116–127.
56. Goldfarb S, Cox M, Singer I, et al. Acute hyperkalemia induced by hyperglycemia: hormonal mechanisms. *Ann Intern Med* 1976; 84(4):426–432.
57. Allon M. Treatment and prevention of hyperkalemia in end-stage renal disease. *Kidney Int* 1993;43(6):1197–1209.
58. Allon M, Copkney C. Albuterol and insulin for treatment of hyperkalemia in hemodialysis patients. *Kidney Int* 1990;38(5): 869–872.
59. Allon M, Shanklin N. Adrenergic modulation of extrarenal potassium disposal in men with end-stage renal disease. *Kidney Int* 1991;40(6):1103–1109.
60. Gifford JD, Rutsky EA, Kirk KA, et al. Control of serum potassium during fasting in patients with end-stage renal disease. *Kidney Int* 1989;35(1):90–94.
61. Montoliu J, Lens XM, Revert L. Potassium-lowering effect of albuterol for hyperkalemia in renal failure. *Arch Intern Med* 1987; 147(4):713–717.
62. Fulop M. Serum potassium in lactic acidosis and ketoacidosis. *N Engl J Med* 1979;300(19):1087–1089.
63. Blumberg A, Weidmann P, Ferrari P. Effect of prolonged bicarbonate administration on plasma potassium in terminal renal failure. *Kidney Int* 1992;41(2):369–374.
64. Massry SG. Renal failure, parathyroid hormone and extrarenal disposal of potassium. *Miner Electrolyte Metab* 1990;16(1): 77–81.
65. Soliman AR, Akmal M, Massry SG. Parathyroid hormone interferes with extrarenal disposition of potassium in chronic renal failure. *Nephron* 1989;52(3):262–267.
66. Sugarman A, Kahn T. Parathyroid hormone impairs extrarenal potassium tolerance in the rat. *Am J Physiol* 1988;254(3 Pt 2): F385–390.
67. Tuck ML, Davidson MB, Asp N, et al. Augmented aldosterone and insulin responses to potassium infusion in dogs with renal failure. *Kidney Int* 1986;30(6):883–890.
68. Hiatt N, Chapman LW, Davidson MB, et al. Adrenal hormones and the regulation of serum potassium in potassium-loaded adrenalectomized dogs. *Endocrinology* 1979;105(1):215–219.
69. Alexander EA, Levinsky NG. An extrarenal mechanism of potassium adaptation. *J Clin Invest* 1968;47(4):740–748.
70. Sugarman A, Brown RS. The role of aldosterone in potassium tolerance: studies in anephric humans. *Kidney Int* 1988;34(3): 397–403.
71. Durand D, Ader JL, Rey JP, et al. Inducing hyperkalemia by converting enzyme inhibitors and heparin. *Kidney Int Suppl* 1988; 25:S196–197.
72. Rabinowitz L. Homeostatic regulation of potassium excretion. *J Hypertens* 1989;7(6):433–442.
73. Giebish G, Malnic G, Berliner R. Renal transport and control of potassium excretion. In: Brenner B, Rector F, eds. *The kidney.* Philadelphia: WB Saunders, 1991:283–317.
74. Choi MJ, Fernandez PC, Patnaik A, et al. Brief report: trimethoprim-induced hyperkalemia in a patient with AIDS. *N Engl J Med* 1993;328(10):703–706.
75. Wilson I, Goetz F. Selective hypoaldosteronism after prolonged heparin administration. *Am J Med* 1984;36:635–639.
76. O'Kelly R, Magee F, McKenna TJ. Routine heparin therapy inhibits adrenal aldosterone production. *J Clin Endocrinol Metab* 1983;56(1):108–112.
77. Martin RS, Panese S, Virginillo M, et al. Increased secretion of potassium in the rectum of humans with chronic renal failure. *Am J Kidney Dis* 1986;8(2):105–110.
78. Simon GE, Bove JR. The potassium load from blood transfusion. *Postgrad Med* 1971;49(6):61–64.
79. Bronson WR, DeVita VT, Carbone PP, et al. Pseudohyperkalemia due to release of potassium from white blood cells during clotting. *N Engl J Med* 1966;274(7):369–375.
80. Don BR, Sebastian A, Cheitlin M, et al. Pseudohyperkalemia caused by fist clenching during phlebotomy. *N Engl J Med* 1990; 322(18):1290–1292.
81. Hartmann R, Auditore J, Jackson D. Studies on thrombocytosis. I. Hyperkalemia due to release of potassium from platelets during coagulation. *J Clin Invest* 1958;37:699–707.
82. Slatopolsky E, Hruska K, Klahr S. Disorders of phosphorus, calcium, and magnesium metabolism. In: Schrier RW, Gottschalk C, eds. *Diseases of the kidney.* Boston: Little, Brown, 1993: 2630–2635.
83. Sutton R, Dirks J. Disturbances of calcium and magnesium metabolism. In: Brenner B, Rector F, eds. *The kidney.* Philadelphia: WB Saunders, 1991:841.
84. Dick M, Evans RA, Watson L. Effect of ethanol on magnesium excretion. *J Clin Pathol* 1969;22(2):152–153.
85. Contiguglia SR, Alfrey AC, Miller N, et al. Total-body magnesium excess in chronic renal failure. *Lancet* 1972;1(7764): 1300–1302.
86. Mitch W, Klahr S. Composition of common foods. In: Mitch W, Klahr S, eds. *Nutrition and the kidney.* Boston: Little, Brown, 1988:331.

19

TRACE ELEMENT METABOLISM IN RENAL DISEASE

RAYMOND VANHOLDER
RITA CORNELIS
ANNEMIEKE DHONDT
NORBERT LAMEIRE

During the last decades, research on uremic toxicity has focused almost exclusively on retention and removal of organic compounds; inorganic compounds, however, may induce biologic, biochemical, and/or functional disturbances as well. Changes in the homeostasis of water and current electrolytes play an important pathophysiologic role, and changes in trace element concentration sometimes have an impact on morbidity as well.

The term "trace element" dates back to the developmental stage of analytical methods (19th century) and refers to all elements in body fluids and tissues that were found in such small amounts that they could not be measured accurately at that time. The terminology persisted, although most trace elements now can be measured very accurately.

Trace elements are divided into two categories: essential and nonessential. The definition of "essential" includes: (a) the element should be present in healthy tissues, (b) deficiency of the element consistently produces functional impairment, (c) the abnormalities induced by the deficiency always are associated with specific biochemical changes, and (d) supplementation of the element prevents or corrects these changes (1).

It sometimes is stated that the term "trace element" bears on elements that under normal conditions occur in the body at concentrations below 50 mg/kg (1). Some elements that are reviewed in this chapter (e.g., iron) do not conform to this definition. In this chapter adherence to a broader definition is preferred and all compounds that currently are referred to in the literature as "trace element concentration in renal failure" are reviewed.

METHODOLOGY FOR THE MEASUREMENT OF TRACE ELEMENT CONCENTRATION

Various analytical techniques can be used to measure trace element concentrations in body fluids and tissues. The sensitivity per element differs substantially from one technique to another. Some elements may be assayed equally well by several methods, but a given technique may show superior characteristics as far as sensitivity, accuracy, or labor intensity are concerned.

Accurate determination of trace element concentrations is essential to allow a correct interpretation of the pathophysiologic events related to their accumulation or deficiency in chronic uremia. Analytical methods for these measurements continued to improve during the last decade. The implementation of additional software to make the well-established methods more user friendly is a major asset in the application of flame/flameless atomic absorption spectrometry, electron microprobe analysis, inductively coupled plasma emission spectrometry, inductively coupled plasma mass spectrometry (ICP-MS), neutron-activation analysis, and x-ray fluorescence. There is an increase in the application of high-resolution ICP-MS because it guarantees analytical data that are practically free of interferences. A remarkable development in reducing spectral interferences has been the dynamic reaction cell for ICD-MS (2,3). The analytical methods at hand should be specific and sensitive and should enable the analysis of trace elements in small tissue samples.

For many elements, such as aluminum, chromium, cobalt, and manganese, which occur in the ng/L or ng/kg range, major difficulties arise already at the stage of sample collection and handling. Because of the very low concentration of these elements, contamination is an important problem. Utmost care should be taken to collect samples in reliable recipients and tubes (4). Some trace elements might be leached out of the collection tubes during one or several of the preparative steps, and specific measures should be taken to prevent this (5).

For single-element analysis, the most commonly available system is flameless atomic absorption spectrometry. For some studies, it may be interesting to use a multielement method that allows the estimation of several trace elements at the same time. Some of these methods, however, necessitate a sophisticated infrastructure and are very labor intensive. The management of large numbers of samples in a relatively limited study period then becomes difficult. Radiochemical neutron activation analysis is an example of such a method. Its value lies in being the pioneer in producing accurate data, and it continues to serve as a very reliable reference method for certification purposes. ICP-MS has superseded all other methods for multiple-element analysis. The introduction of high-resolution ICP-MS also markedly improved the situation for the analysis of the trace elements

TABLE 19.1. CHARACTERISTICS OF TRACE ELEMENTS

Name	Abbreviation	Atomic Weight	Atomic Number	Valence
Aluminum	Al	26.98	13	3
Antimony	Sb	121.75	51	3,5
Arsenic	As	74.92	33	3,5
Barium	Ba	137.34	56	2
Beryllium	Be	9.01	4	2
Boron	B	10.81	5	3
Bromine	Br	79.90	35	1,3,5,7
Cadmium	Cd	112.40	48	2
Cerium	Ce	140.12	58	3,4
Cesium	Cs	132.91	55	1
Chromium	Cr	52.00	24	2,3,5,6
Cobalt	Co	58.93	27	2,3
Copper	Cu	63.55	29	1,2
Europium	Eu	151.96	63	2,3
Fluorine	F	18.99	9	1
Gallium	Ga	69.72	31	2,3
Germanium	Ge	72.59	32	2,4
Gold	Au	196.97	79	1,3
Hafnium	Hf	178.49	72	4
Indium	In	114.82	49	1,2,3
Iodine	I	126.91	53	1,3,5,7
Iridium	Ir	192.22	77	3,4
Iron	Fe	55.85	26	2,3,4,6
Lanthanum	La	138.91	57	3
Lead	Pb	207.20	82	2,4
Lithium	Li	6.94	3	1
Lutetium	Lu	174.97	71	3
Manganese	Mn	54.94	25	2,3,4,6,7
Mercury	Hg	200.59	80	1,2
Molybdenum	Mo	95.94	42	3,4,6
Neodynium	Nd	144.24	60	3
Nickel	Ni	58.71	28	2,3
Palladium	Pd	106.40	46	2,4,6
Platinum	Pt	195.90	78	2,4
Rubidium	Rb	85.47	37	1
Samarium	Sm	150.40	62	2,3
Scandium	Sc	44.96	21	3
Selenium	Se	78.96	34	2,4,6
Silicon	Si	28.08	14	4
Silver	Ag	107.87	47	1
Strontium	Sr	87.62	38	2
Tantalum	Ta	180.95	73	5
Terbium	Tb	158.93	65	3
Thallium	Tl	204.37	81	1,3
Thorium	Th	232.04	90	4
Tin	Sn	118.93	50	2,4
Titanium	Ti	47.90	22	3,4
Tungsten	W	183.85	74	6
Uranium	U	238.03	92	4,6
Vanadium	V	50.94	23	3,5
Zinc	Zn	65.38	30	2
Zirconium	Zr	91.22	40	2,3,4

All elements may have "0" as valence. Only the oxidative condition as it occurs in humans is mentioned.

in body fluids and tissues. There is, however, not a single method that allows the measurement of all possible trace elements both in body fluids and tissues.

Trace elements currently are determined in blood and blood constituents such as plasma, serum, erythrocytes, packed cells, platelets, or leukocytes. In addition, analyses of trace elements in tissues are performed on biopsy and autopsy samples. The latter values are not necessarily representative for those present in circulating blood.

TRACE ELEMENTS

A list of 52 known trace elements is given in Table 19.1. In what follows, we mainly concentrate on those trace elements that have been evaluated in uremia; these include aluminum, arsenic, bromine, cadmium, cesium, chromium, cobalt, copper, germanium, gold, iron, lanthanum, lead, manganese, mercury, molybdenum, nickel, rubidium, selenium, silicon, strontium, vanadium, and zinc.

TRACE ELEMENT CONCENTRATIONS IN UREMIA

The deviation from normal of uremic trace element concentrations in body fluids and tissues depends on many factors; the most important one is the degree of renal failure. Changes in trace element concentration also may be induced by specific renal replacement strategies. In addition, in some patients, end-stage renal failure may be the result of an intoxication with one of the trace elements (e.g., lead).

The lack of uniformity in the reported results is a source of misunderstanding and discrepancy. Sometimes whole blood values are reported, or concentrations in blood constituents such as serum or plasma, packed cells, or erythrocytes are reported. Concentrations in various tissues are in almost all cases markedly different from blood or plasma concentrations (6,7). The kidneys and skin, especially, are known to sequester trace elements (e.g., arsenicum and cadmium). Studies of the kinetics of trace elements show that distribution in the body might be different, depending on the way of their ingestion (8).

Trace element concentrations in uremia that were reported in the 1960s and 1970s might differ from more recently found values because the sensitivity and accuracy of trace element measurement have improved, and the therapeutic interventions (dialysis strategies, nutrition, dialysis adequacy, erythropoietin) have changed substantially.

Table 19.2 gives the range of normal serum concentrations of various trace elements (9–15), and Table 19.3 gives the comparative values in uremia (7,9,10,16–30), together with an indication of whether the values are increased or decreased compared to the reference.

Some elements increase (e.g., arsenicum, cobalt, cesium, chromium, mercury, molybdenum, silicon, strontium) in renal failure, whereas others decrease (e.g., bromine, rubidium, selenium, zinc). The degree of renal failure and the type of renal replacement therapy further influence trace element concentration (e.g., bromine is decreased in patients being treated with hemodialysis or continuous ambulatory peritoneal dialysis [CAPD], but it is elevated in patients with renal failure not yet undergoing renal replacement therapy). Differences may be observed from organ to organ (31), or they also may depend on the area where the patients under study are living (32,33).

TABLE 19.2. TRACE ELEMENTS: RANGE OF THE MEANS OF REFERENCE CONCENTRATIONS AS REPORTED IN NORMAL SERUM/PLASMA

Element	Serum
Aluminum (μg/L)	1.0–6.0
Antimony (μg/L)	<0.01
Arsenic (μg/L)	0.09–5.49
Bromine (mg/L)	2.19–5.00
Cadmium (μg/L)	<0.10–0.20
Cesium (μg/L)	0.45–1.50
Chromium (μg/L)	0.04–0.35
Cobalt (μg/L)	0.04–0.40
Copper (mg/L)	0.98–1.07
Gold (ng/L)	9–12
Iron (mg/L)	0.79–1.63
Manganese (μg/L)	0.38–1.04
Mercury (μg/L)	0.55–2.10
Molybdenum (μg/L)	0.28–1.17
Rubidium (mg/L)	0.095–0.272
Selenium (mg/L)	0.081–0.185
Silicon (mg/L)	0.14–0.20
Strontium (μg/L)	15–30
Vanadium (μg/L)	0.01–1.0
Zinc (mg/L)	0.69–1.21

Normal values extracted from references 9–15.

The authors consider it beyond the scope of this chapter to review in depth reported tissue concentrations of various trace elements, and the reader is referred to the specialized literature. It should be kept in mind that most of the available data have been collected in autopsied cases and that the reported values reflect the trace element status in the terminally ill patient, rather than in the currently treated patient with uremia whose health status is well under control.

As expected, erythropoietin treatment decreases body iron stores. In addition, increases in zinc, nickel, and manganese have been observed (34,35). These changes might be related to an improved nutritional intake and/or metabolic status.

POTENTIAL CONTRIBUTION OF TRACE ELEMENTS TO THE UREMIC SYNDROME

The uremic syndrome is characterized by a complex of symptoms and functional disturbances of biochemical sys-

TABLE 19.3. TRACE ELEMENTS: REPORTED EVOLUTION OF SERUM/PLASMA CONCENTRATIONS IN RENAL FAILURE (RANGE OF MEAN VALUES AS REPORTED IN VARIOUS PAPERS)[a]

		Evolution in Renal Failure		
Element	**References**	**OP**	**HD**	**CAPD**
Aluminum (μg/L)	27,28	50.0–186.3(↑)	50.0–183.6(↑)	105.3(↑)
Antimony (μg/L)	24	—	73.0(=)	—
Arsenic (μg/L)	19–21,24	—	8.5–79.8(↑↓)	—
Bromine (mg/L)	22,23,30	6.9(=)	1.1–1.9(↓)	1.0(↓)
Cadmium (μg/L)	24	—	1.2(=)	—
Cesium (μg/L)	23,24	—	0.6–1.5(=/↑)	1.1(=)
Chromium (μg/L)	18,23	—	—	4.3(↑)
Cobalt (μg/L)	23	—	—	0.3(↑)
Copper (mg/L)	23,24,27,30	0.8–1.3(=/↑)	0.8–1.5(=/↑)	1.1–1.2(=)
Gold (ng/L)	24	—	40.9(=/↑)	—
Iron (mg/L)	23,24,30	0.7(=)	0.9–1.6(=/↑)	1.2(=)
Manganese (μg/L)	23	—	—	0.6(=)
Mercury (μg/L)	24	—	2.5(↑)	—
Molybdenum (μg/L)	17,24	—	2.3–2.7(↑)	—
Rubidium (mg/L)	23,27	—	0.1(↓)	0.2(=)
Selenium (mg/L)	7,23,24	0.2(=)	0.05–0.1(=/↓)	0.06–0.1(↓)
Silicon (mg/L)	16,25,26	1.3(↑)	2.5–4.6(↑)	1.9(↑)
Strontium (μg/L)	9,10	—	25–466(↑)	50–55(↑)
Vanadium (μg/L)	29	—	18.4(↑)	—
Zinc (mg/L)	23,27,30	0.7–0.9(↓)	0.7–0.9(↓)	0.8(↓)

OP, outpatients (chronic renal failure without dialysis); HD, hemodialysis; CAPD, continuous ambulatory peritoneal dialysis.
[a]= points to no significant difference versus the reference value, ↑ and ↓ to a significant increase or decrease. Note that reference values may be different from study to study, and hence they may differ slightly from the reference values outlined in Table 19.2.

tems and organs, which will lead to death if the responsible toxins are not eliminated. Several of the typical functional disturbances of uremia may be the consequence of loss or accumulation of trace elements. A list of trace elements with their potential toxic/depletory side effects is summarized in Table 19.4. In the following section, we discuss the major physiologic systems that are affected during uremia and the potential role of trace elements. It should be stressed that changes in concentration of trace elements are not necessarily the sole pathophysiologic mechanisms for the observed uremic alterations, but other factors such as uremic retention of organic solutes, malnutrition, and dialyzer bioincompatibility may affect the same biochemical/biologic systems to an even more substantial degree.

Finally, the discussed alterations have not necessarily been described in patients with renal failure; in some instances they were observed in subjects with normal renal function but with trace element concentrations, comparable to those obtained in uremia. Therefore, these changes were extrapolated to the uremic status.

Impairment of Renal Function

The progression of renal failure may in part be attributed to the accumulation of nephrotoxic compounds in the body. In healthy individuals, trace elements are partially or totally removed from the body by the healthy kidneys. Because accumulation of some of these trace elements occurs in uremia, and because some of them are potentially nephrotoxic, the presence of supranormal trace element concentrations may be one possible mechanism for the deterioration of renal function. It should be kept in mind, however, that environmental factors (ingestion of food, air pollution, or industrial exposure) may play an equally important role in these accumulation processes.

Aluminum increases the bioavailability and the nephrotoxicity of cyclosporin A in rats (36). This, however, was not confirmed in humans (37).

Arsenic may provoke tubulointerstitial nephritis (38). Arsenic toxicity of the kidney or the liver might be tempered by the presence of selenium, which results in the precipitation of arsenic selenide in the lysosomes, which are eliminated later via the urine (39,40).

Cadmium, copper, and mercury, which accumulate preferentially in kidney tissue (41), may cause multiple renal tubular transport defects resulting in the equivalent of the Fanconi's syndrome (42). Cadmium provokes biochemical changes in lipid and glutamate metabolism that precede classical nephrotoxic effects (43,44), and at a later stage the junctions between tubular cells are disrupted (45). Renal accumulation of cadmium results in cortical and medullary lipid peroxidation (46). Blocking of this lipid peroxidation, however, does not counteract the adverse effect of cadmium on kidney function (46). Itai-itai disease, a disorder characterized by renal tubulopathy and osteomalacia, typically occurs in cadmium-polluted areas (47). Cadmium nephrotox-

TABLE 19.4. TRACE ELEMENTS AND POSSIBLE TOXIC EFFECTS

- Aluminum (↑)
  - Anemia
  - Decreased-affinity PTH receptor
  - Encephalopathy
  - Gastrointestinal dysfunction
  - Increase in nephrotoxicity of cyclosporin A
  - Osteomalacia
  - Suppression PTH-stimulated adenylate cyclase
  - Tumoral calcifications of soft tissues
- Arsenic (↑)
  - Anemia
  - Cancer
  - Cerebrovascular disease
  - Disturbances in lipid peroxidation
  - Hepatotoxicity
  - Nephropathy
- Cadmium (↑)
  - Cancer
  - Disturbances in lipid peroxidation
  - Fanconi's syndrome
  - Inhibition Na-glucose cotransport
  - Inhibition Na-K-ATPase
  - Hypertension
  - Nephropathy
  - Osteomalacia
  - Vascular disease
- Chromium (↑)
  - Hepatotoxicity
  - Nephropathy
- Cobalt (↑)
  - Heart failure
  - Inhibition hepatic gluconeogenesis
  - Production platelet-derived growth factor
- Copper (↑)
  - Atherogenesis
  - Fanconi's syndrome
  - Fever
  - Myocardial infarction
- Copper (↓)
  - Cardiovascular dysfunction
  - Electrical instability of the heart
  - Pancytopenia
  - Superoxide dismutase deficiency
- Germanium (↑)
  - Hepatotoxicity
  - Lactic acidosis
  - Nephropathy
  - Neuropathy
- Iron (↑)
  - Adynamic bone disease
  - Cardiac ischemia
  - DNA damage
  - Generation of free radicals
  - Glucose intolerance
  - Hepatotoxicity
  - Immune deficiency
- Lead (↑)
  - Anemia
  - Fanconi's syndrome
  - Hypertension
  - Inhibition Na-K-ATPase
  - Nephropathy
- Mercury (↑)
  - Fanconi's syndrome
  - Hypertension
  - Inhibition Na-K-ATPase
  - Nephropathy
- Molybdenum (↑)
  - Hypercalcemia
  - Hyperparathyroidism
- Selenium (↓)
  - Anemia
  - Cancer
  - Cardiovascular disease
  - Congestive cardiomyopathy
  - Deficiency antioxidative mechanisms
  - Glutathione peroxidase deficiency
  - Immune dysfunction
  - Peroxidative damage to cells
  - Skeletal myopathy
  - Thyroid dysfunction
- Strontium (↑)
  - Osteomalacia
- Silicon (↑)
  - Hypercalcemia
  - Nephropathy
  - Skin eruptions
  - Wegener's granulomatosis
- TIn (↑)
  - Nephropathy
- Vanadium (↑)
  - Anemia
  - Broadening cardiac action potentials
  - Hypertension
  - Inhibition Na-K-ATPase
  - Negative inotropic effects
- Zinc (↓)
  - Decreased scar formation
  - Decreased smell acuity
  - Decreased taste acuity
  - Hypogonadism
  - Immune dysfunction
  - Sexual dysfunction
  - Superoxide dismutase deficiency

PTH, parathyroid hormone.

icity is accentuated by the simultaneous accumulation of arsenic (48). Long-term follow-up of subjects with moderate environmental exposure to cadmium, however, showed no evolution to progressive renal failure (49).

Chromium affects the viability of kidney epithelial cells and, to a lesser extent, that of hepatic epithelial cells (50). In the working area of chrome workers, elevated airborne chromium concentrations have been found (51). At the same time, an elevation of several urinary markers of potential renal injury was found in this population (52).

Germanium may be administered as a nonprescription drug as prevention of immune deficiency. Ingestion of substantial doses has been associated with renal failure, hepatic failure, and lactic acidosis (53).

Elevated blood lead concentrations have been associated with subtle impairment of renal function in the general population (54). Although exposure to lead causes impaired renal function, it cannot be excluded that the renal impairment results in lead accumulation.

It has been suggested that bone lead generally is increased in patients with overt chronic renal failure and that body burden depends on renal function; some authors, however, found that, except in patients with excessive lead exposure, lead body burden in the uremic population is in the normal range (55). Possible differences can be attributed to environmental factors; the global population with renal failure may contain patients with previously unrecognized lead exposure. Furthermore, if exposure to subtle quantities of lead occurs as a result of contamination of ambient air or transitory forensic contacts, retention may be more pronounced in patients with renal failure. This may result in higher blood lead levels in patients with end-stage renal disease (ESRD) living in urban and/or industrial areas. Similar events may occur for other trace elements that normally are excreted in the urine.

In an extended case-control study, exposure to lead, chromium, copper, tin, mercury, and silicon-containing compounds was shown to be related to an increased risk for chronic renal failure (56).

Inhalation of silicon-containing compounds, such as silica and grain dust, has been related to the development of Wegener's granulomatosis (57). Administration of tetraethoxysilane to normal mice resulted in an increase of blood silicon levels and in the development of tubulointerstitial nephritis (58). In a retrospective cohort study, ESRD was shown to be more prevalent among silica-exposed gold miners, especially after a prolonged exposure time (>10 years) (59). Renal involvement is not uncommon in patients with exposure to silicon and a history of pulmonary silicosis (60).

Susceptibility to Cancer

Several reports associate increased contact with and/or uptake of arsenic to a higher incidence of lung and skin cancer (61–63). Although there is more debate on the role of arsenic in the development of gastrointestinal, urogenital, or hematologic cancers, it should be noted that the incidence of bladder and kidney cancer also is high in areas with high dietary arsenic ingestion (64). In a study extended over a long time period and with a large number of subjects, greater mortality was found for most cancer types in patients exposed to excess arsenic (65). Industrial exposure to arsenic results in a higher incidence of bone, kidney, intestinal, and renal cancers (66). The arsenic metabolite, dimethylarsinic acid, induces carcinogenesis in the rat (67).

The earlier described potential association between cadmium and prostate cancer (68) now is considered to be less probable. However, a high incidence of lung cancer was found in subjects exposed to cadmium (69). Selenium deficiency also has been incriminated to play a role in the induction of cancer (70).

Cardiovascular Disease

In subjects with normal renal function, elevated plasma aluminum and whole blood lead levels are related to essential hypertension (71). Exposure to excess arsenic predisposes to cerebrovascular disease (65). Arsenic has been shown to induce lipid peroxidation (72).

Cadmium promotes lipid peroxidation (73) and blocks antioxidant mechanisms in the rat kidney (74). The latter effect is counterbalanced by the simultaneous administration of selenium.

Copper deficiency is associated with cardiovascular dysfunction (75) and may play an important role in the promotion of electrical instability of the heart (76). Copper excess, however, is related to lipid oxidation, accelerated atherogenesis, and excess risk of acute myocardial infarction (77). Cobalt excess also may play a role in uremic heart failure (78).

Excess iron stores are associated with an increased risk for myocardial infarction (77), even after adjustment for serum cholesterol values (79). This may be attributed to catalization of free radical production, which results in oxidation of lipids and catecholamines. Iron chelators reduce the extent of experimental myocardial ischemia. Also, alterations of glucose metabolism and insulin resistance have been related to iron overload (80).

Mercury, lead, and cadmium all inhibit Na-K-ATPase (sodium-potassium-adenosine triphosphate) (42). Inhibition of this enzyme ultimately will lead to an increased intracellular sodium concentration, which determines vascular wall tension; this in turn results in peripheral vasoconstriction, hypertension, and probably cardiomyopathy.

Selenium deficiency has been associated with an increased risk for cardiovascular complications (81,82). Intravenous application of sodium selenite to patients who have undergone dialysis not only corrects plasma selenium, but also corrects deficiencies of protective antioxidative mechanisms (83). These data suggest a role for selenium in oxidative damage in uremia, which is related to atherogenesis. Vanadium also has been associated with inhibition of Na-K-ATPase activity, resulting in either positive or negative inotropic effects, broadening of heart action potentials (84), and hypertension (85).

Bone Disease

Aluminum intoxication is related to vitamin D–resistant osteomalacia (86). Aluminum also decreases the affinity of parathyroid hormone (PTH) receptors as well as the subsequent activity of PTH-stimulated adenylate cyclase, which possibly accounts for the peripheral resistance to PTH currently observed during aluminum intoxication (87). Clinical symptoms and histologic evidence of aluminum-related bone disease in patients with ESRD disappear after renal transplantation (88).

Exposure to cadmium provokes a strong increase in serum levels of bone γ-carboxyglutamate (Gla)-protein, which is an index of bone damage (89). Cadmium induces osteomalacia in ovariectomized rats (90), and the concentration of cadmium is increased in bone of patients with ESRD (91). Also, the chromium concentration in bone of patients with ESRD is increased (91).

Iron overload may be associated with an unusually high incidence of adynamic bone disease (92). It also may be associated with a state of relative hypoparathyroidism in patients undergoing dialysis (86).

Lanthanum, a rare earth metal, is used as a phosphate binder in the form of its carbonate salt (93). Administration of lanthanum carbonate to uremic rats, however, may lead to the accumulation of lanthanum in the bone.

Molybdenum levels are correlated to PTH, calcemia, and symptoms of dialysis-related arthritis (94) and also are correlated with the duration of the dialysis treatment. Therefore, the question arises whether molybdenum plays a direct pathophysiologic role or whether the increase in its concentration is a secondary consequence of long-term dialysis together with hyperparathyroidism.

Silicon may protect against aluminum-induced bone disease (16). However, silicon overload in patients undergoing dialysis might result in hypercalcemia and nodular skin eruptions (95). Bone strontium is increased in patients with ESRD and is associated with osteomalacia (91,96,97).

Anemia

Hypochromic anemia despite adequate iron status has been associated with aluminum accumulation. Aluminum can blunt the effect of erythropoietin (98), in part by its interference with iron bioavailability (99). This effect can be reversed by aluminum chelation therapy. Furthermore, aluminum overload leads to increased lipid peroxidation in the membranes of erythrocytes, which can reduce red-cell life span (100). Aluminum is also responsible for erythroid ferropenia, even if global body iron stores are normal (101).

Preferential transport of arsenic on transferrin and high bone marrow concentrations as a result of enhanced uptake of this complex may contribute to renal anemia (78,102, 103).

Copper deficiency has been associated with deficient growth of individual cell lines of the bone marrow as well as with pancytopenia (104,105). It should be stressed, however, that the uremic state in general gives rise to copper accumulation, rather than deficiency, except in severely ill patients with prolonged hospitalization. In one single study, a relative copper deficiency was recognized in patients being treated with hemodialysis or CAPD (106), but even then mononuclear cell copper was normal and copper-containing superoxide dismutase activity was high.

Serum vanadium is inversely correlated with red blood cell count and hemoglobin (29).

Encephalopathy, Coma, and Nerve Conduction

Acute trace element intoxication should be considered with any altered mental state (107). Dialysis dementia has been associated especially with aluminum intoxication (108); this complication mainly occurred in dialysis centers with extremely high aluminum concentrations in the water used to prepare dialysate (109), in combination with an inadequate water treatment system.

Hair concentrations of trace elements did not correlate with nerve conduction velocities (110).

Immune Deficiency

Aluminum intoxication is related to the impairment of several markers of immune function (111). Iron overload is one of the potential causes of immune deficiency and especially affects the phagocytic capacity to kill bacteria (112). Reversal of this iron overload (e.g., by erythropoietin) also reverses immune dysfunction (113). Not only iron overload, but also therapeutic measures to correct it, such as chelation with desferrioxamine, may induce immune deficiency (114).

Although iron overload tends to decrease the response of immune cells on stimulation, baseline immune cell activity tends to be enhanced, as illustrated by an increased capacity to produce markers of free radical generation (115). These events might be related to atherogenesis. It has been suggested that intravenous iron administration for treatment of iron deficiency may result in a temporary increase of oxidative reaction (116). In addition, high serum ferritin levels have been related to an enhanced risk for infection (112). It is, however, not always clear whether the increase of ferritin is the cause or the consequence of infection (117). Endocrine dysfunction and cardiomyopathy, related to high serum ferritin, disappear after iron depletion (118,119).

In a study by Golconda et al. it has been suggested that iron plays a role in hydrogen peroxide–induced DNA damage (120).

Selenium deficiency has been related to a deficient elimination of toxic free radical species as a result of underactivity of the selenium-dependent metalloenzymes, such as the superoxide dismutases (121). These free radicals, if not thoroughly neutralized, are toxic toward lipids, proteins, and nucleic acids, resulting in cell destruction and atherogenesis. The involvement of selenium in the immune response is increasingly recognized, cell-mediated immunity being principally affected by selenium deficiency (122). Selenium therapy in patients undergoing hemodialysis results in an improvement of T-cell response to phytohemagglutinin and an increase in delayed-type hypersensitivity (123).

Zinc deficiency is a well known side effect of uremia and of uremic malnutrition (124). It most likely will affect those compartments with high turnover rates such as the liver and peripheral blood cells, including lymphocytes (125).

Zinc substitution results in an increase of tetanus antibody titers, as well as in an increase of soluble interleukin-2 receptor concentration (126). At least one study did not confirm the positive impact of zinc supplementation on immune functional capacity (127).

FACTORS AFFECTING TRACE ELEMENT CONCENTRATION

Trace element deficiencies are the result of inadequate intake, decreased availability, impaired absorption, excessive excretion, extracorporeal losses, and total parenteral nutrition without adequate substitution (Table 19.5). Some trace elements are removed by dialysis because of low concentration in the dialysate (e.g., bromide and zinc) (24). Malnutrition, as reflected by low serum protein, may be one of the causes of low serum zinc, manganese, and nickel (128).

Deficiency of protein-bound trace elements may be aggravated in the presence of substantial urinary protein losses (nephrotic syndrome).

In patients with ESRD and those undergoing dialysis, however, increases of trace element concentration may play the most important pathophysiologic role. An increase in concentration may result from excess intake, increased gastrointestinal uptake, and defective excretion. Because most of the trace elements are eliminated by the kidneys, renal failure will lead to their accumulation. Additional sources of accumulation could be the result of the presence of excess trace elements in the dialysate, implant material, food, topical applications, and/or drugs (129–131). In addition to trace elements, drugs also may change trace element uptake and distribution.

It is conceivable that workers with excessive professional exposure will accumulate trace elements in their body, which will be aggravated by the development of renal failure. The most current examples of industrial contaminants that may accumulate in the body of workers are lead, cadmium, and vanadium (132–134).

Increased uptake also may be the result of inhalation. This may occur because of industrial activities; combustion of fossil fuels; use of agricultural products such as fertilizers, insecticides, or herbicides; or presence of trace elements in cigarette smoke.

There has been debate about the role of dialysis in the excessive accumulation of trace elements in patients who have undergone dialysis. Chromium has been shown to be added from dialysate to the blood of patients undergoing

TABLE 19.5. FACTORS AFFECTING TRACE ELEMENT CONCENTRATION IN UREMIA AND OTHER CONDITIONS

Inadequate intake
Absolute deficiency: protein calorie malnutrition, anorexia, fat diets, low-income diets, diets with alcohol providing the bulk of calories, total parenteral nutrition without adequate supplementation, loss of taste and smell
Increased requirements: rapid growth, pregnancy, lactation, tissue anabolism

Decreased availability
Interactions with other dietary constituents
Gastrointestinal dysfunction: inadequate digestive processes, secondary interactions with unabsorbed dietary constituents
Iatrogenic problems: complexing with drugs, drug-induced alterations of gastrointestinal function

Impaired absorption
Altered binding factors: quantitative or qualitative, congenital or acquired, competitive uptake of other nutrients
Inadequate functional surface: surgical resection, gastrointestinal mucosal disease, competitive uptake of other nutrients, disturbances in vitamin D metabolism → altered uptake, gastrointestinal absorption (especially for divalent cations)
Physiologically appropriate depression of absorption
Impaired mucosal "packaging": inability to store, sequestration

Altered distribution
Defective transport: quantitative or qualitative changes in transport of compounds, competitive displacement, altered tissue receptor sites, altered tissue storage of compounds, inability to store, sequestration
Transient alterations in distribution: infection, myocardial infarction, stress

Excessive losses
Sweat
Menstrual, other forms of blood loss
Urinary, cave: proteinuria for protein-bound elements
Fecal
Pancreatic
Biliary
Gut
Upper gastrointestinal losses: vomiting, nasogastric suction, enterostomies
Dialysis

Excess intake
Drugs: containing trace elements (cave: homeopathy), increasing uptake, altering distribution
Food and water supplies
Contamination dialysate: addition to tap water, excess presence of minerals in soil, environmental contamination
Industrial contact
Inhalation after environmental contamination
Inhalation via cigarette smoke
Parenteral fluids
Increased gastrointestinal uptake

Diminished losses
Renal failure

CAPD if impurities are present in dialysate (23). Lithium, rubidium, and cesium, however, are removed via the dialysate (135). Molybdenum, selenium, and zinc levels decrease during the course of a dialysis session (94,136). If changes occur, they might be most pronounced in patients with a long history of renal failure and/or dialysis treatment.

Most of the available data are related to total trace element concentration, although trace elements may be present in the body as different species (i.e., free in inorganic forms, free in organic forms, bound to various proteins) (20,21). All these variants may have different levels of toxicity. In addition, shifts may occur over time from one form to the other. Generation of various species with divergent potential toxicity might differ depending on the trace element load (137) and the degree of renal failure (138). Uremic retention compounds, such as p-cresol, might influence the toxicity (139) and metabolization of trace elements (140). Protein binding, especially of inorganic trace elements, may play a role in trace element detoxification (21,141). To the extent that some trace elements may be carried by and bound to the same proteins (e.g., aluminum and iron on transferrin) (142), they may compete with each other for these binding sites, resulting in higher free concentrations and hence increased toxicity (143). Competition between aluminum and iron at the level of intestinal absorption and urinary excretion has been described as well (144,145), although after dietary supplementation of aluminum and iron, no interaction could be demonstrated (146). Simultaneous intake of citrate increases intestinal uptake of aluminum (147).

Also, chromium is mainly bound to transferrin, so a similar competition may be possible (148).

Excessive intake of one trace element may influence kinetics and metabolism of other trace elements. An interference between copper, zinc, aluminum, and cadmium has been reported (34). Rubidium depletion influences tissue levels of several other trace elements (149). Selenium might bind 1/1 to mercury, with a detoxifying effect as a consequence (150). Anorganic arsenic species (arsenate and arsenite) provoke an increase of copper accumulation in the kidneys, which is not the case for organic arsenic species (151,152). In the presence of vanadium, aluminum stimulates superoxide dismutase and catalase activities and membrane lipid peroxidation (153).

The bone may act as a reservoir for various trace elements such as aluminum, lead, strontium, cadmium, chromium, zinc, and magnesium (8,91,96). These elements become relatively harmless for other organ systems after their intraosseous sequestration; nevertheless, it is conceivable that slow release from the bone may result in damage to other organs in the long run (e.g., in the case of lead) or that they even may cause acute toxicity on chelation.

Important regional differences might be present in the concentration of specific trace elements in patients with renal failure (9). During the course of evolution, intercompartmental translocation and shifts may occur. For chromium, a preferential glucose-dependent uptake by insulin-sensitive tissues has been described (154) and plasma insulin levels may influence its plasma concentration (155).

SPECIFIC EXAMPLES

Aluminum

Aluminum intoxication first was recognized in patients receiving chronic dialysis with untreated water from municipal sources because aluminum often was added to clarify tap water (109). This excess aluminum from the dialysate readily crossed the semipermeable dialysis membrane to reach the bloodstream (156). Other sources of excess aluminum in dialysate are the use of untreated tap water in areas where the soil is rich in aluminum and in industrial areas with environmental wasting of aluminum-contaminated material. Also the salts used for the preparation of dialysate concentrates may be contaminated with aluminum (157). Dialysate aluminum content and serum levels are closely correlated (157). Although most of these sources of overt aluminum intoxication have been eliminated in both Europe and the United States, this intoxication might persist if water purification facilities are insufficient or show temporary failures (158).

The oral administration of aluminum hydroxide as a phosphate-binding agent is another source of aluminum (159). Therefore, it is preferable to replace it with calcium salts.

Factors playing a possible role in increased gastrointestinal uptake of aluminum may be age, chronic renal failure, PTH, vitamin D, citrate, and fluorine (143,147,160). Coadministration of citrate with aluminum should be avoided because citrate enhances aluminum toxicity especially on brain; citrate modifies the distribution pattern of aluminum in the body with increased predilection for brain (161).

It has been suggested that in hemodialysis, the intravenous administration of citrate to obtain regional anticoagulation is also a source of aluminum, especially if citrate is prepared in glass bottles (162).

Erythropoietin may alter trace element levels, and a decrease of serum aluminum has been demonstrated during erythropoietin treatment (163), in contrast to zinc, nickel, and manganese, where an increase was observed. Desferrioxamine can be applied as a chelator of aluminum to remove the compound and to estimate the accumulated mass (164). For diagnostic purposes, a low dose of the chelator (5 mg/kg) is sufficient (164). Renal transplantation may remove aluminum from the body stores (165). Aluminum is cleared via the urine after successful renal transplantation, possibly through interaction with silicon (166). Also, in patients undergoing dialysis, silicon may prevent the accumulation and subsequent toxicity of aluminum (167).

Arsenic

High arsenic levels may be the result of excessive intake via food and/or cigarette smoke (62). Speciation of arsenic may play a role in the transformation of the compound from more toxic inorganic forms to less toxic organic variants (168,169). Arsenic metabolism may be different in renal failure compared to normal renal function (137,138), with a preferential accumulation of inorganic species.

Chromium

Chromium concentration tends to increase with chronic dialysis treatment. Extra addition to the blood was demonstrated in CAPD (170) and hemodialysis from the impurities present in dialysate (23). A case of chromium intoxication in a patient with chronic renal failure was described after ingestion of over-the-counter chromium picolinate (171).

Iron

Before the availability of erythropoietin, many patients undergoing dialysis suffered from iron overload as a result of excessive iron administration, blood transfusion, and hemolysis. When erythropoietin became available, increased erythropoiesis resulted in a relative iron deficiency in many patients, necessitating even extra iron administration (172). Such an approach results in a decreased need for erythropoietin (173,174).

Lead

Excess lead as a result of forensic contact may be found in workers at battery factories; after contact with fuel additives or exhausts of vehicles; or after contact with pipes, paint, solders, or shielding (175). Intoxication has been related to the use of lead paint, whereby lead toxicity has been described in children eating pealed-off paint (176).

Selenium

Low serum selenium may be related to low selenium mineral contents in soil and food (e.g., grain) (177). Selenium plasma levels are not reduced at the end of a hemodialysis session compared to the start (178).

Silicon

Elevated silicon levels may be the result of excess silicon concentrations in the dialysate as well as of consumption of drinking water that contains excess silicon (16,25,179).

Strontium

Increased serum strontium levels are encountered, especially in developing countries (9). Contamination of dialysate as a result of the presence of strontium in concentrates is a major source. Other, less important, factors are dialytic age, vitamin D supplements, and phosphate binders.

Vanadium

Increased vanadium relates to its use as an alloy in steel industries, as a catalyst in chemical industries, and in the production of semiconductors and ceramics. Therefore, vanadium is found in higher concentrations near industrial settlements (180).

Zinc

Low serum zinc may be related to removal by dialysis (24) and inefficient caloric intake. Although serum zinc tends to increase at the end of dialysis, this must be attributed entirely to the increase in concentration of vector proteins as a result of hemoconcentration (181). Intestinal zinc absorption is not affected by vitamin D metabolites (182).

THERAPEUTIC ASPECTS

One way to prevent excess trace element ingestion is by reducing intake via food and other sources and by reducing contact with environmentally contaminated material. If it can be presumed that excess load can be attributed to presence in dialysate, water purification should be improved by using reverse osmosis and ion-exchange systems (109). Further excess, present in the toxic range, can be removed by chelation (e.g., by desferrioxamine for aluminum and iron or ethylene-diamine-tetra-acetic acid [EDTA] for lead) (183). It, however, should be taken into account that an overzealous chelation may induce enhanced toxicity by itself. Removal of lead from the bone compartment, where it resides in a relatively dormant form, may accelerate progression of renal failure; chelation of aluminum temporarily may induce symptoms of dementia. In renal failure, chelation must be combined with an increase of dialytic removal (179). It should be stressed that chelators may exert toxicity: desferrioxamine has been associated with opportunistic infections such as mucormycosis (184).

It is easier to replace elements that are below the reference levels; this can be accomplished either orally by intravenous administration during hemodialysis or by addition to the dialysate. The latter solution, however, may be too expensive and labor intensive, in view of the large dialysate volumes that cross the dialyzer at the occasion of each dialysis. Oral administration of selenium-supplemented formulas in patients undergoing dialysis results in an increase of plasma selenium (185). Special attention should be paid to patients in intensive care, who are prone to trace element depletion because of prolonged parenteral nutrition.

GENERAL CONCLUSIONS

Trace elements may play an important role in various pathophysiologic events that affect the general condition of patients with uremia. Because trace elements are not measured routinely, they often are overlooked as possible factors contributing to the uremic syndrome. The treatment of uremia by dialysis strategies may further lead to changes in trace element homeostasis. Disturbances in trace element concentration should be considered in any unexplained toxic event in uremia. In a polluted environment (air, water, nutrients), the pathophysiologic importance of trace elements becomes even more prominent.

REFERENCES

1. Mertz W. Trace-element nutrition in health and disease: contributions and problems of analysis. *Clin Chem* 1975;21:468–475.
2. Tanner SD, Baranov VI. A dynamic reaction cell for inductively coupled plasma mass spectrometry (ICP-DRC-MS). II. Reduction of interferences produced within the cell. *J Am Soc Mass Spectrom* 1999;10:1083–1094.
3. Tanner SD, Baranov VI, Vollkopf U. A dynamic reaction cell for inductively coupled mass spectrometry (ICP-DRC-MS)—Part III. Optimization and analytical performance. *J Anal Atom Spectrom* 2000;15:1261–1269.
4. Cornelis R, Heinzow B, Herber RF, et al. Sample collection guidelines for trace elements in blood and urine. IUPAC Commission of Toxicology. *J Trace Elem Med Biol* 1996;10:103–127.
5. Scancar J, Milacic R, Benedik M, et al. Problems related to determination of trace elements in spent continuous ambulatory peritoneal dialysis fluids by electrothermal atomic absorption spectrometry. *Clin Chim Acta* 1999;283:139–150.
6. Schmitt Y. Copper and zinc determination in plasma and corpuscular components of peripheral blood of patients with preterminal and terminal renal failure. *J Trace Elem Med Biol* 1997;11:210–214.
7. Zima T, Mestek O, Nemecek K, et al. Trace elements in hemodialysis and continuous ambulatory peritoneal dialysis patients. *Blood Purif* 1998;16:253–260.
8. O'Flaherty EJ. A physiologically based model of chromium kinetics in the rat. *Toxicol Appl Pharmacol* 1996;138:54–64.
9. Schrooten I, Elseviers MM, Lamberts LV, et al. Increased serum strontium levels in dialysis patients: an epidemiological survey. *Kidney Int* 1999;56:1886–1892.
10. Apostolidis N, Paradellis T, Karydas A, et al. Calcium and strontium metabolic studies in patients on CAPD. *Perit Dial Int* 1998;18:410–414.
11. Versieck J, Barbier F, Speecke A, et al. Manganese, copper, and zinc concentrations in serum and packed blood cells during acute hepatitis, chronic hepatitis, and posthepatitic cirrhosis. *Clin Chem* 1974;20:1141–1145.
12. Cornelis R, Ringoir S, Mees L, et al. Behavior of trace metals during hemoperfusion. *Miner Electrol Metab* 1980;4:123–129.
13. Versieck J, Hoste J, Barbier F, et al. Determination of chromium and cobalt in human serum by neutron activation analysis. *Clin Chem* 1978;24:303–308.
14. Versieck J, Speecke A, Hoste J, Barbier F. Determination of manganese, copper and zinc in serum and packed blood cells by neutron activation analysis. Studies on the metabolism of trace elements. *Z Klin Chem Klin Biochem* 1973;11:193–196.
15. Wester PO. Trace elements in serum and urine from hypertensive patients before and during treatment with chlorthalidone. *Acta Med Scand* 1973;194:505–512.
16. D'Haese PC, Shaheen FA, Huraib SO, et al. Increased silicon levels in dialysis patients due to high silicon content in the drinking water, inadequate water treatment procedures, and concentrate contamination: a multicentre study. *Nephrol Dial Transplant* 1995;10:1838–1844.
17. Hosokawa S, Yoshida O. Role of molybdenum in chronic hemodialysis patients [editorial]. *Int J Artif Organs* 1994;17:567–569.
18. Zima T, Mestek O, Tesar V, et al. Chromium levels in patients with internal diseases. *Biochem Mol Biol Int* 1998;46:365–374.
19. Mayer DR, Kosmus W, Pogglitsch H, et al. Essential trace elements in humans. Serum arsenic concentrations in hemodialysis patients in comparison to healthy controls. *Biol Trace Elem Res* 1993;37:27–38.
20. De Kimpe J, Cornelis R, Mees L, et al. More than tenfold increase of arsenic in serum and packed cells of chronic hemodialysis patients. *Am J Nephrol* 1993;13:429–434.
21. Zhang X, Cornelis R, Mees L, et al. Chemical speciation of arsenic in serum of uraemic patients. *Analyst* 1998;123:13–17.
22. Cornelis R, Ringoir S, Lameire N, et al. Blood bromine in uremic patients. *Miner Electrol Metab* 1979;2:186–192.
23. Wallaeys B, Cornelis R, Mees L, et al. Trace elements in serum, packed cells, and dialysate of CAPD patients. *Kidney Int* 1986;30:599–604.
24. Van Renterghem D, Cornelis R, Vanholder R. Behaviour of 12 trace elements in serum of uremic patients on hemodiafiltration. *J Trace Elem Electrolytes Health Dis* 1992;6:169–174.
25. Gitelman HJ, Alderman F, Perry SJ. Renal handling of silicon in normals and patients with renal insufficiency. *Kidney Int* 1992;42:957–959.
26. Gitelman HJ, Alderman FR, Perry SJ. Silicon accumulation in dialysis patients. *Am J Kidney Dis* 1992;19:140–143.
27. Thomson NM, Stevens BJ, Humphery TJ, et al. Comparison of trace elements in peritoneal dialysis, hemodialysis, and uremia. *Kidney Int* 1983;23:9–14.
28. Marumo F, Tsukamoto Y, Iwanami S, et al. Trace element concentrations in hair, fingernails and plasma of patients with chronic renal failure on hemodialysis and hemofiltration. *Nephron* 1984;38:267–272.
29. Hosokawa S, Yoshida O. Serum vanadium levels in chronic hemodialysis patients. *Nephron* 1993;64:388–394.
30. Tsukamoto Y, Iwanami S, Marumo F. Disturbances of trace element concentrations in plasma of patients with chronic renal failure. *Nephron* 1980;26:174–179.
31. Zevin D, Weinstein T, Levi J, et al. X-ray microanalysis of the fingernails of uremic patients treated by hemodialysis. *Clin Nephrol* 1991;36:302–304.
32. Smythe WR, Alfrey AC, Craswell PW, et al. Trace element abnormalities in chronic uremia. *Ann Intern Med* 1982;96:302–310.
33. Nunnelley LL, Smythe WR, Alfrey AC, et al. Uremic hyperstannum: elevated tissue tin levels associated with uremia. *J Lab Clin Med* 1978;91:72–75.
34. Liu X, Jin T, Nordberg GF, et al. Influence of zinc and copper administration on metal disposition in rats with cadmium-metallothionein-induced nephrotoxicity. *Toxicol Appl Pharmacol* 1994;126:84–90.
35. Hosokawa S, Yoshida O. Effect of erythropoietin (rHuEPO) on trace elements and quality of life (Qol) in chronic hemodialysis patients. *Int J Clin Pharmacol Ther* 1994;32:415–421.
36. Tariq M, Morais C, Sujata B, et al. Aluminum exacerbates cyclosporin induced nephrotoxicity in rats. *Ren Fail* 1999;21:35–48.

37. Reichenspurner H, Meiser BM, Muschiol F, et al. The influence of gastrointestinal agents on resorption and metabolism of cyclosporine after heart transplantation: experimental and clinical results. *J Heart Lung Transplant* 1993;12:987–992.
38. Prasad GV, Rossi NF. Arsenic intoxication associated with tubulointerstitial nephritis. *Am J Kidney Dis* 1995;26:373–376.
39. Berry JP, Galle P. Selenium-arsenic interaction in renal cells: role of lysosomes. Electron microprobe study. *J Submicrosc Cytol Pathol* 1994;26:203–210.
40. Chen CL, Whanger PD. Interaction of selenium and arsenic with metallothionein: effect of vitamin B12. *J Inorg Biochem* 1994;54:267–276.
41. Fowler BA. Mechanisms of kidney cell injury from metals. *Environ Health Perspect* 1993;100:57–63.
42. Kramer HJ, Gonick HC, Lu E. In vitro inhibition of Na-K-ATPase by trace metals: relation to renal and cardiovascular damage. *Nephron* 1986;44:329–336.
43. Griffin JL, Walker LA, Troke J, et al. The initial pathogenesis of cadmium induced renal toxicity. *FEBS Lett* 2000;478:147–150.
44. Kinne RK, Schutz H, Kinne-Saffran E. The effect of cadmium chloride in vitro on sodium-glutamate cotransport in brush border membrane vesicles isolated from rabbit kidney. *Toxicol Appl Pharmacol* 1995;135:216–221.
45. Prozialeck WC, Lamar PC. Effects of glutathione depletion on the cytotoxic actions of cadmium in LLC-PK1 cells. *Toxicol Appl Pharmacol* 1995;134:285–295.
46. Senturk UK, Oner G, Izgut-Uysal VM. Cadmium induced lipid peroxidation in kidney function. *J Basic Clin Physiol Pharmacol* 1994;5:305–313.
47. Yasuda M, Miwa A, Kitagawa M. Morphometric studies of renal lesions in Itai-itai disease: chronic cadmium nephropathy. *Nephron* 1995;69:14–19.
48. Liu J, Liu Y, Habeebu SM, et al. Chronic combined exposure to cadmium and arsenic exacerbates nephrotoxicity, particularly in metallothionein-I/II null mice. *Toxicology* 2000;147: 157–166.
49. Hotz P, Buchet JP, Bernard A, et al. Renal effects of low-level environmental cadmium exposure:5-year follow-up of a subcohort from the Cadmibel study. *Lancet* 1999;354:1508–1513.
50. Dartsch PC, Hildenbrand S, Kimmel R, et al. Investigations on the nephrotoxicity and hepatotoxicity of trivalent and hexavalent chromium compounds. *Int Arch Occup Environ Health* 1998;71 Suppl:S40–S45.
51. Wang X, Qin Q, Xu X, et al. Chromium-induced early changes in renal function among ferrochromium-producing workers. *Toxicology* 1994;90:93–101.
52. Liu CS, Kuo HW, Lai JS, et al. Urinary N-acetyl-beta-glucosaminidase as an indicator of renal dysfunction in electroplating workers. *Int Arch Occup Environ Health* 1998;71:348–352.
53. Takeuchi A, Yoshizawa N, Oshima S, et al. Nephrotoxicity of germanium compounds: report of a case and review of the literature. *Nephron* 1992;60:436–442.
54. Staessen JA, Lauwerys RR, Buchet JP, et al. Impairment of renal function with increasing blood lead concentrations in the general population. The Cadmibel Study Group. *N Engl J Med* 1992;327:151–156.
55. Emmerson BT. Lead stores in patients with renal insufficiency [letter]. *Nephron* 1991;58:233–234.
56. Nuyts GD, Van Vlem E, Thys J, et al. New occupational risk factors for chronic renal failure. *Lancet* 1995;346:7–11.
57. Nuyts GD, Van Vlem E, De Vos A, et al. Wegener granulomatosis is associated to exposure to silicon compounds: a case-control study. *Nephrol Dial Transplant* 1995;10:1162–1165.
58. Nakashima H. Time course of effects of tetraethoxysilane (TEOS) on the kidney and blood silicon concentration in mice. *Arch Toxicol* 1994;69:59–64.
59. Calvert GM, Steenland K, Palu S. End-stage renal disease among silica-exposed gold miners. A new method for assessing incidence among epidemiologic cohorts. *JAMA* 1997;277: 1219–1223.
60. Kallenberg CG. Renal disease—another effect of silica exposure? [editorial]. *Nephrol Dial Transplant* 1995;10:1117–1119.
61. Smith AH, Goycolea M, Haque R, et al. Marked increase in bladder and lung cancer mortality in a region of Northern Chile due to arsenic in drinking water. *Am J Epidemiol* 1998;147: 660–669.
62. Bates MN, Smith AH, Hopenhayn-Rich C. Arsenic ingestion and internal cancers: a review. *Am J Epidemiol* 1992;135: 462–476.
63. Chen CJ, Chen CW, Wu MM, et al. Cancer potential in liver, lung, bladder and kidney due to ingested inorganic arsenic in drinking water. *Br J Cancer* 1992;66:888–892.
64. Engel RR, Receveur O. Re: "Arsenic ingestion and internal cancers: a review" [letter]. *Am J Epidemiol* 1993;138:896–897.
65. Tsai SM, Wang TN, Ko YC. Mortality for certain diseases in areas with high levels of arsenic in drinking water. *Arch Environ Health* 1999;54:186–193.
66. Enterline PE, Day R, Marsh GM. Cancers related to exposure to arsenic at a copper smelter. *Occup Environ Med* 1995;52: 28–32.
67. Yamamoto S, Konishi Y, Matsuda T, et al. Cancer induction by an organic arsenic compound, dimethylarsinic acid (cacodylic acid), in F344/DuCrj rats after pretreatment with five carcinogens. *Cancer Res* 1995;55:1271–1276.
68. Kazantzis G, Blanks RG, Sullivan KR. Is cadmium a human carcinogen? *IARC Sci Publ* 1992;435–446.
69. Waalkes MP. Cadmium carcinogenesis in review. *J Inorg Biochem* 2000;79:241–244.
70. Bonomini M, Mujais SK, Ivanovich P, et al. Selenium in uremia: culprit or bystander? [editorial]. *Nephron* 1992;60: 385–389.
71. Granadillo VA, Tahan JE, Salgado O, et al. The influence of the blood levels of lead, aluminum and vanadium upon the arterial hypertension. *Clin Chim Acta* 1995;233:47–59.
72. Ramos O, Carrizales L, Yanez L, et al. Arsenic increased lipid peroxidation in rat tissues by a mechanism independent of glutathione levels. *Environ Health Perspect* 1995;103 Suppl 1:85–88.
73. Yiin SJ, Chern CL, Sheu JY, et al. Cadmium induced lipid peroxidation in rat testes and protection by selenium. *Biometals* 1999;12:353–359.
74. Nehru LB, Bansal MP. Effect of selenium supplementation on the glutathione redox system in the kidney of mice after chronic cadmium exposures. *J Appl Toxicol* 1997;17:81–84.
75. Klevay LM. Ischemic heart disease: nutrition or pharmacotherapy? *J Trace Elem Electrolytes Health Dis* 1993;7:63–69.
76. Fisler JS. Cardiac effects of starvation and semistarvation diets: safety and mechanisms of action. *Am J Clin Nutr* 1992;56: 230S–234S
77. Salonen JT, Nyyssonen K, Korpela H, et al. High stored iron levels are associated with excess risk of myocardial infarction in eastern Finnish men. *Circulation* 1992;86:803–811.
78. Pehrsson SK, Lins LE. The role of trace elements in uremic heart failure. *Nephron* 1983;34:93–98.
79. Ascherio A, Willett WC, Rimm EB, et al. Dietary iron intake and risk of coronary disease among men. *Circulation* 1994;89: 969–974.
80. Dmochowski K, Finegood DT, Francombe W, et al. Factors determining glucose tolerance in patients with thalassemia major. *J Clin Endocrinol Metab* 1993;77:478–483.
81. Huttunen JK. Selenium and cardiovascular diseases—an update. *Biomed Environ Sci* 1997;10:220–226.

82. Foster LH, Sumar S. Selenium in health and disease: a review. *Crit Rev Food Sci Nutr* 1997;37:211–228.
83. Richard MJ, Ducros V, Foret M, et al. Reversal of selenium and zinc deficiencies in chronic hemodialysis patients by intravenous sodium selenite and zinc gluconate supplementation. Time-course of glutathione peroxidase repletion and lipid peroxidation decrease. *Biol Trace Elem Res* 1993;39:149–159.
84. Hosokawa S, Yoshida O. Vanadium in chronic hemodialysis patients. *Int J Artif Organs* 1990;13:197–199.
85. Boscolo P, Carmignani M, Volpe AR, et al. Renal toxicity and arterial hypertension in rats chronically exposed to vanadate. *Occup Environ Med* 1994;51:500–503.
86. McCarthy JT, Hodgson SF, Fairbanks VF, et al. Clinical and histologic features of iron-related bone disease in dialysis patients. *Am J Kidney Dis* 1991;17:551–561.
87. Pun KK, Ho PW, Lau P. Effects of aluminum on the parathyroid hormone receptors of bone and kidney. *Kidney Int* 1990; 37:72–78.
88. Nordal KP, Dahl E, Halse J, et al. Aluminum metabolism and bone histology after kidney transplantation: a one-year follow-up study. *J Clin Endocrinol Metab* 1992;74:1140–1145.
89. Kido T, Honda R, Tsuritani I, et al. Serum levels of bone Gla-protein in inhabitants exposed to environmental cadmium. *Arch Environ Health* 1991;46:43–49.
90. Katsuta O, Hiratsuka H, Matsumoto J, et al. Cadmium-induced osteomalacic and osteopetrotic lesions in ovariectomized rats. *Toxicol Appl Pharmacol* 1994;126:58–68.
91. D'Haese PC, Couttenye MM, Lamberts LV, et al. Aluminum, iron, lead, cadmium, copper, zinc, chromium, magnesium, strontium, and calcium content in bone of end-stage renal failure patients. *Clin Chem* 1999;45:1548–1556.
92. Van de Vyver FL, Visser WJ, et al. Iron overload and bone disease in chronic dialysis patients. *Nephrol Dial Transplant* 1990;5:781–787.
93. Finn WF, Joy MS, Hladik GA, et al. Results of a randomized, dose-ranging, placebo-controlled study of lanthanum carbonate for reduction of serum phosphate in chronic renal failure patients receiving hemodialysis [abstract]. *J Am Soc Nephrol* 1999; 10:261A
94. Hosokawa S, Yoshida O. Clinical studies on molybdenum in patients requiring long-term hemodialysis. *ASAIO J* 1994;40: M445–M449.
95. Saldanha LF, Gonick HC, Rodriguez HJ, et al. Silicon-related syndrome in dialysis patients. *Nephron* 1997;77:48–56.
96. D'Haese PC, Schrooten I, Goodman WG, et al. Increased bone strontium levels in hemodialysis patients with osteomalacia. *Kidney Int* 2000;57:1107–1114.
97. Schrooten I, Cabrera W, Goodman WG, et al. Strontium causes osteomalacia in chronic renal failure rats. *Kidney Int* 1998;54: 448–456.
98. Donnelly SM, Smith EK. The role of aluminum in the functional iron deficiency of patients treated with erythropoietin: case report of clinical characteristics and response to treatment. *Am J Kidney Dis* 1990;16:487–490.
99. Donnelly SM, Ali MA, Churchill DN. Bioavailability of iron in hemodialysis patients treated with erythropoietin: evidence for the inhibitory role of aluminum. *Am J Kidney Dis* 1990;16: 447–451.
100. Jain SK, Abreo K, Duett J, et al. Lipofuscin products, lipid peroxides and aluminum accumulation in red blood cells of hemodialyzed patients. *Am J Nephrol* 1995;15:306–311.
101. Caramelo CA, Cannata JB, Rodeles MR, et al. Mechanisms of aluminum-induced microcytosis: lessons from accidental aluminum intoxication. *Kidney Int* 1995;47:164–168.
102. Bucher M, Sandner P, Wolf K, et al. Cobalt but not hypoxia stimulates PDGF gene expression in rats. *Am J Physiol* 1996; 271:E451–E457.
103. Pershagen G, Hast R, Lins LE, et al. Increased arsenic concentration in the bone marrow in chronic renal failure. *Nephron* 1982; 30:250–252.
104. Wasa M, Satani M, Tanano H, et al. Copper deficiency with pancytopenia during total parenteral nutrition. *JPEN* 1994;18: 190–192.
105. Tamura H, Hirose S, Watanabe O, et al. Anemia and neutropenia due to copper deficiency in enteral nutrition. *JPEN* 1994; 18:185–189.
106. Emenaker NJ, DiSilvestro RA, Nahman NS Jr, et al. Copper-related blood indexes in kidney dialysis patients. *Am J Clin Nutr* 1996;64:757–760.
107. Mahoney CA, Arieff AI. Uremic encephalopathies: clinical, biochemical, and experimental features. *Am J Kidney Dis* 1982;2: 324–336.
108. Van Landeghem GF, D'Haese PC, et al. Aluminium speciation in cerebrospinal fluid of acutely aluminium-intoxicated dialysis patients before and after desferrioxamine treatment; a step in the understanding of the element's neurotoxicity. *Nephrol Dial Transplant* 1997;12:1692–1698.
109. McGonigle RJ, Parsons V. Aluminium-induced anaemia in haemodialysis patients. *Nephron* 1985;39:1–9.
110. Sasagawa I, Nakada T, Sawamura T, et al. Nerve conduction velocities and hair concentrations of trace elements in haemodialysis patients. *Int Urol Nephrol* 1993;25:191–196.
111. Tzanno-Martins C, Azevedo LS, Orii N, et al. The role of experimental chronic renal failure and aluminium intoxication in cellular immune response. *Nephrol Dial Transplant* 1996;11: 474–480.
112. Boelaert JR, Daneels RF, Schurgers ML, et al. Iron overload in haemodialysis patients increases the risk of bacteraemia: a prospective study. *Nephrol Dial Transplant* 1990;5:130–134.
113. Boelaert JR, Cantinieaux BF, Hariga CF, et al. Recombinant erythropoietin reverses polymorphonuclear granulocyte dysfunction in iron-overloaded dialysis patients. *Nephrol Dial Transplant* 1990;5:504–517.
114. Gaughan WJ, Beserab A, Stein HD, et al. Serum bactericidal activity for Yersinia enterocolitica in hemodialysis patients: effects of iron overload and deferoxamine. *Am J Kidney Dis* 1992; 19:144–148.
115. Patruta SI, Edlinger R, Sunder-Plassmann G, et al. Neutrophil impairment associated with iron therapy in hemodialysis patients with functional iron deficiency. *J Am Soc Nephrol* 1998; 9:655–663.
116. Lim PS, Wei YH, Yu YL, et al. Enhanced oxidative stress in haemodialysis patients receiving intravenous iron therapy. *Nephrol Dial Transplant* 1999;14:2680–2687.
117. Fishbane S. Review of issues relating to iron and infection. *Am J Kidney Dis* 1999;34:S47–S52.
118. el Reshaid K, Seshadri MS, Hourani H, et al. Endocrine abnormalities in hemodialysis patients with iron overload: reversal with iron depletion. *Nutrition* 1995;11:521–526.
119. Liu P, Olivieri N. Iron overload cardiomyopathies: new insights into an old disease. *Cardiovasc Drugs Ther* 1994;8:101–110.
120. Golconda MS, Ueda N, Shah SV. Evidence suggesting that iron and calcium are interrelated in oxidant-induced DNA damage. *Kidney Int* 1993;44:1228–1234.
121. Richard MJ, Arnaud J, Jurkovitz C, et al. Trace elements and lipid peroxidation abnormalities in patients with chronic renal failure. *Nephron* 1991;57:10–15.
122. Bonomini M, Albertazzi A. Selenium in uremia. *Artif Organs* 1995;19:443–448.
123. Bonomini M, Forster S, De Risio F, et al. Effects of selenium supplementation on immune parameters in chronic uraemic

patients on haemodialysis. *Nephrol Dial Transplant* 1995;10: 1654–1661.
124. Erten Y, Kayatas M, Sezer S, et al. Zinc deficiency: prevalence and causes in hemodialysis patients and effect on cellular immune response. *Transplant Proc* 1998;30:850–851.
125. Bonomini M, Manfrini V, Cappelli P, et al. Zinc and cell-mediated immunity in chronic uremia. *Nephron* 1993;65:1–4.
126. Holtkamp W, Brodersen HP, Stollberg T, et al. Zinc supplementation stimulates tetanus antibody formation and soluble interleukin-2 receptor levels in chronic hemodialysis patients. *Clin Investig* 1993;71:537–541.
127. Turk S, Bozfakioglu S, Ecder ST, et al. Effects of zinc supplementation on the immune system and on antibody response to multivalent influenza vaccine in hemodialysis patients. *Int J Artif Organs* 1998;21:274–278.
128. Hosokawa S, Oyamaguchi A, Yoshida O. Trace elements and complications in patients undergoing chronic hemodialysis. *Nephron* 1990;55:375–379.
129. Mathur AK, Gupta BN. Effect of linear alkylbenzene sulphonate on topical absorption of chromium and nickel. *Vet Hum Toxicol* 1999;41:353–354.
130. Pereira MD, Pereira MD, Sousa JP. Individual study of chromium in the stainless steel implants degradation: an experimental study in mice. *Biometals* 1999;12:275–280.
131. Padovese P, Gallieni M, Brancaccio D, et al. Trace elements in dialysis fluids and assessment of the exposure of patients on regular hemodialysis, hemofiltration and continuous ambulatory peritoneal dialysis. *Nephron* 1992;61:442–448.
132. Gerhardsson L, Chettle DR, Englyst V, et al. Kidney effects in long term exposed lead smelter workers. *Br J Ind Med* 1992; 49:186–192.
133. Khalil-Manesh F, Gonick HC, Cohen AH, et al. Experimental model of lead nephropathy. I. Continuous high-dose lead administration. *Kidney Int* 1992;41:1192–1203.
134. Jung K, Pergande M, Graubaum HJ, et al. Urinary proteins and enzymes as early indicators of renal dysfunction in chronic exposure to cadmium. *Clin Chem* 1993;39:757–765.
135. Krachler M, Scharfetter H, Wirnsberger GH. Exchange of alkali trace elements in hemodialysis patients: a comparison with Na(+) and K(+). *Nephron* 1999;83:226–236.
136. Lin TH, Chen JG, Liaw JM, et al. Trace elements and lipid peroxidation in uremic patients on hemodialysis. *Biol Trace Elem Res* 1996;51:277–283.
137. De Kimpe J, Cornelis R, Wittevrongel L, et al. Dose dependent changes in 74As-arsenate metabolism of Flemish Giant rabbits. *J Trace Elem Med Biol* 1999;12:193–200.
138. De Kimpe J, Cornelis R, Mees L, et al. 74As-arsenate metabolism in Flemish Giant rabbits with renal insufficiency. *J Trace Elem Med Biol* 1999;13:7–14.
139. Abreo K, Sella M, Gautreaux S, et al. P-Cresol, a uremic compound, enhances the uptake of aluminum in hepatocytes. *J Am Soc Nephrol* 1997;8:935–942.
140. De Kimpe J, Cornelis R, Vanholder R. In vitro methylation of arsenite by rabbit liver cytosol: effect of metal ions, metal chelating agents, methyltransferase inhibitors and uremic toxins. *Drug Chem Toxicol* 1999;22:613–628.
141. Zhang X, Cornelis R, De Kimpe J, et al. Study of arsenic-protein binding in serum of patients on continuous ambulatory peritoneal dialysis. *Clin Chem* 1998;44:141–147.
142. Soldado Cabezuelo AB, Blanco GE, Sanz-Medel A. Quantitative studies of aluminium binding species in human uremic serum by fast protein liquid chromatography coupled with electrothermal atomic absorption spectrometry. *Analyst* 1997;122: 573–577.
143. Cannata JB, Olaizola IR, Gomez-Alonso C, et al. Serum aluminum transport and aluminum uptake in chronic renal failure: role of iron and aluminum metabolism. *Nephron* 1993;65: 141–146.
144. Kooistra MP, Niemantsverdriet EC, van Es A, et al. Iron absorption in erythropoietin-treated haemodialysis patients: effects of iron availability, inflammation and aluminium. *Nephrol Dial Transplant* 1998;13:82–88.
145. Lin JL, Lim PS, Leu ML. Relationship of body iron status and serum aluminum in chronic renal insufficiency patients not taking any aluminum-containing drugs. *Am J Nephrol* 1995; 15:118–122.
146. Morgan EH, Redgrave TG. Effects of dietary supplementation with aluminum and citrate on iron metabolism in the rat. *Biol Trace Elem Res* 1998;65:117–131.
147. Deng Z, Coudray C, Gouzoux L, et al. Effect of oral aluminum and aluminum citrate on blood level and short-term tissue distribution of aluminum in the rat. *Biol Trace Elem Res* 1998;63: 139–147.
148. Borguet F, Cornelis R, Delanghe J, et al. Study of the chromium binding in plasma of patients on continuous ambulatory peritoneal dialysis. *Clin Chim Acta* 1995;238:71–84.
149. Yokoi K, Kimura M, Itokawa Y. Effect of low dietary rubidium on plasma biochemical parameters and mineral levels in rats. *Biol Trace Elem Res* 1996;51:199–208.
150. Drasch G, Wanghofer E, Roider G, et al. Correlation of mercury and selenium in the human kidney. *J Trace Elem Med Biol* 1996; 10:251–254.
151. Ademuyiwa O, Elsenhans B, Nguyen PT, et al. Arsenic-copper interaction in the kidney of the rat: influence of arsenic metabolites. *Pharmacol Toxicol* 1996;78:154–160.
152. Hunder G, Schaper J, Ademuyiwa O, et al. Species differences in arsenic-mediated renal copper accumulation: a comparison between rats, mice and guinea pigs. *Hum Exp Toxicol* 1999;18: 699–705.
153. Abou-Seif MA. Oxidative stress of vanadium-mediated oxygen free radical generation stimulated by aluminium on human erythrocytes. *Ann Clin Biochem* 1998;35:254–260.
154. Morris BW, Gray TA, MacNeil S. Glucose-dependent uptake of chromium in human and rat insulin-sensitive tissues. *Clin Sci* 1993;84:477–482.
155. Morris BW, MacNeil S, Stanley K, et al. The inter-relationship between insulin and chromium in hyperinsulinaemic euglycaemic clamps in healthy volunteers. *J Endocrinol* 1993;139: 339–345.
156. Alfrey AC. Aluminum toxicity in patients with chronic renal failure. *Ther Drug Monit* 1993;15:593–597.
157. Fernandez-Martin JL, Canteros A, Serrano M, et al. Prevention of aluminium exposure through dialysis fluids. Analysis of changes in the last 8 years. *Nephrol Dial Transplant* 1998;13 Suppl 3:78–81.
158. Drueke TB. Adynamic bone disease, anaemia, resistance to erythropoietin and iron-aluminium interaction. *Nephrol Dial Transplant* 1993;8 Suppl 1:12–16.
159. Salusky IB, Foley J, Nelson P, et al. Aluminum accumulation during treatment with aluminum hydroxide and dialysis in children and young adults with chronic renal disease. *N Engl J Med* 1991;324:527–531.
160. Rudy D, Sica DA, Comstock T, et al. Aluminum-citrate interaction in end-stage renal disease. *Int J Artif Organs* 1991;14: 625–629.
161. van Ginkel MF, van der Voet GB, D'Haese PC, et al. Effect of citric acid and maltol on the accumulation of aluminum in rat brain and bone. *J Lab Clin Med* 1993;121:453–460.
162. Janssen MJ, Deegens JK, Kapinga TH, et al. Citrate compared to low molecular weight heparin anticoagulation in chronic hemodialysis patients. *Kidney Int* 1996;49:806–813.
163. Hosokawa S, Yoshida O. Effects of erythropoietin on trace ele-

ments in patients with chronic renal failure undergoing hemodialysis. *Nephron* 1993;65:414–417.

164. D'Haese PC, Couttenye MM, Goodman WG, et al. Use of the low-dose desferrioxamine test to diagnose and differentiate between patients with aluminium-related bone disease, increased risk for aluminium toxicity, or aluminium overload. *Nephrol Dial Transplant* 1995;10:1874–1884.
165. David-Neto E, Jorgetti V, Soeiro NM, et al. Reversal of aluminum-related bone disease after renal transplantation. *Am J Nephrol* 1993;13:12–17.
166. Bellia JP, Newton K, Davenport A, et al. Silicon and aluminium and their inter-relationship in serum and urine after renal transplantation. *Eur J Clin Invest* 1994;24:703–710.
167. Parry R, Plowman D, Delves HT, et al. Silicon and aluminium interactions in haemodialysis patients. *Nephrol Dial Transplant* 1998;13:1759–1762.
168. Zhang X, Cornelis R, De Kimpe J, et al. Speciation of arsenic in serum, urine, and dialysate of patients on continuous ambulatory peritoneal dialysis. *Clin Chem* 1997;43:406–408.
169. Zhang X, Cornelis R, De Kimpe J, et al. Accumulation of arsenic species in serum of patients with chronic renal disease. *Clin Chem* 1996;42:1231–1237.
170. Borguet F, Wallaeys B, Cornelis R, et al. Transperitoneal absorption and kinetics of chromium in the continuous ambulatory peritoneal dialysis patient—an experimental and mathematical analysis. *Nephron* 1996;72:163–170.
171. Cerulli J, Grabe DW, Gauthier I, et al. Chromium picolinate toxicity. *Ann Pharmacother* 1998;32:428–431.
172. Silva J, Andrade S, Ventura H, et al. Iron supplementation in haemodialysis—practical clinical guidelines. *Nephrol Dial Transplant* 1998;13:2572–2577.
173. Macdougall IC, Tucker B, Thompson J, et al. A randomized controlled study of iron supplementation in patients treated with erythropoietin. *Kidney Int* 1996;50:1694–1699.
174. Sunder-Plassmann G, Hörl WH. Importance of iron supply for erythropoietin therapy. *Nephrol Dial Transplant* 1995;10: 2070–2076.
175. Nolan CV, Shaikh ZA. Lead nephrotoxicity and associated disorders: biochemical mechanisms. *Toxicology* 1992;73:127–146.
176. Price J, Grudzinski AW, Craswell PW, et al. Bone lead measurements in patients with chronic renal disease studied over time. *Arch Environ Health* 1992;47:330–335.
177. Maksimovic ZJ. Selenium deficiency and Balkan endemic nephropathy. *Kidney Int Suppl* 1991;34:S12–S14.
178. Bonomini M, Manfrini V, Marini A, et al. Hemodialysis with regenerated cellulosic membranes does not reduce plasma selenium levels in chronic uremic patients. *Artif Organs* 1995;19: 81–85.
179. Navarro JA, Granadillo VA, Rodriguez-Iturbe B, et al. Removal of trace metals by continuous ambulatory peritoneal dialysis after desferrioxamine B chelation therapy. *Clin Nephrol* 1991; 35:213–217.
180. Tsukamoto Y, Saka S, Kumano K, et al. Abnormal accumulation of vanadium in patients on chronic hemodialysis therapy. *Nephron* 1990;56:368–373.
181. Hachache T, Meftahi H, Foret M, et al. [Short- (1 session) and long-term (6 months) course of the serum level of zinc in 33 hemodialysis patients]. *Nephrologie* 1989;10:87–90.
182. Kiilerich S, Christiansen C, Christensen MS, et al. Zinc metabolism in patients with chronic renal failure during treatment with 1.25-dihydroxycholecalciferol: a controlled therapeutic trial. *Clin Nephrol* 1981;15:23–27.
183. Yokel RA. Aluminum chelation: chemistry, clinical, and experimental studies and the search for alternatives to desferrioxamine. *J Toxicol Environ Health* 1994;41:131–174.
184. Boelaert JR, de Locht M, Van Cutsem J, et al. Mucormycosis during deferoxamine therapy is a siderophore-mediated infection. In vitro and in vivo animal studies. *J Clin Invest* 1993;91: 1979–1986.
185. Temple KA, Smith AM, Cockram DB. Selenate-supplemented nutritional formula increases plasma selenium in hemodialysis patients. *J Ren Nutr* 2000;10:16–23.

20

VITAMIN METABOLISM AND REQUIREMENTS IN RENAL DISEASE AND RENAL FAILURE

CHARLES CHAZOT
JOEL D. KOPPLE

Kidney diseases and renal failure alter the biochemistry, metabolism, and nutritional requirements for many vitamins. Deficiencies and abnormally high levels of vitamins occur in patients with renal failure. These factors may enhance the risk of abnormal vitamin function in renal diseases (1). The causes of altered vitamin levels or function in renal failure include (a) decreased vitamin intake caused by anorexia, unpalatability of prescribed diets, or a dietary prescription that provides insufficient vitamins; (b) increased degradation or endogenous clearance of vitamins from blood; (c) elevated levels of vitamin-binding proteins; (d) losses of vitamins, primarily water soluble, into dialysate; (e) excretion of protein-bound vitamins by nephrotic patients; and (f) interference of medicines with the absorption, excretion, or metabolism of vitamins. An important question, with economic implications, is whether vitamin supplementation should be administered routinely to patients with renal failure. In this chapter, each of the common vitamins will be reviewed briefly for its normal biochemistry and metabolism, the effect of renal diseases and renal failure on these processes, and the clinical spectrum of vitamin disorders in these conditions. The latest recommendations for vitamin requirements will be given (2,3). Guidelines concerning the need for supplementation in renal patients will be proposed. The recent recognition that chronic renal diseases and renal failure are associated with oxidant stress, hyperhomocysteinemia, and cardiovascular risk has refocused interest and research on vitamin nutrition. The nutrition of 1,25-dihydroxycholecalciferol in renal patients is reviewed elsewhere (Chapter 17) and will not be addressed in this chapter.

VITAMIN A

Structure and Metabolism

Several reviews have described the structure and metabolism of vitamin A in normal individuals (4,5). Vitamin A is composed of several compounds including retinol (Table 20.1) and the biologically active retinoids, which have a common structure consisting of four isoprenoid units (20 carbons) with five double bonds. Retinol, retinoic acid, and retinal are the main bioactive retinoic compounds. Several years ago, the accepted units for vitamin A content were changed from International Units (IU) to Retinol Equivalents (RE), where 1 IU = 0.3 μg RE (6). Carotenoids (40 carbon compounds) may be biologically active and are included as vitamin A precursors. Variable quantities of carotenoids are converted to retinol; this conversion is regulated according to body vitamin A levels (5,7,8). The allo-trans-β-carotene is the main bioactive carotenoid. Retinoids and carotenoids are fat soluble and predominantly are found in foods derived from animals for retinyl esters and from vegetables for carotenoids (9).

During digestion, retinyl esters are hydrolyzed in the intestinal lumen by pancreatic lipase. Retinol and carotenoids are incorporated into micelles and absorbed by enterocytes where β-carotene is converted to retinol. Retinol is esterified, combined in chylomicrons, and broken down into chylomicron remnants in the lymphatic system by lipoprotein lipase. The hepatic cells incorporate the chylomicron remnants through apoprotein(E), or apo(E), or apo(B) receptors. A significant part (10% to 40%) of the absorbed retinoids are oxidized or conjugated and excreted into bile and urine. At least 50% of the retinoid compounds are transferred into the perisinusoidal stellate cells of the liver where they are stored as retinyl palmitate and other retinyl esters. In plasma, retinol is bound largely to apo-retinol–binding protein (RBP), a 21.3 kd protein primarily synthesized in the liver. This equimolar complex is bound to one molecule of prealbumin (also called transthyretin) and delivered to the target where it binds to RBP cell-surface receptors. Retinol is incorporated into the cell, whereas apo-RBP is released and catabolized by the kidney.

TABLE 20.1. VITAMIN CHARACTERISTICS

Vitamin	Main Compound	Solubility	MW	Protein Binding in Plasma	HD Losses	Peritoneal Losses	Body Stores	Toxicity[a]
A	Retinol	Lipid	286	RBP+ prealbumin	None	Controversial[b]	Large	Yes
E	α-tocopherol	Lipid	431	Lipoproteins	None	Small	Small	No
K	Phylloquinone (K1)	Lipid	451	Lipoproteins	NA[c]	NA[c]	Small	No
B1	Thiamin	Water	337	Albumin	13–40 mL/min[d]	Low	4–10 days	No
B2	Riboflavin	Water	376	Weak albumin, IgG	27–52 mL/min[d]	High	2–3 months	No
B6	Pyridoxine	Water	169	Albumin	54 mL/min[e]	= or < urinary excretion	3–4 months	Yes
B12	Cyanocobalamin	Water	1355	Transcobalamin II	Controversial[f]	None	Years	NA[c]
C	Ascorbic acid	Water	176	No	80–280 mg/ session[d]	40–56 mg/day	3–4 months	Yes
Folate	Pteroylglutamic acid	Water	441	No	135 mL/min[e]	1/3 of RDA	>1 year	Yes
Niacin	Nicotinic acid Nicotinamide	Water	123	Weak	Very low	NA[c]	2 months	NA[c]
Biotin	Biotin	Water	244	Weak	52 mL/min[d]	NA[c]	5 weeks	None
Pantothenic acid	Pantothenic acid	Water	219	NA[c]	30 mL/min[d]	NA[c]	Several weeks	None

MW, molecular weight; HD, hemodialysis; RBP, retinol binding protein; IgG, immunoglobulin G; RDA, recommended dietary allowance.
[a]For normal individuals.
[b]See Vitamin A section.
[c]Not available.
[d]Values obtained with low-flux/low-efficiency dialysis.
[e]Values obtained with high-flux/high-efficiency dialysis.
[f]Possible effect of convective forces.

Physiologic Role

Vitamin A is necessary for normal nocturnal vision. It also plays a role in the differentiation of epithelial cells and morphogenesis of solid organs, including the kidney, and in the immune response (4,5,10,11). The cellular differentiation effect of 13-cis-retinoic acid has been used to treat acute promyelocytic leukemia (12). Although vitamin A has antioxidant properties (4), two large-scale clinical trials (13,14) failed to demonstrate a benefit of large doses of retinol and carotenoids for the prevention of lung cancer or cardiovascular disease. Furthermore, an increased death rate was reported in the patients given vitamin A supplements, which was attributed to the oxidant effects of carotenoids (8). The physiologic effects of vitamin A are mediated through the nuclear retinoic acid receptor, which belongs to the same nuclear receptor superfamily as the vitamin D receptor. Plasma vitamin A usually is measured by high-pressure liquid chromatography (HPLC) (15), which has replaced older colorimetric methods.

Vitamin A in Kidney Disease

Role of the Kidney in the Homeostasis of Retinoids

The kidney affects vitamin A metabolism in three major ways. These include RBP catabolism, hepatic release of retinol, and retinoic acid synthesis. Many years ago, patients who had been binephrectomized were reported to have higher retinol levels than patients undergoing MHD (16). This argues for a pivotal role of the kidney in the homeostasis of retinoids. Earlier data suggested that serum RBP is modified in renal failure so that the binding of retinol to RBP is diminished (17), but this is not commonly accepted. Using SDS-Page immunoblotting analysis, Jaconi et al. (18) found a loss of C-terminal leucines from RBP in sera of patients undergoing MHD. Whether this change modifies the binding capacity of RBP or its propensity to be catabolized by the kidney is not known. After the delivery of retinol to target tissues, the free RBP can be filtered by the glomerulus and catabolized by the tubular cells. Thus, renal failure results in an increase in plasma RBP as well as in the plasma RBP/prealbumin and RBP/retinol ratios (19). The small proportion (5%) of the RBP-retinol complex that is not bound to transthyretin is filtered by the glomerulus. The complex is captured by the proximal tubular cell by a specific apical receptor, megalin, allowing for retinol recycling into the bloodstream at the basolateral level of the cell. Knockout mice for megalin display a urinary loss of the RBP-retinol complex (20). There is debate as to whether the RBP undergoes lysosomal degradation with *de novo* synthesis of new RBP or whether the RBP simply is transported across the cell (transcytosis) (20,21).

The kidney appears to play a role in the control of retinol

release by the liver. It has been proposed that plasma apo-RBP levels may be a positive feedback signal for increased hepatic release of retinol (22–24). Also, labeled retinyl acetate given intravenously to rats rapidly appears in the kidney as retinoic acid (25). Bhat et al. (26), studying the effects of retinoic acid on retinol metabolism, gave labeled retinol to rats fed a vitamin A–deficient diet for 6 days. Plasma retinol and retinyl esters levels fell and retinyl esters increased in the liver of these rats; labeled retinoic acid was not found in the liver but was present in high concentrations in the kidney. These findings suggest a major role for the kidney in the production of retinoic acid; in parenchymal kidney disease, the transformation of retinol to retinoic acid would be expected to be impaired, and this disorder has been proposed as an explanation for the accumulation of retinol in chronic renal failure (CRF) (27,28). However, at least two authors describe normal plasma retinoic acid levels in patients with CRF (29,30). Therefore, whether this mechanism causes the increase of retinol in patients with CRF is unclear.

Vitamin A Status in Renal Disease

High plasma vitamin A levels and an increased plasma vitamin A level in response to a vitamin A load test was reported in patients with CRF in 1945 (31). The protein-restricted diets usually prescribed to these patients have been found to contain a normal vitamin A content (Table 20.2). In nephrotic patients without renal failure, plasma RBP, retinol, and retinyl esters levels are reported to be increased (32). Many authors subsequently have confirmed elevated plasma concentrations of total vitamin A, RBP-bound vitamin A, and free vitamin A in patients with CRF and patients undergoing MHD, including long-term MHD survivors (27,28,30,33–41). As shown many years ago, hemodialysis (HD) treatment does not change vitamin A levels (41); indeed losses of vitamin A into dialysate would not be expected because of the relatively large size of the vitamin A-RBP-prealbumin complex. However, beta carotene, ubiquinol, and lycopene have been found to be lower in patients undergoing MHD than in controls (36,42), and beta carotene and ubiquinol decrease further after a single HD treatment. There are no published data on the dialysis kinetics of vitamin A and RBP handling in patients undergoing treatment with high-flux membranes. Recently, Rock et al. (43) found racial differences in plasma concentrations of antioxidant vitamins, with higher serum levels of retinol and carotenoids in African-American patients undergoing MHD. White patients had higher levels of α-tocopherol.

The lipid status may influence vitamin A level in patients with CRF and those undergoing chronic dialysis. A relationship between plasma vitamin A and lipid abnormalities has been reported. Smith et al. (44) found that, in individuals without CRF who have type IIa or IIb hyperlipidemia, plasma vitamin A levels correlated significantly with serum total cholesterol but not with serum triglycerides. In 72 patients undergoing MHD, Werb et al. (41) showed a positive correlation between plasma vitamin A levels and both serum total cholesterol and triglycerides. Other investigators have found similar relationships (38,45). Also, individuals without renal failure and with hypertriglyceridemia are reported to be at increased risk of vitamin A toxicity because of increased bioavailability of retinyl esters from lipoproteins (28). Because hypertriglyceridemia occurs commonly in patients with renal failure, it is possible that these latter individuals also may be at increased risk for vitamin A toxic-

TABLE 20.2. CALCULATED VITAMIN CONTENTS OF DIFFERENT DIETS PRESCRIBED TO PATIENTS WITH CHRONIC RENAL FAILURE AND PATIENTS UNDERGOING DIALYSIS[a]

Dietary Protein Intake	Vitamin A (μg RE[b])		Vitamin E (mg)		Vitamin K (μg)		Thiamin (mg)		Riboflavin (mg)		Biotin (μg)		Pyridoxine (mg)		Folic Acid (μg)		Vitamin B12 (μg)		Niacin (mg)		Ascorbic Acid (mg)		Pantothenic Acid (mg)	
	1[c]	2[d]	1	2	1	2	1	2	1	2	1	2	1	2	1	2	1	2	1	2	1	2	1	2
40 g	1245	556		16.0		80	0.6	1.2	0.8	0.8		13.4	1.0	1.4	260	50	2.3	0.6	8.8	9.0	86	107	2.7	3.0
60 g	1299	570		12.0		80	1.0	1.5	1.2	1.4		17.8	1.2	1.5	290	80	3.2	1.2	12.6	10.5	87	88	3.6	4.0
80 g	1548	568		14.0		80	1.1	1.3	1.7	1.2		15.8	1.5	1.8	320	70	5.1	2.5	14.7	15.0	88	60	5.1	3.2
100 g	1770	—		—		—	1.3	—	2.1	—		—	1.6	—	350	—	5.9	—	17.5	—	82	—	5.9	—
RDA[e]	700–900 (67)		15		90–120[f] (67)		1.1–1.2		1.1–1.3		30[f]		1.3–1.7[g]		400		2.4		14–16		75–90[h]		5[f]	

[a]Data refer to 24-hour intake of the nutrient from the diet.
[b]RE, retinol equivalents. Vitamin A values given by Kopple et al. (303) have been converted from interactional units (IU) to μg RE by multiplying IU by 0.3.
[c]Numbers under column 1 are from Kopple (303).
[d]Numbers under column 2 are from Stein (100).
[e]Recommended dietary allowance for healthy, nonpregnant, nonlactating adults.
[f]This value is not a RDA; there is inadequate scientific evidence to allow calculation of RDA. Recommended intake, termed "adequate intake" is used instead. It is derived from experimental data or by an approximation of observed mean intakes, as suggested by the Standing Committee on the Scientific Evaluation of Dietary Reference Intakes (2,67).
[g]In female and male adults younger than age 50, the RDA is 1.3 mg/day. Over the age of 50, the RDA is, respectively, 1.5 and 1.7 mg/day for women and men.
[h]Values of the RDA are for nonsmoking female and male adults. Add 35 mg/day for smokers (3).

ity. However, although one report described a low serum ratio of retinol/RBP in nondialyzed patients with CRF (46), clinical manifestations of vitamin A deficiency have not been reported in patients with CRF and those undergoing maintenance dialysis (MD).

Plasma vitamin A and beta carotene also are elevated in patients undergoing chronic peritoneal dialysis (CPD) (37, 47). The data are conflicting as to whether vitamin A and RBP are present in the effluent peritoneal dialysate (33, 37). After renal transplantation, plasma vitamin A decreases slowly toward normal. Yatzidis et al. reported that more than 20 months may elapse in patients with a well-functioning kidney transplant before plasma vitamin A levels are normal (48). In patients with acute renal failure (ARF), serum vitamin A levels were found to be normal in one study (19), decreased in another study (with normal serum RBP levels) (49), and increased in a third study of patients with ARF receiving total parenteral nutrition (TPN) containing standard retinol supplementation (50).

Clinical Relevance of Increased Plasma Vitamin A Levels in Renal Failure

Whether there is an increased risk of vitamin A toxicity in individuals with CRF and in patients undergoing chronic dialysis is controversial. Many patients with renal failure who have increased plasma vitamin A levels do not show evidence for toxicity (39,40). Elevated plasma vitamin A in renal failure is considered by many authors to be relative as a result of increased plasma RBP and to have no clinical significance as long as the vitamin A/RBP ratio is normal or low. Vitamin A toxicity is believed to occur when plasma retinyl esters in the lipoprotein fractions increase (4,19). Stewart and Fleming have reported mean plasma retinol levels 3.8 times normal values in 38 patients undergoing MHD receiving vitamin A supplements of 5,000 IU per day for 2 years; patients did not show clinical manifestations of vitamin A toxicity (39). After vitamin A supplements were stopped, plasma retinol decreased only slightly over the following 2 years to 3.1 times normal values. Throughout this 4-year period of follow-up, retinyl esters remained within the normal range (39). Whether vitamin A accumulates in solid tissues in patients with renal failure is unclear. Yatzidis et al. (27) found increased liver vitamin A content in two nondialyzed patients with CRF in comparison to published normal values. On the contrary, Stein et al. (38) reported a liver vitamin A content that was much lower in patients with chronic renal failure and patients undergoing MHD than in controls. Vahlquist et al. (40) reported increased skin vitamin A content in patients with CRF who did not have clinical features of vitamin A toxicity. The authors hypothesized that in the absence of increased serum prealbumin, an excess of the vitamin A/RBP complex would bind easily to RBP receptors in tissues, causing toxic effects. In contrast, Delacoux et al. (30) did not find features of vitamin A toxicity in a skin examination of 50 patients undergoing MHD who had elevated serum levels of RBP and retinol, some of whom underwent skin biopsies. Therefore, although it is not known whether the increased vitamin A levels that are commonly found in patients with CRF and those undergoing chronic dialysis are hazardous, there is no clear evidence for toxicity.

However, the risk of developing vitamin A toxicity when vitamin A supplements are given to patients with CRF and those undergoing chronic dialysis is high. Case reports of vitamin A toxicity in patients with CRF and those undergoing chronic dialysis are summarized in Table 20.3. Two of these reports mention vitamin A toxicity in patients with CRF or those undergoing MHD without supplemental vitamin A intake. However, some of the reported clinical features of vitamin A toxicity (i.e., yellowish appearance of the skin and anemia) are nonspecific, especially with regard to patients undergoing dialysis and those with CRF (40,45). The clinical features of retinoid excess are not unique to patients with renal failure and are similar to the syndrome of vitamin A intoxication in patients with normal renal function. The usual signs are cutaneous lesions (fissures, dryness, desquamation), headaches and central nervous system manifestations, joint pains, bone tenderness to palpation, hepatomegaly, and muscle stiffness (4,51). Hair loss ascribed to vitamin A toxicity has been reported in one patient being treated with dialysis (52).

A particularly relevant symptom of vitamin A intoxication in renal patients is hypercalcemia (53–55), and this condition should be considered in the differential diagnosis of hypercalcemia in patients with renal failure. It is intriguing that, in patients with CRF who do not have vitamin A toxicity, a correlation has been reported between plasma vitamin A concentrations and serum calcium levels (41,56). Farrington et al. (56) reported that in patients undergoing MHD, those who were taking vitamin A supplements, 2,500 to 15,000 IU per day, had higher serum vitamin A and calcium concentrations than those who were not. These latter patients, in turn, had higher serum vitamin A levels than normal individuals. Some patients undergoing MHD taking as little as 7,500 IU of vitamin A per day displayed hypercalcemia and increased alkaline phosphatase, which decreased with cessation of the vitamin A supplements. However, such correlations between plasma vitamin A and increased serum calcium or serum alkaline phosphatase have not been found consistently. Cundy et al. (35) found no correlation between the degree of elevation in plasma vitamin A levels and the severity of osteodystrophy in 50 patients undergoing MHD. As indicated earlier, serum alkaline phosphatase is usually at least slightly elevated in vitamin A toxicity (56,57). It is not always clear whether the increased serum alkaline phosphatase is derived from vitamin A–induced bone or liver injury; however, hepatic injury generally occurs only with markedly increased vitamin A intake (e.g., >100,000 IU/day in nonrenal individuals) (51). Also, there is no consensus as to whether elevated hydroxyprolinuria occurs in vitamin A toxicity (56,57). In

TABLE 20.3. VITAMIN A OVERLOAD PATTERNS REPORTED IN PATIENTS WITH RENAL FAILURE

First Author	Patients	Vitamin A Supplement[a]	Clinical Features
Gleghorn (50)	3 ARF	Total parenteral nutrition (4,500 IU/day)	Hypercalcemia, skin and CNS changes
Shmunes (52)	1 HD	Multivitamin supplement (5,000 IU/day)	Alopecia
Farrington (56)			Hypercalcemia
Vahlquist (40)	10 CRF	None	Yellowish appearance of the skin
Ono (45)	27 HD	None	Anemia
Doireau (54)	1 Alagille syndrome	12,000 IU for 2 years	Bone pain, hypercalcemia
Beijer (53)	1 CRF	Retinol palmitate (600 IU), cholecalciferol (200 IU)	Hypercalcemia

ARF, acute renal failure; CNS, central nervous system; CRF, chronic renal failure; HD, hemodialysis.
[a]Vitamin A dose associated with toxicity.

patients with normal or slightly altered renal function, Frame et al. (58) reported impressive periosteal calcifications that disappeared after discontinuation of vitamin A supplements. This radiologic sign has not been found in patients undergoing dialysis by others (56). The mechanism of hypercalcemia with vitamin A toxicity is related to the osteolytic action of the retinoids on bone (57). In most cases of hypercalcemia associated with vitamin A toxicity, vitamin D was present in the supplements, and it is possible that cholecalciferol might contribute to or potentiate the pathogenesis of hypercalcemia associated with increased vitamin A (53,56–58). It is unlikely that vitamin A toxicity contributes to classical renal osteodystrophy.

Erythropoiesis and Vitamin A

The hematocrit has been found to be correlated with the plasma vitamin A/RBP ratio in patients undergoing MD (45). Several studies have addressed the relationship between erythropoietin (EPO) treatment and vitamin A (see Chapter 22). Vitamin A increases EPO production by EPO-producing hepatoma cell cultures in a dependent-dose manner (59). EPO production by isolated perfused rat kidneys also is stimulated by vitamin A, mimicking hypoxic induction (60). In the same study, vitamin A also was able to reverse the inhibitory effect of prooxidant molecules on EPO production (60). Also, EPO treatment for 12 months has been shown to induce a significant decrease of serum vitamin A levels (61).

Vitamin A Effect in Experimental Nephropathies

Based on its antioxidant effect, vitamin A has been used to improve renal lesions in experimental nephropathies. Retinoic acid has been studied *in vitro* as a therapeutic tool against H_2O_2-induced mesangial cell death (62). Also, in rats with anti-Thy1.1-induced glomerulonephritis, all-trans retinoic acid or isotretinoid were shown to decrease significantly the severity of glomerular histopathology (63). Vitamin A has been shown to reduce scarring in experimental pyelonephritis (64,65). Moreover, tretinoic acid treatment given to rats for 3 months is reported to prevent the aging-related loss of glomerular filtration rate (GFR), with evidence of *in vitro* protection against H_2O_2-induced cell lesions (66).

Need for Supplemental Vitamin A

Because plasma levels of vitamin A are elevated in patients with CRF and patients undergoing MD, vitamin A deficiency rarely has been observed, and even small supplements of vitamin A (i.e., 7,500 to 15,000 IU, that is 2,250 to 4,500 μg of RE) may cause vitamin A toxicity (19,56). There is a consensus that supplemental doses of vitamin A larger then the recommended dietary allowance (RDA; see Chapter 23) for vitamin A in normal healthy adults (i.e., 700 to 900 μg of RE) (67) should not be given (1,39,41, 68–70) (Table 20.4). For patients with chronic renal failure who routinely ingest less than two-thirds of the RDA for vitamin A, a vitamin A supplement not to exceed the RDA may be prescribed.

Because patients with the nephrotic syndrome may excrete vitamins that bind to protein, a daily intake of the RDA for vitamin A may be indicated. For renal transplant recipients, vitamin A supplements are not necessary unless patients received their renal transplant more than 1 to 2 years previously, their vitamin A intake is low, and their renal function is not markedly reduced. Vitamin A supplements are probably not necessary for patients with ARF unless patients are given TPN without vitamin supplements for at least 2 to 3 weeks. Given the risks of vitamin A toxicity in patients with CRF and reports of vitamin A toxicity in patients treated with TPN with ARF receiving as little as 1,500 μg of RE per day (50), it is recommended that no more than the RDA for vitamin A (700 to 900 μg/day) RE for nonpregnant, nonlactating adults) should be given for patients with ARF receiving TPN as their sole nutritional source for extended periods.

VITAMIN E

Structure and Metabolism

Vitamin E is a fat-soluble vitamin with a main active compound of α-tocopherol (Table 20.1); other naturally occurring isomers are also present. The main sources of vitamin E are vegetable oils such as corn, soybean, wheat germ, or sunflower oil (71). Animal products are not rich sources of vitamin E. After intestinal absorption of vitamin E conge-

TABLE 20.4. GUIDELINES FOR VITAMIN SUPPLEMENTS IN ADULTS WITH RENAL DISEASE

Vitamin[a]	Nondialyzed Stage 3, 4, or 5 Chronic Kidney Disease	Chronic Hemodialysis	Chronic Peritoneal Dialysis	Acute Renal Failure (TPN)	Nephrotic Syndrome
			Recommended Daily Intakes		
Vitamin A	None	None	None	None	None
Vitamin E	400–800 IU[b]	400–800 IU[b]	400–800 IU[b]	10 IU	400–800 IU[b]
Vitamin K	None[c]	None[c]	None[c]	7.5 mg/week	Unknown
Vitamin B1	1.1–1.2 mg	1.1–1.2 mg	1.1–1.2 mg	2 mg	Unknown
Riboflavin	1.1–1.3 mg	1.1–1.3 mg	1.1–1.3 mg	2 mg	Unknown
Vitamin B6	5 mg[d]	10 mg[d]	10 mg[d]	10 mg[d]	Unknown[e]
Vitamin B12	2.4 μg	2.4 μg	2.4 μg	3 μg	Unknown
Vitamin C	75–90 mg	75–90 mg	75–90 mg	75–90 mg	Unknown
Folic acid	1 mg	1 mg	1 mg	2 mg	Unknown
Niacin	14–16 mg	14–16 mg	14–16 mg	20 mg	Unknown
Biotin	30 μg	30 μg	30 μg	200 μg	Unknown
Pantothenic acid	5 mg	5 mg	5 mg	10 mg	Unknown

TPN, total parenteral nutrition.
[a]Vitamin D is discussed in Chapter 17.
[b]For possible prevention of cardiovascular disease (131).
[c]For clinically stable patients who are ingesting food and not receiving antibiotics.
[d]Amounts indicated refer to pyridoxine hydrochloride. If nondialyzed patients with chronic kidney disease develop a catabolic illness, pyridoxine HCl 10 mg/day is recommended.
[e]Optimal supplementation has not been determined (197,234).

ners, these compounds are transported with fat, mainly through the lymphatic flow, into the venous circulation. In plasma, there is no specific carrier for α-tocopherol, and it is bound to lipoproteins. Alpha-tocopherol exchanges rapidly with cell membranes; this is mediated by high-density lipoprotein (HDL) cholesterol (72). There is substantial evidence that in normal individuals, the dietary vitamin E requirement increases and decreases as the dietary fat intake rises and is reduced (73).

Assessment of nutritional status of vitamin E is difficult. HPLC is used widely to measure serum vitamin E levels (74). The peroxide hemolysis test has been used to assess vitamin E deficiency (74). The cell-membrane concentration of α-tocopherol and/or its antioxidant activity might give more helpful information concerning the activity and adequacy of tissue α-tocopherol levels than the plasma α-tocopherol level itself. Vitamin E is carried in plasma by lipoproteins, and its plasma concentration is affected by the lipid content of blood. Horwitt et al. (75) reported that when plasma cholesterol level was decreased in eight tocopherol-supplemented subjects by administration of L-triiodothyronine, the plasma tocopherol also fell. These authors have recommended that plasma tocopherol levels should be expressed preferably as the α-tocopherol/total plasma lipids ratio; 0.8 mg/g of total lipids was considered to be a normal ratio. The ratio of tocopherol/cholesterol + triglycerides also has been proposed as a method for expression of the plasma tocopherol levels (76). Sokol et al. (77) reported that in three children with clinical vitamin E deficiency and a normal plasma level of tocopherol, the plasma tocopherol/total lipid ratio was a better discriminator for tocopherol deficiency than the plasma tocopherol/cholesterol ratio. Sadowski et al. (78) observed a strong relationship ($r = 0.98$) between the plasma vitamin E level and the quintile distribution of plasma triglycerides. In the same epidemiologic survey, elderly individuals had a higher plasma tocopherol level than did young subjects. This difference disappeared when the tocopherol/triglyceride ratio was used.

Physiologic Role

Vitamin E is the main antioxidant in biologic membranes, protecting phospholipid membranes from oxidative stress. Vitamin E deficiency from intestinal malabsorption has been reported to increase hemolysis by causing membrane fragility (74). In individuals with genetically transmitted hemoglobinopathies, such as glutathione synthetase deficiency, G6PD deficiency or β-thalassemia (79,80), α-tocopherol suppementation may increase erythrocyte life span and decrease the reticulocyte count. It is thought that tocopherol deficiency in premature infants or patients with severe malabsorption syndrome is responsible for the accumulation of lipopigment in certain tissues including the spinal cord and small intestine. Oxidized polyunsaturated fatty acids are thought to be the major constituent of this pigment (74). Vitamin E is also an antiatherogenic agent. Epidemiologic studies have found a reduced risk of coronary heart disease in men and women with higher intakes of vitamin E from foods (81,82). The mechanism of this protective effect is considered to be decreased oxidation of low-density lipoprotein (LDL) cholesterol—a key step in the pathogenesis of the fatty streak, the first step in the development of the atheromatous plaque. However, vitamin E may promote synthesis and secretion of selectin, an adhesion molecule involved in the endothelial attachment of monocytes to endothelial cells—another step in atherogenesis (83).

Vitamin E Status in Kidney Disease

In patients with the nephrotic syndrome, plasma levels of plasma tocopherol are reported to be increased (32,84), normal (85), or decreased (86,87). Fydryk et al. (84) reported a relationship between plasma lipids and vitamin E levels. Warwick et al. (85) found that patients with the nephrotic syndrome had an increased absolute level of plasma vitamin E but had plasma vitamin E/cholesterol ratios that were not different from controls. Also, Mydlik et al. (32) found that in patients with the nephrotic syndrome, the increased tocopherol levels returned to normal values after successful treatment of this condition.

In nondialyzed patients with advanced CRF, plasma vitamin E levels are usually within the normal range (88,89). Protein-restricted diets generally provide a normal and nutritionally sufficient vitamin E intake (Table 20.2). Gentile et al. (88) found a normal serum level of tocopherol in predialysis patients, which remained normal after they ingested 0.6 or 1 g/kg/day protein diets for 6 months. However, no data were given regarding the plasma lipid levels of the patients. Malnutrition also may influence the vitamin E status, and lower serum α-tocopherol levels were found in malnourished patients with CRF than in well-nourished individuals (90). Taccone-Galluchi et al. (91) and Peuchant et al. (92) found decreased α-tocopherol in red blood cells (RBC) from nondialyzed patients with CRF who had increased erythrocyte peroxidation, as determined by elevated intraerythrocyte malonyldialdehyde (MDA) concentrations.

In patients undergoing MHD, serum α-tocopherol levels are reported to be low (42,93–95), normal (80,89,96–99), or increased (100). There is no difference in plasma vitamin E concentrations between predialysis and postdialysis samples (42,95,96), and no tocopherol is found in spent dialysate (94,95), indicating that significant amounts of α-tocopherol are not removed by the dialysis procedure. Pastor et al. (72) did not find differences in the plasma level of tocopherol in patients undergoing MHD or continuous ambulatory peritoneal dialysis (CAPD) when compared to controls and after correction for the serum lipid levels. In 10 long-term MHD survivors treated with MHD for an average of 274 ± 35 (SD) months, Chazot et al. found that serum vitamin E levels were increased but not different from 10 age- and gender-matched patients who were treated with MHD for 51 ± 29 months (34). There are conflicting results with regard to RBC tocopherol concentrations in patients undergoing MHD that have been found to be normal (101) or, more commonly, decreased (72,96,102–104). These findings were interpreted to reflect either increased consumption of tocopherol, possibly as a result of oxidative stress, or a defect in the HDL-mediated transfer of tocopherol from plasma to the RBC membrane. It is noteworthy that low RBC tocopherol levels may occur in patients who have normal plasma tocopherol concentrations (96,102). However, in these latter studies, the tocopherol/lipid ratio was not reported. Nevertheless, Cohen et al. (105) showed that RBC tocopherol concentrations were low in patients undergoing MHD who had sustained hemolysis caused by a high chloramine concentration in the water supply for MHD. The RBC tocopherol level rose after the hemolytic condition was corrected by removal of the chloramine (105).

In patients undergoing CPD, data regarding vitamin E status are conflicting. Blumberg et al. found that plasma tocopherol levels were normal at the onset of CPD and were slightly decreased 3 months later (69). Very low amounts of tocopherol were found in peritoneal dialysate. Boeschoten et al. (33) reported vitamin E deficiency, as determined by low plasma levels, in 13% of patients undergoing CPD. Henderson et al. (106) did not find decreased plasma vitamin E after 12 months of CPD treatment, whereas Mydlik et al. (37) found an increase in plasma vitamin E after 1 year of CPD treatment. None of these studies describe the plasma tocopherol/lipid ratios. More recently, high plasma levels of α-tocopherol were reported in patients undergoing CAPD (47,107). The level of erythrocyte oxidative stress in patients undergoing CPD, as indicated by erythrocyte MDA and tocopherol concentrations, is reported to be similar to control values (72,91).

In renal transplant recipients, McGrath et al. (108) reported a normal plasma vitamin E/lipid ratio in 40 transplant patients, 20 of whom were receiving cyclosporine and 20 of whom were receiving azathioprine and glucocorticoids. Erythrocyte α-tocopherol was found to be decreased in kidney transplant patients with features of chronic rejection (109). Plasma vitamin E levels are decreased in patients with acute renal failure, regardless of whether they are treated with continuous hemofiltration (110).

Oxidative Stress in Kidney Diseases and the Protective Effects of Vitamin E

Experimental Nephropathies

Reactive oxygen species (i.e., H_2O_2, OH—, O═) may contribute to the pathogenesis of many nephropathies. The possible protective effects of vitamin E have been studied in several models of kidney disease. Vitamin E did not improve glycerol-induced acute renal failure (111). Its protective effect in chronic puromycin aminonucleoside and gentamicin nephropathies is controversial (112–114). However, a beneficial effect of vitamin E was described in other models of renal diseases including the aging kidney (115), extracorporeal shock wave lithotripsy–induced renal lesions (116), obstructive nephropathy (65,117), the remnant kidney rat model (118,119), cisplatin nephrotoxicity (120), focal and segmental sclerosis (121), mesangial-proliferative glomerulonephritis (118), immunoglobulin A (122,123), chromate and thallium-induced nephrotoxicity (124), and diabetic nephropathy (125–127).

Nephrotic Syndrome

The nephrotic syndrome appears to be a condition of oxidative stress. Bulucu et al. (128) studied the oxidative status of 20 adults with the nephrotic syndrome with normal serum creatinine levels and without overt inflammatory disease. Compared to healthy control subjects, these patients displayed increased plasma and erythrocyte MDA, decreased plasma selenium and glutathione peroxidase, and reduced erythrocyte superoxide dismutase and glutathione peroxidase, suggesting that they suffered from increased oxidative stress. Similar findings are reported in children with nephrotic syndrome (86,87). However, the susceptibility of LDL to oxidation and the plasma hydroxyperoxide-LDL content were not increased in the nephrotic syndrome (85). Whether this oxidative stress is a cause or the consequence of the nephrotic syndrome is not known. Yoshioka et al. (129) found a serum-dependent down-regulation of manganese-superoxide dismutase gene transcription in patients with active nephrotic syndrome. Also, erythrocyte glutathione peroxidase was found to be decreased during both the active proteinuric and remission phases of the nephrotic syndrome (84). In an open label study, Tahzib et al. (130) gave 11 children with focal glomerulosclerosis and nine children with nonnephrotic nephropathies 400 IU/ day of vitamin E for 2.9 months. There was a significant decrease in the urinary protein/creatinine ratio from 9.7 to 4.1 in the nephrotic children and no change in the nonnephrotic patients. However, serum albumin did not change in either group of patients (130).

Chronic Renal Failure

Much evidence supports the hypothesis that nondialyzed patients with CRF and individuals undergoing MHD or CPD suffer from oxidant stress, as discussed in Chapter 5. Several studies have examined the effects on oxidant stress of vitamin E supplementation given orally, during HD treatment using vitamin E–coated dialyzer membranes, or through dialysate (hemolipodialysis).

Oral Vitamin E

The Secondary Prevention with Antioxidants of Cardiovascular disease in End-stage renal disease (SPACE) study randomized 196 patients undergoing MHD to receive oral vitamin E, 800 IU/day, or placebo in a double-blind prospective clinical trial. Median duration of follow-up was 519 days. All patients previously had an adverse cardiovascular event. Patients undergoing MHD assigned to vitamin E, as compared to those given placebo, had a reduction in subsequent cardiovascular events (RR = 0.46) and myocardial infarction (RR = 0.30) (131). However, in the larger Heart Outcomes Prevention Evaluation (HOPE) trial, individuals with certain risk factors for cardiovascular disease, the majority of whom did not have advanced chronic renal insufficiency, demonstrated a reduction in adverse cardiovascular events with the angiotensin converting enzyme inhibitor ramipril but not with vitamin E supplements (132). The Micro-HOPE study confirmed these findings in patients with diabetes (133); also, there was a reduction in the development of overt diabetic nephropathy with ramipril but not with vitamin E (133). Other studies in small numbers of patients undergoing MHD and/or CAPD have shown that vitamin E therapy had a number of potentially beneficial effects including: (a) enriched vitamin E content of LDL, without affecting monocyte-endothelial adhesion (134); (b) increased erythrocyte life span or reduced EPO dose (96, 99,102,135); (c) decreased MDA in platelets (98,136); (d) reduced LDL susceptibility to oxidation (104,137,138); and (e) decreased oxidative stress from an intravenous iron load (98).

Vitamin E–Coated Hemodialysis Membranes

Vitamin E–coated hemodialysis membranes have been investigated as a method for reducing oxidative stress during MHD treatment. Most trials using these membranes were carried out for at least 3 months and described an increase in plasma or RBC vitamin E levels (139–141) and a decrease in plasma MDA (140,142–144). Other observed potentially beneficial effects of vitamin E–coated membranes include decreased neutrophil activation (145), reduced apoptosis of mononuclear cells (140), greater resistance of HDL to oxidation (139), decreased prooxidant activity of leucocytes (141,144,146,147), reduced intradialytic interleukin-6 production (146), lower oxidized LDL (148), lower heparin (149), reduced EPO requirements (149,150), and reduced oxidative damage to DNA (141). Some studies indicated no improvement in leucocyte count and leucocyte surface molecules (151) and no reduction in oxidized LDL after exposure to vitamin E–coated membranes (142); these studies were of shorter duration (2 to 6 weeks).

Hemolipodialysis

Hemolipodialysis has been proposed by Wratten et al. (151) to reduce the oxidant stress of MHD treatment. Both vitamin C and vitamin E are added to dialysate. Because vitamin E is not very water soluble, it is added to the dialysate in liposomes. These liposomes, which are 250 to 300 nm in diameter, do not cross the hemodialyzer membrane, but they are expected to interfere with the generation of reactive oxygen species and reduce the oxidative burden. Vitamin C is added to prevent vitamin C losses into dialysate and also may promote recycling of vitamin E from tocopheroxyl to α-tocopherol (152).

Transplantation

Oxidative damage is particularly likely to occur at several steps during the course of kidney transplantation. Reperfusion after cold ischemia may lead to marked oxidative bursts. An antioxidant mixture, including 10 mg of α-tocopherol, given 30 minutes before reperfusion, was able to reduce the degree of lipid peroxidation as assessed by the plasma MDA levels (153). Cristol et al. (109) found evidence for increased oxidative stress in 77 kidney transplant recipients, including individuals with and without chronic rejection. Evidence indicated that oxidative stress was greater in the patients with chronic rejection. However, McGrath et al. (108) did not observe differences in plasma TBARS (thiobarbituric acid reactive substances) and plasma vitamin E concentrations in patients receiving cyclosporine or azathioprine when compared to controls. Patients treated with tacrolimus were found to have increased susceptibility to oxidation when compared to patients treated with cyclosporine (154).

Evidence for increased lipid peroxidation has been shown in uninephrectomized rats given cyclosporine; concomitant administration of vitamin E prevented lipid peroxidation and resulted in significantly increased GFR, renal blood flow (RBF), and renal vascular resistance (154). Increased glomerular production of superoxide anion, malondialdehyde, hydrogen peroxide, and thromboxane A_2 were found in rats after a daily intake of 50 mg/kg cyclosporine for 30 days. This production of oxidants was attenuated in rats receiving pretreatment with vitamin E for 15 days (155). These findings have been confirmed in rabbits receiving cyclosporine for 10 days; they presented with decreased tissue antioxidant defense potential and displayed a partial improvement when given supplements of vitamins E and C (156). In another study, rabbits receiving cyclosporine displayed increased messenger RNA expression for COX-1 (cyclooxygenase-1) and transforming growth factor-β, that was blunted when vitamin E was added (157). Barany et al. (158) found that in 12 healthy subjects, the acute reduction of RBF and GFR that occurs after a single dose of cyclosporine (5 mg/kg) was significantly attenuated when the subjects were pretreated with 800 IU of vitamin E for 6 weeks.

Need for Supplemental Vitamin E

It is not clear whether most patients with CRF or those undergoing MD should receive vitamin E supplementation (68,69). In the SPACE study, patients undergoing MHD with preexisting cardiovascular disease who were given 800 IU/day of vitamin E showed a lower incidence of adverse cardiovascular events (131). In individuals without renal disease, platelet dysfunction and interference with the vitamin K–dependent coagulation factors have been reported with pharmacologic doses of vitamin E (159). Moreover, the HOPE study did not show clinical benefit of vitamin E supplements in individuals with or without chronic renal insufficiency (132,133). Nonetheless, because chronic renal disease and CRF are associated with a state of increased oxidant stress and increased cardiovascular risk, and because vitamin E appears to be rather safe and may be beneficial, a supplement of 400 to 800 IU/day of vitamin E may be recommended (Table 20.4).

VITAMIN K

Structure and Metabolism

There are several excellent reviews of vitamin K metabolism (160–162). Two classes of compounds, phylloquinone (K1) and menaquinones (K3), are primarily responsible for vitamin K activity. Phylloquinone (Table 20.1) is found essentially in green and leafy vegetables (e.g., spinach, kale, cabbage, broccoli) and cow's milk. Menaquinones are of bacterial origin and are found in yogurt but are also produced by colonic bacteria. The intestinal absorption of these compounds requires biliary and pancreatic juices and occurs in the small bowel where vitamin K is incorporated in chylomicrons. The importance of intestinal bacterial synthesis of vitamin K (menaquinone) as a vitamin source is still controversial. Its importance had been emphasized because of the frequent vitamin K deficiency states associated with the use of large spectrum antibiotics. However, antibiotic therapy is not necessary for the development of vitamin K deficiency (162). Moreover, certain antibiotics may promote vitamin K deficiency by an independent mechanism. Antibiotics that have a N-methyl-5-thiotetrazole side chain have a warfarin-like effect and interfere directly with the γ-carboxylation of proteins, independently of any suppression of intestinal flora (159). Furthermore, a vitamin K1 deficient state is easily induced experimentally by restricting food for a few days or weeks; this leads to decreased levels of plasma descarboxy-prothrombin and reduced urinary excretion of γ-carboxyglutamic acid (163).

The uptake of vitamin K by the liver depends on β-lipoproteins and the clearance of the chylomicron remnants including its apo(E) component (164). There is no specific carrier for vitamin K in plasma. As has been shown for other fat-soluble vitamins, serum lipid concentrations may affect the bioavailability of vitamin K. Sadowski et al. (78) found a strong direct correlation (r = 0.99) between the quintile distribution of serum triglycerides and serum phylloquinone levels. The plasma phylloquinone/triglyceride ratio may be used as an indicator of vitamin K status. The plasma level of phylloquinone is found to be lower in elderly individuals, as compared to young subjects (78). Vitamin K turnover is rapid, and the body pool is small (Table 20.1). Ferland et al. (165) showed that after injection of radio-labeled phylloquinone into normal humans, up to 30% of the metabolites are excreted in the urine and most of the radioactivity is recovered in the feces. The kidney has no major role in vitamin K metabolism.

The reference method for measuring plasma vitamin K levels is liquid chromatography. There is a seasonal variation in the fasting plasma concentration of vitamin K, with higher levels found at the end of summer. This may be explained by the findings that the vitamin K content of cow's milk is fourfold higher during the summer (166). Thus, a seasonal variation of the phylloquinone intake may account for the fluctuations in the plasma vitamin K level.

Physiologic Role

Vitamin K is a coenzyme for the posttranslational carboxylation of glutamate residues in several proteins that form other proteins with γ-carboxyglutamate (Gla) residues, also called Gla proteins (167). The Gla residue in protein binds to calcium. In the process of forming the Gla residue, vitamin K is transformed from the hydroquinone form (KH_2) to the epoxide form (KO), releasing the amount of energy required to generate the carboxylation reaction. The epoxide form of vitamin K then is recycled back to the hydroquinone form; thus, a rather small quantity of vitamin K can generate a much larger amount of the Gla proteins. Indeed, the urinary excretion of Gla residues is 200 to 500 times greater than the dietary intake of vitamin K. The currently known Gla proteins are found in the coagulation cascade, in bone and dentin, in microsomes of tubular cells (168), and in atherogenic plaques. The importance of vitamin K for the normal coagulation cascade is well known. In fact, the name "vitamin K" reflects this association (K for koagulation). The procoagulant factors that contain Gla residues, and hence require vitamin K for their posttranslational carboxylation, are prothrombin (Factor II), proconvertin (Factor VII), Christmas factor (Factor IX), and Stuart factor (Factor X). The anticoagulation effect of coumarin derivatives is related to the blockade of the dithiol-dependent reductases that are necessary for the recycling of vitamin K. However, the production of several inhibitors of coagulation is also vitamin K dependent, including proteins C, S, and Z. This is the explanation for the uncommon and paradoxic thrombotic complications of coumarin therapy, such as skin necrosis (169).

Two Gla proteins are present in bone: osteocalcin and matrix Gla protein (MGP). Osteocalcin is the most abundant noncollagenous protein of bone and is a specific marker for osteoblast activity. *In vitro*, osteocalcin binds to hydroxyapatite and inhibits its formation. This action requires the vitamin K-dependent carboxylation of the protein (159). The exact role of these carboxylated proteins in bone is not yet well defined, but indirect evidence argues for a key role in bone homeostasis. Women with hip fractures have been found to have lower plasma vitamin K levels (170). It has been suggested that patients receiving warfarin therapy have greater bone density loss, but this remains controversial (171–174). MGP is thought to modulate vascular calcification; MGP knockout mice present with extensive lethal vascular calcifications (175).

Kidney Diseases and Renal Failure

Renal Failure: Risk Factor for Vitamin K Deficiency

Few studies have systematically examined the vitamin K status of patients with CRF. The low-protein diets, often prescribed before starting dialysis, usually provide a normal phylloquinone intake (Table 20.2). However, Alperin (176) and Ansell et al. (162) reported that one-third of hospitalized patients who had vitamin K deficiency with elevated prothrombin times and symptomatic bleeding disorders had CRF. Thus, CRF may be a risk factor for vitamin K deficiency. The mechanism underlying such a relationship is not clear. It is possible that renal impairment could alter the metabolism of the antibiotics often used in such patients. Such an effect either could suppress the gut flora or directly antagonize actions of vitamin K–dependent coagulation factors. Alternatively, suppression of vitamin K–dependent anticoagulants in patients with CRF could lead to thrombotic complications. Soundararajan et al. (177) reported a case of spontaneous skin necrosis related to a vitamin K deficiency state with a low plasma protein C level in a renal transplant recipient who had CRF. These authors suggest that both vitamin K deficiency and altered metabolism of protein C in CRF could lead to the low protein C levels. Moreover, abnormal anticoagulant activity of protein C has been observed in patients undergoing MHD with normal plasma antigen levels and amidolytic activity of this protein (178). This activity of protein C increased after hemodialysis, which suggests that there may be circulating dialyzable inhibitors to protein C in renal failure. However, Robert et al. (179) reported a higher plasma level of phylloquinone in patients undergoing MHD. No data were given regarding the plasma lipid concentrations in these patients, and the biologic effects, if any, of the elevated phylloquinone concentrations are unclear. No data are available concerning vitamin K in patients undergoing CPD.

Vitamin K and Calciuria

Administration of vitamin K1 reduces urinary calcium excretion in postmenopausal women who have increased urinary calcium excretion (i.e., urine Ca/creatinine ratio >0.5) (180). Coumarin derivatives also increase the urinary calcium excretion in young adults (181). The anticalciuric effects of vitamin K may be mediated through the carboxylation of bone proteins (i.e., osteocalcin and other Gla proteins that bind calcium). The reduced bone mineral content found in patients receiving oral anticoagulants supports the possibility that vitamin K antagonists increase urinary calcium by mobilizing bone calcium (174). However, a direct effect of vitamin K or its antagonists on the kidney cannot be ruled out. In some patients with nephrolithiasis, the lack of inhibition of calcium oxalate crystal growth by their urine has been linked to the presence in the urine of defective glycoproteins that do not contain the normal Gla residues (182).

Vitamin K as a Risk Factor for Ectopic Calcification

Two reports have described a relationship between high plasma vitamin K levels and ectopic soft-tissue calcification in patients undergoing MHD (170,177). It is possible that high levels of vitamin K, by stimulating the formation of the Gla proteins that have a high affinity for calcium, may promote calcium deposits in soft tissues. It is pertinent that in both of the forgoing studies, the patients had a high serum calcium–phosphorus product (179,183), which also might have promoted the calcium deposits in soft tissues.

Vitamin K and Renal Osteodystrophy

Administration of a pharmacologic dose of vitamin K2 (45 mg/day) for 1 year has been found to prevent loss of bone mass in patients undergoing MHD with bone disease characterized by low bone turnover (184). Moreover, an inverse relationship between a history of bone fractures and the plasma phylloquinone levels or the proportion of carboxylated versus noncarboxylated osteocalcin in plasma has been reported in patients undergoing MHD (185). Also, in the same study, parathyroid hormone levels were found to be high (>300 ng/L) only in patients with low plasma phylloquinone concentrations. These latter patients also had an abnormally high incidence of an apo(E) phenotype that may indicate impaired tissue uptake of phylloquinone from chylomicrons. The authors suggested that this impaired clearance may reduce delivery of phylloquinone to osteoblasts that produce osteocalcin and that this may be related to their apo(E) genotype (186).

Need for Vitamin K Supplements

Because patients with CRF or undergoing dialysis generally do not have evidence for vitamin K deficiency, vitamin K supplements generally have not been recommended (1, 100). Vitamin K supplements have been proposed for these patients when they are eating poorly and receiving antibiotics, particularly for extended periods, because they are probably at risk for developing vitamin K deficiency (1,187). At the least, the prothrombin time and proteins C and S should be monitored in these latter individuals. Alternatively, such patients simply can be given vitamin K supplements. Further research should determine whether vitamin K supplementation or inhibition may help to prevent the formation of calcium stones and to prevent or treat osteodystrophy and soft-tissue or vascular calcifications.

VITAMIN B1 (THIAMIN)

Structure and Metabolism

It has been stated that the syndrome of beriberi has been recognized for more than 4,000 years (188). In 1911, an antiberiberi principle was discovered in rice bran extracts, and in 1934 the structure of thiamin was identified (188). Vitamin B1 or thiamin (Table 20.1) is a compound formed by the condensation of pyrimidine and thiazole rings. Thiamin forms esters with phosphate, functionally the most important of which are thiamin pyrophosphate (TPP), monophosphate, and triphosphate. Thiamin is rather labile and may be destroyed by heat, high pH (above 8), oxidants, and ultraviolet irradiation. Thiamin is abundant in only a few foods of animal and vegetable origin. These foods include lean pork, yeast, and legumes. Because thiamin is water soluble, foods cooked with water can be leached of significant amounts of thiamin. Thiamin is absorbed from the small intestine by active and passive processes. In plasma, thiamin mainly is bound to albumin. Most thiamin in the body is present as thiamin pyrophosphate. The availability or activity of thiamin is inhibited by alcohol, thiaminases, folate deficiency, and protein-energy malnutrition. Catabolism of thiamin produces many metabolites that are excreted in the urine. Urinary thiamin excretion is flow dependent, and diuretic agents induce a dose-dependent, significant increase in urinary thiamin excretion (189).

In vivo, thiamin stores can be assessed indirectly by measuring the erythrocyte transketolase activity (ETKA), before ($ETKA_o$) and after ($ETKA_s$) stimulation by TPP (190). The ETKA stimulation index (αETKA) (i.e., the ETKA after addition of TPP × 100, divided by $ETKA_o$) is considered to be a more sensitive and reliable indicator of thiamin deficiency than either the $ETKA_o$ or $ETKA_s$. HPLC has become the preferred method for measuring thiamin status in many laboratories (191,192). It measures whole blood thiamin and RBC TPP, the active functional form of thiamin (193).

Physiologic Role

TPP, in association with coenzyme A (CoA), flavine adenine nucleotide (FAD), and nicotinamide adenine nucleotide

(NAD), is a coenzyme for the oxidative decarboxylation of α-ketoacids. TPP is a coenzyme for many other enzymes and particularly those involved with carbohydrate metabolism, including pyruvate dehydrogenase. This enzyme catalyzes the conversion of pyruvate to acetyl CoA; hence, thiamin deficiency may impair lactate utilization and lead to thiamin-responsive lactic acidosis (194,195). As indicated earlier, thiamin is also a coenzyme for the transketolase reaction, which is an integral part of the pentose phosphate pathway. Transketolase is found abundantly in myelinated structures of nervous tissues (196). This may account for the peripheral neuropathy that occurs in beriberi. Independent of its activity as a coenzyme for transketolase, it has been suggested that thiamin may play a role in nerve impulse transmission by interacting with sodium channels (188).

Thiamin and Kidney Disease

Thiamin Status in Renal Disease

Mydlik and Derzsiova investigated 33 nephrotic patients without CRF and found erythrocyte thiamin pyrophosphate to be in the normal range (197). Lonergan et al. reported a dialyzable compound in uremic serum that inhibited ETKA and suggested that it might be guanidosuccinic acid (198). This inhibitory effect of uremic sera was alleviated by dialysis. However, Kopple et al. (199) did not find any relationship between ETKA or the ETKA stimulation index and the level of renal function. The ETKA stimulation index was also normal in 15 predialysis patients with CRF (199). These patients were receiving about 1 mg of supplemental thiamin hydrochloride daily. Those individuals who were ingesting a low protein intake were marginally close to having thiamin deficiency but did not satisfy the criterion for this disorder as assessed by the ETKA stimulation index. None of the patients prescribed 1 g protein/kg/day had a high ETKA stimulation index (i.e., an ETKA index indicating thiamin deficiency); the thiamin content of their diets was presumably greater. Hence, patients with CRF ingesting a low-protein diet, but less likely if they ingest a usual protein diet, may have a deficient thiamin intake as determined by the RDA for healthy volunteers (2). Indeed, Porrini et al. described evidence for thiamin deficiency in 6% to 10% of patients with CRF ingesting such diets (200).

The thiamin status of patients undergoing chronic dialysis remains unclear. In 28 of 30 children treated with CAPD or MHD, the spontaneous thiamin intake was reported to be lower than the RDA (201). In the early years of dialysis therapy, Kopple et al. (199) did not find that ETKA changed acutely during a single hemodialysis treatment. However, Sterzel et al. (202) reported that transketolase activity of nervous tissue was inhibited by plasma and cerebrospinal fluid and by a low molecular weight (MW) fraction (<500 kd) contained in dialysate. Kuriyama et al. observed a low basal ETKA ($ETKA_o$) or stimulated ETKA ($ETKA_s$) in a group of 72 MHD, CPD, and nondialyzed patients with CRF, although they had high blood thiamin levels associated with the ingestion of supplements (203). No correlation between ETKA and clinical manifestations of uremic neuropathy or motor-nerve conduction velocity was found. Most studies described little or no incidence of thiamin deficiency in patients undergoing MHD (68,199, 204–207). In initial studies, thiamin clearance was reported to be 13 mL/min (205) and 40 mL/min (208) with cuprophan dialyzers. The blood flow was 200 mL/min in the latter study (208). However, in some of these studies, patients were receiving supplemental thiamin hydrochloride. In 43 unsupplemented patients undergoing MHD, Descombes et al. found low or marginal $ETKA_o$ in 56%, and the ETKA stimulation index was increased in 21% of the patients (209). In $ETKA_o$-deficient patients, whole blood thiamin was normal. The deficiency was reversed with large amounts of thiamin hydrochloride (100 mg postdialysis). In the same study, patients undergoing MHD with a polyacrylonitrile membrane dialyzer had lower $ETKA_o$ than those treated with cellulose acetate. Hence, highly permeable membranes may increase the risk of thiamin deficiency in patients undergoing MHD, presumably by increasing the thiamin losses from hemodialysis. Thirty-three patients undergoing MHD treated with high-flux membranes and receiving 100 mg of thiamin hydrochloride postdialysis were found to have normal $ETKA_o$ and αETKA (210).

Blumberg et al. (69) and Boeschoten et al. (33) reported thiamin deficiency in 50% and 26% of patients undergoing CPD who were not receiving thiamin supplements. Losses of this vitamin into the peritoneal dialysate were substantially lower than the normal daily urine excretion of thiamin (33). Dietary thiamin intake was reduced below the RDA in most patients in the two studies (33,69). When patients undergoing CPD received supplemented thiamin hydrochloride, 1.5 mg/day in children and 2 or 5 mg/day in adults, no thiamin deficiency was detected (37,106,211).

Clinical Relevance

Clinical manifestations of thiamin deficiency rarely have been described in patients with CRF. Beriberi has been reported twice in patients undergoing MHD (212,213). Case reports of Wernicke's encephalopathy are increasing and have been described in 12 patients undergoing CPD or MHD (214–216) but frequently may be overlooked because the classical triad of this syndrome (confusional state, ataxia, ophthalmoplegia) is present in only 20% of the cases (215). In this latter study, typical pathologic lesions of Wernicke's encephalopathy were found in five patients who had received some other diagnosis such as uremic encephalopathy, dysequilibrium syndrome, dialysis dementia, or brainstem hemorrhage. Also, chorea has been reported in two cases of thiamin deficiency (217). The same author found thiamin deficiency in 10 patients undergoing dialysis presenting with mental disturbances. Nine out of 10 recovered with intravenous thiamin supplementation (218). Infection, surgery, and large glucose loads may increase the nutritional needs for thiamin and precipitate clinical manifestations of thiamin deficit.

Need for Supplemental Thiamin

The recommended amount of thiamin for supplementation of patients undergoing MHD and CPD range from 1 to 45 mg daily. Niwa et al. did not find low plasma blood thiamin levels in 10 patients undergoing MHD who ingested 2 to 3 mg/day of vitamin B1 in the diet (219). Descombes et al. obtained normal ETKA in 33 patients undergoing MHD treated with high-flux dialysis and who received 100 mg of thiamin hydrochloride after hemodialysis three times per week (300 mg/week) (210). However, these investigators did not examine whether lower thiamin doses also would maintain a normal ETKA stimulation index. Moreover, only two patients (5%) had a high ETKA stimulation index, and seven patients had a marginal index before thiamin treatment was commenced. Blumberg et al. (69) found low or borderline $ETKA_o$ but with normal ETKA stimulation indices in five of 10 patients undergoing CAPD. After these patients received 8 mg/day of thiamin hydrochloride, the $ETKA_o$ remained low in five patients and the ETKA stimulation index remained normal in all individuals. Because the ETKA stimulation index and serum thiamin levels are frequently normal in patients with CRF and in patients undergoing MHD or CPD and measures of thiamin deficiency, when present, are readily corrected with feeding low quantities of thiamin, we recommend that these patients should take a daily supplement providing the RDA for thiamin (i.e., 1.1 to 1.2 mg/day of the thiamin base given as thiamin hydrochloride; Table 20.4). This daily supplement is taken in addition to the thiamin intake from foods, which averages about 0.6 to 1.5 mg/day in patients with CRF or those undergoing MHD or CPD.

RIBOFLAVIN

Structure, Metabolism, and Physiologic Role

Riboflavin (vitamin B2) is an alloxazine derivative with a MW of 376.4 (Table 20.1). The vitamin undergoes modification to an orthophosphate ester in the flavin mononucleotide (FMN), which can be combined in a more complex structure with a pyrophosphate-bridged adenylate moiety, an activated adenosine monophosphate (AMP), to form FAD. Riboflavin is modestly soluble in aqueous solutions, heat stable, and photosensitive. It is present in many plant and animal products, such as milk, eggs, bread, cereals, lean meats, and broccoli (220). An active sodium and glucose-dependent absorption pathway for riboflavin is present in the proximal jejunum and is important for the transport of small quantities of this vitamin. Large amounts are absorbed by passive diffusion. Bile salts appear to facilitate uptake of riboflavin.

Rats with CRF have impaired intestinal absorption of riboflavin as determined by *in vitro* experiments (221). However, the same investigators were unable to confirm these results in *in vivo* studies (221). After cellular uptake, riboflavin is transformed by the action of flavokinase and FAD synthetase to FMN and FAD to form functional flavoproteins. Riboflavin metabolites are excreted in urine. Flavoenzymes are involved in numerous oxidation-reduction reactions that are necessary for many metabolic pathways including energy production. The erythrocyte glutathione reductase (EGR) activity without (EGR_o) and with the saturation of this enzyme with FAD has been used to assess riboflavin status (190). The ratio of EGR with FAD $\times$ 100 divided by EGR_o indicates the EGR stimulation index (α-EGR). The α-EGR is a reproducible and sensitive test; a high α-EGR indicates riboflavin deficiency. Riboflavin may be measured directly by a fluorometric method and by HPLC, which has been used in studies of patients with CRF (222).

Riboflavin and Human Kidney Disease

In nephrotic patients without renal insufficiency, the α-EGR was found to be normal by Mydlik et al. (197). In predialysis patients with CRF, using a fluorometric measurement of riboflavin, Marumo et al. did not identify low plasma levels of riboflavin, although the patients were ingesting a low-protein diet (208). In contrast, Porrini et al. (200) found a high α-EGR in 8% to 25% of patients with CRF. Patients were prescribed a 1.0-g protein/kg/day diet, and over the next 24 months, the number who demonstrated evidence for riboflavin deficiency (i.e., abnormally high α-EGR) increased from 8% to 22%. For patients prescribed an 0.6-g protein/kg/day diet, the percentage of patients with evidence for riboflavin deficiency increased from 25% to 41%. These authors, as well as others (88,100,223), found that low-protein diets may have a nutritionally inadequate riboflavin content (Table 20.2).

Most adult patients undergoing MHD or CPD appear to have a sufficient dietary intake of riboflavin (33,68,69). Dietary riboflavin intake in pediatric patients undergoing CPD may be inadequate, although blood riboflavin levels were not diminished (211). Recently, Pereira et al. (201) found that the spontaneous riboflavin intake in 22 of 30 children treated with CAPD or MHD was lower than the RDA. Most studies have shown normal or excess riboflavin in plasma of patients undergoing MHD and CPD (33,69, 209,211,224); in only two of these studies (33,211) were patients receiving riboflavin supplements. However,

Mackenzie et al. reported a low plasma riboflavin level in six patients undergoing MHD when compared to normal patients and pointed out that there may be a high dialysance of riboflavin (52 mL/min with Kiil dialyzers) (205). These data were published in 1968, at a time when malnutrition may have been more prevalent. Marumo et al. reported a lower hemodialysis clearance of riboflavin (27 mL/min), but no information on the dialysis technique was given (208). Boeschoten et al. reported high losses of riboflavin into peritoneal dialysate (33). In summary, riboflavin deficiency does not appear to be common in patients undergoing MD, despite the losses from dialysis. No clinical syndromes associated with riboflavin excess or deficiency have been reported in patients with CRF.

Needs for Supplemental Riboflavin

Recommendations concerning riboflavin supplementation vary from no supplement (33,69,208,209) to an amount equivalent to the RDA (68,70). Mydlik et al. found a normal α-EGR in patients undergoing CAPD receiving 2 mg/day of supplemental riboflavin and stated that the supplement could be decreased to 1 mg/day (37). Because riboflavin supplements are safe and because riboflavin deficiency may occur in patients with renal failure who are eating poorly, a daily supplement equal to the RDA (respectively, 1.3 and 1.1 mg/day for men and women [2]) is recommended (Table 20.4).

VITAMIN B6

Structure and Metabolism

Normal vitamin B6 metabolism has been reviewed by Leklem (225). Vitamin B6 is composed of three derivatives of the pyridine ring: pyridoxine, pyridoxal, and pyridoxamine. Some characteristics of vitamin B6 are listed in Table 20.1. Phosphorylation in the 5 position is necessary for the biologic activity of vitamin B6. Pyridoxal-5′-phosphate (PLP) and pyridoxamine-5′-phosphate are the active coenzyme forms. Pyridoxine mainly is found in plant foods (especially wheat bran, avocado, banana, lentils, walnuts, cooked soybean, and potatoes), and pyridoxal and pyridoxamine primarily are obtained from animal products (e.g., canned tuna, raw chicken breast, ground beef). These compounds are absorbed by a nonsaturable, passive process in the jejunum. These three vitamers are phosphorylated in the liver by pyridoxine kinase, which requires zinc and adenosine triphosphate. PLP is derived from the other vitamers by the action of a FMN oxidase and is transported bound to albumin in plasma and bound to hemoglobin in red cells. The major pool of PLP is in the skeletal muscle, where it is bound to glycogen phosphorylase. In liver, PLP and the other phosphorylated forms of vitamin B6 are dephosphorylated by alkaline phosphatase, leading first to pyridoxal and then 4-pyridoxic acid (4-PA) by the irreversible action of a FAD-dependent aldehyde oxidase.

Functional tests have been used to assess vitamin B6 deficiency. Erythrocyte glutamate oxaloacetate transaminase (EGOT) or erythrocyte glutamic pyruvate transaminase (EGPT) activity is measured in the basal state ($EGOT_o$, $EGPT_o$) and after stimulation by adding an excess of PLP. The ratio of the stimulated to basal activity is the activation coefficient or index (α-EGOT and α-EGPT). If stores of the coenzyme (PLP) are adequate, the addition of an excess of the coenzyme will cause little or no increase in the apoenzyme activity, and the ratio will be close to 1.0. If there is deficiency of PLP, the apoenzyme will be more greatly stimulated by the addition of the coenzyme and the index value will be higher (225).

The nutritional status of vitamin B6 also may be assessed by direct measurement of total pyridoxine by microbiologic tests or by measurement of the urinary metabolites of tryptophan or methionine, particularly after a load of the respective amino acid is given (225–227). More recently, plasma levels of PLP and other B6 compounds are measured using HPLC (225). Several parameters influence the plasma PLP level. People older than age 65 years have lower plasma levels of PLP than younger individuals (225). Females have lower levels than males. One explanation for these findings could be the differences in muscle mass. Plasma PLP levels are inversely correlated with dietary protein intake. Tobacco smoking decreases plasma B6 levels. A large epidemiologic study in normal individuals confirmed higher plasma vitamin B6 levels in young people as compared to the elderly; it also confirmed the association of increased serum acute-phase proteins, alkaline phosphatase activity, and impaired renal function with lower plasma B6 levels (228). Also, many medicines interfere with the actions or metabolism of vitamin B6 (see Chapter 33). Many of these medicines are taken by patients with CRF (Table 20.5). For example,

TABLE 20.5. MEDICINES AND OTHER SUBSTANCES INTERFERING WITH VITAMIN B6 AND FOLIC ACID METABOLISM THAT MAY CONTRIBUTE TO VITAMIN DEFICIENCY

Vitamin B6	Folic Acid
Isoniazide	Salicylazosulfapyridine
Hydralazine	Ethanol
Iproniazide	Diphenylhydantoin
Penicillamine	Methotrexate
Oral contraceptives	Pyrimethamine
Cycloserine	Pentamidine
Thyroxine	Trimethoprim
Theophylline	Triamterene
Caffeine	Cycloserine
Ethanol	Mysoline
	Primidone
	Barbiturates
	Yeasts, beans

theophylline decreases PLP by inhibition of pyridoxal kinase (229). The intake of these medicines must be considered when evaluating studies indicating the dietary requirements for vitamin B6 or when prescribing vitamin B6 intake.

Physiologic Role

PLP forms a Schiff base with the ϵ-amino group of lysine in the enzyme. The Schiff base alters the charge of the rest of the PLP molecule and strongly increases its reactivity, particularly to other amino acids. PLP is known to be a coenzyme for almost 100 enzymatic reactions, and particularly for those enzymes involved with the metabolism of amino acids and some lipids. Vitamin B6 is essential for gluconeogenesis, by facilitating transamination and glycogen phosphorylation; for niacin formation, via the PLP-dependent kynureninase, which transforms tryptophan to niacin; and for normal erythrocyte metabolism, by acting as coenzyme for transaminase and influencing the O_2 affinity of hemoglobin. Vitamin B6 facilitates the synthesis of several neurotransmitters and modulates the action of certain hormones through the binding of PLP to steroid receptors (225).

Vitamin B6 in Kidney Diseases

Experimental Data

Chronic renal failure and vitamin B6 deficiency share such common features as peripheral neuropathy, normochromic anemia, depression of the immune response, increased risk of infection, central nervous system disturbances, improvement with low-protein diet, and increased body oxalate levels (227,230,231). Thus, it would not be surprising if vitamin B6 deficiency contributes to some of the manifestations of advanced CRF. Wolfson et al. studied the combined effect of CRF and vitamin B6 deficiency in rats (232). Chronically azotemic and sham-operated rats were pair-fed diets containing either no vitamin B6 or a surfeit of vitamin B6. Weight gain was blunted after 4 weeks in all azotemic rats but significantly more so in the B6-deficient azotemic group. Also, both rats with CRF and sham-operated rats with B6 deficiency displayed low levels of plasma serine, alanine, and asparagine and a higher plasma glycine/serine ratio. Plasma serine was lowest in the azotemic B6-depleted rats. Because PLP is a cofactor for enzymes involved in the metabolism of these amino acids, it is possible that vitamin B6 deficiency could contribute to some of the amino acid disturbances described in uremia. Moreover, after the subtotal extirpation of renal tissue to cause CRF, the B6-deficient rats did not show the same subsequent compensatory increase in GFR as the B6-replete rats, arguing for a defect in the adaptive renal hypertrophy. Barbari et al. described reduced jejunal sac absorption of pyridoxine *in vivo* in azotemic rats, but *in vitro* studies using everted jejunal sacs indicated increased intestinal transport in the rats with CRF (233).

Vitamin B6 Status and Human Kidney Disease

Few studies have addressed vitamin B6 status in the nephrotic syndrome. Labadarios et al. (234) found low levels of plasma PLP in both nephrotic and nonnephrotic patients with glomerulonephritis. There was no correlation between plasma PLP and plasma albumin concentrations. Mydlik et al. (197) reported significantly decreased plasma PLP in 33 adults with the nephrotic syndrome. In children with the nephrotic syndrome receiving supplemental pyridoxine, plasma PLP was correlated with plasma albumin (235); this may reflect the binding of PLP to albumin in these patients. Most surveys detected a high incidence of vitamin B6 deficiency in both adult and pediatric patients with CRF or those undergoing MHD or CPD (33,69,100,209,227, 229–231,236–239). The frequency of B6 deficiency may increase with duration of MHD treatment (209,230) but not with duration of CPD treatment (226). However, in 10 long-term MHD survivors treated for an average of 304 months without vitamin supplementation, three patients had plasma PLP below the normal range, whereas in 10 age-, gender-, and height-matched patients treated for an average of 51 months with MHD and without B6 supplements, four patients had deficient plasma PLP levels (34). However, several studies in patients undergoing MHD, including one in patients treated with high-flux MHD without B6 supplements (240), reported normal plasma and/or red-cell vitamin PLP levels (208,240–242).

Methodologic differences in the measurement of vitamin B6 could explain this discrepancy. Some studies that reported an increased incidence of vitamin B6 deficiency used red-cell transaminase activity ($EGOT_o$ or $EGPT_o$) as the criterion for deficiency (33,208,209,227,231,236,237,240, 241). Assessment of B6 status by erythrocyte transaminase activity has been criticized because of the shortened life span of red cells in CRF and the higher activities of some enzymes in younger erythrocytes (243). However, each study that assessed plasma PLP concentrations also found decreased levels in dialyzed and nondialyzed patients with CRF (226, 227,230,236,244), and plasma vitamin B6 measured by microbiologic assay was found to be normal in individuals with low plasma PLP levels (226,227). In a cohort of 119 kidney transplant patients, plasma PLP deficiency was found in 65% of the cases (238). However, these results were obtained before the cyclosporine era and need to be reexamined with the newer medicinal regimens given to transplant recipients.

Causes for Vitamin B6 Deficiency in Chronic Renal Failure

The causes of vitamin B6 deficiency in CRF are probably multifactorial. Vitamin B6 intake is often low, according to the dietary surveys of patients undergoing MD (68,69, 226). In patients undergoing MHD and CPD and individuals with advanced CRF, Kopple found, respectively, a mean vitamin B6 intake of 1.4, 1.6, and 1.2 mg per day (237), whereas the RDA for normal healthy, nonpregnant, nonlactating adults is 1.3 to 1.7 mg/day (2). Low vitamin B6 intakes were reported in 120 children with CRF (245). Stockberger et al. (246) found daily vitamin B6 intake to be lower than 59% of the RDA in 67% of children undergoing CAPD. Low-protein diets are generally low in B6 content (Table 20.2).

Many years ago, Spannuth et al. (244) reported increased metabolic clearance of PLP in patients with CRF. They measured the plasma clearance of intravenously injected PLP in patients with CRF, most of whom were undergoing MHD, and normal controls. Their observations are somewhat difficult to interpret because the vitamin B6 status or intake of the two groups of subjects were not well defined. It is possible that the patients with CRF were vitamin B6 deficient, a not uncommon finding, and that this deficiency might have increased the rate of removal of PLP from plasma. Also, two factors, often present in CRF, might enhance PLP clearance: a high level of alkaline phosphatase, engendered by the high incidence of secondary hyperparathyroidism (226), and increased quantities of bacteria in the small intestine, which may more readily take up and possibly metabolize PLP. Circulating inhibitors of vitamin B6 in CRF also could lead to measurement of vitamin B6 deficiency, particularly when biologic activity of vitamin B6 is measured (e.g., enzyme activities or stimulation indices). Consistent with this possibility are the initial studies by Dobbelstein et al. (231) that hemodialysis improved EGOT activity. However, these investigators did not find that incubation of normal red cells with uremic plasma altered EGOT activity.

Removal of vitamin B6 by dialysis may contribute to vitamin B6 deficiency. Lacour et al. (238) did not find PLP in the hemodialysis ultrafiltrate. This is not surprising because PLP is bound to albumin. Also, Teehan et al. (230) did not find arteriovenous differences for PLP during the hemodialysis procedure nor significant differences between plasma PLP levels obtained predialysis and postdialysis. However, more recent studies argue for a significant decrease in PLP during MHD treatment. Kasama et al. (247), in six patients undergoing MHD, surprisingly observed a high blood PLP clearance of 86 mL/min with cuprophan dialyzers. After changing from cuprophan to higher flux cellulose triacetate hemodialyzers, a significant reduction of serum PLP in patients undergoing MHD occurred with the PLP clearance increasing from 86 to 173 mL/min. Leblanc et al. (248) reported a lower blood PLP clearance of 54.4 mL/min in 36 patients undergoing MHD using comparable high-flux membranes and dialysis treatment characteristics. The explanation for these discrepant results is unclear.

Boeschoten et al. reported that the quantity of PLP lost into peritoneal dialysate, assessed by HPLC, is similar to the normal urinary vitamin B6 excretion (33). In another study, much lower losses of PLP, as assessed by the L-tyrosine decarboxylase apoenzyme assay, were reported (226). In children, PLP losses during peritoneal dialysis appeared negligible (246), but the authors of this study emphasized that additional PLP bound to proteins may be lost into dialysate. The amount of glucose in peritoneal dialysis solution was not found to affect the peritoneal clearance of PLP (249).

Mydlik et al. (61) studied a subgroup of 30 patients undergoing MHD who received EPO treatment for 1 year and found decreased erythrocyte vitamin B6 content. A low dose of furosemide increased the urinary excretion of vitamin B6 both in healthy subjects and in patients with advanced CRF (250). In patients with acute renal failure treated with continuous venovenous hemofiltration or hemodiafiltration, plasma PLP decreased and the calculated PLP loss was 80 nmol/day (251); the PLP clearance was about 49% of the urea clearance.

Vitamin B6 Deficiency in Renal Disease: Clinical Relevance

Immune Function

Vitamin B6 deficiency in experimental animals and humans is associated with many alterations in immune function. These include reduced numbers of blood granulocytes and lymphocytes, decreased lymphocyte maturation, reduced blastogenic response of lymphocytes to mitogenic stimuli, delayed cutaneous hypersensitivity, and decreased antibody production. These findings suggest that some of the alterations in immune function in advanced CRF might be caused by vitamin B6 deficiency. Many years ago, Dobbelstein et al. (231) were able to reverse decreased reactivity in mixed lymphocyte culture by giving patients undergoing MHD 300 mg/day of pyridoxine HCl for 2 weeks. Casciato et al. (236) improved immunologic function of polymorphonuclear neutrophils and lymphocytes in eight patients undergoing MHD, most of whom had vitamin B6 deficiency, by giving 50 mg/day of pyridoxine hydrochloride for 3 to 5 weeks. Moreover, there was an increase in lymphocyte transformation in response to mitogens in three of these patients who received supplemental pyridoxine and who had low transformation activity prior to treatment (236). Kleiner et al. (252) did not find differences of lymphocyte reactivity to concanavalin A between patients undergoing MHD and control subjects, and they found no effect on this parameter of 2 weeks of pyridoxine HCl supplementation, 300 mg/day. However, the patients probably were not vitamin B6 deficient because their EGOT indices were not different from controls. Nonetheless, these investigators reported that some plasma amino acid concentrations that were low in patients undergoing MHD increased after they were given the 300 mg/day of pyridoxine HCl (252). Mydlik et al. (253) were able to improve the reduced T-lymphocyte count in 30 stable patients undergoing MHD who received 50 mg/day of pyridoxine HCl for 3 months.

Oxalate Metabolism

Plasma oxalate concentrations virtually always are increased in nondialyzed and dialyzed patients with advanced CRF (254–262). Plasma oxalate may be increased several times above normal values, close to the level found in primary hyperoxaluria (254). Calcium oxalate deposits are described in several tissues in CRF and appear to be most pronounced in kidneys, heart, blood vessels, thyroid, and skin. There seems to be a higher incidence of soft-tissue oxalate deposits in both patients undergoing CPD and longstanding nondialyzed patients with CRF as compared to patients undergoing MHD (261,263–266). Moreover, oxalate retention seems to increase with the duration of MHD therapy (260,266). Mydlik et al. (250) showed that in healthy subjects and nondialyzed patients with CRF the excretion of vitamins B6 and C and oxalate increases with water diuresis or furosemide administration.

There are probably several causes for the increased plasma and tissue oxalate concentrations in renal failure. Decreased clearance of oxalate because of impaired renal function, increased ascorbic acid intake (see vitamin C section), and vitamin B6 deficiency are three such causes. Increased oxalate synthesis also has been described in CRF (267). However, gastrointestinal absorption of ^{14}C-oxalate appears to be normal in azotemic rats (268). Vitamin B6 is the coenzyme for the transamination of glyoxylate to glycine (Fig. 20.1). Because vitamin B6 deficiency is not uncommon in CRF, this might contribute to increased plasma oxalate levels. However, Costello et al. (268) found an increased plasma clearance rate of oxalate from patients undergoing MHD in comparison to normal individuals, suggesting increased biosynthesis of oxalate in these patients. Plasma oxalate clearance was similar in patients undergoing CPD and normal individuals. These investigators found no association between the vitamin B6 status and the oxalate removal rate in patients undergoing either MHD or CPD (268), suggesting that B6 deficiency is not the primary cause of increased endogenous oxalate production or plasma oxalate levels in these individuals.

It is possible that large doses of pyridoxine HCl may suppress oxalate synthesis and plasma or tissue levels even if vitamin B6 deficiency, measured by standard techniques, is not associated with the reduced removal rate or increased body burden of oxalate (268). Several attempts have been made to decrease plasma oxalate levels with pharmacologic doses of pyridoxine HCl. Conflicting results were obtained. Tomson et al. (269) did not obtain a significant decrease in oxalemia in 21 patients undergoing MD treated for 4 months with pyridoxine HCl, 100 mg/day. In contrast, a 46% decrease in plasma oxalate was observed by Balcke et al. (270) after 1 month of treatment with pyridoxine HCl, 600 mg/day orally or 600 mg three times per week given intravenously after hemodialysis. However, the plasma oxalate level remained elevated and in the supersaturation range (256). Also, Morgan et al. (254) reported a 35% decrease in plasma oxalate after 1 month of supplementation with a large dose of pyridoxine HCl, 800 mg/day. But in a controlled study, Costello was unable to reduce plasma oxalate levels after 6 months of treatment with 100 mg/day of pyridoxine HCl or after 4 weeks of therapy with 750 mg/day of pyridoxine HCl (267). The reason for these discrepant results is not clear. Descombes et al. (210) reported a high plasma oxalic acid level in 33 patients receiving high-flux dialysis and 50 mg of pyridoxine after each dialysis treatment, indicating that current dialysis techniques and vitamin B6 supplementation are not sufficient to normalize oxalic acid levels. Patients with type I or type II primary hyperoxaluria (Fig. 20.1) have been treated with different doses of pyridoxine (25 to 1,000 mg/day), also with variable results (271–273).

Mydlik et al. (249) reported increased plasma oxalic acid in 32 patients undergoing CAPD (23.6 ± 7.4 mmol/L;

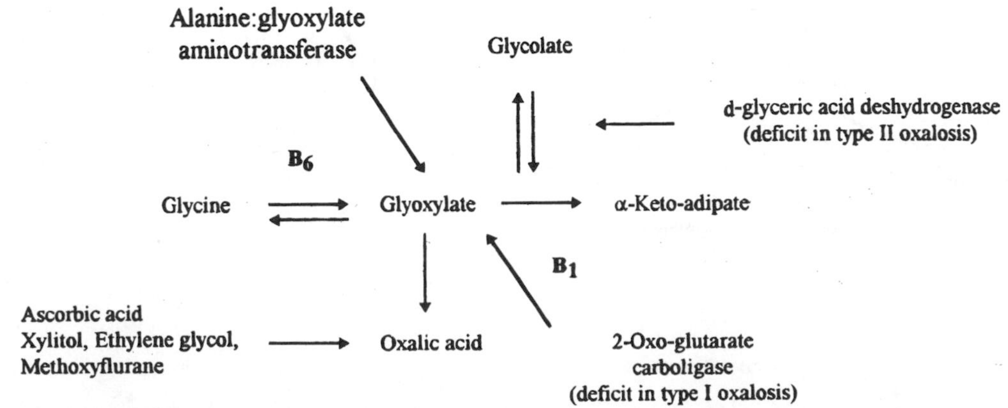

FIGURE 20.1. Oxalic acid production pathways and sites of intervention of vitamins.

normal range: 2 to 5.5 mmol/L) despite a large peritoneal clearance. Also, in 15 patients undergoing MHD, plasma oxalate was increased (40.3 ± 9.8 mmol/L) and oxalate clearance was greater with postdilutional hemofiltration (74.2% of urea clearance) than with conventional hemodialysis (58.1%) or postdilutional hemodiafiltration (69%) (274). There was a large discrepancy between oxalate clearances in children undergoing CAPD (7.14 mL/min, n = 15) as compared to MHD (115.6 mL/min, n = 10) (275). Nonetheless, the weekly elimination of oxalate was similar, and blood oxalic acid levels remained high and not different between the two groups.

Homocysteine

Homocysteine (Hcy) is discussed in the folic acid section later in this chapter and in Chapters 7 and 12. The formation of cysteine from methionine requires vitamin B6 (Fig. 20.2). PLP is a coenzyme for cystathionine synthase, which transforms methionine to cystathionine, and for cystathionase, which cleaves cystathionine to form cysteine. Hcy is an intermediate in the formation of cystathionine from methionine. As suggested in Fig. 20.2, PLP deficiency could participate in the pathogenesis of increased plasma Hcy in patients with CRF and those undergoing MD. However, Shemin et al. (276) did not find evidence for vitamin B6 deficiency in 24 patients undergoing MD with high plasma levels of Hcy. Also, Chauveau et al. (277) did not find any effect of treatment on plasma Hcy levels in nondialyzed patients with CRF given pyridoxine HCl, 70 mg/day for 3 months. Moreover, Arnadottir et al. reported a slight increase in plasma Hcy after 4 months of treatment with pyridoxine HCl, 300 mg/day (278). A placebo-controlled 8-week trial was conducted in 27 patients undergoing MHD, where the patients received 15 mg of folic acid, 100 mg of pyridoxine HCl, and 1 mg of vitamin B12 daily (279). Plasma Hcy was reduced significantly (by 29.8%) after 4 weeks and by 25.8% after 8 weeks. Most of the other studies giving large doses of vitamin B6 also included folic acid supplementation (280–283), making it difficult to interpret the influence of vitamin B6 on the plasma Hcy levels of renal patients. (See folic acid section and Chapter 7.)

Miscellaneous

It has been suggested that the low serum alanine and aspartate aminotransferase (transaminase) activities in patients undergoing MHD may be the result of vitamin B6 deficiency because plasma PLP levels correlate with these plasma transaminase activities (284) and oral pyridoxine HCl, 30 mg/day, may increase plasma aminotransferase in patients with low plasma enzyme values (285). However, not all studies confirm a correlation between serum aminotransferase activities and serum PLP levels (284). It also has been suggested that low serum transaminase activities in CRF are artifactual and the result of the failure to add PLP to the laboratory assay (286). This explanation does not explain why normal controls have higher measured transaminase activities using the same laboratory techniques and why these low levels can be obtained in patients with CRF when serum vitamin B6 and PLP measurements are normal. The effects of vitamin B6 on serum lipids are conflicting. Kleiner

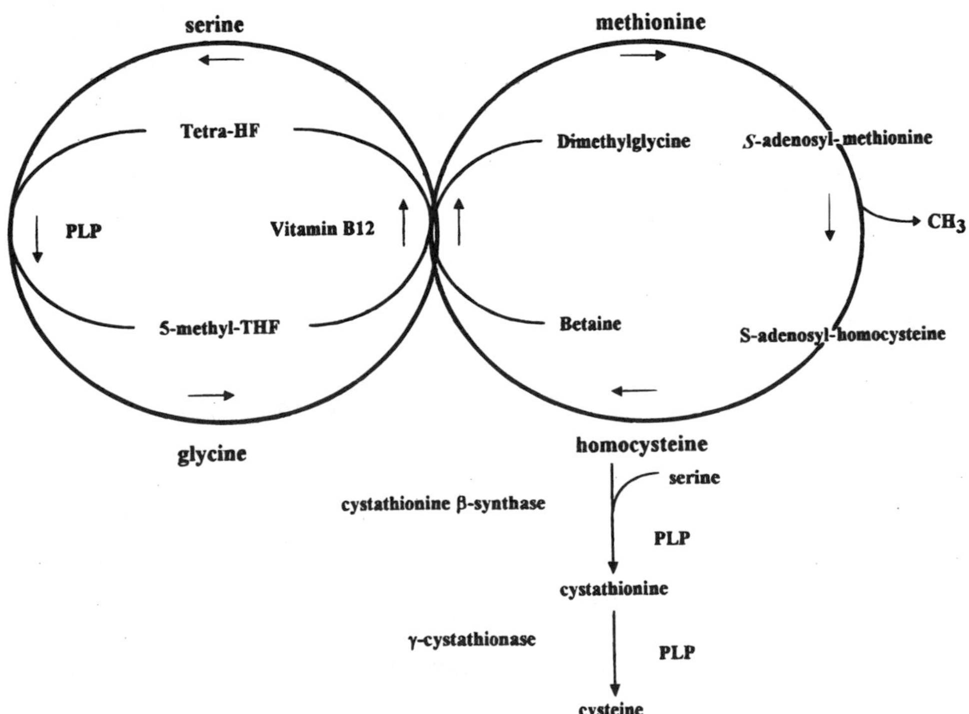

FIGURE 20.2. Role of vitamins in homocysteine metabolism.

et al. (252) reported that in 15 patients undergoing MHD serum high-density lipoproteins increased significantly after they were given pyridoxine HCl, 300 mg/day for 14 days; no effect was found on serum triglycerides or total cholesterol. These patients had a normal EGOT index with low levels of basal EGOT ($EGOT_o$). Arnadottir et al. gave the same dose of pyridoxine HCl for 4 months to patients undergoing MHD and CPD and observed a slight but statistically significant reduction in serum total cholesterol (by 7%) and LDL concentrations (by 5.6%) (278).

Nankivell described a sideroblastic anemia in a patient undergoing MHD who was vitamin B6 depleted that responded to pyridoxine HCl, 25 mg daily (287). Toriyama et al. (288) gave 180 mg/day of pyridoxine HCl for 20 weeks to nine patients undergoing MHD with microcytic hypochromic anemia who had serum iron-binding saturation and ferritin levels that were not low. The hematocrit in these patients increased significantly from 26.2 ± 3.8% (standard error of the mean) to 28.3 ± 3.2% ($p < 0.05$). No patient was receiving EPO during the study, and serum vitamin B6 levels were normal (288). However, a prospective, controlled study found that both 50 and 100 mg/day of pyridoxine HCl failed to raise the hematocrit above 33% in EPO-resistant patients (241). In a randomized, blinded, prospective clinical trial in 26 patients undergoing MHD with symptoms of peripheral neuropathy, there was improvement of symptoms in 14 patients who received pyridoxine HCl, 60 mg/day, for 4 weeks but not in 12 patients who received vitamin B12, 500 μg/day orally, although the initial serum PLP was only slightly, and not significantly, lower than in controls (240).

Need for Supplemental Vitamin B6

Most workers in the field agree that there is a need for routine pyridoxine supplementation in patients undergoing MHD (68,209,230,231,236–238) or CPD (33,37,69,106, 226,246) and probably patients with the nephrotic syndrome (197,234,235). Recommended supplemental pyridoxine HCl doses vary from 2 mg/day to 50 mg/day. There are few data concerning the dose for supplemental vitamin B6 needed in nondialyzed patients with CRF. Kopple et al. (237) described normalization of the EGPT index in all nondialyzed patients with CRF given a supplement of 5 mg/day of pyridoxine HCl (4.1 mg/day of the pyridoxine base); in patients with CRF given a lower amount of pyridoxine HCl, the EGPT index became normal more slowly or did not normalize at all. In patients undergoing MHD, various doses of pyridoxine HCl have normalized one or more parameters of vitamin B6 status. However, the lowest pyridoxine HCl supplement that consistently has normalized a parameter of vitamin B6 deficiency (i.e., the EGPT index) in patients undergoing MHD is 10 mg per day (1, 237). In patients undergoing CAPD, the lowest pyridoxine HCl dose that normalized vitamin B6 nutriture (i.e., serum PLP levels) was also 10 mg per day (226). However, these latter investigators did not examine whether a lower dose also would normalize vitamin B6 nutriture. Until further data indicate otherwise, 10 mg/day of pyridoxine HCl are recommended for adult patients undergoing MHD and CPD because this is the lowest dose that has been shown to normalize a parameter of B6 nutriture. In eight children undergoing CPD, 10 mg daily of free pyridoxine increased serum PLP to twice the normal control levels (211); lower doses of pyridoxine HCl probably would be adequate for this pediatric population. In patients undergoing MHD, Mydlik et al. (61) recommend 20 mg/day of pyridoxine HCl to correct or prevent a decrease in RBC vitamin B6 levels that may occur after several months of EPO treatment. In renal transplant recipients, no supplementation trials have been reported.

Pyridoxine has been given as pyridoxylate, which is a vasodilator that has been used to treat coronary artery and peripheral circulatory insufficiency. This medicine can cause oxalate nephropathy and end-stage renal disease (ESRD) (289,290). Also, very high doses of pyridoxine HCl (i.e., 200 to 600 mg/day) occasionally have been associated with peripheral neuropathy in patients without renal disease (291,292). The mechanism of this possible effect is not known but could be the result of inhibition by a metabolite of B6. Because patients with CRF may have impaired ability to excrete metabolites of vitamin B6, it is possible that these metabolites may accumulate and interfere with the normal, active metabolites of B6. Indeed, 4-pyridoxic acid, the main metabolite of vitamin B6, is excreted primarily in the urine and might be expected to accumulate in patients with renal failure, particularly in those taking vitamin B6 supplements. Therefore, until more information is available, caution should be exercised when prescribing very large doses of pyridoxine HCl to nondialyzed patients with CRF and to patients undergoing MD (e.g., 100 mg/day or greater) for extended periods.

VITAMIN C

Structure and Metabolism

Vitamin C (ascorbic acid, Table 20.1), which prevents scurvy, is oxidized to dehydroascorbic acid (DHAA), which also possesses antiscorbutic activity. Ascorbic acid mainly is found in fresh fruits (e.g., black currant, strawberry, lemon, orange, lime) and vegetables (e.g., broccoli, Brussels sprouts, cauliflower, cabbage). Ascorbic acid in food can be degraded by heat or extracted in cooking water. Intestinal absorption of ascorbic acid is an active, energy-requiring, and saturable process. About 70% to 90% of the usual dietary vitamin C intake is absorbed, but this fraction decreases substantially when large loads of ascorbic acid are ingested. In plasma, vitamin C is nonprotein bound and is present in a reduced form (293). Ascorbic acid enters the cell by active transport. The average half-life of ascorbic acid in normal adult humans is about 16 to 20 days. The body ascorbic acid pools are regulated by intestinal absorption, renal tubule reabsorption, and the catabolism of ascorbic acid (294). Excess ascorbic acid is filtered at the glomerulus and excreted intact in the urine. The catabolic rate for ascorbic acid is directly related to the body pool size. Ascorbic acid can be oxidized to DHAA and then to a variety of compounds, including L-xylose, threonic acid, and oxalic acid, that are excreted in urine. Oxalic acid represents 5% to 10% of the metabolites of ascorbic acid.

The methods for assessment of ascorbic acid have evolved in the last years. Colorimetric methods, based on the reductive properties of ascorbic acid, have been supplanted by HPLC technology, which is sensitive and specific (295). Ascorbic acid is measured in plasma, which reflects recent dietary intake, and in leucocytes, which gives a more accurate estimate of the body pool of ascorbic acid. Women usually have higher plasma ascorbic acid levels than men; smokers and elderly individuals have lower values of plasma ascorbic acid. Also, the oxidized form of ascorbic acid, the ascorbyl free radical (AFR), can be detected by electron paramagnetic resonance spectroscopy. The AFR/ascorbic acid ratio is used as an index of oxidant stress (89).

Physiologic Role

The function of ascorbic acid is largely the result of its reversible reducing power. For instance, ascorbic acid plays an important role in metal catalyzed hydroxylations by reducing the metal catalyst and by allowing the metal-enzyme complex to reconstitute after it is oxidized. Perhaps the most well-recognized activities of ascorbic acid are collagen synthesis via lysyl and prolyl hydroxylations, hydroxylations of peptidyl proline, enhanced secretion of procollagen that contains hydroxyproline, carnitine synthesis, hydroxylation of dopamine to form norepinephrine and of tryptophan to form serotonin, amidation of peptide hormones, intestinal iron absorption, and antioxidant protection of folates and vitamin E. Potential immune activities, actions on cholesterol metabolism, and anticancer effects of ascorbic acid are still the subjects of investigation.

Vitamin C and Renal Disease

Vitamin C Status in Renal Disease

Rajbala et al. (86) found decreased serum vitamin C in 45 children presenting with the nephrotic syndrome. This was confirmed by Fydryk et al. (84), who found decreased blood vitamin C during relapse of steroid-dependent nephrotic syndrome in 18 children. Recently, 29 patients with the nephrotic syndrome were studied with regard to their vitamin C and E status and compared with 25 patients with hematuria (85). Plasma vitamin C and the ascorbate/vitamin E ratio were significantly lower in the patients with the nephrotic syndrome. However, these did not show an increase in susceptibility to LDL oxidation. Few studies of vitamin C status are available for predialysis patients with CRF. Low-protein diets do not necessarily provide a low vitamin C intake (Table 20.2). It was surprising that Marumo et al. found low plasma ascorbic acid levels in patients with mild to moderate CRF but not in nondialyzed individuals with advanced CRF or in patients undergoing MHD (208). Bohm et al. (296) reported an adequate vitamin C intake and normal plasma ascorbic acid concentrations in patients with CRF. In contrast, Clermont et al. (89) found decreased vitamin C levels, with an increased ascorbyl free radical/ascorbic acid ratio in patients with CRF. Intravenous furosemide increases urinary vitamin C excretion in patients with CRF (250). Also, concomitant administration of vitamin C and furosemide in dogs increased the diuretic and natriuretic effects of the latter drug (121).

In the early days of MHD treatment, Sullivan and Eisenstein described ascorbic acid deficiency in patients undergoing MHD (297). These authors found that five of 11 patients undergoing MHD not receiving vitamin C supplements had severely reduced serum ascorbic acid levels and that the severity of the deficiency increased with the duration of MHD therapy. In these patients, plasma ascorbic acid levels decreased by 40% during a single dialysis treatment. Patients receiving 250 or 500 mg of ascorbic acid supplements for 2 months had markedly elevated serum vitamin C levels; discontinuing the vitamin C supplements led to a rapid decrease in plasma ascorbic acid concentrations in 3 months (297). Several more recent reports confirm a high incidence of vitamin C deficiency in patients undergoing MHD not given vitamin C supplements (34, 68,89,94,298–300). However, Tarng et al. (301) found normal vitamin C levels in a group of 65 nonsupplemented patients treated with MHD for a mean of 48.7 months. It was surprising that some patients undergoing MHD receiving vitamin C, 200 mg 3 times per week, have been reported to have vitamin C deficiency (209) and discontinuation of supplementation may quickly lead to abnormally low plasma ascorbic acid levels (300,302). However, Ramirez et al. (207) monitored plasma ascorbic acid levels for 1 year after discontinuing vitamin C supplements. A dramatic decrease of plasma ascorbic acid was observed, but no patient reached a deficient level (207). The daily dietary vitamin C intake of their patients was not reported. Also, the patients studied by Ramirez et al. (207) had been undergoing MHD treatment for less than 38 months and, as indicated earlier, the risk of vitamin C deficiency appears to increase with the duration of time spent on dialysis therapy. Chazot et al. (34) found significantly lower mean plasma vitamin C levels and a higher frequency of low plasma vitamin C values in 10 long-term MHD survivors treated for a mean of 304 months as compared to a group of patients undergoing MHD matched for age, gender, and height treated for an average of 51.0 months.

There are two main causes for vitamin C deficiency in patients undergoing MHD: low intake and ascorbic acid losses in dialysate. In contrast to Kopple et al. (303) and Stein et al. (100) (Table 20.2), Allman et al. (68) showed a low spontaneous intake of vitamin C in their patients undergoing MHD (69% consumed less than two-thirds of the RDA). In children undergoing MHD, the vitamin C intake was 51% of the RDA (201). A prescription of a low potassium diet is likely to reduce intake of vitamin C–containing foods. Both ascorbic acid and potassium are abundant in fresh fruits and leafy vegetables. Hence, a restriction in foods high in potassium will reduce the intake of ascorbic acid and may predispose to vitamin deficiency (297). Indeed, the average ascorbic acid intake in the patients undergoing MHD reported by Sullivan and Eisenstein (297) was 34 mg/day, whereas the adult RDA for ascorbic acid is respectively 75 mg and 90 mg/day in nonsmoking female and male adults (3). Moreover, prolonged soaking and boiling of vegetables, which may be used to reduce the potassium content of food, may leech out or degrade ascorbic acid as well. A reduced food intake, because of anorexia or illness, will decrease further the quantity of ascorbic acid ingested.

Ascorbic acid is a small (MW: 176) and nonprotein-bound molecule that is readily dialyzable. In initial studies, the quantity of ascorbic acid recovered in dialysate was found proportional to the blood flow rate (297) and the ascorbic acid lost in hemodialysate varied from 80 to 280 mg in patients not receiving vitamin C supplements (297). Bohm et al. (296) measured the amount of vitamin C in dialysate and found it to range from 92 to 334 mg per treatment, with a 50% decrease in plasma ascorbic acid during a HD treatment and a return to predialysis levels by 44 hours (296). Hultqvist et al. (94) found a 40% decrease in plasma ascorbic acid during a 3-hour HD treatment. During a single HD treatment, vitamin C clearance was 212 mL/min and blood vitamin C fell by 33% (300). In 15 patients undergoing MHD with a Kt/V of 1.6, vitamin C clearance was 134 mL/min with a pre-post dialysis vitamin C reduction of 45.5% (274). Descombes et al. (209) found lower plasma ascorbic acid levels in patients hemodialyzed with high-flux polyacrylonitrile membranes as compared to patients hemodialyzed with cellulose acetate membranes. More recently, the same authors reported normal plasma ascorbic acid in 33 patients receiving high-flux MHD who were given 500 mg of vitamin C at the end of each HD treatment (210).

Vitamin C deficiency also is described in patients undergoing peritoneal dialysis. Boeschoten et al. found low plasma ascorbic acid levels in at least 25% of 44 patients who were either undergoing CAPD training or were established on CPD treatment (33). The vitamin C intake of these patients was similar to the RDA; but 56 mg of ascorbic acid were recovered in the 24-hour peritoneal dialysate effluent (33). Henderson et al. studied nine patients undergoing CAPD who were taking a 100 mg/day ascorbic acid supplement. Plasma and leucocyte vitamin C levels were normal. However, when the supplement was stopped, their mean plasma ascorbic acid value fell to the lower limit of normal in 6 months (106). Blumberg found that three of 10 patients treated with CAPD for less than 1 year and who were not receiving ascorbic acid supplements had low plasma ascorbate levels (69). Two of the 10 patients had a low vitamin C intake. These authors reported that the ascorbic acid losses into peritoneal dialysate during the overnight exchange averaged 4.8 mg/L (69). Roob et al. (304) reported that in 17 patients undergoing CAPD not taking supplements, plasma ascorbic acid levels were significantly below normal. On the contrary, Mydlik et al. (249) have found normal plasma vitamin C levels in 32 patients undergoing CAPD not receiving ascorbic acid supplements. The peritoneal transfer of ascorbic acid was 136.4 mmol/6 hours with 1.5% glucose in dialysate and increased to 175.8 mmol/6 hours with 2.5% dialysate glucose (249). In 23 children receiving CAPD, the vitamin C intake was 77% of the RDA (201). Bohm et al. (296) reported that renal transplant recipients have a vitamin C intake equal to or greater than the RDA and normal plasma vitamin C levels.

Vitamin C Deficiency: Clinical Relevance

Whereas low plasma ascorbic acid levels are not reported infrequently in patients undergoing MHD and CPD who do not receive vitamin C supplements, scurvy has been described only rarely in patients with CRF. Ihle and Gillies reported a patient undergoing MHD with cutaneous symptoms (pruritus, bruising, and ecchymoses), impaired platelet function, a low vitamin C intake, and decreased plasma and leukocyte ascorbic acid levels (305). The defect in platelet function was similar to that reported with scurvy. Treatment with 1 g of vitamin C per day for a few days rapidly corrected the ecchymoses, prolonged bleeding time, and platelet dysfunction (305). Ganguly et al. studied 12 patients undergoing MHD before and after they received 300 mg/day of vitamin C (302). One month after stopping the supplements, plasma ascorbic acid was abnormally low, although monocyte ascorbic acid was not significantly below normal values. One to 2 months following the discontinuation of vitamin C, several parameters of immune function had not changed significantly. The authors concluded that vitamin C supplements are unnecessary in patients undergoing MHD ingesting an adequate diet; these conclusions should be qualified because the duration of follow-up was short and the sample size of the MHD and control groups were small (302).

Role of Ascorbic Acid in Oxalate Metabolism

As shown in Fig. 20.1, oxalate is a metabolic end product of ascorbic acid. In normal humans, urinary excretion of oxalate increases when these individuals are fed an ascorbic acid load (306). However, the relationship between ascorbic acid intake and urinary oxalate excretion is not linear, and only a fraction of the ascorbic acid ingested is normally recovered in the urine as oxalate (307). CRF appears to greatly increase the risk of secondary oxalosis, as indicated earlier (see Vitamin B6 section). There is strong evidence that excessive vitamin C intake may contribute to hyperoxalemia and to oxalate deposition in soft tissues of patients with CRF. Acute oxalate nephropathy has been reported in a patient without severely impaired renal function who received a single intravenous dose of 45 g of ascorbic acid (308). Plasma oxalate levels increase in patients undergoing MHD given oral supplements of 0.5 to 1 g/day of ascorbic acid (309–311) and in those treated with a hemodialysate supplemented with ascorbic acid (312); cessation of ascorbic acid supplements results in a decrease in plasma oxalate (311, 313). The association between the plasma ascorbic acid and oxalate levels in patients undergoing MHD is more controversial. Pru et al. (312) and Ono (309) found a significant correlation between these two compounds in plasma, but this was not confirmed by Costello et al. (258) or Rolton et al. (310). Hyperoxalemia also is associated with ascorbic acid supplementation in patients undergoing CPD (314).

Ott et al. (315) report bone oxalate deposits in a bone biopsy from a patient who had undergone MHD for 23 years and who had ingested 2.6 g/day of ascorbic acid for 7 years. A bone biopsy in the same patient obtained before commencing ascorbic acid supplements showed no evidence for bone oxalate deposits. Calcium oxalate deposits in kidneys and pancreas have been reported in a pediatric patient with the hemolytic uremic syndrome who received 500 mg/day of ascorbic acid by parenteral nutrition (316). In a patient with mild renal failure treated by total parenteral nutrition, Swartz et al. (317) estimated that 12% of the parenterally given ascorbic acid is transformed into oxalate. The mechanism of oxalate accumulation with low doses of ascorbic acid is related to the decrease or absence of renal function. In such circumstances, excess ascorbic acid and the oxalate subsequently produced cannot be eliminated in the urine, unlike in normal subjects who can tolerate much higher intakes of ascorbic acid without oxalate accumulation (262,318). A case of acute renal failure with oxalosis has been reported in a young adult taking vitamin C tablets (319).

Vitamin C, EPO Effect, and Iron Status

There has been much interest concerning the potential value of ascorbic acid as an adjuvant therapy to EPO to increase hemoglobin and reduce the cost of erythropoietin therapy, particularly in patients undergoing MHD or CPD with erythropoietin-resistant anemia (see Chapter 22). Tarng et al. (301) reported that iron therapy is ineffective for improving anemia in patients undergoing MHD who are hyporesponsive to erythropoietin and who have a hematocrit less than 30%, ferritin greater than 500 mmol/L, and transferrin saturation less than 30%. In contrast, 300 mg of vitamin C given at the end of dialysis for 8 weeks raised the hematocrit and allowed a decrease in the EPO dose and an increase in transferrin saturation (301). The same authors found that in a group of 46 EPO-hyporesponsive patients undergoing MHD treated with vitamin C, 18 patients had a dramatic improvement in anemia parameters, whereas 19 patients did not respond. The plasma vitamin C level was normal in all the patients before vitamin C treatment, and plasma oxalate levels increased slightly, but not to a statistical significant degree, during the vitamin C therapy (301). Giancaspro et al. (320) confirmed the beneficial effect of vitamin C therapy in EPO-hyporesponsive patients who had high levels of serum ferritin.

Ascorbic Acid and Intestinal Aluminum Absorption

Domingo et al. (321) showed that in both rats and healthy human volunteers, ingestion of ascorbic acid enhances the intestinal absorption of aluminum. In animals, a combination of dietary ascorbic acid and $Al(OH)_3$ increases concentrations of aluminum in brain, liver, and bone. In humans, the dose of ascorbic acid that augmented aluminum accumulation was 2 g/day. Thus, it appears important to avoid oral ascorbic acid supplements, at least in large doses, in patients ingesting aluminum-containing preparations.

Miscellaneous

Ascorbic acid currently is being studied as a therapeutic agent for a number of clinical and experimental disorders involving the kidney or hypertension. It has been postulated that some of these possible benefits of ascorbic acid may be the result of its antioxidant properties. A dramatic decrease in blood pressure has been observed in spontaneously hypertensive rats (SHRs) that were supplemented with ascorbic acid (322). Vasdev et al. (323) reported a similar decrease in blood pressure and also a reduction of hypertension-induced smooth-muscle–cell hyperplasia in vitamin C–supplemented SHRs. Americans of Chinese ancestry without known renal disease have been shown to display an inverse correlation between their blood pressure and plasma ascorbic acid levels (324). Halimi and Mimran (325) studied the systemic and renal effects of nicotine and/or vitamin C in 10 healthy nonsmokers. Nicotine decreased the GFR, renal plasma flow (RPF), and urinary cyclic guanosine 3′:5′5-cyclic monophosphate (cGMP). Ascorbic acid alone had no effect on any of these parameters and did not prevent the nicotine suppressive effect on GFR and RPF, whereas it did maintain the urinary excretion of cGMP. It is hypothesized that vitamin C prevented the reactive oxygen species-induced degradation of nitric oxide triggered by nicotine.

Ascorbic acid (1 g) has been used in association with other antioxidant agents to reduce reperfusion injury in transplanted organs successfully (152). However, the specific contribution of ascorbic acid to this effect is not known. Vitamin C has been shown to correct the increased susceptibility to LDL oxidation in tacrolimus-treated renal transplant recipients (153). Ascorbic acid also has ameliorated renal injury in several experimental animal models of cadmium, cisplatinum, chromium (124), and cyclosporine (156) nephrotoxicity and extracorporeal shock-wave lithotripsy-induced renal injury (116).

Need for Supplemental Vitamin C

Taken together, the forgoing studies suggest that a substantial subset of patients undergoing MHD and CPD may be at risk for vitamin C deficiency if they do not receive supplements, and several authors have recommended various amounts of daily ascorbic acid supplements. The combination of insufficient dietary intake of vitamin C and dialysate losses appears to be primarily responsible for the risk of deficiency. However, there is no clear evidence that the dietary vitamin requirement is increased in patients undergoing MD, at least with regard to the amount necessary to maintain normal plasma ascorbic acid levels. Indeed, the lack of urinary vitamin C excretion will at least to some extent offset the dialysate losses. However, larger doses of vitamin C have been associated with increased oxalate concentrations in plasma and probably soft tissues. Thus, at the present time, it is recommended that nondialyzed patients with CRF and those undergoing MHD and CPD should be prescribed the RDA for ascorbic acid recommended for normal, nonpregnant, nonlactating adults: 75 to 90 mg/day (Table 20.4) (3). It is possible that the ascorbic acid clearance with high efficiency and/or high-flux hemodialyzers may increase the dietary requirement for vitamin C. However, considering the small size of ascorbic acid, it is not likely that highly permeable dialyzers will markedly increase the dialysis losses of vitamin C. The data also suggest that a 2-month trial of ascorbic acid, 300 mg/day by mouth at the end of each MHD treatment, may be indicated in EPO-hyporesponsive patients undergoing MHD with high serum ferritin levels (>500 mmol/L) and low serum transferrin saturation (<25%).

FOLIC ACID

Structure and Metabolism

Folic acid (pteroylglutamic acid) is composed of three subunits: a pteridine moiety, paraaminobenzoic acid, and glutamic acid (Table 20.1). Reduced forms of folic acid are present both in foods and in the human body, usually as tetrahydrofolate (THF). Folic acid is ubiquitous in foods and is present in large amounts in polyglutamate forms, usually of THFs or dihydrofolates, in yeast, liver, meats, green vegetables, and fruits. Very sensitive to oxidation, folate is readily destroyed by extensive cooking and also by food processing such as canning or refining (326). Intestinal absorption, reviewed by Fowler (327), occurs mainly in the proximal one-third of the small bowel. For intestinal transport, polyglutamates require the action of conjugases, present in the brush border of enterocytes, to be transformed to folate monoglutamates, such as 5-methyl-THF, formyl-THF, or dihydrofolates (328). Another enzyme, the glutamate carboxypeptidase II anchored in the intestinal brush border, participates in polyglutamate catabolism. Devlin et al. (329) identified a H475Y DNA variant coding for this enzyme; low folate levels and hyperhomocysteinemia are associated with a 53% reduction of the enzyme activity. Cellular transport relies on specific folate membrane receptors, carriers, and cellular exit pumps (327). Folates are stored in the body as polyglutamates and require the action of conjugases, which are present in many tissues, to yield the biologically active monoglutamate form (328). However, polyglutamates may have physiologic actions themselves. Actions of conjugases can be inhibited by various substances, including medicines. Indeed, many medicines may inhibit the actions of folate, including ones that commonly are prescribed for patients with CRF (Table 20.5) (see Chapter 33). Folic acid in plasma is mainly free or loosely bound to nonspecific carriers. Delivery of folic acid to the cell requires a specific cell-membrane receptor protein (326). Also, vitamin B12, involved in transmethylation reactions, is necessary for cellular transport and storage of folate (326). Excretion of the free form and metabolites of folic acid occurs in urine and bile. There is an enterohepatic cycle that helps to preserve the body pool of folates, and that is impaired by alcohol consumption.

Folate nutriture is assessed mainly by measuring serum, plasma, or red-cell folate levels. This formerly was performed by a microbiologic assay using *Lactobacillus casei.* Antibiotic administration may alter the results of the microbiologic assay. Currently, a radioimmunologic measurement more commonly is used, which is able to detect nanogram quantities of 5-methyl THF (326).

Physiologic Role

The fundamental action of folate can be summarized as one carbon unit transfers (326,327). Folic acid is required for DNA synthesis. The 5,10-methylene THF (requiring the vitamin B12–dependent transmethylation of homocysteine–methionine) delivers its methyl group to deoxyuridylate, which is transformed to thymidylate and is necessary for DNA synthesis. A defect in this step in DNA synthesis leads to megaloblastosis, which occurs in all replicating cells in the body but is most striking in bone-marrow cells (326,327). Folic acid plays a role in amino acid metabolism, particularly for those amino acids that are methyl donors, and a number of the amino acid reactions that folate catalyzes yield methyl groups that then participate in other biochemical processes. Metabolic processes involving amino acids catalyzed by folic acid that involve methyl groups include the interconversion of glycine and serine, the transformation of Hcy to methionine (Fig. 20.2), and the conversion of histidine to glutamic acid. Moreover, folic acid is required for purine synthesis in the methylation of transfer RNA. Unlike vitamin B12, folate is not involved in myelin synthesis, and therefore folate deficiency does not cause neurologic disease.

Folic Acid and Kidney Diseases

Folate Metabolism in Uremia

Folate metabolism appears to be altered in uremia. CRF may impair the intestinal absorption of THF. Using *in vivo* perfusion of the jejunum, Said et al. (330) showed that azotemic rats had significantly lower absorption of 5-methyl THF than sham-operated controls. Also, these authors found that using an *in vitro* everted jejunal sac technique, predialysis sera obtained from patients undergoing MHD suppressed intestinal absorption of 5-methyl THF, whereas postdialysis sera caused significantly less suppression (330). However, many years ago, Mackenzie et al. (205) did not find impaired absorption of folic acid in six patients undergoing MHD, whereas Jennette and Goldman reported that anions retained in uremic sera may inhibit the transport of folate across cell membranes (331). Livant et al. (328) reported that plasma conjugase activity was reduced in predialysis sera and increased to normal levels posthemodialysis. The authors suggest that there are one or more circulating heat-stable compounds in uremic plasma, possibly including sulfate, which may inhibit plasma folate conjugase activity (328). Paine et al. (332) described increased serum folic acid-binding protein levels in patients with CRF who were not receiving hemodialysis. These authors suggested that the elevated level of this binding protein could falsely reduce serum folate concentrations, measured by radioimmunoassay, but should not impair the delivery of folate to tissues.

Folic Acid Status in Renal Diseases

In nondialyzed patients with CRF, older reports suggested a high incidence of folate deficiency, as evidenced by megaloblastic bone-marrow changes (333) and hypersegmented polymorphonuclear leucocytes (334), which could be corrected with folic acid supplements. However, Paine et al. (332) described normal folate levels in patients with CRF. It was not stated whether these patients were receiving folic acid supplements. More recently, Marumo et al. (208) reported that in patients with CRF who were not receiving folate supplements, serum folic acid was normal in those with mild to moderate CRF and increased to above normal in patients with advanced CRF not undergoing MHD. In 18 children with moderate to advanced CRF, Litwin et al. (335) found normal levels of serum folic acid. Diets recommended for nondialyzed patients with CRF are likely to contain amounts of folic acid that are below the RDA (400 μg/day; Table 20.2) (100,303).

From the 1960s to 1980s, reports regarding folic acid status in patients undergoing MHD were contradictory, describing both normal (209,336–338) and deficient (204, 205,333) status. Lasker et al. (204) described low serum folate levels that were related to low food intake and the duration of the uremic state. Mackenzie et al. (205) also reported a daily folate intake in these patients that was below the RDA. However, Pereira et al. (201) found adequate folic acid intake in 30 children treated with MHD or CPD. Many studies have examined folate status in patients undergoing MHD who either were receiving (68,209,328) or recently had received (207,339–341) folic acid supplements. Marked increases in plasma and red-cell folate levels have been found in patients receiving folate supplements (68,339,342).

Normal folate pools are believed to be sufficiently large to satisfy folic acid requirements for at least 1 year (209). Thus, at least several months, if not more than 1 year, of follow-up after interruption of supplementation may be necessary to assess the risk of folate depletion. Moreover, most of these studies were conducted before the advent of high flux/high dialysis, which appears to have increased dramatically the risk of folic acid deficiency in patients undergoing MHD. Livant et al. (328) found that in 32 patients undergoing MHD treated with high-flux polysulfone dialyzers, five had reduced predialysis plasma folate concentrations and four had decreased red-cell folate concentrations. The incidence of folate deficiency might have been greater if 20 of the patients had not been prescribed folate supplements. Leblanc et al. (248) reported the folic acid clearance with high-flux/high-efficiency MHD to be at 134.7 ± 22.2 mL/min, with a 26.3% decrease in plasma folic acid during MHD treatment. The risk of folic acid depletion with high-flux membrane has been confirmed by Lasseur et al. (343), who reported a significant decrease in plasma folate levels after nonsupplemented patients undergoing MHD were transferred to high-flux membrane. However, De Vecchi et al. (344) and Tremblay et al. (239) have reported normal folic acid status in large cohorts of patients receiving high-efficiency/high-flux MHD. In veno-venous continuous renal replacement therapy for acute renal failure, the amount of folic acid removed has been estimated by Fortin et al. (251) to be 650 nmol/day, with a clearance as high as 76% of urea clearance.

The incidence of folate deficiency in patients undergoing CPD is controversial. Whereas Boeschoten et al. (33) and Blumberg et al. (69) found that 11% and 40%, respectively, of nonsupplemented patients undergoing CPD had low plasma folic acid levels, Henderson et al. (106), Salahudeen et al. (345), and De Vecchi et al. (344) found normal serum and/or red folate levels in their nonsupplemented patients undergoing CPD. The methyltetrahydrofolate reductase (MTHFR) genotype may influence the folic acid level in patients undergoing CPD, as reported by Vychytil et al. (346), who found low folic acid concentrations in patients with the T/T genotype. As with patients undergoing MHD, folic acid supplements led to high levels of serum and red-cell folic acid (69). Pediatric patients undergoing CPD receiving 800 μg/day of folate also developed high levels of serum folic acid (211). In patients undergoing CAPD, folate losses into peritoneal dialysate averaged 107 μg/day in one study (33).

Low serum folate was encountered in 29% of 52 renal transplant recipients, even after a prolonged period of good graft function (340). Intestinal folate absorption was decreased in two out of 10 of these patients. This was attributed to intestinal mucosa injury caused by azathioprine treatment. Folic acid levels did not correlate with the presence or absence of macrocytosis. Han et al. (347) reported low plasma folate level in 47% of 91 stable renal transplant patients. However, Stein et al. (348) found normal serum folic acid in 50 renal transplant patients. Also, the MTHFR genotypes, labeled 677 and 1298, have been shown to significantly influence plasma folic acid levels in a group of 733 renal transplant patients; the 677TT/1298AA group had a lower plasma folic acid level (349).

Folate Status in Erythropoietin-Treated Patients

EPO treatment may transiently increase folic acid needs during the time that the hemoglobin is increasing rapidly. It has been suggested that failure to provide sufficient supplemental folate to patients with marginal endogenous folate stores may impair the response to EPO. Mydlik et al. (61) reported a significant decrease of erythrocyte folic acid after 1 year of EPO therapy in 15 patients undergoing MHD. Ono and Hisasue (342) found that the hematologic response to EPO therapy in patients undergoing MHD who discontinued their folic acid supplement when EPO treatment was commenced was no different from that of patients who continued to receive folic acid supplements. However, all of the patients had received large doses of folate (15 mg/week) before the study began, and the patients' predialysis plasma and red-cell folate concentrations before commencing EPO treatment were much higher than normal. Indeed, 12 months later, predialysis serum and red-cell folate had fallen from high levels to normal values in these patients. Thus, the body pools in the patients no longer receiving the supplement appeared to be sufficient to maintain normal folate levels and an adequate hematologic response to EPO, at least for this 12-month period. Pollock et al. (350) did not find any difference in folate concentrations before and after 18 months of EPO treatment in 81 patients undergoing MHD; information is lacking as to whether these patients were receiving supplemental folate. In 31 patients undergoing CPD treated with EPO for 18 months, there also were no significant changes in serum folate concentrations (350). Again, no information was given concerning folic acid supplements in these patients.

Hyperhomocysteinemia

In the normal population, elevated plasma Hcy is a risk factor for adverse cardiovascular events. Because plasma Hcy usually is increased in patients with ESRD, there has been much research concerning plasma Hcy levels and methods for decreasing these levels in CRF, MD, and renal transplant patients. Homocysteine metabolism is discussed in detail in Chapter 7.

Homocysteine in Kidney Disease

Arnadottir et al. (351) reported lower Hcy concentrations in patients with the nephrotic syndrome than in nonnephrotic patients with membranous nephropathy. The plasma Hcy level was positively correlated with serum creatinine and albumin levels and negatively correlated with GFR, as measured by iohexol clearance, and urinary protein excretion. Thus, the nephrotic syndrome appears to be associated with a reduction of plasma Hcy; the mechanism for this phenomenon is unknown but may be because some Hcy in plasma is protein bound and, hence, may be lost in increased amounts in the urine. Plasma Hcy is increased in nondialyzed patients with advanced CRF (352–360), in patients undergoing CPD (276,346,356,361,362), in patients undergoing MHD (276,344,355,356,363,364), and in renal transplant recipients (347,348,358,365–367). Plasma Hcy levels tend to be two to four times higher than in healthy controls and correlate inversely with the GFR. Plasma Hcy also is increased in nondialyzed children with CRF and in children undergoing MHD (335). Arnadottir et al. (368) found that 6 months after renal transplantation plasma Hcy decreased by an average of 14% but that plasma Hcy was significantly higher in the transplant patients as compared to a control group matched for renal function (24-hour endogenous creatinine clearances, respectively, at 51 ± 21 and 52 ± 16 mL/min). Urinary excretion of Hcy is low even in humans with normal renal function (369). Patients with CRF and those undergoing MHD who have normal levels of folate, cobalamin, and PLP still manifest increased plasma Hcy (344,370).

Clinical Relevance of Increased Homocysteine in Renal Patients

Elevated plasma Hcy now is recognized as an independent risk factor for vascular disease in nonuremic individuals and generally also in patients with CRF (371–374). In a prospective study in patients with proven coronary heart disease and normal renal function, the risk of dying from a cardiovascular cause increased continuously with plasma Hcy level (375). In 2001 Pinto et al. (376) reported that plasma Hcy increased the risk ratio for premature coronary artery disease (RR = 3.2 for plasma Hcy greater than the 90th percentile), and Morris et al. (377) found an association between hyperhomocysteinemia and altered short-delayed recall tests. Jungers et al. (357) found higher plasma Hcy in nondialyzed patients with CRF who had clinical evidence of occlusive arterial disease. Sakurabayashi et al. (378) reported that by multiple regression analysis, the factors significantly associated with increased carotid intima-medial thickness in 168 patients undergoing MHD were age, smoking, systolic blood pressure, and plasma Hcy. Manns et al. (379) found a significant relationship between Hcy plasma levels and atherosclerotic vascular disease only in male patients undergoing MHD. However, in nondialyzed CRF, CPD, MHD, and renal transplant patients, plasma Hcy levels were not found to be associated with coronary heart disease (358). Moreover, Gale et al. (380) found in 128 men and women an association between carotid atherosclerosis and declining renal function that was not explained by plasma Hcy levels (see also Chapter 12). Two prospective studies described an association between plasma Hcy and cardiovascular risk in patients with renal failure. Moustapha et al. (381) followed 167 patients with ESRD for a 17-month period and reported an increased cardiovascular morbidity and mortality risk of 1% for each mmol increase in plasma Hcy. In patients undergoing MHD and CPD, Bostom et al. (382) found a relative risk for nonfatal and fatal cardiovascular events of 3.0 and 4.4, respectively, when comparing the highest quartile versus the lower three quartiles of plasma Hcy levels during a follow-up period of 17 months. Tamura et al. (383) did not find higher plasma Hcy levels in vascular access thrombosis-prone patients.

Dialysis Handling of Homocysteine

Several studies examined the role of the dialyzer membrane on Hcy clearance. Despite a greater intradialytic decrease in plasma Hcy (42% versus 32% with high-flux versus low-flux membranes), there was no difference in predialysis plasma Hcy levels with the two types of membranes during a 3-month period (384). Lasseur et al. (343) did not find any change in plasma Hcy levels after 12 patients had been changed from low-flux dialysis to treatment with high-flux dialysis for 2 months. A close correlation between predialysis and postdialysis plasma Hcy levels was reported by Biasioli et al. (385). Also, Van Tellingen et al. (386) reported that superflux dialyzers with optimized convective transport and increased numbers and/or optimized distribution of dialyzer pores was associated with lower predialysis plasma Hcy levels when compared to conventional high-flux dialyzers. Vychytil et al. (346) studied peritoneal excretion of Hcy in 39 patients undergoing CPD. Daily peritoneal Hcy losses (38.9 ± 20.8 mmol) were correlated with plasma Hcy levels, effluent volume, and the D/P creatinine ratio. Free Hcy represented 47.5% and 75.2% of total Hcy in plasma and dialysate, respectively. Hirose et al. (387) reported similar findings; the daily Hcy elimination with CAPD was 40.6 ± 28.4 mmol in 20 patients. These two authors concluded that CPD is too inefficient to normalize Hcy plasma levels.

Homocysteine Lowering Trials in Renal Failure Patients

Most of these trials are reported in Table 20.6. The effects of therapy on plasma Hcy levels may be summarized as follows. The usual effect is a 30% to 50% decrease in Hcy with folic acid therapy but with few patients attaining normal plasma Hcy levels. The magnitude of the lowering effect of folic acid is positively related to the pretreatment plasma Hcy level and negatively associated with the RBC folic acid concentration. Folinic acid is not superior to folic acid for plasma Hcy–lowering therapy (388). In 14 stable patients undergoing hemodialysis followed for four consecutive 6-week periods, Arnadottir et al. (389) reported that an increase of folic acid dose to more than 15 mg/week provided no additional benefit in lowering plasma Hcy in patients undergoing dialysis. Most clinical trials using low doses (2.5 to 5 mg/d) of folic acid treatment to lower plasma Hcy levels in patients with advanced CRF or undergoing MD (360,390–394) show a similar magnitude of reduction as compared to trials using larger doses of folic acid (208,388, 395–397). Bostom et al. (398) reported a more effective lowering effect of plasma Hcy with a combination of folic acid, vitamin B6, and vitamin B12 in renal transplant recipients than in patients undergoing MHD. A Veterans Administration–sponsored large-scale cooperative clinical trial in the United States currently is examining the effect of a combination of folic acid, pyridoxine HCl, and vitamin B12 treatment on plasma Hcy levels and clinical outcome in patients undergoing MHD. Vitamin B6 decreased plasma Hcy levels by 22% after a methionine loading test in stable renal transplant patients (399). N-acetylcysteine did not lower plasma Hcy in patients undergoing MHD (400).

Need for Supplemental Folic Acid

There is no consensus concerning the need for folate supplementation in patients with CRF not receiving dialysis as well as those undergoing MHD or CPD. Many authors have argued either that folate supplements are important (1,33,69,205,209,328,401,402) or are not necessary (207, 332,338,339,342,345). Folic acid supplements appear to be safe for such patients, even at the range of doses pre-

TABLE 20.6. FOLIC ACID TRIALS TO REDUCE HYPERHOMOCYSTEINEMIA IN RENAL PATIENTS

First Author	Subjects	*n*	Folic Acid or Folinic Acid Dose (mg)[b]	Vitamin B6 Dose (mg)	B12 Dose (μg)	Average Decrease in Plasma Hcy (%)	Patients Who Achieved Normal Hcy	Duration of Study	Comments
Jansen (430)	HD and CAPD	20	FA 5 mg/d			56,9 (HD) 58,4 (PD)		6 weeks	
Wilcken (360)	CRF	21	FA 5 mg/d			47		15 days	
Arnadottir (278)	HD and CAPD	18	FA 5 mg/d	300 mg		33		4 months	
Chauveau (277)	CRF	37	10 mg/d	70 mg/d		0		3 months	
Yango (395)	MHD	24	FA 5 mg/d			20,7	8,3	12 weeks	
		24	FNA 17 mg/d			22,1	9,1		
Van Guldener (431)	MHD	41	FA 1–5 mg/d			53,1	?	52 weeks	No effect on carotid artery stiffness
Tremblay (239)	MHD	128	FA 1 mg/d ± 30 mg/w	10 mg/d	6 μg/d	34,8	3,1	52 weeks	No difference at 52 weeks between the two folic acid regimens
Touam (280)	MHD	37	FNA:50 mg/w IV	750 mg/w IV		67,0	78	7,5–17 months	
Sunder-Plassmann[a] (396)	MHD	150	FA 15 or 30 or 60 mg/d			32,1 vs. 29,9 vs. 37,8		4 weeks	Hcy rebound after 30 and 60 mg FA are stopped
Suliman (283)	MHD	10	FA 15 mg/d	200 mg/d		28	0		
Stanford (393)	MHD	28	FA 5 mg/d			38,9	35,7	6 weeks	No effect of atherosclerotic lesion on Hcy decrease
Schroder (432)	Children on MHD and CPD	21	FA 2,5 mg/d			59,5		4 weeks	
Naruszewicz (281)	MHD	21	FA 15 mg/d	150 mg/d	1 mg/w	30		4 weeks	
McGregor (394)	MHD and CAPD	21	FA 5 mg			33		3 months	
Kaplan (413)	MHD	12			1 mg/4 weeks	10,9		12 weeks	Return to baseline level for Hcy 7 months after the last injection
House (433)	MHD	11	FA 1 mg	10 mg	6 μg	23,7		3 weeks	RBC folate levels increased by 60%
Hauser[a] (397)	MHD	66	FA 15 mg IV vs. FNA 16.1 mg IV 3 times/week			32,2 (FA) vs. 34,1 (FNA)	30,3 (FA) vs. 18,2 (FNA)	4 weeks	Increased response in MTHFR 677TT/1298AA genotypes and low FA RBC
Dierkes (406)	MHD	14			1 mg/week	35		4 weeks	Low B12 at start (<180 pm/L); 47% reduction in serum FA levels
Dierkes[a] (434)	MHD	61	FA 1.6 vs. 0.32 mg 3 times a week	20 mg 3 times a week in both groups	12 vs. 0 μg 3 times a week	48,2 vs. 28,3 (21,6 in placebo)		12 weeks	
Dierkes (390)	MHD	70	FA 2.5 vs. 5 mg 3 × week			68 vs. 69	16	12 weeks	Increased response in MTHFR 677TT genotype
	CPD	12	FA 2.5 mg 3 × week			64	50	12 weeks	
Bostom (282)	MHD	50	FA 15 mg/d vs. 17 mg FNA	50 mg/day	1 mg/day	14,8 vs. 17	0 vs. 8	12 weeks	
Beaulieu (435)	Renal transplant	60	FA 2.4 vs. 0.4 vs. 0	50 mg/day	0.4 mg/day	32,3 vs. 23,4 vs. 19,1	50 vs. 9 vs. 0	12 weeks	

FA, folic acid; FNA, folinic acid; HD, hemodialysis; CAPD, continuous ambulatory peritoneal dialysis; PD, peritoneal dialysis; CRF, chronic renal failure; MHD, maintenance hemodialysis; IV, intravenous; RBC, red blood cell; MTHFR, methyltetrahydrofolate reductase.
[a]Randomized and placebo-controlled.
[b]Vitamins given orally, unless otherwise specified.

scribed to reduce plasma Hcy levels. Exceptions are the possibility that folate treatment could mask the neurologic disturbances associated with vitamin B12 deficiency or that metabolites of folate might be toxic, possibly by inhibiting cellular transport of folate. Possible mild side effects of folate, such as nausea, headache, or vivid dreams, have been reported, usually with the 5 mg/day dose (340). Although many of the more recent studies indicate that plasma and red-cell folate levels are usually normal in patients with CRF and those undergoing MD, some patients still have low folate concentrations (328). High-efficiency/high-flux dialysis increases the risk of folate deficiency. Also, as indicated earlier, there may be endogenous as well as exogenous (i.e., from medicines) inhibitors of folic acid in renal failure, and this inhibition may not be reflected in the plasma or red-cell folate levels. Thus, it seems prudent to add folic acid, at least 1.0 mg/day, to prevent the possibility of folate deficiency in nondialyzed patients with CRF and those undergoing MHD and CPD, although clear clinical benefits of this treatment have not been demonstrated. The consistent findings from several clinical trials that 5 or 10 mg/day supplements of folate may decrease plasma Hcy levels (although usually not to normal values) suggest that patients with CRF and those undergoing MD perhaps routinely should be prescribed 5 to 10 mg/day of folic acid.

VITAMIN B12

Structure and Metabolism

Vitamin B12 or cobalamin (Table 20.1) has been identified as the "extrinsic factor" (i.e., present in food) that, when combined with the "intrinsic factor" (elaborated in gastric juice), results in the absorption of the antipernicious anemia factor. The molecule of vitamin B12 is constituted by a corrin nucleus, a nucleotide, and a cobalt atom. Cobalamins are unstable in light and destroyed by strong oxidizing and reducing agents. Cyanocobalamin, the pharmaceutical form of vitamin B12, has been isolated from liver extracts. Coenzyme B12 and methylcobalamin are the metabolically active forms, but all forms of vitamin B12 are equipotent when used in large doses (401). Cobalamins are present in animal tissues, mostly liver, meat, and seafood, but also can be found in lesser amounts in egg yolk and milk. Very small amounts are present in fruits and vegetables. Physiologic intestinal absorption follows several steps: free cobalamin is combined with a salivary peptide binder, then is released in small intestine by trypsin and is combined again with the intrinsic factor, a glycoprotein molecule of gastric origin. Absorption of the vitamin B12-intrinsic factor complex occurs after binding to a receptor on the brush border of mucosal cells in the ileum. However, large pharmacologic doses of cobalamins may be absorbed by the small intestine via a passive diffusion process. Three binding proteins (transcobalamins I, II, and III) participate in cobalamin transport in plasma and also in the storage of vitamin B12. Several milligrams of vitamin B12 can be stored and may prevent vitamin B12 deficiency from occurring for several years after intestinal absorption ceases (209) (Table 20.1). Vitamin B12 is not catabolized and is excreted in urine and bile, with an efficient enterohepatic cycle (403).

Vitamin B12 assessment is performed using microbiologic and, more recently, radioassay methods. Radioassays are not modified by antibiotic treatment. When pure intrinsic factor is used as a ligand for the radioassay, it is possible to separate cobalamin from corrinoid analogues. These analogues have various degrees of biologic activity and may jeopardize the early detection of vitamin B12 deficiency if they are detected by the assay (403).

Physiologic Role

Vitamin B12 plays a key role in folic acid metabolism. Its essential function is the demethylation of methyltetrahydrofolate and methylation of Hcy (Fig. 20.2). This step is essential for regeneration of THF, which is involved in DNA synthesis by thymidylate synthesis, and for folate delivery to tissues. In the absence of demethylation, signs of folate deficiency may occur (403). Furthermore, vitamin B12 is required for myelin synthesis, as demonstrated by the severe neurologic disturbances experienced in pernicious anemia. However, the exact mechanism of cobalamin action on myelin is unknown.

Vitamin B12 and Kidney Disease

Contradictory data have been reported concerning the vitamin B12 status of patients with renal failure. From the early years of dialysis therapy until the present, plasma vitamin B12 usually has been observed to be within the normal range in patients with CRF, those undergoing MD, and renal transplant recipients (106,204,205,209,340,345,401,404,405). In patients undergoing MHD not receiving vitamin B12, abnormally low plasma vitamin B12 has been reported in 4.6% to 31.6% of the cases (248,405,406) Also, plasma vitamin B12 was found to decrease with the time spent on MHD treatment (407). In patients receiving monthly parenteral vitamin B12 supplementation, withdrawal for 9 months was followed by a significant decrease in plasma cobalamin, reaching the lower range of normal levels in two patients (408). However, most frequently, normal plasma vitamin B12 values are reported in patients undergoing MHD not receiving supplements (204,205,209,244,334,337). Several factors may favor the development of vitamin B12 deficiency in renal failure. Vitamin B12 intake with low-protein diets is reported to be normal (303) or low (100). Chandna et al. (409) found low vitamin B12 intake in 16% of patients undergoing MHD. Intestinal absorption of vitamin B12 in patients undergoing MHD is not impaired according to $Co^{57,58}$-labeled-cobalamin studies (405,409). Also, because cobalamin is protein-bound, losses of vitamin B12 in dialysate should be low. Many years ago, predialysis and postdialysis serum levels of cobalamin were found to be either not modified at all or only slightly decreased by HD (205). In 11 patients undergoing MHD, Marumo et al. (208) measured the vitamin B12 clearance at 11 mL/min with low-efficiency hemodialysis (time: 4 to 5 hours; average membrane area: 1.2 m^2; blood flow: 200 mL/min; dialysate flow: 500 mL/min). In 1997, with high-flux/high-efficiency dialysis in 67 patients, Chandna et al. (409) reported a similar value of vitamin B12 clearance at 9.1 mL/min. In the same study, no $Co^{57,58}$-labeled cobalamin was absorbed onto the dialysis membrane (409); however, serum vitamin B12 decreased during a 6-month follow-up period, and 22 patients were prescribed vitamin B12 supplements. In patients undergoing CPD, no cobalamin was recovered in peritoneal fluid by Boeschoten et al. (33).

The clinical relevance of potential vitamin B12 deficiency in patients undergoing chronic dialysis is unknown. In initial studies, Bastow et al. (407) reported low serum cobalamin levels in four patients undergoing HD. None of the patients displayed megaloblastosis in bone-marrow aspirates. Normocytic or microcytic anemia was present in the four patients. A single injection of 1,000 μg of vitamin B12 was sufficient to obtain a dramatic and sustained improvement of the hematocrit in those patients who did not have a vitamin B12 absorptive defect. These observations suggest that vitamin B12 deficiency may occur in patients with CRF and those undergoing MHD, even if macrocytosis is lacking. Moreover, serum vitamin B12 concentrations were significantly and directly correlated with nerve-conduction velocities in 51 patients undergoing MHD (405). In six of these patients undergoing MHD with low serum vitamin B12 levels, reversal of slow conduction velocities was obtained with a loading dose of 1,000 μg followed by doses of 100 μg of vitamin B12 at the end of each dialysis treatment for 4 to 6 months. In other studies, vitamin B12 therapy also was reported to be beneficial (410) or inefficient (240) for treatment of peripheral neuropathy. It has been speculated that EPO therapy enhances vitamin B12 needs for patients undergoing dialysis. Pollock et al. (350) followed 53 patients undergoing MHD and CPD for 13.1 ± 0.6 months after commencing EPO treatment. Serum vitamin B12 levels did not change significantly during the follow-up; but no information was given concerning vitamin B12 supplements in these patients.

Because of its effect on folate metabolism, vitamin B12 affects Hcy metabolism (see Chapter 7). A negative correlation between plasma Hcy and vitamin B12 levels is described in patients undergoing MHD and CPD and renal transplant recipients (344,349,362). The MTHFR genotype has not been found to influence plasma vitamin B12 levels (349,411). Most of the Hcy-lowering trials using vitamin B12 have given B12 in conjunction with folic acid and/or pyridoxine (Table 20.6). An effect of vitamin B12 alone was reported in 2000. In a cross-sectional study, Hoffer et al. (412) compared plasma Hcy levels in patients undergoing MHD treated in two different dialysis facilities. In one facility, the patients were given 6 mg daily of folic acid, and in the other facility, the patients received 1 mg of vitamin B12 intravenously each month. Predialysis and postdialysis plasma Hcy levels were significantly lower in the patients receiving vitamin B12 (412). Also, parenteral vitamin B12 given monthly at a dose of 1 mg was shown to decrease plasma Hcy by an average of 10.9% after 3 months (413).

Need for Supplemental Vitamin B12

Because vitamin B12 deficiency is unusual in patients with CRF and those undergoing MD, most authors do not think that vitamin B12 supplementation is necessary (33,209,242, 345,401). Moreover, very high levels of cobalamin were reported in 106 patients undergoing MHD receiving 2,500 μg of vitamin B12 three times per week (401). Although no side effects were reported in these patients, the safety of this treatment was questioned by the authors (401). Because vitamin B12 intake has been found to be below the RDA in some patients undergoing CPD (69) and MHD (205, 405), several cases of vitamin B12 deficiency have been reported in high-flux/high-efficiency patients undergoing MHD. Also, because the long-term effects of EPO therapy on vitamin B12 stores are unknown, it seems safe to recommend a daily vitamin B12 supplement equivalent to the RDA for adults (i.e., 2.4 μg/day) (2) in patients with CRF and those undergoing MHD and CPD. Moreover, even in patients undergoing MHD with normal cobalamin stores, the therapeutic use of pharmacologic amounts of vitamin B12 has been reported to improve nerve-conduction velocities (405) and autonomic neuropathy (414) or to lower plasma Hcy (406,413). Further research will be necessary to assess the benefits of such therapy.

NIACIN

Structure and Metabolism

Niacin has been identified as the therapeutic agent for pellagra, a condition described initially in maize-eating populations (415). Niacin is a generic term including nicotinic acid and nicotinamide (Table 20.1). Active coenzymes are pyridine nucleotides, NAD, and NAD phosphate (NADP). High amounts of NAD and NADP (main forms of niacin intake) are present in meat, fish, legumes, coffee, and tea. These compounds are hydrolyzed in the intestine to yield nicotinamide and then nicotinic acid. However, niacin bioavailability may be reduced because of its binding to carbohydrate and peptide macromolecules. Intestinal absorption by diffusion is efficient, even for large doses of niacin. Tryptophan, requiring vitamin B6 and riboflavin, is a precursor for niacin, and tryptophan intake alone may be sufficient to provide the RDA for nicotinic acid. Niacin is removed quickly from plasma by tissues (mainly by liver and RBC) where it is converted to coenzyme forms. Storage, mostly in the liver, is limited, and signs of pellagra may occur within 50 to 60 days in humans fed a corn diet deficient in niacin (415). Excess niacin is methylated in the liver, and the methylated metabolites are excreted in the urine. Niacin status is assessed by measuring nicotinic acid and nicotinamide in blood and red cells, using microbiologic or, more recently, chemical assays or HPLC. The NAD/NADP ratio in red cells, which is decreased in niacin deficiency, may be used as a marker of niacin depletion in patients with renal failure.

Physiologic Role

Pyridine nucleotides are involved in many enzymatic reactions (at least 200). These may include NAD, which is mainly involved in catabolic reactions (such as oxidation of fuel molecules), and NADP, which primarily is concerned with synthesis (such as for steroids). These coenzymes are key elements for carbohydrate, fatty-acid, and amino acid metabolism. There is a close relationship between the metabolism of niacin and other vitamins. Vitamin B6 and riboflavin are necessary for niacin synthesis from tryptophan. Niacin is necessary for the synthesis of active forms of vitamin B6, riboflavin, and folic acid. Pharmacologic doses of nicotinic acid decrease total cholesterol, LDL and very–low-density lipoprotein fractions, and triglycerides and increase the HDL-cholesterol fraction (416).

Niacin and Kidney Diseases

Few data are available regarding niacin status in nondialyzed and dialyzed patients with CRF. Niacin intake with low-protein diets has been found to be below (205) or equivalent to (68,100,303) the RDA. Because of its rapid metabolic clearance, losses of niacin in dialysate are expected to be low. Many years ago, plasma clearance of niacin was estimated as low as 4 mL/min by Mackenzie et al. (205). Ramirez et al. (207) did not find any difference between predialysis and postdialysis red-cell niacin concentrations in patients undergoing MHD. No data are available on niacin losses in peritoneal dialysate.

DeBari et al. reported low concentrations of niacin in leucocytes but normal niacin content in red cells of patients undergoing MHD (242). Lasker et al. (204) found low blood levels of niacin in two of five patients undergoing MHD and in three patients treated with CPD. One of the patients with low niacin blood levels had a burning feet syndrome that improved with high doses of niacin. However, Ramirez et al. (207,243) did not find evidence of low niacin levels in whole blood or erythrocytes of patients undergoing MHD who were not receiving supplements or in whom supplements had been stopped for at least 1 year. Pellagra (characterized by diarrhea, dementia, and dermatitis) never has been reported in patients with CRF, but niacin deficiency has been suggested as the cause of onycholysis in patients undergoing MHD (416). Also, it has been suggested that niacin may decrease lipoprotein a in patients undergoing MHD (417). In 12 renal transplant recipients with dyslipidemia, nicotinic acid was found to be as effective as lovastatin in improving the lipid profile; nicotinic acid was even associated with an increase in the HDL fraction, whereas lovastatin was not (418).

Need for Supplemental Niacin

Because a low-protein diet may provide a small amount of niacin and some studies have demonstrated niacin deficiency in patients undergoing dialysis, it appears safe to recommend a daily supplement of niacin that is equivalent to the RDA for nonpregnant, nonlactating, normal adults (i.e., 14 to 16 mg/day of niacin equivalents) (2) in nondialyzed patients with CRF and those undergoing MD. There is currently not sufficient scientific data to evaluate whether pharmacologic doses of niacin for the treatment of lipid disturbances in patients with renal failure is beneficial.

BIOTIN

Structure and Metabolism

Biotin or vitamin B8 is a bicyclic compound containing an ureido ring and a tetrahydrothiophene ring (Table 20.1). Biotin is synthesized by intestinal flora. It is controversial as to whether this source of biotin can satisfy the daily need for this vitamin in humans (419). Major biotin sources are liver, egg yolk, soybean, and yeast. Cereals, legumes, and nuts contain moderate amounts of biotin; fruits and vegetables are poor sources of biotin, except for cauliflower and mushrooms. Biotin absorption occurs mainly in the jejunum and requires the release of biocytin (biotinyl lysine) from ingested proteins and the action of biotinidase to free lysine and biotin, which each are absorbed by a diffusive saturable process. Long-term anticonvulsant therapy may interfere with the binding of biotin to biotinidase. The presence of avidin, a glycoprotein that strongly binds to biotin, may impair biotin absorption. Free biotin and its metabolites are excreted in the urine. Biotin stores appear sufficient to cover the biotin needs for about 1 month. Biotin is assessed in plasma by microbiologic assays.

Physiologic Role

Biotin mainly acts as a "CO_2 carrier" being the coenzyme for carboxylases (acetyl CoA carboxylase, pyruvate carboxylase, propionyl CoA carboxylase, B methylcrotonyl CoA carboxylase). Biotin is bound covalently to the ϵ-amino group of a lysine residue of carboxylases. Thus, it plays an important role in the metabolism of carbohydrates, fatty acids, and some amino acids. Uremic toxins have been shown to impair tubuline polymerization, which leads to microtubule formation (420); biotin counteracts the effects of uremic toxins on tubulin (420).

Experimental biotin deficiency has been induced in seven healthy human volunteers who were given a biotin-free diet and an excessive intake of raw egg white (rich in avidin) (421). In 5 weeks, the subjects developed mild depression, somnolence, muscle pains, hyperesthesia, anorexia, and later a maculosquamous dermatitis with greyish palor and fine desquamation. All symptoms disappeared within 5 days of starting biotin injections (421). Alopecia is also a common feature of biotin deficiency (421).

Biotin and Kidney Diseases

Several observations suggest that patients with CRF and those undergoing MD are at risk for biotin deficiency. Intestinal absorption of biotin is impaired in rats with CRF (422). Biotin intake in patients with CRF prescribed low-protein diets has been estimated to be much lower than the RDA (205) (Table 20.2). Many years ago, Lasker et al. reported two patients (one receiving MHD and one undergoing CPD) with low plasma biotin levels but did not mention any clinical signs of biotin deficiency in these patients (204). Mackenzie et al. (205) measured biotin clearance at 52 mL/min with a Kiil dialyzer. However, Lasker et al. (204) found an inconsistent decrease in plasma biotin during the hemodialysis procedure. No data are available concerning biotin losses in patients undergoing CPD.

However, several studies did not find biotin deficiency in patients with renal failure. Biotin concentrations in plasma, leucocytes, or RBC were found to be high in patients undergoing MHD (204,205,423,424) and even higher in patients undergoing MHD treated for longer periods and in anuric patients (209). In 23 patients undergoing MHD, Jung et al. (423) found that the predialysis plasma biotin concentrations were increased up to four to six times normal levels, with a 30% decrease in plasma biotin during HD treatment (425). The plasma biotin level was not influenced by the type of dialyzer (low-flux versus high-flux) or the blood flow rate. In the same study, no biotin deficiency was observed in nondialyzed patients with CRF and renal transplant recipients. Biotin is excreted in the urine. Reduced or absent renal function could compensate for the low biotin intake and/or impaired intestinal absorption and the dialysate losses and could explain the absence of biotin deficiency in these patients.

Ten mg of biotin given daily for 1 to 4 years was reported to improve neurologic symptoms in nine patients undergoing MHD who were diagnosed with uremic encephalopathy and neuropathy (425). However, no changes in the electroencephalographic patterns or nerve-conduction velocities occurred, and these observations should be interpreted with caution. Also, the same dose of biotin was reported to improve or eradicate malignant hiccups in seven patients undergoing MHD (426). Biotin also may improve the oral glucose tolerance test in patients undergoing MHD (427).

Need for Supplemental Biotin

There is no RDA for biotin intake in healthy subjects, but there is an estimation of the dietary need called the "Adequate Intake" (2). (See Table 20.2 and Chapter 23.) Some investigators contend that for patients with CRF the biotin requirements are not known (68) or that there is no need for biotin supplementation (209). Because there appear to have been some cases of biotin deficiency in patients undergoing MHD, it seems prudent to recommend a biotin supplement for patients with CRF and those undergoing MHD and CPD equivalent to the adequate intake (i.e., 30 μg/day). It will require further studies to determine whether this is the optimal dose of biotin for patients with renal failure.

PANTOTHENIC ACID

Structure and Metabolism

Pantothenic acid or "chick antidermatitis factor" is formed from the combination of pantoic acid and β-alanine. Some of the characteristics of this vitamin are given in Table 20.1. Pantothenic acid, after passing through several biochemical steps, is incorporated into the CoA macromolecule, which is comprised of pantothenic acid, AMP, and β-mercaptoethylamine. Pantothenic acid is ubiquitous and is present in large amounts in many foods, especially liver, kidney, egg yolk, fresh vegetables, royal bee jelly, and ovaries of tuna and cod (428). After CoA hydrolysis, pantothenic acid is liberated and excreted in the urine. Pantothenic acid is assessed by microbiologic assays, or, currently, by radioimmunoassay.

Physiologic Role

Pantothenic acid, through CoA, is necessary for the synthesis of many compounds including fatty acids, cholesterol, steroid hormones, molecules containing isoprenoid units (e.g., vitamins A and D), δ-aminolevulinic acid, and some neurotransmitters and amino acids. Pantothenic acid is necessary for energy extraction during the β-oxidation of fatty acids and oxidation of amino acids. Also, pantothenic acid and CoA play a central role in the acetylation of proteins, microtubules, and histones and in the acylation of proteins with fatty acids, mainly myristic and palmitic acids. The acetylation and acylation of proteins affect both their structure and activity.

In animals, pantothenic acid deficiency results in retarded growth, neuromuscular disorders, abnormalities of skin and hair, and gastrointestinal symptoms. In young men fed a pantothenic-free diet for 9 weeks, their main complaint was fatigue (429).

Pantothenic Acid and Kidney Diseases

There are few data concerning the pantothenic acid status of patients with renal failure. Low-protein diets have lower pantothenic acid content (1,205). More than 30 years ago, the clearance of pantothenic acid by hemodialysis was measured at 30 mL/min by Mackenzie et al. (205) using low-efficiency dialysis techniques. Lasker et al. reported a decrease in plasma pantothenic acid during hemodialysis (204). Conflicting data have been reported regarding the pantothenic acid status of patients undergoing MHD. DeBari et al. (242) found in 12 nonsupplemented patients undergoing MHD that pantothenic acid concentrations in plasma, leucocytes, and red cells were significantly higher than in normal controls. Lasker et al. (204) reported normal or high concentrations of pantothenic acid in blood of six MHD and three CPD patients who were not receiving vitamin supplements. However, Mackenzie et al. (205) reported low concentrations of plasma pantothenic acid in six patients undergoing MHD who were not receiving supplemental pantothenic acid.

Need for Supplemental Pantothenic Acid

There are few data on which to base recommendations concerning the needs, if any, for supplemental pantothenic acid. Because the reported dialyzer clearance of pantothenic acid in older reports was not negligible and the clearances with high-flux and/or high-efficiency dialysis are unknown, and because low concentrations of pantothenic acid have been found in one study in nonsupplemented dialysis patients, it appears prudent to recommend a pantothenic acid supplement equivalent to 5 mg/day for patients undergoing MHD or CPD. As with biotin, this recommendation is not based on RDA data but is derived from the "Adequate Intake" estimation (2). (See Table 20.2.)

CONCLUSIONS

It should be clear from the foregoing discussion that the nutritional requirements for many vitamins are not well defined for patients with renal disease or renal failure. Indeed, we currently do not know how to assess the nutritional status for many vitamins in renal patients. The blood or plasma concentrations of vitamins may be poor indicators of their functional activities. The effects of renal failure or uremic toxins on the metabolism and actions of vitamins are largely unknown. The use of pharmacologic doses of vitamins in renal patients barely has begun to be investigated. It therefore can be concluded that the field of vitamin metabolism and nutriture in renal disease and renal failure should be a fruitful one for both basic and clinical research.

REFERENCES

1. Kopple J. Dietary considerations in patients with advanced chronic renal failure, acute renal failure, and transplantation. In: Shills M, Olson JA, Shike M, et al, eds. *Diseases of the kidney.* Baltimore: Williams & Wilkins, 1998:3167–3210.
2. Dietary Reference Intakes for thiamin, riboflavin, niacin, vitamin B6, folate, pantothenic acid, biotin and cholin. Washington, DC: National Academy Press, 1998.
3. Dietary References Intakes for vitamin C, vitamin E, selenium and carotenoids. Washington, DC: National Academy Press, 2000.
4. Ross A. Vitamin A and retinoids. In: Shills M, Olson JA, Shike M, et al, eds. *Modern nutrition in health and disease.* Baltimore: Williams & Wilkins, 1998:305–327.
5. Bates CJ. Vitamin A. *Lancet* 1995;345:31–35.
6. Norum KR, Blomhoff R. McCollum Award Lecture, 1992: vitamin A absorption, transport, cellular uptake, and storage. *Am J Clin Nutr* 1992;56:735–744.
7. Olson JA. Carotenoids. In: Shills M, Olson JA, Shike M, et al, eds. *Modern nutrition in health and disease*, 9th ed. Baltimore: Williams & Wilkins, 1998:525–541.
8. Russell RM. The vitamin A spectrum: from deficiency to toxicity. *Am J Clin Nutr* 2000;71:878–884.
9. Blomhoff R, Wake K. Perisinusoidal stellate cells of the liver: important roles in retinol metabolism and fibrosis. *Faseb J* 1991; 5:271–277.
10. Burrow CR. Retinoids and renal development. *Exp Nephrol* 2000;8:219–225.
11. Gilbert T, Merlet-Benichou C. Retinoids and nephron mass control. *Pediatr Nephrol* 2000;14:1137–1144.
12. Randolph TR. Acute promyelocytic leukemia (AML-M3)—Part 1: Pathophysiology, clinical diagnosis, and differentiation therapy. *Clin Lab Sci* 2000;13:98–105.
13. Omenn GS, Goodman GE, Thornquist MD, et al. Effects of a combination of beta carotene and vitamin A on lung cancer and cardiovascular disease. *N Engl J Med* 1996;334:1150–1155.
14. Kushi LH, Folsom AR, Prineas RJ, et al. Dietary antioxidant vitamins and death from coronary heart disease in postmenopausal women. *N Engl J Med* 1996;334:1156–1162.
15. McCormick AM, Napoli JL, Deluca HF. High-pressure liquid chromatographic resolution of vitamin A compounds. *Anal Biochem* 1978;86:25–33.
16. Vahlquist A, Peterson PA, Wibell L. Metabolism of the vitamin A transporting protein complex. I. Turnover studies in normal persons and in patients with chronic renal failure. *Eur J Clin Invest* 1973;3:352–362.
17. Peterson PA. Demonstration in serum of two physiological forms of the human retinol binding protein. *Eur J Clin Invest* 1971;1:437–444.
18. Jaconi S, Rose K, Hughes GJ, et al. Characterization of two post-translationally processed forms of human serum retinol-binding protein: altered ratios in chronic renal failure. *J Lipid Res* 1995;36:1247–1253.
19. Smith FR, Goodman DS. Vitamin A transport in human vitamin A toxicity. *N Engl J Med* 1976;294:805–808.

20. Christensen EI, Moskaug JO, Vorum H, et al. Evidence for an essential role of megalin in transepithelial transport of retinol. *J Am Soc Nephrol* 1999;10:685–695.
21. Marino M, Andrews D, Brown D, et al. Transcytosis of retinol-binding protein across renal proximal tubule cells after megalin (gp 330)-mediated endocytosis. *J Am Soc Nephrol* 2001;12: 637–648.
22. Gerlach TH, Zile MH. Upregulation of serum retinol in experimental acute renal failure. *Faseb J* 1990;4:2511–2517.
23. Gerlach TH, Zile MH. Metabolism and secretion of retinol transport complex in acute renal failure. *J Lipid Res* 1991;32: 515–520.
24. Gerlach TH, Zile MH. Effect of retinoic acid and apo-RBP on serum retinol concentration in acute renal failure. *Faseb J* 1991; 5:86–92.
25. Kleiner-Bossaler A, Deluca HF. Formation of retinoic acid from retinol in the kidney. *Arch Biochem Biophys* 1971;142:371–377.
26. Bhat PV, Lacroix A. Effects of retinoic acid on the concentrations of radioactive metabolites of retinol in tissues of rats maintained on a retinol-deficient diet. *Can J Physiol Pharmacol* 1991; 69:826–830.
27. Yatzidis H, Digenis P, Fountas P. Hypervitaminosis A accompanying advanced chronic renal failure. *Br Med J* 1975;3: 352–353.
28. Ellis S, DePalma J, Cheng A, et al. Vitamin A supplements in hemodialysis patients. *Nephron* 1980;26:215–218.
29. De Bevere VO, De Paepe M, De Leenheer AP, et al. Plasma vitamin A in haemodialysis patients. *Clin Chim Acta* 1981;114: 249–256.
30. Delacoux E, Evstigneeff T, Leclercq M, et al. Skin disorders and vitamin A metabolism disturbances in chronic dialysis patients: the role of zinc, retinol-binding protein, retinol and retinoic acid. *Clin Chim Acta* 1984;137:283–289.
31. Popper H, Steigman F, Dyniewicz H. Plasma vitamin A level in renal diseases. *Am J Clin Pathol* 1945;15:272–277.
32. Mydlik M, Derzsiova K, Bratova M, et al. Serum vitamin A, retinyl esters and vitamin E in nephrotic syndrome. *Int Urol Nephrol* 1991;23:399–405.
33. Boeschoten EW, Schrijver J, Krediet RT, et al. Deficiencies of vitamins in CAPD patients: the effect of supplementation. *Nephrol Dial Transplant* 1988;3:187–193.
34. Chazot C, Laurent G, Charra B, et al. Malnutrition in long-term haemodialysis survivors. *Nephrol Dial Transplant* 2001; 16:61–69.
35. Cundy T, Earnshaw M, Heynen G, et al. Vitamin A and hyperparathyroid bone disease in uremia. *Am J Clin Nutr* 1983;38: 914–920.
36. Ha TK, Sattar N, Talwar D, et al. Abnormal antioxidant vitamin and carotenoid status in chronic renal failure. *Qjm* 1996; 89:765–769.
37. Mydlik M, Derzsiova K, Valek A, et al. Vitamins and continuous ambulatory peritoneal dialysis (CAPD). *Int Urol Nephrol* 1985;17:281–286.
38. Stein G, Schone S, Geinitz D, et al. No tissue level abnormality of vitamin A concentration despite elevated serum vitamin A of uremic patients. *Clin Nephrol* 1986;25:87–93.
39. Stewart WK, Fleming LW. Plasma retinol and retinol binding protein concentrations in patients on maintenance haemodialysis with and without vitamin A supplements. *Nephron* 1982; 30:15–21.
40. Vahlquist A, Berne B, Berne C. Skin content and plasma transport of vitamin A and beta-carotene in chronic renal failure. *Eur J Clin Invest* 1982;12:63–67.
41. Werb R, Clark WF, Lindsay RM, et al. Serum vitamin A levels and associated abnormalities in patients on regular dialysis treatment. *Clin Nephrol* 1979;12:63–68.
42. de Cavanagh EM, Ferder L, Carrasquedo F, et al. Higher levels of antioxidant defenses in enalapril-treated versus non-enalapril-treated hemodialysis patients. *Am J Kidney Dis* 1999;34: 445–455.
43. Rock CL, Jahnke MG, Gorenflo DW, et al. Racial group differences in plasma concentrations of antioxidant vitamins and carotenoids in hemodialysis patients. *Am J Clin Nutr* 1997;65: 844–850.
44. Smith DK, Greene JM, Leonard SB, et al. Vitamin A in hypercholesterolemia. *Am J Med Sci* 1992;304:20–24.
45. Ono K, Waki Y, Takeda K. Hypervitaminosis A: a contributing factor to anemia in regular dialysis patients. *Nephron* 1984;38: 44–47.
46. Ford D, Stall C, Volinsky J, et al. Vitamin A restriction in end stage renal disease (ESRD) challenged (abstract). *J Am Soc Nephrol* 1994;5:491(20P).
47. Bonnefont-Rousselot D, Jaudon MC, Issad B, et al. Antioxidant status of elderly chronic renal patients treated by continuous ambulatory peritoneal dialysis. *Nephrol Dial Transplant* 1997; 12:1399–1405.
48. Yatzidis H, Digenis P, Koutsicos D. Hypervitaminosis A in chronic renal failure after transplantation. *Br Med J* 1976;2: 1075.
49. Druml W, Schwarzenhofer M, Apsner R, et al. Fat-soluble vitamins in patients with acute renal failure. *Miner Electrolyte Metab* 1998;24:220–226.
50. Gleghorn EE, Eisenberg LD, Hack S, et al. Observations of vitamin A toxicity in three patients with renal failure receiving parenteral alimentation. *Am J Clin Nutr* 1986;44:107–112.
51. Muenter MD, Perry HO, Ludwig J. Chronic vitamin A intoxication in adults. Hepatic, neurologic and dermatologic complications. *Am J Med* 1971;50:129–136.
52. Shmunes E. Hypervitaminosis A in a patient with alopecia receiving renal dialysis. *Arch Dermatol* 1979;115:882–883.
53. Beijer C, Planken EV. [Hypercalcemia due to chronic vitamin A use by an elderly patient with renal insufficiency]. *Ned Tijdschr Geneeskd* 2001;145:90–93.
54. Doireau V, Macher MA, Brun P, et al. [Vitamin A poisoning revealed by hypercalcemia in a child with kidney failure]. *Arch Pediatr* 1996;3:888–890.
55. Wieland RG, Hendricks FH, Amat y Leon F, et al. Hypervitaminosis A with hypercalcaemia. *Lancet* 1971;1:698.
56. Farrington K, Miller P, Varghese Z, et al. Vitamin A toxicity and hypercalcaemia in chronic renal failure. *Br Med J (Clin Res Ed)* 1981;282:1999–2002.
57. Katz CM, Tzagournis M. Chronic adult hypervitaminosis A with hypercalcemia. *Metabolism* 1972;21:1171–1176.
58. Frame B, Jackson CE, Reynolds WA, et al. Hypercalcemia and skeletal effects in chronic hypervitaminosis A. *Ann Intern Med* 1974;80:44–48.
59. Jelkmann W, Pagel H, Hellwig T, et al. Effects of antioxidant vitamins on renal and hepatic erythropoietin production. *Kidney Int* 1997;51:497–501.
60. Neumcke I, Schneider B, Fandrey J, et al. Effects of pro- and antioxidative compounds on renal production of erythropoietin. *Endocrinology* 1999;140:641–645.
61. Mydlik M, Derzsiova K. [Vitamin levels in the serum and erythrocytes during erythropoietin therapy in hemodialyzed patients]. *Bratisl Lek Listy* 1999;100:426–431.
62. Manzano VM, Munoz JC, Jimenez JR, et al. Human renal mesangial cells are a target for the anti-inflammatory action of 9-cis retinoic acid. *Br J Pharmacol* 2000;131:1673–1683.
63. Wagner J, Dechow C, Morath C, et al. Retinoic acid reduces glomerular injury in a rat model of glomerular damage. *J Am Soc Nephrol* 2000;11:1479–1487.
64. Kavukcu S, Soylu A, Turkmen M, et al. The role of vitamin A

in preventing renal scarring secondary to pyelonephritis. *BJU Int* 1999;83:1055–1059.

65. Bennett RT, Mazzaccaro RJ, Chopra N, et al. Suppression of renal inflammation with vitamins A and E in ascending pyelonephritis in rats. *J Urol* 1999;161:1681–1684.
66. Moreno-Manzano V, Rodriguez-Puyol M, Arribas-Gomez I, et al. Prevention by tretinoin (all-trans-retinoic acid) of age-related renal changes. *Int J Vitam Nutr Res* 1997;67:427–431.
67. Dietary Reference Intakes for vitamin A, vitamin K, arsenic, boron, chromium, copper, iodine, iron, manganese, molybdenum, nickel, silicon, vanadium and zinc. Washington, DC: National Academy Press, 2001.
68. Allman MA, Truswell AS, Tiller DJ, et al. Vitamin supplementation of patients receiving haemodialysis. *Med J Aust* 1989; 150:130–133.
69. Blumberg A, Hanck A, Sander G. Vitamin nutrition in patients on continuous ambulatory peritoneal dialysis (CAPD). *Clin Nephrol* 1983;20:244–250.
70. Makoff R. Vitamin replacement therapy in renal failure patients. *Miner Electrolyte Metab* 1999;25:349–351.
71. Meydani M. Vitamin E. *Lancet* 1995;345:170–175.
72. Pastor MC, Sierra C, Bonal J, et al. Serum and erythrocyte tocopherol in uremic patients: effect of hemodialysis versus peritoneal dialysis. *Am J Nephrol* 1993;13:238–243.
73. *Recommended dietary allowances*, 10th ed. Washington, DC: National Academic Press, 1989.
74. Farrell P, Roberts R. Vitamin E. In: Shills M, Olson J, Shike M, eds. *Modern nutrition in health and disease.* Philadelphia: Lea & Febiger, 1993:326–341.
75. Horwitt MK, Harvey CC, Dahm CH Jr, et al. Relationship between tocopherol and serum lipid levels for determination of nutritional adequacy. *Ann N Y Acad Sci* 1972;203:223–236.
76. Thurnham DI, Davies JA, Crump BJ, et al. The use of different lipids to express serum tocopherol: lipid ratios for the measurement of vitamin E status. *Ann Clin Biochem* 1986;23:514–520.
77. Sokol RJ, Heubi JE, Iannaccone ST, et al. Vitamin E deficiency with normal serum vitamin E concentrations in children with chronic cholestasis. *N Engl J Med* 1984;310:1209–1212.
78. Sadowski JA, Hood SJ, Dallal GE, et al. Phylloquinone in plasma from elderly and young adults: factors influencing its concentration. *Am J Clin Nutr* 1989;50:100–108.
79. Spielberg SP, Boxer LA, Corash LM, et al. Improved erythrocyte survival with high-dose vitamin E in chronic hemolyzing G6PD and glutathione synthetase deficiencies. *Ann Intern Med* 1979; 90:53–54.
80. Giardini O, Cantani A, Donfrancesco A. Vitamin E therapy in homozygous beta-thalassemia. *N Engl J Med* 1981;305:644.
81. Rimm EB, Stampfer MJ, Ascherio A, et al. Vitamin E consumption and the risk of coronary heart disease in men. *N Engl J Med* 1993;328:1450–1456.
82. Stampfer MJ, Hennekens CH, Manson JE, et al. Vitamin E consumption and the risk of coronary disease in women. *N Engl J Med* 1993;328:1444–1449.
83. Faruqi R, de la Motte C, DiCorleto PE. Alpha-tocopherol inhibits agonist-induced monocytic cell adhesion to cultured human endothelial cells. *J Clin Invest* 1994;94:592–600.
84. Fydryk J, Jacobson E, Kurzawska O, et al. Antioxidant status of children with steroid-sensitive nephrotic syndrome. *Pediatr Nephrol* 1998;12:751–754.
85. Warwick GL, Waller H, Ferns GA. Antioxidant vitamin concentrations and LDL oxidation in nephrotic syndrome. *Ann Clin Biochem* 2000;37:488–491.
86. Rajbala A, Sane AS, Zope J, et al. Oxidative stress status in children with nephrotic syndrome. *Panminerva Med* 1997;39: 165–168.
87. Kinra S, Rath B, Kabi BC. Indirect quantification of lipid peroxidation in steroid responsive nephrotic syndrome. *Arch Dis Child* 2000;82:76–78.
88. Gentile MG, Manna GM, D'Amico G, et al. Vitamin nutrition in patients with chronic renal failure and dietary manipulation. *Contrib Nephrol* 1988;65:43–50.
89. Clermont G, Lecour S, Lahet J, et al. Alteration in plasma antioxidant capacities in chronic renal failure and hemodialysis patients: a possible explanation for the increased cardiovascular risk in these patients. *Cardiovasc Res* 2000;47:618–623.
90. Stenvinkel P, Heimburger O, Paultre F, et al. Strong association between malnutrition, inflammation, and atherosclerosis in chronic renal failure. *Kidney Int* 1999;55:1899–1911.
91. Taccone-Gallucci M, Giardini O, Lubrano R, et al. Red blood cell lipid peroxidation in predialysis chronic renal failure. *Clin Nephrol* 1987;27:238–241.
92. Peuchant E, Delmas-Beauvieux MC, Dubourg L, et al. Antioxidant effects of a supplemented very low protein diet in chronic renal failure. *Free Radic Biol Med* 1997;22:313–320.
93. Nenov D, Paskalev D, Yankova T, et al. Lipid peroxidation and vitamin E in red blood cells and plasma in hemodialysis patients under rhEPO treatment. *Artif Organs* 1995;19: 436–439.
94. Hultqvist M, Hegbrant J, Nilsson-Thorell C, et al. Plasma concentrations of vitamin C, vitamin E and/or malondialdehyde as markers of oxygen free radical production during hemodialysis. *Clin Nephrol* 1997;47:37–46.
95. De Bevere VO, Nelis HJ, De Leenheer AP, et al. Vitamin E levels in hemodialysis patients. *JAMA* 1982;247:2371.
96. Cristol JP, Bosc JY, Badiou S, et al. Erythropoietin and oxidative stress in haemodialysis: beneficial effects of vitamin E supplementation. *Nephrol Dial Transplant* 1997;12:2312–2317.
97. Nguyen-Khoa T, Massy ZA, Witko-Sarsat V, et al. Critical evaluation of plasma and LDL oxidant-trapping potential in hemodialysis patients. *Kidney Int* 1999;56:747–753.
98. Roob JM, Khoschsorur G, Tiran A, et al. Vitamin E attenuates oxidative stress induced by intravenous iron in patients on hemodialysis. *J Am Soc Nephrol* 2000;11:539–549.
99. Inal M, Kanbak G, Sen S, et al. Antioxidant status and lipid peroxidation in hemodialysis patients undergoing erythropoietin and erythropoietin-vitamin E combined therapy. *Free Radic Res* 1999;31:211–216.
100. Stein G, Sperschneider H, Koppe S. Vitamin levels in chronic renal failure and need for supplementation. *Blood Purif* 1985; 3:52–62.
101. Paul JL, Sall ND, Soni T, et al. Lipid peroxidation abnormalities in hemodialyzed patients. *Nephron* 1993;64:106–109.
102. Ono K. Effects of large dose vitamin E supplementation on anemia in hemodialysis patients. *Nephron* 1985;40:440–445.
103. Ongajooth L, Ongajyooth S, Likidlilid A, et al. Role of lipid peroxidation, trace elements and anti-oxidant enzymes in chronic renal disease patients. *J Med Assoc Thai* 1996;79: 791–800.
104. Giardini O, Taccone-Gallucci M, Lubrano R, et al. Effects of alpha-tocopherol administration on red blood cell membrane lipid peroxidation in hemodialysis patients. *Clin Nephrol* 1984; 21:174–177.
105. Cohen JD, Viljoen M, Clifford D, et al. Plasma vitamin E levels in a chronically hemolyzing group of dialysis patients. *Clin Nephrol* 1986;25:42–47.
106. Henderson I, Leung A, Shenkin A. Vitamin status in continuous ambulatory peritoneal dialysis. *Perit Dial Bull* 1984;4:143–145.
107. Nikolakakis N, Kounali D, Tornaritis M, et al. Adipose tissue fatty acid composition, serum lipids, and serum alpha-tocopherol in continuous ambulatory peritoneal dialysis patients living on the island of Crete. *Perit Dial Int* 1999;19:154–159.
108. McGrath LT, Treacy R, McClean E, et al. Oxidative stress in

cyclosporin and azathioprine treated renal transplant patients. *Clin Chim Acta* 1997;264:1–12.
109. Cristol JP, Vela C, Maggi MF, et al. Oxidative stress and lipid abnormalities in renal transplant recipients with or without chronic rejection. *Transplantation* 1998;65:1322–1328.
110. Story DA, Ronco C, Bellomo R. Trace element and vitamin concentrations and losses in critically ill patients treated with continuous venovenous hemofiltration. *Crit Care Med* 1999; 27:220–223.
111. Akpolat T, Akpolat I, Ozturk H, et al. Effect of vitamin E and pentoxifylline on glycerol-induced acute renal failure. *Nephron* 2000;84:243–247.
112. Abdel-Naim A, Abdel-Wahab M, Attia F. Protective effects of vitamin E and probucol against gentamicin-induced nephrotoxicity in rats. *Pharmacol Res* 1999;40:183–187.
113. Drukker A, Eddy AA. Failure of antioxidant therapy to attenuate interstitial disease in rats with reversible nephrotic syndrome. *J Am Soc Nephrol* 1998;9:243–251.
114. Trachtman H, Schwob N, Maesaka J, et al. Dietary vitamin E supplementation ameliorates renal injury in chronic puromycin aminonucleoside nephropathy. *J Am Soc Nephrol* 1995;5: 1811–1819.
115. Reckelhoff JF, Kanji V, Racusen LC, et al. Vitamin E ameliorates enhanced renal lipid peroxidation and accumulation of F2-isoprostanes in aging kidneys. *Am J Physiol* 1998;274: R767–R774.
116. Biri H, Ozturk HS, Buyukkocak S, et al. Antioxidant defense potential of rabbit renal tissues after ESWL: protective effects of antioxidant vitamins. *Nephron* 1998;79:181–185.
117. Saborio P, Krieg RJ Jr, Kuemmerle NB, et al. Alpha-tocopherol modulates lipoprotein cytotoxicity in obstructive nephropathy. *Pediatr Nephrol* 2000;14:740–746.
118. Otani H, Mune M, Yukawa S, et al. Vitamin E treatment of experimental glomerular disease in rats. *Kidney Int Suppl* 1999; 71:S66–S69.
119. Hahn S, Kuemmerle NB, Chan W, et al. Glomerulosclerosis in the remnant kidney rat is modulated by dietary alpha-tocopherol. *J Am Soc Nephrol* 1998;9:2089–2095.
120. Appenroth D, Frob S, Kersten L, et al. Protective effects of vitamin E and C on cisplatin nephrotoxicity in developing rats. *Arch Toxicol* 1997;71:677–683.
121. Lee HS, Jeong JY, Kim BC, et al. Dietary antioxidant inhibits lipoprotein oxidation and renal injury in experimental focal segmental glomerulosclerosis. *Kidney Int* 1997;51:1151–1159.
122. Chan W, Krieg RJ Jr, Norkus EP, et al. Alpha-tocopherol reduces proteinuria, oxidative stress, and expression of transforming growth factor beta 1 in IgA nephropathy in the rat. *Mol Genet Metab* 1998;63:224–229.
123. Kuemmerle NB, Krieg RJ Jr, Chan W, et al. Influence of alpha-tocopherol over the time course of experimental IgA nephropathy. *Pediatr Nephrol* 1999;13:108–112.
124. Appenroth D, Winnefeld K. Vitamin E and C in the prevention of metal nephrotoxicity in developing rats. *Exp Toxicol Pathol* 1998;50:391–396.
125. Craven PA, DeRubertis FR, Kagan VE, et al. Effects of supplementation with vitamin C or E on albuminuria, glomerular TGF-beta, and glomerular size in diabetes. *J Am Soc Nephrol* 1997;8:1405–1414.
126. Douillet C, Bost M, Accominotti M, et al. Effect of selenium and vitamin E supplements on tissue lipids, peroxides, and fatty acid distribution in experimental diabetes. *Lipids* 1998;33: 393–399.
127. Kim SS, Gallaher DD, Csallany AS. Vitamin E and probucol reduce urinary lipophilic aldehydes and renal enlargement in streptozotocin-induced diabetic rats. *Lipids* 2000;35: 1225–1237.
128. Bulucu F, Vural A, Aydin A, et al. Oxidative stress status in adults with nephrotic syndrome. *Clin Nephrol* 2000;53: 169–173.
129. Yoshioka T, Iwamoto N, Tsunoda Y, et al. Down-regulation of manganese-superoxide dismutase gene expression in idiopathic nephrotic syndrome. *J Pediatr* 1997;130:800–807.
130. Tahzib M, Frank R, Gauthier B, et al. Vitamin E treatment of focal segmental glomerulosclerosis: results of an open-label study. *Pediatr Nephrol* 1999;13:649–652.
131. Boaz M, Smetana S, Weinstein T, et al. Secondary prevention with antioxidants of cardiovascular disease in endstage renal disease (SPACE): randomised placebo-controlled trial. *Lancet* 2000;356:1213–1218.
132. Yusuf S, Sleight P, Pogue J, et al. Effects of an angiotensin-converting-enzyme inhibitor, ramipril, on cardiovascular events in high-risk patients. The Heart Outcomes Prevention Evaluation Study Investigators. *N Engl J Med* 2000;342:145–153.
133. Effects of ramipril on cardiovascular and microvascular outcomes in people with diabetes mellitus: results of the HOPE study and MICRO-HOPE substudy. Heart Outcomes Prevention Evaluation Study Investigators. *Lancet* 2000;355:253–259.
134. O'Byrne D, Devaraj S, Islam KN, et al. Low-density lipoprotein (LDL)-induced monocyte-endothelial cell adhesion, soluble cell adhesion molecules, and autoantibodies to oxidized-LDL in chronic renal failure patients on dialysis therapy. *Metabolism* 2001;50:207–215.
135. Yalcin AS, Yurtkuran M, Dilek K, et al. The effect of vitamin E therapy on plasma and erythrocyte lipid peroxidation in chronic hemodialysis patients. *Clin Chim Acta* 1989;185:109–112.
136. Taccone-Gallucci M, Giardini O, Lubrano R, et al. Red blood cell membrane lipid peroxidation in continuous ambulatory peritoneal dialysis patients. *Am J Nephrol* 1986;6:92–95.
137. Islam KN, O'Byrne D, Devaraj S, et al. Alpha-tocopherol supplementation decreases the oxidative susceptibility of LDL in renal failure patients on dialysis therapy. *Atherosclerosis* 2000; 150:217–224.
138. Bonnefont-Rousselot D, Lehmann E, Jaudon MC, et al. Blood oxidative stress and lipoprotein oxidizability in haemodialysis patients: effect of the use of a vitamin E-coated dialysis membrane. *Nephrol Dial Transplant* 2000;15:2020–2028.
139. Tarng DC, Huang TP, Liu TY, et al. Effect of vitamin E-bonded membrane on the 8-hydroxy 2′-deoxyguanosine level in leukocyte DNA of hemodialysis patients. *Kidney Int* 2000; 58:790–799.
140. Sommerburg, Sostmann K, Grune T, et al. Oxidative stress in hemodialysis patients treated with a dialysis membrane which has alpha-tocopherol bonded to its surface. *Biofactors* 1999;10: 121–124.
141. Galli F, Canestrari F, Buoncristiani U. Biological effects of oxidant stress in haemodialysis: the possible roles of vitamin E. *Blood Purif* 1999;17:79–94.
142. Shimazu T, Kondo S, Toyama K, et al. Effect of vitamin E-modified regenerative cellulose membrane on neutrophil superoxide anion radical production and lipid peroxidation. *Contrib Nephrol* 1999;127:251–260.
143. Omata M, Higuchi C, Demura R, et al. Reduction of neutrophil activation by vitamin E modified dialyzer membranes. *Nephron* 2000;85:221–231.
144. Buoncristiani U, Galli F, Rovidati S, et al. Oxidative damage during hemodialysis using a vitamin-E-modified dialysis membrane: a preliminary characterization. *Nephron* 1997;77:57–61.
145. Girndt M, Lengler S, Kaul H, et al. Prospective crossover trial of the influence of vitamin E-coated dialyzer membranes on T-cell activation and cytokine induction. *Am J Kidney Dis* 2000; 35:95–104.
146. Galli F, Rovidati S, Benedetti S, et al. Lipid peroxidation, leuko-

cyte function and apoptosis in hemodialysis patients treated with vitamin E-modified filters. *Contrib Nephrol* 1999;127: 156–171.

147. Mune M, Yukawa S, Kishino M, et al. Effect of vitamin E on lipid metabolism and atherosclerosis in ESRD patients. *Kidney Int Suppl* 1999;71:S126–S129.
148. Huraib S, Tanimu D, Shaheen F, et al. Effect of vitamin-E-modified dialysers on dialyser clotting, erythropoietin and heparin dosage: a comparative crossover study. *Am J Nephrol* 2000; 20:364–368.
149. Usberti M, Bufano G, Lima G, et al. Increased red blood cell survival reduces the need of erythropoietin in hemodialyzed patients treated with exogenous glutathione and vitamin E-modified membrane. *Contrib Nephrol* 1999;127:208–214.
150. Dhondt A, Vanholder R, Glorieux G, et al. Vitamin E-bonded cellulose membrane and hemodialysis bioincompatibility: absence of an acute benefit on expression of leukocyte surface molecules. *Am J Kidney Dis* 2000;36:1140–1146.
151. Wratten ML, Navino C, Tetta C, et al. Haemolipodialysis. *Blood Purif* 1999;17:127–133.
152. Rabl H, Khoschsorur G, Colombo T, et al. A multivitamin infusion prevents lipid peroxidation and improves transplantation performance. *Kidney Int* 1993;43:912–917.
153. Varghese Z, Fernando RL, Turakhia G, et al. Calcineurin inhibitors enhance low-density lipoprotein oxidation in transplant patients. *Kidney Int Suppl* 1999;71:S137–S140.
154. Wang C, Salahudeen AK. Lipid peroxidation accompanies cyclosporine nephrotoxicity: effects of vitamin E. *Kidney Int* 1995; 47:927–934.
155. Parra T, de Arriba G, Conejo JR, et al. Cyclosporine increases local glomerular synthesis of reactive oxygen species in rats: effect of vitamin E on cyclosporine nephrotoxicity. *Transplantation* 1998;66:1325–1329.
156. Durak I, Karabacak HI, Buyukkocak S, et al. Impaired antioxidant defense system in the kidney tissues from rabbits treated with cyclosporine. Protective effects of vitamins E and C. *Nephron* 1998;78:207–211.
157. Jenkins JK, Huang H, Ndebele K, et al. Vitamin E inhibits renal mRNA expression of COX II, HO I, TGFbeta, and osteopontin in the rat model of cyclosporine nephrotoxicity. *Transplantation* 2001;71:331–334.
158. Barany P, Stenvinkel P, Ottosson-Seeberger A, et al. Effect of 6 weeks of vitamin E administration on renal haemodynamic alterations following a single dose of neoral in healthy volunteers. *Nephrol Dial Transplant* 2001;16:580–584.
159. Olson JA. Vitamin K. In: Shills M, Olson JA, Shike M, et al, eds. *Modern nutrition in health and disease*, 9th ed. Baltimore: Williams & Wilkins, 1998:363–380.
160. Vermeer C, Hamulyak K. Pathophysiology of vitamin K-deficiency and oral anticoagulants. *Thromb Haemost* 1991;66: 153–159.
161. Shearer MJ. Vitamin K. *Lancet* 1995;345:229–234.
162. Ansell JE, Kumar R, Deykin D. The spectrum of vitamin K deficiency. *JAMA* 1977;238:40–42.
163. Suttie JW, Mummah-Schendel LL, Shah DV, et al. Vitamin K deficiency from dietary vitamin K restriction in humans. *Am J Clin Nutr* 1988;47:475–480.
164. Saupe J, Shearer MJ, Kohlmeier M. Phylloquinone transport and its influence on gamma-carboxyglutamate residues of osteocalcin in patients on maintenance hemodialysis. *Am J Clin Nutr* 1993;58:204–208.
165. Ferland G, Sadowski JA, O'Brien ME. Dietary induced subclinical vitamin K deficiency in normal human subjects. *J Clin Invest* 1993;91:1761–1768.
166. Fournier B, Sann L, Guillaumont M, et al. Variations of phylloquinone concentration in human milk at various stages of lactation and in cow's milk at various seasons. *Am J Clin Nutr* 1987; 45:551–558.
167. Price PA. Role of vitamin-K-dependent proteins in bone metabolism. *Annu Rev Nutr* 1988;8:565–583.
168. Friedman PA, Mitch WE, Silva P. Localization of renal vitamin K-dependent gamma-glutamyl carboxylase to tubule cells. *J Biol Chem* 1982;257:11037–11040.
169. Scandling J, Walker BK. Extensive tissue necrosis associated with warfarin sodium therapy. *South Med J* 1980;73: 1470–1472.
170. Hodges SJ, Akesson K, Vergnaud P, et al. Circulating levels of vitamins K1 and K2 decreased in elderly women with hip fracture. *J Bone Miner Res* 1993;8:1241–1245.
171. Jamal SA, Browner WS, Bauer DC, et al. Warfarin use and risk for osteoporosis in elderly women. Study of Osteoporotic Fractures Research Group. *Ann Intern Med* 1998;128:829–832.
172. Sato Y, Honda Y, Kunoh H, et al. Long-term oral anticoagulation reduces bone mass in patients with previous hemispheric infarction and nonrheumatic atrial fibrillation. *Stroke* 1997;28: 2390–2394.
173. Rosen HN, Maitland LA, Suttie JW, et al. Vitamin K and maintenance of skeletal integrity in adults. *Am J Med* 1993;94: 62–68.
174. Fiore CE, Tamburino C, Foti R, et al. Reduced axial bone mineral content in patients taking an oral anticoagulant. *South Med J* 1990;83:538–542.
175. Shanahan CM, Proudfoot D, Tyson KL, et al. Expression of mineralisation-regulating proteins in association with human vascular calcification. *Z Kardiol* 2000;89:63–68.
176. Alperin JB. Coagulopathy caused by vitamin K deficiency in critically ill, hospitalized patients. *JAMA* 1987;258:1916–1919.
177. Soundararajan R, Leehey DJ, Yu AW, et al. Skin necrosis and protein C deficiency associated with vitamin K depletion in a patient with renal failure. *Am J Med* 1992;93:467–470.
178. Sorensen PJ, Knudsen F, Nielsen AH, et al. Protein C assays in uremia. *Thromb Res* 1989;54:301–310.
179. Robert D, Jorgetti V, Leclercq M, et al. Does vitamin K excess induce ectopic calcifications in hemodialysis patients? *Clin Nephrol* 1985;24:300–304.
180. Knapen MH, Jie KS, Hamulyak K, et al. Vitamin K-induced changes in markers for osteoblast activity and urinary calcium loss. *Calcif Tissue Int* 1993;53:81–85.
181. Jie KS, Gijsbers BL, Knapen MH, et al. Effects of vitamin K and oral anticoagulants on urinary calcium excretion. *Br J Haematol* 1993;83:100–104.
182. Nakagawa Y, Abram V, Parks JH, et al. Urine glycoprotein crystal growth inhibitors. Evidence for a molecular abnormality in calcium oxalate nephrolithiasis. *J Clin Invest* 1985;76: 1455–1462.
183. Chawki M, Rainfray M, Meyrier A. Calcifications ectopiques des dialysés: rôle de l'hypervitaminose K. In: Dialyse SF, ed. Réunion annuelle. Montpelier, France, 1994.
184. Akiba T, Kurihara S, Tachibana K, et al. Vitamin K increased bone mass in hemodialysis patients with low turnover bone disease. *J Am Soc Nephrol* 1991;2:608.
185. Kohlmeier M, Saupe J, Shearer MJ, et al. Bone health of adult hemodialysis patients is related to vitamin K status. *Kidney Int* 1997;51:1218–1221.
186. Kohlmeier M, Saupe J, Schaefer K, et al. Bone fracture history and prospective bone fracture risk of hemodialysis patients are related to apolipoprotein E genotype. *Calcif Tissue Int* 1998; 62:278–281.
187. Makoff R. Vitamin supplementation in patients with renal disease. *Dialysis and Transplantation* 1992;21:18–36.
188. Tanphaichitr V. Thiamin. In: Shills M, Olson JA, Shike M,

et al, eds. *Modern nutrition in health and disease.* Baltimore: Williams & Wilkins, 1998.

189. Lubetsky A, Winaver J, Seligmann H, et al. Urinary thiamine excretion in the rat: effects of furosemide, other diuretics, and volume load. *J Lab Clin Med* 1999;134:232–237.
190. Vuilleumier JP, Keller HE, Rettenmaier R, et al. Clinical chemical methods for the routine assessment of the vitamin status in human populations. Part II: The water-soluble vitamins B1, B2 and B6. *Int J Vitam Nutr Res* 1983;53:359–370.
191. Laschi-Loquerie A, Vallas S, Viollet J, et al. High performance liquid chromatographic determination of total thiamine in biological and food products. *Int J Vitam Nutr Res* 1992;62: 248–251.
192. Lynch PL, Young IS. Determination of thiamine by high-performance liquid chromatography. *J Chromatogr A* 2000;881: 267–284.
193. Floridi A, Pupita M, Palmerini CA, et al. Thiamine pyrophosphate determination in whole blood and erythrocytes by high performance liquid chromatography. *Int J Vitam Nutr Res* 1984; 54:165–171.
194. Nakasaki H, Ohta M, Soeda J, et al. Clinical and biochemical aspects of thiamine treatment for metabolic acidosis during total parenteral nutrition. *Nutrition* 1997;13:110–117.
195. Luft FC. Lactic acidosis update for critical care clinicians. *J Am Soc Nephrol* 2001;12 Suppl 17:S15–S19.
196. Sterzel RB, Semar M, Lonergan ET, et al. Effect of hemodialysis on the inhibition of nervous tissue transketolase and on uremic neuropathy. *Trans Am Soc Artif Intern Organs* 1971;17:77–79.
197. Mydlik M, Derzsiova K. Erythrocyte vitamin B1, B2 and B6 in nephrotic syndrome. *Miner Electrolyte Metab* 1992;18: 293–294.
198. Lonergan ET, Semar M, Sterzel RB, et al. Erythrocyte transketolase activity in dialyzed patients. A reversible metabolic lesion of uremia. *N Engl J Med* 1971;284:1399–1403.
199. Kopple JD, Dirige OV, Jacob M, et al. Transketolase activity in red blood cells in chronic uremia. *Trans Am Soc Artif Intern Organs* 1972;18:250–256.
200. Porrini M, Simonetti P, Ciappellano S, et al. Thiamin, riboflavin and pyridoxine status in chronic renal insufficiency. *Int J Vitam Nutr Res* 1989;59:304–308.
201. Pereira AM, Hamani N, Nogueira PC, et al. Oral vitamin intake in children receiving long-term dialysis. *J Ren Nutr* 2000;10: 24–29.
202. Sterzel RB, Semar M, Lonergan ET, et al. Relationship of nervous tissue transketolase to the neuropathy in chronic uremia. *J Clin Invest* 1971;50:2295–2304.
203. Kuriyama M, Mizuma A, Yokomine R, et al. Erythrocyte transketolase activity in uremia. *Clin Chim Acta* 1980;108:169–177.
204. Lasker N, Harvey A, Baker H. Vitamin levels in hemodialysis and intermittent peritoneal dialysis. *Trans Am Soc Art Int Organs* 1963;9:51–56.
205. Mackenzie J, Ford J, Waters A, et al. Erythropoiesis in patients undergoing regular dialysis treatment without transfusion. *Proc Eur Dial Transplant Assoc* 1968;5:172–178.
206. Niwa T, Ito T, Matsui E. Plasma thiamine levels with hemodialysis. *JAMA* 1971;218:885–886.
207. Ramirez G, Chen M, Boyce HW Jr, et al. Longitudinal follow-up of chronic hemodialysis patients without vitamin supplementation. *Kidney Int* 1986;30:99–106.
208. Marumo F, Kamata K, Okubo M. Deranged concentrations of water-soluble vitamins in the blood of undialyzed and dialyzed patients with chronic renal failure. *Int J Artif Organs* 1986;9: 17–24.
209. Descombes E, Hanck AB, Fellay G. Water soluble vitamins in chronic hemodialysis patients and need for supplementation. *Kidney Int* 1993;43:1319–1328.
210. Descombes E, Boulat O, Perriard F, et al. Water-soluble vitamin levels in patients undergoing high-flux hemodialysis and receiving long-term oral postdialysis vitamin supplementation. *Artif Organs* 2000;24:773–778.
211. Kriley M, Warady BA. Vitamin status of pediatric patients receiving long-term peritoneal dialysis. *Am J Clin Nutr* 1991;53: 1476–1479.
212. Gotloib L, Servadio C. A possible case of beriberi heart failure in a chronic hemodialyzed patient. *Nephron* 1975;14:293–298.
213. Cage JB, Wall BM. Shoshin beriberi in an AIDS patient with end-stage renal disease. *Clin Cardiol* 1992;15:862–865.
214. Ihara M, Ito T, Yanagihara C, et al. Wernicke's encephalopathy associated with hemodialysis: report of two cases and review of the literature. *Clin Neurol Neurosurg* 1999;101:118–121.
215. Jagadha V, Deck JH, Halliday WC, et al. Wernicke's encephalopathy in patients on peritoneal dialysis or hemodialysis. *Ann Neurol* 1987;21:78–84.
216. Sandoval E, Borja H, Gatica A. [Wernicke's encephalopathy as a complication of chronic hemodialysis: report of one case]. *Rev Med Chil* 1997;125:582–585.
217. Hung SC, Hung SH, Tarng DC, et al. Chorea induced by thiamine deficiency in hemodialysis patients. *Am J Kidney Dis* 2001;37:427–430.
218. Hung SC, Hung SH, Tarng DC, et al. Thiamine deficiency and unexplained encephalopathy in hemodialysis and peritoneal dialysis patients. *Am J Kidney Dis* 2001;38:941–947.
219. Niwa T, Ito T, Matsui E, et al. Plasma level and transfer capacity of thiamin in patients undergoing long-term hemodialysis. *Am J Clin Nutr* 1975;28:1105–1109.
220. McCormick D. Riboflavin. In: Shills M, Olson JA, Shike M, et al, eds. *Modern nutrition in health and disease.* Baltimore: Williams & Wilkins, 1998:391–399.
221. Vaziri ND, Said HM, Hollander D, et al. Impaired intestinal absorption of riboflavin in experimental uremia. *Nephron* 1985; 41:26–29.
222. Mohammed HY, Veening H, Dayton DA. Liquid chromatographic determination and time—concentration studies of riboflavin in hemodialysate from uremic patients. *J Chromatogr* 1981;226:471–476.
223. Kopple JD, Swendseid ME, Holliday MA, et al. Recommendations for nutritional evaluation of patients on chronic dialysis. *Kidney Int Suppl* 1975:249–252.
224. Ito T, Niwa T, Matsui E, et al. Plasma flavin levels of patients receiving long-term hemodialysis. *Clin Chim Acta* 1972;39: 125–129.
225. Leklem J. Vitamin B6. In: Shills M, Olson JA, Shike M, et al, eds. *Modern nutrition in health and disease.* Baltimore: Williams & Wilkins, 1998.
226. Ross EA, Shah GM, Reynolds RD, et al. Vitamin B6 requirements of patients on chronic peritoneal dialysis. *Kidney Int* 1989;36:702–706.
227. Stone WJ, Warnock LG, Wagner C. Vitamin B6 deficiency in uremia. *Am J Clin Nutr* 1975;28:950–957.
228. Bates CJ, Pentieva KD, Prentice A. An appraisal of vitamin B6 status indices and associated confounders, in young people aged 4–18 years and in people aged 65 years and over, in two national British surveys. *Public Health Nutr* 1999;2:529–535.
229. Ubbink JB, Delport R, Becker PJ, et al. Evidence of a theophylline-induced vitamin B6 deficiency caused by noncompetitive inhibition of pyridoxal kinase. *J Lab Clin Med* 1989;113:15–22.
230. Teehan BP, Smith LJ, Sigler MH, et al. Plasma pyridoxal-5′-phosphate levels and clinical correlations in chronic hemodialysis patients. *Am J Clin Nutr* 1978;31:1932–1936.
231. Dobbelstein H, Korner WF, Mempel W, et al. Vitamin B6 deficiency in uremia and its implications for the depression of immune responses. *Kidney Int* 1974;5:233–239.

232. Wolfson M, Kopple JD. The effect of vitamin B6 deficiency on food intake, growth, and renal function in chronically azotemic rats. *JPEN J Parenter Enteral Nutr* 1987;11:398–402.
233. Barbari A, Vaziri ND, Benavides I, et al. Intestinal transport of pyridoxine in experimental renal failure. *Life Sci* 1989;45: 663–669.
234. Labadarios D, Shephard GS, Mineur LG, et al. Biochemical vitamin B6 deficiency in adults with chronic glomerulonephritides with and without the nephrotic syndrome. *Int J Vitam Nutr Res* 1984;54:313–319.
235. van Buuren AJ, Louw ME, Shephard GS, et al. The effect of pyridoxine supplementation on plasma pyridoxal-5′-phosphate levels in children with the nephrotic syndrome. *Clin Nephrol* 1987;28:81–86.
236. Casciato DA, McAdam LP, Kopple JD, et al. Immunologic abnormalities in hemodialysis patients: improvement after pyridoxine therapy. *Nephron* 1984;38:9–16.
237. Kopple JD, Mercurio K, Blumenkrantz MJ, et al. Daily requirement for pyridoxine supplements in chronic renal failure. *Kidney Int* 1981;19:694–704.
238. Lacour B, Parry C, Drueke T, et al. Pyridoxal 5′-phosphate deficiency in uremic undialyzed, hemodialyzed, and non-uremic kidney transplant patients. *Clin Chim Acta* 1983;127:205–215.
239. Tremblay R, Bonnardeaux A, Geadah D, et al. Hyperhomocysteinemia in hemodialysis patients: effects of 12-month supplementation with hydrosoluble vitamins. *Kidney Int* 2000;58: 851–858.
240. Okada H, Moriwaki K, Kanno Y, et al. Vitamin B6 supplementation can improve peripheral polyneuropathy in patients with chronic renal failure on high-flux haemodialysis and human recombinant erythropoietin. *Nephrol Dial Transplant* 2000;15: 1410–1413.
241. Weissgarten J, Modai D, Oz D, et al. Vitamin B(6) therapy does not improve hematocrit in hemodialysis patients supplemented with iron and erythropoietin. *Nephron* 2001;87:328–332.
242. DeBari VA, Frank O, Baker H, et al. Water soluble vitamins in granulocytes, erythrocytes, and plasma obtained from chronic hemodialysis patients. *Am J Clin Nutr* 1984;39:410–415.
243. Ramirez G, Chen M, Boyce HW Jr, et al. The plasma and red cell vitamin B levels of chronic hemodialysis patients: a longitudinal study. *Nephron* 1986;42:41–46.
244. Spannuth CL Jr, Warnock LG, Wagner C, et al. Increased plasma clearance of pyridoxal 5′-phosphate in vitamin B6-deficient uremic man. *J Lab Clin Med* 1977;90:632–637.
245. Foreman JW, Abitbol CL, Trachtman H, et al. Nutritional intake in children with renal insufficiency: a report of the growth failure in children with renal diseases study. *J Am Coll Nutr* 1996;15:579–585.
246. Stockberger R, Parrot K, Alexander S, et al. Vitamin B-6 status of children undergoing continuous ambulatory peritoneal dialysis. *Nutr Res* 1987;7:1021–1030.
247. Kasama R, Koch T, Canals-Navas C, et al. Vitamin B6 and hemodialysis: the impact of high-flux/high-efficiency dialysis and review of the literature. *Am J Kidney Dis* 1996;27:680–686.
248. Leblanc M, Pichette V, Geadah D, et al. Folic acid and pyridoxal-5′-phosphate losses during high-efficiency hemodialysis in patients without hydrosoluble vitamin supplementation. *J Ren Nutr* 2000;10:196–201.
249. Mydlik M, Derzsiova K, Svac J, et al. Peritoneal clearance and peritoneal transfer of oxalic acid, vitamin C, and vitamin B6 during continuous ambulatory peritoneal dialysis. *Artif Organs* 1998;22:784–788.
250. Mydlik M, Derzsiova K, Zemberova E. Influence of water and sodium diuresis and furosemide on urinary excretion of vitamin B(6), oxalic acid and vitamin C in chronic renal failure. *Miner Electrolyte Metab* 1999;25:352–356.
251. Fortin MC, Amyot SL, Geadah D, et al. Serum concentrations and clearances of folic acid and pyridoxal-5-phosphate during venovenous continuous renal replacement therapy. *Intensive Care Med* 1999;25:594–598.
252. Kleiner MJ, Tate SS, Sullivan JF, et al. Vitamin B6 deficiency in maintenance dialysis patients: metabolic effects of repletion. *Am J Clin Nutr* 1980;33:1612–1619.
253. Mydlik M, Derzsiova K, Zemberova E. Metabolism of vitamin B6 and its requirement in chronic renal failure. *Kidney Int Suppl* 1997;62:S56–S59.
254. Morgan SH, Purkiss P, Watts RW, et al. Oxalate dynamics in chronic renal failure. Comparison with normal subjects and patients with primary hyperoxaluria. *Nephron* 1987;46: 253–257.
255. Marangella M, Petrarulo M, Mandolfo S, et al. Plasma profiles and dialysis kinetics of oxalate in patients receiving hemodialysis. *Nephron* 1992;60:74–80.
256. Worcester EM, Nakagawa Y, Bushinsky DA, et al. Evidence that serum calcium oxalate supersaturation is a consequence of oxalate retention in patients with chronic renal failure. *J Clin Invest* 1986;77:1888–1896.
257. McConnell KN, Rolton HA, Modi KS, et al. Plasma oxalate in patients with chronic renal failure receiving continuous ambulatory peritoneal dialysis or hemodialysis. *Am J Kidney Dis* 1991;18:441–445.
258. Costello JF, Sadovnic MJ, Cottington EM. Plasma oxalate levels rise in hemodialysis patients despite increased oxalate removal. *J Am Soc Nephrol* 1991;1:1289–1298.
259. Boer P, van Leersum L, Hene RJ, et al. Plasma oxalate concentration in chronic renal disease. *Am J Kidney Dis* 1984;4: 118–122.
260. Tomson CR, Channon SM, Ward MK, et al. Plasma oxalate concentration, oxalate clearance and cardiac function in patients receiving haemodialysis. *Nephrol Dial Transplant* 1989;4: 792–799.
261. Thomson C, Weinman E. The secondary oxalosis of renal failure. *Seminars in Dialysis* 1988;1:94–99.
262. Ramsay AG, Reed RG. Oxalate removal by hemodialysis in end-stage renal disease. *Am J Kidney Dis* 1984;4:123–127.
263. Salyer WR, Keren D. Oxalosis as a complication of chronic renal failure. *Kidney Int* 1973;4:61–66.
264. Nakazawa R, Hamaguchi K, Hosaka E, et al. Cutaneous oxalate deposition in a hemodialysis patient. *Am J Kidney Dis* 1995; 25:492–497.
265. op de Hoek CT, Diderich PP, Gratama S, et al. Oxalosis in chronic renal failure. *Proc Eur Dial Transplant Assoc* 1980;17: 730–735.
266. Fayemi AO, Ali M, Braun EV. Oxalosis in hemodialysis patients: a pathologic study of 80 cases. *Arch Pathol Lab Med* 1979;103:58–62.
267. Costello JF, Sadovnic MC, Smith M, et al. Effect of vitamin B6 supplementation on plasma oxalate and oxalate removal rate in hemodialysis patients. *J Am Soc Nephrol* 1992;3:1018–1024.
268. Costello JF, Smith M, Stolarski C, et al. Extrarenal clearance of oxalate increases with progression of renal failure in the rat. *J Am Soc Nephrol* 1992;3:1098–1104.
269. Tomson CR, Channon SM, Parkinson IS, et al. Effect of pyridoxine supplementation on plasma oxalate concentrations in patients receiving dialysis. *Eur J Clin Invest* 1989;19:201–205.
270. Balcke P, Schmidt P, Zazgornik J, et al. Effect of vitamin B6 administration on elevated plasma oxalic acid levels in haemodialysed patients. *Eur J Clin Invest* 1982;12:481–483.
271. Chlebeck PT, Milliner DS, Smith LH. Long-term prognosis in primary hyperoxaluria type II (L-glyceric aciduria). *Am J Kidney Dis* 1994;23:255–259.
272. Yendt ER, Cohanim M. Response to a physiologic dose of pyri-

doxine in type I primary hyperoxaluria. *N Engl J Med* 1985; 312:953–957.
273. Will EJ, Bijvoet OL. Primary oxalosis: clinical and biochemical response to high-dose pyridoxine therapy. *Metabolism* 1979;28: 542–548.
274. Mydlik M, Derzsiova K. Renal replacement therapy and secondary hyperoxalemia in chronic renal failure. *Kidney Int Suppl* 2001;78:S304–S307.
275. Hoppe B, Graf D, Offner G, et al. Oxalate elimination via hemodialysis or peritoneal dialysis in children with chronic renal failure. *Pediatr Nephrol* 1996;10:488–492.
276. Shemin D, Gohh R, Dworkin L. Prevalence and determinants of hyperhomocysteinemia in chronic renal failure (Abstract). *J Am Soc Nephrol* 1994;5:503.
277. Chauveau P, Chadefaux B, Coude M, et al. Long-term folic acid (but not pyridoxine) supplementation lowers elevated plasma homocysteine level in chronic renal failure. *Miner Electrolyte Metab* 1996;22:106–109.
278. Arnadottir M, Brattstrom L, Simonsen O, et al. The effect of high-dose pyridoxine and folic acid supplementation on serum lipid and plasma homocysteine concentrations in dialysis patients. *Clin Nephrol* 1993;40:236–240.
279. Bostom AG, Shemin D, Lapane KL, et al. High dose-B-vitamin treatment of hyperhomocysteinemia in dialysis patients. *Kidney Int* 1996;49:147–152.
280. Touam M, Zingraff J, Jungers P, et al. Effective correction of hyperhomocysteinemia in hemodialysis patients by intravenous folinic acid and pyridoxine therapy. *Kidney Int* 1999;56: 2292–2296.
281. Naruszewicz M, Klinke M, Dziewanowski K, et al. Homocysteine, fibrinogen, and lipoprotein(a) levels are simultaneously reduced in patients with chronic renal failure treated with folic acid, pyridoxine, and cyanocobalamin. *Metabolism* 2001;50: 131–134.
282. Bostom AG, Shemin D, Bagley P, et al. Controlled comparison of L-5-methyltetrahydrofolate versus folic acid for the treatment of hyperhomocysteinemia in hemodialysis patients. *Circulation* 2000;101:2829–2832.
283. Suliman ME, Divino Filho JC, Barany P, et al. Effects of high-dose folic acid and pyridoxine on plasma and erythrocyte sulfur amino acids in hemodialysis patients. *J Am Soc Nephrol* 1999; 10:1287–1296.
284. Chimata M, Masaoka H, Fujimaki M, et al. Low serum aminotransferase activity in patients undergoing regular hemodialysis. *Nippon Jinzo Gakkai Shi* 1994;36:389–395.
285. Ono K, Ono T, Matsumata T. The pathogenesis of decreased aspartate aminotransferase and alanine aminotransferase activity in the plasma of hemodialysis patients: the role of vitamin B6 deficiency. *Clin Nephrol* 1995;43:405–408.
286. Yasuda K, Okuda K, Endo N, et al. Hypoaminotransferasemia in patients undergoing long-term hemodialysis: clinical and biochemical appraisal. *Gastroenterology* 1995;109:1295–1300.
287. Nankivell BJ. Vitamin B6 deficiency on hemodialysis causing sideroblastic anemia. *Nephron* 1991;59:674–675.
288. Toriyama T, Matsuo S, Fukatsu A, et al. Effects of high-dose vitamin B6 therapy on microcytic and hypochromic anemia in hemodialysis patients. *Nippon Jinzo Gakkai Shi* 1993;35: 975–980.
289. Mousson C, Justrabo E, Rifle G, et al. Piridoxilate-induced oxalate nephropathy can lead to end-stage renal failure. *Nephron* 1993;63:104–106.
290. Vigeral P, Kenouch S, Chauveau D, et al. Piridoxilate-associated nephrocalcinosis: a new form of chronic oxalate nephropathy. *Nephrol Dial Transplant* 1987;2:275–278.
291. Schaumburg H, Kaplan J, Windebank A, et al. Sensory neuropathy from pyridoxine abuse. A new megavitamin syndrome. *N Engl J Med* 1983;309:445–448.
292. Parry GJ, Bredesen DE. Sensory neuropathy with low-dose pyridoxine. *Neurology* 1985;35:1466–1468.
293. Levine M. New concepts in the biology and biochemistry of ascorbic acid. *N Engl J Med* 1986;314:892–902.
294. Jacob R. Vitamin C. In: Shills M, Olson JA, Shike M, et al, eds. *Modern Nutrition in Health and Disease*. Baltimore: Williams & Wilkins, 1998.
295. Jacob RA. Assessment of human vitamin C status. *J Nutr* 1990; 120 Suppl 11:1480–1485.
296. Bohm V, Tiroke K, Schneider S, et al. Vitamin C status of patients with chronic renal failure, dialysis patients and patients after renal transplantation. *Int J Vitam Nutr Res* 1997;67: 262–266.
297. Sullivan JF, Eisenstein AB. Ascorbic acid depletion in patients undergoing chronic hemodialysis. *Am J Clin Nutr* 1970;23: 1339–1346.
298. Bakaev VV, Efremov AV, Tityaev II. Low levels of dehydroascorbic acid in uraemic serum and the partial correction of dehydroascorbic acid deficiency by haemodialysis. *Nephrol Dial Transplant* 1999;14:1472–1474.
299. Papastephanidis C, Agroyannis B, Tzanatos-Exarchou H, et al. Re-evaluation of ascorbic acid deficiency in hemodialysed patients. *Int J Artif Organs* 1987;10:163–165.
300. Wang S, Eide TC, Sogn EM, et al. Plasma ascorbic acid in patients undergoing chronic haemodialysis. *Eur J Clin Pharmacol* 1999;55:527–532.
301. Tarng DC, Wei YH, Huang TP, et al. Intravenous ascorbic acid as an adjuvant therapy for recombinant erythropoietin in hemodialysis patients with hyperferritinemia. *Kidney Int* 1999; 55:2477–2486.
302. Ganguly R, Ramirez G, Fuller S, et al. Immunologic competence of hemodialysis patients following withdrawal of vitamin C supplement. *Nephron* 1987;47:299–304.
303. Kopple JD, Swendseid ME. Vitamin nutrition in patients undergoing maintenance hemodialysis. *Kidney Int Suppl* 1975: 79–84.
304. Roob JM, Rabold T, Hayn M, et al. Ex vivo low-density lipoprotein oxidizability and in vivo lipid peroxidation in patients on CAPD. *Kidney Int Suppl* 2001;78:S128–S136.
305. Ihle BU, Gillies M. Scurvy and thrombocytopathy in a chronic hemodialysis patient. *Aust N Z J Med* 1983;13:523.
306. Mitch WE, Johnson MW, Kirshenbaum JM, et al. Effect of large oral doses of ascorbic acid on uric acid excretion by normal subjects. *Clin Pharmacol Ther* 1981;29:318–321.
307. Tsao CS, Salimi SL. Effect of large intake of ascorbic acid on urinary and plasma oxalic acid levels. *Int J Vitam Nutr Res* 1984; 54:245–249.
308. Lawton JM, Conway LT, Crosson JT, et al. Acute oxalate nephropathy after massive ascorbic acid administration. *Arch Intern Med* 1985;145:950–951.
309. Ono K. Secondary hyperoxalemia caused by vitamin C supplementation in regular hemodialysis patients. *Clin Nephrol* 1986; 26:239–243.
310. Rolton HA, McConnell KM, Modi KS, et al. The effect of vitamin C intake on plasma oxalate in patients on regular haemodialysis. *Nephrol Dial Transplant* 1991;6:440–443.
311. Balcke P, Schmidt P, Zazgornik J, et al. Ascorbic acid aggravates secondary hyperoxalemia in patients on chronic hemodialysis. *Ann Intern Med* 1984;101:344–345.
312. Pru C, Eaton J, Kjellstrand C. Vitamin C intoxication and hyperoxalemia in chronic hemodialysis patients. *Nephron* 1985; 39:112–116.
313. Ono K. The effect of vitamin C supplementation and with-

drawal on the mortality and morbidity of regular hemodialysis patients. *Clin Nephrol* 1989;31:31–34.

314. Tomson CR, Channon SM, Parkinson IS, et al. Plasma oxalate in patients receiving continuous ambulatory peritoneal dialysis. *Nephrol Dial Transplant* 1988;3:295–299.
315. Ott SM, Andress DL, Sherrard DJ. Bone oxalate in a long-term hemodialysis patient who ingested high doses of vitamin C. *Am J Kidney Dis* 1986;8:450–454.
316. Friedman AL, Chesney RW, Gilbert EF, et al. Secondary oxalosis as a complication of parenteral alimentation in acute renal failure. *Am J Nephrol* 1983;3:248–252.
317. Swartz RD, Wesley JR, Somermeyer MG, et al. Hyperoxaluria and renal insufficiency due to ascorbic acid administration during total parenteral nutrition. *Ann Intern Med* 1984;100: 530–531.
318. Wandzilak TR, D'Andre SD, Davis PA, et al. Effect of high dose vitamin C on urinary oxalate levels. *J Urol* 1994;151:834–837.
319. Mashour S, Turner JF Jr, Merrell R. Acute renal failure, oxalosis, and vitamin C supplementation: a case report and review of the literature. *Chest* 2000;118:561–563.
320. Giancaspro V, Nuzziello M, Pallotta G, et al. Intravenous ascorbic acid in hemodialysis patients with functional iron deficiency: a clinical trial. *J Nephrol* 2000;13:444–449.
321. Domingo JL, Gomez M, Llobet JM, et al. Influence of citric, ascorbic and lactic acids on the gastrointestinal absorption of aluminum in uremic rats. *Nephron* 1994;66:108–109.
322. Yoshioka M, Aoyama K, Matsushita T. Effects of ascorbic acid on blood pressure and ascorbic acid metabolism in spontaneously hypertensive rats (SH rats). *Int J Vitam Nutr Res* 1985; 55:301–307.
323. Vasdev S, Ford CA, Parai S, et al. Dietary vitamin C supplementation lowers blood pressure in spontaneously hypertensive rats. *Mol Cell Biochem* 2001;218:97–103.
324. Choi ES, McGandy RB, Dallal GE, et al. The prevalence of cardiovascular risk factors among elderly Chinese Americans. *Arch Intern Med* 1990;150:413–418.
325. Halimi JM, Mimran A. Systemic and renal effect of nicotine in non-smokers: influence of vitamin C. *J Hypertens* 2000;18: 1665–1669.
326. Herbert V. Folic acid. In: Shills M, Olson JA, Shike M, et al, eds. *Modern nutrition in health and disease,* 9th ed. Baltimore: Williams & Wilkins, 1998:433–446.
327. Fowler B. The folate cycle and disease in humans. *Kidney Int Suppl* 2001;78:S221–S229.
328. Livant E, Tamura T, Johnston K, et al. Plasma folate conjugase activities and folate concentrations in patients receiving hemodialysis. *J Nutr Biochem* 1994;5:504–508.
329. Devlin AM, Ling EH, Peerson JM, et al. Glutamate carboxypeptidase II: a polymorphism associated with lower levels of serum folate and hyperhomocysteinemia. *Hum Mol Genet* 2000;9: 2837–2844.
330. Said HM, Vaziri ND, Kariger RK, et al. Intestinal absorption of 5-methyltetrahydrofolate in experimental uremia. *Acta Vitaminol Enzymol* 1984;6:339–346.
331. Jennette JC, Goldman ID. Inhibition of the membrane transport of folates by anions retained in uremia. *J Lab Clin Med* 1975;86:834–843.
332. Paine CJ, Hargrove MD Jr, Eichner ER. Folic acid binding protein and folate balance in uremia. *Arch Intern Med* 1976; 136:756–760.
333. Hampers CL, Streiff R, Nathan DG, et al. Megaloblastic hematopoiesis in uremia and in patients on long-term hemodialysis. *N Engl J Med* 1967;276:551–554.
334. Siddiqui J, Freeburger R, Freeman RM. Folic acid, hypersegmented polymorphonuclear leukocytes and the uremic syndrome. *Am J Clin Nutr* 1970;23:11–16.
335. Litwin M, Abuauba M, Wawer ZT, et al. [Sulphur amino acids, vitamin B12 and folic acid in children with chronic renal failure]. *Pol Merkuriusz Lek* 2000;8:268–269.
336. Cunningham J, Sharman VL, Goodwin FJ, et al. Do patients receiving haemodialysis need folic acid supplements? *Br Med J (Clin Res Ed)* 1981;282:1582.
337. Whitehead VM, Comty CH, Posen GA, et al. Homeostasis of folic acid in patients undergoing maintenance hemodialysis. *N Engl J Med* 1968;279:970–974.
338. Sharman VL, Cunningham J, Goodwin FJ, et al. Do patients receiving regular haemodialysis need folic acid supplements? *Br Med J (Clin Res Ed)* 1982;285:96–97.
339. Westhuyzen J, Matherson K, Tracey R, et al. Effect of withdrawal of folic acid supplementation in maintenance hemodialysis patients. *Clin Nephrol* 1993;40:96–99.
340. Zazgornik J, Druml W, Balcke P, et al. Diminished serum folic acid levels in renal transplant recipients. *Clin Nephrol* 1982;18: 306–310.
341. Swainson CP, Winney RJ. Do dialysis patients need extra folate? *Lancet* 1983;1:239.
342. Ono K, Hisasue Y. Is folate supplementation necessary in hemodialysis patients on erythropoietin therapy. *Clin Nephrol* 1992; 38:290–292.
343. Lasseur C, Parrot F, Delmas Y, et al. Impact of high-flux/high-efficiency dialysis on folate and homocysteine metabolism. *J Nephrol* 2001;14:32–35.
344. De Vecchi AF, Bamonti-Catena F, Finazzi S, et al. Homocysteine, vitamin B12, and serum and erythrocyte folate in peritoneal dialysis and hemodialysis patients. *Perit Dial Int* 2000;20: 169–173.
345. Salahudeen AK, Varma SR, Karim T, et al. Anaemia, ferritin, and vitamins in continuous ambulatory peritoneal dialysis. *Lancet* 1988;1:1049.
346. Vychytil A, Fodinger M, Wolfl G, et al. Major determinants of hyperhomocysteinemia in peritoneal dialysis patients. *Kidney Int* 1998;53:1775–1782.
347. Han H, Dwyer JT, Selhub J, et al. Determinants of plasma total homocysteine levels in Korean chronic renal transplant recipients. *J Ren Nutr* 2000;10:202–207.
348. Stein G, Muller A, Busch M, et al. Homocysteine, its metabolites, and B-group vitamins in renal transplant patients. *Kidney Int Suppl* 2001;78:S262–S265.
349. Fodinger M, Buchmayer H, Heinz G, et al. Effect of MTHFR 1298A→C and MTHFR 677C→T genotypes on total homocysteine, folate, and vitamin B(12) plasma concentrations in kidney graft recipients. *J Am Soc Nephrol* 2000;11:1918–1925.
350. Pollock CA, Wyndham R, Collett PV, et al. Effects of erythropoietin therapy on the lipid profile in end-stage renal failure. *Kidney Int* 1994;45:897–902.
351. Arnadottir M, Hultberg B, Berg AL. Plasma total homocysteine concentration in nephrotic patients with idiopathic membranous nephropathy. *Nephrol Dial Transplant* 2001;16:45–47.
352. Chauveau P, Chadefaux B, Coude M, et al. Hyperhomocysteinemia, a risk factor for atherosclerosis in chronic uremic patients. *Kidney Int Suppl* 1993;41:S72–S77.
353. Bostom AG, Kronenberg F, Gohh RY, et al. Chronic renal transplantation: a model for the hyperhomocysteinemia of renal insufficiency. *Atherosclerosis* 2001;156:227–230.
354. Robinson K. Homocysteine, B vitamins, and risk of cardiovascular disease. *Heart* 2000;83:127–130.
355. Hong SY, Yang DH, Chang SK. Plasma homocysteine, vitamin B6, vitamin B12 and folic acid in end-stage renal disease during low-dose supplementation with folic acid. *Am J Nephrol* 1998; 18:367–372.
356. Hultberg B, Andersson A, Arnadottir M. Reduced, free and total fractions of homocysteine and other thiol compounds in

plasma from patients with renal failure. *Nephron* 1995;70: 62–67.
357. Jungers P, Chauveau P, Bandin O, et al. Hyperhomocysteinemia is associated with atherosclerotic occlusive arterial accidents in predialysis chronic renal failure patients. *Miner Electrolyte Metab* 1997;23:170–173.
358. Klusmann A, Ivens K, Schadewaldt P, et al. [Is homocysteine a risk factor for coronary heart disease in patients with terminal renal failure?]. *Med Klin* 2000;95:189–194.
359. Thambyrajah J, Landray MJ, McGlynn FJ, et al. Does folic acid decrease plasma homocysteine and improve endothelial function in patients with predialysis renal failure? *Circulation* 2000;102:871–875.
360. Wilcken DE, Dudman NP, Tyrrell PA, et al. Folic acid lowers elevated plasma homocysteine in chronic renal insufficiency: possible implications for prevention of vascular disease. *Metabolism* 1988;37:697–701.
361. van Guldener C, Janssen MJ, Lambert J, et al. Folic acid treatment of hyperhomocysteinemia in peritoneal dialysis patients: no change in endothelial function after long-term therapy. *Perit Dial Int* 1998;18:282–289.
362. De Vecchi AF, Bamonti-Catena F, Finazzi S, et al. Homocysteine, vitamin B12, serum and erythrocyte folate in peritoneal dialysis patients. *Clin Nephrol* 2001;55:313–317.
363. Smolin LA, Laidlaw SA, Kopple JD. Altered plasma free and protein-bound sulfur amino acid levels in patients undergoing maintenance hemodialysis. *Am J Clin Nutr* 1987;45:737–743.
364. Brunetti M, Terracina L, Timio M, et al. Plasma sulfate concentration and hyperhomocysteinemia in hemodialysis patients. *J Nephrol* 2001;14:27–31.
365. Arnadottir M, Hultberg B, Vladov V, et al. Hyperhomocysteinemia in cyclosporine-treated renal transplant recipients. *Transplantation* 1996;61:509–512.
366. Ducloux D, Fournier V, Rebibou JM, et al. Hyperhomocyst(e)inemia in renal transplant recipients with and without cyclosporine. *Clin Nephrol* 1998;49:232–235.
367. Machado DJ, Paula FJ, Sabbaga E, et al. Hyperhomocyst(e)inemia in chronic stable renal transplant patients. *Rev Hosp Clin Fac Med Sao Paulo* 2000;55:161–168.
368. Arnadottir M, Hultberg B, Wahlberg J, et al. Serum total homocysteine concentration before and after renal transplantation. *Kidney Int* 1998;54:1380–1384.
369. Refsum H, Guttormsen AB, Fiskerstrand T, et al. Hyperhomocysteinemia in terms of steady-state kinetics. *Eur J Pediatr* 1998; 157 Suppl 2:S45–S49.
370. Moustapha A, Gupta A, Robinson K, et al. Prevalence and determinants of hyperhomocysteinemia in hemodialysis and peritoneal dialysis. *Kidney Int* 1999;55:1470–1475.
371. Clarke R, Stansbie D. Assessment of homocysteine as a cardiovascular risk factor in clinical practice. *Ann Clin Biochem* 2001; 38:624–632.
372. Boushey CJ, Beresford SA, Omenn GS, et al. A quantitative assessment of plasma homocysteine as a risk factor for vascular disease. Probable benefits of increasing folic acid intakes. *JAMA* 1995;274:1049–1057.
373. Bachmann J, Tepel M, Raidt H, et al. Hyperhomocysteinemia and the risk for vascular disease in hemodialysis patients. *J Am Soc Nephrol* 1995;6:121–125.
374. Robinson K, Gupta A, Dennis V, et al. Hyperhomocysteinemia confers an independent increased risk of atherosclerosis in end-stage renal disease and is closely linked to plasma folate and pyridoxine concentrations. *Circulation* 1996;94:2743–2748.
375. Nygard O, Nordrehaug JE, Refsum H, et al. Plasma homocysteine levels and mortality in patients with coronary artery disease. *N Engl J Med* 1997;337:230–236.
376. Pinto X, Vilaseca MA, Garcia-Giralt N, et al. Homocysteine and the MTHFR 677C→T allele in premature coronary artery disease. Case control and family studies. *Eur J Clin Invest* 2001; 31:24–30.
377. Morris MS, Jacques PF, Rosenberg IH, et al. Hyperhomocysteinemia associated with poor recall in the third National Health and Nutrition Examination Survey. *Am J Clin Nutr* 2001;73: 927–933.
378. Sakurabayashi T, Fujimoto M, Takaesu Y, et al. Association between plasma homocysteine concentration and carotid atherosclerosis in hemodialysis patients. *Jpn Circ J* 1999;63: 692–696.
379. Manns BJ, Burgess ED, Hyndman ME, et al. Hyperhomocyst(e)inemia and the prevalence of atherosclerotic vascular disease in patients with end-stage renal disease. *Am J Kidney Dis* 1999; 34:669–677.
380. Gale CR, Ashurst H, Phillips NJ, et al. Renal function, plasma homocysteine and carotid atherosclerosis in elderly people. *Atherosclerosis* 2001;154:141–146.
381. Moustapha A, Naso A, Nahlawi M, et al. Prospective study of hyperhomocysteinemia as an adverse cardiovascular risk factor in end-stage renal disease. *Circulation* 1998;97:138–141.
382. Bostom AG, Shemin D, Verhoef P, et al. Elevated fasting total plasma homocysteine levels and cardiovascular disease outcomes in maintenance dialysis patients. A prospective study. *Arterioscler Thromb Vasc Biol* 1997;17:2554–2558.
383. Tamura T, Bergman SM, Morgan SL. Homocysteine, B vitamins, and vascular-access thrombosis in patients treated with hemodialysis. *Am J Kidney Dis* 1998;32:475–481.
384. House AA, Wells GA, Donnelly JG, et al. Randomized trial of high-flux vs low-flux haemodialysis: effects on homocysteine and lipids. *Nephrol Dial Transplant* 2000;15:1029–1034.
385. Biasioli S, Schiavon R, Petrosino L, et al. Do different dialytic techniques have different atherosclerotic and antioxidant activities? *Asaio J* 2001;47:516–521.
386. Van Tellingen A, Grooteman MP, Bartels PC, et al. Long-term reduction of plasma homocysteine levels by super-flux dialyzers in hemodialysis patients. *Kidney Int* 2001;59:342–347.
387. Hirose S, Kim S, Matsuda A, et al. [Effects of folic acid supplementation on hyperhomocysteinemia in CAPD patients: effects on unsaturated fatty acids]. *Nippon Jinzo Gakkai Shi* 1998;40: 8–16.
388. Bostom AG, Shemin D, Gohh RY, et al. Treatment of hyperhomocysteinemia in hemodialysis patients and renal transplant recipients. *Kidney Int Suppl* 2001;78:S246–S252.
389. Arnadottir M, Gudnason V, Hultberg B. Treatment with different doses of folic acid in haemodialysis patients: effects on folate distribution and aminothiol concentrations. *Nephrol Dial Transplant* 2000;15:524–528.
390. Dierkes J, Domrose U, Ambrosch A, et al. Response of hyperhomocysteinemia to folic acid supplementation in patients with end-stage renal disease. *Clin Nephrol* 1999;51:108–115.
391. Janssen MJ, van den Berg M, van Guldener C, et al. Withdrawal of folic acid supplementation in maintenance hemodialysis patients. *Clin Nephrol* 1994;42:136–137.
392. van Guldener C, Robinson K. Homocysteine and renal disease. *Semin Thromb Hemost* 2000;26:313–324.
393. Stanford JL, Molina H, Phillips J, et al. Oral folate reduces plasma homocyst(e)ine levels in hemodialysis patients with cardiovascular disease. *Cardiovasc Surg* 2000;8:567–571.
394. McGregor D, Shand B, Lynn K. A controlled trial of the effect of folate supplements on homocysteine, lipids and hemorheology in end-stage renal disease. *Nephron* 2000;85:215–220.
395. Yango A, Shemin D, Hsu N, et al. Rapid communication: L-folinic acid versus folic acid for the treatment of hyperhomocysteinemia in hemodialysis patients. *Kidney Int* 2001;59: 324–327.

396. Sunder-Plassmann G, Fodinger M, Buchmayer H, et al. Effect of high dose folic acid therapy on hyperhomocysteinemia in hemodialysis patients: results of the Vienna multicenter study. *J Am Soc Nephrol* 2000;11:1106–1116.
397. Hauser AC, Hagen W, Rehak PH, et al. Efficacy of folinic versus folic acid for the correction of hyperhomocysteinemia in hemodialysis patients. *Am J Kidney Dis* 2001;37:758–765.
398. Bostom AG, Gohh RY, Beaulieu AJ, et al. Treatment of hyperhomocysteinemia in renal transplant recipients. A randomized, placebo-controlled trial. *Ann Intern Med* 1997;127:1089–1092.
399. Bostom AG, Gohh RY, Tsai MY, et al. Excess prevalence of fasting and postmethionine-loading hyperhomocysteinemia in stable renal transplant recipients. *Arterioscler Thromb Vasc Biol* 1997;17:1894–1900.
400. Bostom AG, Shemin D, Yoburn D, et al. Lack of effect of oral N-acetylcysteine on the acute dialysis-related lowering of total plasma homocysteine in hemodialysis patients. *Atherosclerosis* 1996;120:241–244.
401. Mangiarotti G, Canavese C, Salomone M, et al. Hypervitaminosis B12 in maintenance hemodialysis patients receiving massive supplementation of vitamin B12. *Int J Artif Organs* 1986;9: 417–420.
402. Minar E, Zazgornik J, Bayer PM, et al. [Hematologic changes in patients under long-term hemodialysis and hemofiltration treatment with special reference to serum concentrations of folic acid and vitamin B 12]. *Schweiz Med Wochenschr* 1984;114: 48–53.
403. Weir D, Scott J. Vitamin B12 "Cobalamin." In: Shills M, Olson JA, Shike M, et al, eds. *Modern nutrition in health and disease.* Baltimore, 1998:447–458.
404. Litwin M, Abuauba M, Wawer ZT, et al. Folate, vitamin B12, and sulfur amino acid levels in patients with renal failure. *Pediatr Nephrol* 2001;16:127–132.
405. Rostand SG. Vitamin B12 levels and nerve conduction velocities in patients undergoing maintenance hemodialysis. *Am J Clin Nutr* 1976;29:691–697.
406. Dierkes J, Domrose U, Ambrosch A, et al. Supplementation with vitamin B12 decreases homocysteine and methylmalonic acid but also serum folate in patients with end-stage renal disease. *Metabolism* 1999;48:631–635.
407. Bastow MD, Woods HF, Walls J. Persistent anemia associated with reduced serum vitamin B12 levels in patients undergoing regular hemodialysis therapy. *Clin Nephrol* 1979;11:133–135.
408. Moelby L, Rasmussen K, Ring T, et al. Relationship between methylmalonic acid and cobalamin in uremia. *Kidney Int* 2000; 57:265–273.
409. Chandna SM, Tattersall JE, Nevett G, et al. Low serum vitamin B12 levels in chronic high-flux haemodialysis patients. *Nephron* 1997;75:259–263.
410. Kuwabara S, Nakazawa R, Azuma N, et al. Intravenous methylcobalamin treatment for uremic and diabetic neuropathy in chronic hemodialysis patients. *Intern Med* 1999;38:472–475.
411. Lee HA, Choi JS, Ha KS, et al. Influence of 5,10-methylenetetrahydrofolate reductase gene polymorphism on plasma homocysteine concentration in patients with end-stage renal disease. *Am J Kidney Dis* 1999;34:259–263.
412. Hoffer LJ, Bank I, Hongsprabhas P, et al. A tale of two homocysteines—and two hemodialysis units. *Metabolism* 2000;49: 215–219.
413. Kaplan LN, Mamer OA, Hoffer LJ. Parenteral vitamin B12 reduces hyperhomocysteinemia in end-stage renal disease. *Clin Invest Med* 2001;24:5–11.
414. Taniguchi H, Ejiri K, Baba S. Improvement of autonomic neuropathy after mecobalamin treatment in uremic patients on hemodialysis. *Clin Ther* 1987;9:607–614.
415. Cervantes-Laurean D, McElvaney G, Moss J. Niacin. In: Shills M, Olson JA, Shike M, et al, eds. *Modern nutrition in health and disease.* Baltimore: Williams & Wilkins, 1998:401–411.
416. Henkin Y, Oberman A, Hurst DC, et al. Niacin revisited: clinical observations on an important but underutilized drug. *Am J Med* 1991;91:239–246.
417. Saika Y, Kodama N, Kimura K, et al. [Plasma nicotinic acid levels in hemodialysis patients after the administration of niceritrol]. *Nippon Jinzo Gakkai Shi* 1999;41:430–435.
418. Lal SM, Hewett JE, Petroski GF, et al. Effects of nicotinic acid and lovastatin in renal transplant patients: a prospective, randomized, open-labeled crossover trial. *Am J Kidney Dis* 1995; 25:616–622.
419. Tanaka K. New light on biotin deficiency. *N Engl J Med* 1981; 304:839–840.
420. Braguer D, Gallice P, Yatzidis H, et al. Restoration by biotin of the in vitro microtubule formation inhibited by uremic toxins. *Nephron* 1991;57:192–196.
421. Mock D. Biotin. In: Shills M, Olson JA, Shike M, et al, eds. *Modern nutrition in health and disease.* Baltimore: Williams & Wilkins, 1998:459–466.
422. Said HM, Vaziri ND, Oveisi F, et al. Effect of chronic renal failure on intestinal transport of biotin in the rat. *J Lab Clin Med* 1992;120:471–475.
423. Jung U, Helbich-Endermann M, Bitsch R, et al. Are patients with chronic renal failure (CRF) deficient in Biotin and is regular Biotin supplementation required? *Z Ernahrungswiss* 1998; 37:363–367.
424. Livaniou E, Evangelatos GP, Ithakissios DS, et al. Serum biotin levels in patients undergoing chronic hemodialysis. *Nephron* 1987;46:331–332.
425. Yatzidis H, Koutsicos D, Alaveras AG, et al. Biotin for neurologic disorders of uremia. *N Engl J Med* 1981;305:764.
426. Jones W, Nidus B. Biotin and hiccups in chronic dialysis patients. *J Renal Nutr* 1991;1:80–83.
427. Koutsikos D, Fourtounas C, Agroyannis B, et al. Glucose metabolism in normoglucaemic haemodialysis patients: a possible role for biotin? *Nephrol Dial Transplant* 1995;10:1256–1257.
428. Plesofsky-Vig N. Pantothenic acid. In: Shills M, Olson JA, Shike M, et al, eds. *Modern nutrition in health and disease.* Baltimore: Williams & Wilkins, 1998:423–432.
429. Fry PC, Fox HM, Tao HG. Metabolic response to a pantothenic acid deficient diet in humans. *J Nutr Sci Vitaminol* 1976;22: 339–346.
430. Janssen MJ, van Guldener C, de Jong GM, et al. Folic acid treatment of hyperhomocysteinemia in dialysis patients. *Miner Electrolyte Metab* 1996;22:110–114.
431. van Guldener C, Lambert J, ter Wee PM, et al. Carotid artery stiffness in patients with end-stage renal disease: no effect of long-term homocysteine-lowering therapy. *Clin Nephrol* 2000; 53:33–41.
432. Schroder CH, de Boer AW, Giesen AM, et al. Treatment of hyperhomocysteinemia in children on dialysis by folic acid. *Pediatr Nephrol* 1999;13:583–585.
433. House AA, Donnelly JG. Effect of multivitamins on plasma homocysteine and folate levels in patients on hemodialysis. *Asaio J* 1999;45:94–97.
434. Dierkes J, Domrose U, Bosselmann KP, et al. Homocysteine lowering effect of different multivitamin preparations in patients with end-stage renal disease. *J Ren Nutr* 2001;11:67–72.
435. Beaulieu AJ, Gohh RY, Han H, et al. Enhanced reduction of fasting total homocysteine levels with supraphysiological versus standard multivitamin dose folic acid supplementation in renal transplant recipients. *Arterioscler Thromb Vasc Biol* 1999;19: 2918–2921.

21

CARNITINE IN RENAL FAILURE

GIANFRANCO GUARNIERI
GIANNI BIOLO
GABRIELE TOIGO
ROBERTA SITULIN

Carnitine is a water-soluble zwitterionic quaternary amine (β-hydroxy-gamma trimethylaminobutyric acid, molecular weight: 161.2 daltons), biologically active only in the "L" isoform, which is a natural constituent of cells of animal origin (from prokaryotic to eukaryotic ones) (1). L-carnitine is involved in the transesterification reactions, catalyzed by a number of carnitine acyltransferase enzymes, which allow the reversible transfer of fatty acids from coenzyme A (CoA) to the carnitine hydroxyl:

$$\text{Carnitine} + \text{Acyl-CoA} \rightleftarrows \text{Acyl-carnitine} + \text{CoA}$$

By these reactions carnitine can exert its roles in the regulation of several metabolic pathways, in the maintenance of a normal structure of cell membrane phospholipids (as has been shown in erythrocytes) and in the removal of acyl moieties excess (1–9). Disease states characterized by inborn errors of carnitine metabolism were first described in 1973 (7). Besides the use of carnitine therapy in these specific clinical conditions, the study of the effects of carnitine supplementation in several situations of carnitine insufficiency is still an area of growing interest in sports medicine (e.g., to improve performance), cardiology (e.g., to protect the ischemic heart from reperfusion injury or to treat patients with angina), neurology (e.g., to improve mental function in Alzheimer's disease), infectious diseases (e.g., to improve immune defense in patients with the human immunodeficiency virus), and nephrology (e.g., to improve anemia in patients undergoing hemodialysis) (1,5,7,10).

This chapter will review the metabolism of carnitine in the physiologic state and describe the conditions of carnitine deficiencies and insufficiencies. It then will focus on carnitine pathophysiology in uremia and on the effects of carnitine supplementation in patients undergoing dialysis.

CARNITINE METABOLISM AND FUNCTION IN THE NORMAL INDIVIDUAL

Biosynthesis, Intake, Transport, and Excretion

Carnitine homeostasis depends on the equilibrium among endogenous biosynthesis, dietary intake, efficiency of renal reabsorption, and transmembrane transport exchange (Fig. 21.1).

Biosynthesis

In humans, carnitine is synthesized in the liver, brain, and kidney, starting with protein-bound lysine, at a rate of up to 1.2 μmol/kg body weight/day (Fig. 21.1) (1,2,5,7). The lysine residues are three-methylated, and the methyl groups are provided by three methionine molecules. After protein hydrolysis, trimethyllysine undergoes other reactions before finally being converted into butyrobetaine by the enzyme butyrobetaine hydroxylase. Skeletal and heart muscles cannot synthesize carnitine because they lack this final enzyme step. Therefore, these tissues are entirely dependent on carnitine uptake from the blood. The biosynthesis of carnitine is also dependent on a number of cofactors such as Fe^{2+} (iron), niacin, ascorbate, pyridoxal phosphate, and 2-oxoglutarate. However, the synthesis rate seems to be regulated only by the availability of trimethyllysine (7).

Dietary Intake and Absorption

Major dietary sources of carnitine are meat, poultry, fish, and dairy products (1). Darker meats, compared to white meats, have a higher carnitine content. Vegetables contain limited amounts of carnitine. A typical omnivorous diet provides from 100 up to 1,000 μmol/day, whereas a vegetarian diet contains only 50 to 100 μmol/day (Fig. 21.1). Nonetheless, the latter diet usually provides enough precursor lysine and methionine to support endogenous carnitine synthesis adequately. In vegetarian adults, plasma carnitine levels are about 10% lower than in omnivorous subjects (1). Normally, about 60% to 75% of the carnitine present in a mixed diet rapidly is absorbed from the intestinal lumen across the mucosal membrane by passive- and active-transport mechanisms. However, in the case of oral carnitine supplementation the bioavailability of this compound decreases to 15% or less (11). The absorbed carnitine reaches the liver through the portal bed and is released into the

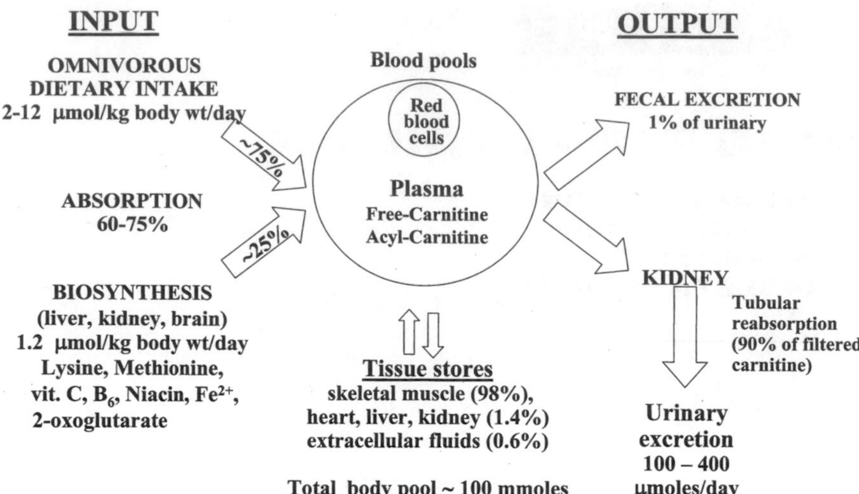

FIGURE 21.1. Carnitine metabolism in normal subjects.

systemic circulation to be taken up by the tissues. The rate of endogenous carnitine synthesis is inversely related to the amount of absorbed dietary carnitine. In the absence of dietary carnitine intake, carnitine requirements are fulfilled completely by endogenous biosynthesis.

Plasma and Tissue Carnitine Levels

Specific transport systems located at the cell membrane levels actively take up carnitine from the extracellular space and maintain a concentration gradient between the extracellular and intracellular pools ranging from 10-fold to 100-fold in the different tissues (2,3,5,7). In the fasting state, carnitine uptake by the liver is increased. Skeletal muscle contains the largest carnitine pool in the body, accounting for about 98% of the total carnitine pool (i.e., about 90 and about 110 mmol in women and men, respectively) (3,5,7).

The liver, kidney, and heart account for about 1.4% of total carnitine; the remaining 0.6% can be found in plasma and in the other extracellular fluids. In all intracellular and extracellular compartments, carnitine is present both in the free and in the esterified (acyl) form. The proportion of esterified carnitine may vary considerably with nutritional conditions, exercise level, and disease states. Under normal conditions acylcarnitine esters account for about 18.5% of total carnitine in serum, about 13% in muscle and liver, and as much as 50% to 60% in the urine. Therefore, carnitine fractions appear to be highly compartmentalized in the human body. The kinetics of carnitine exchange between plasma and the intracellular carnitine pools vary in the different tissues (5,10,12,13). The liver is characterized by very fast carnitine exchange kinetics with plasma, whereas in skeletal muscle such exchange is very slow. For this reason, the concentrations of plasma carnitine fractions may reflect more the liver carnitine–acylcarnitine distribution than the muscle pattern.

Renal Excretion

Plasma carnitine levels mainly are regulated by the kinetics of carnitine reabsorption by the kidney (2,3,5,7,14). At normal plasma concentrations, the proximal renal tubule reabsorbs more than 90% of filtered carnitine. The apparent renal excretory threshold for free carnitine is 40 micromol/L, which is close to the normal plasma carnitine concentration (i.e., 50 μmol/L). The percentage distribution of total urinary carnitine in normal subjects was found to be about 45% for free carnitine, about 10% for acetylcarnitine, about 30% for short-chain acylcarnitines, and 15% for long-chain acylcarnitines (3). The mean tubular maximum for total carnitine reabsorption is 74 micromol/L of glomerular filtration rate (GFR) and is reached at a plasma concentration of 126 micromol/L (2). The renal clearance of acylcarnitines is four to eight times higher than that of free carnitine because of the preferential tubular reabsorption of free carnitine; therefore, the acyl to free carnitine ratio in the urine of healthy subjects is around 1, whereas the same ratio in plasma is about 0.2 to 0.3 (2,3). In states of increased lipolysis, accelerated ketogenesis or protein catabolism (e.g., starvation, insulin deficiency, cortisol excess, strenuous exercise, hyperthyroidism, trauma, sepsis, burns, surgery), the urinary excretion of both free and esterified carnitine is increased (3).

THE PHYSIOLOGIC ROLE OF CARNITINE

The carnitine system refers to the free and esterified carnitines and the carnitine-related enzymes (1,5,7,8,9). The acylcarnitine translocases are involved in the transport of carnitine or acylcarnitines across the inner mitochondrial membranes. The carnitine acyltransferases, located at different cellular sites, are involved in the transesterification reactions. They are characterized by substrate specificities for the fatty acids of different chain length, with some overlap among the various forms. Eight different mammalian carnitine acyltransferases have been characterized. Five of them have been cloned and sequenced (8). These enzymes allow the exchange of acyl moieties among at least four distinct intracellular pools of acyl-CoA (i.e., the cytosol, the endoplasmic reticulum, the peroxisomes, and the mitochondrial matrix). This mechanism allows substrate exchange among the lipid metabolic pathways located in different cellular compartments. The acetyltransferases react with short-chain acyl-esters. The mitochondrial long-chain acyltransferases generally are called carnitine palmitoyl transferases (CPT). There are two membrane-bound enzymes, CPT-I and CPT-II, located in the inner sites of the outer and the inner mitochondrial membranes, respectively. Only CPT-I is sensitive to the malonyl-CoA–inhibitory action. The peroxisomal acyltransferases, also named octanoyltransferases, have greater specificity for the medium-chain fatty acids, whereas the peroxisomal acetyltransferase is specific for the short-chain fatty acids. In the peroxisomes the incomplete oxidation of very long–chain fatty acids takes place. The peroxisomal acyltransferases together with the peroxisomal acetyltransferases allow the transport of the partially oxidized shortened fatty acids from the peroxisomes to the mitochondria, where their oxidation is completed (2,5,7). The oxidation is possible even if the translocases are saturated because the medium- and the short-chain fatty acids can cross the mitochondrial membranes without being carried by carnitine.

The carnitine system is involved in the following physiologic functions:

- Transport of long-chain fatty acids into the mitochondrial matrix for β-oxidation to provide cellular energy (Fig. 21.2) (1,2,5,7,9). The inner mitochondrial mem brane is impermeable to CoA esters, so the transport of the activated long-chain fatty acids, as carnitine esters, in the mitochondrial matrix is essential to fuel β-oxidation. CPT-I exchanges the acyl moieties of acyl-CoAs with carnitine. These acylcarnitines are transported across the inner mitochondrial membrane into the matrix by the translocase through a 1:1 exchange with free carnitine. Then, CPT II converts the acylcarnitines back to acyl-CoAs. The acetyl-CoA produced from the β-oxidation reactions can enter the citric-acid cycle to complete the fatty-acid oxidation process. In skeletal and heart muscles β-oxidation and the citric-acid cycle are strictly associated, like in a cog wheel, whereas in the liver the acetyl-CoA also can be used for ketone body synthesis. The K_m of CPT I and II increase with higher cytoplasmic long-chain acyl-CoA concentrations. This allows a slower entrance of fatty acid into the mitochondria, thereby avoiding excessive mitochondrial free CoA consumption. Carnitine (through the action of a carnitine acetyltransferase) also may shuttle acetyl groups from the mitochondria and the peroxisomes into the cytosol, where fatty-acid and triglyceride synthesis take place. The carnitine-mediated transport of acetyl-CoA from the mitochondria

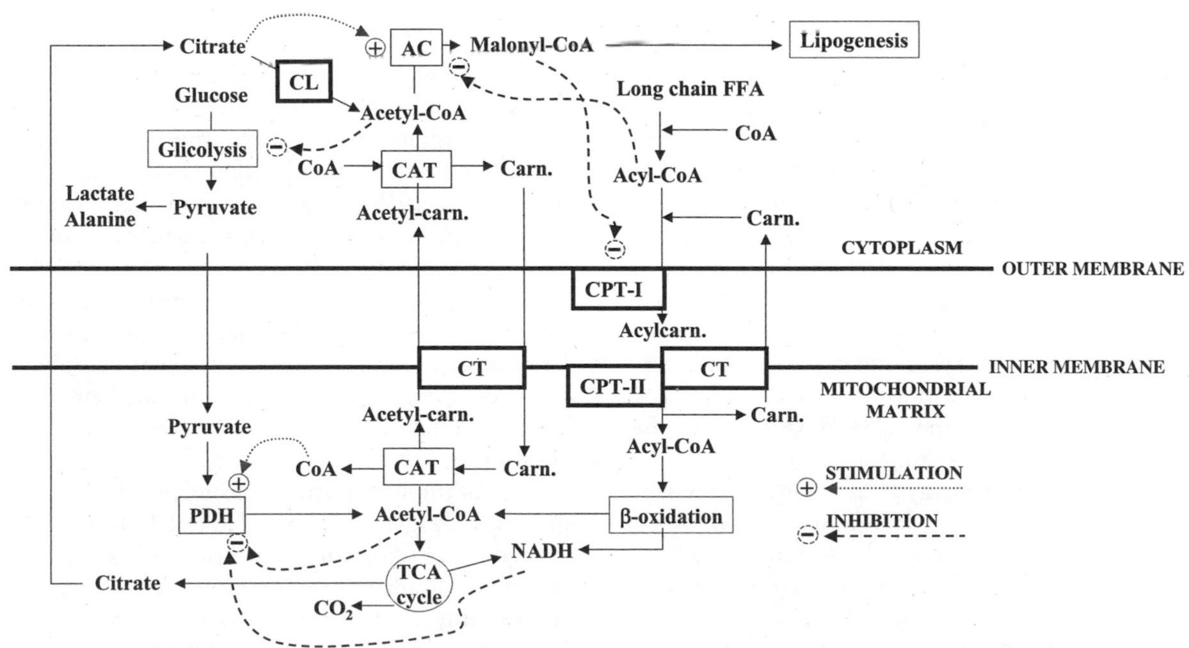

FIGURE 21.2. Free fatty-acid–glucose interactions and the carnitine system. Carn., L-carnitine; FFA, free fatty acids; TCA, tricarboxylic acids; PDH, pyruvate dehydrogenase; CT, carnitine-acylcarnitine translocase; CAT, carnitine acyltransferase; AC, acetyl-CoA carboxylase; CPT, carnitine palmitoyl transferase; CL, citrate lyase.

to the cytosol is inexpensive because it does not utilize energy, unlike the citrate pathway, which requires adenosine triphosphate (ATP) (Fig. 21.2). In the cytoplasm, acetyl-CoA can be converted to malonyl-CoA through the action of the acetyl-CoA carboxylase. Increased levels of malonyl-CoA inhibit CPT-I activity and esterified fatty-acid transport into the mitochondria, thereby favoring fatty-acid synthesis in the cytoplasm (7,9).

- Transport of partially oxidized fatty-acid from peroxisomes to mitochondria (see earlier).
- Modulation of the intramitochondrial acyl-CoA/free CoA ratio (2,3,5,7,8). In the mitochondria short- and medium-chain fatty acids can accumulate as a result of normal or abnormal metabolism. Carnitine can reduce the acyl-CoA/CoA ratio by exporting them from the mitochondria into the cytosol. Thus, by buffering CoA availability, carnitine can exert a regulatory role in the numerous CoA-dependent metabolic pathways (3,8). By this mechanism carnitine regulates β-oxidation itself at the level of the thiolase or the activation of fatty acid by acyl-CoA synthetase, the citric acid cycle at the level of 2-oxoglutarate dehydrogenases, the oxidative decarboxylation of lactate/pyruvate at the level of the pyruvate dehydrogenase complex, and the catabolism of many amino acids. Therefore carnitine can increase pyruvate dehydrogenase activity, improve insulin-mediated glucose utilization, and reduce lactate production. Such carnitine action of buffering the acyl-CoA/CoA ratio is especially important whenever the availability of acyl-CoA esters is higher than their utilization in the citric-acid cycle (7). This condition can be observed in the liver during starvation, in skeletal muscle during exercise, and possibly during hemodialysis (3).
- Export from the mitochondria of the branched-chain acyl groups. This process is critical in the catabolism of the branched-chain amino acids and may secondarily contribute to the regulation of protein kinetics (5).
- Detoxifying action. Carnitine is involved in the trapping and excretion of unphysiologic acyl groups, such as valproic acid and those that accumulate in organic acid disorders (5,7). Acyl groups at lower levels exert toxic effects on the cells through enzyme inhibition (e.g., adenine nucleotide transferase), and acyl groups at higher concentrations exert a detergentlike action (7). Carnitine acts as a sink and allows a shift of the "acyl pressure" from the mitochondria to the cytoplasm.
- Storage and transport of energy. Tissue carnitine content is much higher than tissue CoA content. Thus, acylcarnitines may serve as storage of acyl moieties ready to form the energy-rich acyl-CoA without any further ATP need (2,5,7). Cytoplasmic acylcarnitines also may leave the cells, enter the bloodstream, and reach other tissues. Therefore, it has been suggested that carnitine is also important for energy transport between different compartments within a cell and between different tissues. The erythrocyte acylcarnitine pool may represent an important reservoir of stored energy (15).
- Regulation of membrane phospholipids. Carnitine may serve as a transporter and reservoir of the fatty acids needed for the synthesis of membrane phospholipids and their repair (e.g., after oxidative damage) (4).
- Other functions. Carnitine also has osmolyte functions that might be relevant for the protection of cells and tissues from osmotic stress (16). In the endoplasmic reticulum carnitine is involved in the acylation-deacylation of such lipoproteins as very–low-density lipoproteins (VLDLs) or of phospholipids (6). Carnitine might have a regulatory role in cytokine production and function and is potentially useful in systemic inflammatory conditions (7,17). Experimental evidence also suggests that carnitine may improve sperm count and sperm motility (7). Carnitine can be detected at the nuclear level, where it could influence gene transcription by modulating acyl-CoA content (18).

CARNITINE DEFICIENCY AND INSUFFICIENCY

Carnitine *deficiency* indicates conditions in which carnitine concentrations in plasma or tissues are below the requirements for the normal function of the organism. Carnitine *insufficiency* indicates conditions in which there is a relative lack of carnitine compared to an increased metabolic need.

Carnitine deficiencies can be primary (systemic and myopathic) or secondary (7). Primary carnitine deficiencies are the consequence of alterations in the intestinal, renal, or intracellular transport of carnitine or rarely decreased carnitine synthesis as a result of genetic disorders. Secondary deficiency can be the consequence of genetically determined metabolic errors involving excessive production of short-chain organic acids or of acquired conditions (7). These may involve a decreased biosynthesis (e.g., liver cirrhosis, chronic renal disease, extreme prematurity), a decreased intake (malnutrition, vegetarian diets), increased requirements (pregnancy, puerperium, severe trauma or infections, burns), or increased losses (Fanconi's syndrome, renal tubular acidosis, hypercatabolism). Iatrogenic conditions of carnitine deficiency or insufficiency include hemodialysis and administration of valproic acid, pivalic acid derivatives, and zidovudine.

In conditions of carnitine insufficiency an excess of acyl groups, arising from either decreased β-oxidation or increased fatty-acid administration or production, overwhelms the availability of free CoA. Consequently, the acyl/free carnitine ratio increases because a larger amount of free carnitine is esterified to acylcarnitines to "buffer" the excess of acyl groups (2,3,5,7). In these situations carnitine supplements may contribute to regenerate the sequestrated free CoA, thereby maintaining normal metabolic processes.

TABLE 21.1. SERUM CARNITINE LEVELS IN PATIENTS WITH CHRONIC UREMIA

	Conservative Treatment	MHD	CAPD
Total car	↑	↔	↔
Free car	↑	↓	↓
Acyl car	↑	↑	↑
SCAC		↑	
LCAC		↔	
Free car/Total car	↓	↓	↓
Free car/Acyl car	↓	↓	↓

MHD, maintenance hemodialysis; CAPD, continuous ambulatory peritoneal dialysis; ↑, increased versus control group; ↓, decreased versus control group; ↔, unchanged versus control group; car, carnitine; SCAC, short-chain acylcarnitine; LCAC, long-chain acylcarnitine.

The potential consequences of carnitine deficiency/insufficiency are the following: (a) accumulation in the cells of toxic acyl moieties that may have a detergentlike action; (b) accumulation of acetyl-CoA in the mitochondria, which has been shown to inhibit several enzymes (see earlier); (c) impaired export of the excess of organic acids; (d) reduced efficiency of energy production from lipids and glucose; (e) impaired amino acid metabolism (mainly of the branched-chain amino acids) and, possibly, worsening nitrogen balance.

ABNORMALITIES OF CARNITINE METABOLISM IN THE PATIENT WITH UREMIA

In uremia carnitine homeostasis is altered. There also are disturbances not only in the plasma and tissue absolute carnitine levels but also in the relative proportions of the different carnitine fractions (Tables 21.1 and 21.2) (3,7,19–22).

In chronically uremic patients receiving conservative treatment, carnitine clearance decreases proportionally to the decline in GFR (20). Consequently, the concentrations of all plasma carnitine fractions may be increased slightly. The relative proportion of acylcarnitines to free carnitine increases because deterioration of renal function is associated with a reduction in the tubular excretion of the esterified fraction. In addition, during caloric deprivation these patients exhibit an exaggerated increase in the plasma short-chain acylcarnitines that is paralleled by a blunted ketone body production (23). These findings suggest an abnormal handling of long-chain fatty acids in these noncarnitine-depleted patients. We previously have observed a reduced utilization of exogenously administered acetate and pyruvate in chronically uremic patients, and this suggests that the defect may be at the level of acetyl-CoA disposal (24).

In patients undergoing maintenance hemodialysis, predialysis serum levels of total carnitine are normal or increased, whereas free carnitine is reduced and acylcarnitines (especially the short-chain acylcarnitines) are increased (3, 19–22). Consequently, the ratio between acylcarnitines and free carnitine is increased greatly (above 0.4). This ratio has been proposed as a clinical indicator of carnitine insufficiency. Nonetheless, plasma carnitine levels are not always representative of tissue carnitine content, especially that of skeletal muscle (10). In this latter tissue total carnitine levels have been found to be either normal or low. In fact, whereas muscle free carnitine concentrations usually are reduced, acylcarnitines may be either increased or reduced (3,20,21, 25–28). Such discrepancies may be because the carnitine values assessed by various authors are difficult to compare mainly because of the differences in the measured fractions and in the ways of normalizing results (wet weight, dry weight, or content of noncollagen proteins).

Carnitine insufficiency and, sometimes, deficiency in dialysis can have multiple causes (Fig. 21.3). First, it can be the consequence of carnitine losses through dialysis membranes. In fact, during each 4- to 5-hour dialysis session about 600 to 700 μmoles of carnitine are lost in the dialysate, leading to a rapid decline of plasma carnitine concentrations of about 50% to 70% (20,27,28). In contrast to

TABLE 21.2. SERUM CARNITINE LEVELS IN PATIENTS UNDERGOING MAINTENANCE HEMODIALYSIS. AVERAGE VALUES OF DATA REPORTED IN 28 STUDIES (μmol/L)

	Controls	MHD
Total car	50.12	49.80
Free car	42.20	31.51
Acyl car	9.41	17.42
SCAC	7.40	15.90
LCAC	2.91	3.08
Free car/Total car	0.82	0.65
Acyl/Free car	0.22	0.55

MHD, maintenance hemodialysis; car, carnitine; SCAC, short-chain acylcarnitine; LCAC, long-chain acylcarnitine.

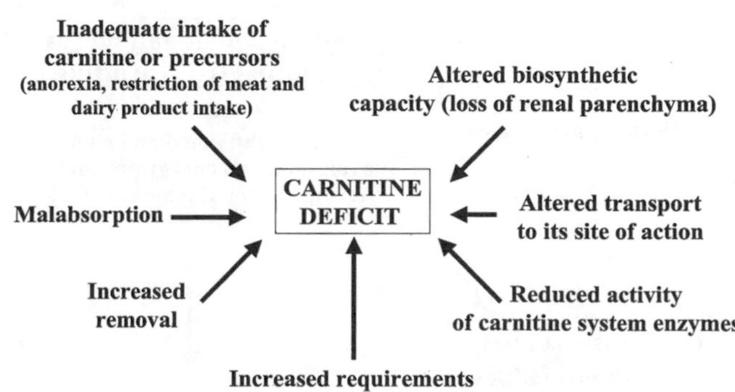

FIGURE 21.3. Potential causes of carnitine deficit in patients undergoing hemodialysis.

the physiologic carnitine handling by the normal kidney, hemodialysis favors the loss of free carnitine as compared to the loss of the esterified fractions, which have a lower dialyzer clearance. The carnitine losses in dialysate are compensated for by dietary intake, by increased endogenous synthesis, and by carnitine efflux from the intracellular pools. Even if the carnitine balance usually is maintained over a short period, the rapid changes of carnitine content in different compartments may adversely affect metabolism, especially at the skeletal muscle level. Despite optimal nutritional support, skeletal muscle carnitine content tends to become depleted over the long term, proportionally to the dialytic age of the patient (26,29).

In addition to carnitine removal with the dialysate, other factors may contribute to the carnitine depletion of these patients (3,20). Exogenous carnitine availability may decrease as a result of reduced carnitine or carnitine precursor intake or intestinal malabsorption. Cellular requirements may be increased by intercurrent illnesses. Renal tissue loss may contribute to the reduced synthetic capacity. The carnitine precursor, trimethyllysine, accumulates in uremia with levels increasing up to fourfold; this metabolite can directly inhibit carnitine transporters (3,20). Finally, patients undergoing dialysis may have reduced activities of key enzymes of carnitine metabolism, such as carnitine palmitoyltransferases (which may be directly inhibited by parathyroid hormone) and glycerophospholipid acyltransferase (15).

Besides carnitine depletion, patients undergoing dialysis also are characterized by a decreased free carnitine to acylcarnitine ratio mainly as a result of the preferential removal of free carnitine during dialysis (see earlier). Other factors contributing to this alteration may include (3,20): (a) impaired acetyl-CoA disposal; or (b) enhanced carnitine acylation secondary to increased fatty-acid availability as a result of fat-enriched diet, starvation, heparin administration, or acetate administration in the past. Acetate administration during dialysis could have been responsible for the preferential increase of short-chain acylcarnitines often observed in these patients in less recent studies (3).

The described alterations of the carnitine system in hemodialysis (i.e., the association of carnitine depletion with increased acylcarnitine/free carnitine ratio) may lead to several metabolic disturbances at the cellular level (Fig. 21.4), including accumulation of toxic acyl moieties, inhibition of key enzymes of metabolic pathways, and impairment of fatty-acid and glucose oxidation and energy production (see earlier). These metabolic abnormalities may contribute to several clinical alterations often observed in patients undergoing hemodialysis (Fig. 21.4), such as muscle weakness and myopathy, loss of body protein and cachexia, insulin resistance and glucose intolerance, dyslipidemia, anemia refractory to erythropoietin treatment, cardiomyopathy, and intradialytic symptoms (muscle cramps, hypotension, cardiac arrhythmias) (2,5,7,20).

The alterations of the carnitine system observed in patients undergoing hemodialysis are similar to those seen in patients undergoing continuous ambulatory peritoneal dialysis (CAPD) (5,20). In these patients an even greater decrease in free carnitine serum concentrations is observed, with a parallel increase of esterified carnitine, which represents about 75% of total carnitine. These changes alter the acylcarnitine/free carnitine ratio substantially, inducing a severe state of carnitine insufficiency.

CARNITINE THERAPY IN RENAL DISEASE

The rationale for carnitine supplementation in patients with renal failure is based on a number of theoretic considerations. First, carnitine metabolism and homeostasis are altered profoundly by uremia and replacement therapy. Second, carnitine has a regulatory role in intermediate

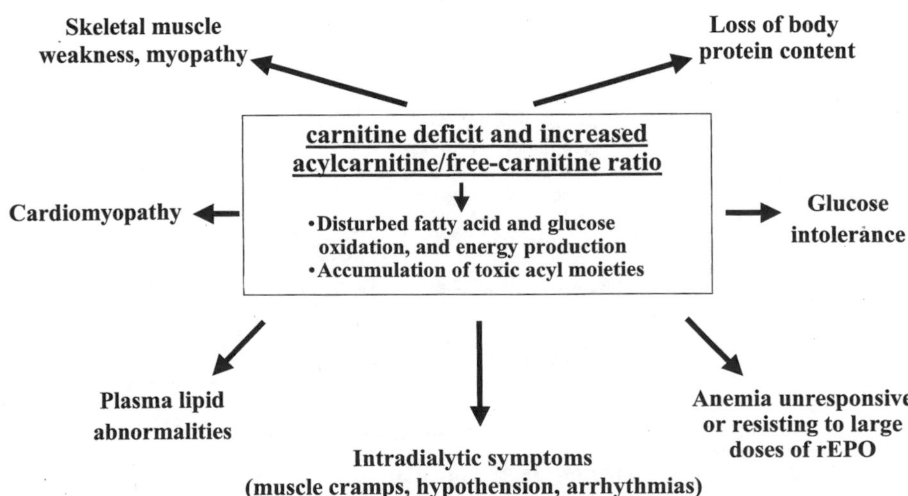

FIGURE 21.4. Potential consequences of carnitine deficit in patients undergoing hemodialysis.

metabolism, a detoxifying action, and a direct influence on cell membrane regeneration and stability. Third, some of the alterations observed in primary carnitine deficiencies are similar to those observed in patients undergoing dialysis. Based on these considerations, on several animal and *in vitro* studies, and on the positive safety profile of carnitine, a large number of studies have been performed in the last decades to evaluate the clinical efficacy of carnitine supplementations in patients undergoing hemodialysis and in particular whether carnitine may positively affect some of the clinical and metabolic alterations usually observed in patients undergoing dialysis such as dyslipidemia, insulin resistance, body protein catabolism, anemia, myopathy, and cardiomyopathy.

Pharmacokinetics of Carnitine Supplementation

The removal of carnitine by hemodialysis is extremely efficient, leading to a 50% to 70% reduction of plasma carnitine concentrations at the end of each session (see earlier). During the interdialytic interval, plasma carnitine levels slowly are restored with a biphasic temporal pattern (5,10, 12,13). In the first phase, carnitine moves into the circulation from the rapidly equilibrating pools (i.e., those tissues exhibiting a fast carnitine turnover—mainly the liver). In the second phase, carnitine is released into the circulation from the slowly equilibrating pools (mainly from skeletal muscle). This process may lead to a progressive depletion, mainly of the slowly equilibrating tissues with the development of a secondary deficiency status. When supplemental carnitine is administered parenterally at the end of the dialysis session, carnitine levels in plasma and in the other rapidly equilibrating pools are restored immediately. In contrast, restoration of the carnitine pools in the slowly equilibrating tissues is more difficult. In fact, evidence indicates that at least 2 months of carnitine supplementation given at a dose of 20 mg/kg after each dialysis session are required to achieve an apparent steady state in the slowly equilibrating pools and possibly prevent a progressive carnitine depletion. Carnitine supplementation increases both free and esterified carnitine levels. However, the acylcarnitine to free carnitine ratio is only slightly modified by carnitine supplementation (20).

The dosage of carnitine and the route of administration also may be relevant. Oral supplementation may be effective in delivering carnitine to the liver because of the first-pass effect (13). The bioavailability of the enterally administered carnitine is only 15% or even lower (11). Nonetheless, low carnitine doses also may be effective because the carnitine transport systems are saturable. In fact, in some cases low carnitine doses have been shown to be more efficient than higher levels of carnitine administration (see later in this chapter).

Effects on Erythrocyte Function and Anemia

The reduced erythropoietin (EPO) synthesis by the kidney is the main cause of anemia in patients with uremia (15). The administration of recombinant human EPO (rEPO) therefore has become a standard treatment in chronically uremic patients (30). Many patients, however, exhibit variable degrees of rEPO resistance, thereby often requiring very high doses of this hormone (i.e., >300 IU/kg/week) (31). This abnormality can be related to the fact that anemia in these patients can be the consequence of multiple factors besides low EPO synthesis (30). Furthermore, carnitine depletion may reduce red blood cell survival, anemia being a common feature of primary carnitine deficiencies. In patients undergoing dialysis a negative correlation has been observed between serum-free and esterified carnitine and erythrocyte osmotic fragility or rEPO requirements (15,32). Low carnitine content in red blood cells can reduce the acyl flow needed to maintain red blood cell membrane structure, function, and stability (4). Evidence indicates that carnitine administration in these patients may restore the reduced erythrocyte CPT activity, improve red blood cell osmotic and mechanical fragility, and increase the erythrocyte sodium-potassium-adenosine triphosphate activity, thereby increasing red blood cell survival (15,33,34). Before rEPO therapy availability, some studies suggested a potential carnitine efficacy in increasing hematocrit values (15). More recently, several studies have been designed to evaluate the ability of carnitine supplementation in reducing rEPO requirement (15,30,35).

The two available metaanalyses evaluating results obtained in randomized controlled trials on the clinical carnitine effects did not achieve consistent conclusions (28,36). The first metaanalysis (28) showed a significant positive carnitine effect on increasing hematocrit levels as well as on reducing rEPO dosage (with an average reduction of about 30% in the rEPO dosage). The second larger metaanalysis was not able to confirm these positive results (36). However, when prospective cohort trials were included in this second analysis, beneficial effects of carnitine on hematologic indexes were observed. Thus, although definitive conclusions cannot be drawn, the available data suggest that carnitine administration in patients undergoing dialysis is likely to improve the hematologic indexes and reduce the rEPO dosages, thereby lowering treatment costs (37). Both the American Association of Kidney Patients (38) and the National Kidney Foundation Consensus (39) concluded that carnitine supplementation should not be a routine practice, but it should be administered to selected patients unresponsive to or requiring large doses of rEPO at a dosage of 1 g intravenously at the end of the dialysis session or daily, per os. A pragmatic approach is suggested using a trial supplementation period to exclude L-carnitine deficiency as a cause of rEPO resistance (30). It has been suggested that patients with elevated serum parathyroid hormone or C-reactive protein, as well as those with aluminum toxicity or megaloblastosis, should not be treated with carnitine (30).

Effects on Lipid Metabolism

Hypertriglyceridemia, as well as high serum LDL cholesterol and low HDL (high-density lipoprotein) cholesterol levels are common findings in patients undergoing hemodialysis. The pathogenesis of the abnormal lipid profile is multifactorial and can be the consequence of one of the following: (a) reduced triglyceride clearance as a result of decreased activity of lipases or lecithin-cholesterol acyltransferases (3); (b) a lower β-oxidation rate from reduced carnitine levels; (c) or increased lipid synthesis from excessive carbohydrate or fat intake and, in the past, from the acetate added to the dialysate. Carnitine supplementation could decrease triglyceride and cholesterol levels by stimulating the oxidation of long-chain fatty acids. However, the results of the trials on the effects of carnitine supplementation on triglyceride and cholesterol levels are quite inconsistent (3,21,28,36,40–46). This could be the consequence not only of differences in study designs but also of other factors, such as differences in duration or modality of carnitine supplementation (e.g., the previous use of the DL-isomer of carnitine instead of the present use exclusively of the more physiologic L-isomer) or in dialysis techniques (e.g., the previous use of acetate instead of the more recent use of bicarbonate in the dialysate). Some studies have included subjects with both normal and pathologic profiles. Furthermore, differences in carnitine dosage and route of administration also may contribute to the lack of homogeneous results.

A dual response on serum triglyceride levels has been observed after the administration of different carnitine dosages, with a paradoxical increase in triglyceride levels following the administration of the higher dosages (3,40). Such a paradoxical response may be the consequence of the fact that in the presence of an excess of exogenous carnitine, fatty acids are no longer trapped as acyl-CoA in cell organelles but are shuttled as acetylcarnitine from the mitochondria and the peroxisome to the cytosol, where fatty-acid and triglyceride synthesis takes place (3). A number of studies in adults and children have obtained a lipid-lowering effect through low-dose carnitine supplementation (5 to 10 mg/kg/day) (41–45). For example, we have observed in patients with hypertriglyceridemia undergoing hemodialysis a reduction in the triglyceride levels after a trial of intravenous (IV) administration of D-L carnitine (the D and the L isoforms were present with a 1:1 ratio) (41). Carnitine was given at the end of each dialysis session at the dosages of 0.5 g for 8 weeks and then of 1 g for the following 6 weeks. The effective dose was even lower than the total supplemented amount because only the L-isomer is biologically active. In other studies, when carnitine was given orally a greater triglyceride-lowering effect was observed as compared to the observations made during parenteral carnitine administration (13,36). Thus, considering the low bioavailability of oral carnitine, these results might represent an indirect evidence of the greater efficacy of low carnitine dosages on lipid metabolism.

The effects of carnitine supplementation on the lipid profile also seem to be related to plasma or erythrocyte carnitine levels (42,47). Furthermore, the basal lipid profile also may influence the carnitine response. For example, we observed a cholesterol-reducing effect of carnitine supplementation only in patients with hypercholesterolemia (48). The presence of low levels of HDL and apoprotein-A (apo-A) in patients with hypertriglyceridemia allows the identification of responders from nonresponders (49). The two recent metaanalyses of the available randomized controlled studies of carnitine supplementation showed no effect of carnitine on plasma triglyceride levels, whereas the lowering effect on cholesterol concentrations was significant (28,36). In addition, before considering this compound as not useful for the treatment of triglyceride abnormalities in patients undergoing hemodialysis, more attention should be paid to issues such as the dosage of carnitine (41–45,50), the selection of patients (42,47–49), or the choice of adequate indicators. In another study by our group, carnitine supplementation induced some changes in lipoprotein composition, with the synthesis of less atherogenic VLDL even in patients that would have been considered nonresponders, if only the changes in total serum cholesterol and triglyceride levels had been evaluated (22).

Effects on Glucose and Protein Metabolism

Carnitine plays a fundamental role in the regulation of energy production from both lipids and glucose (Fig. 21.2) (3,5,7). This may explain the observed carnitine-mediated improvements of both insulin resistance and protein balance. These carnitine actions may be particularly advantageous for patients with uremia who may have both impaired insulin sensitivity and accelerated protein catabolism. The insulin actions on glucose metabolism can be assessed *in vivo* by the euglycemic insulin clamp or by the "minimal model" techniques. Using these methods carnitine has been shown to directly improve insulin sensitivity in both normal subjects and diabetics (7). A similar effect has been observed in dialyzed chronically uremic patients using different approaches (51). From a clinical point of view, carnitine therapy in hemodialysis tends to decrease insulin concentrations without significantly affecting glucose concentrations. Carnitine regenerates the free CoA necessary for the oxidative decarboxylation of pyruvate (and lactate) and oxoglutarate (50). Furthermore, the carnitine-mediated decrease in the ratio between acetyl-CoA to free CoA in the mitochondria directly activates the enzyme pyruvate dehydrogenase, thereby favoring pyruvate oxidation and glucose utilization (3,5,7). This mechanism also accounts for the reduced blood lactate levels observed after carnitine supplementation in patients undergoing hemodialysis by us and other groups (50, 52).

In patients undergoing hemodialysis several significant associations have been found between altered carnitine levels and indexes of protein-energy malnutrition, such as protein intake; serum albumin levels; relative body weight; and the diameter of type I, mitochondrial-rich, oxidative skeletal muscle fibers (53–55a). A carnitine-mediated improvement of nitrogen balance has been observed both in experimental conditions and in the clinical setting (e.g., in trauma patients, low–birth-weight infants) (56). In a randomized controlled trial carnitine administration in patients undergoing dialysis (20 mg/kg/body weight IV at the end of each dialysis session) improved some potential indexes of protein homeostasis such as the serum predialysis concentrations of urea, creatinine, and phosphate and the mid-arm muscle area (53). Other studies in smaller numbers of subjects have shown beneficial effects of carnitine on protein intake and serum levels of albumin and transferrin in patients undergoing hemodialysis, and on nitrogen balance and body fat in patients undergoing CAPD (55,55a). Some of these findings, however, have not been confirmed in other studies (57).

Effects on Skeletal Muscle Functions and on Quality of Life

In normal subjects the skeletal muscle is the largest body carnitine pool. Skeletal muscles at rest and during low-intensity exercise preferentially use fat as an energy source. Carnitine is essential for fatty-acid β-oxidation. The use of fat as a main fuel, by sparing the skeletal muscle glycogen stores during exercise, may delay the development of fatigue. Furthermore, carnitine, as shown in the hypoxic heart model in the rat, also may favor a shift from fat to glucose oxidation through the reduction of the acetyl-CoA/CoA ratio and the activation of pyruvate dehydrogenase. By this mechanism, carnitine could produce a greater amount of ATP per unit of oxygen and reduce lactate production (10). Furthermore, exercise itself decreases skeletal muscle carnitine levels in normal subjects. On the basis of these premises, healthy subjects were given carnitine supplements, with the rationale of improving exercise performance. The available data on the effects of carnitine on exercise metabolism or performance, however, did not allow definitive conclusions (10). Although carnitine supplementation did not unequivocally improve performance in athletes, this rationale has been extended to patients with uremia with the aim of improving their poor exercise tolerance and intradialytic symptoms such as asthenia and muscle cramps. Patients undergoing hemodialysis are characterized by a depletion of muscle carnitine content, structural changes of skeletal muscle with fiber atrophy, reduced exercise capacity, weakness, and muscle cramps (5,7, 20,53,54). These problems may limit the range of daily activity and greatly deteriorate their quality of life. Carnitine, by improving muscle metabolism, could increase strength and improve symptoms such as fatigue, intradialytic weakness, and cramps. In patients undergoing dialysis, exercise tolerance shows an inverse correlation with plasma carnitine levels (26). In these patients, carnitine administration has been shown to improve muscle strength and morphology (increased diameter of type I and type IIa fibers), maximal oxygen consumption, electromyographic power, intradialytic weakness or cramps, exercise duration, and quality of life (20, 25,28,29,36,53,54,58). Other authors, however, have not confirmed these findings (57,59). Two metaanalyses of the available randomized controlled studies on carnitine supplementation in dialysis have confirmed the positive effects on muscle cramp intensity and frequency as well as on exercise capacity (28,36).

Possibly related to the improvement of skeletal muscle function is the amelioration of quality of life reported by carnitine-supplemented patients. Such perceived improvement of well-being appears to be a short-term effect of carnitine, being observed only during the first months of therapy (58). Furthermore, the low reliability of subjective indicators of well-being must be kept in mind.

Effects on Heart Functions

The heart muscle produces energy mainly from fatty acids. Carnitine, therefore, should play a crucial role in heart metabolism both in physiologic and pathologic conditions (5, 7). In nonuremic patients, carnitine supplementation has been shown to reduce the rate and severity of anginal episodes and rhythm disorders and to improve left ventricular function and exercise tolerance. Carnitine levels in heart tissue have been assessed only in two patients undergoing hemodialysis with severe cardiomyopathy and were found to be reduced (20). In patients undergoing hemodialysis with cardiomyopathy, carnitine levels showed an inverse correlation with the cardiothoracic ratio (60). Carnitine supplementation in patients undergoing hemodialysis reduced the incidence and the severity of intradialytic arrhythmias and hypotension, reduced left-ventricular mass, and improved left-ventricular ejection fraction (20,36,53, 60–63). Nonetheless, these studies of the effects of carnitine on the heart in uremia have been performed on a limited number of patients; some of them could have been biased by the inclusion of both symptomatic and asymptomatic patients, and the results were not always consistent (57). The American Association of Kidney Patients suggests carnitine treatment for patients with cardiomyopathy who do not respond adequately to standard therapy (38). The U.S. National Kidney Foundation guidelines also state that the evidence to support supplementation to improve cardiac function is not sufficient to justify routine use and recommend that standard therapy be attempted first (39).

CONCLUSIONS

Experimental studies demonstrated consistent effects of carnitine on several metabolic pathways. Many human studies have assessed the efficacy of carnitine supplementation either in patients with chronic renal failure undergoing dialysis or in other pathologic conditions. Whereas many of these studies demonstrated clinical improvements during carnitine therapy, others showed negative or inconsistent results. Differences in experimental design, sample size, patient selection (e.g., severity of carnitine deficiency or insufficiency before therapy), and carnitine dosage (e.g., low-dosage carnitine supplementation could be more beneficial on the plasma lipid profile) may account for such discrepancies among published studies.

Two metaanalyses indicate that carnitine supplementation in patients undergoing hemodialysis may improve: (a) the hematologic status by increasing hematocrit or allowing a reduction of erythropoietin dosage, (b) the exercise tolerance by increasing the aerobic capacity and decreasing cramp occurrence, (c) the plasma lipid profile by decreasing cholesterol, and (d) the patients' overall "well-being" (28, 36). The latter results may be related to the overall detoxifying action of carnitine in patients who have an accumulation of acyl moieties in their body compartments. Carnitine therapy may reduce not only patient morbidity but also the costs of patient care in dialysis (possibly as a result of reduced erythropoietin requirements).

Working groups of the U.S. National Kidney Foundation and the European Renal Association-European Dialysis and Transplant Association developed clinical practice guidelines for the treatment of chronically uremic patients (30,39). With regard to carnitine supplementation in hemodialysis, both groups concluded that there are insufficient data to support the *routine* use of carnitine in unselected patients. Furthermore, serum carnitine levels should not be used necessarily to identify carnitine depletion (e.g., free carnitine <20 mmol/L; acylcarnitine/free carnitine ratio >0.4) because they are not readily available and not sufficiently representative of tissue carnitine content. Therefore, they suggested that a trial with carnitine supplementation should be recommended for certain conditions in selected patients undergoing dialysis who do not respond adequately to standard therapy. These conditions are severe and persistent muscle cramps or hypotension during dialysis, lack of energy affecting the quality of life, skeletal muscle weakness or myopathy, cardiomyopathy, and anemia of uremia unresponsive to or requiring large doses of erythropoietin. A dose of 20 mg/kg of body weight of carnitine should be administered intravenously after each dialysis session. However, oral carnitine or IV carnitine at doses less than 20 mg/kg or the addition of carnitine in the dialysis bath also may be effective for a variety of these disorders. The U.S. Food and Drug Administration (Jan. 5th, 2000, page 11, No. 2391) considered the effects of carnitine supplementation together with the very positive risk/benefit ratio of this compound and extended the approval of IV levocarnitine use in patients undergoing hemodialysis not only to the *treatment* but also to the *prevention* of carnitine deficiency. This expanded indication applies only to the IV formulation—not to the oral formulations of the drug.

REFERENCES

1. Rebouche CH. Carnitine. In: Shills ME, Olson JA, Shike M, eds. *Modern nutrition in health and disease.* 9th ed. Philadelphia: Lea & Febiger, 2000:505–512.
2. Borum PR, ed. *Clinical aspects of human carnitine deficiency.* New York: Pergamon Press, 1986.
3. Guarnieri G, Toigo G, Crapesi L, et al. Carnitine metabolism in chronic renal failure. *Kidney Int* 1987;32(Suppl 22):S116–S127.
4. Arduini A, Mancinelli G, Radatti GL, et al. Role of carnitine and carnitine palmitoyltransferase as integral components of the pathway for membrane phospholipid fatty acid turnover in intact human erythrocytes. *J Biol Chem* 1992;267:673–681.
5. Ferrari R, DiMauro S, Sherwood G, eds. *L-Carnitine and its role in medicine: from function to therapy.* London: Academic Press, 1992.
6. Broadway NM, Saggerson ED. Microsomal carnitine acyltransferases. *Biochem Soc Trans* 1995;23:490–494.
7. De Simone C, Famularo G, eds. *Carnitine today.* Heidelberg: Springer-Verlag, 1997.
8. Ramsey RR. The carnitine acyltransferases: modulators of acyl-CoA-dependent reactions. *Biochem Soc Trans* 2000;28:182–186.
9. Kerner J, Hoppel C. Fatty acid transport into mitochondria. *Biochim Biophys Acta* 2000;1486:1–17.
10. Brass EP. Supplemental carnitine and exercise. *Am J Clin Nutr* 2000;72(Suppl 2):S618–S623.
11. Harper P, Elwin CE, Cederblad G. Pharmacokinetics of bolus intravenous and oral doses of L-carnitine in healthy subjects. *Eur J Clin Pharmacol* 1988;35:69–75.
12. Evans AM, Faull R, Fornasini G, et al. Pharmacokinetics of L-carnitine in patients with end-stage renal disease undergoing long-term hemodialysis. *Clin Pharmacol Ther* 2000;68:238–249.
13. Brass EP. Pharmacokinetic considerations for the therapeutic use of carnitine in hemodialysis patients. *Clin Ther* 1995;17: 176–185.
14. Rebouche CJ, Lombard KA, Chenard CA. Renal adaptation to dietary carnitine in humans. *Am J Clin Nutr* 1993;58:660-665.
15. Kletzmayr J, Mayer G, Legenstein E, et al. Anemia and carnitine supplementation in hemodialysis patients. *Kidney Int* 1999; 55(Suppl.69):S93–S106.
16. Peluso G, Barbarisi A, Savica V, et al. Carnitine: an osmolite that plays a metabolic role. *J Cell Biochem* 2000;80(1):1–10.
17. Famularo G, DeSimone C. A new era for carnitine? *Immunol Today* 1995;16:211–213.
18. Park EA, Cook G. Differential regulation in the heart of mitochondrial carnitine palmitoyltransferase-I muscle and liver isoforms. *Mol Cell Biochem* 1998;180:27–32.
19. Wanner C, Horl WH. Carnitine abnormalities in patients with renal insufficiency. *Nephron* 1988;50:89–102.
20. Golper TA, Ahmad S. L-carnitine administration to hemodialysis patients: has its time come? *Semin Dial* 1992;5:94–98.
21. Golper TA, Wolfson M, Ahmah S, et al. Multicenter trial of

carnitine in maintenance hemodialysis patients. I. Carnitine concentrations and lipid effects. *Kidney Int* 1990;38:904–911.

22. Guarnieri G, Fonda M, Situlin R, et al. Effects of L-Carnitine supplementation in the dialysate on serum lipoprotein composition of hemodialysis patients. In: Guarnieri G, Panzetta G, Toigo G, eds. *Metabolic and nutritional abnormalities in kidney disease. Contributions to Nephrology.* Basel: Karger, 1992;98:36–43.
23. Ricanati ES, Tserng K, Hoppel CL. Abnormal fatty acid utilization during prolonged fasting in chronic uremia. *Kidney Int* 1987; 32(Suppl 22):S145– S148.
24. Guarnieri GF, Carretta R, Toigo G, et al. Acetate intolerance in chronic uremic patients. *Nephron* 1979;24:212–216.
25. Siami G, Clinton ME, Mrak R, et al. Evaluation of the effect of intravenous l-carnitine therapy on function, structure and fatty acid metabolism of skeletal muscle in patients receiving chronic hemodialysis. *Nephron* 1991;57:306-313.
26. Hiatt WR, Koziol BJ, Shapiro JI, et al. Carnitine metabolism during exercise in patients on chronic hemodialysis. *Kidney Int* 1992;41(6):1613–1619.
27. Bulla M, Glogler A, Rossle C, et al. Dysregulation of carnitine metabolism in renal insufficiency: a summary of findings in adults and children. In: Seim H, Loster H, eds. *Carnitine—Pathobiochemical basics and clinical applications.* Bochum: Ponte Press, 1996:177–193.
28. Hurot JM, Cucherat M, Haugh M, et al. Effects of L-carnitine supplementation in maintenance hemodialysis patients: a systematic review. *J Am Soc Nephrol* 2002;13:708–714.
29. Bellinghieri G, Savica V, Mallamace A, et al. Correlation between increased serum and tissue carnitine levels and improved muscle symptoms in hemodialyzed patients. *Am J Nutr* 1983;38: 523–531.
30. Hörl WH. Is there a role for adjuvant therapy in patients being treated with epoietin? *Nephrol Dial Transplant* 1999;14(Suppl. 2):S50–S60.
31. Hörl WH, Jacobs C, Macdougall IC, et al. European best practice guidelines 14–16. Inadequate response to epoietin. *Nephrol Dial Transplant* 2000;15(Suppl 4):S43–S50.
32. Matsumura M, Hatakeyama S, Koni I, et al. Correlation between serum carnitine levels and erythrocyte osmotic fragility in hemodialysis patients. *Nephron* 1996;72:574–578.
33. De Los Reyes B, Perez Garcia R, Liras A. L-Carnitine normalizes the reduced carnitine palmitoyl transferase activity in red cells from haemodialysis patients. *Nephrol Dial Transplant* 1997;12: 1300–1301.
34. Labonia WD. L-Carnitine effects on anemia in hemodialyzed patients treated with erythropoietin. *Am J Kidney Dis* 1995;26: 757–764.
35. Cianciaruso B, Torraca S, De Blasio A, et al. Carnitine as adjuvant therapy in the management of renal anemia. *Contrib Nephrol* 2002;137:426–430.
36. Amato A, Muenz L, Kim C, et al. L-carnitine therapy in hemodialysis patients: a meta-analysis based review. 2001; *(submitted for publication)* (personal communication).
37. Mantovani LG, Belisari A. L-carnitine use in hemodialyzed patients. *Am J Kidney Dis* 1999;34:400–403.
38. Ahmad S, Brass EP, Hoppel C, et al. (Consensus Group) Role of L-Carnitine in treating renal dialysis patients. *Dial Transplant* 1994;23:177–181.
39. Kopple JD. K/DOQIT clinical practice guidelines for nutrition in chronic renal failure. *Am J Kidney Dis* 2000;35(Suppl 2): S54–S55.
40. Chan MK, Persaud JW, Varghese, et al. Response patterns to DL-carnitine in patients on maintenance hemodialysis. *Nephron* 1982;30:240–243.
41. Guarnieri G, Ranieri F, Toigo G, et al. Lipid-lowering effect of carnitine in chronically uremic patients treated with maintenance hemodialysis. *Am J Clin Nutr* 1980;33:1489–1492.
42. Wanner C, Wieland H, Wackerle B, et al. Ketogenic and antiketogenic effects of L-carnitine in hemodialysis patients. *Kidney Int* 1989;36(Suppl 27):S264–S268.
43. Elisaf M, Bairaktari E, Katopodis K, et al. Effect of L-Carnitine supplementation on lipid parameters in hemodialysis patients. *Am J Nephrol* 1998;18(5):416–421.
44. Glöggler A, Bulla M, Furst P. Effect of low dose supplementation of L-carnitine on lipid metabolism in hemodialyzed children. *Kidney Int* 1989;36 (Suppl 27):S256–S258.
45. Böhles H, Michalk D, Von Wendt Goknur E. Effect of l-carnitine supplementation on lipid metabolism of renal failure, dialysis-dependent children and adolescents. *Infusionstherapie* 1991; 18(5):224–226.
46. Savica V, Bellinghieri G. Carnitine and lipid profile in uremia. *Clin Ther* 1997;148(5–6):229–236.
47. Mayer G, Graf H, Legenstain E, et al. L-Carnitine substitution in patients on chronic hemodialysis. *Nephron* 1989;52:295–299.
48. Toigo G, Situlin R, Dardi F, et al. Results of a multicenter study on the effect on serum triglycerides and cholesterol administration of carnitine in chronic uremia patients undergoing periodic hemodialysis treatment. *G Clin Med* 1982;63:841–849.
49. Vacha GM, Giorcelli G, Siliprandi N, et al. Favorable effects of L-carnitine treatment on hypertriglyceridemia in hemodialysis patients: decisive role of low levels of high density lipoprotein cholesterol. *Am J Clin Nutr* 1983;38:532–540.
50. Guarnieri G, Toigo G, Crapesi L, et al. Metabolic effects of supplementation of L-carnitine in the dialysate of patients treated with acetate hemodialysis. *Kidney Int* 1989;36(Suppl 27): S247–S255.
51. Gunal AI, Celiker H, Donder E, et al. The effect of l-carnitine on insulin resistance in hemodialysed patients with chronic renal failure. *J Nephrol* 1999;12:38–40.
52. Wanner C, Forstner Wanner S, et al. Serum free carnitine, carnitine esters and lipids in patients on peritoneal dialysis and hemodialysis. *Am J Nephrol* 1986;6:208–211.
53. Ahmad S, Robertson HT, Golper TA, et al. Multicenter trial of L-carnitine in maintenance hemodialysis patients. II. Clinical and biochemical effects. *Kidney Int* 1990;38:912–918.
54. Giovenali P, Fenocchio D, Montanari G, et al. Selective trophic effect of L-carnitine in type I and IIa skeletal muscle fibers. *Kidney Int* 1994;46:1616–1619.
55. Trovato GM, Iannetti E, Murgo AM, et al. Body composition and long-term L-carnitine supplementation. *Clin Ther* 1998;149: 209–214.

55a. Kopple JD, Qing D-P. Effect of L-carnitine on nitrogen balance in CAPD patients. *J Am Soc Nephrol* 1999;10:264A.

56. Toigo G, Biolo G, Ciocchi B, et al. Modulation of protein metabolism in acutely ill patients: effects of carnitine and glutamine dipeptides. In: Tessari P, Soeters PB, Pittoni G, et al, eds. *Amino acid and protein metabolism in health and disease: nutritional implications.* London: Smith-Gordon, 1997:253–260.
57. Thomas S, Fischer FP, Mettang T, et al. Effects of L-carnitine on leukocyte function and viability in hemodialysis patients: a double-blind randomized trial. *Am J Kidney Dis* 1999;34(4): 678–687.
58. Sloan RS, Kastan B, Rice SI, et al. Quality of life during and between hemodialysis treatments: role of L-carnitine supplementation. *Am J Kidney Dis* 1998;32:265–272.
59. Semeniuk J, Shalanski KF, Taylor N, et al. Evaluation of the effects of intravenous L-carnitine on quality of life in chronic hemodialysis patients. *Clin Nephrol* 2000;54:470–477.
60. Kudoh Y, Shoji T, Oimatsu H, et al. The role of carnitine in the pathogenesis of cardiomegaly in patients with chronic hemodialysis. *Jpn Circ J* 1983;47:1391–1397.

61. Van Es A, Henny FC, Kooistra MP. Amelioration of cardiac function by l-carnitine administration in patients on haemodialysis. In: Guarnieri G, Panzetta G, Toigo G, eds. *Metabolic and nutritional abnormalities in kidney disease. Contribution to nephrology.* Basel: Karger, 1992;98:28–35.
62. Sakurabayashi T, Takaesu Y, Haginoshita S, et al. Improvement of myocardial fatty acid metabolism through l-carnitine administration to chronic hemodialysis patients. *Am J Nephrol* 1999;19: 480–484.
63. Matsumoto-Y, Sato-M, Ohashi-H, et al. Effects of L-carnitine supplementation on cardiac morbidity in hemodialyzed patients. *Am J Nephrol* 2000;20:201–207.

22

NUTRITION AND ANEMIA IN END-STAGE RENAL DISEASE

RAJNISH MEHROTRA
JOEL D. KOPPLE

Erythropoietin deficiency is a hallmark of progressive renal failure and is the most important cause for anemia in individuals undergoing maintenance dialysis (MD). The development of recombinant human erythropoietin (rHuEpo) has revolutionized anemia management in this patient population. However, other nutrients and factors may facilitate the process of erythropoiesis. Hence, an understanding of their role in anemia management is critical to ensure the optimal utilization of rHuEpo therapy; some of these may be required to replace deficits and others may need to be provided in surfeit (Table 22.1). We present a review of the potential role of key nutrients and growth factors in the management of anemia associated with end-stage renal disease (ESRD).

IRON

The need to prevent, identify, and treat iron deficiency in patients undergoing MD, particularly those being treated with rHuEpo, is well established. Clinical practice guidelines formulated in the United States and Europe recommend routine evaluation and management of available body iron stores in patients undergoing MD receiving treatment with rHuEpo (1–3).

Role in Anemia of Renal Failure

Iron is essential for hemoglobin formation in health and disease. Hence, an adequate supply of iron is necessary to ensure an optimal response to rHuEpo therapy.

Status in Renal Failure

Iron deficiency commonly is present at the time of initiation of MD therapy (4,5). Moreover, patients undergoing MD have a higher than normal amount of iron loss, which is the result of blood loss during the hemodialysis procedure, oozing of blood from the gastrointestinal tract, and frequent venipuncture. Indeed, one study has estimated that patients undergoing maintenance hemodialysis (MHD) may lose 3 L of blood annually from the dialysis procedure and venipuncture alone (6). Finally, rHuEpo therapy increases the rate of erythropoiesis and, hence, the demand for iron. Thus, it is no surprise that dietary intake of iron is insufficient to maintain adequate available iron stores in most individuals undergoing MD.

Evidence and Recommendations

Numerous studies have demonstrated that oral iron therapy is usually ineffective for either correcting the iron deficiency or reducing the rHuEpo dose requirements in patients undergoing MD (7–15). However, several studies consistently have demonstrated the ability of intravenous (IV) iron treatment to correct the iron deficiency as well as to reduce the rHuEpo requirements (9,13,15–24). Hence, IV therapy forms the cornerstone of iron supplementation in patients undergoing MD.

Three IV iron preparations are available for clinical use: iron dextran, ferric sodium gluconate, and iron sucrose (2). Iron dextran is associated with dose-related arthralgias and myalgias and dose-unrelated anaphylactoid reactions in a small proportion of patients; although rare, these latter reactions may be fatal (2,25–29). However, ferric sodium gluconate and iron sucrose are not reported to be associated with the anaphylactoid reaction and are likely to be more widely used (2,30,31).

The percent serum transferrin saturation (TSAT) and serum ferritin levels are the most widely used parameters for the diagnosis of absolute and relative iron deficiency in individuals undergoing MD (2). Absolute iron deficiency in this patient population is defined by the National Kidney Foundation-Kidney/Dialysis Outcome Quality Initiative (NKF-K/DOQI) Clinical Practice Guidelines on Anemia as either a TSAT of less than 20% or a serum ferritin of less than 100 ng/mL, and the goal of iron therapy is to maintain the two parameters above these levels (2). Individ-

TABLE 22.1. THE RATIONALE FOR THE ROLE OF VARIOUS NUTRIENTS AND GROWTH FACTORS IN THE TREATMENT OF ANEMIA ASSOCIATED WITH END-STAGE RENAL DISEASE

Nutrient	Replace Deficit	Give Surfeit
Iron	✓	✓
Folate	✓	
Vitamin B12	✓	
Ascorbic acid		✓
Protein	✓	✓
1,25-di(OH) D3[a]	✓	✓
L-carnitine[a]	✓	✓
Growth hormone, insulinlike growth factor-I[a]	✓	✓

[a]Not clear if the benefit is by replacing a deficit or giving a surfeit.

uals undergoing treatment with rHuEpo also may develop functional iron deficiency. This occurs when the iron requirements exceed the rate at which iron can be released from the reticuloendothelial cells and often is characterized by a low TSAT with a normal serum ferritin level (2,13, 32). However, there are significant limitations to the use of TSAT and serum ferritin for the assessment of iron status: serum transferrin is a negative acute-phase reactant, whereas serum ferritin is a positive acute-phase reactant (33,34). The serum concentrations of these proteins may be modified by inflammatory disorders. Moreover, there is no single value of either TSAT or serum ferritin that accurately identifies individuals in need of iron supplementation (13,15,22,23, 35–37). Other noninvasive tests, such as zinc protoporphyrin, reticulocyte hemoglobin, soluble transferrin receptors, and percent hypochromic red cells, appear more promising, but they have not been widely tested and are not available for clinical use (38–41). Thus, it is necessary to combine clinical judgment with a routine evaluation of laboratory parameters when making decisions regarding either the need to provide or to withhold iron supplementation.

Concern has been raised about the safety of routine use of IV iron in the MD patient population. There are two major potential risks associated with iron therapy. First, iron is known to enhance the pathogenicity of a large number of infectious microbes. Some investigators have identified a high serum ferritin level in patients undergoing MHD as a risk factor for bacteremia, particularly related to catheter sepsis (42,43). In a more recent study conducted by Hoen et al., anemia—and not an elevated serum ferritin—emerged as a risk factor for bacteremia (44). As pointed out earlier, serum ferritin is also an acute-phase reactant, and an elevated serum ferritin may be a marker of processes that increase the susceptibility of patients undergoing MD to infection. Furthermore, there is no direct evidence that causally links iron therapy with an increased risk of infection in patients undergoing MD. Indeed, two groups have failed to demonstrate an increased incidence of peritonitis following single-dose infusion of iron in patients undergoing chronic peritoneal dialysis (CPD) (45,46). Second, administration of large IV doses of iron may increase oxidative stress, and concern has been raised that this may accelerate atherosclerosis and increase cardiovascular morbidity or mortality. Keeping these concerns in mind, the NKF-K/DOQI Anemia Workgroup recommends that iron therapy be withheld when either the TSAT is 50% or more or the serum ferritin is 800 ng/mL or more.

To conclude, individuals with either a TSAT of less than 20% or serum ferritin of less than 100 ng/mL can be considered to have absolute iron deficiency, and they should be given 500 to 1,000 mg intravenously (2). The regimen depends on whether the patient is undergoing MHD or CPD. Individuals with apparent rHuEpo resistance or with TSAT between 20% and 50% and with serum ferritin between 100 and 800 ng/mL may have functional iron deficiency and also should receive a trial of IV iron therapy (2). Maintenance, weekly IV iron should be administered to patients undergoing MHD to maintain TSAT between 20% and 50% and serum ferritin between 100 and 800 ng/mL (2). There is no evidence to support the use of maintenance doses of iron for patients undergoing CPD.

VITAMIN C

Role in Anemia of Renal Failure

Vitamin C is emerging as an important adjuvant for rHuEpo therapy in patients undergoing MD because it maintains iron in a reduced state. This, in turn, potentiates the intestinal absorption of iron and the enzymatic incorporation of iron into protoporphyrin (47), an intermediate in heme biosynthesis.

Status in Patients Undergoing Maintenance Dialysis

Subclinical vitamin C deficiency may exist in some patients undergoing MHD (48,49). The deficiency is most likely the result of an insufficient dietary intake and increased losses during the dialysis procedure. Hence, some investigators have recommended a daily oral intake of 150 to 200 mg/day of ascorbic acid for patients undergoing MHD (50).

Evidence and Recommendations

Over the last few years, several studies have demonstrated that vitamin C may overcome rHuEpo hyporesponsiveness in patients undergoing MD (51–54). However, these studies enrolled a relatively small number of patients. The maximum duration of follow-up was 12 weeks; most of these studies were observational, and one used a randomized crossover design. Extending these observational findings,

Tarng et al. reported that two indices predicted the response to IV supplementation of ascorbic acid: an erythrocyte zinc-protoporphyrin level greater than 105 μmol/mol heme and a TSAT less than 25% (53). Based on these studies, in 1999 a workgroup recommended the following vitamin C supplementation for MHD patients with rHuEpo hyporesponsiveness: 1 to 1.5 g/day orally or 300 mg intravenously, three times weekly (55). There are no studies that define the potential role of vitamin C in individuals undergoing CPD (see also Chapters 20 and 25).

Care needs to be exercised because vitamin C supplements can lead to oxalate accumulation in patients undergoing MD (56,57). The available data suggest that the total daily dose of ascorbic acid should not exceed 150 mg/day in individuals with chronic renal failure. Some investigators suggest the recommended dietary allowance for normal, nonpregnant, nonlactating adult individuals—70 mg/day (see Chapters 20 and 25). Short-term studies with this dose, for up to 8 weeks, have not demonstrated any increase in serum oxalate levels (53). Moreover, preliminary data suggests that giving vitamin B6 supplements can prevent this hazard (58). There is additional concern that vitamin C may behave as an oxidant and enhance cellular toxicity in individuals with iron overload. However, two studies, one in healthy humans and the other in individuals with ESRD, failed to demonstrate any increase in DNA damage in the presence of iron overload (59,60).

In summary, adjuvant therapy with vitamin C may potentiate the response to erythropoietin in individuals undergoing MHD with hyperferritinemia. Also, erythrocyte zinc protoporphyrin greater than 105 μmol/mol heme and a TSAT less than 25% should be considered for adjuvant vitamin C therapy.

VITAMIN D

Role in Anemia of Renal Failure

The contribution of secondary hyperparathyroidism to the anemia of renal failure has been investigated over the last three decades. The beneficial effect of vitamin D for treating anemia appears to be because of two factors. First, it may be a result of the amelioration of secondary hyperparathyroidism. The marrow fibrosis associated with secondary hyperparathyroidism correlates with resistance to rHuEpo (61) and parathyroidectomy may be associated with an increase in hematocrit with or without a decrease in rHuEpo dose (62–67). Indeed, parathyroidectomy may be followed by a reticulocytosis and a several-fold increase in serum erythropoietin (65). Moreover, there is evidence that parathyroid hormone (PTH) directly inhibits erythropoiesis and also increases osmotic fragility of red cells, and this could explain the rapid increase in hemoglobin concentrations observed in some individuals after parathyroidectomy (68–71). However, not all investigators have confirmed the inhibitory effect of PTH on erythropoiesis (72). Second, there appears to be a direct effect of vitamin D on hematopoiesis (73). This may explain the observation that hemoglobin levels may increase without a concomitant decrease in serum PTH in patients undergoing MD treated with high-dose alfacalcidol (74–76). Addition of calcium and 1,25-dihydroxy-cholecalciferol to cell cultures has been shown to attenuate the uremia-associated decline in the growth rate of erythroid burst- and colony-forming units (77). This finding is supported by the increase in hemoglobin observed in individuals with myelodysplastic syndrome, but without renal failure, on treatment with high-dose alfacalcidol (78).

Status in Patients Undergoing Maintenance Dialysis

Because the 1-α hydroxylation of vitamin D occurs in the kidney, ESRD is characterized by a deficiency of 1,25-dihydroxycholecalciferol. Vitamin D deficiency plays an important role in the genesis of secondary hyperparathyroidism in chronic renal failure.

Evidence and Recommendations

Three studies have described the beneficial effect of vitamin D supplementation on anemia in patients undergoing MHD. Two of these studies used α-calcidiol, and one study used calcitriol, with durations of follow-up ranging between 4 and 18 months (74–76). Thus, current evidence suggests that aggressive treatment of hyperparathyroidism with or without vitamin D supplementation may have a beneficial effect on the anemia associated with ESRD. However, no randomized controlled trials have investigated the potential benefit of calcitriol or α-calcidiol in patients undergoing MHD, and we are not aware of any studies of vitamin D on treatment of anemia in patients undergoing CPD.

FOLIC ACID

Role in Anemia of Renal Failure

Like iron, folic acid is a key nutrient required for erythropoiesis. It serves as a cofactor for DNA synthesis, and its requirements are increased in the face of increased cell turnover.

Status in Patients Undergoing Maintenance Dialysis

Folic acid, a water-soluble vitamin, is lost during dialytic therapy, particularly with high-flux hemodialysis (79). Hence, folic-acid deficiency may develop in the absence of supplementation (80). Several recent reports have indicated that there is variable prevalence of folate deficiency in the dialysis population; most studies, however, report a low prevalence of folic-acid deficiency in such individuals if they do not receive folate supplementation (4,48,81–89).

Evidence and Recommendations

Several published reports have suggested a role for folic-acid deficiency in mediating rHuEpo resistance in individuals being treated with MD (80,90). Moreover, several reports have indicated the development of macrocytosis in individuals undergoing rHuEpo treatment who do not receive folic-acid therapy. This macrocytosis is prevented with routine folate supplementation (91,92). However, it appears that routine supplementation is not necessary to optimize the response to rHuEpo therapy (93). Hence, in 1999 a workgroup recommended folate supplementation (2 to 3 mg/week) for patients undergoing MD and rHuEpo therapy (55). The use of folic acid to treat hyperhomocysteinemia and the rationale for daily folate supplementation is discussed in Chapters 7, 20, 23, and 25.

VITAMIN B6 (PYRIDOXINE)

Role in Anemia of Renal Failure

Vitamin B6 is a cofactor in the formation of δ-amino levulinic acid, a rate-limiting step in heme biosynthesis. Vitamin B6 also plays a potentially important role in the incorporation of iron into protoporphyrin, the final step in heme synthesis. Hence, vitamin B6 is an important nutrient for erythropoiesis.

Status in Patients Undergoing Maintenance Dialysis

There is evidence that in the absence of supplementation, there is a high prevalence of vitamin B6 deficiency. Vitamin B6 metabolism is altered in individuals with ESRD. The metabolism of pyridoxal phosphate (the major active metabolite of vitamin B6) also is impaired, and there are substantial vitamin B6 losses in the dialysate, particularly with high-flux hemodialysis (48,82,94–97). More importantly, evidence suggests that vitamin B6 is consumed during treatment with rHuEpo, and oral supplementation prevents the depletion of erythrocyte vitamin B6 (98,99).

Evidence and Recommendations

There are at least two studies that have evaluated the role of vitamin B6 supplementation on hematocrit of patients undergoing MD and rHuEpo therapy. In the first study, vitamin B6 supplementation alone or with IV iron therapy resulted in a significant increase in the hematocrit in patients undergoing MHD who had microcytic and hypochromic anemia, although they had normal plasma pyridoxine levels (100). In a more recent study, vitamin B6 supplementation of individuals undergoing MHD with normal plasma pyridoxine levels failed to result in an increase in hematocrit (101).

A workgroup has recommended that patients undergoing MD and treatment with rHuEpo should be given supplemental pyridoxine hydrochloride, 100–150 mg/week. Other daily doses of vitamin B6, and particularly its most prevalent form pyridoxine hydrochloride, for the treatment of patients with chronic renal failure, also are proposed (see Chapters 20, 23, and 25).

VITAMIN B12

Status in Patients Undergoing Maintenance Dialysis

Vitamin B12 deficiency is unusual in patients with chronic renal failure and patients undergoing MD because it is a large compound, is largely protein bound in serum (and poorly dialyzable), and the usual urinary losses do not occur in chronic renal failure and ESRD (4,50,80,82,89,102, 103).

Evidence and Recommendations

Although vitamin B12 is necessary for normal erythropoiesis, there is no direct evidence for the benefits of vitamin B12 supplementation in individuals undergoing MD and rHuEpo therapy. It, however, may be prudent to consider the recommendations of a workgroup to give low-dose vitamin B12 supplementation (0.25 mg/month) to patients undergoing MD and rHuEpo treatment (55). A more detailed discussion of vitamin B12 needs in patients with CRF and patients undergoing MD is given in Chapters 20, 23, and 25.

CARNITINE

Role in Anemia of Renal Failure

Although the most important cause for the anemia associated with chronic renal failure is erythropoietin deficiency, increased osmotic fragility leading to reduced red blood cell survival also appears to play a role (104,105). Because L-carnitine plays a key role in lipid metabolism, several investigators have postulated that a deficiency of L-carnitine or alteration in carnitine metabolism may contribute to the reduction in red blood cell survival observed in uremia. Indeed, a direct correlation has been demonstrated between the rHuEpo dose and total or free plasma carnitine in patients undergoing MD (106,107). Matsumura et al. demonstrated an increased red cell osmotic fragility, as measured by coil planet centrifuge, in individuals with low carnitine levels (107). Finally, administration of L-carnitine has been associated with an improvement in the red cell membrane fragility, measured *in vitro*, in some but not all studies of patients being treated with MHD (108–110).

Status in Patients Undergoing Maintenance Dialysis

L-carnitine is dialyzable, and hence, serum levels of free carnitine frequently have been found to be deficient in patients undergoing MD (111). Moreover, uremia is associated with an increased acylcarnitine to free carnitine ratio as a result of impaired urinary excretion of acylcarnitine (111). Free carnitine also is reduced in skeletal muscle of some patients undergoing MHD, particularly in those who have been undergoing MHD for longer periods.

Evidence and Recommendations

Before erythropoietin was introduced into clinical practice, several studies, including two randomized trials in patients undergoing MHD, demonstrated a beneficial effect of L-carnitine supplementation on hematocrit levels (112–116). In a 2002 metaanalysis, these three studies resulted in a statistically significant common size effect of 0.50 ($p < 0.01$) (111). Numerous studies have evaluated the effect of L-carnitine supplementation on rHuEpo requirements (108, 110,117–126); only six of these were randomized trials (110,120–124). In four of these six trials, there occurred a significant reduction in the rHuEpo dose required to maintain a similar target hematocrit level (110,120,121,124). Moreover, in three of four evaluable trials, there was a significant decline in the rHuEpo resistance index (110,123,124). Finally, in a metaanalysis of the effect of L-carnitine supplementation on the rHuEpo dose requirements, a common effect size of -0.75 was observed, indicating an overall statistically significant benefit (111,127). Indeed, this latter analysis identified resistance to erythropoietin as the most well-established indication for L-carnitine therapy in patients undergoing MHD (111,127).

Thus, there is suggestive evidence supporting a role for L-carnitine supplementation for individuals undergoing MD who have rHuEpo resistance in the absence of other known causes of this condition. However, there is a need to conduct a large, randomized controlled trial to address this issue more definitively. In the meantime, L-carnitine supplementation should be considered for some patients with rHuEpo resistance who have not responded to other standard treatment (55). This is consistent with the recommendations of the NKF-K/DOQI Guidelines on Nutrition (127). Chapters 21 and 25 discuss the physiology and potential uses of carnitine therapy in greater detail.

GROWTH HORMONE AND INSULINLIKE GROWTH FACTOR-I (IGF-I)

Role in Anemia of Renal Failure

In humans, insulinlike growth factor-I (IGF-I) is a key mediator of the anabolic actions of growth hormone. There is increasing *in vitro* evidence that recombinant human IGF-I stimulates erythropoiesis (128–132), and *in vivo* studies in rats suggest an important role for IGF-I in erythropoiesis, particularly during accelerated growth (133,134). Moreover, studies in humans with ESRD suggest that the hematocrit correlates with the serum level of IGF-I, rather than with the serum level of erythropoietin (135,136). Furthermore, there is emerging evidence that suggests a causal role for IGF-I in post–kidney transplant erythrocytosis as well as in the genesis of spontaneous erythrocytosis that occasionally occurs in patients undergoing MD (136,137).

In humans with growth-hormone deficiency, treatment with recombinant human growth hormone (rhGH) may lead to an increase in erythropoiesis, an increase in total blood volume, and an increase in total body water (138). This change may occur without a concomitant increase in serum erythropoietin levels. However, when anemic patients with chronic renal failure are treated with rhGH, the reticulocytosis that occurs is associated with an increase in serum erythropoietin levels (139). Finally, studies in mice with chronic renal failure suggest that the administration of IGF-I may have a synergistic effect on the response of anemia to erythropoietin therapy (140).

Evidence and Recommendations

There are no studies that have evaluated the effect of rhGH or IGF-I administration on either the response to rHuEpo therapy or the dose requirements of rHuEpo necessary to achieve the target hematocrit in patients undergoing MD. Hence, there is a need for prospective, randomized clinical trials to examine the role for rhGH and IGF-I treatment in individuals undergoing MD and rHuEpo therapy. Growth hormone and IGF-I are discussed in more detail in Chapters 25, 29, 30, and 32.

REFERENCES

1. National Kidney Foundation-Dialysis Outcomes Quality Initiative. Clinical Practice Guidelines: Anemia of Chronic Renal Failure. *Am J Kidney Dis* 1997;30:S190–S240.
2. National Kidney Foundation Kidney Disease Outcome Quality Initiative. Clinical Practice Guidelines for Anemia of Chronic Kidney Disease: Update 2000. *Am J Kidney Dis* 2001;37: S182–S238.

3. Horl WH, Jacobs C, MacDougall IC, et al. European best practice guidelines 14–16: inadequate response to epoetin. *Nephrol Dial Transplant* 2000;15:43–50.
4. Hutchinson FN, Jones WJ. A cost-effectiveness analysis of anemia screening before erythropoietin in patients with end-stage renal disease. *Am J Kidney Dis* 1997;29:651–657.
5. Mehrotra R, Berman N, Alistwani A, et al. Improvement of nutritional status after initiation of maintenance hemodialysis. *Am J Kidney Dis* 2002;40:133–142.
6. Moore LW, Acchiardo S, Sargent JA, et al. Incidence, causes, and treatment of iron deficiency anemia in haemodialysis patients. *J Ren Nutr* 1992;3:105–112.
7. Bergmann M, Grutzmacher P, Heuser J, et al. Iron metabolism under rEPO therapy in patients on maintenance hemodialysis. *Int J Artif Organs* 1990;13:109–112.
8. Horl WH, Dreyling K, Steinhauer HB, et al. Iron status of dialysis patients under rHuEPO therapy. *Contrib Nephrol* 1990; 87:78–86.
9. Allegra V, Mengozzi G, Vasile A. Iron deficiency in maintenance hemodialysis patients: assessment of diagnosis criteria and of three different iron treatments. *Nephron* 1991;57:175–182.
10. Kooistra MP, van Es A, Struyvenberg A, et al. Iron metabolism in patients with the anaemia of end-stage renal disease during treatment with recombinant human erythropoietin. *Br J Haematol* 1991;79:634–639.
11. Anastassiades EG, Howarth D, Howarth J, et al. Monitoring of iron requirements in renal patients on erythropoietin. *Nephrol Dial Transplant* 1993;8:846–853.
12. Dunea G, Swagel MA, Bodiwala U, et al. Intra-dialytic oral iron therapy. *Int J Artif Organs* 1994;17:261–264.
13. Fishbane S, Frei GL, Maesaka J. Reduction in recombinant human erythropoietin doses by the use of chronic intravenous iron supplementation. *Am J Kidney Dis* 1995;26:41–46.
14. Wingard RL, Parker RA, Ismail N, et al. Efficacy of oral iron therapy in patients receiving recombinant human erythropoietin. *Am J Kidney Dis* 1995;25:433–439.
15. Macdougall IC, Tucker B, Thompson J, et al. A randomized controlled study of iron supplementation in patients treated with erythropoietin. *Kidney Int* 1996;50:1694–1699.
16. Macdougall IC, Hutton RD, Cavill I, et al. Poor response to treatment of renal anaemia with erythropoietin corrected by iron given intravenously. *BMJ* 1989;299:157–158.
17. Suh H, Wadhwa NK. Iron dextran treatment in peritoneal dialysis patients on erythropoietin. *Adv Perit Dial* 1992;8: 464–466.
18. Sunder-Plassmann G, Horl WH. Importance of iron supply for erythropoietin therapy. *Nephrol Dial Transplant* 1995;10: 2070–2076.
19. Senger JM, Weiss RJ. Hematologic and erythropoietin responses to iron dextran in the hemodialysis environment. *Anna J* 1996;23:319–323; discussion 324–325.
20. Sepandj F, Jindal K, West M, et al. Economic appraisal of maintenance parenteral iron administration in treatment of anaemia in chronic haemodialysis patients. *Nephrol Dial Transplant* 1996;11:319–322.
21. Silverberg DS, Blum M, Peer G, et al. Intravenous ferric saccharate as an iron supplement in dialysis patients. *Nephron* 1996; 72:413–417.
22. Taylor JE, Peat N, Porter C, et al. Regular low-dose intravenous iron therapy improves response to erythropoietin in haemodialysis patients. *Nephrol Dial Transplant* 1996;11:1079–1083.
23. Charytan C, Levin N, Al-Saloum M, et al. Efficacy and safety of iron sucrose for iron deficiency in patients with dialysis-associated anemia: North American Clinical Trial. *Am J Kidney Dis* 2001;37:300–307.
24. Prakash S, Walele A, Dimkovic N, et al. Experience with a large dose (500 mg) of intravenous iron dextran and iron saccharate in peritoneal dialysis patients. *Perit Dial Int* 2001;21:290–295.
25. Hamstra RD, Block MH, Schocket AL. Intravenous iron dextran in clinical medicine. *JAMA* 1980;243:1726–1731.
26. Fishbane S, Ungureanu VD, Maesaka JK, et al. The safety of intravenous iron dextran in hemodialysis patients. *Am J Kidney Dis* 1996;28:529–534.
27. Ahsan N. Intravenous infusion of total dose iron is superior to oral iron in treatment of anemia in peritoneal dialysis patients: a single center comparative study. *J Am Soc Nephrol* 1998;9: 664–668.
28. Auerbach M, Chaudhry M, Goldman H, et al. Value of methylprednisolone in prevention of the arthralgia-myalgia syndrome associated with the total dose infusion of iron dextran: a double blind randomized trial. *J Lab Clin Med* 1998;131:257–260.
29. Auerbach M, Winchester J, Wahab A, et al. A randomized trial of three iron dextran infusion methods for anemia in EPO-treated dialysis patients. *Am J Kidney Dis* 1998;31:81–86.
30. Faich G, Strobos J. Sodium ferric gluconate complex in sucrose: safer intravenous iron therapy than iron dextrans. *Am J Kidney Dis* 1999;33:464–470.
31. Fishbane S, Wagner J. Sodium ferric gluconate complex in the treatment of iron deficiency for patients on dialysis. *Am J Kidney Dis* 2001;37:879–883.
32. Eschbach JW, Egrie JC, Downing MR, et al. Correction of the anemia of end-stage renal disease with recombinant human erythropoietin. Results of a combined phase I and II clinical trial. *N Engl J Med* 1987;316:73–78.
33. Gunnell J, Yeun JY, Depner TA, et al. Acute-phase response predicts erythropoietin resistance in hemodialysis and peritoneal dialysis patients. *Am J Kidney Dis* 1999;33:63–72.
34. Van Wyck DB, Bailie G, Aronoff G. Just the FAQs: Frequently Asked Questions about iron and anemia in patients with chronic kidney disease. *Am J Kidney Dis* 2002;39:426–432.
35. Tarng DC, Chen TW, Huang TP. Iron metabolism indices for early prediction of the response and resistance to erythropoietin therapy in maintenance hemodialysis patients. *Am J Nephrol* 1995;15:230–237.
36. Rosenlof K, Kivivuori SM, Gronhagen-Riska C, et al. Iron availability is transiently improved by intravenous iron medication in patients on chronic hemodialysis. *Clin Nephrol* 1995;43: 249–255.
37. Fishbane S, Kowalski EA, Imbriano LJ, et al. The evaluation of iron status in hemodialysis patients. *J Am Soc Nephrol* 1996; 7:2654–2657.
38. Fishbane S, Lynn RI. The utility of zinc protoporphyrin for predicting the need for intravenous iron therapy in hemodialysis patients. *Am J Kidney Dis* 1995;25:426–432.
39. Macdougall IC, Cavill I, Hulme B, et al. Detection of functional iron deficiency during erythropoietin treatment: a new approach. *BMJ* 1992;304:225–226.
40. Schaefer RM, Schaefer L. The hypochromic red blood cell: A new parameter for monitoring iron supplementation during rEpo therapy. *J Perinatol Med* 1995;23:83–88.
41. Mittman N, Sreedhara R, Muschnick R, et al. Reticulocyte hemoglobin content predicts functional iron deficiency in hemodialysis patients receiving rHuEpo. *Am J Kidney Dis* 1997; 30:912–922.
42. Seifert A, von Herrath D, Schaefer K. Iron overload, but not treatment with desferrioxamine favours the development of septicemia in patients on maintenance hemodialysis. *Q J Med* 1987; 65:1015–1024.
43. Hoen B, Kessler M, Hestin D, et al. Risk factors for bacterial infections in chronic haemodialysis adult patients: a multicentre prospective survey. *Nephrol Dial Transplant* 1995;10:377–381.
44. Hoen B, Paul-Dauphin A, Hestin D, et al. EPIBACDIAL: a

multicenter prospective study of risk factors for bacteremia in chronic hemodialysis patients. *J Am Soc Nephrol* 1998;9: 869–876.
45. Allen JR, Troidle LK, Juergensen PH, et al. Incidence of peritonitis in chronic peritoneal dialysis patients infused with intravenous iron dextran. *Perit Dial Int* 2000;20:674–678.
46. Mehrotra R, Marwaha T, Appel M, et al. Reduced the incidence of peritonitis in a peritoneal dialysis program: the impact of exit site mupirocin and single-dose infusion of iron. *Perit Dial Int* 2001;20:S37.
47. Goldberg A. The enzymatic formation of haem by incorporation of iron into protoporphyrin; Importance of ascorbic acid, ergothioneine and glutathione. *Brit J Hematol* 1959;5:150–157.
48. Boeschoten EW, Schrijver J, Krediet RT, et al. Deficiencies of vitamins in CAPD patients: the effect of supplementation. *Nephrol Dial Transplant* 1988;3:187–193.
49. Sullivan JF, Eisenstein AB. Ascorbic acid depletion in patients undergoing chronic hemodialysis. *Am J Clin Nutr* 1970;23: 1339–1346.
50. Descombes E, Hanck AB, Fellay G. Water soluble vitamins in chronic hemodialysis patients and need for supplementation. *Kidney Int* 1993;43:1319–1328.
51. Gastaldello K, Vereerstraeten A, Nzame-Nze T, et al. Resistance to erythropoietin in iron-overloaded haemodialysis patients can be overcome by ascorbic acid administration. *Nephrol Dial Transplant* 1995;10:44–47.
52. Tarng DC, Huang TP. A parallel, comparative study of intravenous iron versus intravenous ascorbic acid for erythropoietin-hyporesponsive anaemia in haemodialysis patients with iron overload. *Nephrol Dial Transplant* 1998;13:2867–2872.
53. Tarng DC, Wei YH, Huang TP, et al. Intravenous ascorbic acid as an adjuvant therapy for recombinant erythropoietin in hemodialysis patients with hyperferritinemia. *Kidney Int* 1999; 55:2477–2486.
54. Petrarulo F, Giancaspro V. Intravenous ascorbic acid in haemodialysis patients with functional iron deficiency. *Nephrol Dial Transplant* 2000;15:1717–1718.
55. Horl WH. Is there a role for adjuvant therapy in patients being treated with epoetin? *Nephrol Dial Transplant* 1999;14:50–60.
56. Pru C, Eaton J, Kjellstrand C. Vitamin C intoxication and hyperoxalemia in chronic hemodialysis patients. *Nephron* 1985; 39:112–116.
57. Alkhunaizi AM, Chan L. Secondary oxalosis: a cause of delayed recovery of renal function in the setting of acute renal failure. *J Am Soc Nephrol* 1996;7:2320–2326.
58. Rolton HA, McConnell KM, Modi KS, et al. The effect of vitamin C intake on plasma oxalate in patients on regular haemodialysis. *Nephrol Dial Transplant* 1991;6:440–443.
59. Proteggente AR, Rehman A, Halliwell B, et al. Potential problems of ascorbate and iron supplementation: pro-oxidant effect in vivo? *Biochem Biophys Res Commun* 2000;277:535–540.
60. Tarng DC, Huang TP, Wei YH. Erythropoietin and iron: the role of ascorbic acid. *Nephrol Dial Transplant* 2001;16:35–39.
61. Rao DS, Shih MS, Mohini R. Effect of serum parathyroid hormone and bone marrow fibrosis on the response to erythropoietin in uremia. *N Engl J Med* 1993;328:171–175.
62. Shasha SM, Better OS, Winaver J, et al. Improvement in the anemia of hemodialyzed patients following subtotal parathyroidectomy. Evidence for the role of secondary hyperparathyroidism in the etiology of the anemia of chronic renal failure. *Isr J Med Sci* 1978;14:328–332.
63. Zingraff J, Drueke T, Marie P, et al. Anemia and secondary hyperparathyroidism. *Arch Intern Med* 1978;138:1650–1652.
64. Barbour GL. Effect of parathyroidectomy on anemia in chronic renal failure. *Arch Intern Med* 1979;139:889–891.
65. Urena P, Eckardt KU, Sarfati E, et al. Serum erythropoietin and erythropoiesis in primary and secondary hyperparathyroidism: effect of parathyroidectomy. *Nephron* 1991;59:384–393.
66. Garcia-Canton C, Palomar R, Moreno A, et al. Evolution of anemia of chronic renal failure after the treatment of hyperparathyroidism. *Nephron* 1996;74:444–445.
67. Goicoechea M, Gomez-Campdera F, Polo JR, et al. Secondary hyperparathyroidism as cause of resistance to treatment with erythropoietin: effect of parathyroidectomy. *Clin Nephrol* 1996; 45:420–421.
68. Meytes D, Bogin E, Ma A, et al. Effect of parathyroid hormone on erythropoiesis. *J Clin Invest* 1981;67:1263–1269.
69. McGonigle RJ, Wallin JD, Husserl F, et al. Potential role of parathyroid hormone as an inhibitor of erythropoiesis in the anemia of renal failure. *J Lab Clin Med* 1984;104:1016–1026.
70. Bogin E, Massry SG, Levi J, et al. Effect of parathyroid hormone on osmotic fragility of human erythrocytes. *J Clin Invest* 1982; 69:1017–1025.
71. Malachi T, Bogin E, Gafter U, et al. Parathyroid hormone effect on the fragility of human young and old red blood cells in uremia. *Nephron* 1986;42:52–57.
72. Delwiche F, Garrity MJ, Powell JS, et al. High levels of the circulating form of parathyroid hormone do not inhibit in vitro erythropoiesis. *J Lab Clin Med* 1983;102:613–620.
73. Munker R, Norman A, Koeffler HP. Vitamin D compounds. Effect on clonal proliferation and differentiation of human myeloid cells. *J Clin Invest* 1986;78:424–430.
74. Albitar S, Genin R, Fen-Chong M, et al. High-dose alfacalcidol improves anaemia in patients on haemodialysis. *Nephrol Dial Transplant* 1997;12:514–518.
75. Argiles A, Mourad G, Lorho R, et al. Medical treatment of severe hyperparathyroidism and its influence on anaemia in end-stage renal failure. *Nephrol Dial Transplant* 1994;9:1809–1812.
76. Goicoechea M, Vazquez MI, Ruiz MA, et al. Intravenous calcitriol improves anaemia and reduces the need for erythropoietin in haemodialysis patients. *Nephron* 1998;78:23–27.
77. Carozzi S, Ramello A, Nasini MG, et al. Ca++ and 1,25(OH)2D3 regulate in vitro and in vivo the response to human recombinant erythropoietin in CAPD patients. *Adv Perit Dial* 1990;6:312–315.
78. Kelsey SM, Newland AC, Cunningham J, et al. Sustained haematological response to high-dose oral alfacalcidol in patients with myelodysplastic syndromes. *Lancet* 1992;340: 316–317.
79. Lasseur C, Parrot F, Delmas Y, et al. Impact of high-flux/high-efficiency dialysis on folate and homocysteine metabolism. *J Nephrol* 2001;14:32–35.
80. Hampers CL, Streiff R, Nathan DG, et al. Megaloblastic hematopoiesis in uremia and in patients on long-term hemodialysis. *N Engl J Med* 1967;276:551–554.
81. Hemmeloff Andersen KE. Folic acid status of patients with chronic renal failure maintained by dialysis. *Clin Nephrol* 1977; 8:510–513.
82. Ramirez G, Chen M, Boyce HW Jr, et al. Longitudinal follow-up of chronic hemodialysis patients without vitamin supplementation. *Kidney Int* 1986;30:99–106.
83. Westhuyzen J, Matherson K, Tracey R, et al. Effect of withdrawal of folic acid supplementation in maintenance hemodialysis patients. *Clin Nephrol* 1993;40:96–99.
84. Hong SY, Yang DH, Chang SK. Plasma homocysteine, vitamin B6, vitamin B12 and folic acid in end-stage renal disease during low-dose supplementation with folic acid. *Am J Nephrol* 1998; 18:367–372.
85. Bamonti-Catena F, Buccianti G, Porcella A, et al. Folate measurements in patients on regular hemodialysis treatment. *Am J Kidney Dis* 1999;33:492–497.

86. Lee EY, Kim JS, Lee HJ, et al. Do dialysis patients need extra folate supplementation? *Adv Perit Dial* 1999;15:247–250.
87. Tremblay R, Bonnardeaux A, Geadah D, et al. Hyperhomocysteinemia in hemodialysis patients: effects of 12-month supplementation with hydrosoluble vitamins. *Kidney Int* 2000;58: 851–858.
88. McDonald SP, Whiting MJ, Tallis GA, et al. Relationships between homocysteine and related amino acids in chronic hemodialysis patients. *Clin Nephrol* 2001;55:465–470.
89. Billion S, Tribout B, Cadet E, et al. Hyperhomocysteinaemia, folate and vitamin B12 in unsupplemented haemodialysis patients: effect of oral therapy with folic acid and vitamin B12. *Nephrol Dial Transplant* 2002;17:455–461.
90. Breen CP, MacDougall IC. Correction of epoetin-resistant megaloblastic anaemia following vitamin B(12) and folate administration. *Nephron* 1999;83:374–375.
91. Pronai W, Riegler-Keil M, Silberbauer K, et al. Folic acid supplementation improves erythropoietin response. *Nephron* 1995; 71:395–400.
92. Polak VE, Lorch JA, Means RT Jr. Unanticipated favorable effects of correcting iron deficiency in chronic hemodialysis patients. *J Investig Med* 2001;49:173–183.
93. Ono K, Hisasue Y. Is folate supplementation necessary in hemodialysis patients on erythropoietin therapy. *Clin Nephrol* 1992; 38:290–292.
94. Kopple JD, Mercurio K, Blumenkrantz MJ, et al. Daily requirement for pyridoxine supplements in chronic renal failure. *Kidney Int* 1981;19:694–704.
95. Blumberg A, Hanck A, Sander G. Vitamin nutrition in patients on continuous ambulatory peritoneal dialysis (CAPD). *Clin Nephrol* 1983;20:244–250.
96. Kasama R, Koch T, Canals-Navas C, et al. Vitamin B6 and hemodialysis: the impact of high-flux/high-efficiency dialysis and review of the literature. *Am J Kidney Dis* 1996;27:680–686.
97. Leblanc M, Pichette V, Geadah D, et al. Folic acid and pyridoxal-5′-phosphate losses during high-efficiency hemodialysis in patients without hydrosoluble vitamin supplementation. *J Ren Nutr* 2000;10:196–201.
98. Mydlik M, Derzsiova K. Erythrocyte vitamins B1, B2 and B6 and erythropoietin. *Am J Nephrol* 1993;13:464–466.
99. Mydlik M, Derzsiova K, Zemberova E. Metabolism of vitamin B6 and its requirement in chronic renal failure. *Kidney Int Suppl* 1997;62:S56–59.
100. Toriyama T, Matsuo S, Fukatsu A, et al. Effects of high-dose vitamin B6 therapy on microcytic and hypochromic anemia in hemodialysis patients. *Nippon Jinzo Gakkai Shi* 1993;35: 975–980.
101. Weissgarten J, Modai D, Oz D, et al. Vitamin B(6) therapy does not improve hematocrit in hemodialysis patients supplemented with iron and erythropoietin. *Nephron* 2001;87:328–332.
102. Zachee P, Chew SL, Daelemans R, et al. Erythropoietin resistance due to vitamin B12 deficiency. Case report and retrospective analysis of B12 levels after erythropoietin treatment. *Am J Nephrol* 1992;12:188–191.
103. De Vecchi AF, Bamonti-Catena F, Finazzi S, et al. Homocysteine, vitamin B12, serum and erythrocyte folate in peritoneal dialysis patients. *Clin Nephrol* 2001;55:313–317.
104. Rosenmund A, Binswanger U, Straub PW. Oxidative injury to erythrocytes, cell rigidity, and splenic hemolysis in hemodialyzed uremic patients. *Ann Intern Med* 1975;82:460–465.
105. Zachee P, Ferrant A, Daelemans R, et al. Oxidative injury to erythrocytes, cell rigidity and splenic hemolysis in hemodialyzed patients before and during erythropoietin treatment. *Nephron* 1993;65:288–293.
106. Kooistra MP, Struyvenberg A, van Es A. The response to recombinant human erythropoietin in patients with the anemia of end-stage renal disease is correlated with serum carnitine levels. *Nephron* 1991;57:127–128.
107. Matsumura M, Hatakeyama S, Koni I, et al. Correlation between serum carnitine levels and erythrocyte osmotic fragility in hemodialysis patients. *Nephron* 1996;72:574–578.
108. Berard E, Iordache A. Effect of low doses of L-carnitine on the response to recombinant human erythropoietin in hemodialyzed children: about two cases. *Nephron* 1992;62:368–369.
109. Nikolaos S, George A, Telemachos T, et al. Effect of L-carnitine supplementation on red blood cells deformability in hemodialysis patients. *Ren Fail* 2000;22:73–80.
110. Labonia WD. L-carnitine effects on anemia in hemodialyzed patients treated with erythropoietin. *Am J Kidney Dis* 1995;26: 757–764.
111. Hurot JM, Cucherat M, Haugh M, et al. Effects of L-carnitine supplementation in maintenance hemodialysis patients: a systematic review. *J Am Soc Nephrol* 2002;13:708–714.
112. Torvato G, Ginardi V, Di Marco V, et al. Long term L-carnitine treatment of chronic anemia of patients with end-stage renal failure. *Curr Ther Res* 1982;31:1042–1049.
113. Bellinghieri G, Savica V, Mallamace A, et al. Correlation between increased serum and tissue L-carnitine levels and improved muscle symptoms in hemodialyzed patients. *Am J Clin Nutr* 1983;38:523–531.
114. Fagher B, Cederblad G, Monti M, et al. Carnitine and left ventricular function in haemodialysis patients. *Scand J Clin Lab Invest* 1985;45:193–198.
115. Fagher B, Cederblad G, Eriksson M, et al. L-carnitine and haemodialysis: double blind study on muscle function and metabolism and peripheral nerve function. *Scand J Clin Lab Invest* 1985;45:169–178.
116. Nilsson-Ehle P, Cederblad G, Fagher B, et al. Plasma lipoproteins, liver function and glucose metabolism in haemodialysis patients: lack of effect of L-carnitine supplementation. *Scand J Clin Lab Invest* 1985;45:179–184.
117. Albertazzi A, Capelli P, Di Paolo B, et al. Endocrine-metabolic effects of L-carnitine in patients on regular dialysis treatment. *Proc Eur Dial Transplant Assoc* 1983;19:302–307.
118. Donatelli M, Terrizzi C, Zummo G, et al. Effects of L-carnitine on chronic anemia and erythrocyte adenosine triphosphate concentration in hemodialyzed patients. *Curr Ther Res* 1987;41: 620–624.
119. Boran M, Dalva I, Gonenc F, et al. Response to recombinant human erythropoietin (r-Hu EPO) and L-carnitine combination in patients with anemia of end-stage renal disease. *Nephron* 1996;73:314–315.
120. Patrikarea A, Stamatelow K, Ntaountaki I, et al. The effect of combined L-carnitine and erythropoietin administration on the anaemia and on the lipid profile of patients on hemodialysis (abstract). *Nephrol Dial Transplant* 1996;11:A262.
121. Megrie K, Trombert J, Zannier A. Effect de la L-carnitine chez les patients en hemodialyse chronique traitee par erythropoietine recombinante (abstract). *Nephrologie* 1998;19:171.
122. Caruso U, Leone L, Cravotto E, et al. Effects of L-carnitine on anemia in aged hemodialysis patients treated with recombinant human erythropoietin: A pilot study. *Dial Transplant* 1998;27: 498–506.
123. Altmann P, Thompson C, Graham K, et al. Randomized, placebo controlled study on intravenous L-carnitine supplementation in hemodialysis patients—no benefit in vivo magnetic resonance spectroscopic assessment of muscle. International Congress of Nephrology. Buenos Aires, Argentina, 1999.
124. Kletzmayr J, Mayer G, Legenstein E, et al. Anemia and carnitine supplementation in hemodialyzed patients. *Kidney Int Suppl* 1999;69:S93–106.
125. Kawabata M, Kasuga S, Hara H, et al. Erythropoietin-resistant

refractory renal anemia: effects of oral L-carnitine supplementation. *Clin Nephrol* 2001;55:265–266.

126. Matsumoto Y, Amano I, Hirose S, et al. Effects of L-carnitine supplementation on renal anemia in poor responders to erythropoietin. *Blood Purif* 2001;19:24–32.
127. National Kidney Foundation, Kidney-Dialysis Outcome Quality Initiative. Clinical Practice Guidelines for nutrition in chronic renal failure. *Am J Kidney Dis* 2000;35:S1–S140.
128. Kurtz A, Jelkmann W, Bauer C. A new candidate for the regulation of erythropoiesis. Insulin-like growth factor I. *FEBS Lett* 1982;149:105–108.
129. Akahane K, Tojo A, Urabe A, et al. Pure erythropoietic colony and burst formations in serum-free culture and their enhancement by insulin-like growth factor I. *Exp Hematol* 1987;15: 797–802.
130. Claustres M, Chatelain P, Sultan C. Insulin-like growth factor I stimulates human erythroid colony formation in vitro. *J Clin Endocrinol Metab* 1987;65:78–82.
131. Merchav S, Tatarsky I, Hochberg Z. Enhancement of erythropoiesis in vitro by human growth hormone is mediated by insulin-like growth factor I. *Br J Haematol* 1988;70:267–271.
132. Correa PN, Eskinazi D, Axelrad AA. Circulating erythroid progenitors in polycythemia vera are hypersensitive to insulin-like growth factor-1 in vitro: studies in an improved serum-free medium. *Blood* 1994;83:99–112.
133. Kurtz A, Zapf J, Eckardt KU, et al. Insulin-like growth factor I stimulates erythropoiesis in hypophysectomized rats. *Proc Natl Acad Sci U S A* 1988;85:7825–7829.
134. Kurtz A, Matter R, Eckardt KU, et al. Erythropoiesis, serum erythropoietin, and serum IGF-I in rats during accelerated growth. *Acta Endocrinol (Copenh)* 1990;122:323–328.
135. Urena P, Bonnardeaux A, Eckardt KU, et al. Insulin-like growth factor I: a modulator of erythropoiesis in uraemic patients? *Nephrol Dial Transplant* 1992;7:40–44.
136. Shih LY, Huang JY, Lee CT. Insulin-like growth factor I plays a role in regulating erythropoiesis in patients with end-stage renal disease and erythrocytosis. *J Am Soc Nephrol* 1999;10: 315–322.
137. Brox AG, Mangel J, Hanley JA, et al. Erythrocytosis after renal transplantation represents an abnormality of insulin-like growth factor-I and its binding proteins. *Transplantation* 1998;66: 1053–1058.
138. Christ ER, Cummings MH, Westwood NB, et al. The importance of growth hormone in the regulation of erythropoiesis, red cell mass, and plasma volume in adults with growth hormone deficiency. *J Clin Endocrinol Metab* 1997;82:2985–2990.
139. Sohmiya M, Ishikawa K, Kato Y. Stimulation of erythropoietin secretion by continuous subcutaneous infusion of recombinant human GH in anemic patients with chronic renal failure. *Eur J Endocrinol* 1998;138:302–306.
140. Brox AG, Zhang F, Guyda H, et al. Subtherapeutic erythropoietin and insulin-like growth factor-1 correct the anemia of chronic renal failure in the mouse. *Kidney Int* 1996;50:937–943.

23

NUTRITIONAL MANAGEMENT OF NONDIALYZED PATIENTS WITH CHRONIC RENAL FAILURE

JOEL D. KOPPLE

ALTERED HANDLING OF NUTRIENTS IN PATIENTS WITH CHRONIC RENAL FAILURE

The patient with chronic renal failure (CRF) has alterations in both the dietary requirements and the tolerance for most nutrients. The causes of these disorders include the following: decreased (or occasionally increased) urinary, intestinal, and dermal excretion and intestinal absorption and/or altered metabolism of individual nutrients or their metabolites or products. A list of these abnormalities include the following:

1. Decreased renal clearance of water, sodium, potassium, calcium, magnesium, phosphorus, some trace elements, organic and inorganic acids, and other organic compounds (1,2)
2. Accumulation of certain proteins, peptides, and amino acids and retention of products of protein, peptide, nucleic acid, and amino acid metabolism (3); carbohydrate intolerance that is usually mild and that partly improves with hemodialysis therapy; and accumulation of some products of carbohydrate metabolism (4–7)
3. Decreased intestinal absorption of calcium (8,9) and possibly iron (10,11), riboflavin (12), folate (13), vitamin D_3 (14), and certain amino acids (intestinal dipeptide absorption appears to be normal (15))
4. Possibly increased metabolic clearance of plasma pyridoxine hydrochloride (16)
5. Antagonism to the actions of several vitamins (in part resulting from medicines ingested and possibly from the accumulation of metabolic products that antagonize these vitamins) and a high risk for developing deficiencies of certain vitamins, especially for folic acid, vitamin B_6, vitamin C, and 1,25-dihydroxycholecalciferol (the most potent metabolite of vitamin D) (17,18) (see Chapter 20)
6. Increased cytosolic calcium concentrations (19,20)

Patients with CRF also may accumulate potential toxins that normally are eaten in small amounts and are excreted readily by the kidneys; notable among these is aluminum (21).

Nondialyzed patients with advanced CRF display a high incidence of type IV hyperlipoproteinemia with elevated serum triglycerides, low serum high–density lipoprotein (HDL) cholesterol, and increased serum low–density lipoprotein (LDL) and intermediate–density lipoprotein (IDL) cholesterol levels (22–26) (see Chapter 3). Serum lipoprotein (a) (Lp(a)) concentrations are often high (i.e., >30 mg/dL). High serum Lp(a) is associated with a high risk for coronary artery atherosclerosis, cerebrovascular arteriosclerosis, and stenosis of saphenous vein bypass grafts (26). The serum concentrations of certain lipoproteins are altered in uremia. In addition, the proportions of individual lipids and apolipoproteins in the lipoprotein molecules may differ from normal (22–24,26). It has been suggested that this abnormal serum lipoprotein and apolipoprotein pattern contributes to the increased risk of atherosclerosis and coronary artery disease (22,24). Synthesis of triglycerides usually is normal, but the metabolic clearance of triglycerides is impaired (27). The patient with advanced kidney failure is often in a state of oxidant (Chapter 5) and carbonyl (Chapter 6) stress and often suffers from protein-energy malnutrition (PEM) (Chapters 11 and 12) and inflammation (Chapter 13).

THE PROBLEM OF MALNUTRITION IN THE PATIENT WITH CHRONIC RENAL FAILURE

Virtually every survey of the nutritional status of patients with chronic advanced renal failure and patients undergoing maintenance hemodialysis (MHD) or chronic peritoneal dialysis (CPD) (i.e., continuous ambulatory peritoneal dialysis or automated peritoneal dialysis) indicates that they frequently suffer from PEM (28–37). There are much fewer studies of the incidence of malnutrition in patients with advanced CRF as compared to patients undergoing MHD or CPD. However, the prevalence and severity of PEM in patients with CRF who are commencing chronic dialysis therapy appear to be similar to that of patients who are well established on MHD or CPD (28,29,33). Moreover, the nutritional status at the onset of MHD or peritoneal dialysis appears to be a strong predictor of nutritional status 1 or 2 years later. This relationship has been observed both in children (Chapter 29) and adults (33,38), although some improvement in nutritional status may be observed following the commencement of maintenance dialysis (39). Thus, to avoid malnutrition in patients undergoing maintenance dialysis, it would seem important to prevent it from developing before patients with chronic renal disease develop end-stage renal disease (ESRD).

In this regard, recent data suggest that nutritional status of patients with CRF may begin to deteriorate long before patients develop ESRD (40,41). The nutritional status of approximately 1,700 patients entering the baseline period of the Modification of Diet in Renal Disease (MDRD) study was compared to their glomerular filtration rate (GFR), measured as the ^{131}I-iothalamate clearance (41). This was a cross-sectional study in which each nutritional parameter from each individual constituted a single data point. The results showed that a number of indictors of protein-energy nutritional status began to decline as the GFR fell toward 10 mL/min/1.73 m^2. This decline was noted for dietary protein and energy intake and also for serum albumin and transferrin, body weight, midarm muscle circumference, and percent body fat. Some parameters of nutrition status began to decrease when the GFR was 21 to 37 mL/min/1.73 m^2 or higher. It should be emphasized that the patients were not malnourished—indeed, frank malnutrition was a criterion for exclusion from the MDRD study—but there clearly was a statistically significant trend toward worsening nutritional status as the GFR decreased. For comparison, a GFR of 30 mL/min/1.73 m^2, on average, is associated with a measured true serum creatinine (essentially exclusive of noncreatinine chromagen) of roughly 1.7 mg/dL (42). The foregoing results may be particularly noteworthy because the patients in the MDRD study were almost certainly a healthier subset of patients with chronic renal insufficiency because of the study's exclusionary criteria. However, a number of studies indicate that patients with CRF who are prescribed low-protein diets and whose nutritional intake and clinical condition are monitored carefully can maintain good nutritional status as they develop ESRD (38,41,43–45).

The causes for PEM and methods for assessing malnutrition in patients with CRF are discussed in Chapters 11 and 15. The causes for malnutrition in nondialyzed patients with CRF include (a) reduced nutrient intake, (b) chronic comorbid conditions (e.g., diabetes mellitus, lupus erythematosus, other causes of the nephrotic syndrome, congestive heart failure, emphysema), (c) acute intercurrent illnesses, (d) inflammation without clinically apparent associated illnesses (Chapter 13), (e) the altered hormonal milieu (including resistance to the anabolic hormones—insulin, growth hormone, and insulin-like growth factor 1) and elevated levels of the catabolic hormones (glucagon and parathyroid hormone), and possibly (f) accumulation of toxic uremic metabolites, and (g) loss of the metabolic activity of the kidney (46).

Reduced nutrient intake may be a particularly important cause of PEM. Decreased food intake may be caused by anorexia (as a result of renal failure itself, emotional depression, intercurrent illnesses), anorexigenic cytokines associated with inflammation (e.g., tumor necrosis factor α, interleukin-6) (Chapter 13), superimposed catabolic diseases (e.g., vomiting from diabetic gastropathy, infection), loss of dentures, or inability to purchase or prepare foods. Anorexia appears to occur frequently and relatively early in the course of renal failure.

Although several studies indicate that patients with CRF who are not in need of dialysis therapy often have a low dietary intake of many nutrients, including protein (40,41, 47–49), they are particularly likely to have a decreased energy intake (41,43,47–51) (Chapter 11). In almost all studies of dietary energy intake in individuals with stage 3, 4, or 5 chronic kidney disease (i.e., individuals with chronic kidney disease and GFRs of 30 to 59, 15 to 29, and less than 15 mL/min/1.73 m^2, respectively) (51), their energy intake averaged less than 30 kcal/kg/day (Chapter 11). Their energy intake was usually 10% to 30% lower than the recommended dietary allowances (RDAs) of the Food and Nutrition Board, National Research Council, for dietary energy intake of healthy nonpregnant, nonlactating adults engaging in light to moderate physical activity. These latter values were, respectively, 40 and 38 kcal/kg/day for men and women 19 to 24 years old; 37 and 36 kcal/kg/day, respectively, for men and women 25 to 50 years old; and 30 kcal/kg/day for both men and women 51 years or older. Even in clinically stable individuals with GFRs of 45 to 55 mL/min/1.73 m^2, the mean dietary energy intake was less than 30 kcal/kg/day (41). Because the foregoing intakes represent mean values, approximately one-half of these men and women with stage 3 to 5 chronic kidney disease have even lower dietary energy intakes.

Dietary protein intakes in individuals with stages 3 to 5 chronic kidney disease also are reduced, usually averaging around 0.8 to 1.0 g/kg/day (40,41,48,49) (Chapter 11). Dietary protein intake tends to fall to roughly 0.8 g/kg/day as people approach end-stage kidney failure (40,41). This reduction occurs even in people with chronic kidney disease who report not having received any medical or dietetic counseling to reduce their dietary protein. The dietary intake of 0.8 g protein/kg/day is the RDA for protein of mixed biologic value in healthy adult humans (52,53), but, again, approximately half of the patients with stage 5 chronic kidney disease may be ingesting less than this quantity of daily protein intake (41).

Although the nutritional disorder most commonly associated with CRF is PEM, other nutritional deficiencies frequently occur if the patient does not receive supplemental nutrients. Particularly common in patients with CRF not receiving dialysis therapy who do not take nutritional supplements are deficiencies for 1,25-dihydroxycholecalciferol, vitamin B_6, folic acid, vitamin C, iron, and zinc (10,11,17, 18,54–57) (Chapters 19 and 20).

The nutritional status of the patient undergoing MHD or CPD is a powerful predictor of morbidity and mortality (58–64) (see Chapter 12). Low serum albumin, transferrin, transthyretin (prealbumin), cholesterol, body weight-for-height, subjective global nutritional assessment, bioelectrical impedance, and dietary protein intake (as indicated by decreased normalized protein equivalent of total nitrogen appearance [nPNA], also referred to as normalized protein catabolic rate [nPCR]) (65) all have been associated with increased mortality in patients undergoing MHD or CPD (58–64) (Chapter 12).

These data do not prove that malnutrition itself causes the high morbidity and mortality. It is possible that the same comorbid conditions that engender these measures of PEM independently cause fatality. Indeed, much data indicate that measures of inflammation, such as serum C-reactive protein (CRP), commonly are increased in patients undergoing maintenance dialysis; in both patients undergoing maintenance dialysis (66–68) and normal individuals (69,70) increased serum CRP levels are associated with adverse cardiovascular events and cardiovascular and all-cause mortality. The relation between low serum albumin, transferrin, prealbumin, and adverse outcome has been related to the fact that these proteins are negative acute-phase proteins and are lowered by inflammation as well as PEM (71–73) (Chapter 13). Inflammatory states not only are associated with an increased catabolic state but also with anorexia. Thus, the possibility remains that inflammation actually may engender morbidity and mortality by causing PEM. Also, PEM, by lowering host resistance, may predispose to inflammation. It is pertinent that one prospective study indicated that patients undergoing MHD improved their nutritional status when they received intradialytic parenteral nutrition (IDPN) (74), and two retrospective analyses of rather large patient populations indicated improved survival rates in malnourished patients undergoing MHD who were given IDPN (75,76). These results are consistent with the thesis that protein-calorie malnutrition does contribute to the adverse outcomes and that increasing the nutrient intake of these malnourished patients undergoing MHD does improve survival.

TRAINING AND MONITORING THE PATIENT UNDERGOING DIETARY THERAPY

Adherence to renal failure diets is frequently a difficult and frustrating endeavor for patients and their families. Usually the patient must make fundamental changes in behavior patterns and forsake some of the traditional sources of daily pleasure. Patients often must obtain special foods, prepare special recipes, forego or severely limit their intake of favorite foods, or eat foods that they may not desire. Demands are made on the patient's time and daily activities and on the emotional support system of the family or close associates. Therefore, it is incumbent on the physician not to prescribe radical changes in the patient's diet unless there is good reason to believe that these modifications may be beneficial. To ensure successful dietary therapy, patients with renal disease must undergo extensive training concerning the principles of nutritional therapy and the design and preparation of diets, and they need to be encouraged continuously to adhere to the prescribed diet. They usually require repeated training regarding their nutritional therapy. Without careful monitoring of nutritional intake; frequent retraining and encouragement; and sensitivity to their cultural background, psychosocial condition, and lifestyle, the patients will be less likely to adhere to their dietary prescription. They may eat too little rather than too much. A systematic, problem-oriented approach to dietary compliance can improve compliance substantially (77–80). These issues are discussed in greater detail in Chapter 36.

Recipes and meal plans should be designed specifically for the individual tastes of the patient. A team approach, including participation of the physician, dietitian, close family members, the nursing staff, and (when available) social workers or psychiatrists, may improve adherence. Because the prescribed diet for patients with renal failure is complicated, and because obtaining an accurate diet history and maximizing dietary compliance for these individuals is a complex and subtle art, it is important for the physician to work with a dietitian who is knowledgeable and experienced in nephrology dietetics (see Chapter 36). It is often advantageous to organize the dietetic program in a medical center so that the dietitians who treat nephrology patients work exclusively or primarily in this specialty.

Because diets prescribed for patients with renal insufficiency are often marginally low in some nutrients (e.g., protein) and high in others (e.g., calcium) and malnutrition is not infrequent, it is important to evaluate the adequacy of the diet and the patient's nutritional status periodically (Table 23.1). The National Kidney Foundation Kidney Disease Outcomes Quality Initiative (NKF-K/DOQI) Clinical Practice Guidelines for Nutrition in Chronic Renal Failure states that "for individuals with CRF and a GFR less than 20 mL/min, protein-energy nutritional status should be evaluated by serial measurements of a panel of

TABLE 23.1. MINIMAL REQUIREMENTS FOR ASSESSMENT OF NUTRITIONAL STATUS OF PATIENTS WITH STAGE 3, 4, OR 5 CHRONIC KIDNEY DISEASE NOT RECEIVING DIALYSIS TREATMENT[a]

Every 1–3 months[b]
Patient reviews diet with dietitian
Blood hemoglobin or hematocrit taken
Serum measured
- Urea
- Creatinine
- Sodium
- Potassium
- Chloride
- Bicarbonate
- Albumin and/or transthyretin (prealbumin)

Edema-free body weight, percent standard body weight[c] assessed
Recent change in body weight determined
Subjective global nutritional assessment performed

Every 3–6 months
Dietary interview by dietitian and 3-day diary of daily nutrient intake[d] or normalized protein equivalent of total nitrogen appearance (see text) assessed

Every 12 months
Serum or plasma measured
- Total cholesterol
- Low–density-lipoprotein cholesterol
- High–density-lipoprotein cholesterol
- Triglycerides
- Homocysteine
- C-reactive protein

Anthropometry[e] performed

[a]Glomerular filtration rate levels with stages of kidney disease: stage 3, 30–59 mL/min/1.73 m^2; stage 4, 15–29 mL/min/1.73 m^2; stage 5, <15 mL/min/1.73 m^2.
[b]This frequency of monitoring is more important for people with stage 5 chronic kidney disease.
[c]Standard body weight is the median body weight of normal persons of the same age range, gender, height, and skeletal frame size as the patient as determined from the NHANES II data (81, 82).
[d]This constitutes a more formal, in-depth assessment of daily nutrient intake than is obtained at the 1- to 3-month intervals.
[e]Anthropometry is optional and dependent on the availability of a trained anthropometrist. See Chapter 15 for listing of anthropometric measurements.

markers including at least one value from each of the following clusters: 1) serum albumin; 2) edema-free actual body weight, percent standard (NHANES II) body weight, or subjective global assessment (SGA); and 3) normalized protein nitrogen appearance (nPNA) or dietary interviews and diaries" (81). NHANES II refers to the second National Health and Nutrition Evaluation Survey (82,83).

The NKF-K/DOQI guidelines recommend that if patients are clinically stable, serum albumin and actual or percent standard body weight and/or SGA should be measured every 1 to 3 months and dietary interviews and diaries and/or nPNA should be performed every 3 to 4 months. For patients with more advanced CRF (i.e., GFR 15 mL/min or lower—essentially stage 5 chronic kidney disease), concomitant illness, inadequate nutrient intake, deteriorating nutritional status, or frank malnutrition, more frequent monitoring may be necessary (81). Recent reevaluation of the usefulness of serum transthyretin (i.e., serum prealbumin) suggests that, like serum albumin, it is affected by both nutrition and inflammation, but it is an independent risk factor for mortality in patients undergoing MHD, and monitoring of serum transthyretin may be substituted for albumin (63,84).

Changes in body weight and history of weight loss are often very helpful. To assess intake of other nutrients, 24-hour urine excretion of sodium, potassium, and phosphorus often are helpful (see Chapter 18). Roughly 60% to 70% of ingested phosphorus is excreted in the urine in patients with CRF (85). Other measures of nutritional assessment and indications for their use are discussed in Chapter 15.

Dietitians are often best qualified to perform anthropometric measurements of nutritional status because of their experience and training, interest in nutritional therapy, and access to the patient. Whichever individual performs the anthropometry must be trained and shown to be able to obtain precise and reproducible measurements. Otherwise, the anthropometric values almost certainly will be too inaccurate to be useful. Good equipment for performing the anthropometry is a necessity. Fortunately, this equipment is not expensive. If the resources for obtaining these anthropometric measurements are not available, assessment of the edema-free weight, height, and bicondylar width will enable percent relative and desirable body weights and the BMI to be calculated. The creatinine appearance is reported to correlate with the muscle mass in patients undergoing CPD (86), although a number of factors may impair the precision of this measurement (87).

More technology-based methods for assessing body composition are available. Dual-energy x-ray absorptiometry (DEXA); bioelectrical impedance; near-infrared interactance; and measurements of total body nitrogen, potassium, and carbon are among the more popular of the high technology methods. Each technique has advantages and limitations (see Chapter 15), and many of these can be expensive to use. Moreover, it has not yet been demonstrated that the use of these methods will lead to improvement in the nutritional or clinical status of the patient, other than perhaps for assessing bone mineralization by the DEXA procedure. At present these techniques appear to be most useful for research studies.

In general, to maintain good dietary compliance and to monitor closely the patient's clinical, fluid and electrolyte, and nutritional status, patients with stage 4 or 5 chronic kidney disease should be seen approximately monthly by the physician and the dietitian. Patients with slowly progressive or less severe renal insufficiency who are clinically stable and adhere well to the diet probably can be seen by a physician less frequently. To maximize compliance to the diet, most patients should continue to see the dietitian frequently, often monthly. In one study in patients with CRF, frequent clinic visits, apparently independent of dietary prescription, led to a slowing in the rate of progression of renal insufficiency (88).

In many but not all patients with progressive renal failure, the creatinine clearance decreases more or less linearly with time (89,90). Transposing the clearance equation, it can be predicted that the log of the serum creatinine or the ratio of 1.0/serum creatinine also should decrease linearly with time. This has been confirmed in several studies (89, 90); approximately 60% to 80 of patients with chronic progressive kidney disease lose creatinine clearance in a roughly linear fashion. Thus, for patients with CRF, the creatinine clearance and/or the ratio of 1.0/serum creatinine periodically should be plotted against time. If the rate of progression slows, it may indicate that treatment is beneficial. However, an increase in the rate of progression may indicate the superimposition of another condition that has impaired renal function. These conditions may include worsening hypertension, urinary-tract obstruction, infection, intake of nonsteroidal antiinflammatory medicines, an adverse reaction to another medicinal intake, or increased activity of the underlying renal disease.

It is well established that the creatinine clearance is not as precise a measure of the GFR as is the clearance of inulin, iothalamate, or several other solutes and may give misleading results (91,92). This is primarily the result of variability in the renal tubular secretion of creatinine (93) and because common techniques for serum creatinine measurements are often not entirely specific. Indeed, the creatinine clearance largely has been invalidated as a measure of GFR for clinical or laboratory research studies (92). Nonetheless, the creatinine clearance is often helpful for the clinical management of patients, particularly when serial measurements are taken, and under some circumstances it may give a more precise estimate of the actual GFR than does the serum creatinine. In patients with a GFR less than about 20 mL/min/1.73 m^2, the mean of the creatinine and urea clearances may give a more accurate measure of the GFR than the creatinine clearance alone (94).

Because the nutritional status of patients with chronic progressive renal disease may begin to deteriorate when the GFR decreases to somewhere below 55 mL/min/1.73 m^2 (40,41), careful attention to nutritional status should commence at this time or earlier. Patients with chronic kidney disease appear to be at greatest risk for malnutrition from the time that the GFR falls below 10 mL/min until the patient is established on maintenance dialysis therapy (38, 41). Hence, particular effort should be given to preventing malnutrition as the patient approaches dialysis therapy and during the first few weeks of maintenance dialysis treatment. These efforts should be directed toward maintaining a good nutritional intake during this period, rapidly instituting therapy for superimposed illnesses, and maintaining good nutritional intake during such illnesses.

Urea Nitrogen Appearance and the Serum Urea Nitrogen: Serum Creatinine Ratio

Because the control of protein intake is central to the nutritional management of patients with acute or chronic renal failure, it is important to monitor nitrogen intake accurately. Fortunately, this is feasible for most patients with the use of the total nitrogen appearance (TNA) or urea nitrogen appearance (UNA). TNA is the sum of all measured nitrogen outputs (e.g., urine, feces, dialysate, emesis, tube or fistula drainage) and the change in body urea nitrogen. Change in body urea nitrogen is calculated as follows:

$$\begin{aligned}\text{Change in body urea nitrogen (g/day)}\\ &= (\text{SUN}_f - \text{SUN}_i,\ \text{g/L/day}) \times \text{BW}_i\ \text{(kg)}\\ &\times (0.60\ \text{L/kg}) + (\text{BW}_f - \text{BW}_i,\ \text{kg/day})\\ &\times \text{SUN}_f\ \text{(g/L)} \times (1.0\ \text{L/kg}) \qquad \text{[Eq. 1]}\end{aligned}$$

where i and f are the initial and final values for the period of measurement; SUN is serum urea nitrogen (grams per liter); BW is body weight (kilograms); 0.60 is an estimate of the fraction of body weight that is water; and 1.0 is the volume of distribution of urea in the weight that is gained or lost. The estimated proportion of body weight that is water may be increased in patients who are edematous or lean and decreased in individuals who are obese or very young. Changes in body weight during the 1- to 3-day period of measurement of UNA are assumed to result entirely from changes in body water.

Patients who are in neutral nitrogen balance usually will have a TNA that is equal to nitrogen intake minus about 0.5 g nitrogen per day from such unmeasured losses as sweat; respiration; flatus; blood drawing; and growth of skin, hair, and nails (95). Thus, TNA should correlate closely with nitrogen intake in patients who are more or less in nitrogen balance. For the degree of precision needed for the clinical management of patients, a nitrogen balance that is slightly positive or negative will not alter substantially the reliability of the TNA measurement as an estimate of nitrogen intake. In patients who are in very positive or negative nitrogen balance (e.g., during mid or late pregnancy or severe infection), the TNA may not reflect intake. However, when the patient is in very positive or negative balance, there is usually an accompanying alteration in the patient's clinical status that is readily apparent to the physician.

The measurement of TNA is too laborious and expensive to be widely applied for clinical uses. However, because urea is the major nitrogenous product of protein and amino acid degradation, the UNA can be used to estimate total nitrogen output and hence nitrogen intake (96–98). UNA is the amount of urea nitrogen that appears or accumulates in body fluids and all outputs (e.g., urine, dialysate, fistula drainage). The term UNA is used rather than urea production or urea generation because some urea is degraded in the intestinal tract; the ammonia released from urea largely is transported to the liver and converted back to urea (99, 100). Thus, the enterohepatic urea cycle leads to an increase in absolute urea synthesis but has little effect on serum urea levels or total nitrogen economy, and this cycle can be ignored without compromising the accuracy of the UNA for estimating total nitrogen output or intake. This offers an important advantage because the recycling of urea cannot be measured without costly and time-consuming isotope studies.

UNA is calculated as follows:

$$\text{UNA (g/day)} = \text{urinary urea nitrogen (g/day)} + \text{dialysate urea nitrogen (g/day)} + \text{change in body urea nitrogen (g/day)} \quad \text{[Eq. 2]}$$

In our experience, the relationship between UNA and TNA in patients with CRF not undergoing dialysis is as follows (98):

$$\text{TNA (g/day)} = 1.19\ \text{UNA (g/day)} + 1.27 \quad \text{[Eq. 3]}$$

If the individual is approximately in neutral nitrogen balance, the UNA also will correlate closely with nitrogen intake. Equation 4 describes our observed relationship between UNA and dietary nitrogen intake in clinically stable, nondialyzed patients with CRF (98):

$$\text{Dietary nitrogen intake (g/day)} = 1.20\ \text{UNA (g/day)} + 1.74 \quad \text{[Eq. 4]}$$

When both nitrogen intake and UNA are known, nitrogen balance can be estimated from the difference between nitrogen intake and nitrogen output estimated from the UNA. If the patient is markedly anabolic, such as in pregnancy or in a young person with anorexia nervosa who is being re-fed, equation 4 will underestimate nitrogen intake. In patients who have large protein losses (e.g., from the nephrotic syndrome or peritoneal dialysis) or who are acidemic and have sufficient kidney function to excrete large quantities of ammonia, equations 3 and 4 will underestimate both TNA and nitrogen intake. In most circumstances, however, these conditions are not present, and the UNA provides a powerful tool for monitoring nitrogen output and intake or for estimating balance. Other investigators have described similar approaches to monitoring nitrogen intake and output (97,101), and indeed the terms nPNA or PCR are based on analogous estimates of UNA (65,102).

One cautionary note concerning prediction of dietary protein intake from the urea nitrogen appearance: the data are incontrovertible that in clinically stable patients, the UNA accurately predicts TNA. However, for several reasons, TNA is not equal to dietary nitrogen intake in these individuals. First, because there are a number of unmeasured nitrogen outputs, TNA is not quite equal to the sum of the change in body urea nitrogen and total nitrogen output. These unmeasured losses of nitrogen include the nitrogen lost in sweat, epidermal and nail growth, saliva, feces on toilet paper, and debris left on toothpaste or toothbrushes and from respiration and probably flatus. An estimate of these losses, obtained experimentally from clinically stable patients with advanced renal failure, can be approximated by comparing equation 3 to equation 4. The level of nitrogen loss in these individuals is probably approximately 0.50 g/day. In individuals with larger protein or amino acid intakes, these unmeasured nitrogen losses appear to increase, and the discrepancy between the UNA and total nitrogen intake (or between TNA and total nitrogen intake) becomes greater. Second, individuals, including those who apparently are clinically stable, are commonly in slightly positive or negative nitrogen balance, and this phenomenon also will cause discrepancies between the TNA and dietary nitrogen intake. These factors have been discussed and reviewed extensively elsewhere (95,98,103).

The ratio of the SUN to serum creatinine also correlates fairly closely with dietary protein or amino acid intake in nondialyzed patients with CRF (104). This relationship can be used to estimate the recent daily intake of these patients. Although the SUN/serum creatinine ratio is not as precise as the UNA and is influenced by a number of clinical factors (104), it is easy and inexpensive to measure. For clinically stable, nondialyzed, chronically uremic patients, this ratio also can be used to estimate the level at which the SUN will stabilize for any given dietary protein intake and GFR.

ASSESSMENT OF CARDIOVASCULAR, CEREBROVASCULAR, AND PERIPHERAL VASCULAR RISK

The most common causes of death in patients undergoing maintenance dialysis therapy are cardiovascular, cerebrovascular, and peripheral vascular disease. These disorders include coronary artery disease, myocardial infarction, and sudden death, presumably associated with coronary artery disease. Many factors dispose to cardiac and vascular diseases and are reviewed in Chapters 3, 5, 6, 7, 10, 12, and 13. Many of these predisposing factors are also present in patients with chronic kidney disease who are not undergoing maintenance dialysis therapy. Moreover, recent studies indicate that patients with diabetes and stage 3, 4, or 5 chronic kidney disease have abnormally high degrees of coronary artery calcification (105,106). These findings suggest that it is important to evaluate cardiovascular risk factors even in individuals with chronic kidney disease who are not in need of dialysis therapy.

At present, there is a paucity of data indicating that modification of these risk factors will improve outcome. However, because modification of these risk factors in patients without chronic renal insufficiency does seem to be protective, unless scientific evidence emerges to the contrary, it would seem reasonable to try to modify cardiovascular risk factors in individuals with chronic kidney disease as well. Thus, it would seem important to periodically perform the following measurements in individuals with stage 2, 3, 4, or 5 chronic kidney disease: serum total cholesterol, LDL cholesterol, HDL cholesterol, triglycerides, CRP (possibly serum albumin or transthyretin may be substituted for CRP), and plasma or serum homocysteine and microalbuminuria and macroalbuminuria. These measurements probably should be obtained at least every 12 months and in general more frequently if they are abnormal and especially when therapy for these abnormalities is inaugurated or changed. Other measures of oxidant or carbonyl stress may be measured, but it can be argued that their relevance for clinical management is less well established at this time (Chapters 5 and 6).

DIETARY THERAPY FOR NONDIALYZED PATIENTS WITH CHRONIC RENAL DISEASE OR CHRONIC RENAL FAILURE

The pervasive nutritional and metabolic alterations, high prevalence of malnutrition, and research studies indicating that diets may retard the rate of progression of CRF (see Chapter 16) indicate that dietary treatment should be a key component of the management of chronic renal disease. Nutritional therapy has four aims:

1. To maintain good nutritional status
2. To arrest or slow the progression of renal failure
3. To prevent or reduce metabolic disorders (e.g., sodium, chloride, and water overload; hyperkalemia; hyperphosphatemia; hypertension) and uremic toxicity
4. To prevent or retard the development of cardiovascular, cerebrovascular, or peripheral vascular disease; hyperparathyroidism; and possibly other life-threatening or debilitating diseases

Protein, Amino Acids, and Ketoacids—Background Information

Because modification of protein intake may help to advance the first three of these nutritional aims, a brief description of the past experience with various protein diets may be indicated. Low-protein diets have been prescribed for many decades to reduce the accumulation of potentially toxic metabolites of protein metabolism in patients with CRF (78, 107–120) (Chapter 16). For about the past 40 years, nephrologists also have prescribed essential amino acid diets or very-low-protein diets (approximately 0.28 g protein/kg/day) supplemented with either essential amino acids or ketoacid or hydroxy acid analogues of essential amino acids to increase the efficiency of nitrogen utilization (78, 121–132) and to reduce the generation of potential uremic toxins while attempting to maintain good nutrition. There is considerable evidence that dietary intake of mixtures of small quantities of essential amino acids or ketoacids and essential amino acids can conserve protein mass more efficiently than diets containing similar quantities of protein in patients with CRF (121–123,125–127,130,133–136).

Substitution of α-ketoacid analogues for some essential amino acids was proposed to further reduce nitrogen intake while maintaining good nutrition. Alpha-ketoacids contain a keto group instead of an amino group on the α-carbon; α-hydroxy acids contain a hydroxyl group on this carbon. When the ketoacid or hydroxy acid analogue of most essential amino acids (with the exception of lysine and threonine) is fed or infused, some of the compounds are oxidized and some rapidly are converted to amino acids (128,129,136). Administering them is almost tantamount to giving amino acids without increasing the nitrogen load. Several investigators showed that in normal subjects and subjects with CRF, nitrogen balance may be improved by adding ketoacid analogues of phenylalanine, valine, or tryptophan to diets deficient in these essential amino acids (124,125,134–136). Leucine and its ketoacid analogue, α-ketoisocaproate acid, actually may promote protein anabolism (137,138). Hydroxy acid analogues also have been shown to substitute adequately for essential amino acids to varying degrees in patients or animals with CRF.

Walser et al. (125,129,131) administered low-protein diets usually supplemented with the ketoacid salts of five essential amino acids and the other four essential L-amino acids—threonine, lysine, histidine, and tryptophan—to patients with far advanced renal failure. Urea appearance was remarkably low in many patients, and nitrogen balance was often neutral or positive even with nitrogen intakes of less than 4.0 g/day. Some studies suggested that low-protein, low-phosphorus diets may retard the progression of CRF. These observations were consistent with research performed in the first half of the 20th century indicating that low-protein diets could retard the progression of renal failure in animals (120).

In recent years there have been three types of low-nitrogen diets that commonly have been used for the treatment of patients with CRF: (a) a low-protein diet providing about 0.55 to 0.60 g protein/kg body weight/day (78,110–120); (b) a very-low-protein diet providing approximately 16 to 20 g/day of protein of miscellaneous quality (i.e., about 0.28 gm protein/kg/day) supplemented with about 10 to 20 g/day of the nine L-essential amino acids (127,133,139, 140); and (c) a similar 16 to 20 g protein diet generally supplemented with four essential amino acids–histidine, lysine, threonine, and tryptophan—and the ketoacid or hydroxy acid analogues of the other five essential amino acids sometimes with a few other amino acids added (78,125, 129,131,132,141–143). There is strong evidence that histidine is an essential amino acid for both normal individuals and patients with CRF (144), and for this reason histidine or its ketoacid analogue is included in all amino acid and ketoacid preparations. The 0.55 to 0.60 g protein/kg/day diet contains primarily high biologic value protein (i.e., protein containing a high fraction of the essential amino acids proportioned roughly according to the daily dietary requirements for humans). Because the diets with very low protein content (0.28 g/kg/day) are supplemented with essential amino acids or ketoacids, it is not important that the protein be of high biologic value.

Clinical trials concerning whether very-low-protein and phosphorus diets (e.g., 0.30 g protein/kg/day) supplemented with essential amino acids and ketoacids will retard the rate of progression of renal failure more effectively than low-protein and low-phosphorus diets (e.g., 0.55 to 0.60 g protein/kg/day) have given mixed results (78,141–143,145, 146). These trials are discussed in more detail in Chapter 16. The largest and most thorough examination of whether dietary control will retard the rate of progression of renal disease was the National Institutes of Health–funded Modification of Diet in Renal Disease (MDRD) Study (78,146). This project investigated, in an intention-to-treat analysis, the effects of three levels of dietary protein and phosphorus intakes and two blood pressure management goals on the progression of chronic renal disease. For the study, 840 adults with various types of renal disease, but excluding insulin-dependent diabetes mellitus, were divided into two study groups according to their GFR.

Study A included 585 patients with a GFR, measured by ^{131}I-iothalamate clearances, of 25 to 55 mL/min/1.73 m^2. They were randomly assigned to either a usual-protein, usual-phosphorus diet (1.3 g protein/kg standard body weight/day and 16 to 20 mg phosphorus/kg/day) or to a low-protein, low-phosphorus diet (0.58 g protein/kg/day and 5 to 10 mg phosphorus/kg/day) and also to either a moderate or strict blood pressure goal (mean arterial blood pressure 107 mm Hg [113 mm Hg for those 61 years of age or older] or 92 mm Hg [98 mm Hg for those 61 years of age or older]). In study B, 255 patients with a baseline GFR of 13 to 24 mL/min/1.73 m^2 were randomly assigned to the low-protein and low-phosphorus diet or to a very-low-protein and low-phosphorus diet (0.28 g protein/kg/day and 4 to 9 mg/phosphorus/kg/day) with a ketoacid–amino acid supplement (0.28 g/kg/day). They also were randomly assigned to either the moderate or strict blood pressure control groups, as in Study A. The adherence to the dietary protein prescription in the different diet groups was excellent (78–80).

Among participants in Study A, those prescribed the low-protein diet had significantly faster declines in GFR during the first 4 months than those on the usual-protein diet. Thereafter, the rate of decline of the GFR in the low-protein, low-phosphorus group was significantly slower than in the group fed the usual-protein and usual-phosphorus diet. Over the course of the entire treatment period, there was no difference in the overall rate of progression of renal failure in the two diet groups. However, it is likely that the initial greater fall in GFR in the patients prescribed the low-protein diet may reflect a hemodynamic response to the reduction in protein intake, rather than a greater rate of progression of the parenchymal renal disease. In fact, this might be beneficial, reflecting a reduction of intrarenal hyperfiltration and intrarenal hypertension. If this explanation is correct—and it is not established that it is correct—the subsequent slower rate of progression of disease after the first 4 months of dietary treatment is consistent with a beneficial effect of this intervention in renal disease. In Study B, the very-low-protein group had a marginally slower decline of GFR than the low-protein group; the average rate of decline did not differ significantly between the two groups ($p = 0.066$).

In a secondary analysis of Study B in which the decrease in GFR was compared with the actual quantity of protein ingested, there was no effect of ingesting the low-protein diet versus the very-low-protein diet supplemented with ketoacids–amino acids on the progression of renal failure (146). However, if the two diet groups were analyzed together and the protein intake of the latter diet was considered to be the sum of the protein and ketoacid–amino acid supplement ingested, a significantly lower rate of decline in GFR was found in the patients who actually ingested lower protein diets (146). The actual dietary protein intake associated with a slower rate of progression was 0.75 g/kg/day, but it is possible that more data would have shown that lower protein diets might have retarded progression even more effectively (146). These findings suggest that a lower total protein intake, but not the specific ketoacid–amino acid preparation itself, retarded the rate of progression of renal failure.

It should be emphasized that in the MDRD study, the very-low-protein ketoacid–amino acid–supplemented diet was not compared to the usual protein intake. Also, it is possible that the lack of significant effect of the low-protein diet on the progression of renal failure might reflect the rather short mean duration of treatment in the MDRD study—2.2 years. Indeed, if the trend toward slower progression of renal failure in the low-protein diet groups present at the termination of the MDRD study had persisted during a longer follow-up period, statistically significantly slower progression would have been observed with the 0.60 g/kg protein diet in Study A and the very-low-protein, ketoacid–amino acid–supplemented diet in Study B. Other possible causes for the lack of effect of the diet include the high percentage of patients that had adult polycystic kidney disease (about 25% of the total), which is probably particularly refractory to dietary therapy; the fact that some patients in the study did not progress regardless of dietary prescription; and the rather small sample size for an intention-to-treat study of this kind.

Another possible reason for the failure to demonstrate a benefit with the ketoacid-supplemented very-low-protein diet is the fact that tryptophan was added to the supplement for the main clinical trial. This was done because the tryptophan content of the original ketoacid preparation was low and there was concern that this supplement, in association with a very-low-protein intake, might engender protein malnutrition. Recently, Niwa and Ise reported that metabolites of tryptophan and particularly indoxyl sulfate (147) may be nephrotoxic. Rats fed indoxyl sulfate develop more rapid progression of renal failure (147), whereas oral sorbents that lower serum levels of indoxyl sulfate (and other compounds as well) retard progression of renal failure in both animals and humans (148–150). In addition, in a *post hoc* analysis of the data from the pilot and feasibility phase of the MDRD study, in which the ketoacid supplement contained the lower tryptophan content, there was a trend for a slower rate of progression of kidney failure among the patients prescribed the ketoacid-supplemented diet (145).

Several metaanalyses have concluded that low-protein diets delay the commencement of renal replacement therapy in patients with chronic renal insufficiency (118,151–153). Fouque et al. reported a relative risk of renal death with protein-restricted diets of 0.54 (118). In another study involving 1,413 patients, the relative risk of renal death with the low-protein diet decreased to 0.67 (151). A third metaanalysis involving 1,919 patients described a reduction in the rate of loss of GFR of 6% (152). It should be noted that low-protein diets may delay the onset of renal replacement therapy not only by slowing the rate of decline in GFR but also by reducing the rate of generation of potentially toxic metabolites that accumulate in renal failure. In a fourth metaanalysis, also conducted by Fouque et al. (153) and involving 1,494 patients, there was a 61% relative risk of renal death with low-protein intakes.

There are fewer and smaller size studies of the effects of low-protein diets on progression of renal failure in patients with diabetes mellitus (151,152,154–158). Pedrini et al. reported in a metaanalysis of five studies in 108 patients with insulin-dependent diabetes and chronic renal disease that a low-protein diet reduced the increase in urine albumin excretion or the decrease in GFR or creatinine clearance (relative risk, 0.56) (151). Another analysis of six studies, including that of Pedrini et al. (151), in 357 patients with type I or type II diabetes and renal disease indicated that one study showed no benefit, whereas three studies showed a benefit of the low-protein diet on the rate of progression of renal failure and two studies were not conclusive (158). The approximate mean GFR in the two inconclusive studies was 70.4 and 71.2 mL/min, respectively, whereas in the three studies that described a beneficial effect, the approximate mean GFR in each study varied from 47 to 50 mL/min (158).

In the MDRD study, the dietary and blood pressure treatments generally were well tolerated, safe, and acceptable to patients. As has been shown in other studies, the mean blood pressure attained during follow-up also correlated directly with the rate of decrease in GFR (159) This was particularly evident for those individuals with 1.0 g/day or more of proteinuria. However, there was a tendency for some patients to develop worsening parameters of protein-energy nutritional status (43). This was particularly evident during the first 4 months of therapy in the patients prescribed the low-protein and very-low-protein diets. It is possible that the lower dietary energy intakes may have contributed to this phenomenon (156). It should be emphasized that no treatment group developed evidence for frank PEM during the study, serum albumin levels remained the same or rose significantly in the diet groups, and the development of a PEM endpoint in individual patients during the study was very uncommon.

Thus, the four meta-analyses of the effects of protein-restricted diets on the rate of progression of renal failure in nondiabetics, three of which involved the MDRD study data, can be interpreted to indicate that the ingestion of diets low in protein and phosphorus will delay the need for dialysis therapy and probably retard the rate of progression of renal failure in patients with chronic progressive renal disease. On average, this effect, although confirmed by a composite of randomized, prospective studies, is not dramatic and often requires many months of treatment to become evident. In conjunction with blood pressure control and other medical management, dietary protein and phosphorus restriction appears to offer the patient with chronic renal disease another method for slowing the rate of loss of renal function and delaying the need for renal replacement therapy.

As indicated earlier, the data regarding the use of dietary protein restriction in patients with type I or type II diabetes mellitus are inconclusive. There are fewer randomized prospective clinical trials in individuals with diabetic renal disease, and these studies generally were carried out in smaller numbers of patients for shorter periods. Metaanalyses of some of these clinical trials suggest that low-protein diets may retard progression of CRF (151,158).

It also should be emphasized that the specific effects of low-protein, low-phosphorus diets on the rate of progression of renal failure in patients who adhere precisely to those diets, as opposed to those individuals who follow them but less compliantly, have not been well tested. As indicated by the MDRD study secondary analyses (146), it is possible that for those individuals who will comply closely with such diets, they offer substantial benefits with regard to progression.

However, some of the same physiologic changes that are observed with ingestion of low-protein diets also occur when angiotensin converting enzyme (ACE) inhibitors or angiotensin-I receptor blockers (ARBs) are given. It is therefore possible that with aggressive management with ACE inhibitors and/or ARBs there will be less beneficial effect of protein restriction on retardation of renal failure. In this regard, Hansen et al. studied 82 patients with type I diabetes and progressive diabetic renal disease, about 88% of whom received ACE inhibitors during the study (160). Patients were randomized to a prescription of a 0.6 g protein/kg/day diet or to no dietary protein restriction. The estimated protein intake during the study averaged 0.89 g/kg/day (95% confidence interval; 0.83 to 0.95) and 1.02 g/kg/day (0.95 to 1.10) with the low- and usual-protein diets. The rate of decline of GFR was not different in those prescribed the low-protein versus the usual-protein diets and averaged 3.8 and 3.9 mL/min/year, respectively. ESRD or death occurred in 10% of patients prescribed the low-protein diet and in 27% of patients on the usual-protein diet ($p = 0.042$). Because almost all of these patients were receiving ACE inhibitors, the data suggest that in individuals with type I diabetes mellitus and progressive diabetic renal disease, the combination of an ACE inhibitor and a low-protein diet is more beneficial than an ACE inhibitor without dietary protein restriction.

Other Types of Low-Protein Intakes

A number of studies have examined the potential benefit of plant-based protein diets in nondiabetic or diabetic patients with chronic renal disease or the nephrotic syndrome. In general, cereal and soya protein were used as the primary source of protein. These plant-based diets tend to be lower in phosphorus and cholesterol and have a higher ratio of energy to protein, energy to phosphorus, and polyunsaturated to saturated fatty acids (161). Studies suggest that the soya-based, low-protein diets may be as effective at retarding the progression of renal failure (162) and are at least as effective at reducing urinary albumin excretion as are low-protein diets based on animal protein; the soya protein may be more effective at reducing serum total cholesterol levels in both individuals with and without diabetes (156, 161–166). It has been suggested that the soya-based protein diet or a rotation between soya- and animal-based protein diets (167) may be more satisfying to the patient because of the increased variety of foods offered with this regimen.

Reducing dietary tryptophan intake or oral intake of sorbents that bind potentially toxic metabolites of tryptophan has been proposed as another method for slowing the rate of decline in renal function (147–150,168–172) (also see earlier in this chapter). The tryptophan metabolite, indole, is increased in serum of rats with CRF (147,168). Indoxyl sulfate is increased in serum and renal tubular cells of nondiabetic and diabetic rats with renal insufficiency (150,172). The indole metabolite, indoxyl sulfate, is believed to stimulate synthesis of transforming growth factor β-1 (TGF–β1) synthesis in the kidney, which, in turn, increases the renal expression of tissue inhibitor of metalloproteinase and type 1 collagen and thereby promotes fibrosis in the kidney (170, 171). An oral sorbent (AST-120) decreases serum and renal levels of indoxyl sulfate and gene expression of TGF-β1 (150,169,172).

Dietary supplements of L-arginine also have been proposed as a method for slowing the rate of progression of renal failure (173–176). L-arginine is converted in tissue to a number of compounds including nitric oxide, polyamines, L-proline, and agmatine. Some of these metabolites of arginine may induce renal pathology (176). The release of small amounts of nitric oxide from endothelial tissue also can induce vasodilation (177). However, in larger amounts, nitric oxide may promote immunologic injury in the kidney (176–178). Polyamines and L-proline may induce cell proliferation and enhancement of fibrotic matrix (176–178).

Some studies in rats indicate that arginine supplementation may be beneficial (173,174), particularly in rats that have glomerular hypertension. In animals with immunologic renal injury, dietary L-arginine restriction was protective of the kidney and L-arginine supplementation increased renal injury (176). Short-term studies in humans with chronic renal disease have not yet consistently shown renal-protective benefits to arginine supplementation (175,179).

Recommended Nutrient Intakes (Table 23.2)

Expression of Body Weights

When the recommended nutrient intake is given in terms of body weight, the latter generally refers to the edema-free standard or normal body weight as determined from the National Health and Nutrition Evaluation Survey (NHANES) data (82,83). The author prefers to use the NHANES II data published in 1984 (81) because Americans have been becoming more obese. The standard or normal body weight is the median body weight of normal Americans of the same height, gender, skeletal frame size and age range, as the individual in question. For patients who are obese or very lean (e.g., relative body weight less than 90% or greater than 120%), the use of the edema-free adjusted body weight is often preferable (65). This latter weight is defined as follows (81):

Adjusted edema-free body weight (kg)
= patient's edema-free body weight (kg)
+ (standard or normal body weight (kg)
− patient's edema-free body weight (kg) × 0.25)

where standard or normal body weight is determined as the median values for normal weights obtained from the NHANES II data (82).

Protein

Glomerular Filtration Rate Greater Than 70 mL/min/1.73 m^2

There is almost no information concerning the most desirable dietary protein and phosphorus prescription for patients with chronic renal disease and mild impairment in renal function. Indeed, almost all of the studies of the effect of low-protein diets on the rate of progression of renal failure have examined patients with stage 3, 4, or 5 chronic kidney disease (i.e., serum creatinine of about 1.4 to 1.7 or greater). It is recommended that protein (and phosphorus)

TABLE 23.2. RECOMMENDED DIETARY NUTRIENT INTAKE FOR PATIENTS WITH STAGE 4 OR 5 CHRONIC KIDNEY DISEASE NOT UNDERGOING DIALYSIS[a,b,c]

Protein		Vitamins	
Low protein diet (g/kg/day)	0.55–0.60 to 0.75 including ≥ 50% of high biologic value protein		Diet may be supplemented with these quantities
Energy (kcal/kg/day)	60 years old, less than 35; 60 years old or greater, 30–35; unless the patient's relative body weight is greater than 120% or the patient gains or is afraid of gaining unwanted weight	Thiamin (mg/day)	1.1–1.2
		Riboflavin (mg/day)	1.1–1.3
		Biotin (mg/day)	30
		Pantothenic acid (mg/day)	5
		Niacin (mg/day)	14–16
		Pyrldoxine HCl (mg/day)[k]	5 or 10
		Vitamin B_{12} (μg/day)	2.4
Total fat (% of total energy intake)[d,e]	25–35	Vitamin C (mg/day)	75–90
		Folic acid (mg/day)[l]	1 to 10
Saturated fat (% of total energy intake)[e]	< 7%	Vitamin A	None (see text)
		Vitamin D	See text
Polyunsaturated–saturated fatty acids (% of total calories)[e]	up to 10	Vitamin E (IU/day)[m]	400–800
		Vitamin K[n]	None
Monounsaturated fatty acids (% of total calories)[e]	up to 20		
Carbohydrate[e,f]	Rest of nonprotein calories		
Total fiber (g/day)[e]	20–30		
Minerals (range of intake)			
Sodium (mg/day)[g]	1,000 to 3,000		
Potassium (mEq/day)	40 to 70		
Phosphorus (mg/kg/day)	≤ 10[h]		
Calcium (mg/day)[i]	1,400 to 1,600		
Magnesium (mg/day)	200 to 300		
Iron (mg/day)[j]	≥ 10 to 18		
Zinc (mg/day)	15		
Water (mL/day)[g]	Up to 3,000 as tolerated		

[a]Glomerular filtration rate less than 30 mL/min/1.73 m^2 (see text for discussion of dietary intake for patients with less severe renal insufficiency).
[b]The protein intake is increased by 1.0 g per day of high biologic value protein for each gram per day of urinary protein loss.
[c]When recommended intake is expressed per kilogram body weight, this refers to the median values for body weight of a normal person of the same age range, height, gender, and skeletal frame size, as determined from the NHANES II data (119).
[d]Refers to percent of total energy intake; if triglyceride levels are very high, the percentage of fat in the diet may be increased to about 35 percent of total calories; otherwise 25% to 30% of total calories is preferable. Intake of trans-fatty acids should be kept low because they raise low–density-lipoprotein cholesterol (see text [200]).
[e] Although important for health, these dietary recommendations are considered less crucial than the others. They are only emphasized if the patient has a specific disorder that may benefit from this modification or has expressed interest in this dietary prescription and is complying well to more important aspects of the dietary treatment (see text).
[f]Should be primarily complex carbohydrates.
[g]Can be higher in patients who have greater urinary losses.
[h]Phosphate binders (sevelamer HCl, calcium carbonate or acetate, or aluminum carbonate or hydroxide) often are needed to maintain normal serum phosphorus levels.
[i]Dietary intake usually must be supplemented to provide these levels. Higher daily calcium intakes sometimes are ingested because of the use of calcium binders of phosphate.
[j]≥ 10 mg/day for males and nonmenstruating females; ≥ 18 mg/day for menstruating females.
[k]When individuals develop catabolic illnesses, 10 mg/day of pyridoxine HCl may be preferable.
[l]At least 1 mg/day of folic acid should be routine, but up to 10 mg/day may be given to reduce elevated plasma homocysteine levels.
[m]Vitamin E, 400 or 800 IU day, may be given to reduce oxidative stress and prevent cardiovascular disease, but the value of these supplements is controversial (see text and Chapter 20).
[n]Vitamin K supplements may be needed for patients who are not eating and who receive antibiotics.

intake be restricted for patients with GFR greater than 70 mL/min/1.73 m^2 only if there is evidence that renal function is decreased for the patient's age and that it is continuing to decline. In this situation, the patient is treated as indicated in the next paragraph.

Glomerular Filtration Rate 30 to 70 mL/min/1.73 m^2

It is recognized that the evidence is not conclusive that a low-protein diet is beneficial for patients with chronic kidney disease, and the information is particularly sparse as to whether nondiabetic individuals who are taking ACE inhibitors and/or ARBs will show additional benefits from low-protein diets. Indeed, the NKF-K/DOQI clinical practice guidelines for nutrition in chronic kidney disease concluded that there was insufficient evidence to recommend routinely a low-protein diet (e.g., 0.60 g/kg/day) for patients with chronic kidney disease, and they recommended individual decision making after a discussion of risks and benefits with the patient (51). However, four out of four rigorous metaanalyses have demonstrated at least some ability of these diets to delay the onset of end-stage renal failure, if not retard progressive renal disease (118,151–153). It is also noteworthy that a *post hoc* analysis of the MDRD study indicated that ingestion of 0.75 g protein/kg/day does retard progression (146). Indeed, the relationship between the actual dietary protein intake and the rate of decline in GFR suggests the possibility that slightly lower protein diets might have an even greater suppressive effect on the decline in GFR (146). Therefore, it is the author's policy to discuss with the patient the evidence that low-protein, low-phosphorus diets may retard progression and to indicate that the data, although not definitive, are sufficiently convincing to justify prescription of a protein- and phosphorus-restricted diet.

If the patient agrees to dietary therapy, he is offered a diet providing 0.60 g protein/kg/day, of which at least 50% of the protein is of high biologic value to ensure a sufficient intake of the essential amino acids. Many nitrogen-balance studies (111,112,130,180) as well as clinical experience with outpatients (43,110,113) indicate that this quantity of protein should maintain neutral or positive nitrogen balance in most patients with CRF as long as sufficient calories are ingested. For many patients this diet should not be excessively burdensome. If an individual will not adhere to such a low-protein diet or is unable to maintain sufficient dietary energy intake with this low-protein diet, the dietary protein intake may be increased up to 0.75 g protein/kg/day. At least 50% of the protein should be of high biologic value. This recommendation is consistent with the NKF-K/DOQI guidelines for nondialyzed patients with a GFR less than 25 mL/min (Table 23.3) (81). At present, ketoacid preparations are not available in the United States for therapeutic use.

TABLE 23.3. NKF-K/DOQI GUIDELINE 24: DIETARY PROTEIN INTAKE FOR NONDIALYZED PATIENTS WITH STAGE 4 OR 5 CHRONIC KIDNEY DISEASE

For individuals with chronic renal failure (glomerular filtratlon rate less than 25 mL/min) who are not undergoing maintenance dialysis, the institution of a planned low-protein diet providing 0.60 g protein/kg/day should be considered. For individuals who will not accept such a diet or who are unable to maintain adequate dietary energy intake with such a diet, an intake of up to 0.75 g protein/kg/day may be prescribed. (*Evidence and opinion*)

- When properly implemented and monitored, low-protein, high-energy diets maintain nutritional status while limiting the generation of potentially toxic nitrogenous metabolites, the development of uremic symptoms, and the occurrence of other metabolic complications.
- Evidence suggests that low-protein diets may retard the progression of renal failure or delay the need for dialysis therapy.
- At least 50% of the dietary protein should be of high biologic value.
- When patients with chronic renal failure consume uncontrolled diets, a decline in protein intake and in indices of nutritional status is often observed.

From National Kidney Foundation Clinical practice guidelines for nutrition in chronic renal failure, K/DOQI, *Am J Kidney Dis* 2000;35 (6 Suppl 2):S1–140, with permission.

Glomerular Filtration Rate Less Than 30 mL/min/1.73 m^2

At this level of renal insufficiency, the potential advantages to using a low-protein, low phosphorus diet become more compelling for the following reasons. First, at this degree of renal failure, potentially toxic products of nitrogen metabolism begin to accumulate in substantial quantities. The low-protein diet will generate less nitrogenous compounds. Second, because the low-protein diet generally contains less phosphorus and potassium, the intake of these minerals can be lowered more readily with this diet (see following sections on recommended phosphorus and potassium intakes). Third, some patients with chronic renal insufficiency eat too little protein rather than too much. Specific training and encouragement to follow a prescribed diet may increase the likelihood that the patient will not ingest too little protein. Patients should be prescribed 0.60 g protein/kg/day. This diet generally will maintain neutral or positive protein and nitrogen balance as long as energy intake is not deficient (Table 23.2) and should generate a low UNA (Table 23.4) (97,98,112,181). For patients who will not accept such a diet or who are unable to maintain an adequate energy intake with such a diet, an intake of up to 0.75 g protein/kg/day may be prescribed. At least 50% of the dietary protein should be of high biologic value. These recommendations are consistent with the NKF-K/DOQI Guidelines for Nutrition in Chronic Renal Failure (Table 23.3). The protein content of this diet should be increased by 1.0 g/day of high biologic value protein for each gram of protein excreted in the urine each day.

When the GFR falls below 5 mL/min/1.73 m^2, there is no conclusive evidence that patients fare as well with low-nitrogen diets as with regular dialysis therapy and higher protein intakes. Because these patients may be at high risk for malnutrition (38,40,41), it is recommended that maintenance dialysis treatment or renal transplantation be inaugurated at this time.

Energy

In many studies, the average dietary energy intake of patients with stage 3, 4, or 5 kidney disease is reported to be reduced. The mean dietary energy intake generally is about 24 to 27 kcal/kg/day (41,43,50) (Chapter 11). These intakes are far below the recommended dietary energy intakes by the Food and Nutrition Board, National Academy of

TABLE 23.4. COMPARISON OF LOW-PROTEIN AND KETOACID- OR AMINO ACID–SUPPLEMENTED DIETS[a]

	Low Protein (0.55–0.60 g protein/kg/day)	Very Low Protein with Essential Amino Acids	Very Low Protein with an Essential Amino Acid and Ketoacid Formulation
Intake (g/day)			
Protein	39	20	20
Amino acids		20.7	2.3
Ketoacid formulation			13.9
Total nitrogen	6.2	5.8	3.8
Urea nitrogen appearance (g nitrogen/day)	3.6	2.8	1.8
Estimated SUN (mg/dL) for a given urea clearance[b]			
3 mL/min	83	65	42
6 mL/min	42	32	21

SUN, serum urea nitrogen.

[a]The data in this table should be given as approximate values for a 68- to 72-kg person who is ingesting 0.55–0.60 g/kg/day of primarily high biologic value protein or about 0.28 g/kg/day of miscellaneous quality protein and about 21 g per day of an essential amino acid preparation or a ketoacid–amino acid formulation.

[b]These values are calculated from the urea nitrogen appearance data and the urea clearance equation:

$$\text{Serum urea nitrogen (mg/dL)} = \frac{\text{Urea nitrogen appearance (mg/min)} \times 100}{\text{Urea clearance (mL/min)}}$$

Values are calculated for steady-state conditions when SUN should be unchanging and hence the urea nitrogen appearance should equal the urine urea nitrogen (see text on calculation of urea nitrogen appearance).

From Kopple JD. *Dietary considerations in patients with advanced chronic renal failure, acute renal failure and transplantation in Diseases of the Kidney*, 6th ed. Schrier RW, Gottschalk CW, eds. Boston: Little, Brown and Company, 1996, with permission.

Sciences for normal individuals participating in light to moderate physical activity (52,53). However, there is a body of evidence indicating that nondialyzed patients with stage 3 to 5 chronic kidney disease have normal or possibly increased resting energy expenditure. In nondialyzed patients with CRF, energy expenditure, measured by indirect calorimetry, appears to be normal or near normal during resting and during sitting quietly in an easy chair (Fig. 23.1), after ingestion of a standard meal, and with a defined quantity of work from riding a stationary bicycle (Chapter 11) (180, 182,183). However, Kuhlmann et al., using direct calorimetry, found an inverse relation between resting energy expenditure and creatinine clearance in nondiabetic patients with stage 3, 4, or 5 chronic kidney disease (184). There was no comparison made in this study of the resting energy expenditure in these patients to normal individuals. Moreover, in a study of 241 men and women with type I or type II diabetes mellitus and mild to moderate CRF (serum creatinine, 2.6 + 1.5 (SD) mg/dL) who did not have evidence for PEM, resting energy expenditure, measured by indirect calorimetry, was increased by an average of 12.5% in comparison to 24 age- and gender-matched individuals with similar levels of chronic renal insufficiency ($p = 0.004$) (185).

Dietary energy requirements also were assessed by conducting nitrogen-balance studies in six nondialyzed patients with CRF ingesting 0.55 to 0.60 g protein/kg/day who lived in a metabolic balance unit and ingested a diet that provided a constant intake of 0.55 to 0.60 g protein/kg/day and were fed, in random order, a diet providing 25, 35, or 45 kcal/kg/day (180). Two of the six patients also were fed a diet providing 15 kcal/kg/day. Each of the dietary energy intakes were fed for a mean of 23.7 + 5.7 days. The change in body weight with each diet (Fig. 23.2) and the nitrogen balance were each directly correlated with the dietary energy intake. Nitrogen balance, adjusted for unmeasured changes in body urea nitrogen but not for estimated unmeasured losses of about 0.58 g/day from respiration, flatus, sweat, exfoliated skin, nail and hair growth, and blood drawing, was negative in both patients fed 15 kcal/kg/day, in three of five patients ingesting 25 kcal/kg/day, in one of five patients fed 35 kcal/kg/day, and in one of four patients ingesting 45 kcal/kg/day (Fig. 23.3). The UNA divided by the daily nitrogen intake (Fig. 23.4) and the plasma concentrations of several amino acids, determined after an overnight fast, each correlated inversely with dietary energy intake. The data suggest that a dietary energy intake of about 35 kcal/kg/day was more likely to maintain or increase body mass, maintain neutral or positive nitrogen balance, and decrease the UNA (Figs. 23.2–23.4) (180).

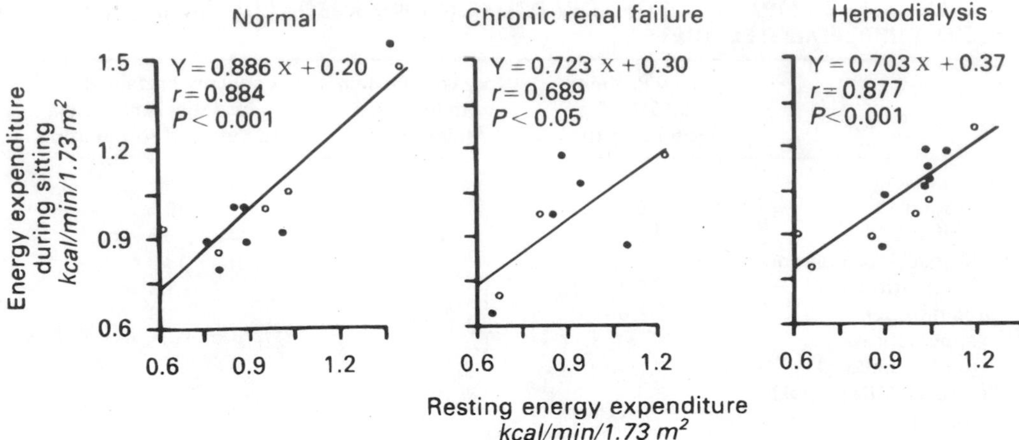

FIGURE 23.1. The direct correlation between energy expenditure during the basal resting state and while sitting quietly in an easy chair in normal subjects, nondialyzed patients with advanced chronic renal failure, and patients undergoing hemodialysis. Energy expenditure was measured by indirect calorimetry. M, men; F, women. (From Monteon FJ, Laidlaw SA, Shaib JK, et al. Energy expenditure in patients with chronic renal failure. *Kidney Int* 1986;30:741–747, with permission.)

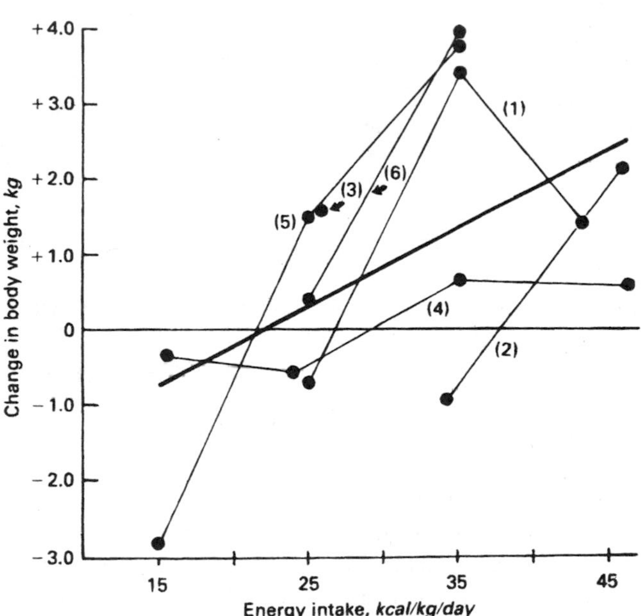

FIGURE 23.2. The direct correlation between the change in edema-free body weight and energy intake in six clinically stable nondialyzed patients with advanced chronic renal failure who were fed diets providing 45, 35, 25, or 15 kcal/kg/day in a clinical research center. All diets provided about 0.55 to 0.60 g protein/kg/day. Any given patient was prescribed the same dietary protein intake with each of the diets. Change in body weight was measured as the difference between the weight at the termination and the onset of a given energy intake. The thin lines connect data obtained from the same patient. Numbers in parentheses indicate the patient from whom data was obtained. The heavy diagonal line represents the least squares regression equation. $Y = 0.10x - 2.31$; $r = 0.542$; $p < 0.05$. (From Kopple JD, Monteon FJ, Shaib JK, et al. Effect of energy intake on nitrogen metabolism in nondialyzed patients with chronic renal failure. *Kidney Int* 1986;29:734–742, with permission.)

Children with CRF also have low energy intakes (186) (see Chapter 29). In nondialyzed patients with stages 4 and 5 chronic kidney disease, decreased body fat is one of the more prominent alterations in nutritional status. Moreover, in the author's experience, most patients commencing dialysis therapy who have not been edematous describe recent weight loss. These observations support the contention that patients with advanced CRF require more energy than they usually ingest (30). Food preferences and eating habits are altered in patients undergoing maintenance dialysis therapy (187,188). Hence, the mechanisms underlying reduced energy intake may be more complex than simply anorexia.

It is recommended that nondialyzed patients with stage 3, 4, or 5 chronic kidney disease ingest at least 35 kcal/kg/day if they are younger than 60 years of age and 30-35 kcal/kg/day if they are older than 60 years of age (Table 23.2). This is consistent with the NKF-K/DOQI guidelines concerning energy intake for patients with chronic kidney disease and a GFR less than 25 mL/min (81).

A vexing problem is that it seems to be more difficult to maintain adequate energy intakes on low-protein diets (e.g., 0.60 to 0.75 g protein/kg/day). This was observed in the MDRD study where those patients prescribed the 0.60 g protein/kg/day diet or the very-low-protein diet supplemented with ketoacids/essential amino acids were observed to have lower energy intakes and to have a slight decline in measures of somatic protein mass in comparison to individuals prescribed a more normal protein intake (43). However, no group of patients with chronic kidney disease in the MDRD study developed PEM, and the serum albumin actually remained the same or increased with the 0.60 g protein/kg/day or a ketoacid-supplemented very-low-protein diet. Moreover, in many but not all studies, patients prescribed either of these diets maintained normal serum

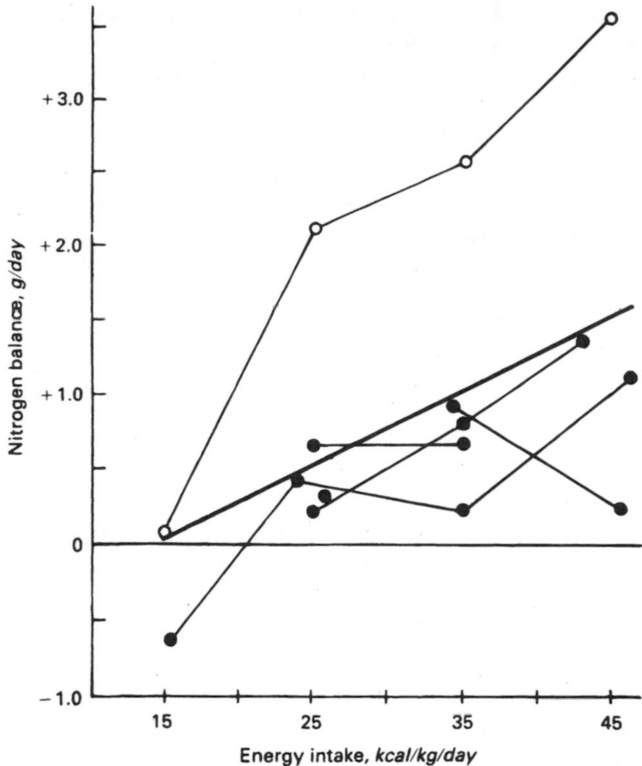

FIGURE 23.3. The direct correlation between nitrogen balance and energy intake in six clinically stable nondialyzed patients with advanced chronic renal failure. The conditions under which these patients were studied are described in the legend to Figure 23.2. Nitrogen balance was obtained after metabolic equilibration and is adjusted for changes in body urea nitrogen but not for unmeasured losses, which are estimated to be about 0.58 g/day. The open circles represent Patient 5, who had the lowest resting energy expenditure. The thin lines that connect the circles indicate the balance data from the same individual during different energy intakes. The heavy diagonal line represents the least squares regression equation. The heavy horizontal line represents zero balance not adjusted for unmeasured nitrogen losses. $Y = 0.52x - 0.73$; $r = 0.505$; $p < 0.05$. (From Kopple JD, Monteon FJ, Shaib JK, et al. Effect of energy intake on nitrogen metabolism in nondialyzed patients with chronic renal failure. *Kidney Int* 1986;29: 734–742, with permission.)

albumin levels and/or somatic body composition (45,189). It is possible that these discrepancies in the response of protein-energy nutritional status to low-protein diets in patients with advanced CRF are the result of differences in the degree to which the health care workers emphasize the importance of maintaining high energy intakes.

It seems clear, however, that for patients prescribed low-protein diets, careful monitoring of dietary energy intake and nutritional status is mandatory. This recommendation was put forth both by the NKF-K/DOQI *Guidelines on Nutrition in Chronic Renal Failure* (81) (Table 23.1) and *Chronic Kidney Disease: Evaluation, Classification, and Stratification* (51). Adjustments must be made according to the individual clinical and metabolic needs of the patient and whether the patient is obese or underweight. Patients who are obese with an edema-free body weight greater than 120% of desirable body weight may be treated with lower energy intakes. Some patients, particularly those with more mild renal insufficiency and young or middle-aged women, may become obese on this energy intake or may refuse to ingest the recommended calories out of fear of obesity. These individuals may require a lower energy prescription.

The optimal weight for the patient with advanced CRF has not been well defined. In normal individuals there is a linear relationship between BMI and increasing mortality with a possible J-curve at the lowest levels of BMI (61, 190,191). In contrast, in patients undergoing maintenance dialysis, the relationship between BMI or weight-for-height and mortality is reversed (61,192). This has given rise to the concept of a reversal of certain risk factors or reverse epidemiology in patients undergoing maintenance dialysis (192) (Chapter 12). Individuals who are underweight at the commencement of maintenance dialysis therapy are also at risk for increased mortality (see Chapter 12). Thus, it is possible that for individuals with advanced renal failure as well as those undergoing dialysis, the desirable or optimal body weight may be greater than for normal individuals. In the absence of randomized prospective clinical trials to resolve the question of the optimal body mass for patients

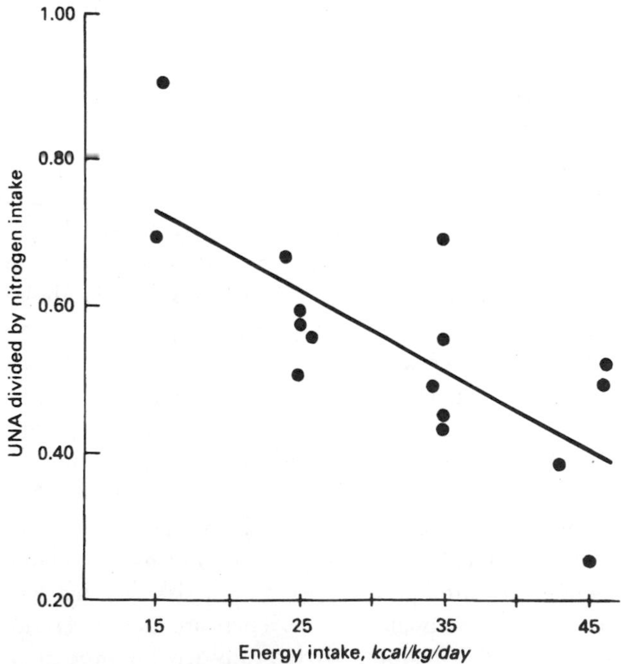

FIGURE 23.4. The negative correlation between the urea nitrogen appearance (UNA) divided by the dietary nitrogen intake ("fractional UNA") and energy intake in six clinically stable patients with advanced chronic renal failure. Symbols are described in the legend to Figure 23.2. $Y = 0.89 - 0.011x$; $r = -0.736$; $p < 0.005$. (From Kopple JD, Monteon FJ, Shaib JK, et al. Effect of energy intake on nitrogen metabolism in nondialyzed patients with chronic renal failure. *Kidney Int* 1986;29:734–742, with permission.)

with stage 3, 4, and 5 chronic kidney disease, it is recommended that these individuals maintain normal body weight for their height, gender, age range, and skeletal frame size, as determined from the NHANES II data (81).

Because the dietary energy (and protein) intake begins to decrease when the GFR falls somewhere below about 55 mL/min/1.73 m^2 (see earlier) (41,43), it is important to monitor dietary intake and to treat inadequate intakes, even in clinically stable healthy-appearing adults, when the GFR decreases to this level. This level of GFR may be associated with a serum creatinine as low or lower than 1.8 to 2.5 mg/dL in an adult patient. For patients who have difficulty in meeting their energy needs by ingesting normal foods, there are many commercially available high-calorie foodstuffs that are low in protein, sodium, and potassium. The renal dietitian can recommend these products as well as other low-protein, high-calorie foods that can be prepared easily at home (see Chapters 36 and 37).

LIPIDS AND CARDIOVASCULAR RISK MANAGEMENT

The pattern of abnormal serum lipid and lipoprotein concentrations in patients with CRF and the causes for these disorders are reviewed extensively in Chapter 3. These alterations may contribute to the high incidence of atherosclerosis and cardiovascular, cerebrovascular, and peripheral vascular diseases in patients with CRF, and attention has been directed toward reducing serum LDL cholesterol and triglyceride levels and increasing serum HDL cholesterol. Elevated serum triglyceride levels in kidney failure are caused primarily by impaired catabolism of triglyceride-rich lipoproteins (27,193,194). There are reduced activities of plasma and hepatic lipoprotein lipase and lecithin cholesterol acyltransferase, which may lead to impaired clearance of plasma triglycerides (22,23). Also, because diets for patients with renal failure usually are restricted in protein, sodium, potassium, and water, it is often difficult to provide sufficient energy without resorting to a large intake of purified sugars that may increase triglyceride production.

Alterations in serum cholesterol–carrying lipoproteins are of greater concern because in the normal population these abnormalities pose a much greater risk than hypertriglyceridemia for vascular disease. There are increased serum levels of apoB-containing triglyceride-rich lipoproteins in very–low-density lipoprotein (VLDL) and IDL cholesterol and reduced levels in HDL cholesterol (195). These alterations may occur early in the course of chronic kidney disease (194,195). A key characteristic of the altered lipoprotein levels is a decreased ratio of apoA-I to apoC-III. Serum Lp(a), a strong risk factor for coronary artery events, is increased in patients with as early as stage 2 to 3 chronic kidney disease, and it appears to increase progressively as GFR decreases (194). In particular, Lp(a) with high–molecular-weight isoforms of the apo(a) protein is likely to be elevated in serum at stage 2 to 3 chronic kidney disease (194). However, the third National Health and Nutrition Examination Survey (NHANES III), conducted from 1991 to 1994, showed a significant but only modest association between reduced GFR and an increase in serum Lp(a) levels in individuals with chronic kidney disease (196). Patients with the nephrotic syndrome most commonly have increased serum total and LDL cholesterol and serum triglycerides (197–200) (Chapter 3).

Measures to reduce the risk of coronary heart disease are described in Chapter 3 and are summarized in the Executive Summary of the Third Report of the National Cholesterol Education Program (NCEP) Expert Panel (200). In view of evidence that CRF (i.e., GFR below 20 to 30 mL/min/1.73 m^2) is a state of increased oxidative and carbonyl stress (Chapters 5 and 6) and is associated with many risk factors for accelerated vascular disease (Chapters 3–7, 10, 12, 13), it should be viewed as constituting a coronary heart disease risk equivalent (200). The goals concerning serum lipids therefore should be to maintain serum LDL cholesterol below 100 mg/dL, HDL cholesterol above 40 mg/dL and (if possible) 60 mg/dL or greater, and serum triglycerides probably below 200 mg/dL.

One approach to the management and treatment of altered lipid levels and cardiovascular risk is as follows (see also Chapters 3 and 10). Patients with stage 3, 4, or 5 chronic kidney disease should be monitored for coronary heart disease risk factors every 6 to 12 months, depending on their past history of such risk factors. Such monitoring should include, at a minimum, serum total, LDL, and HDL cholesterol and total triglycerides; BMI and/or total body fat; daily physical activity; and dietary intake of the components of the therapeutic lifestyle changes (TLC) diet (200), as discussed later in this chapter. In general, patients with a past history of increased risk for coronary heart disease, with borderline increased risk for this condition, or who recently have been inaugurated on or have had major changes in treatment of these risk factors, should be monitored every 6 months or more frequently as needed. Plasma homocysteine and serum CRP should be monitored every 12 months or more frequently as indicated.

In general, all patients with stage 3, 4, or 5 chronic kidney disease are urged to follow the NCEP TLC Diet (200): Saturated fat should be less than 7% of total calories; polyunsaturated fat should be up to 10% of total calories; monounsaturated fat should be up to 20% of total calories; fiber should be 20 to 30 g/day; cholesterol should be less than 200 mg/day; and total fat should be 25% to 35% of total calories. The particular dietary protein needs of the chronic kidney disease patient (see earlier) will determine the proportions of the remaining ingested calories that are derived from protein and carbohydrates. Total calories should be targeted to maintain desirable body weight and to prevent weight gain above this level. Carbohydrates should be derived primarily from foods that are rich in complex carbohydrates including grains (particularly whole grains), fruits, and vegetables. Trans fatty acids tend to increase LDL cholesterol and should be kept low.

Management of other risk factors for individuals with chronic kidney disease include strict blood pressure control; no smoking; routine use of ACE inhibitors or angiotensin receptor-2 blockers (201–207); reduction of hyperhomocysteinemia (Chapters 7 and 20); avoidance of excess calcium intake; hypercalcemia and a serum calcium-phosphorus product above 55 (Chapter 17, see later in this chapter); daily aspirin intake (about 81 mg/day); aggressive management to avoid chronic inflammation (e.g., from chronic osteomyelitis); frequent exercise; and, if the patient does not have an addictive propensity or liver disease, daily intake of one glass of an alcoholic beverage, red wine preferably (208,209).

If serum cholesterol or triglycerides are elevated, an evaluation of potential underlying causes of this condition is conducted (e.g., obesity, diabetes mellitus, hypothyroidism, glucocorticoid therapy, use of thiazide diuretics, or excessive alcohol intake). If the serum LDL cholesterol is greater than 100 mg/dL on two consecutive occasions separated by 1 month and prescription of the NCEP TLC diet (see earlier) is not effective or expected to be sufficiently effective at lowering the serum cholesterol (e.g., because of poor compliance), it is the author's policy to prescribe a hydroxymethyl-glutaryl coenzyme A (HMG-CoA) reductase inhibitor (a statin). HMG-CoA inhibitors block cholesterol synthesis and lower serum levels of LDL cholesterol and certain apolipoproteins in patients with hypercholesterolemia and the nephrotic syndrome or renal failure (210). The reduction in serum total and LDL cholesterol and in apolipoprotein B100 in these individuals averages approximately 30% (range, 18% to 55%) (200). Statins also may increase serum HDL cholesterol by 5% to 15% and decrease serum triglycerides by 7% to 30% (200). Statins may cause a myopathy and increase liver enzymes and are contraindicated in liver disease.

A randomized, double-blind, placebo-controlled clinical trial was conducted in 1,711 individuals with chronic renal insufficiency and a creatinine clearance of 75 mL/min or lower as determined by the Cockcroft-Gault equation (211). Median follow-up was 58.9 months. The results indicated a significant reduction in the incidence of the primary endpoint (death from coronary disease or symptomatic nonfatal myocardial infarction) in the individuals receiving pravastatin as compared to placebo (adjusted hazard ratio, 0.72, $p = 0.02$). The incidence of other secondary outcomes also were reduced significantly in the pravastatin-treated group.

Bile-acid sequestrants, such as cholestyramine, colestipol, and colesevelam, will lower serum LDL by about 5% to 25% and increase HDL by 3% to 5% (200). Serum triglycerides are unchanged or increase slightly. These medicines commonly cause gastrointestinal distress and constipation and may decrease intestinal absorption of other medicines. Nicotinic acid may lower serum LDL cholesterol and triglycerides and increase HDL cholesterol. Flushing often makes this medicine difficult to tolerate, and increased serum glucose or uric acid, gastrointestinal distress, or liver injury may occur. Fibric acids (e.g., gemfibrozil) also may be used. These medicines are effective at lowering serum LDL (by 5% to 20%) and triglycerides (by 20% to 50%) and increasing HDL (by 20% to 50%) (200,212). The pharmacokinetics of fibric acids are altered in patients with kidney failure and should not be used in severe kidney or liver failure (200,213). Ingestion of activated charcoal has been reported to lower serum cholesterol and triglycerides in chronically azotemic rats (214).

Elevated serum triglycerides are a less hazardous risk factor. It is our current plan to use serum triglyceride–lowering medicines when the serum triglyceride level is about 500 mg/dL or greater. Serum triglycerides may be lowered by feeding a diet in which the carbohydrate content is reduced to about 35% of total calories, the fat content is increased to about 55% of total calories, and the polyunsaturated/saturated fatty acid ratio is raised to about 1.5:1.0 (27,193). However, the evidence that high cholesterol and fat intakes enhance the risk for arteriosclerotic vascular disease indicates that such a diet is inadvisable, particularly because hypertriglyceridemia is a weak risk factor for atherosclerotic vascular disease. Nonetheless, a reduction in total carbohydrate intake and provision of a high proportion of dietary carbohydrates in the complex form may lower serum triglyceride levels. These modifications often lower the palatability of the diet. Therefore, the patient's total energy intake must be monitored closely to ensure that it does not fall. Ethanol intake is reduced to no more than one drink per day. Ethanol and exercise may increase serum HDL cholesterol. In obese individuals with hypertriglyceridemia or hypercholesterolemia weight reduction is particularly important.

Omega-3 fatty acids (e.g., eicosapentaenoic acid and docosahexaenoic acid, which are found in fish oil) lower serum triglycerides and have more variable effects on serum LDL cholesterol and HDL cholesterol (215). Fish oil also decreases platelet aggregation and appears to exert antiinflammatory effects (216), and omega-3 fatty acids may enhance immune function. Low-fat diets and lipid-lowering medicines retard the rate of progression of renal failure in animal models (217,218). In humans, some research suggests that omega-3 fatty acids may lower the progression of renal failure in renal transplant recipients (219). A preponderance of studies suggests that omega-3 fatty acids given as fish oil may retard the rate of progression of immunoglobulin A (IgA) nephropathy (220–223).

Abnormal carnitine metabolism (see later in this chapter) has been implicated as a cause of hypertriglyceridemia in

CRF. However, the many clinical trials of carnitine treatment of hypertriglyceridemia in patients undergoing maintenance dialysis are almost equally divided between those that show carnitine lowers serum triglycerides and those that show no change or, rarely, an increase in serum triglycerides (224,225).

It should be pointed out that there are no long-term prospective interventional clinical trial data on the effects of modifying dietary fat and carbohydrate intake, lowering obesity, or changing serum lipid levels on the clinical course of patients with specific renal diseases, the nephrotic syndrome, or renal failure. The recommendations given here are based largely on epidemiologic data, on the effects of long-term clinical trials on survival or adverse vascular disease events in populations without renal disease, on the fact that there is a high incidence of abnormal serum lipid and lipoprotein levels and atherosclerotic vascular disease in patients with renal disease or renal failure, and on research in experimental animals with chronic renal disease indicating that high lipid intakes or elevated lipoprotein levels may accelerate the rate of progression of renal failure.

Carbohydrates

Patients should be encouraged to eat complex rather than purified carbohydrates to reduce triglyceride synthesis and to improve glucose tolerance if it is abnormal (200). However, it has been proposed that ingestion of fermentable carbohydrates may increase fecal nitrogen excretion, thereby decreasing the nitrogen load for patients with CRF (226).

Carnitine

Carnitine is a naturally occurring compound that is essential for life. It is discussed in detail in Chapter 21. Although relative or absolute carnitine deficiency may occur in patients undergoing maintenance dialysis therapy (see Chapters 21 and 25), there is no evidence that patients with chronic renal disease who are not undergoing chronic dialysis therapy develop carnitine deficiency or benefit from L-carnitine supplements. Indeed, serum carnitine levels are generally normal or slightly increased in nondialyzed patients with stage 3 to 5 chronic kidney disease.

Sodium and Water

Normally, the renal tubules reabsorb more than 99% of the filtered sodium (227). As renal insufficiency progresses, both the glomerular filtration and the fractional reabsorption of sodium fall progressively. Thus, many patients with stage 3, 4, or 5 kidney disease are able to maintain sodium balance with a normal sodium intake. In both normal individuals and people with CRF, only about 1 to 3 mEq per day of sodium are excreted in the feces, and in the absence of visible sweating, only a few mEq per day of sodium are lost through the skin. Despite the adaptive reduction in the renal tubular reabsorption of sodium, patients with advanced renal failure may be unable to excrete the quantity of sodium ingested, and they may develop edema, hypertension, and congestive heart failure. This syndrome is particularly likely to occur when the GFR is below 4 to 10 mL per minute. When congestive heart failure, the nephrotic syndrome, or advanced liver disease complicates renal insufficiency, the propensity for sodium retention is increased. In patients with renal failure, hypertension often is controlled more easily when they are sodium restricted, and hypertension may be accentuated by an increased sodium intake, probably because of expanded extracellular fluid volume (228) and possibly because of an altered intracellular electrolyte composition within arteriolar smooth muscle cells that increases contractility. When the ability to excrete sodium decreases below usual intake or extracellular fluid volume becomes expanded, restriction of sodium and water intake and/or the use of diuretic medications becomes necessary.

However, nondialyzed patients with advanced CRF often have an inability to conserve sodium normally (1). A low sodium intake may not be sufficient to replace urinary and extrarenal sodium losses, and the patient may develop sodium depletion; a decrease in extracellular fluid volume, blood volume, and renal blood flow; and a further reduction in GFR (i.e., prerenal insufficiency superimposed on CRF). Volume depletion may be difficult to recognize. Unexplained weight loss or reduction in blood pressure may be signs of volume depletion. If the nondialyzed patient with CRF does not have evidence of fluid overload, hypertension, or heart failure, he cautiously may be given a greater sodium intake to determine whether the GFR can be improved somewhat by extracellular volume expansion.

Usually, when sodium balance is well controlled, the thirst mechanism will regulate water balance adequately. However, when the GFR falls below about 2 to 5 mL/min, the risk of overhydration increases, and water intake should be controlled independently of sodium to prevent overhydration. In patients with diabetes mellitus, hyperglycemia also may increase thirst and enhance positive water balance. For patients with far advanced renal failure whose total body water is considered appropriate (as indicated by normal or near normal blood pressure, absence of edema, and normal serum sodium), urine volume may be a good guide to water intake; the daily water intake should equal the urine output plus approximately 500 mL to replace insensible losses.

For most nondialyzed patients with advanced renal failure, a daily intake of 1,000 to 3,000 mg (about 40 to 130 mEq) of sodium and 1,500 to 3,000 mL of fluid will maintain sodium and water balance. The requirements for sodium and water vary markedly, and each patient must be managed individually. For nondialyzed patients with CRF who gain excessive sodium or water despite attempts at dietary restriction, a potent loop diuretic, such as furosemide or bumetanide, may be tried to increase urinary sodium and water excretion. The diuretic metolazone may potentiate the actions of loop diuretics.

Observational data in individuals with chronic kidney disease, primarily stage 4 or 5, who were prescribed low-protein diets suggest that those ingesting low-sodium diets, as indicated by urine sodium excretion less than 100 mEq/day had a slower rate of progression of renal failure as compared to those with a urine sodium excretion greater than 200 mEq/day (229). It is also important to keep in mind that in patients with proteinuria, the antiproteinuric effects of ACE inhibitors are attenuated substantially when their urinary sodium excretion exceeds roughly 100 to 150 mEq/day (2.3 to 3.4 g/day) (230,231). Coadministration of a thiazide diuretic reestablishes the antiproteinuric effects of ACE inhibitors even when urinary sodium excretion continues to exceed 100 mEq/day (232). It is assumed, but not yet documented, that loop diuretics will have the same effect under these circumstances as thiazide diuretics.

Potassium

The kidney normally is the major vehicle for potassium excretion. In renal failure, potassium retention may occur and cause fatal hyperkalemia. Three factors act to prevent this adverse effect of CRF. First, as renal failure progresses, the tubular secretion of potassium per unit GFR tends to increase as long as the urine volume is approximately 1,000 mL per day or greater. Thus, the renal potassium clearance does not fall as markedly as the GFR. Second, the fecal excretion of potassium increases, probably owing to enhanced intestinal secretion (112,233). Third, potassium intake tends to fall as a result of anorexia and also in response to dietary counseling.

Thus, patients with CRF usually do not become hyperkalemic unless there is (a) excessive intake of potassium; (b) acidemia, oliguria, hypoaldosteronism (e.g., secondary to decreased renin secretion by the diseased kidney or renal tubular resistance to the actions of aldosterone); (c) catabolic stress; or (d) possibly hypoinsulinism or use of medicines such as potassium-sparing diuretics, nonsteroidal antiinflammatory drugs, ACE inhibitors, angiotensin receptor 2 blockers, or beta-receptor blockers (234). Patients with diabetes mellitus are especially likely to develop hyperkalemia. Individuals with stage 4 or 5 chronic kidney disease generally should receive no more than 70 mEq of potassium per day. For most patients, this quantity of potassium should maintain potassium balance without causing hyperkalemia, and it will not render a low-protein diet unpalatable. Some patients, particularly those with less advanced renal failure, may tolerate higher potassium intakes; these individuals can be identified by liberalizing the dietary potassium and monitoring their serum potassium carefully.

Magnesium

In nondialyzed patients with stage 4 or 5 chronic kidney disease, there is a net absorption of about 40% to 50% of ingested magnesium from the intestinal tract (net absorption is the difference between dietary intake and fecal excretion) (85,233). Because the absorbed magnesium is excreted primarily by the kidney, hypermagnesemia may occur in patients with renal failure (189). Magnesium also commonly accrues in bone in renal failure and may contribute to the pathogenesis of renal osteodystrophy (235). The restricted diets of patients with renal failure are low in magnesium (usually about 100 to 300 mg/day for a 40-g protein diet). Thus, the serum magnesium levels of patients with CRF are usually normal or only slightly elevated unless the patient takes medicines that contain large quantities of magnesium, such as magnesium-containing antacids and laxatives (85,189). Nondialyzed individuals with stage 4 or 5 chronic kidney disease require about 200 mg/day of magnesium to maintain neutral magnesium balance (85).

Phosphorus and Phosphate Binders

The rationale for controlling dietary phosphorus and the use of gastrointestinal binders of phosphate to prevent and treat hyperphosphatemia, a high serum calcium-phosphorus product, calcium-phosphate deposition in soft tissue, and hyperparathyroidism are discussed in Chapters 16 and 17. This section will consider the prescription of dietary phosphorus intake and phosphate binders. In patients with renal failure, a large dietary phosphorus intake can lead to a high plasma calcium-phosphorus product with increased risk of calcium and phosphate deposition in soft tissues. Also, animal and human studies suggest the possibility that a low phosphorus intake may reduce the rate of progression of renal failure in individuals with chronic renal disease (236–239) (see earlier in this chapter and Chapter 16).

There are little data concerning the optimal level of phosphorus restriction for minimizing or preventing hyperparathyroidism, retarding the progression of renal failure, or preventing calcium and phosphate deposition. One approach for nondialyzed patients is to maintain a sufficiently low phosphorus intake so that serum phosphorus will be within the normal range even at normal levels of renal tubular reabsorption of phosphorus. This will reduce the propensity to stimulate parathyroid hormone secretion and the resultant elevation in serum parathyroid hormone levels. This approach requires a very low phosphorus intake, lower than usually can be obtained with the combination of a low-phosphorus diet and phosphate binders, unless ketoacid or essential amino acid–supplemented very-low-protein diets are used and the GFR is higher than 15 mL/min (i.e., stage 2, 3, or 4 chronic kidney disease). Another less aggressive approach is to maintain the morning fasting serum phosphorus concentrations within the normal range. Because there is a rough correlation between the protein and phosphorus content of the diet, it is much easier to reduce phosphorus intake if a lower protein diet is used.

For patients who have a GFR between 25 and 70 mL/min/1.73 m^2 or who have a higher GFR with a documented progressive loss of renal function, 8 to 10 mg phosphorus/kg/day may be prescribed with the 0.55 to 0.60 g protein/kg/day diet. These individuals generally are not given phosphate binders unless the serum phosphorus rises above normal levels. For nondialyzed patients with a GFR below 25 mL/min/1.73 m^2 who are prescribed a 0.55 to 0.60 g/kg/day protein diet, the phosphorus intake can be maintained at about 5 to 10 mg/kg/day, although the lower end of this range of phosphorus intake may be burdensome for many individuals. Without phosphate binders, there is a net intestinal phosphate absorption (diet minus fecal phosphorus) of roughly 60% of the phosphorus intake (85). Therefore, this level of dietary phosphorus restriction usually will not maintain normal serum phosphorus levels in patients with a GFR of less than about 15 mL per minute, even with a substantial reduction in the renal tubular reabsorption of phosphorus, unless phosphate binders also are used. Because amino acid and ketoacid formulations do not contain phosphorus, one advantage of very-low-protein diets supplemented with these preparations is the greater ease with which the phosphorus intake can be reduced, often to as low as 4 to 6 mg/kg/day.

In the 1960s and 1970s, the two most commonly used phosphate binders were aluminum carbonate and aluminum hydroxide. Usually, two to four 500-mg capsules taken three to four times per day with meals are needed. Larger doses may be used if necessary. Evidence that aluminum-induced osteomalacia, anemia, and other toxicities can be caused by the intake of aluminum phosphate binders led nephrologists to use calcium salts to bind phosphate (240–243). Calcium carbonate, calcium acetate, and calcium citrate have been used for this purpose (244–247). Of these three compounds, calcium acetate may have the greatest binding affinity to phosphate (247–249). Intestinal phorus, one advantage of very-low-protein diets suppleacetate (247–249). Hypercalcemia is reported to be less common with calcium acetate as compared to calcium carbonate (247). However, calcium acetate appears to cause more symptoms such as nausea, abdominal distention, diarrhea, or constipation (249). This may be the cause of poorer compliance described with calcium acetate tablets. Calcium citrate enhances the intestinal absorption of aluminum (246). It probably should not be ingested by patients with renal failure and definitely should not be given if individuals are taking aluminum salts.

The calcium content is 40% for calcium carbonate, 25% for calcium acetate, 21% for calcium citrate, 18% for calcium lactate, and 9% for calcium gluconate. In general, calcium chloride should not be given to patients with CRF because of its acidifying characteristics. Calcium is usually given in two or three doses daily with meals. Typical starting doses are calcium carbonate 750 mg or calcium acetate 667 mg, two tablets three times daily with meals. To avoid precipitation of calcium and phosphate in soft tissues, these compounds should not be prescribed if the serum phosphorus level is very high (e.g., greater than 6.5 mg/dL). Thus, patients with hyperphosphatemia may be treated with an aluminum or other noncalcium binder of phosphate (see later in this chapter) until serum phosphorus falls to normal or near normal. At that time the regimen may be changed to a calcium binder.

In the last several years, several noncalcium, nonaluminum binders of phosphate have been developed. The most popular and well accepted among these is sevelamer hydrochloride, which was approved by the U.S. Food and Drug Administration in 1998. This binder is roughly as effective as calcium acetate in its ability to bind phosphorus or control the serum phosphorus level. Sevelamer HCl, in comparison to calcium-containing binders of phosphate, causes less hypercalcemia and less oversuppression of parathyroid hormone (250–252). Sevelamer HCl also has the unusual advantage of lowering serum total cholesterol, primarily by reducing serum LDL levels; serum HDL cholesterol concentrations either do not change or increase (250–252). Side effects with sevelamer HCl include bloating, flatulence, and sometimes diarrhea.

Other binders of phosphate that have been used and shown to be effective include magnesium carbonate (often used with calcium acetate) (253), lanthanum carbonate (254), and a series of iron compounds including polynuclear iron hydroxide and ferric polymaltose (255–257). These more recently investigated phosphate binders appear to be effective in limited studies, and more research is needed to more fully define their safety and effectiveness. With each of these metallic binders of phosphate, it is important to ensure that patients do not receive excessive amounts of the metal. This may be of particular concern for magnesium carbonate because serum magnesium levels may not be an accurate measure of total body magnesium.

Aluminum and probably iron toxicity can cause a syndrome of low bone turnover that has been referred to as aplastic bone disease and that is characterized by low serum parathyroid hormone levels, decreased bone osteoblasts, and markedly reduced bone turnover (242,243,258). It has been suggested that the large calcium intake from dietary calcium supplements or dialysate may also cause this syndrome of low bone turnover (259) and also cause calcium deposits in soft tissues. Indeed, patients undergoing MHD given calcium-containing binders of phosphate, in comparison to those given sevelamer HCl, are reported to develop more coronary artery calcification, as determined by electron-beam computerized tomography (260).

In the past, some practitioners have prescribed such large doses of calcium binders of phosphorus that patients ingested 3 to 5 g/day or more of elemental calcium. Because of the risk of calcification of blood vessels, patients with stage 3 to 5 chronic kidney disease probably should not receive more than about 1.5 g/day of elemental calcium from calcium binders of phosphate. Some clinicians suggest that, given the high prevalence of vascular disease in patients with CRF, these individuals should not be prescribed calcium binders of phosphorus except as a last resort and that sevelamer hydrochloride or noncalcium, nonaluminum binders should be the initial treatment for serum phosphorus control. Unfortunately, the differences in the cost of these various binders will influence prescribing patterns for the present time.

It is important to keep in mind that all phosphate binders have a limited ability to bind phosphate in the intestinal tract. The maximum quantity of phosphate bound is probably somewhere around 300 to 400 mg/day. Considering that a normal person may eat 1,600 to 2,400 mg/day, it is clear that phosphate binders usually will not allow a patient with advanced chronic kidney failure to eat a normal phosphorus intake and still maintain normal serum phosphorus levels. Hence, dietary phosphorus restriction is still an important component of phosphorus control. Patients with severe hyperparathyroidism may develop increased serum phosphorus levels from release of phosphate from bone. This is particularly likely to happen in patients with advanced CRF and particularly those undergoing MHD or peritoneal dialysis. If the serum phosphorus of these individuals cannot be controlled with diet, phosphorus binders, and vitamin D analogues (e.g., paricalcitol) (see Chapter 17), subtotal parathyroidectomy may be indicated.

At present, there is no well-defined safe lower limit for the serum phosphorus level in patients with renal failure. Experience suggests that if the fasting serum phosphorus level is maintained above the lower limit of normal, patients will not develop clinical manifestations of phosphate depletion. More research is required to ascertain whether this view is correct.

Calcium

Nondialyzed patients with CRF have an increased dietary requirement for calcium because they have vitamin D deficiency and resistance to the actions of vitamin D. These abnormalities, which are discussed in greater detail in Chapter 17, impair the intestinal absorption of calcium. The risk of calcium deficiency in these patients is enhanced because the diets prescribed for patients with renal failure are almost always low in calcium. Foods high in calcium content are usually high in phosphorus (e.g., dairy products) and therefore are restricted for patients with stage 3 to 5 chronic kidney disease. For example, a 40-g protein diet generally provides only about 300 to 400 mg/day of calcium, whereas the RDA for healthy, nonpregnant, nonlactating adults is about 800 to 1,200 mg/day (53,261).

Balance studies indicate that nondialyzed patients with stage 4 or 5 chronic kidney disease usually require about 1,200 to 1,600 mg/day of calcium for neutral or positive calcium balance (85). Total daily calcium intake (diet plus supplement) therefore should be maintained at about 1,400 to 1,600 mg/day (Table 23.2). Thus, the low-protein diets should be supplemented with about 1,000 to 1,200 mg/day of elemental calcium. As indicated earlier, slightly higher intakes (up to 1,500 mg/day) of elemental calcium may be given as calcium carbonate or acetate to bind phosphate in the intestinal tract. To prevent calcium-phosphate deposition in soft tissues, supplemental calcium should not be given unless the serum phosphorus concentration is normal or near normal (e.g., 5.5 mg/dL or lower). Treatment with 1,25-dihydroxycholecalciferol (calcitriol) will decrease the daily calcium requirement by enhancing intestinal calcium absorption (8,262). For patients receiving calcitriol or calcium supplements or phosphate binders, the serum calcium should be monitored because hypercalcemia may develop, particularly if serum phosphorus falls to low normal or low levels.

Trace Elements

Trace element metabolism in CRF is discussed more extensively in Chapter 19, and this section will focus on dietary requirements. A number of factors in patients with renal failure tend to either increase or decrease the body burden of certain trace elements. Many trace elements are excreted primarily in the urine and may accumulate with renal failure (263,264). Elements such as iron, zinc, and copper, which are protein bound, may be lost in excessive quantities when there are large urinary protein losses (e.g., the nephrotic syndrome) (265). Occupational exposure or pica may increase the burden of some trace elements. The effect of the altered dietary intake of the patient with CRF on body pools of trace elements is unknown (264).

Assessment of trace element burden in patients with renal failure is difficult because the binding-protein concentrations in serum may be decreased (e.g., by PEM), thereby lowering serum trace element levels, and the binding characteristics of these proteins may be altered in renal failure. Also, red-cell concentrations of trace elements may not reflect levels in other tissues. Trace element supplementation should be undertaken with caution because impaired urinary excretion of trace elements increases the risk of overdosage.

Dietary requirements for trace elements have not been well defined in patients with renal failure (see Table 23.2). Oral iron supplements often are given to patients who are iron deficient or as a routine treatment for patients who have a propensity to develop iron deficiency (e.g., individuals who frequently have marginal or low serum iron, percent saturation of the iron binding capacity, or ferritin levels). Iron requirements increase when erythropoietin therapy is started and hemoglobin synthesis rises. Moreover, higher serum iron concentrations appear to enhance the responsiveness to erythropoietin (266) (Chapter 22). Oral iron salts, such as ferrous sulfate, 300 mg three times per day one-half hour after meals, may be tried. Patients with a chronic but small need for iron supplements sometimes require only one or two iron doses per day. Some patients develop anorexia, nausea, constipation, or abdominal pain with ferrous sulfate; these individuals sometimes tolerate other iron compounds better, such as ferrous fumarate, gluconate, or lactate. Patients who are intolerant to oral iron supplements, who have iron deficiency, or who have iron needs not adequately responsive to oral supplements (e.g., with erythropoietin therapy) may be best treated with intravenous iron.

Although the zinc content of most tissues is normal in patients with renal failure (264), usually serum and hair zinc are reported to be low and red-cell zinc is increased (263,267–269). In nondialyzed chronically uremic patients the fractional urinary excretion of zinc is increased; however, because the GFR is reduced, total urinary excretion of zinc may be normal or reduced (263). Fecal zinc is increased (269), and a dietary zinc intake greater than the recommended dietary allowance (53,270) may be necessary to maintain normal body zinc pools. Further studies are needed to confirm this. Some reports indicate that dysgeusia, poor food intake, and impaired sexual function, which are common problems of patients with advanced renal failure, may be improved by giving them zinc supplements. This has been shown particularly for patients undergoing MHD (54,267,269,271). Other studies, however, have not confirmed this (272). Intestinal absorption of zinc is not affected by administration of 1,25-dihydroxycholecalciferol (273).

Vitamins

Vitamin metabolism and nutrition in patients with CRF are discussed in greater depth in Chapter 20. Patients with stage 4 or 5 chronic kidney disease are at high risk for relative or absolute vitamin deficiencies. These are the result of several factors. First, in renal failure, 1,25-dihydroxycholecalciferol production is diminished in the diseased kidney (17). Second, vitamin intake often is decreased in patients with CRF because of anorexia and reduced food intake. Intercurrent illnesses, which occur frequently in patients with advanced renal failure (274,275), also impair food intake. Many foods that have a high content of water-soluble vitamins are restricted for patients with renal failure because of the elevated protein or potassium content of these foods; hence, the diets prescribed for nondialyzed CRF patients frequently contain less than the recommended daily allowances for certain water-soluble vitamins (18,276). Third, renal failure appears to alter the absorption, metabolism, or activity of some vitamins. Animal studies indicate that intestinal absorption of riboflavin, folate, and vitamin D_3 is impaired in renal failure (12–14). The metabolism of pyridoxine appears to be abnormal in CRF (16). Fourth, certain medicines may interfere with the intestinal absorption, metabolism, or actions of vitamins (18) (see Chapters 20 and 33).

In patients with CRF, vitamin deficiencies have been observed with particular frequency for 1,25-dihydroxycholecalciferol; folic acid; vitamin B_6; vitamin C; and to a lesser extent, other water-soluble vitamins (18,55,277–280). Dietary folic acid requirements increase in patients with CRF during the time when they commence erythropoietin therapy and undergo a major increase in their hemoglobin levels. Also, pharmacologic doses of folic acid have been shown to reduce elevated plasma homocysteine, although not to normal levels (281,282). Plasma total homocysteine is elevated in about 85% to 90% of patients with ESRD and those undergoing maintenance dialysis (283,284) (see Chapters 7 and 20).

Elevated plasma homocysteine is a risk factor for adverse cardiovascular events in the non–renal failure population (285,286); evidence supporting this relationship in the renal failure population is somewhat more equivocal (192). Treatment with folic acid or the combination of folic acid and pyridoxine HCl has decreased plasma homocysteine levels in patients with CRF (281,282). However, supplements of pyridoxine HCl alone have not been shown to reduce plasma homocysteine (282), so the beneficial effects are most likely the result of folic acid. Generally, 5 to 10 mg/day of folic acid appears to have the maximum homocysteine-lowering effects. A national clinical trial in the United States is being conducted to examine the effects of large doses of a combination of vitamin B_{12}, pyridoxine HCl, and folic acid on plasma homocysteine levels and clinical outcome in patients undergoing MHD. The results of this trial should be available in several years.

Pyridoxine hydrochloride, 5 mg/day, is reported to induce a normal red-cell erythrocyte glutamate–pyruvate transaminase activation index in nondialyzed, clinically stable patients with stage 4 or 5 chronic kidney disease (55). Ten mg per day of pyridoxine hydrochloride may be necessary to normalize this index when such individuals sustain superimposed infection (55).

Vitamin B_{12} deficiency is uncommon in patients with CRF (277,278) because the recommended intakes for normal nonpregnant, nonlactating adults for this vitamin are small (e.g., 2.4 μg/day) (53) and the body stores large quantities of this vitamin. Moreover, although vitamin B_{12} is water soluble, it is protein bound in plasma; hence, in individuals with normal plasma levels, little vitamin B_{12} is excreted in the urine, particularly when such people have CRF.

Except for vitamin D, deficiency of the fat-soluble vitamins is less common in patients with CRF. Serum retinol-binding protein, total vitamin A, and non–protein-bound vitamin A are increased in patients with renal failure (287,

288). Elevated liver vitamin A was described in two patients with CRF (289), although other investigators did not confirm elevated vitamin A levels in solid tissues (288). In nondialyzed individuals with advanced CRF, normal plasma vitamin E levels have been reported (57,290,291), but decreased red-cell α-tocopherol has been observed (57,292). Although protein-restricted diets generally provide adequate amounts of vitamin E (Chapter 20), malnourished patients with CRF appear to have lower serum α-tocopherol concentrations as compared to well-nourished individuals. Low levels of α-tocopherol in erythrocytes of patients with CRF have been associated with increased red-cell peroxidation as indicated by increased red-cell malonyldialdehyde levels (292).

Patients with advanced chronic kidney disease are at increased risk for oxidative injury (Chapter 5); therefore, it is important to examine whether vitamin E supplements providing an excess of vitamin E will be beneficial for these individuals. Vitamin E supplements are protective against oxidative stress in many (293–297) but not all experimental models (298) of renal disease. The SPACE (Secondary Prevention with Antioxidants of Cardiovascular Disease in End-stage Renal Disease) Study showed a reduction in the incidence of adverse cardiovascular events in patients at increased risk for these disorders who were given 800 IU/day of vitamin E (299). However, neither the HOPE (Heart Outcomes Prevention Evaluation) nor the MicroHOPE Study showed a clinical benefit from vitamin E supplements in older individuals without advanced CRF who had increased risk factors for cardiovascular events (201,202). Other smaller-scale studies have shown that vitamin E may decrease oxidative stress in patients undergoing MHD or peritoneal dialysis (300–302), and dialysis treatment using vitamin E–bound hemodialysis membranes appears to reduce oxidative activity in many (303–306) but not all (307, 308) studies. Vitamin E generally is safe to administer in doses of 400 to 800 IU/day. Because patients with stage 3, 4, and 5 chronic kidney disease may be in a state of increased oxidative stress and have increased risk factors for cardiovascular disease, it would seem reasonable to prescribe these doses of vitamin E to such individuals.

Vitamin K deficiency is uncommon (18). Patients who do not eat (and hence do not ingest foods containing vitamin K) and who are receiving antibiotics that suppress intestinal bacteria for extended periods may require supplemental vitamin K to prevent deficiency of this vitamin (309).

A number of clinical syndromes associated with inadequate vitamin intake or vitamin excess in patients with CRF are described in Chapters 17 and 20. The following are among the more common syndromes. Excessive intake of 1,25-dihydroxycholecalciferol may cause hypercalcemia. Patients with chronic renal failure taking 1,25-dihydroxycholecalciferol for extended periods may experience a reduction in their tolerance for this compound, leading to hypercalcemia. This may occur because as bone calcium becomes repleted, bone may stop serving as a sink for calcium and excess calcium absorbed from the intestinal tract may accumulate in plasma. Increased plasma oxalate in patients with renal failure appears to be largely the result of impaired urinary excretion, although large doses of vitamin C (ascorbic acid), a precursor of oxalate, may increase oxalate production (see later in this chapter). Glyoxylate, a metabolic precursor of oxalate, also may be transaminated to form glycine. Vitamin B_6 is a cofactor for the enzyme that catalyzes this step. Vitamin B_6 deficiency increases urinary oxalate excretion in rats with experimental renal insufficiency as well as in normal individuals (310). In patients with CRF, treatment with large doses of pyridoxine HCl may decrease plasma oxalate levels, although not to normal values (311,312); some clinical trials have not confirmed these findings (313,314).

Some authors have suggested that patients undergoing MHD (and, by inference, nondialyzed patients with CRF) who do not receive vitamin supplementation may not develop water-soluble vitamin deficiencies (315–317). They have recommended that vitamin supplements should not be prescribed routinely to patients undergoing maintenance dialysis. However, in the studies indicating that patients undergoing maintenance dialysis may maintain normal plasma or blood cell levels of vitamins without supplements, patients generally were followed for less than 1 year; it is possible that with longer periods, the incidence of vitamin deficiency may increase. Moreover, in these studies, some water-soluble vitamins fell to borderline low levels in a number of patients.

Many of the studies that indicate a need for routine vitamin supplementation in nondialyzed patients with CRF and those undergoing maintenance dialysis were carried out in the 1960s and early 1970s when the incidence of poor nutritional intake of these individuals might have been greater than it is today (18). Nonetheless, poor vitamin intake is still common in patients with renal failure (276,316,318), and recent reports continue to show that substantial numbers of patients with renal failure show evidence for vitamin deficiencies (279,290,317–319). For the nondialyzed patient with CRF, more severe dietary protein or potassium restriction might enhance the need for vitamin supplements. Indeed, the vitamin content of renal failure diets that provide about 0.55 to 0.60 g protein/kg/day is not uncommonly below the RDAs. It is not known at what point in the course of renal failure vitamin supplements become indicated. Because the water-soluble vitamin supplements generally are safe, it would seem prudent to use them routinely for people with stage 4 or 5 chronic kidney disease until these issues are resolved more completely.

The nutritional requirements for most vitamins are not well defined in patients with CRF, and it is likely that they will be modified in the future. There is evidence that, in addition to vitamin intake from foods, the following daily supplements of vitamins will prevent or correct vitamin deficiency (Table 23.2): pyridoxine hydrochloride, 5 mg in nondialyzed patients (10 mg during times of intercurrent catabolic illness); folic acid, 1.0 mg and up to 10 mg if patients have hyperhomocysteinemia; and the recommended intakes (Food and Nutrition Board, Institute of Medicine, National Academies) for normal individuals for the other water-soluble vitamins (53,320). Because there may be competitive interference with the actions of folic acid in CRF (321) and the competitive compound(s) may be a folate metabolite, patients taking these larger doses of folic acid should be monitored for potential signs of folate toxicity. A supplement of only 75 to 90 mg/day of vitamin C (the RDA) (313,320) is advised because ascorbic acid can be metabolized to oxalate. Large doses of ascorbic acid have been associated with increased plasma oxalate levels in patients with renal failure (322,323). Oxalate is highly insoluble, and high plasma oxalate concentrations might lead to precipitation in soft tissues, including the kidney, possibly causing further impairment in renal function in the nondialyzed patient with renal insufficiency. However, Gaede et al. reported that patients with type II diabetes with urine albumin losses of 30 to 300 mg/day who were given vitamin C, 1,250 mg/day, and vitamin E, 680 IU/day, for 4 weeks sustained a 19% decrease in urine albumin excretion (324).

Supplemental vitamin A is not recommended unless the patient's daily dietary vitamin A intake is less than the recommended intake for normal adults (313). Under these conditions, a supplement to raise dietary vitamin A to the recommended allowance for normal adults may be used (53). In patients with CRF, serum vitamin A levels are increased, and there appears to be a high risk of vitamin A toxicity with supplements as low as 2,250 retinol equivalents (7,500 IU of vitamin A) (289,325). It is not clear whether vitamin E supplements are necessary (290), but a supplement of the recommended allowance for vitamin E α-tocopherol equivalents (10 mg/day for men; 8 mg/day for women) (53,320) would appear to be safe. Additional vitamin K is not needed unless the patient is not eating and is receiving antibiotics that suppress intestinal bacteria that synthesize vitamin K. Recommendations for intake of vitamin D or its analogues are given in Chapter 17.

Alkalinizing Agents

Nondialyzed patients with advanced CRF frequently develop metabolic acidosis associated with an increased anion gap because there is impaired ability of the kidney to excrete acidic metabolites. In the earlier stages of CRF, and sometimes with advanced renal failure, hyperchloremic metabolic acidosis also may be caused by excessive renal losses of bicarbonate. Ingestion of low-nitrogen diets may prevent or decrease the severity of the acidosis because the endogenous generation of acidic products of protein metabolism will be reduced. Because in clinically stable patients with CRF the rate of acid production is usually normal or below normal, alkalinizing medicines are usually very effective for preventing or treating the acidosis. Research indicates that metabolic acidemia may engender protein and amino acid catabolism, suppress albumin synthesis, and promote protein wasting and bone loss (326–330).

Sodium bicarbonate or citrate are effective treatments for acidosis. They may be administered orally or intravenously. If the patient with CRF is not oliguric and is not particularly likely to develop edema, sodium is usually readily excreted when it is given as sodium bicarbonate. Because the exact level of acidemia at which net protein loss or bone reabsorption is stimulated is not well defined, it would seem prudent to prevent any degree of chronic acidemia. Therefore, alkali therapy probably should be initiated if the arterial pH is below 7.35. The NKF-K/DOQI guidelines recommend that serum bicarbonate be maintained at or above 22 mmol/L (81). This appears to be a reasonable recommendation for individuals with stage 4 or 5 chronic kidney disease although maintaining a normal serum bicarbonate may be a preferable goal. In general, treatment may be given with oral bicarbonate or citrate salts, although the latter may enhance the intestinal absorption of aluminum (246). Patients may be started with 30 or 40 mEq/day of sodium bicarbonate or citrate, and the dose may be increased or reduced according to the patient's response. Sodium bicarbonate tablets, 325 mg (3.9 mEq), may be taken. For many patients, Shohl's solution, containing one mEq of alkali per mL, is a convenient method for taking alkali. If acidosis is severe and is not controlled by the foregoing measures, hemodialysis or peritoneal dialysis may be used.

Fiber

Research in normal individuals suggests that a high dietary fiber intake may lower the incidence of constipation, irritable bowel syndrome, diverticulitis, and neoplasia of the colon and possibly improve glucose tolerance (331). In patients with CRF, a high dietary fiber intake also may reduce SUN by decreasing colonic bacterial ammonia generation and enhancing fecal nitrogen excretion (332). Because it seems reasonable that the benefits of a high dietary fiber intake in normal people also would occur in nondialyzed patients with CRF, a high dietary fiber intake of 20 to 25 gm/day is recommended (200).

MANAGEMENT OF THE PATIENT WITH DIABETIC NEPHROPATHY

Diabetes mellitus is the most common cause of ESRD in the United States and accounts for approximately 43% of patients commencing maintenance dialysis therapy (275). Renal failure is more likely to occur in individuals with type I diabetes, but because type II diabetes is much more prevalent, most patients who develop kidney disease from diabetic nephropathy have type II diabetes mellitus. The prevalence of diabetes mellitus in the United States as well as worldwide has reached epidemic proportions (333). There are about 13 million individuals in the United States with diabetes mellitus (333). This epidemic is engendered by increasing dietary energy intakes, obesity, and reduction in physical activity. Increasing numbers of older people and individuals with a genetic predisposition also contribute to the increasing prevalence of diabetes mellitus in the United States.

Development of microalbuminuria is considered to be a precursor of clinical diabetic nephropathy (334,335). There is now clear evidence that the intensive control of plasma glucose will prevent or retard the development of microalbuminuria, macroalbuminuria, and frank diabetic nephropathy and retinopathy and prevent the occurrence of diabetic neuropathy (336,337). Strict blood pressure control (systolic and diastolic blood pressures of 130 and 80 mm Hg, respectively (338) may retard progression of renal failure more successfully. Lower blood pressures (less than 125/75 mm Hg) have been recommended for individuals with proteinuria of 1.0 g/24 hours or greater and renal insufficiency (159,338). ACE inhibitors and angiotensin 2 receptor blockers each may reverse microalbuminuria and reduce macroalbuminuria, and they are associated with a slower rate of progression of renal failure even when compared to patients with similar blood pressure levels (339–341). The National Kidney Foundation recommends that ACE inhibitors should be used in patients with diabetes and microalbuminuria even if elevated blood pressure is not present (342). Once diabetic renal disease has become established, intensive control of the plasma glucose will not reverse the renal disease, and it is unclear as to how effectively strict glucose control will retard the rate of progression of renal failure (343–345). Several studies and metaanalyses indicate that low-protein diets may retard the progression of renal failure in patients with insulin-dependent diabetes mellitus (see earlier) (151,154–158,346–349). The prescribed low-protein diets in these studies usually provided 0.6 to 0.8 g protein/kg/day.

The question of whether the protective effects of dietary protein restriction and treatment with ACE inhibitors and/or angiotensin 2 receptor blockers are additive is just beginning to be examined (160). In several studies, low-protein diets also were associated with a reduction in urine albumin or total protein excretion (155,346–349). Although low-protein diets have been reported to be associated with decreased insulin needs in patients with diabetes and renal failure, these changes have not been controlled for weight loss (350). Other investigators have not shown changes in insulin requirements in patients with insulin-dependent diabetes mellitus treated with low-protein diets (351).

It is recommended that the specific goals for the nutritional therapy of patients with diabetes mellitus, with or without insulin dependency, are to maintain physiologic plasma glucose concentrations and optimal plasma lipid concentrations, retard the development and progression of CRF, prevent or retard the occurrence of other complications of diabetes mellitus, and manage the nutritional and metabolic complications of CRF (352). Patients with diabetic nephropathy who develop CRF sustain a high incidence of PEM (352). The prevalence of malnutrition in patients with diabetes undergoing MHD appears to be similar to that of nondiabetic patients undergoing MHD (353).

The approach to the patient with diabetes and chronic renal disease should include careful dietary, metabolic, and blood pressure control; medical treatment of the nephropathy; and exercise (342,354,355) (see Chapter 34). The Professional Practice Committee of the American Diabetes Association recommends that for type I and type II diabetes, 60% to 70% of total dietary energy intake should be distributed between carbohydrate and monounsaturated fat based on nutritional assessment and treatment goals (355). Polyunsaturated fatty acids should be about 10% of energy intake. Less than 10% of energy intake should be derived from saturated fats. Foods containing carbohydrates from whole grains, fruits, vegetables, and low-fat milk are important components of the diet (355). Diabetic individuals with microalbuminuria should reduce protein intake to 0.8 to 1.0 g/kg/day; those with overt nephropathy should ingest 0.8 g protein/kg/day (355). (This recommendation is discrepant with the somewhat lower recommended protein intake proposed earlier in this chapter for patients with chronic progressive renal disease of any type [Table 23.2].) If protein intake is reduced, it would seem reasonable to increase the percent of energy intake derived from carbohydrate and monounsaturated fat. Weight reduction in overweight or obese patients with diabetes should be encouraged strongly. As indicated by the results of the Diabetic Control and Complications Trial, intensive glucose control should be instituted to reduce the incidence of microalbuminuria and to slow the progression of diabetic renal disease (337). Normalization of blood glucose and HbA1c (glycosylated hemoglobin) concentrations is ideal. However, any improvement in blood glucose control may be beneficial (354).

When chronic progressive renal failure is established, a 0.55 to 0.60 g protein/kg/day diet is recommended. At least 0.35 g/kg/day should be protein of high biologic value. Prescription of other nutrients is essentially as described in Table 23.2. Patients must be monitored carefully to ensure that malnutrition does not occur. If patients will not accept this degree of protein restriction, cannot maintain their prescribed energy intake with this low-protein diet, or show evidence for developing PEM (e.g., falling serum albumin, weight loss, or muscle weakness), dietary protein intake may be increased up to 0.75 g/kg/day. Protein intake also should be increased for proteinuria as follows: 1 g/day of high biologic value protein intake for each gram per day of urine protein excretion. For patients ingesting 0.55 to 0.60 g protein/kg/day, protein intake should be increased starting at any urine protein excretion above zero; for individuals ingesting 0.75 g protein/kg/day, the increment in protein intake should commence with urine protein excretion above 5 g/kg/day.

The reduction in dietary protein intake and the restriction of dietary fat to no more than 30% of calories can lead to a substantial increase in the total carbohydrate content of the diet (to as high as 63% of total calories). Brodsky has pointed out that this diet may be associated with an increase in plasma triglycerides and VLDL triglycerides and a decrease in HDL cholesterol both in patients with insulin-dependent and non–insulin-dependent diabetes mellitus (351). A modest (6%) decrease in apolipoprotein D also has been reported after 1 month of treatment with such diets.

Effort should be made to control the altered lipid metabolism in patients with diabetes. This may be approached by the dietary modifications indicated earlier and by careful glycemic control by diet and insulin treatment and pharmacologic therapy, as indicated earlier and in Chapter 3. Nutritional assessment of patients with diabetes should be similar to that of nondiabetic patients with chronic renal disease (see earlier and Chapter 15), in addition to the periodic measurements of serum glucose and blood HbA1c concentrations.

Prioritizing Dietary Goals

The magnitude of the prescribed changes in the dietary intake for patients with stage 3, 4, and 5 chronic kidney disease is so great that if they all were presented to the patient at once, the patient could become demoralized and lose his motivation to comply with the diet. Therefore, we prioritize goals for dietary treatment. Usually we emphasize the importance of controlling the protein, phosphorus, sodium, energy, potassium, and magnesium intake and the need to take calcium and vitamin supplements. However, unless the patient has diabetes mellitus or a lipid disorder that carries a particularly high risk of atherosclerotic disease, the recommended quantity and types of dietary carbohydrate, fat, and fiber are discussed with the patient, but adherence to these dietary guidelines is not as strongly emphasized. Once the patient has complied well with the other more critical elements of dietary therapy, if the patient has diabetes mellitus or a specific lipid disorder that may benefit from dietary therapy or has expressed an interest in modifying fat, carbohydrate, or fiber intake, then the modification of the dietary intake of these latter nutrients is explored more intensively with the patient. At some point the value of the therapeutic lifestyle changes approach is discussed with the patient (200).

NUTRITIONAL MANAGEMENT DURING CATABOLIC STRESS

It is not uncommon for patients with CRF to sustain acute catabolic illnesses. If the hypercatabolic state persists for more than a few days, nutritional support must be considered. The techniques of nutritional support and methods of administration of nutrients are discussed in Chapter 26, 30, and 31. The discussion in Chapters 30 and 31 primarily is devoted to treatment of acute renal failure, but the principles apply to the patient with CRF as well.

The intensity of nutritional support and of the amino acid or protein intake should be determined by the catabolic status of the patient, which usually is assessed by the UNA and estimated or measured energy expenditure (see earlier and Chapter 15). However, the GFR of the patient also may influence the nutritional prescription. If the patient has a GFR higher than 30 mL/min, the nutritional support may be more similar to the treatment of the acutely ill patients with little or no renal failure. If the GFR is 10 to 15 mL/min or less, the patient temporarily may require intermittent hemodialysis or continuous ultrafiltration with or without dialysis to manage the nitrogen, water, and mineral loads. Sometimes dialysis or ultrafiltration treatment may be avoided in these latter patients by using essential amino preparations and restricting water and mineral intake as necessary (see Chapter 30).

USE OF GROWTH FACTORS

Recombinant human growth hormone (rhGH) and recombinant human insulinlike growth factor-1 (rhIGF-1) have been used in recent years to improve growth or nutritional status in patients with CRF. rhGH has been used extensively in children with chronic kidney disease to treat growth retardation (356) (Chapters 29 and 32) and now is considered a standard therapy. Studies in adult patients with CRF and PEM indicate that rhGH and rhIGF-1 can induce anabolism, at least for short periods (357–360) (Chapter 32). The anabolic steroid, nandrolone decanoate, 100 mg injected intramuscularly once per week for 6 months in protein-energy malnourished patients undergoing MHD or peritoneal dialysis who were not acutely ill, resulted in significantly increased lean body mass, serum creatinine levels, and physical functioning (361). Virtually all studies that have examined the anabolic effects of rhGH, rhIGF-1, or anabolic steroids in adults with CRF have been carried out in patients undergoing MHD or chronic peritoneal dialysis and not in nondialyzed patients with CRF.

rhIGF-1 has been used to increase GFR in patients with advanced CRF and thus delay the need for maintenance dialysis therapy (362). At the present time, the use of rhGH or rhIGF-1 to treat nondialyzed adult patients with CRF or adult patients who are undergoing MHD or chronic peritoneal dialysis must be considered experimental.

Two prospective studies in critically ill patients living in intensive care units who may or may not have renal disease found increased mortality in those patients randomized to rhGH treatment (363). It seems reasonable, therefore, to not give rhGH to severely ill patients with renal failure. However, studies in patients hospitalized in a surgical intensive care unit for more than 5 days indicate that intensive insulin infusions to maintain blood glucose between 80 and 110 mg/dL was associated with lower mortality (364,365). It is possible that the increased mortality of severely ill individuals given rhGH treatment may be the result of the increased insulin resistance and hyperglycemia that may be induced by growth hormone. Insulin also may reduce the catabolic status of sick patients (366,367).

NUTRITIONAL INDICATIONS FOR COMMENCING RENAL REPLACEMENT THERAPY

Although clinical indications for inaugurating renal replacement therapy are discussed in a number of texts (368,369), a statement concerning nutritional indications may be appropriate here. Because patients with CRF commencing renal replacement therapy often have PEM and this condition is associated with increased risk of mortality (370–374), the workgroup that developed the NKF-K/DOQI *Clinical Practice Guidelines for Nutrition in Chronic Renal Failure* considered it appropriate to develop indications for renal replacement therapy (81). These indications are listed in Table 23.5 along with a quotation abstracted from the Rationale for this guideline that expands on and qualifies this guideline. It should be emphasized that there are no randomized prospective clinical trials that have examined whether commencement of renal replacement therapy, as indicated in this guideline (Table 23.5), will result in decreased morbidity or mortality. However, a number of retrospective analyses have shown that late onset of chronic dialysis treatments are associated with increased mortality (373,374).

TABLE 23.5. NKF-K/DOQI GUIDELINE 27: INDICATIONS FOR RENAL REPLACEMENT THERAPY[a,b]

In patients with chronic renal failure (e.g., glomerular filtration rate < 15 to 20 mL/min) who are not undergoing maintenance dialysis, if protein-energy malnutrition develops or persists despite vigorous attempts to optimize protein and energy intake and there is no apparent cause for malnutrition other than low nutrient intake, initiation of maintenance dialysis or a renal transplant is recommended. (*Opinion*)

"Although the following criteria are not considered rigid or definitive, initiation of renal replacement therapy should be considered if, despite vigorous attempts to optimize protein and energy intake, any of the following nutritional indicators show evidence of deterioration: (1) more than a 6% involuntary reduction in edema-free usual body weight (% UBW) or to less than 90% of standard body weight (NHANES II) in less than 6 months; (2) a reduction in serum albumin by greater than or equal to 0.3 g/dL and to less to than 4.0 g/dL (Guideline 3), in the absence of acute infection or inflammation, confirmed by repeat laboratory testing; or (3) a deterioration in SGA (viz., Subjective Global Assessment) by one category (i.e., normal, mild, moderate, or severe; Guideline 9 and Appendix VI)."

[a]This guideline refers to nutritional indications for commencing renal replacement therapy.
[b]From National Kidney Foundation K/DOQI Clinical practice guidelines for nutrition in chronic renal failure. *Am J Kidney Dis* 2000;35(Suppl 2): S1–140, with permission.

REFERENCES

1. Gonick HC, Maxwell MH, Rubini ME, et al. Functional impairment in chronic renal disease. I. Studies of sodium-conserving ability. *Nephron* 1966;3(3):137–152.
2. Bricker NS. On the pathogenesis of the uremic state. An exposition of the "trade-off hypothesis." *N Engl J Med* 1972;286: 1093.
3. Kopple JD. Amino acid and protein metabolism in chronic renal failure. Massry SG, Glassock RJ, eds. In: *Textbook of nephrology*, 4th ed. 2001, Baltimore: Lippincott Williams & Wilkins, 2001;1356–1361.
4. Westervelt FJ, Schreiner GE. The carbohydrate intolerance of uremic patients. *Ann Intern Med* 1962;57:266.
5. Hutchings R, Hegstrom RM, Scribner BH. Glucose intolerance in patients on long-term intermittent dialysis. *Ann Intern Med* 1966;65:275.
6. Horton E, Johnson C, Lebovitz HE. Carbohydrate metabolism in uremia. *Ann Intern Med* 1968;68:63.
7. Bergstrom J, Hultman E. Glycogen content of skeletal muscle in patients with renal failure. *Acta Med Scand* 1969;186(3): 177–181.
8. Coburn JW, Hartenbower DL, Massry SG. Intestinal absorption of calcium and the effect of renal insufficiency. *Kidney Int* 1973;4(2):96–104.
9. Coburn JW, Hartenbower DL, Brickman AS, et al. Intestinal absorption of calcium, magnesium and phosphorus in chronic renal insufficiency. In: David DS, ed. *Perspectives in hypertension and nephrology-calcium metabolism in renal disease.* New York: Wiley, 1977;77–109.
10. Delano BG, Manis JG, Manis T. Iron absorption in experimental uremia. *Nephron* 1977;19(1):26–31.
11. Lawson DH, Boddy K, King PC, et al. Iron metabolism in patients with chronic renal failure on regular dialysis treatment. *Clin Sci* 1971;41(4):345–351.
12. Vaziri ND, Said HM, Hollander D, et al. Impaired intestinal absorption of riboflavin in experimental uremia. *Nephron* 1985; 41(1):26–29.
13. Said HM, Vaziri ND, Kariger RK, et al. Intestinal absorption of 5-methyltetrahydrofolate in experimental uremia. *Acta Vitaminol Enzymol* 1984;6(4):339–346.
14. Vaziri ND, Hollander D, Hung EK, et al. Impaired intestinal absorption of vitamin D3 in azotemic rats. *Am J Clin Nutr* 1983;37(3):403–406.
15. Sterner G, Lindberg T, Denneberg T. In vivo and vitro absorption of amino acids and dipeptides in the small intestine of uremic rats. *Nephron* 1982;31(3):273–276.
16. Spannuth CL Jr, Warnock LG, Wagner C, et al. Increased plasma clearance of pyridoxal 5′-phosphate in vitamin B6-deficient uremic man. *J Lab Clin Med* 1977;90(4):632–637.
17. Gray RW, Weber HP, Dominguez JH, et al. The metabolism of vitamin D3 and 25-hydroxyvitamin D3 in normal and anephric humans. *J Clin Endocrinol Metab* 1974;39(6):1045–1056.
18. Kopple JD, Swendseid ME. Vitamin nutrition in patients

undergoing maintenance hemodialysis. *Kidney Int Suppl* 1975(2):79–84.
19. Massry SG, Fadda GZ. Chronic renal failure is a state of cellular calcium toxicity. *Am J Kidney Dis* 1993;21(1):81–86.
20. Smogorzewski M, Zayed M, Zhang YB, et al. Parathyroid hormone increases cytosolic calcium concentration in adult rat cardiac myocytes. *Am J Physiol* 1993;264(6 Pt 2):H1998–2006.
21. Ott SM, Maloney NA, Coburn JW, et al. The prevalence of bone aluminum deposition in renal osteodystrophy and its relation to the response to calcitriol therapy. *N Engl J Med* 1982; 307(12):709–713.
22. Appel G. Nephrology forum: Lipid abnormalities in renal disease. *Kidney Int* 1991;39(1):169–183.
23. Attman PO. Hyperlipoproteinaemia in renal failure: pathogenesis and perspectives for intervention. *Nephrol Dial Transplant* 1993;8(4):294–295.
24. Krol E, Rutkowski B, Wroblewska M, et al. Classification of lipid disorders in chronic hemodialyzed patients. *Miner Electrolyte Metab* 1996;22(1–3):13–15.
25. Cocchi R, Viglino G, Cancarini G, et al. Prevalence of hyperlipidemia in a cohort of CAPD patients. Italian Cooperative Peritoneal Dialysis Study Group (ICPDSG). *Miner Electrolyte Metab* 1996;22(1–3):22–25.
26. Wanner C, Bartens W, Nauck M, et al. Lipoprotein(a) in patients with the nephrotic syndrome: influence of immunosuppression and proteinuria. *Miner Electrolyte Metab* 1996; 22(1–3):26–30.
27. Sanfelippo ML, Swenson RS, Reaven GM. Reduction of plasma triglycerides by diet in subjects with chronic renal failure. *Kidney Int* 1977;11(1):54–61.
28. Guarnieri G, Faccini L, Lipartiti T, et al. Simple methods for nutritional assessment in hemodialyzed patients. *Am J Clin Nutr* 1980;33(7):1598–1607.
29. Attman PO, Ewald J, Isaksson B. Body composition during long-term treatment of uremia with amino acid supplemented low-protein diet. *Am J Clin Nutr* 1980;33(4):801–810.
30. Young GA, Kopple JD, Lindholm B, et al. Nutritional assessment of continuous ambulatory peritoneal dialysis patients. *Am J Kidney Dis* 1991;17:462–471.
31. Cianciaruso B, Brunori G, Kopple JD, et al. Cross-sectional comparison of malnutrition in continuous ambulatory peritoneal dialysis and hemodialysis patients. *Am J Kidney Dis* 1995; 26:475–486.
32. Laidlaw SA, Berg RL, Kopple JD, et al. Patterns of fasting plasma amino acid levels in chronic renal insufficiency: results from the feasibility phase of the Modification of Diet in Renal Disease Study. *Am J Kidney Dis* 1994;23(4):504–513.
33. Kopple JD. McCollum Award Lecture, 1996: Protein-energy malnutrition in maintenance dialysis patients. American Society for Clinical Nutrition, 1997;65:1544–1557.
34. Kalantar-Zadeh K, Kleiner M, Dunne E, et al. Total iron-binding capacity-estimated transferrin correlates with the nutritional subjective global assessment in hemodialysis patients. *Am J Kidney Dis* 1998;31(2):263–272.
35. Kalantar-Zadeh K, Dunne E, Nixon K, et al. Near infra-red interactance for nutritional assessment of dialysis patients. *Nephrol Dial Transplant* 1999;14(1):169–175.
36. Kalantar-Zadeh K, Kleiner M, Dunne E, et al. A modified quantitative subjective global assessment of nutrition for dialysis patients. *Nephrol Dial Transplant* 1999;14(7):1732–1738.
37. Fung F, Sherrard DJ, Gillen DL, et al. Increased risk for cardiovascular mortality among malnourished end-stage renal disease patients. *Am J Kidney Dis* 2002;40(2):307–314.
38. Kopple JD. Nutrition in renal failure. Causes of catabolism and wasting in acute or chronic renal failure. In: Robinson RR, ed. *Nephrology. Proceedings of the IXth International Congress of Nephrology*. New York: Springer-Verlag, 1984;1498–1515.
39. Mehrotra R, Berman N, Alistwani A, et al. Improvement of nutritional status after initiation of maintenance hemodialysis. *Am J Kidney Dis* 2002;40(1):133–142.
40. Ikizler TA, Greene JH, Wingard RL, et al. Spontaneous dietary and protein intake during progression of chronic renal failure. *J Am Soc Nephrol* 1995;6:1386–1391.
41. Kopple JD, Greene T, Chumlea WC, et al. Relationship between nutritional status and the glomerular filtration rate: Results from the MDRD study. *Kidney Int* 2000;57:1688–1703.
42. Shemesh O, Golbetz H, Kriss JP, et al. Limitations of creatinine as a filtration marker in glomerulopathic patients. *Kidney Int* 1985;28:830–838.
43. Kopple JD, Levey AS, Greene T, et al. Effect of dietary protein restriction on nutritional status in the Modification of Diet in Renal Disease Study. *Kidney Int* 1997;52(3):778–791.
44. Walser M, Hill S. Can renal replacement be deferred by a supplemented very low protein diet? *J Am Soc Nephrol* 1999;10(1): 110–116.
45. Aparicio M. Low protein diets and outcome of renal patients. *J Nephrol* 2001;14:433–439.
46. Kuhlmann MK, Kopple JD. Amino acid metabolism in the kidney. *Semin Nephrol* 1990;10(5):445–457.
47. Aparicio M, Chauveau P, De Précigout V, et al. Nutrition and outcome on renal replacement therapy of patients with chronic renal failure treated by a supplemented very low protein diet. *J Am Soc Nephrol* 2000;11(4):708–716.
48. Park JS, Jung HH, Yang WS, et al. Protein intake and the nutritional status in patients with pre-dialysis chronic renal failure on unrestricted diet. *Korean J Intern Med* 1997;12(2): 115–121.
49. Pollock CA, Ibels LS, Zhu FY, et al. Protein intake in renal disease. *J Am Soc Nephrol* 1997;8(5):777–783.
50. Chauveau P, Barthe N, Rigalleau V, et al. Outcome of nutritional status and body composition of uremic patients on a very low protein diet. *Am J Kidney Dis* 1999;34:500–507.
51. National Kidney Foundation. K/DOQI clinical practice guidelines for chronic kidney disease: evaluation, classification, and stratification. *Am J Kidney Dis* 2002;39(2 Suppl 1):S1–266.
52. Institute of Medicine. Dietary Reference Intakes for energy, carbohydrate fiber, fat, fatty acids, cholesterol, protein and amino acids. Food and Nutrition Board. Washington, D.C.: National Academy Press, 2003.
53. Trumbo P, Schlicker S, Yates AA, et al. Dietary reference intakes for energy, carbohydrate, fiber, fat, fatty acids, cholesterol, protein and amino acids. *J Am Diet Assoc* 2002;102(11): 1621–1630.
54. Mahajan SK, Prasad AS, Lambujon J, et al. Improvement of uremic hypogeusia by zinc: a double-blind study. *Am J Clin Nutr* 1980;33(7):1517–1521.
55. Kopple JD, Mercurio K, Blumenkrantz MJ, et al. Daily requirement for pyridoxine supplements in chronic renal failure. *Kidney Int* 1981;19(5):694–704.
56. Sprenger KB, Bundschu D, Lewis K, et al. Improvement of uremic neuropathy and hypogeusia by dialysate zinc supplementation: a double-blind study. *Kidney Int Suppl* 1983;16: S315–S318.
57. Clermont G, Lecour S, Lahet J, et al. Alteration in plasma antioxidant capacities in chronic renal failure and hemodialysis patients: a possible explanation for the increased cardiovascular risk in these patients. *Cardiovasc Res* 2000;47(3):618–623.
58. Churchill DN, Taylor DW, Cook RJ, et al. Canadian hemodialysis morbidity study. *Am J Kidney Dis* 1992;19:214–234.
59. Kalantar-Zadeh K, Kopple JD. Relative contributions of nutri-

tion and inflammation to clinical outcome in dialysis patients. *Am J Kidney Dis* 2001;38(6):1343–1350.

60. Kalantar-Zadeh K, Lehn R, McAllister C, et al. Normalized protein nitrogen appearance is correlated with hospitalization and mortality in hemodialysis patients with Kt/V greater than 1.20. *J Ren Nutr* 2003;13(1):15–25.
61. Kopple JD, Zhu X, Lew NL, et al. Body weight-for-height relationships predict mortality in maintenance hemodialysis patients. *Kidney Int* 1999;56(3):1136–1148.
62. Chertow GM, Jacobs D, Lazarus J, et al. Phase angle predicts survival in hemodialysis patients. *J Ren Nutr* 1997;7(4): 204–207.
63. Chertow GM, Ackert K, Lew NL, et al. Prealbumin is as important as albumin in the nutritional assessment of hemodialysis patients. *Kidney Int* 2000;58(6):2512–2517.
64. Iseki K, Yamazato M, Tozawa M, et al. Hypocholesterolemia is a significant predictor of death in a cohort of chronic hemodialysis patients. *Kidney Int* 2002;61(5):1887–1893.
65. Kopple JD, Jones MR, Keshaviah PR, et al. A proposed glossary for dialysis kinetics. *Am J Kidney Dis* 1995;26(6):963–981.
66. Owen WF, Lowrie EG. C-reactive protein as an outcome predictor for maintenance hemodialysis patients. *Kidney Int* 1998; 54:627–636.
67. Yeun JY, Levine RA, Mantadilok V, et al. C-reactive protein predicts all-cause and cardiovascular mortality in hemodialysis patients. *Am J Kidney Dis* 2000;35(3):469–476.
68. Noh H, Lee SW, Kang SW, et al. Serum C-reactive protein: a predictor of mortality in continuous ambulatory peritoneal dialysis patients. *Perit Dial Int* 1998;18:387–394.
69. Koenig W, Sund M, Frohlich M, et al. C-reactive protein, a sensitive marker of inflammation, predicts future risk of coronary heart disease in initially healthy middle aged men: results from the MONICA (Monitoring Trends and Determinants in Cardiovascular Disease) Asugsburg Study, 1984 to 1992. *Circulation* 1999;237–242.
70. Ridker PM, Rifai N, Rose L, et al. Comparison of C-reactive protein and low-density lipoprotein cholesterol levels in the prediction of first cardiovascular events. *N Engl J Med* 2002; 347(20):1557–1565.
71. Bergstrom J, Lindholm B, Lacson E Jr, et al. What are the causes and consequences of the chronic inflammatory state in chronic dialysis patients? *Semin Dial* 2000;13(3):163–175.
72. Bologa RM, Levine DM, Parker TS, et al. Interleukin-6 predicts hypoalbuminemia, hypocholesterolemia, and mortality in hemodialysis patients. *Am J Kidney Dis* 1998;32:107–114.
73. Kaysen GA, Chertow GM, Adhikarla R, et al. Inflammation and dietary protein intake exert competing effects on serum albumin and creatinine in hemodialysis patients. *Kidney Int* 2001;60:333–340.
74. Mortelmans AK, Vanholder R. Intradialytic parenteral nutrition in malnourished hemodialysis patients. Review of the literature. *Miner Electrolyte Metab* 1999;25(4–6):324–332.
75. Chertow GM, Ling J, Lew NL, et al. The association of intradialytic parenteral nutrition administration with survival in hemodialysis patients. *Am J Kidney Dis* 1994;24(6):912–920.
76. Capelli JP, Kushner H, Camiscioli TC, et al. Effect of intradialytic parenteral nutrition on mortality rates in end-stage renal disease care. *Am J Kidney Dis* 1994;23(6):808–816.
77. Russell ML. *Behavioral counseling in medicine: strategies for modifying at-risk behavior.* New York: Oxford University Press, 1986.
78. Klahr S, Levey AS, Beck GJ, et al. The effects of dietary protein restriction and blood-pressure control on the progression of chronic renal disease. Modification of Diet in Renal Disease Study Group. *N Engl J Med* 1994;330(13):877–884.
79. Gillis BP, Caggiula AW, Chiavacci AT, et al. Nutrition intervention program of the Modification of Diet in Renal Disease Study: a self-management approach. *J Am Diet Assoc* 1995; 95(11):1288–1294.
80. Milas NC, Nowalk MP, Akpele L, et al. Factors associated with adherence to the dietary protein intervention in the Modification of Diet in Renal Disease Study. *J Am Diet Assoc* 1995; 95(11):1295–1300.
81. National Kidney Foundation. National Kidney Foundation K/DOQI clinical practice guidelines for nutrition in chronic renal failure. *Am J Kidney Dis* 2000;35(suppl 2):S1–S140.
82. Frisancho AR. New standards of weight and body composition by frame size and height for assessment of nutritional status of adults and the elderly. *Am J Clin Nutr* 1984;40(4):808–819.
83. Najjar MF, Rowland M. Anthropometric reference data and prevalence of overweight, United States, 1976–80. *Vital Health Stat 11* 1987(238):1–73.
84. Kopple JD, Mehrotra R, Supasyndh O, et al. Transthyretin in patients with renal failure. *Clin Chem Lab Med* 2003;40(12): 1308–1312.
85. Kopple JD, Coburn JW. Metabolic studies of low protein diets in uremia. II. Calcium, phosphorus and magnesium. *Medicine (Baltimore)* 1973;52(6):597–607.
86. Keshaviah PR, Nolph KD, Moore HL, et al. Lean body mass estimation by creatinine kinetics. *J Am Soc Nephrol* 1994;4(7): 1475–1485.
87. Lo WK, Prowant BF, Gamboa SB, et al. How reproducible is daily creatinine recovery in chronic peritoneal dialysis? *Perit Dial Int* 1994;14(3):286–288.
88. Bergstrom J, Alvestrand A, Bucht H, et al. Progression of chronic renal failure in man is retarded with more frequent clinical follow-ups and better blood pressure control. *Clin Nephrol* 1986;25(1):1–6.
89. Mitch WE, Walser M, Buffington GA, et al. A simple method of estimating progression of chronic renal failure. *Lancet* 1976; 2(7999):1326–1328.
90. Rutherford WE, Blondin J, Miller JP, et al. Chronic progressive renal disease: rate of change of serum creatinine concentration. *Kidney Int* 1977;11(1):62–70.
91. Perrone RD, Steinman TI, Beck GJ, et al. Utility of radioisotopic filtration markers in chronic renal insufficiency: simultaneous comparison of 125I-iothalamate, 169Yb-DTPA, 99mTc-DTPA, and inulin. The Modification of Diet in Renal Disease Study. *Am J Kidney Dis* 1990;16(3):224–235.
92. Levey AS, Greene T, Schluchter MD, et al. Glomerular filtration rate measurements in clinical trials. Modification of Diet in Renal Disease Study Group and the Diabetes Control and Complications Trial Research Group. *J Am Soc Nephrol* 1993; 4(5):1159–1171.
93. Levey AS, Berg RL, Gassman JJ, et al. Creatinine filtration, secretion and excretion during progressive renal disease. Modification of Diet in Renal Diseases (MDRD) Study Group. *Kidney Int Suppl* 1989;27:S73–S80.
94. Lavender S, Hilton PJ, Jones NF. The measurement of glomerular filtration-rate in renal disease. *Lancet* 1969;2(7632): 1216–1218.
95. Calloway DH, Odell AC, Margen S. Sweat and miscellaneous nitrogen losses in human balance studies. *J Nutr* 1971;101(6): 775–786.
96. Grodstein GP. Urea nitrogen appearance, a simple and practical indicator of total nitrogen output. *Kidney Int* 1979;16:953.
97. Maroni BJ, Steinman TI, Mitch WE. A method for estimating nitrogen intake of patients with chronic renal failure. *Kidney Int* 1985;27(1):58–65.
98. Kopple JD, Gao XL, Qing DP. Dietary protein, urea nitrogen appearance and total nitrogen appearance in chronic renal failure and CAPD patients. *Kidney Int* 1997;52(2):486–494.

99. Walser M. Urea metabolism in chronic renal failure. *J Clin Invest* 1974;53(5):1385–1392.
100. Varcoe R, Halliday D, Carson ER, et al. Efficiency of utilization of urea nitrogen for albumin synthesis by chronically uraemic and normal man. *Clin Sci Mol Med* 1975;48(5):379–390.
101. Bergstrom J, Furst P, Alvestrand A, et al. Protein and energy intake, nitrogen balance and nitrogen losses in patients treated with continuous ambulatory peritoneal dialysis. *Kidney Int* 1993;44(5):1048–1057.
102. Sargent JA, Gotch FA. Mass balance: a quantitative guide to clinical nutritional therapy. I. The predialysis patient with renal disease. *J Am Diet Assoc* 1979;75(5):547–551.
103. Kopple JD. Uses and limitations of the balance technique. *JPEN J Parenter Enteral Nutr* 1987;11(5 Suppl):79S–85S.
104. Kopple JD, Coburn JW. Evaluation of chronic uremia. Importance of serum urea nitrogen, serum creatinine, and their ratio. *JAMA* 1974;227(1):41–44.
105. Merjanian R, Budoff M, Adler S, et al. Coronary artery calcification in non-dialyzed patients with diabetic renal disease. *J Am Soc Nephrol* 2002;13:647A.
106. Mehrotra R, Budoff M, Ipp E, et al. High prevalence and severity of coronary calcification in non-dialyzed patients with diabetic nephropathy (DN): No correlation with risk factors for atherosclerosis or Ca-P metabolism. *J Am Soc Nephrol* 2002;13:648A.
107. Addis T. *Glomerular Nephritis Diagnosis and Treatment*. 1948, Macmillan: New York.
108. Borst JGG. Protein metabolism in uraemia; effects of protein-free diet, infections and blood-transfusions. *Lancet* 1948;1:824.
109. Berlyne GM, Shaw AB, Nilwarangkur S. Dietary treatment of chronic renal failure. Experiences with a modified Giovannetti diet. *Nephron* 1965;2(3):129–147.
110. Kopple JD, Sorensen MK, Coburn JW, et al. Controlled comparison of 20-g and 40-g protein diets in the treatment of chronic uremia. *Am J Clin Nutr* 1968;21(6):553–564.
111. Ford J, Phillips ME, Toye FE, et al. Nitrogen balance in patients with chronic renal failure on diets containing varying quantities of protein. *Br Med J* 1969;1(646):735–740.
112. Kopple JD, Coburn JW. Metabolic studies of low protein diets in uremia. I. Nitrogen and potassium. *Medicine* 1973;52(6):583–595.
113. Maschio G, Oldrizzi L, Tessitore N, et al. Effects of dietary protein and phosphorus restriction on the progression of early renal failure. *Kidney Int* 1982;22(4):371–376.
114. Rossman JB, Meijer S, Sluiter WJ, et al. Prospective randomised trial of early dietary protein restriction in chronic renal failure. *Lancet* 1984;2:1291.
115. Locatelli F, Alberti D, Graziani G, et al. Prospective, randomised, multicentre trial of effect of protein restriction on progression of chronic renal insufficiency. Northern Italian Cooperative Study Group. *Lancet* 1991;337(8753):1299–1304.
116. Williams PS, Stevens MD, Fass G, et al. A randomized trial of the effects of protein and phosphate restriction on the progression of chronic renal failure. *Nephrol Dial Transplant* 1987;7:285.
117. Ihle BU, Becker GJ, Whitworth JA, et al. The effect of protein restriction on the progression of renal insufficiency. *N Engl J Med* 1989;321(26):1773–1777.
118. Fouque D, Laville M, Boissel JP, et al. Controlled low protein diets in chronic renal insufficiency: meta-analysis. *Br Med J* 1992;304(6821):216–220.
119. D'Amico G, Gentile MG, Fellin G, et al. Effect of dietary protein restriction on the progression of renal failure: a prospective randomized trial. *Nephrol Dial Transplant* 1994;9(11):1590–1594.
120. Kopple JD. History of dietary protein therapy for the treatment of chronic renal disease from the mid 1800s until the 1950s. *Am J Nephrol* 2002;22(2–3):278–283.
121. Giordano C. Use of exogenous and endogenous urea for protein synthesis in normal and uremic subjects. *J Lab Clin Med* 1963;62:231.
122. Giovannetti S, Maggiore Q. A low nitrogen diet with proteins of high biological value for severe chronic uraemia. *Lancet* 1964;1:1000.
123. Bergstrom J, Furst P, Josephson B, et al. Factors affecting the nitrogen balance in chronic uremic patients receiving essential amino acids intravenously or by mouth. *Nutr Metab* 1972;14:162–170.
124. Giordano C, Phillips ME, De Santo NG, et al. Utilisation of ketoacid analogues of valine and phenylalanine in health and uraemia. *Lancet* 1972;1(7743):178–182.
125. Walser M, Coulter AW, Dighe S, et al. The effect of keto-analogues of essential amino acids in severe chronic uremia. *J Clin Invest* 1973;52(3):678–690.
126. Kopple JD, Swendseid ME. Nitrogen balance and plasma amino acid levels in uremic patients fed an essential amino acid diet. *Am J Clin Nutr* 1974;27(8):806–812.
127. Bergstrom J, Furst P, Noree LO. Treatment of chronic uremic patients with protein-poor diet and oral supply of essential amino acids. I. Nitrogen balance studies. *Clin Nephrol* 1975;3(5):187–194.
128. Richards P, Brown CL, Lowe SM. Synthesis of tryptophan from 3-indolepyruvic acid by a healthy woman. *J Nutr* 1972;102(11):1547–1549.
129. Walser M. Ketoacids in the treatment of uremia. *Clin Nephrol* 1975;3(5):180–186.
130. Kopple JD. Treatment with low protein and amino acid diets in chronic renal failure. In: Barcelo R, Bergeron M, Carriere S, et al., eds. *Proceedings VIIth International Congress of Nephrology*. Basel: S. Karger, 1978:497–507.
131. Walser M, Mitch WE, Abras E. Supplements containing amino acids and keto acids in the treatment of chronic uremia. *Kidney Int Suppl* 1983;16:S285–S289.
132. Jungers P, Chauveau P, Ployard F, et al. Comparison of keto-acids and low protein diet on advanced chronic renal failure progression. *Kidney Int Suppl* 1987;22:S67–S71.
133. Noree LO, Bergstrom J. Treatment of chronic uremic patients with protein-poor diet and oral supply of essential amino acids. II. Clinical results of long-term treatment. *Clin Nephrol* 1975;3(5):195–203.
134. Gallina DL, Dominguez JM, Hoschoian JC, et al. Maintenance of nitrogen balance in a young woman by substitution of alpha-ketoisovaleric acid for valine. *J Nutr* 1971;101(9):1165–1167.
135. Rudman D. Capacity of human subjects to utilize keto analogues of valine and phenylalanine. *J Clin Invest* 1971;50(1):90–96.
136. Walser M, Lund P, Ruderman NB, et al. Synthesis of essential amino acids from their alpha-keto analogues by perfused rat liver and muscle. *J Clin Invest* 1973;52(11):2865–2877.
137. Buse MG, Reid SS. Leucine. A possible regulator of protein turnover in muscle. *J Clin Invest* 1975;56(5):1250–1261.
138. Mitch WE, Walser M, Sapir DG. Nitrogen sparing induced by leucine compared with that induced by its keto analogue, alpha-ketoisocaproate, in fasting obese man. *J Clin Invest* 1981;67(2):553–562.
139. Furst P, Alvesstrand A, Bergstrom J. Effects of nutrition and catabolic stress on intracellular amino acid pools in uremia. *Am J Clin Nutr* 1980;33(7):1387–1395.
140. Alvestrand A, Ahlberg M, Bergstrom J. Retardation of the progression of renal insufficiency in patients treated with low-protein diets. *Kidney Int Suppl* 1983;16:S268–S272.
141. Mitch WE, Abras E, Walser M. Long-term effects of a new

ketoacid-amino acid supplement in patients with chronic renal failure. *Kidney Int* 1982;22(1):48–53.

142. Barsotti G, Morelli E, Giannoni A, et al. Restricted phosphorus and nitrogen intake to slow the progression of chronic renal failure: a controlled trial. *Kidney Int Suppl* 1983;16:S278–S284.
143. Mitch WE, Walser M, Steinman TI, et al. The effect of a keto acid-amino acid supplement to a restricted diet on the progression of chronic renal failure. *N Engl J Med* 1984;311(10): 623–629.
144. Kopple JD, Swendseid ME. Evidence that histidine is an essential amino acid in normal and chronically uremic man. *J Clin Invest* 1975;55(5):881–891.
145. Teschan PE, Beck GJ, Dwyer JT, et al. Effect of a ketoacid-aminoacid-supplemented very low protein diet on the progression of advanced renal disease: a reanalysis of the MDRD feasibility study. *Clin Nephrol* 1998;50(5):273–283.
146. Levey AS, Adler S, Caggiula AW, et al. Effects of dietary protein restriction on the progression of advanced renal disease in the Modification of Diet in Renal Disease Study. *Am J Kidney Dis* 1996;27(5):652–663.
147. Niwa T, Ise M. Indoxyl sulfate, a circulating uremic toxin, stimulates the progression of glomerular sclerosis. *J Lab Clin Med* 1994;124(1):96–104.
148. Niwa T, Nomura T, Sugiyama S, et al. The protein metabolite hypothesis, a model for the progression of renal failure: an oral adsorbent lowers indoxyl sulfate levels in undialyzed uremic patients. *Kidney Int Suppl* 1997;62:S23–S28.
149. Sanaka T, Sugino N, Teraoka S, et al. Therapeutic effects of oral sorbent in undialyzed uremia. *Am J Kidney Dis* 1988;12(2): 97–103.
150. Aoyama I, Niwa T. An oral adsorbent ameliorates renal overload of indoxyl sulfate and progression of renal failure in diabetic rats. *Am J Kidney Dis* 2001;37(1 Suppl 2):S7–S12.
151. Pedrini MT, Lau J, Levey AS. Effect of dietary protein restriction on the progression of non-diabetic renal disease: Meta-analysis. *J Am Soc Nephrol (abs)* 1995;6:399.
152. Kasiske BL, Lakatua JD, Ma JZ, et al. A meta-analysis of the effects of dietary protein restriction on the rate of decline in renal function. *Am J Kidney Dis* 1998;31(6):954–961.
153. Fouque D, Wang P, Laville M, et al. Low protein diets delay end-stage renal disease in non-diabetic adults with chronic renal failure. *Nephrol Dial Transplant* 2000;15(12):1986–1992.
154. Zeller KR. Low-protein diets in renal disease. *Diabetes Care* 1991;14:856–866.
155. Raal FJ, Kalk WJ, Lawson M, et al. Effect of moderate dietary protein restriction on the progression of overt diabetic nephropathy: A 6-mo prospective study. *Am J Clin Nutr* 1994;60(4): 57–85.
156. Anderson JW, Blake JE, Turner J, et al. Effects of soy protein on renal function and proteinuria in patients with type 2 diabetes. *Am J Clin Nutr* 1998;68(6 Suppl):1347S–1353S.
157. Barsotti G, Cupisti A, Barsotti M, et al. Dietary treatment of diabetic nephropathy with chronic renal failure. *Nephrol Dial Transplant* 1998;13(Suppl 8):49–52.
158. Meloni C, Morosetti M, Suraci C, et al. Severe dietary protein restriction in overt diabetic nephropathy: benefits or risks? *J Ren Nutr* 2002;12(2):96–101.
159. Peterson JC, Adler S, Burkart JM, et al. Blood pressure control, proteinuria, and the progression of renal disease. The Modification of Diet in Renal Disease Study. *Ann Intern Med* 1995; 123(10):754–762.
160. Hansen HP, Tauber-Lassen E, Jensen BR, et al. Effect of dietary protein restriction on prognosis in patients with diabetic nephropathy. *Kidney Int* 2002;62(1):220–228.
161. Barsotti G, Morelli E, Cupisti A, et al. A low-nitrogen low-phosphorus vegan diet for patients with chronic renal failure. *Nephron* 1996;74(2):390–394.
162. Soroka N, Silverberg DS, Greemland M, et al. Comparison of a vegetable-based (soya) and an animal-based low-protein diet in predialysis chronic renal failure patients. *Nephron* 1998;79: 173–180.
163. Barsotti G, Morelli E, Cupisti A, et al. A special, supplemented 'vegan' diet for nephrotic patients. *Am J Nephrol* 1991;11(5): 380–385.
164. D'Amico G, Gentile MG, Manna G, et al. Effect of vegetarian soy diet on hyperlipidaemia in nephrotic syndrome. *Lancet* 1992;339(8802):1131–1134.
165. Gentile MG, Fellin G, Cofano F, et al. Treatment of proteinuric patients with a vegetarian soy diet and fish oil. *Clin Nephrol* 1993;40(6):315–320.
166. Jibani MM, Bloodworth LL, Foden E, et al. Predominantly vegetarian diet in patients with incipient and early clinical diabetic nephropathy: effects on albumin excretion rate and nutritional status. *Diabet Med* 1991;8(10):949–953.
167. Cupisti A, Morelli E, Meola M. Vegetarian diet alternated with conventional low-protein diet for patients with chronic renal failure. *J Ren Nutr* 2002;12(1):32–37.
168. Niwa T, Ise M, Miyazaki T. Progression of glomerular sclerosis in experimental uremic rats by administration of indole, a precursor of indoxyl sulfate. *Am J Nephrol* 1994;14(3):207–212.
169. Aoyama I, Shimokata K, Niwa T. An oral adsorbent downregulates renal expression of genes that promote interstitial inflammation and fibrosis in diabetic rats. *Nephron* 2002;92(3): 635–651.
170. Miyazaki T, Ise M, Hirata M, et al. Indoxyl sulfate stimulates renal synthesis of transforming growth factor-beta 1 and progression of renal failure. *Kidney Int Suppl* 1997;63:S211–S214.
171. Miyazaki T, Ise M, Seo H, et al. Indoxyl sulfate increases the gene expressions of TGF-beta 1, TIMP-1 and pro-alpha 1(I) collagen in uremic rat kidneys. *Kidney Int Suppl* 1997;62: S15–S22.
172. Miyazaki T, Aoyama I, Ise M, et al. An oral sorbent reduces overload of indoxyl sulphate and gene expression of TGF-beta 1 in uraemic rat kidneys. *Nephrol Dial Transplant* 2000;15(11): 1773–1781.
173. Reyes AA, Purkerson ML, Karl I, et al. Dietary supplementation with L-arginine ameliorates the progression of renal disease in rats with subtotal nephrectomy. *Am J Kidney Dis* 1992;20: 168–176.
174. Katoh T, Takahashi K, Klahr S, et al. Dietary supplementation with L-arginine ameliorates glomerular hypertension in rats with subtotal nephrectomy. *J Am Soc Nephrol* 1994;4:1690–1694.
175. Wolf SC, Erley CM, Kenner S, et al. Does L-arginine alter proteinuria and renal hemodynamics in patients with chronic glomerulonephritis and hypertension? *Clin Nephrol* 1995;43: S42–S46.
176. Peters H, Border WA, Noble NA. From rats to man: a perspective on dietary L-arginine supplementation in human renal disease. *Nephrol Dial Transplant* 1999;14:1640–1650.
177. Moncada S. Nitric oxide in the vasculature: physiology and pathophysiology. *Ann NY Acad Sci* 1997;811:60–67.
178. Kone BC. Nitric oxide in renal health and disease. *Am J Kidney Dis* 1997;30:311–333.
179. De Nicola L, Bellizzi V, Minutolo R, et al. Randomized, double-blind, placebo-controlled study of arginine supplementation in chronic renal failure. *Kidney Int* 1999;56(2):674–684.
180. Kopple JD, Monteon FJ, Shaib JK. Effect of energy intake on nitrogen metabolism in nondialyzed patients with chronic renal failure. *Kidney Int* 1986;29(3):734–742.
181. Tom K, Young VR, Chapman T, et al. Long-term adaptive

responses to dietary protein restriction in chronic renal failure. *Am J Physiol* 1995;268:E668–E677.

182. Monteon FJ, Laidlaw SA, Shaib JK, et al. Energy expenditure in patients with chronic renal failure. *Kidney Int* 1986;30(5): 741–747.
183. Schneeweiss B, Graninger W, Stockenhuber F, et al. Energy metabolism in acute and chronic renal failure. *Am J Clin Nutr* 1990;52:596–601.
184. Kuhlmann U, Schwickardi M, Trebst R, et al. Resting metabolic rate in chronic renal failure. *J Ren Nutr* 2001;11(4):202–206.
185. Avesani CM, Cuppari L, Silva AC, et al. Resting energy expenditure in pre-dialysis diabetic patients. *Nephrol Dial Transplant* 2001;16(3):556–565.
186. Ratsch IM, Catassi C, Verrina E, et al. Energy and nutrient intake of patients with mild-to-moderate chronic renal failure compared with healthy children: an Italian multicentre study. *Eur J Pediatr* 1992;151(9):701–705.
187. Hylander B, Barkeling B, Rossner S. Eating behavior in continuous ambulatory peritoneal dialysis and hemodialysis patients. *Am J Kidney Dis* 1992;20(6):592–597.
188. Dobell E, Chan M, Williams P, et al. Food preferences and food habits of patients with chronic renal failure undergoing dialysis. *J Am Diet Assoc* 1993;93(10):1129–1135.
189. Randall RE, Cohen MD, Spray CC Jr. Hypermagnesemia in renal failure: Etiology and toxic manifestations. *Ann Intern Med* 1964;61:73.
190. Byers T. Body weight and mortality. *N Engl J Med* 1995; 333(11):723–724.
191. Manson JE, Willett WC, Stampfer MJ, et al. Body weight and mortality among women. *N Engl J Med* 1995;333:677–685.
192. Kalantar-Zadeh K, Block G, Humphreys MH, et al. Reverse epidemiology of cardiovascular risk factors in maintenance dialysis patients. *Kidney Int* 2003;63.
193. Sanfelippo ML, Swenson RS, Reaven GM. Response of plasma triglycerides to dietary change in patients on hemodialysis. *Kidney Int* 1978;14(2):180–186.
194. Parsons DS, Reaveley DA, Pavitt DV, et al. Relationship of renal function to homocysteine and lipoprotein(a) levels: the frequency of the combination of both risk factors in chronic renal impairment. *Am J Kidney Dis* 2002;40(5):916–923.
195. Samuelsson O, Attman PO, Knight-Gibson C, et al. Lipoprotein abnormalities without hyperlipidaemia in moderate renal insufficiency. *Nephrol Dial Transplant* 1994;9(11):1580–1585.
196. Kovesdy CP, Astor BC, Longenecker JC, et al. Association of kidney function with serum lipoprotein(a) level: The Third National Health and Nutrition Examination Survey (1991–1994). *Am J Kidney Dis* 2002;40(5):899–908.
197. Joven J, Villabona C, Vilella E, et al. Abnormalities of lipoprotein metabolism in patients with the nephrotic syndrome. *N Engl J Med* 1990;323(9):579–584.
198. Ohta T, Matsuda I. Lipid and apolipoprotein levels in patients with nephrotic syndrome. *Clin Chim Acta* 1981;117(2): 133–143.
199. Gherardi E, Rota E, Calandra S, et al. Relationship among the concentrations of serum lipoproteins and changes in their chemical composition in patients with untreated nephrotic syndrome. *Eur J Clin Invest* 1977;7(6):563–570.
200. Executive Summary of The Third Report of The National Cholesterol Education Program (NCEP) Expert Panel on Detection, Evaluation, and Treatment of High Blood Cholesterol In Adults (Adult Treatment Panel III). *JAMA* 2001;285(19):2486–2497.
201. Yusuf S, Sleight P, Pogue J, et al. Effects of an angiotensin-converting-enzyme inhibitor, ramipril, on cardiovascular events in high-risk patients. The Heart Outcomes Prevention Evaluation Study Investigators. *N Engl J Med* 2000;342(3):145–153.
202. No author. Effects of ramipril on cardiovascular and microvascular outcomes in people with diabetes mellitus: results of the HOPE study and MICRO-HOPE substudy. Heart Outcomes Prevention Evaluation Study Investigators. *Lancet* 2000; 355(9200):253–259.
203. Maschio G, Alberti D, Janin G, et al. Effect of the angiotensin-converting-enzyme inhibitor benazepril on the progression of chronic renal insufficiency. The Angiotensin-Converting-Enzyme Inhibition in Progressive Renal Insufficiency Study Group. *N Engl J Med* 1996;334(15):939–945.
204. Ruggenenti P, Perna A, Gherardi G, et al. Renal function and requirement for dialysis in chronic nephropathy patients on long-term ramipril: REIN follow-up trial. Gruppo Italiano di Studi Epidemiologici in Nefrologia (GISEN). Ramipril Efficacy in Nephropathy. *Lancet* 1998;352(9136):1252–1256.
205. Mann JF, Gerstein HC, Pogue J, et al. Renal insufficiency as a predictor of cardiovascular outcomes and the impact of ramipril: the HOPE randomized trial. *Ann Intern Med* 2001;134(8): 629–636.
206. Lewis EJ, Hunsicker LG, Clarke WR, et al. Renoprotective effect of the angiotensin-receptor antagonist irbesartan in patients with nephropathy due to type 2 diabetes. *N Engl J Med* 2001;345(12):851–860.
207. Brenner BM, Cooper ME, de Zeeuw D, et al. Effects of losartan on renal and cardiovascular outcomes in patients with type 2 diabetes and nephropathy. *N Engl J Med* 2001;345(12): 861–869.
208. Wollin SD, Jones PJ. Alcohol, red wine and cardiovascular disease. *J Nutr* 2001;131(5):1401–1404.
209. Mukamal KJ, Conigrave KM, Mittleman MA, et al. Roles of drinking pattern and type of alcohol consumed in coronary heart disease in men. *N Engl J Med* 2003;348(2):109–118.
210. Thomas ME, Harris KPG, Ramaswamy C. Simvastatin therapy for hypercholesterolemic patients with nephrotic syndrome or significant proteinuria. *Kidney Int* 1993;44:1124–1129.
211. Tonelli M, Moye L, Sacks FM, et al. Pravastatin for secondary prevention of cardiovascular events in persons with mild chronic renal insufficiency. *Ann Intern Med* 2003;138(2):98–104.
212. Expert Panel on Detection, Evaluation, and Treatment of High Blood Cholesterol in Adults. Summary of the Second Report of the National Cholesterol Education Program (NCEP) (Adult Treatment Panel II). *JAMA* 1993;269:3015–3023.
213. Pierides AM, Alvarez-Ude F, Kerr DN. Clofibrate-induced muscle damage in patients with chronic renal failure. *Lancet* 1975;2(7948):1279–1282.
214. Manis T, Deutsch J, Feinstein EI. Charcoal sorbent-induced hypolipidemia in uremia and diabetes. *Am J Clin Nutr* 1980; 33:1485.
215. Pagenkemper JJ. Attaining nutritional goals for hyperlipidemic and obese renal patients. In: Renal Nutrition, Report of the Eleventh Ross Round-Table on Medical Issues. Columbus: Ross Laboratories, 1991;26–33.
216. Leaf A, Weber PC. Cardiovascular effects of n-3 fatty acids. *N Engl J Med* 1988;318:549.
217. Kasiske BL, O'Donnell MP, Cleary MP, et al. Treatment of hyperlipidemia reduces glomerular injury in obese Zucker rats. *Kidney Int* 1988;33(3):667–672.
218. Keane WF, O'Donnell MP, Kasiske BL. Lipids and the progression of renal disease. *J Am Soc Nephrol* 1990;1:S69.
219. Homan van der Heide JJ, Bilo HJ, Tegzess AM, et al. The effects of dietary supplementation with fish oil on renal function in cyclosporine-treated renal transplant recipients. *Transplantation* 1990;49(3):523–527.
220. Hamazaki T, Tateno S, Shishido H. Eicosapentaenoic acid and IgA nephropathy. *Lancet* 1984;1:1017 (letter to the editor).
221. Bennett WM, Walker RG, Kincaid-Smith P. Treatment of IgA

nephropathy with eicosapentanoic acid (EPA): a two-year prospective trial. *Clin Nephrol* 1989;31(3):128–131.

222. Donadio JVJ, Holman RT, Holub BF. Effects of omega (ω)-3 polyunsaturated fatty acids (PUFA) in mesangial IgA nephropathy. *Kidney Int* 1990;37:255 (abstract).
223. Donadio JV Jr, Bergstralh EJ, Offord KP, et al. A controlled trial of fish oil in IgA nephropathy. Mayo Nephrology Collaborative Group. *N Engl J Med* 1994;331(18):1194–1199.
224. Guarnieri G, Toigo G, Crapesi L, et al. Carnitine metabolism in chronic renal failure. *Kidney Int Suppl* 1987;22:S116–S127.
225. Wanner C, Horl WH. Carnitine abnormalities in patients with renal insufficiency. Pathophysiological and therapeutical aspects. *Nephron* 1988;50(2):89–102.
226. Younes H, Alphonse JC, Behr SR, et al. Role of fermentable carbohydrate supplements with a low-protein diet in the course of chronic renal failure: experimental bases. *Am J Kidney Dis* 1999;33(4):633–646.
227. Pitts RF. Physiology of the kidney and body fluids. Chicago: Year Book Medical Publishers, 1974.
228. Koomans HA, Ross JC, Boer P. Salt sensitivity of blood pressure in chronic renal failure. Evidence for renal control of body fluid distribution in man. *Hypertension* 1982;4:190.
229. Cianciaruso B, Bellizzi V, Minutolo R, et al. Salt intake and renal outcome in patients with progressive renal disease. *Miner Electrolyte Metab* 1998;24(4):296–301.
230. Heeg JE, de Jong PE, van der Hem GK, et al. Efficacy and variability of the antiproteinuric effect of ACE inhibition by lisinopril. *Kidney Int* 1989;36(2):272–279.
231. Jerums G, Allen TJ, Tsalamandris C, et al. Angiotensin converting enzyme inhibition and calcium channel blockade in incipient diabetic nephropathy. The Melbourne Diabetic Nephropathy Study Group. *Kidney Int* 1992;41(4):904–911.
232. Buter H, Hemmelder MH, Navis G, et al. The blunting of the antiproteinuric efficacy of ACE inhibition by high sodium intake can be restored by hydrochlorothiazide. *Nephrol Dial Transplant* 1998;13(7):1682–1685.
233. Blumenkrantz MJ, Kopple JD, Moran JK, et al. Metabolic balance studies and dietary protein requirements in patients undergoing continuous ambulatory peritoneal dialysis. *Kidney Int* 1982;21(6):849–861.
234. DeFronzo RA, Smith JD. Clinical disorders of hyperkalemia. In: Narins RG, ed. *Maxwell & Kleeman's clinical disorders of fluid and electrolyte metabolism*. New York: McGraw-Hill, 1994; 697–754.
235. Wallach S. Effects of magnesium on skeletal metabolism. *Magnes Trace Elem* 1990;9(1):1–14.
236. Tomford RC, Karlinsky ML, Buddington B, et al. Effect of thyroparathyroidectomy and parathyroidectomy on renal function and the nephrotic syndrome in rat nephrotoxic serum nephritis. *J Clin Invest* 1981;68(3):655–664.
237. Ibels LS, Alfrey AC, Huffer WE, et al. Calcification in end-stage kidneys. *Am J Med* 1981;71(1):33–37.
238. Barsotti G, Giannoni A, Morelli E, et al. The decline of renal function slowed by very low phosphorus intake in chronic renal patients following a low nitrogen diet. *Clin Nephrol* 1984;21(1): 54–59.
239. Lumlertgul D, Burke TJ, Gillum DM, et al. Phosphate depletion arrests progression of chronic renal failure independent of protein intake. *Kidney Int* 1986;29(3):658–666.
240. Cannata JB, Briggs JD, Junor BJ, et al. Aluminium hydroxide intake: real risk of aluminium toxicity. *Br Med J (Clin Res Ed)* 1983;286(6382):1937–1938.
241. Sedman AB, Miller NL, Warady BA, et al. Aluminum loading in children with chronic renal failure. *Kidney Int* 1984;26(2): 201–204.
242. Kaye M. Oral aluminum toxicity in a non-dialyzed patient with renal failure. *Clin Nephrol* 1983;20(4):208–211.
243. Norris KC, Crooks PW, Nebeker HG, et al. Clinical and laboratory features of aluminum-related bone disease: differences between sporadic and "epidemic" forms of the syndrome. *Am J Kidney Dis* 1985;6(5):342–347.
244. Addison JF, Foulks CJ. Calcium carbonate: An effective phosphorus binder in patients with chronic renal failure. *Curr Ther Res* 1985;38:241.
245. Hercz G, Coburn JW. Prevention of phosphate retention and hyperphosphatemia in uremia. *Kidney Int Suppl* 1987;22: S215–S220.
246. Nolan CR, Califano JR, Butzin CA. Influence of calcium acetate or calcium citrate on intestinal aluminum absorption. *Kidney Int* 1990;38(5):937–941.
247. Schaefer K, Scheer J, Asmus G, et al. The treatment of uraemic hyperphosphataemia with calcium acetate and calcium carbonate: a comparative study. *Nephrol Dial Transplant* 1991;6(3): 170–175.
248. Mai ML, Emmett M, Sheikh MS, et al. Calcium acetate, an effective phosphorus binder in patients with renal failure. *Kidney Int* 1989;36(4):690–695.
249. Pflanz S, Henderson IS, McElduff N, et al. Calcium acetate versus calcium carbonate as phosphate-binding agents in chronic haemodialysis. *Nephrol Dial Transplant* 1994;9(8): 1121–1124.
250. Slatopolsky EA, Burke SK, Dillon MA. RenaGel, a nonabsorbed calcium- and aluminum-free phosphate binder, lowers serum phosphorus and parathyroid hormone. The RenaGel Study Group. *Kidney Int* 1999;55(1):299–307.
251. Chertow GM, Burke SK, Lazarus JM, et al. Poly(allylamine hydrochloride) (RenaGel): a noncalcemic phosphate binder for the treatment of hyperphosphatemia in chronic renal failure. *Am J Kidney Dis* 1997;29(1):66–71.
252. Chertow GM, Burke SK, Dillon MA, et al. Long-term effects of sevelamer hydrochloride on the calcium x phosphate product and lipid profile of haemodialysis patients. *Nephrol Dial Transplant* 1999;14(12):2907–2914.
253. Delmez JA, Kelber J, Norword KY, et al. Magnesium carbonate as a phosphorus binder: a prospective, controlled, crossover study. *Kidney Int* 1996;49(1):163–167.
254. Dewberry K, Fox J, Stewart J, et al. Lanthanum carbonate: A novel non-calcium containing phosphate binder. *J Am Soc Nephrol* 1997;8:A2610.
255. Hsu CH, Patel SR, Young EW. New phosphate binding agents: ferric compounds. *J Am Soc Nephrol* 1999;10(6):1274–1280.
256. Hergesell O, Ritz E. Stabilized polynuclear iron hydroxide is an efficient oral phosphate binder in uraemic patients. *Nephrol Dial Transplant* 1999;14(4):863–867.
257. Chang JM, Hwang SJ, Tsai JC, et al. Effect of ferric polymaltose complex as a phosphate binder in haemodialysis patients. *Nephrol Dial Transplant* 1999;14(4):1045–1047.
258. Van de Vyver FL, Visser WJ, D'Haese PC. Iron overload and bone disease in chronic dialysis patients. *Nephrol Dial Transplant* 1990;5:781.
259. Hercz G, Pei Y, Greenwood C, et al. Aplastic osteodystrophy without aluminum: the role of "suppressed" parathyroid function. *Kidney Int* 1993;44(4):860–866.
260. Chertow GM, Burke SK, Raggi P. Sevelamer attenuates the progression of coronary and aortic calcification in hemodialysis patients. *Kidney Int* 2002;62(1):245–252.
261. Institute of Medicine. Dietary Reference Intakes for calcium, phosphorus, magnesium, vitamin D, and fluoride. Food and Nutrition Board. Washington, DC: National Academy Press, 1997.
262. Brickman AS, Coburn JW, Friedman GR, et al. Comparison

of effects of 1 alpha-hydroxy-vitamin D3 and 1,25-dihydroxy-vitamin D3 in man. *J Clin Invest* 1976;57(6):1540–1547.

263. Chen SM. Renal excretion of zinc in patients with chronic uremia. *Taiwan I Hsueh Hui Chih* 1990;89:220.
264. Rudolph H, Alfrey AC, Smythe WR. Muscle and serum trace element profile in uremia. *Trans Am Soc Artif Intern Organs* 1973;19:456–465.
265. Cartwright GE, Gubler CJ, Wintrobe MM. Studies on copper metabolism in the nephrotic syndrome. *J Clin Invest* 1954;33: 685.
266. Fishbane S, Frei GL, Maesaka J. Reduction in recombinant human erythropoietin doses by the use of chronic intravenous iron supplementation. *Am J Kidney Dis* 1995;26(1):41–46.
267. Mahajan SK, Abraham J, Hessburg T, et al. Zinc metabolism and taste acuity in renal transplant recipients. *Kidney Int Suppl* 1983;16:S310–S314.
268. Atkin-Thor E, Goddard BW, O'Nion J, et al. Hypogeusia and zinc depletion in chronic dialysis patients. *Am J Clin Nutr* 1978; 31(10):1948–1951.
269. Mahajan SK, Bowersox EM, Rye DL, et al. Factors underlying abnormal zinc metabolism in uremia. *Kidney Int Suppl* 1989; 27:S269–S273.
270. Institute of Medicine. Dietary Reference Intakes for vitamin A, vitamin K, arsenic, boron, chromium, copper, iodine, iron, manganese, molybdenum, nickel, silicon, vanadium, and zinc. Food and Nutrition Board. Washington, DC, National Academy Press, 2001.
271. Antoniou LD, Shalhoub RJ, Sudhakar T, et al. Reversal of uraemic impotence by zinc. *Lancet* 1977;2(8044):895–898.
272. Rodger RS, Sheldon WL, Watson MJ, et al. Zinc deficiency and hyperprolactinaemia are not reversible causes of sexual dysfunction in uraemia. *Nephrol Dial Transplant* 1989;4(10): 888–892.
273. Kiilerich S, Christiansen C, Christensen MS, et al. Zinc metabolism in patients with chronic renal failure during treatment with 1.25-dihydroxycholecalciferol: a controlled therapeutic trial. *Clin Nephrol* 1981;15(1):23–27.
274. Keane WF, Collins AJ. Influence of co-morbidity on mortality and morbidity in patients treated with hemodialysis. *Am J Kidney Dis* 1994;24(6):1010–1018.
275. United States Renal Data System. *USRDS 2002 Annual Data Report: atlas of end-stage renal disease in the United States.* Bethesda, MD: National Institutes of Health, National Institute of Diabetes and Digestive and Kidney Diseases, 2002.
276. Stein G, Sperschneider H, Koppe S. Vitamin levels in chronic renal failure and need for supplementation. *Blood Purif* 1985; 3(1–3):52–62.
277. Hampers CL, Streiff R, Nathan DG, et al. Megaloblastic hematopoiesis in uremia and in patients on long-term hemodialysis. *N Engl J Med* 1967;276(10):551–554.
278. Milman N. Serum vitamin B12 and erythrocyte folate in chronic uraemia and after renal transplantation. *Scand J Haematol* 1980;25(2):151–157.
279. Porrini M, Simonetti P, Ciappellano S, et al. Thiamin, riboflavin and pyridoxine status in chronic renal insufficiency. *Int J Vitam Nutr Res* 1989;59(3):304–308.
280. Marumo F, Kamata K, Okubo M. Deranged concentrations of water-soluble vitamins in the blood of undialyzed and dialyzed patients with chronic renal failure. *Int J Artif Organs* 1986;9(1): 17–24.
281. Wilcken DE, Dudman NP, Tyrrell PA, et al. Folic acid lowers elevated plasma homocysteine in chronic renal insufficiency: possible implications for prevention of vascular disease. *Metabolism* 1988;37(7):697–701.
282. Arnadottir M, Brattstrom L, Simonsen O, et al. The effect of high-dose pyridoxine and folic acid supplementation on serum lipid and plasma homocysteine concentrations in dialysis patients. *Clin Nephrol* 1993;40(4):236–240.
283. Hultberg B, Andersson A, Arnadottir M. Reduced, free and total fractions of homocysteine and other thiol compounds in plasma from patients with renal failure. *Nephron* 1995;70(1): 62–67.
284. Thambyrajah J, Landray MJ, McGlynn FJ, et al. Does folic acid decrease plasma homocysteine and improve endothelial function in patients with predialysis renal failure? *Circulation* 2000;102(8):871–875.
285. Nygard O, Nordrehaug JE, Refsum H, et al. Plasma homocysteine levels and mortality in patients with coronary artery disease. *N Engl J Med* 1997;337(4):230–236.
286. Meleady RA, Graham IM. Homocysteine as a risk factor for coronary artery disease. *J Cardiovasc Risk* 1995;2(3):216–221.
287. Smith FR, Goodman DS. The effects of diseases of the liver, thyroid, and kidneys on the transport of vitamin A in human plasma. *J Clin Invest* 1971;50(11):2426–2436.
288. Stein G, Schone S, Geinitz D, et al. No tissue level abnormality of vitamin A concentration despite elevated serum vitamin A of uremic patients. *Clin Nephrol* 1986;25(2):87–93.
289. Yatzidis H, Digenis P, Fountas P. Hypervitaminosis A accompanying advanced chronic renal failure. *Br Med J* 1975;3(5979): 352–353.
290. Taccone-Gallucci M, Lubrano R, Del Principe D, et al. Platelet lipid peroxidation in haemodialysis patients: effects of vitamin E supplementation. *Nephrol Dial Transplant* 1989;4(11): 975–978.
291. Gentile MG, Manna GM, D'Amico G, et al. Vitamin nutrition in patients with chronic renal failure and dietary manipulation. *Contrib Nephrol* 1988;65:43–50.
292. Peuchant E, Delmas-Beauvieux MC, Dubourg L, et al. Antioxidant effects of a supplemented very low protein diet in chronic renal failure. *Free Radic Biol Med* 1997;22(1–2):313–320.
293. Saborio P, Krieg RJ Jr, Kuemmerle NB, et al. Alpha-tocopherol modulates lipoprotein cytotoxicity in obstructive nephropathy. *Pediatr Nephrol* 2000;14(8–9):740–746.
294. Appenroth D, Frob S, Kersten L, et al. Protective effects of vitamin E and C on cisplatin nephrotoxicity in developing rats. *Arch Toxicol* 1997;71(11):677–683.
295. Lee HS, Jeong JY, Kim BC, et al. Dietary antioxidant inhibits lipoprotein oxidation and renal injury in experimental focal segmental glomerulosclerosis. *Kidney Int* 1997;51(4): 1151–1159.
296. Kuemmerle NB, Krieg RJ Jr, Chan W, et al. Influence of alpha-tocopherol over the time course of experimental IgA nephropathy. *Pediatr Nephrol* 1999;13(2):108–112.
297. Kim SS, Gallaher DD, Csallany AS. Vitamin E and probucol reduce urinary lipophilic aldehydes and renal enlargement in streptozotocin-induced diabetic rats. *Lipids* 2000;35(11): 1225–1237.
298. Trachtman H, Schwob N, Maesaka J, et al. Dietary vitamin E supplementation ameliorates renal injury in chronic puromycin aminonucleoside nephropathy. *J Am Soc Nephrol* 1995;5(10): 1811–1819.
299. Boaz M, Smetana S, Weinstein T, et al. Secondary prevention with antioxidants of cardiovascular disease in endstage renal disease (SPACE): randomised placebo-controlled trial. *Lancet* 2000;356(9237):1213–1218.
300. O'Byrne D, Devaraj S, Islam KN, et al. Low-density lipoprotein (LDL)-induced monocyte-endothelial cell adhesion, soluble cell adhesion molecules, and autoantibodies to oxidized-LDL in chronic renal failure patients on dialysis therapy. *Metabolism* 2001;50(2):207–215.
301. Taccone-Gallucci M, Giardini O, Lubrano R, et al. Red blood

cell membrane lipid peroxidation in continuous ambulatory peritoneal dialysis patients. *Am J Nephrol* 1986;6(2):92–95.

302. Bonnefont-Rousselot D, Lehmann E, Jaudon MC, et al. Blood oxidative stress and lipoprotein oxidizability in haemodialysis patients: effect of the use of a vitamin E-coated dialysis membrane. *Nephrol Dial Transplant* 2000;15(12):2020–2028.
303. Galli F, Canestrari F, Buoncristiani U. Biological effects of oxidant stress in haemodialysis: the possible roles of vitamin E. *Blood Purif* 1999;17(2–3):79–94.
304. Galli F, Buoncristiani U, Rovidati S, et al. Lipoperoxidation and glutathione-dependent enzymes in uremic anemia of CAPD patients. *Nephron* 1997;76(3):363.
305. Girndt M, Lengler S, Kaul H, et al. Prospective crossover trial of the influence of vitamin E-coated dialyzer membranes on T-cell activation and cytokine induction. *Am J Kidney Dis* 2000; 35(1):95–104.
306. Mune M, Yukawa S, Kishino M, et al. Effect of vitamin E on lipid metabolism and atherosclerosis in ESRD patients. *Kidney Int Suppl* 1999;71:S126–S129.
307. Shimazu T, Kondo S, Toyama K, et al. Effect of vitamin E-modified regenerative cellulose membrane on neutrophil superoxide anion radical production and lipid peroxidation. *Contrib Nephrol* 1999;127:251–260.
308. Wratten ML, Navino C, Tetta C, et al. Haemolipodialysis. *Blood Purif* 1999;17(2–3):127–133.
309. Udall JA. Human sources and absorption of vitamin K in relation to anticoagulation stability. *JAMA* 1965;194(2):127–129.
310. Wolfson M, Kopple JD. The effect of vitamin B6 deficiency on food intake, growth, and renal function in chronically azotemic rats. *JPEN J Parenter Enteral Nutr* 1987;11(4):398–402.
311. Balcke P, Schmidt P, Zazgornik J, et al. Effect of vitamin B6 administration on elevated plasma oxalic acid levels in haemodialysed patients. *Eur J Clin Invest* 1982;12(6):481–483.
312. Morgan SH, Purkiss P, Watts RW, et al. Oxalate dynamics in chronic renal failure. Comparison with normal subjects and patients with primary hyperoxaluria. *Nephron* 1987;46(3): 253–257.
313. Tomson CR, Channon SM, Parkinson IS, et al. Effect of pyridoxine supplementation on plasma oxalate concentrations in patients receiving dialysis. *Eur J Clin Invest* 1989;19(2): 201–205.
314. Costello JF, Sadovnic MC, Smith M, et al. Effect of vitamin B6 supplementation on plasma oxalate and oxalate removal rate in hemodialysis patients. *J Am Soc Nephrol* 1992;3(4): 1018–1024.
315. Anderson KEH. Folic acid status of patients with chronic renal failure maintained by dialysis. *Clin Nephrol* 1977;8:510.
316. Sharman VL, Cunningham J, Goodwin FJ, et al. Do patients receiving regular haemodialysis need folic acid supplements? *Br Med J (Clin Res Ed)* 1982;285(6335):96–97.
317. Descombes E, Hanck AB, Fellay G. Water soluble vitamins in chronic hemodialysis patients and need for supplementation. *Kidney Int* 1993;43(6):1319–1328.
318. Ross EA, Shah GM, Reynolds RD, et al. Vitamin B6 requirements of patients on chronic peritoneal dialysis. *Kidney Int* 1989;36(4):702–706.
319. Mydlik M, Derzsiova K, Valek A, et al. Vitamins and continuous ambulatory peritoneal dialysis (CAPD). *Int Urol Nephrol* 1985;17(3):281–286.
320. Dietary Reference Intakes for vitamin C, vitamin E, selenium and carotenoids. Food and Nutrition Board. Washington DC: National Academy Press, 2000.
321. Jennette JC, Goldman ID. Inhibition of the membrane transport of folates by anions retained in uremia. *J Lab Clin Med* 1975;86(5):834–843.
322. Balcke P, Schmidt P, Zazgornik J, et al. Ascorbic acid aggravates secondary hyperoxalemia in patients on chronic hemodialysis. *Ann Intern Med* 1984;101(3):344–345.
323. Pru C, Eaton J, Kjellstrand C. Vitamin C intoxication and hyperoxalemia in chronic hemodialysis patients. *Nephron* 1985; 39(2):112–116.
324. Gaede P, Poulsen HE, Parving HH, et al. Double-blind, randomised study of the effect of combined treatment with vitamin C and E on albuminuria in Type 2 diabetic patients. *Diabet Med* 2001;18(9):756–760.
325. Farrington K, Miller P, Varghese Z, et al. Vitamin A toxicity and hypercalcaemia in chronic renal failure. *Br Med J (Clin Res Ed)* 1981;282(6281):1999–2002.
326. Reaich D, Channon SM, Scrimgeour CM, et al. Ammonium chloride-induced acidosis increases protein breakdown and amino acid oxidation in humans. *Am J Physiol* 1992;263(4 Pt 1):E735–E739.
327. Mitch WE, Medina R, Grieber S, et al. Metabolic acidosis stimulates muscle protein degradation by activating the adenosine triphosphate-dependent pathway involving ubiquitin and proteasomes. *J Clin Invest* 1994;93(5):2127–2133.
328. Challa A, Chan W, Kreig RJ Jr, et al. Effect of metabolic acidosis on the expression of insulin-like growth factor and growth hormone receptor. *Kidney Int* 1993;44:1224–1227.
329. Ballmer PE, McNurlan MA, Hulter HN, et al. Chronic metabolic acidosis decreases albumin synthesis and induces negative nitrogen balance in humans. *J Clin Invest* 1995;95(1):39–45.
330. Graham KA, Reaich D, Channon SM, et al. Correction of acidosis in hemodialysis decreases whole-body protein degradation. *J Am Soc Nephrol* 1997;8(4):632–637.
331. Symposium on role of dietary fiber in health. *Am J Clin Nutr* 1978;31:S1.
332. Rampton DS, Cohen SL, Crammond VD, et al. Treatment of chronic renal failure with dietary fiber. *Clin Nephrol* 1984;21(3): 159–163.
333. Mokdad AH, Ford ES, Bowman BA, et al. Diabetes trends in the U.S.: 1990–1998. *Diabetes Care* 2000;23(9):1278–1283.
334. Mogensen CE. Microalbuminuria predicts clinical proteinuria and early mortality in maturity-onset diabetes. *N Engl J Med* 1984;310(6):356–360.
335. Siegel JE, Krolewski AS, Warram JH, et al. Cost-effectiveness of screening and early treatment of nephropathy in patients with insulin-dependent diabetes mellitus. *J Am Soc Nephrol* 1992;3(4 Suppl):S111–S119.
336. The KROC Collaborative Study Group. Blood glucose control and the evolution of diabetic retinopathy and albuminuria. A preliminary multicenter trial. *N Engl J Med* 1984;311:365–372.
337. The effect of intensive treatment of diabetes on the development and progression of long-term complications in insulin-dependent diabetes mellitus. The Diabetes Control and Complications Trial Research Group. *N Engl J Med* 1993;329:977–986.
338. Bakris GL, Williams M, Dworkin L, et al. Preserving renal function in adults with hypertension and diabetes: a consensus approach. National Kidney Foundation Hypertension and Diabetes Executive Committees Working Group. *Am J Kidney Dis* 2000;36(3):646–661.
339. Marre M, Chatellier G, Leblanc H, et al. Prevention of diabetic nephropathy with enalapril in normotensive diabetics with microalbuminuria. *Br Med J* 1988;297(6656):1092–1095.
340. Slomowitz LA, Bergamo R, Grosvenor M, et al. Enalapril reduces albumin excretion in diabetic patients with low levels of microalbuminuria. *Am J Nephrol* 1990;10(6):457–462.
341. Lewis EJ, Hunsicker LG, Bain RP, et al. The effect of angiotensin-converting-enzyme inhibition on diabetic nephropathy. The Collaborative Study Group. *N Engl J Med* 1993;329(20): 1456–1462.
342. Bennett PH, Haffner S, Kasiske BL, et al. Screening and man-

agement of microalbuminuria in patients with diabetes mellitus: recommendations to the Scientific Advisory Board of the National Kidney Foundation from an ad hoc committee of the Council on Diabetes Mellitus of the National Kidney Foundation. *Am J Kidney Dis* 1995;25(1):107–112.

343. Viberti GC, Bilous RW, Mackintosh D, et al. Long term correction of hyperglycaemia and progression of renal failure in insulin dependent diabetes. *Br Med J (Clin Res Ed)* 1983;286(6365): 598–602.
344. Wiseman MJ, Saunders AJ, Keen H, et al. Effect of blood glucose control on increased glomerular filtration rate and kidney size in insulin-dependent diabetes. *N Engl J Med* 1985;312(10): 617–621.
345. Feldt-Rasmussen B, Mathiesen ER, Hegedus L, et al. Kidney function during 12 months of strict metabolic control in insulin-dependent diabetic patients with incipient nephropathy. *N Engl J Med* 1986;314(11):665–670.
346. Ciavarella A, Di Mizio G, Stefoni S, et al. Reduced albuminuria after dietary protein restriction in insulin-dependent diabetic patients with clinical nephropathy. *Diabetes Care* 1987;10(4): 407–413.
347. Viberti GC. Low-protein diet and progression of diabetic kidney disease. *Nephrol Dial Transplant* 1988;3(3):334–339.
348. Walker JD, Dodds RA, Murrells TJ. Restriction of dietary protein and progression of renal failure in diabetic nephropathy. *Lancet* 1989;2:1411–1414.
349. Zeller K, Whittaker E, Sullivan L, et al. Effect of restricting dietary protein on the progression of renal failure in patients with insulin-dependent diabetes mellitus. *N Engl J Med* 1991; 324(2):78–84.
350. Barsotti G, Ciardella F, Morelli E, et al. Nutritional treatment of renal failure in type 1 diabetic nephropathy. *Clin Nephrol* 1988;29(6):280–287.
351. Brodsky IG. Nutritional therapy for patients with diabetic nephropathy. In: Renal Nutrition. Report of the Eleventh Ross Roundtable on Medical Issues. Columbus, OH: Ross Laboratories, 1991;46–50.
352. Anderson JW, Geil PB. Nutritional management of diabetes mellitus. In: Shils ME, Olson JA, Shike M, eds. *Modern nutrition in health and disease.* Philadelphia: Lea & Febiger, 1994; 1259–1286.
353. Kopple JD, Grodstein GP, Roberts CE, et al. Nutritional status of the diabetic patient with chronic uremia. In: Friedman EA, L'Esperance FA Jr, eds. *Diabetic renal-retinal syndrome.* New York: Grune & Stratton, 1980;239–252.
354. Consensus Development Conference on the diagnosis and management of nephropathy in patients with diabetes mellitus. American Diabetes Association and the National Kidney Foundation. *Diabetes Care* 1994;17:1357–1361.
355. Franz MJ, Bantle JP, Beebe CA, et al. Evidence-based nutrition principles and recommendations for the treatment and prevention of diabetes and related complications. *Diabetes Care* 2002; 25(1):148–198.
356. Hokken-Koelega AC, Stijnen T, de Muinck Keizer-Schrama SM, et al. Placebo-controlled, double-blind, cross-over trial of growth hormone treatment in prepubertal children with chronic renal failure. *Lancet* 1991;338(8767):585–590.
357. Ziegler TR, Lazarus JM, Young LS, et al. Effects of recombinant human growth hormone in adults receiving maintenance hemodialysis. *J Am Soc Nephrol* 1991;2(6):1130–1135.
358. Kopple JD. The rationale for the use of growth hormone or insulin-like growth factor I in adult patients with renal failure. *Miner Electrolyte Metab* 1992;18(2–5):269–275.
359. Schulman G, Wingard RL, Hutchison RL, et al. The effects of recombinant human growth hormone and intradialytic parenteral nutrition in malnourished hemodialysis patients. *Am J Kidney Dis* 1993;21(5):527–534.
360. Peng S, Fouque D, Kopple JD. Insulin-like growth factor-I (IGF-I) causes anabolism in malnourished CAPD patients. *J Am Soc Nephrol* 1993;3:414.
361. Johansen KL, Mulligan K, Schambelan M. Anabolic effects of nandrolone decanoate in patients receiving dialysis: a randomized controlled trial. *JAMA* 1999;281(14):1275–1281.
362. Miller SB, Moulton M, O'Shea M, et al. Effects of IGF-I on renal function in end-stage chronic renal failure. *Kidney Int* 1994;46(1):201–207.
363. Takala J, Ruokonen E, Webster NR, et al. Increased mortality associated with growth hormone treatment in critically ill adults. *N Engl J Med* 1999;341(11):785–792.
364. van den Berghe G, Wouters P, Weekers F, et al. Intensive insulin therapy in the critically ill patients. *N Engl J Med* 2001;345(19): 1359–1367.
365. Letters to the Editor. *N Engl J Med* 2002;346(20):1589.
366. Hinton P, Allison SP, Littlejohn S, et al. Insulin and glucose to reduce catabolic response to injury in burned patients. *Lancet* 1971;1(7703):767–769.
367. Woolfson AM, Heatley RV, Allison SP. Insulin to inhibit protein catabolism after injury. *N Engl J Med* 1979;300(1):14–17.
368. Tattersall J, Greenwood R, Farrington K. Urea kinetics and when to commence dialysis. *Am J Nephrol* 1995;15(4): 283–289.
369. NKF-K/DOQI Clinical Practice Guidelines for Peritoneal Dialysis Adequacy: 2000 Update. *Am J Kidney Dis* 2001;37(1 Suppl 1):S65–S136.
370. Iseki K, Uehara H, Nishime K, et al. Impact of the initial levels of laboratory variables on survival in chronic dialysis patients. *Am J Kidney Dis* 1996;28:541–548.
371. Churchill DN, Taylor DW, Keshaviah PR, et al. Adequacy of dialysis and nutrition in continuous peritoneal dialysis: Association with clinical outcomes. *J Am Soc Nephrol* 1996;7:198–207.
372. Mailloux LU, Napolitano B, Bellucci AG, et al. The impact of co-morbid risk factors at the start of dialysis upon the survival of ESRD patients. *ASAIO J* 1996;42:164–169.
373. Obrador GT, Arora P, Kausz AT, et al. Pre-end-stage renal disease care in the United States: A state of disrepair. *J Am Soc Nephrol* 1998;9(Suppl 12):S44–S54.
374. Obrador GT, Pereira BJG. Initiation of dialysis: current trends and the case for timely initiation. *Perit Dial Int* 2000;20(Suppl 2):S142–S149.

24

NUTRITIONAL AND NONNUTRITIONAL MANAGEMENT OF THE NEPHROTIC SYNDROME

BURL R. DON
GEORGE A. KAYSEN

The nephrotic syndrome is a consequence of the urinary loss of albumin and other plasma proteins of similar size and is characterized by hypoalbuminemia, hyperlipidemia, and edema formation (1–4). Although albumin is the principal protein found in the urine, comprising between 75% and 90% of urinary protein, many other proteins are lost as well. These include transferrin, ceruloplasmin, and the binding proteins for vitamin D (5). Albumin is the main zinc-carrying protein in plasma. Thus, iron, zinc, copper, and a key metabolite that regulates calcium metabolism all may be lost in the urine in significant amounts (6–8).

Lipoprotein metabolism is also greatly disturbed, either as a consequence of urinary protein loss (9) or of altered plasma colloid osmotic pressure. Hyperlipidemia in the nephrotic syndrome is characterized by increased levels of low-density lipoprotein (LDL) (10) and either a normal or reduced level of high-density lipoprotein (11). The atherogenic lipoprotein, Lp(a), also is increased (12). Thus, disordered lipid metabolism imposes at least the potential for atherogenic risk to this patient population.

What role, if any, does dietary management play in the treatment of the nephrotic syndrome? The major rationale(s) for changing a patient's diet is to blunt manifestations of the syndrome, such as edema; to replace nutrients lost in the urine; or to reduce risks either of progression of renal disease as might be caused by a high-protein diet or of atherosclerosis that might be a consequence of altered lipid metabolism. It also may be possible that specific allergens contained in food may cause renal disease in some patients (13–17). In this case dietary modification may prove curative.

The principal physiologic role of the kidney is to maintain internal solute balance within narrow limits despite wide differences in the intake of water, minerals, electrolytes, protein, and other nutrients. Fulfillment of this role requires renal function to change in response to variations in diet. Clearly the kidney must be able to respond quickly to changes in water, sodium, or potassium ingestion; however, changes in dietary protein also cause functional adaptations in the kidney.

Renal blood flow, glomerular filtration rate (GFR) (18, 19), and the permselective properties of the glomerular capillary (20–23) increase quickly following an augmentation in dietary protein intake. Renal hypertrophy also occurs (24–26). Ingestion of protein results in the release of a cascade of hormones and vasoactive substances, including growth hormone (27), insulin (27), glucagon (28), kinins (29), prostaglandins (30), dopamine (31,32) and insulinlike growth factor 1 (33,34). In addition, the renin-angiotensin system has been implicated as being one of the mediators of protein-induced hyperfiltration (35). Dietary protein intake stimulates renin secretion (23), and the secondary formation of angiotensin II will, by its effect on efferent arteriolar vasoconstriction, increase intraglomerular capillary pressure and GFR (36). The potent vasodilator, nitric oxide (NO), also has been proposed as a potential mediator of protein-induced hyperfiltration. NO is formed by the vascular endothelium from the guanidino group of arginine by the action of the enzyme NO synthase. Endothelial-derived NO plays a role in maintaining both afferent and efferent arteriolar vasodilation (37–39). It is not surprising, therefore, that the expression of a variety of renal diseases can be modified by changes in dietary protein (Fig. 24.1).

DIETARY PROTEIN

In superficial ways, the nephrotic syndrome is similar to protein-calorie malnutrition, also known as kwashiorkor. In both cases albumin concentration is reduced, plasma volume is expanded, and albumin pools shift from the extravascular to the vascular compartment. Metabolic abnormalities in the nephrotic syndrome include depletion of plasma (21, 22,40–43) and tissue protein pools (44–46); however, in

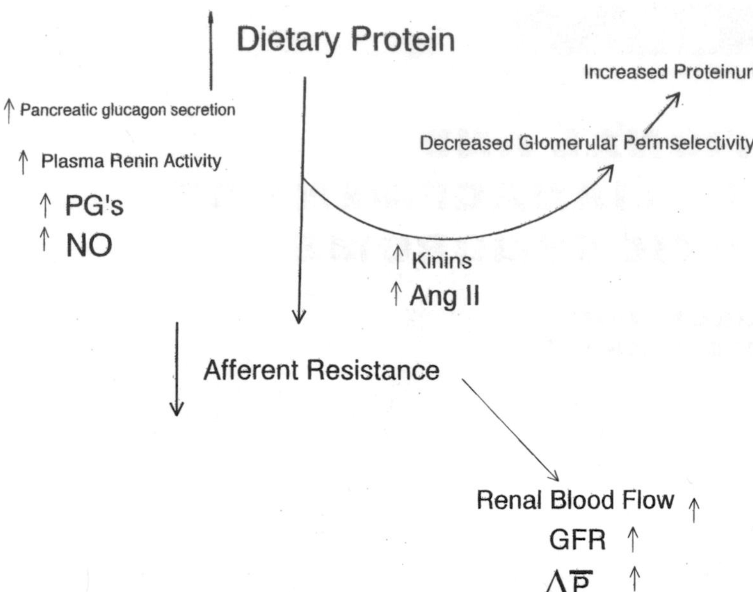

FIGURE 24.1. Effect of dietary protein on renal function. Dietary protein augmentation causes increased secretion of glucagon by the pancreas, alters activity of the renin-angiotensin axis, increases release of nitric oxide, and augments renal prostaglandin (PG) synthesis (30). These, and perhaps other hormones as well, increase renal blood flow; increase glomerular filtration rate (GFR); and, under some circumstances, increase hydraulic pressure across the glomerular capillary. These processes combine to decrease the selectivity of the glomerular capillary and increase proteinuria. Pharmacologic intervention that blocks either kinin or angiotensin II (Ang II) prevents the increase in proteinuria (20, 44,47,68,113).

the case of protein malnutrition it is possible to correct all of the manifestations by providing the needed protein and calories. This is not the case in the nephrotic syndrome. Although average values for proteinuria are approximately 6 to 8 g/day (21,41,47,48)—the amount contained in a hen's egg—simply increasing dietary protein by much more than that amount is of little demonstrable benefit. In fact, dietary protein supplementation causes a greater defect in the filtration barrier of the glomerular capillary (22,23) resulting in increased urinary protein losses (Figs. 24.1 and 24.2). Protein restriction, in contrast, reduces urinary protein excretion and may have a salutary effect on the rate of progression of the renal disease (49).

ALBUMIN HOMEOSTASIS IN THE NEPHROTIC SYNDROME

Albumin is the most abundant protein in plasma. The most notable change in plasma protein composition in the nephrotic syndrome is a decrease in plasma albumin concentration. In patients with the nephrotic syndrome, the primary causes of hypoalbuminemia are urinary losses of albumin and an inappropriate increase in the fractional catabolic rate of albumin (50,51). Although the albumin synthetic rate is increased in the nephrotic syndrome, it is insufficient to replace the losses of albumin resulting from urinary excretion and catabolism. Albumin is important in

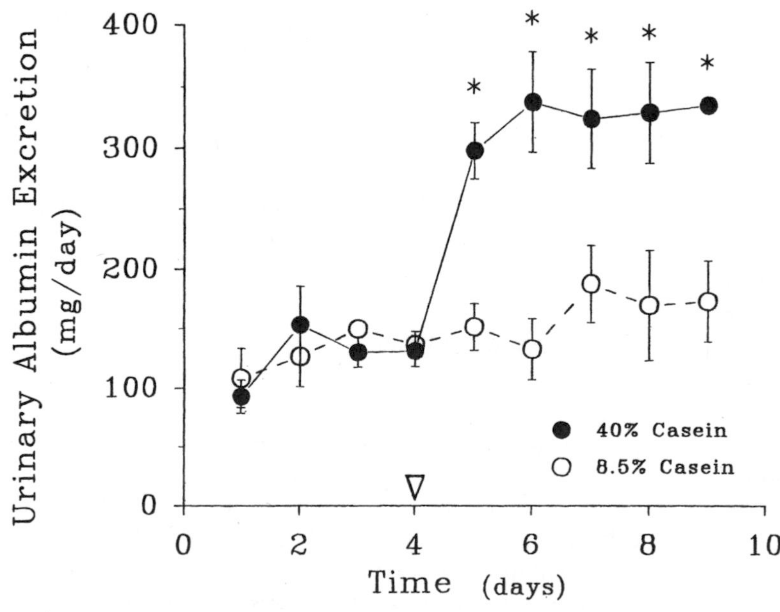

FIGURE 24.2. Effect of dietary protein augmentation on urinary albumin excretion in rats with Heymann nephritis. Eighteen rats were rendered nephrotic by intraperitoneal injection of antibodies to FX-1A (passive Heymann nephritis) (22). All rats remained on an 8.5% protein diet as casein for 11 days, after which each animal was placed in a metabolic cage for urinary albumin collection. After 4 days in the metabolic cages, 10 animals had dietary protein intake augmented to 40% with casein (Purina-purified protein diet 5769) (*solid circles, solid line*) whereas eight remained on 8.5% casein as time controls (*open circles, broken line*). An inverted triangle connotes the day that dietary protein was changed in the high-protein group. Data are mean ± standard error of the mean (SEM). * $p < 0.05$ versus 8.5% protein. Albumin was measured as described (22).

maintaining plasma oncotic pressure because of its relatively low molecular weight and great abundance. Hypoalbuminemia therefore may play a role in the pathogenesis of the edema formation frequently observed in patients with the nephrotic syndrome. Clinical efforts usually are directed at increasing plasma albumin concentration in patients with the nephrotic syndrome to alleviate edema. High-protein diets have been recommended in the past (52) in an effort to maximize the rate of albumin synthesis, replace urinary albumin losses, and thus increase plasma albumin levels. Although the rate of albumin synthesis is regulated in part by dietary protein (53,54), there is no evidence to support this therapy as effective. In fact, as noted earlier, high-protein diets actually worsen proteinuria. The detrimental effects of an increased protein intake on the manifestations of the nephrotic syndrome and renal disease in general may involve both hemodynamic and nonhemodynamic mechanisms.

Dietary Protein and Renal Hemodynamics

Protein supplementation is followed promptly by an increase in both renal and splanchnic blood flow, by an increase in GFR in both humans (27) and animals (19, 55–57), and by increased permeability of the glomerular capillary to protein. As a consequence, urinary albumin excretion increases when patients or animals with the nephrotic syndrome are fed a high-protein diet (21,22,58–60) (Fig. 24.2). The increase in albuminuria is not a consequence of increased plasma albumin levels. Plasma albumin levels either remain the same or decrease following dietary protein augmentation, and in the rat plasma albumin invariably increases when dietary protein is restricted (20,22,44, 59,61). The fractional rate of albumin catabolism (the fraction of the plasma pool catabolized per hour) also increases in patients with the nephrotic syndrome fed a high-protein diet (21). Although it is unknown whether the increased fractional rate of protein catabolism is a direct effect of dietary protein intake on albumin catabolic rate on catabolic sites throughout the body or instead is a consequence of increased renal filtration of albumin followed by increased uptake and catabolism of a greater amount of filtered albumin that occurs in patients eating a high-protein diet, the increased fractional rate of albumin catabolism will tend to reduce albumin levels and negate the positive effect of increased albumin synthesis. Thus, dietary protein augmentation causes three independent processes that may change plasma albumin concentration in proteinuric subjects: (a) an increase in the rate of albumin synthesis, tending to increase albumin mass; (b) an increase in the fractional rate of albumin catabolism, tending to decrease albumin mass; and (c) an increase in urinary loss, tending to deplete albumin pools. There are two possible mechanisms whereby increasing dietary protein intake worsens proteinuria. First, dietary protein intake increases glomerular capillary hydraulic pressure, which will facilitate greater protein passage across the glomerular capillary wall; second, dietary protein may alter the permselectivity of the glomerular basement pore structure, favoring larger pores. Chan et al. (36) demonstrated that dietary protein increases glomerular ultrafiltration pressure in patients with the nephrotic syndrome but did not alter glomerular permselectivity. This would suggest that glomerular porosity is not affected by dietary protein and that increased capillary pressure is the culprit for worsening of proteinuria. Rosenberg et al. (58), however, did show that dietary protein intake affected glomerular permselectivity in patients with proteinuria and renal insufficiency. Thus, it may be that dietary protein worsens proteinuria both by increased glomerular pressures and by greater porosity of the glomerular basement membrane. In summary, proteinuria worsens and serum albumin concentration actually may decrease in either patients with the nephrotic syndrome (21) or animals (22) following dietary protein augmentation.

The physiologic effect of amino acids on renal hemodynamics appears to depend on the specific amino acids fed or infused. Infusion of branched-chain amino acids, for example, fails to increase GFR or renal blood flow in normal rats (62) or humans (27), whereas infusion of arginine causes marked changes in renal hemodynamics (55). The renal hemodynamic response to dietary protein therefore may depend on specific amino acids rather than on the solute or nitrogen intake.

Because the increase in GFR and renal blood flow can be prevented by somatostatin (57), it is hypothesized that changes in renal function induced by protein or amino acid administration are, in part, hormonally mediated. Dietary protein augmentation causes an increased secretion of glucagon (19), growth hormone (56), corticosteroids (63,64), and dopamine (32) and alters expression of the renin-angiotensin system (23), which in turn stimulates prostaglandin synthesis (30). Increased pancreatic glucagon secretion seems to be necessary for the increase in GFR and renal blood flow (19) that follows dietary protein augmentation; however, infusion of even large amounts of glucagon exerts no effect on urinary albumin excretion (61). Paller and Hostetter demonstrated that high-protein diets augment expression of the renin-angiotensin system in the rat (23) and that dietary protein augmentation resulted in altered glomerular permselectivity in humans with the nephrotic syndrome (58). This observation also has been noted in patients (47). There is, however, some conflicting data on the effect of a low-protein diet on renal renin secretion. Martinez-Maldonado et al. suggest that renal angiotensin II activity is increased during dietary protein restriction (35,65) and contributes to renal vasoconstriction and reduced GFR. This observation has not been corroborated by other studies, and most clinical and experimental studies suggest that protein administration increases renin activity (23,47,58,66). It generally is agreed that dietary protein intake leads to activation of the renin-angiotensin system, increased renal blood flow and GFR, and worsening of proteinuria in patients with preexisting proteinuria. Moreover, it is well appreciated that inhibition of the renin-angiotensin system with angiotensin converting enzyme (ACE) inhibitors can blunt or prevent the proteinuric effect of dietary protein in experimental renal diseases (20,49,67,68) and in patients with the nephrotic syndrome (47,48).

The hormonal response to the infusion of amino acids, like the renal hemodynamic changes, is dependent, in part, on the specific amino acids infused. Infusion of either a mixture of amino acids or arginine causes a prompt increase in the secretion of growth hormone (56) and glucagon (55), whereas infusion of branched-chain amino acids does not (27,62,69). In correlating the changes in GFR with an amino acid infusion, the plasma levels of insulin, growth hormone, and glucagon all increase in response to the infusion, but only changes in glucagon exhibited a significant temporal relationship with changes in GFR (27).

A potential mediator of arginine-induced renal vasodilation may be NO, inasmuch as arginine is the substrate for NO production. In experimental animals, however, arginine supplementation actually ameliorates both proteinuria and hyperfiltration in diabetic rats and has no effect on urinary albumin excretion in rats with passive Heymann nephritis (70). Thus, like the protein-renin interaction outlined earlier, there are conflicting data regarding the relationship between arginine and renal hemodynamics.

Dietary Protein and Renal Injury

By increasing the filtered load of protein, dietary protein supplementation may be worsening renal injury. It is becoming more appreciated that proteinuria may be damaging the renal interstitium directly (71) (Table 24.1). Several proteins, including albumin (72) and transferrin (73), have been implicated. Glomerular damage and the concomitant increased glomerular permeability result in a marked increase in protein filtration and initially in augmented proximal tubular reabsorption of protein. Filtered proteins are reabsorbed, carrying iron (74,75), complement components (76), and biologically active lipids (77) into the renal interstitial space and causing injury. Consequently, tubular protein overload occurs, leading to tubular cell injury, which leads to interstitial fibrosis (78). This process probably involves the induction of cytokines and other proinflammatory molecules such as monocyte chemoattractant protein-1, osteopontin, and platelet-derived growth factor (PDGF) (79). The trafficking and deposition of excess filtered protein may be a link between the initial glomerular injury and the subsequent development of tubulointerstitial disease. The resulting tubulointerstitial disease is a better predictor of the GFR and long-term prognosis than is the severity of glomerular damage in almost all chronic progressive glomerular diseases, including immunoglobulin A (IgA) nephropathy, membranous nephropathy, membranoproliferative glomerulonephritis, and lupus nephritis (80,81). Furthermore, diets that are high in protein are also high in acid content, obligating the kidney to increase ammoniagenesis. Accelerated rates of renal ammonia production resulting from increased dietary acid loads accompanying a high protein diet may also lead to renal injury, possibly by the activation of complement (82,83). The reduction in urinary protein excretion that follows dietary protein restriction potentially can have a salutary effect on progressive renal injury through any or all of these mechanisms. Thus, any process that reduces urinary protein losses should be encouraged.

TABLE 24.1. ADVERSE EFFECTS OF PROTEINURIA: INCREASED TUBULAR REABSORPTION OF PROTEIN

Increased tubular exposure to filtered components of the complement cascade Increased tubular exposure to reabsorbed iron Increased tubular exposure to biologically active lipids	Recruitment of macrophages Increased TGF-β Increased PDGF
Increased tubular exposure to filtered growth factors	

TGF, transforming growth factor; PDGF, platelet-derived growth factor.

Dietary protein restriction also reduces the synthesis and/or gene expression of several proteins thought to play a role in progression of renal injury, such as transforming growth factor-β (84), PDGF (85), and fibrinogen (86). It is unknown whether decreased expression of these genes is a direct consequence of dietary protein restriction, a consequence of secondary effects of a protein-restricted diet (such as decreased proteinuria with reduced contact of the interstitium to filtered plasma constituents), or a consequence of reduced renal ammoniagenesis (Table 24.1). In patients with the nephrotic syndrome, the rate of fibrinogen synthesis is increased in proportion to the increased synthesis of albumin (87), and hyperfibrinogenemia may contribute to increased thrombosis associated with the nephrotic syndrome. Moreover, hyperfibrinogenemia may accelerate the progression of renal disease (88). It is interesting to note that dietary protein restriction reduces the synthesis of both albumin and fibrinogen in patients with the nephrotic syndrome; however, the serum levels of albumin tend to increase, whereas serum fibrinogen levels decrease (87). Thus, dietary protein restriction appears to have a favorable effect on both albumin and fibrinogen metabolism in patients with the nephrotic syndrome.

Several studies suggest that the composition of dietary protein may be as important as the absolute nitrogen content. In experimental studies in rats, dietary protein augmentation with a mixture of amino acids causes a prompt increase in urinary albumin excretion (61), whereas other amino acids, specifically branched-chain amino acids, arginine, proline, glutamine, glutamate, aspartate, or asparagine, are devoid of any effect on proteinuria (70). Studies by D'Amico et al. (89) and Walser (90) suggest that dietary protein composition also may be of importance in humans with renal disease. D'Amico et al. found that when patients with the nephrotic syndrome were fed a vegetarian soy diet, urinary protein excretion and blood lipid levels decreased (89). The diet was also low in fat (28% of calories) and of low protein content (0.71 g/kg ideal body weight). The salutary effects of soy diets in patients with the nephrotic syndrome may be a consequence of the amino composition in those diets, although differences in lipid composition or in protein absorption also may explain the apparent benefit of these diets. In a subsequent study, fish oil was added to the vegetarian soy diet; the addition of fish oil did not give any additional benefit (91). Walser has shown that supplementing a very–low-protein diet (0.3 g/kg/day) with essential amino or keto acids not only will reduce proteinuria in patients with nephrotic syndrome, but it also will maintain or improve GFR. In fact, this regimen may induce a prolonged remission, even if the patients resume ingesting a normal diet. As noted by the investigators, the mechanism for this response is not known (92).

EFFECTS OF THE NEPHROTIC SYNDROME ON SOLID-TISSUE PROTEINS

Although it is more difficult to quantitate the losses of tissue protein, marked muscle wasting (46,93), sometimes obscured by edema, has been described in patients with continuous massive proteinuria. Rats with Heymann nephritis gain weight at a rate significantly less than normal rats do (44). Although increasing dietary protein from 8.5% to 40% casein causes a significant increase in growth velocity in normal rats, dietary protein augmentation causes significantly less improvement in growth rate in rats with Heymann nephritis. In fact, nephrotic rats fed 40% protein gain weight more slowly than do normal rats fed 8.5% protein (44), although the difference in protein intake between 8.5% and 40% is many times greater than the urinary protein lost in the nephrotic group. When dietary protein is increased from 8.5% to 40% protein, total carcass (muscle) protein pools are increased in normal rats. In contrast, none of the increase in weight of nephrotic rats fed 40% protein is found in muscle; instead it is in viscera, namely liver and kidney (44). Most of the increased protein nitrogen consumed when high-protein diets are fed to these animals is excreted in the urine as urea (61,94).

Nephrotic rats have a reduced rate of muscle protein synthesis (45) and an increased rate of hepatic protein synthesis, providing a mechanism for growth impairment in these animals. Total body protein synthesis is the same in nephrotic and healthy rats (95), yet the nephrotic animals must replace the vast amounts of protein lost in the urine, which they do through increased hepatic protein synthesis (45). In part, amino acid oxidation is reduced in nephrotic animals to compensate for urinary protein losses (95). Although patients with the nephrotic syndrome may have loss of muscle mass (46,96), it is unknown whether this represents an alteration in muscle metabolism similar to that seen in the rat.

These observations have supported the notion that dietary protein augmentation does not replete protein pools that have been depleted in animals or patients with the nephrotic syndrome; however, in addition, high-protein diets are detrimental in that they cause progressive renal injury in a variety of experimental renal diseases in animals (49,67,97) and in humans (98–100). *Because dietary protein supplementation is of no benefit in patients with the nephrotic syndrome or animals, a diet supplemented with protein or completely unrestricted with regard to protein intake is not recommended.*

The long-term safety of a low-protein diet is uncertain. Using leucine turnover rates as a marker of protein breakdown, Lim et al. (101) noted that patients with the nephrotic syndrome maintained positive nitrogen balance and had lower rates of protein degradation on a modestly restricted protein diet (0.9 g/kg/day) over a period of 35 days. Similarly, Maroni et al. (102) demonstrated that patients with the nephrotic syndrome ingesting 0.8 g/kg/day over a period of 24 days maintained positive nitrogen balance. The principal compensatory response to dietary protein restriction was a decrease in amino acid oxidation. In addition, the investigators noted an inverse correlation between leucine oxidation and the degree of proteinuria, suggesting that proteinuria is the stimulus to conserve dietary essential amino acids. Thus, modest protein restriction may be a safe and effective therapy in reducing proteinuria. However, there are no data on the effect of long-term restriction of protein to amounts much less than 0.8 g/kg/day in patients with the nephrotic syndrome. *It is, therefore, probably not justifiable to place patients who are heavily proteinuric on diets that contain less that 0.8 g/kg/day except on an experimental basis.*

Urinary urea excretion should be monitored to assure that patients are not eating more (or less) protein than recommended and that proteinuria decreases (and plasma albumin and protein concentration do not decrease) when protein intake is restricted. Dietary protein intake can be estimated because, in steady state, protein intake is equal to the protein catabolic rate. If total body urea pools do not change in any 24-hour period (blood urea nitrogen, or BUN, is neither decreasing nor increasing), it is possible to estimate the amount of protein that has been eaten by the following formula:

$$\text{Protein catabolic rate} = (10.7 + \text{24-hour urinary urea excretion}/0.14)\ \text{g/day} + \text{urinary protein excretion}$$

If there is variance from the prescribed diet, an accurate nutritional history should be obtained, and the diet should be adjusted accordingly.

It is still not known whether specific protein sources are clinically superior to others. The amino acid composition of the protein may turn out to be as important as the quantity of protein in the diet, but no specific recommendations can be made at this time, although clearly it is unlikely to be harmful to place patients on a largely vegetarian diet, considering the low fat content and the excellent results reported by D'Amico (89).

DIETARY PROTEINS AS POTENTIAL ALLERGENS RESPONSIBLE FOR RENAL DISEASE

The etiologic agents responsible for many diseases that cause the nephrotic syndrome are unknown. In some patients with minimal change nephrotic syndrome or patients with mesangial proliferation, exposure to specific dietary proteins, such as cow's milk, has been implicated as causal (13–17,103). Bovine serum albumin and casein also have been identified as an allergen in a patient with immune complex glomerulonephritis. In these cases clinical remission followed removal of the offending agent from the diet. Lagrue et al. systematically evaluated 42 patients with steroid-resistant nephrotic syndrome, and ultimately seven of their patients entered remission following removal of offending antigens from their diet (15). Interpretation of these data is made difficult because these studies were not randomized prospective trials and proteinuria may remit spontaneously without treatment in the nephrotic syndrome (15). There is an association of gluten enteropathy IgA deposition in the glomeruli and the development of IgA nephropathy, this may be the result of an allergic reaction to gluten in the diet (104). Overall, it is unclear what fraction of patients with the nephrotic syndrome have food allergy as a causative factor. Nevertheless, the possibility that food allergy might be responsible for the development of specific renal diseases rarely is considered by most clinicians and may be of overlooked importance.

DIETARY FAT

Hyperlipidemia is common in the nephrotic syndrome, as is a consequence of both increased synthesis of lipids and apolipoproteins (105) and their decreased catabolism (Fig. 24.3) (106,107). The characteristic disorder in blood lipid composition in patients with the nephrotic syndrome is an increase in the LDL, very–low-density lipoprotein (VLDL) (10), and/or intermediate-density lipoprotein (IDL) fractions but no change (10) or a decrease in HDL (11), resulting in an increased LDL/HDL cholesterol ratio. The IDL fraction probably arises as VLDL and chylomicron remnants and is atherogenic (108). The atherogenic lipoprotein Lp(a) also increases in patients with the nephrotic syndrome (12). All of these changes in the lipid profile in the nephrotic syndrome are characteristic of those associated with accelerated atherogenesis in other clinical settings.

VLDL levels are increased predominantly because of decreased VLDL clearance/catabolism or delipidation in both patients with the nephrotic syndrome and rats (9,109,110). One determinant of VLDL catabolism is endothelial-bound lipoprotein lipase (LPL). LPL is synthesized in mesenchymal tissue such as adipose tissue and muscle cells and then is secreted and bound initially to the surface of mesenchymal tissue (111). The endothelial-bound pool is reduced in the nephrotic syndrome (106) but also in the condition of hereditary analbuminemia, suggesting that it is hypoalbuminemia rather than proteinuria that causes the depletion in this important lipase pool (112). Although hereditary analbuminemia indeed does increase lipid levels, the degree of hyperlipidemia is far less than seen in the nephrotic syndrome, both in humans and in experimental models of renal disease in the rat. These finding suggest that an additional factor, most likely proteinuria, contributes substantially to hyperlipidemia in the nephrotic syndrome. We postulated that the combined decrease in endothelial-bound LPL and altered VLDL structure together led to the profound defect in clearance of triglyceride-rich lipoproteins as well as the massive increase in triglyceride levels seen in the nephrotic syndrome.

Supporting this hypothesis is the observation (113) that reduction in urinary protein excretion in patients with the nephrotic syndrome leads to a decrease in serum lipid levels even if serum albumin concentration is not increased. The clinical message from these observations is that all efforts must be targeted at reducing proteinuria.

Although diminished catabolism may be the major mechanism underlying the elevations in VLDL, increases in LDL appear to be primarily the result of increased hepatic synthesis in patients with the nephrotic syndrome. It has been demonstrated clearly that the synthesis of LDL apolipoprotein B 100 is increased in patients with the nephrotic syndrome (110). It is not clear what the stimulus might be for augmentation in apo B 100 synthesis. In addition to increased synthesis, decreased hepatic uptake of LDL particles may account, in part, for elevations of this lipoprotein (114). There are conflicting data on whether clearance of LDL is reduced in the nephrotic syndrome; however, a new study has noted decreased expression of the LDL receptor in nephrotic rats, suggesting a mechanism for impaired clearance of this lipoprotein (115).

Total HDL levels are usually normal or decreased in nephrotic humans (116), whereas it is increased in nephrotic rats (117). Although HDL levels may be normal, there appears to be a greater percentage of immature HDL_3 in the circulation of patients with the nephrotic syndrome (118).

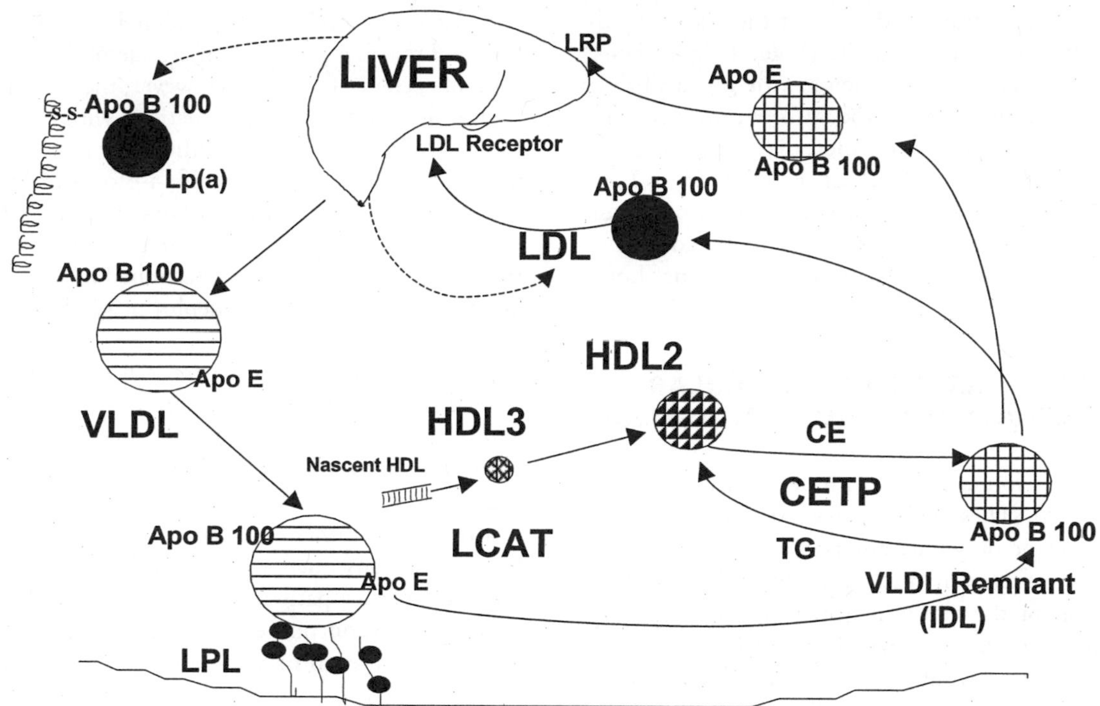

FIGURE 24.3. Metabolism of very–low-density lipoprotein (VLDL). VLDL is secreted by the liver and then hydrolyzed on the vascular endothelium by LPL. LPL (*small filled circles*), is bound electrostatically to heparan sulfate and removes triglycerides (TG) from VLDL facilitated by the presence of apolipoprotein C-II on the surface of VLDL. LPL is important in binding of VLDL to the vascular endothelium (Figure 23.3). High-density lipoprotein (HDL) begins as a nascent particle synthesized in the gut and liver composed of phospholipids and apolipoprotein A-I. As VLDL is metabolized, the surface constituents of VLDL, including apolipoprotein, free cholesterol, and phospholipids, contribute to the formation of HDL. Free cholesterol on the surface of nascent HDL is esterified by lecithin cholesterol ester transferase (LCAT) to form cholesterol esters. These sink into the core as nascent HDL is converted to HDL_3, and finally into cholesterol ester (CE)-rich HDL_2. HDL_2 can be processed by lipases back to HDL_3 to continue the cycle. The TG-depleted VLDL remnant particle is released from the endothelial surface and then either is taken up by the liver directly via the remnant receptor (LRP), which recognizes apo E, or interacts with CE-rich HDL_2. In that interaction, catalyzed by cholesterol ester transfer protein (CETP), the CE-rich core of HDL_2 is exchanged for the TG-rich core of the VLDL remnant, yielding a TG-rich HDL molecule (*not shown*) and LDL. LDL also may be formed by direct synthesis in the liver and thus can arise by pathways other than through the delipidation of VLDL. The LDL receptor on hepatocytes recognizes apolipoprotein B 100 on the surface on LDL and is responsible for uptake of this lipoprotein. Lp(a) also is synthesized by the liver. In the nephrotic syndrome, VLDL levels are increased predominantly because of decreased VLDL clearance/catabolism or delipidation, whereas increases in both LDL and Lp(a) are due primarily to increased synthesis (see text for details). Broken lines connote pathways believed to have increased synthesis in patients with the nephrotic syndrome.

This may be because there is impaired maturation of HDL as a result of a defect in the activity of the enzyme lethicin: cholesterol acyltransferase, which promotes the accumulation of cholesterol on the developing HDL particle.

Lp(a) is a specialized form of LDL in which a single molecule of apolipoprotein(a), or apo(a), is linked covalently to the apo B 100 moiety via a disulfide bridge (119). The apo(a) chain contains domains or kringles, and the structure consists of a single kringle V domain with multiple kringle IV repeats (120). The structure of apo(a) is quite homologous to plasmin but lacks proteolytic activity (121). Synthesis of the apo B 100 moiety associated with Lp(a) may be regulated entirely separately from the pool of apo B 100 that is necessary for secretion of VLDL or LDL. The number of kringle IV repeats and consequently the size of apo(a) in Lp(a) is determined genetically (122). In addition, the synthetic rates and plasma levels of Lp(a) vary inversely with the molecular weight of the isoform encoded (123). Individuals having the largest apo(a) subtypes are most common and have the lowest plasma concentration of Lp(a). Other genetic factors may play a role in establishing Lp(a) levels as well as the number of kringle IV domains expressed

(122); however, alteration in diet or of the use of lipid-lowering agents has no effect on Lp(a) levels in patients. Lp(a) levels are increased in patients with the nephrotic syndrome (12,124) regardless of the isoform expressed. The elevated Lp(a) levels result from increased synthesis alone (124), whereas the increased levels of the other apo B lipoproteins (VLDL, IDL, LDL) in patients with the nephrotic syndrome are predominantly the result of decreased catabolism. During remission of the nephrotic syndrome, Lp(a) levels decrease.

THE EFFECT OF ALTERED GLOMERULAR PERMSELECTIVITY ON LIPID METABOLISM

Hyperlipidemia is found in rats with hereditary analbuminemia (9,51,125). These animals have a reduced plasma oncotic pressure and only trace amounts of albumin in their plasma because of a seven nucleotide deletion isolated to the MN intron of the albumin gene, creating a splicing defect during albumin messenger RNA processing (126). Although this finding would suggest that reduced plasma oncotic pressure or reduced plasma albumin concentration alone is the signal to induce the lipid abnormalities described earlier, the catabolism of both VLDL and chylomicrons is normal in these animals (9). A severe defect in catabolism of both of these lipoproteins follows the onset of proteinuria (113), suggesting that proteinuria plays a role in the pathogenesis of disordered lipid metabolism independent of the serum albumin levels or oncotic pressure. Supporting this hypothesis are the observations that reducing albuminuria by administering ACE inhibitors or dietary protein restriction reduces blood lipid levels (9,127,113) even if neither plasma albumin concentration nor plasma oncotic pressure are increased. The mechanism by which proteinuria is able to induce a reduction in the catabolism of VLDL is an alteration in VLDL structure that decreases its binding to LPL. The specific link between VLDL structural changes and urinary protein losses remains to be elucidated.

CARDIOVASCULAR EFFECTS OF HYPERLIPIDEMIA IN THE NEPHROTIC SYNDROME

Accelerated atherosclerosis occurs in patients with proteinuria and hyperlipidemia and is probably responsible for the sharply increased incidence of cardiovascular disease and stroke (128,129). One study reported an 85-fold increase in the incidence of ischemic heart disease in patients with the nephrotic syndrome (130). This is not surprising when one considers that HDL, specifically the HDL_2 fraction, is reduced (11,118), whereas LDL, IDL, and VLDL fractions are increased.

It is not yet known what the biologic significance is of the increased levels of Lp(a) seen in the nephrotic syndrome. Lp(a) is a powerful atherosclerotic risk factor when it occurs genetically (131). However, these high Lp(a) concentrations occur in combination with low–molecular weight isoform. Thus, it is difficult to know whether it is the concentration or the specific isoform of Lp(a) present that promotes atherogenesis. Newer studies suggest that low–molecular weight isoform may confer atherosclerotic risk (132). It remains to be determined if the elevated levels of Lp(a) in patients with the nephrotic syndrome are responsible for the increased rate of atherosclerosis seen in this population. Although the plasma concentration of most intermediate-sized proteins is reduced, the concentration of many larger proteins, such as fibrinogen and prothrombin (133), are increased, playing a potential role in the hypercoagulable state associated with this syndrome (134) and contributing to atherosclerosis. Hyperlipidemia, therefore, is a serious consequence of proteinuria and should be addressed to protect patients from atherosclerosis. Hyperlipidemia also may contribute to progression of the renal disease (135,136) and even may initiate renal injury (137,138).

EFFECTS OF LIPIDS ON RENAL DISEASE

It generally is accepted that both qualitative and quantitative alterations in blood lipids cause macrovascular disease, and hyperlipidemia caused by the nephrotic syndrome is no less dangerous than hyperlipidemia of other causes. In the process of atherogenesis, lipid-laden macrophages accumulate in the vessel wall, followed by intimal hyperplasia and ultimately by atherosclerosis. Studies from several laboratories (135,137,139) suggest that similar changes may occur in the microvasculature of the kidney, specifically the glomerular mesangium. Al-Shebeb et al. (137) found that focal glomerular sclerosis occurred in guinea pigs fed a high-cholesterol diet for 70 days. The animals developed proteinuria and hematuria. Rats fed a high-cholesterol diet developed albuminuria, accelerated focal glomerulosclerosis, and increased glomerular capillary pressure (135).

The obese Zucker rat develops spontaneous hyperlipidemia, proteinuria, and progressive glomerulosclerosis. These processes can be attenuated by cholesterol-lowering drugs (135,140). It is interesting to note that glomerular capillary pressure and single-nephron GFR are within the normal range, suggesting that hyperfiltration does not mediate glomerular injury caused by hyperlipidemia (135). Diamond and Karnovsky (139) found that rats with the nephrotic syndrome induced by puromycin aminonuleoside (PAN) had more proteinuria and a lower GFR when fed a high-cholesterol diet compared to nephrotic rats eating a regular diet. The glomeruli in rats fed a high-cholesterol diet were more sclerotic and had mesangial cell proliferation and foam cells. Lowering plasma cholesterol by administration of cholestyramine resin attenuated both acute and chronic proteinuria in these animals (135). It has been hypothesized that increased blood lipid levels, from dietary cholesterol or secondary to hyperlipidemia caused by the renal disease, may play an important role in intensifying the rate at which established renal diseases progress (135,136) and may even initiate glomerular injury (137,138). These changes could be mediated either hemodynamically or after direct injury caused by the uptake of lipids by the glomerulus.

The oxidation of circulating lipids may play a role in progressive renal injury. Glomerular macrophages endocytose LDL through specific LDL receptors and through the nonspecific scavenger system. It is known that hyperlipidemia activates mesangial cells (which have LDL receptors), leading to stimulation of mesangial cell proliferation and to increased production of macrophage chemotactic factors, fibronectin (a component of the extracellular matrix), and reactive oxygen species (141–143). Both increased mesangial lipid deposition and enhanced expression of LDL receptors on mesangial and epithelial cells have been demonstrated in patients with chronic glomerular diseases. Unregulated absorption of oxidized LDL then may lead to an uncontrolled increase in intracellular cholesterol (144) because oxidized lipids bypass the protective mechanism regulating LDL uptake. After endocytosis, cholesterol is esterified by acetyl CoA (coenzyme A) cholesterol acyl transferase to form the insoluble cholesterol oleate ester may (144). This process results in creation of foam cells in the glomerulus analogous to that of early atherosclerosis in blood vessels. Thus, the oxidative state of lipids also may play a role in their nephrotoxicity, and antioxidant drugs may prove protective.

These studies in animals are supported in part by further, albeit uncontrolled, observations in patients in which reducing lipid levels with a HMG-CoA (hydroxy-methyl-glutaryl coenzyme A) reductase inhibitor reduces proteinuria or slows the rate of progressive injury (145). Hypercholesterolemia is also a separate independent risk factor for progression of renal injury in patients with diabetes (146).

Lipids represent a wide variety of substances, including steroids, saturated and unsaturated fatty acids, phospholipids, and other compounds, many of which are either directly biologically active or are precursors of important biologically active metabolites. Much attention has been focused on the effect of polyunsaturated fatty acids on renal hemodynamics and on expression or renal injury.

POLYUNSATURATED FATTY ACIDS

Prostaglandins and thromboxane are products of metabolism of polyunsaturated fatty acids. They include both vasoconstrictors, such as thromboxane A_2, and vasodilators, such as PGE_2 or PGI_2, and exert important hemodynamic effects. The effects of oxidized lipoproteins also may be mediated by these autocoids (147).

Eicosanoids are derived from dietary polyunsaturated fatty acids (PUFA) because PUFA cannot be synthesized by mammals. Thus, eicosanoid metabolism can be manipulated nutritionally. Lipids derived from marine sources are enriched with omega-3 PUFA (e.g., eicosapentaenoic acid), whereas those derived from vegetable oils are enriched with omega-6 PUFA (e.g., arachidonic acid). Eicosapentaenoic acid competes with arachidonic acid as a substrate for cyclooxygenase and lipooxygenase. Cyclooxygenase converts arachidonic acid and eicosapentaenoic acid to the diene (e.g., PGI_2, TXA_2 [thromboxane]) and triene metabolites (e.g., PGI_3, TXA_3), respectively (148,149). Lipooxygenase converts arachidonic acid and eicosapentaenoic acid to the four and five series of leukotrienes, respectively (150, 151). TXA_2, an arachidonic acid metabolite, is a potent vasoconstrictor, whereas TXA_3, a metabolite of eicosapentaenoic acid, is biologically inert (152). In contrast, the vasodilators PGI_2 and PGI_3 are equipotent (148).

Alterations in the generation of both vasodilatory prostaglandins (PGE_2, PGI_2) and vasoconstricting cyclooxygenase metabolites (thromboxane A_2, TXA_2) can occur during renal injury or physiologic stress, such as plasma volume contraction. Although changes in eicosanoid metabolism can support GFR in adapting to renal injury or plasma volume contraction, they also may play a pathogenic role. Because of the differences in biologic activity of their vasoconstrictive and vasodilatory metabolites, substitution of eicosapentaenoic acid for arachidonic acid in the diet may alter the expression of renal injury.

The effect of dietary PUFA, particularly fish oil, has been studied in a variety of experimental models of renal disease including the nephrotic syndrome (153–155). In adriamycin-induced nephrosis in the rat, Ito et al. (156) found that plasma cholesterol and triglycerides, proteinuria, and plasma creatinine were significantly lower in rats fed fish oil than in rats fed beef tallow. Glomerular hyalinosis and endothelial swelling were also less in the fish oil–fed rats and were correlated with the changes in plasma triglycerides and cholesterol.

In a subsequent study of the same model, dietary fish oil induced a dose-dependent reduction in glomerular synthesis of dienoic eicosanoids, PGE_2, 6-keto-$PGF_{1\alpha}$ (a stable metabolite of PGI_2), and TXB_2 (a stable product of TXA_2). Fish oil also decreased the generation of TXB_2 from platelets. In studies of the rat with nephrotic syndrome induced by adriamycin, Barcelli et al. (157) studied the effect of dietary fish oil (a source of omega-3 PUFA), evening primrose oil (a source of omega-6 PUFA), or a mixture of reduced plasma triglyceride and cholesterol levels compared to rats fed beef tallow. The fatty-acid composition of the kidney was different in each dietary group, but neither the magnitude of proteinuria nor changes in plasma creatinine were affected by dietary fish oil. In another model of progressive renal injury in the rat—partial renal ablation—Scharschmidt et al. found that diets supplemented with fish oil accelerated the course of renal injury (154) and caused increased mortality.

In studies involving human subjects, Gentile et al. (91) added 5 g of fish oil per day to the diet of patients with the nephrotic syndrome who had maintained on a soy vegetarian diet and found no beneficial effect on either proteinuria or on blood lipids when compared to patients maintained on the soy diet without fish oil supplementation. In contrast, Hall et al. (158) found that 15 g of fish oil per day caused a decrease in total triglycerides and LDL triglycerides and an increase in LDL cholesterol. Donadio et al. (159) treated 55 patients with IgA nephropathy and proteinuria with 12 g of fish oil per day in a prospective randomized placebo-controlled study and found a significant reduction in the rate of progression of renal disease using a 50% increase in serum creatinine concentration as a study endpoint. However, there was no significant effect on proteinuria or blood pressure. These studies suggest that although alterations in dietary PUFA may alter some manifestations of the nephrotic state; the effects are dependent on the model being investigated and still should be viewed with caution. These agents may be neither predictable nor salutary for all patients with renal disease.

Harrs et al. (160) reported that a diet entirely devoid of essential fatty acids provided renal protection by inhibiting macrophage function. Although vasoactive lipids probably play a role in altering the course of a variety of renal diseases, specific alterations in the composition and amounts of dietary PUFAs on the course of renal diseases in humans are not completely known. For this reason, there is no strong reason at this time to recommend the dietary supplements to patients with the nephrotic syndrome, with the possible exception of heavily proteinuric patients with IgA nephropathy.

DERANGEMENTS IN DIVALENT CATION METABOLISM IN THE NEPHROTIC SYNDROME

Some abnormalities in divalent cations can be traced directly to the urinary loss of proteins that either carry divalent cations or in some way regulate their metabolism. Transferrin, a glycoprotein whose principal function is to transport iron (161), is lost in the urine (162,163), providing a potential mechanism for a microcytic hypochromic anemia found uncommonly in patients with the nephrotic syndrome (162, 163). Transferrin turnover rate also is increased in patients with the nephrotic syndrome (40,164). Reduced plasma iron in the presence of a hypochromic microcytic anemia may result from urinary iron loss in patients with the nephrotic syndrome.

Complicating this paradigm are the observations of Alfrey and Hammond (74,75) suggesting that increased delivery of iron to the renal interstitium by filtered transferrin, a protein that binds up to 2 mols of iron per mole of protein, may be of importance in causing the interstitial inflammation that ultimately destroys the kidney. Therefore, the decision to provide iron supplementation to these patients may not be a trivial one.

Anemia also may be a consequence of the urinary loss of another glycoprotein that is of a size likely to pass the glomerular filtration barrier in the nephrotic syndrome—erythropoietin (165–167). Indeed, plasma levels of this protein are reduced in both patients with the nephrotic syndrome (165) and rats (166), and it doesn't appear that synthesis of erythropoietin is increased in response to its urinary loss (166). There are no prospective randomized studies of the effect of administration of either iron (potentially harmful) or erythropoietin (expensive and inconvenient) to patients with anemia and the nephrotic syndrome to guide clinical practice.

Copper, like iron, also is bound to a circulating plasma protein—ceruloplasmin. Although the urinary loss of this 151-kDa protein may cause a decrease in blood copper (6, 8), it results in no clinically recognized manifestations (168). The most important zinc-binding protein is albumin, with the greatest losses occurring in the nephrotic syndrome. Documented zinc deficiency was probably a consequence of reduced absorption of zinc in conjunction with excessive urinary loss (169). The effect of proteinuria on zinc metabolism has been largely ignored, and it is not known to what extent zinc depletion plays a role in the clinical manifestations of the nephrotic syndrome.

Hypocalcemia is well recognized in patients with the nephrotic syndrome (170–173) and includes reduced ionized and total calcium. Hypocalcemia does not result entirely from a reduction in the fraction of calcium bound to albumin; it also results from a reduction in ionized calcium because plasma vitamin D is reduced (5,170,174,175) and the decrease in serum 25 $(OH)_2$ D_3 correlates with urinary albumin excretion (170). Plasma albumin and vitamin D concentrations correlate closely. Vitamin D–binding protein is present in the urine of patients with the nephrotic syndrome (5,175), and vitamin D levels normalize when proteinuria resolves (175,176). Labeled vitamin D appears rapidly in the urine of nephrotic subjects (177), suggesting that urinary vitamin D loss is the cause of hypovitaminosis D in these patients. Hypovitaminosis D is not the result of loss of renal mass because plasma vitamin D levels are also low in patients with the nephrotic syndrome with normal renal function (170–172). The hypovitaminosis D of the nephrotic syndrome may result in rickets, especially in children (173,177). Patients with the nephrotic syndrome malabsorb calcium (170), a defect that can be corrected by exogenously administered vitamin D (177). It is not known whether synthesis of vitamin D–binding protein is altered in response to its urinary loss or is modulated by dietary protein intake. However, unlike many of the other manifestations of the nephrotic syndrome, hypovitaminosis D can be managed with replacement therapy.

DERANGEMENTS IN SALT AND WATER METABOLISM IN THE NEPHROTIC SYNDROME (VOLUME HOMEOSTASIS)

Edema formation is one of the most bothersome symptoms of the nephrotic syndrome. There are two basic steps in edema formation: (a) there is an alteration in capillary hemodynamics that favors movement of fluid from the vascular space into the interstitium, and (b) there is a pathologic retention of salt and water. The classic model of edema formation in the nephrotic syndrome assumed that a decrease in plasma albumin concentration inevitably would lead to a decrease in difference between interstitial and plasma oncotic pressure (delta oncotic pressure) and lead to plasma volume contraction (Fig. 24.4). Ultimately, edema occurs when the amount of fluid filtered into the interstitium exceeded maximal lymph flow, decreasing the circulatory volume resulting from plasma ultrafiltrate left behind in the interstitium (178). One would predict that plasma volume contraction would activate the renin-angiotensin aldosterone axis and lead to secondary (via plasma volume depletion) renal sodium retention—the so-called "underfill" edema. Because plasma volume contraction also causes an increase in vasopressin secretion, one would anticipate that water also would be retained, leading to hyponatremia (as seen in other edema-forming states, specifically congestive heart failure and liver disease).

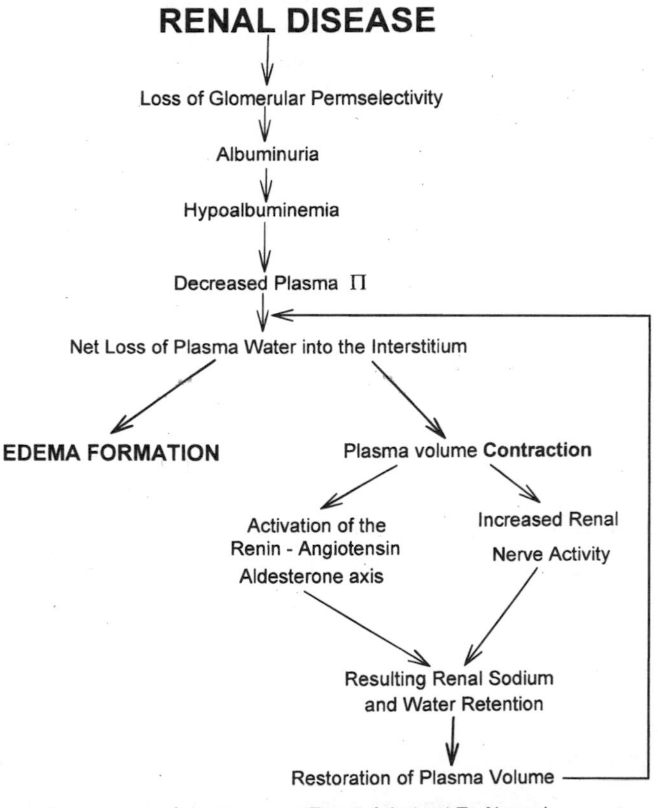

FIGURE 24.4. Primary edema formation and renal sodium retention. Hypoalbuminemia leads to increased transudation of fluid into the interstitium resulting in plasma-volume contraction with secondary activation of the renin-angiotensin aldosterone axis and subsequent renal sodium retention. Because a normal plasma volume cannot be maintained in the presence of hypoalbuminemia, a positive feedback cycle occurs. The reabsorbed salt and water also enter the interstitial space. Edema formation is a direct consequence of hypoalbuminemia, and salt and water retention is a consequence of the plasma-volume contraction that results.

The classic or "underfill" model of edema formation in the nephrotic syndrome has been challenged by a number of observations. It is important to note that when one looks at Starling forces, it is the transcapillary oncotic pressure gradient between the vascular and interstitial compartment that drives fluid movement and not simply the plasma oncotic pressure. In the setting of nephrotic syndrome, with the fall in plasma albumin concentration and oncotic pressure, there is a concomitant fall in interstitial oncotic pressure (179). Thus, there are probably only minor changes in the transcapillary oncotic gradient, and hypoalbuminemia is not the primary step in edema formation. In patients with minimal change disease going into remission with corticosteroid treatment, the maximum recovery diuresis occurs before there has been a substantial increase in plasma albumin concentration (180). Dorhout-Mees et al. (3) found that both plasma and blood volume is decreased in individual patients with minimal change nephrotic syndrome entering remission, providing strong evidence that even (adult) patients with minimal change nephrotic syndrome were apparently plasma volume expanded during their "nephrotic" phase. Furthermore, they found no correlation between plasma volume and renin activity or between plasma albumin and blood volume (181). The lack of a relationship between plasma renin activity and blood volume, or between plasma albumin and blood volume, characterized both patients with minimal change nephrotic syndrome and patients with other kidney diseases. The two groups were indistinguishable (181). These observations raised important questions about the proposed mechanism of edema formation in the nephrotic syndrome.

An alternative explanation to the "underfill" model of edema formation proposes that renal disease induces primary sodium and water retention leading to plasma volume expansion and increased capillary hydrostatic pressure. The sodium avidity is intrinsic to the nephrotic kidney itself and unrelated to systemic volume needs. Strong evidence for this hypothesis is provided by studies using unilateral proteinuric renal disease. In unilateral kidney models of the nephrotic syndrome, impaired sodium excretion is intrinsic to the nephrotic kidney and does not reflect plasma volume regulation. In one such study, Perico et al. (182) demonstrated inability of the proteinuric kidney to excrete fluid or sodium in response to infused atrial natriuretic peptide (ANP), although GFR increased similarly in both the proteinuric and normal, contralateral kidney. Ichikawa et al. found that the proteinuric kidney avidly reabsorbed filtered salt in the distal part of the nephron in PAN-induced nephrotic syndrome in the rat, whereas the normal contralateral kidney did not (183). Clearly, both the normal kidney and the contralateral proteinuric kidney were exposed to the same oncotic pressure and circulating hormones.

Both experimental and human studies have suggested relative resistance to ANP. This defect may result, in part, from increased phosphodiesterase activity in the nephrotic kidney leading to more rapid degradation of cGMP (cyclic guanosine 3′:5′-cyclic monophosphate), which is the second messenger for ANP. Valentin et al. (184) found that the normal increase in urinary cGMP that follows saline infusion was blunted in nephrotic rats because of increased phosphodiesterase in the inner medullary collecting duct cells. Treatment with a phosphodiesterase inhibitor reverses this defect and restores the normal natriuretic response to volume expansion. Thus, an increase in phosphodiesterase activity in the nephrotic syndrome was proposed to accelerate hydrolysis of cGMP resulting in impaired natriuresis. These observations provide a cellular basis for the observations of Perico et al. (182) and Ichikawa et al. (183). The proteinuric kidney avidly reabsorbs filtered salt in the distal nephron and is not responsive to increased ANP that should normally cause a natriuresis when plasma volume is expanded (183). In addition, there is increased activity of the sodium-potassium ATPase (adenosine triphosphate) pump in the cortical-collecting duct in nephrotic rats (185).

In the setting of primary renal sodium retention, the systemic capillary bed is faced with increased hydrostatic pressure at the very time that defense mechanisms normally used to counteract edema formation (increased lymphatic flow and decreased interstitial protein concentration) already have been maximized. Edema results from the combined effect of primary renal salt and water retention coupled with urinary losses of proteins of intermediate-weight causing a decrease in both plasma and interstitial oncotic pressure (Fig. 24.5). These processes deprive the lymphatic system of the capacity to respond to increased hydrostatic pressure. Because sodium retention is frequently, at least in part, a direct result of the renal disease itself and not a consequence of plasma volume contraction, dietary sodium restriction is indicated. Hyponatremia is unlikely to occur in patients with the nephrotic syndrome in the absence of diuretic use and is not often encountered in patients with the nephrotic syndrome.

The relative role of primary sodium retention versus "underfill" in the development of edema in the nephrotic syndrome is not clear and may be variable depending on the underlying cause of the renal disease. Based on their studies in patients with the nephrotic syndrome, Meltzer et al. (4) proposed that patients with the nephrotic syndrome with edema could be divided into two groups. One group was termed "nephrotic" and was made up predominantly of those with minimal change with low plasma volume and high plasma renin. The cause of their edema would fit more with the "underfill" model. The other patients were classified as "nephritic" and comprised those with glomerulone-

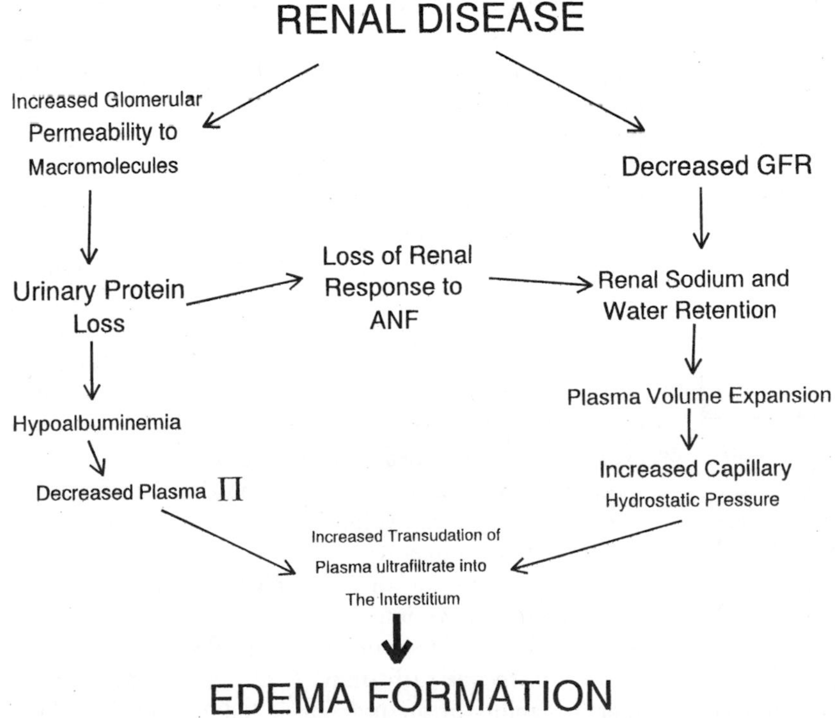

FIGURE 24.5. Primary renal sodium retention with edema formation. Renal salt and water retention occur as a result of the renal disease itself, causing plasma-volume expansion. This produces increased capillary hydrostatic pressure, which, in conjunction with the increased transcapillary flux of fluid resulting from hypoalbuminemia, causes edema. Edema formation is not a direct consequence of reduced oncotic pressure alone. Renal salt and water retention is primarily a consequence of an unresponsiveness of the kidney to atrial natriuretic peptide (ANP).

phritis or diabetes. These patients had normal or expanded plasma volume and reduced plasma renin activity, despite a profound reduction in plasma oncotic pressure. Patients with an elevated intravascular volume tend to have lower GFRs (<50%) and higher serum albumin concentration. Patients with so-called "underfill" edema tend to have normal GFR and more severe hypoalbuminemia, the prototype of this being minimal change disease. Many of the studies evaluating the overflow versus primary sodium retention models have been conflicting, and it is possible that either or both mechanisms may be operational in a given patient dependent on their underlying renal disease and other factors.

It is possible for patients with the nephrotic syndrome to become plasma-volume contracted. This must be detected, guarded against, and treated. It is, however, impossible to predict the plasma volume of a patient with the nephrotic syndrome by measuring plasma protein or albumin concentration or by measuring plasma renin activity (181). Therefore, it is important to determine the intravascular volume state of each patient individually by measuring orthostatic blood pressure, observing neck vein distention, and evaluating BUN relative to creatinine. Patients who show no evidence of plasma volume contraction should respond to the gentle use of diuretics. Patients who have plasma volume contraction should not be treated with diuretics, but their volume deficit should be treated by bed rest, wearing support hose, or even fluid replacement if necessary.

RECOMMENDATIONS FOR NUTRITIONAL AND NONNUTRITIONAL TREATMENT OF THE NEPHROTIC SYNDROME

The treatment of the nephrotic syndrome begins with identifying the specific cause of the proteinuria and treatment of the underlying disorder if possible. There are, however, general nutritional and nonnutritional management issues in patients with the nephrotic syndrome.

Proteinuria

Reducing proteinuria should be a primary objective in the treatment of the nephrotic syndrome. As detailed in this chapter, proteinuria may contribute to further renal damage by promoting tubulointerstitial inflammation and fibrosis. The notion here is that "proteinuria begets more proteinuria." Moreover, reducing proteinuria improves the hyperlipidemia and edema of the nephrotic syndrome. Although the nephrotic syndrome results from the loss of plasma proteins in the urine, dietary protein augmentation is ineffective in correcting the metabolic consequences of urinary protein loss. Furthermore, diets rich in protein increase proteinuria and may accelerate the course of a variety of renal diseases. *Thus, dietary protein supplementation should be avoided.* As detailed in this chapter, dietary protein restriction not only reduces proteinuria but preserves serum albumin concentration. Moreover, modest protein restriction (0.8 g/kg/day) has been shown to maintain nitrogen balance. The studies using an extremely low protein diet (0.3 g/kg/day) supplemented with essential amino acids are provocative but need to be verified by larger controlled trials. The safest recommendation would be to prescribe a diet that contains 0.8 to 1 g/kg/day of protein and 35 kCal/kg and is low in fat, high in complex carbohydrate, and restricted in sodium chloride. Based on the studies with soy protein, vegetarian diets may be especially useful. Modest protein restriction also may be beneficial in attenuating the progression of the primary renal disease by its effect in reducing intraglomerular pressure. Administration of ACE inhibitors (186,187) or angiotensin receptor blockers (188, 189) have been shown to reduce proteinuria as well as slow the progression of the primary renal disease and now has become part of the standard therapy for most all proteinuric conditions.

Hyperlipidemia

Hyperlipidemia in the nephrotic syndrome poses a danger for accelerated atherosclerosis and progressive renal injury. Reductions in plasma lipid levels have been accomplished using therapies such a low-fat diet (89) and fish oil supplements (158). Dietary therapy with a low-fat diet, however, is generally of only minimal benefit, and there is no long-term experience with the use of a low-fat diet in the treatment of the hyperlipidemia of the nephrotic syndrome. In addition, there is no compelling reason to prescribe unsaturated fatty-acid supplements (such as fish oil) until results from controlled studies are available. It is best to avoid cholesterol and saturated fats as much as possible. It has been shown that reducing proteinuria using drugs such as ACE inhibitors lowers blood lipid levels in nephrotic animals (9) and humans (190). Keilani et al. (190) demonstrated a 10% to 20% decrease in the plasma levels of total and LDL cholesterol and Lp(a) with the use of an ACE inhibitor. The magnitude of these changes appears to be related to the degree of reduction in proteinuria. The angiotensin II receptor antagonist, losartan, appears to have a similar beneficial effect on the lipid profile in patients with the nephrotic syndrome (191). Thus, therapy directed at reducing the increased renal clearance of macromolecules has a salutary effect on improving the hyperlipidemia associated with the nephrotic syndrome. Pharmacologic agents, such as probucol (192,193), gemfibrozil (194), or HMG-CoA reductase inhibitors (195–197), may prove useful in reducing blood lipid levels in these patients. Use of these agents may engender some morbidity, such as rhabdomyolysis with lovastatin (198) especially in combination with gemfibrozil (199), and hepatoxicity.

Edema

Dietary sodium restriction remains the cornerstone of the management of edema of the nephrotic syndrome. Edema refractory to treatment with dietary sodium restriction frequently is treated with diuretic drugs. Diuretic therapy begins with the use of loop diuretics in increasing doses to achieve the desired natriuresis. Resistance to diuretics is seen in patients with the nephrotic syndrome. Most diuretics are highly protein bound, and this limits diuretics to the vascular space and optimizes delivery of the drug to the kidney. In the setting of the nephrotic syndrome with hypoalbuminemia, protein binding is reduced and there is less delivery of drug to the kidney (200). It this setting, it has been proposed to infuse the loop diuretic with salt-poor albumin solutions to help improve delivery of the drug to the kidney (201). Resistance to diuretics also may result from filtered proteins binding the diuretic in the tubular lumen, thus limiting the action of the drug (202). The addition of a thiazide diuretic to a loop diuretic may be beneficial in resistant cases of nephrotic edema.

ACKNOWLEDGMENTS

This work was supported in part by a grant from the National Institutes of Health 1-RO1 DK 42297-01 and in part by the research service of the United States Department of Veterans Affairs.

REFERENCES

1. Earley LC, Farland M. Nephrotic syndrome, 3rd ed. In: Strauss MB, Welt LG, eds. *Diseases of the kidney.* Boston: Little, Brown Co., 1979:765–813.
2. Earley LE, Havel RJ, Hopper J, et al. Nephrotic syndrome. *Calif Med* 1971;115:23–41.
3. Dorhout-Mees EJ, Roos JC, Boer P, et al. Observations on edema formation in the nephrotic syndrome in adults with minimal lesions. *Am J Med* 1979;67:378–384.
4. Meltzer JI, Keim HJ, Laragh JH, et al. Nephrotic syndrome: Vasoconstriction and hypervolemia types indicated by renin sodium profiling. *Ann Intern Med* 1979;67:387–384.
5. Barragry JM, France MW, Carter ND, et al. Vitamin D metabolism in nephrotic syndrome. *Lancet* 1977;2:629–632.
6. Pedraza-Chaverri J, Torres-Rodriguez GA, Cruz C, et al. Copper and zinc metabolism in aminonucleoside-induced nephrotic syndrome. *Nephron* 1994;6:87–92.
7. Perrone L, Gialanella G, Giordano V, et al. Impaired zinc metabolic status in children affected by idiopathic nephrotic syndrome. *Eur J Ped* 1990;149:438–440.
8. Stec J, Podracka L, Pavkovcekova O, et al. Zinc and copper metabolism in nephrotic syndrome. *Nephron* 1990;56: 186–187.
9. Davies RW, Staprans I, Hutchison FN, et al. Proteinuria not altered albumin metabolism affects hyperlipidemia in the nephrotic rat. *J Clin Invest* 1990;86:600–605.
10. Joven J, Villabona C, Vilella E, et al. Abnormalities of lipoprotein metabolism in patients with the nephrotic syndrome. *N Engl J Med* 1990;323:579–584.
11. Gherardi E, Rota E, Calandra S, et al. Relationship among the concentrations of serum lipoproteins and changes in their chemical composition in patients with untreated nephrotic syndrome. *Eur J Clin Invest* 1977;7:563–570.
12. Wanner C, Rader D, Bartens W, et al. Elevated plasma lipoprotein a in patients with the nephrotic syndrome. *Ann Intern Med* 1993;119:263–269.
13. Sieniawska M, Szymanik-Grzelak H, Kowalewska M, et al. The role of cow's milk protein intolerance in steroid-resistant nephrotic syndrome. *Acta Paediatrica* 1992;81:1007–1012.
14. Laurent J, Lagrue G. Dietary manipulation for idiopathic nephrotic syndrome. A new approach to therapy. *Allergy* 1989; 44:599–603.
15. Lagrue G, Laurent J, Rostoker G. Food allergy and idiopathic nephrotic syndrome. *Kidney Int Suppl* 1989;27:S147–S151.
16. Laurent J, Rostoker G, Robeva R, et al. Is adult idiopathic nephrotic syndrome food allergy? Value of oligoantigenic diets. *Nephron* 1987;47(1):7–11.
17. Lagrue G, Heslan JM, Belghiti D, et al. Basophil sensitization for food allergens in idiopathic nephrotic syndrome. *Nephron* 1986;42:123–127.
18. Lee KE, Summerill RA. Glomerular filtration rate following administration of individual amino acids in conscious dogs. *Q J Exp Physiol* 1982;67:459–465.
19. Premen AJ, Hall JE, Smith MJ. Postprandial regulation of renal hemodynamics role of pancreatic glucagon. *Am J Physiol* 1985; 248(5 Pt 2):F656–F662.
20. Hutchison FN, Martin VI, Jones H Jr, et al. Differing actions of dietary protein and enalapril on renal function and proteinuria. *Am J Physiol* 1990;258(1 Pt 2):F126–F132.
21. Kaysen GA, Gambertoglio J, Jiminez I, et al. Effect of dietary protein intake on albumin homeostasis in nephrotic patients. *Kidney Int* 1986;29:572–577.
22. Kaysen GA, Kirkpatrick WG, Couser WG. Albumin homeostasis in the nephrotic rat nutritional considerations *Am J Physiol* 1984;247(1 Pt 2):F192–F202.
23. Paller MS, Hostetter TH. Dietary protein increases plasma renin and reduces pressor reactivity to angiotensin II. *Am J Physiol* 1986;251(1 Pt 2):F34–F39.
24. Fine L. The biology of renal hypertrophy. *Kidney Int* 1986;29: 619–634.
25. Kaysen GA, Rosenthal C, Hutchison FN. GFR increases before renal mass or ODC activity increase in rats fed high protein diets. *Kidney Int* 1989;36:441–446.
26. Kenner CH, Evan AP, Blomgren AP, et al. Effect of protein intake on renal function and structure in partially nephrectomized rats. *Kidney Int* 1985;27:739–750.
27. Wada L, Don BR, Schambelan M. Hormonal mediators of amino-acid induced glomerular hyperfiltration in humans. *Am J Physiol* 1991;260(6 Pt 2):F787–F792.
28. Woods LL. Mechanisms of renal hemodynamic regulation in response to protein feeding. *Kidney Int* 1993;44:659–675.
29. Jaffa AA, Vio CP, Silva RH, et al. Evidence for renal kinins as mediators of amino acid-induced hyperperfusion and hyperfiltration in the rat. *J Clin Invest* 1992;89:1460–1468.
30. Don BR, Blake S, Hutchison FN, et al. Dietary protein intake modulates glomerular eicosanoid production in the rat. *Am J Physiol* 1989;256(4 Pt 2):F711–F718.
31. El Sayed AA, Haylor J, El Nahas AM. Mediators of the direct effects of amino acids on the rat kidney. *Clin Sci* 1991;81: 427–432.
32. Williams M, Young JB, Rosa RM, et al. Effect of protein ingestion on urinary dopamine excretion. Evidence for the functional importance of renal decarboxylation of circulating 3 4-dihydroxyphenylalanine in man. *J Clin Invest* 1986;78:1687–1693.
33. Straus DS, Takemoto CD. Effect of dietary protein deprivation

on insulin-like growth factor (IGF)-I and -II, IGF binding protein-2, and serum albumin gene expression in rat. *Endocrinology* 1990;127:1849–1860.
34. Lemozy S, Pucilowska JB, Underwood LE. Reduction of insulin-like growth factor-I IGF-I in protein-restricted rats is associated with differential regulation of IGF-binding protein messenger ribonucleic acids in liver and kidney and peptides in liver and serum. *Endocrinology* 1994;135:617–623.
35. Martinez-Maldonado M, Benabe JE, Wilcox JN, et al. Renal renin angiotensinogen and angiotensin I-converting-enzyme gene expression influence of dietary protein. *Am J Physiol* 1993; 264:F981–F988.
36. Chan YM, Cheng M-LL, Keil LC, et al. Functional response of healthy and diseased glomeruli to a large protein meal. *J Clin Invest* 1988;81:245–254.
37. Palmer RMJ, Ferrige AG, Moncada S. Nitric oxide release accounts for the biological activity of endothelium-derived relaxing factor. *Nature* 1987;327:524–526.
38. Tolins JP, Raij L. Effects of amino acid infusion on renal hemodynamics. *Hypertension* 1991;17:1045–1051.
39. Ito S, Juncos LA, Nushiro N, et al. Endothelium-derived relaxing factor modulates endothelin action in afferent arterioles. *Hypertension* 1991;17:1052–1056.
40. Gitlin D, Janeway CA, Farr LE. Studies on the metabolism of plasma proteins in nephrotic syndrome. I. Albumin gamma globulin and iron-binding globulin. *J Clin Invest* 1956;35: 44–55.
41. Jensen H, Rossing N, Anderson SB, et al. Albumin metabolism in the nephrotic syndrome in adults. *Clin Sci* 1967;33:445–457.
42. Kaitz AL. Albumin metabolism in nephrotic adults. *J Lab Clin Med* 1959;53:186–194.
43. Yssing M, Jensen H, Jarnum S. Albumin metabolism and gastrointestinal protein loss in children with nephrotic syndrome. *Acta Paediat Scand* 1969;58:109–115.
44. Kaysen GA, Davies RW, Hutchison FN. Effect of dietary protein intake and angiotensin converting enzyme inhibition in Heymann nephritis. *Kidney Int* 1989;36:S154–S162.
45. Kaysen GA, Carstensen A, Martin VI. Muscle protein synthesis is impaired in nephrotic rats. *Miner Electrol Metab* 1992;18: 228–232.
46. Keutmann EH, Bassett SH. Dietary protein in hemorrhagic Bright's disease. II. The effect of diet on serum proteins proteinuria and tissue proteins. *J Clin Invest* 1935;14:871–888.
47. Don BR, Kaysen GA, Hutchison FN, et al. The effect of angiotensin-converting enzyme inhibition and dietary protein restriction in the treatment of proteinuria. *Am J Kidney Dis* 1991;17: 10–17.
48. Heeg JE, de Jong PE, van der Hem GK, et al. Angiotensin II does not acutely reverse the reduction of proteinuria by long-term ACE inhibition. *Kidney Int* 1991;40:734–741.
49. Brenner BM, Meyer TW, Hostetter TH. Dietary protein intake and the progressive nature of kidney disease The role of hemodynamically mediated glomerular injury in the pathogenesis of progressive glomerular sclerosis in aging renal ablation and intrinsic renal disease. *N Engl J Med* 1982;307:652–659.
50. Kaysen GA. Albumin turnover in renal disease. *Miner Electrol Metab* 1998;24:55–63.
51. Ando S, Kon K, Tanaka Y, et al. Characterization of hyperlipidemia in Nagase analbuminemia rat (NAR). *J Biochem (Tokyo)* 1980;87:1859–1892.
52. Blainey JD. High protein diets in the treatment of the nephrotic syndrome *Clin Sci* 1954;13:567–581.
53. Kirsch R, Frith L, Black E, et al. Regulation of albumin synthesis and catabolism by alteration of dietary protein. *Nature* 1968; 217:578–579.
54. Rothschild MA, Oratz M, Evans CD, et al. Albumin synthesis. In: Rosemoer M, Oratz M, Rothschild A, eds. *Albumin structure, function, and uses.* New York: Pergamon Press, 1977:227–255.
55. Hirschberg RR, Zipser RD, Slomowitz LA, et al. Glucagon and prostaglandins are mediators of amino acid-induced rise in renal hemodynamics. *Kidney Int* 1988;33:1147–1155.
56. Hirschberg R, Kopple JD. Role of growth hormone in the amino acid-induced acute rise in renal function in man. *Kidney Int* 1987;32:382–387.
57. Premen AJ. Potential mechanisms mediating postprandial renal hyperemia and hyperfiltration. *FASEB J* 1988;2:131–137.
58. Rosenberg ME, Swanson JE, Thomas BL, et al. Glomerular and hormonal responses to dietary protein intake in human renal disease. *Am J Physiol* 1987;253(6 Pt 2):F1083–F1090.
59. Kaysen GA, Jones H Jr, Martin V, et al. A low protein diet restricts albumin synthesis in nephrotic rats. *J Clin Invest* 1989; 83:1623–1629.
60. Farr LE. The assimilation of protein by young children with the nephrotic syndrome. *Am J Med Sci* 1938;195:70–83.
61. Kaysen GA, al-Bander H, Martin VI, et al. Branched-chain amino acids augment neither albuminuria nor albumin synthesis in nephrotic rats. *Am J Physiol* 1991;260(2 Pt 2):R177–184.
62. Claris-Appiani A, Assael BM, Tirelli AS, et al. Lack of glomerular hemodynamic stimulation after infusion of branch-chain amino acids. *Kidney Int* 1988;33:91–94.
63. Anderson KE, Rosner W, Khan MS, et al. Diet-hormone interactions: Protein/carbohydrate ratio alters reciprocally the plasma levels of testosterone and cortisol and their respective binding globulins in man. *Life Sci* 1987;40:1761–1768.
64. Ishizuka B, Quigley ME, Yen SSC. Pituitary hormone release in response to food ingestion: evidence for neuroendocrine signals from gut to brain. *J Clin Endocrinol Metab* 1983;57: 1111–1116.
65. Benabe JE, Wang S, Wilcox JN, et al. Modulation of angiotensin II receptor and its mRNA in normal rat by low-protein feeding. *Am J Physiol* 1993;265:F660–F669.
66. Correa-Rotter R, Hostetter TH, Rosenberg ME. Effect of dietary protein on renin and angiotensinogen gene expression after renal ablation. *Am J Physiol* 1992;262:F631–638.
67. Zatz R, Meyer TW, Rennke HG, et al. Predominance of hemodynamic rather than metabolic factors in the pathogenesis of diabetic glomerulopathy. *Proc Natl Acad Sci* 1985;82: 5963–5967.
68. Hutchison FN, Martin VI. Effects of modulation of renal kallikrein-kinin system in the nephrotic syndrome. *Am J Physiol* 1990;258(1 Pt 2):F1237–F1244.
69. Brouhard BH, LeGrone LF, Richards GE, et al. Somatostatin limits rise in glomerular filtration rate after a protein meal. *J Pediatr* 1987;110:729–734.
70. Kaysen GA, Martin VI, Jones H Jr. Arginine augments neither albuminuria nor albumin synthesis caused by high-protein diets in nephrosis. *Am J Physiol* 1992;263:F907–F917.
71. Eddy AA, McCulloch L, Liu E, et al. A relationship between proteinuria and acute tubulointerstitial disease in rats with experimental nephrotic syndrome. *Am J Pathol* 1991;138: 1111–1123.
72. Thomas ME, Schreiner GF. Contribution of proteinuria to progressive renal injury: consequences of tubular uptake of fatty acid bearing albumin. *Am J Nephrol* 1993;13:385–398.
73. Cooper MA, Buddington B, Miller NL, et al. Urinary iron speciation in nephrotic syndrome. *Am J Kidney Dis* 1995;25: 314–319.
74. Alfrey AC. Role of iron and oxygen radicals in the progression of chronic renal failure. *Am J Kidney Dis* 1994;23:183–187.
75. Alfrey AC, Hammond WS. Renal iron handling in the nephrotic syndrome. *Kidney Int* 1990;37:1409–1413.
76. Nath KA, Hostetter MK, Hostetter TH. Increased ammonia-

genesis as a determinant of progressive renal injury. *Am J Kidney Dis* 1991;17:654–657.

77. Thomas ME, Schreiner GF Jr. Contribution of proteinuria to progressive renal injury consequences of tubular uptake of fatty acid bearing albumin. *Am J Nephrol* 1993;13:385–398.
78. Abbate M, Zoja C, Corna D, et al. In progressive nephropathies overload of tubular cells with filtered proteins translates glomerular permeability dysfunction into cellular signals of interstitial inflammation. *J Am Soc Nephrol* 1998;9:1213–1224.
79. Burton CJ, Combe C, Walls J, et al. Secretion of chemokines by human tubular epithelial cells in response to proteins. *Nephrol Dial Transplant* 1999;14:2628–2633.
80. Nath KD. Tubulointerstitial changes as a major determinant in the progression of renal damage. *Am J Kidney Dis* 1992;20: 1–17.
81. Alexopoulos E, Seron D, Hartley RB, et al. Lupus nephritis Correlation of interstitial cells with glomerular function. *Kidney Int* 1990;37:100–109.
82. Clark EC, Nath KA, Hostetter MK, et al. Role of ammonia in tubulointerstitial injury. *Miner Electrol Metab* 1990;16: 315–321.
83. Agarwal A, Nath KA. Effect of proteinuria on renal interstitium effect of products of nitrogen metabolism. *Am J Nephrol* 1993; 13:376–384.
84. Eddy AA. Protein restriction reduces transforming growth factor-beta and interstitial fibrosis in nephrotic syndrome. *Am J Physiol* 1994;266:F884–F893.
85. Fukui M, Nakamura T, Ebihara I, et al. Low-protein diet attenuates increased gene expression of platelet-derived growth factor and transforming growth factor-beta in experimental glomerular sclerosis. *J Lab Clin Med* 1993;121:224–234.
86. Giordano M, De Feo P, Lucidid P, et al. Effects of dietary protein restriction on fibrinogen and albumin metabolism in nephrotic patients. *Kidney Int* 2001;60:235–242.
87. de Sain-van der Velden MGM, Kaysen GA, De Meer K, et al. Proportionate increase of fibrinogen and albumin synthesis in nephrotic patients: measurement with stable isotopes. *Kidney Int* 1998;53:181–188.
88. Vaziri ND, Gonzales E, Barton CH, et al. Factor XIII and its substrates, fibronectin, fibrinogen, and alpha 2-antiplasmin in plasma and urine of patients with nephrosis. *J Lab Clin Med* 1991;117:152–156.
89. D'Amico G, Gentile MG, Manna G, et al. Effect of vegetarian soy diet on hyperlipidaemia in nephrotic syndrome. *Lancet* 1992;339:1131–1134.
90. Walser M. Does prolonged protein restriction preceding dialysis lead to protein malnutrition at the onset of dialysis? *Kidney Int* 1993;44:1139–1144.
91. Gentile MG, Fellin G, Cofano F, et al. Treatment of proteinuric patients with a vegetarian soy diet and fish oil. *Clin Nephrol* 1993;40(6):315–320.
92. Walser M, Hill S, Tomalis EA. Treatment of nephrotic adults with a supplemented very low protein diet. *Am J Kidney Dis* 1996;28:354–364.
93. Peters JP, Bulger HA. The relation of albuminuria to protein requirement in nephritis. *Arch Intern Med* 1926;37:153–185.
94. Al-Bander H, Kaysen GA. Ineffectiveness of dietary protein augmentation in the management of the nephrotic syndrome. *Pediatr Nephrol* 5:482–486, 1991.
95. Choi EJ, Bailey J, May RC, et al. Metabolic responses to nephrosis effect of a low-protein diet. *Am J Physiol* 1994;266: F432–F438.
96. Katoh T, Takahashi K, Klahr S, et al. Dietary supplementation with L-arginine ameliorates glomerular hypertension in rats with subtotal nephrectomy. *J Am Soc Nephrol* 1994;4:1690–1694.
97. Klahr S, Buerhert J, Purkerson ML. Role of dietary factors in the progression of chronic renal disease. *Kidney Int* 1983;24: 579–587.
98. Evanoff G, Thompson C, Brown H, et al. Prolonged dietary protein restriction in diabetic nephropathy. *Arch Intern Med* 1989;149:1129–1133.
99. Jireidine KF, Hogg RJ, van Renen MJ, et al. Evaluation of long-term aggressive dietary management of chronic renal failure in children. *Pediatr Nephrol* 1990;4:1–10.
100. Zeller K, Whittaker E, Sullivan L, et al. Effect of restricting dietary protein on the progression of renal failure in patients with insulin dependent diabetes mellitus. *N Engl J Med* 1991; 324:78–84.
101. Lim VS, Wolfson M, Yarasheski KE, et al. Leucine turnover in patients with the nephrotic syndrome evidence suggesting body protein conservation. *J Am Soc Nephrol* 1998;9:1067–1073.
102. Maroni BJ, Staffeld C, Young VR, et al. Mechanisms permitting nephrotic patients to achieve nitrogen equilibrium with a protein-restricted diet. *J Clin Invest* 1997;99:2479–2487.
103. McCrory WW, Becker CG, Cunningham-Rundles C, et al. Immune complex glomerulopathy in a child with food hypersensitivity. *Kidney Int* 1986;30:592–598.
104. Coppo R, Amore A, Roccatello D. Dietary antigens and primary immunoglobulin A nephropathy. *J Am Soc Nephrol* 1992;2: S173–S180.
105. Marsh JB. Lipoprotein metabolism in experimental nephrosis. *J Lipid Res* 1984;25:1619–1623.
106. Garber DW, Gottlieb BA, Marsh JB, et al. Catabolism of very low density lipo-proteins in experimental nephrosis. *J Clin Invest* 1984;74:1375–1383.
107. Staprans I, Felts JM, Couser WG. Glycosaminoglycans and chylomicron metabolism in control and nephrotic rats. *Metabolism* 1987;36:496–501.
108. Chung BH, Segrest JP, Smith K, et al. Lipolytic surface remnants of triglyceride-rich lipoproteins are cytotoxic to macrophages but not in the presence of high density lipoprotein A possible mechanism of atherogenesis. *J Clin Invest* 1989;83: 1363–1374.
109. Demant T, Mathes C, Gutlich K, et al. A simultaneous study of the metabolism of apolipoprotein B and albumin in nephrotic patients. *Kidney Int* 1998;54:2064–2080.
110. de Sain-van der Velden MG, Kaysen GA, Barrett HA, et al. Increased VLDL in nephrotic patients results from a decreased catabolism while increased LDL results from increased synthesis. *Kidney Int* 1998;53:994–1001.
111. Blanchette-Mackie EJ, Masuno H, Dwyer NK, et al. Lipoprotein lipase in myocytes and capillary endothelium of heart immunocytochemical study. *Am J Physiol* 1989;256:E818–E828.
112. Shearer GC, Stevenson FT, Atkinson DN, et al. Hypoalbuminemia and proteinuria contribute separately to reduced lipoprotein lipase in the nephrotic syndrome. *Kidney Int* 2001;59(1): 179–189.
113. Kaysen GA, Don B, Schambelan M. Proteinuria albumin synthesis and hyperlipidemia in the nephrotic syndrome. *Nephrol Dial Transplant* 1991;6:141–149.
114. Warwick GL, Packard CJ, Demant T, et al. Metabolism of B-containing lipoproteins in subject with nephrotic-range proteinuria. *Kidney Int* 1991;40:129–138.
115. Vaziri ND, Liang KH. Down regulation of hepatic LDL receptor in experimental nephrosis. *Kidney Int* 1996;50:887–893.
116. Appel G. Lipid abnormalities in renal disease. *Kidney Int* 1991; 39:169–183.
117. Sun X, Jones H Jr, Joles JA, et al. Apolipoprotein gene expression in analbuminemic rats and in rats with Heymann nephritis. *Am J Physiol* 1992;262:F755–F761.
118. Muls E, Rosseneu M, Daneels R, et al. Lipoprotein distribution and composition in the human nephrotic syndrome. *Atherosclerosis* 1985;54:225–237.

119. Steyrer E, Durovic S, Frank S, et al. The role of lecithin cholesterol acyltransferease for lipoprotein a assembly. Structural integrity of low density lipoproteins is a prerequisite for Lp a formation in human plasma. *J Clin Invest* 1994;94:2330–2340.
120. McLean JW, Tomlinson JE, Kuang WJ, et al. cDNA sequence of human apolipoprotein a is homologous to plasminogen. *Nature* 1987;330:132–137.
121. Loscalzo J, Weinfeld M, Fless GM, et al. Lipoprotein(a), fibrin binding, and plasminogen activation. *Arteriosclerosis* 1990;10: 240–245.
122. Kraft HG, Lingenhel A, Pang RW, et al. Frequency distributions of apolipoprotein a kringle IV repeat alleles and their effects on lipoprotein a levels in Caucasian Asian and African populations: the distribution of null alleles is non-random. *Eur J Human Gen* 1996;4:74–87.
123. Gavish D, Azrolan N, Breslow J. Plasma Lp a concentration is inversely correlated with the ratio of kringle IV kringle V encoding domains in the apo a gene. *J Clin Invest* 1989;84: 2021–2027.
124. de Sain-Van Der Velden MG, Reijngoud DJ, Kaysen GA, et al. Evidence for increased synthesis of Lipoprotein a in the nephrotic syndrome. *J Am Soc Nephrol* 1998;9:1474–1481.
125. Takahashi M, Kusumi K, Shumiya S, et al. Plasma lipid concentrations and enzyme activities in Nagase analbuminemia rats (NAR). *Exp Anim* 1983;32:39–46.
126. Esumi H, Takahashi Y, Sekiya T, et al. Presence of albumin mRNA precursors in nuclei of analbuminemic rat liver lacking cytoplasmic albumin mRNA. *Proc Natl Acad Sci* 1982;79: 734–738.
127. Kaysen GA, Davies RW. Reduction in proteinuria attenuates hyperlipidemia in the nephrotic syndrome. *J Am Soc Nephrol* 1990;1:S75–S79.
128. Mallick NP, Short CD. The nephrotic syndrome and ischaemic heart disease. *Nephron* 1981;27:54–57.
129. Wheeler DC, Bernard DB. Lipid abnormalities in the nephrotic syndrome: causes, consequences, and treatment. *Am J Kidney Dis* 1994;23:331–346.
130. Berlyne GM, Mallick NP. Ischemic heart disease as a complication of nephrotic syndrome. *Lancet* 1969;2:399–400.
131. Schreiner PJ, Heiss G, Tyroler HA, et al. Race and gender differences in the association of Lp(a) with carotid artery wall thickness. The Atherosclerosis Risk in Communities (ARIC) Study. *Arterioscler Thromb Vasc Biol* 1996;16:471–478.
132. Sechi LA, Kronenberg F, De Carli S, et al. Association of serum lipoprotein(a) levels and apolipoprotein(a) size polymorphism with target-organ damage in arterial hypertension. *JAMA* 1997; 277:1689–1695.
133. Girot R, Jaubert F, Leon M, et al. Albumin, fibrinogen, prothrombin and antithrombin III variations in blood urines and liver in rat nephrotic syndrome (Heymann nephritis). *Thromb Haemost* 1983;49:13–17.
134. Llach F. Nephrotic syndrome: hypercoagulability, renal vein thrombosis and other thromboembolic complications. In: Brenner BM, Stein JH, eds. *Contemporary issues in nephrology.* New York: Churchill Livingstone, 1982:121–144.
135. Schmitz PG, Kasiske BL, O'Donnell MP, et al. Lipids and progressive renal injury. *Semin Nephrol* 1989;9:354–369.
136. Wellman KF, Volk BW. Renal changes in experimental hypercholesterolemia in normal and subdiabetic rabbits I. Short term studies. *Lab Invest* 1970;22:36–48.
137. Al-Shebeb T, Frohlich J, Magil AB. Glomerular disease in hypercholesterolemic guinea pigs: a pathogenetic study. *Kidney Int* 1988;33:498–507.
138. Drevon CA, Hoving T. The effects of cholesterol fat feeding on lipid levels and morphological structures in liver kidney and spleen in guinea pigs. *Acta Pathol Micro Immunol Scand* 1977; 85:1–18.
139. Diamond JR, Karnovsky MJ. Exacerbation of chronic aminonucleoside nephrosis by dietary cholesterol supplementation. *Kidney Int* 1987;31:671–677.
140. Kasiske BL, O'Donnell MP, Garvis WJ, et al. Pharmacologic treatment of hyperlipidemia reduces glomerular injury in rat 5/6 nephrectomy model of chronic renal failure. *Circ Res* 1988; 62:367–374.
141. Keane WF. Lipids and the kidney. *Kidney Int* 1994;46: 910–920.
142. Rovin BH, Tan LC. LDL stimulates mesangial fibronectin production and chemoattractant expression. *Kidney Int* 1993;43: 218–225.
143. Keane WF, O'Donnell MP, Kasiske BL, et al. Oxidative modification of low-density lipoproteins by mesangial cells. *J Am Soc Nephrol* 1993;4:187–194.
144. Grone HJ, Walli AK, Grone E, et al. Receptor mediated uptake of apo B and apo E rich lipoproteins by human glomerular epithelial cells. *Kidney Int* 1990;37:1449–1459.
145. Rabelink AJ, Hene RJ, Erkelens DW, et al. Partial remission of nephrotic syndrome in patients on long-term simvastatin. *Lancet* 1990;335:1045–1046.
146. Ravid M, Brosh D, Ravid-Safran D, et al. Main risk factors for nephropathy in type 2 diabetes mellitus are plasma cholesterol levels, mean blood pressure, and hyperglycemia. *Arch Intern Med* 1998;158:998–1004.
147. Kaplan R, Aynedjian HS, Schlondorff D, et al. Renal vasoconstriction caused by short-term cholesterol feeding is corrected by thromboxane antagonist or probucol. *J Clin Invest* 1990;86: 1707–1714.
148. Culp BR, Titus BG, Lands WEM. Inhibition of prostaglandin biosynthesis by eicosapentaenoic acid. *Prostaglandin Med* 1979; 3:269–278.
149. Zoja C, Benigni A, Verroust P, et al. Indomethacin reduces proteinuria in passive Heymann nephritis in rats. *Kidney Int* 1987;31:1335–1343.
150. Remuzzi G, Imberti L, Rossini M, et al. Increased glomerular thromboxane synthesis as a possible cause of proteinuria in experimental nephrosis. *J Clin Invest* 1985;75:94–101.
151. Spector AA, Kaduce TL, Figard PH, et al. Eicosapentaenoic acid and prostaglandin production by cultured human endothelial cells. *J Lipid Res* 1983;24:1595–1604.
152. Needleman P, Raz A, Minkes MS, et al. Triene prostaglandins prostacyclin and thromboxane biosynthesis and unique biological properties. *Proc Natl Acad Sci* 1979;76:944–948.
153. Prickett JD, Robinson DR, Steinberg AD. Dietary enrichment with the polyunsaturated fatty acids eicosapentaenoic acid prevents proteinuria and prolongs survival in NZB x NZW f1 mice. *J Clin Invest* 1981;68:556–559.
154. Scharschmidt LA, Gibbons NB, McGarry L, et al. Effects of dietary fish oil on renal insufficiency in rats with subtotal nephrectomy. *Kidney Int* 1987;32:700–709.
155. Sinclair HM. Essential fatty acids in perspective. *Hum Nutr Clin Nutr* 1984;38:245–260.
156. Ito Y, Yamashita W, Barcelli U, et al. Dietary fat in experimental nephrotic syndrome: beneficial effects of fish oil on serum lipids and, indirectly, on the kidney. *Life Sci* 1987;40:2317–2324.
157. Barcelli UO, Beach DC, Thompson M, et al. A diet containing n-3 and n-6 fatty acids favorably alters the renal phospholipids, eicosanoid synthesis, and plasma lipids in nephrotic rats. *Lipids* 1988;23:1059–1063.
158. Hall AV, Parbtani A, Clark WF, et al. Omega-3 fatty acid supplementation in primary nephrotic syndrome effects on plasma lipids and coagulopathy. *J Am Soc Nephrol* 1992;36: 1321–1329.
159. Donadio JV Jr, Bergstralh EJ, Offord KP, et al. A controlled

trial of fish oil in IgA nephropathy. *N Engl J Med* 1994;331:1194–1199.

160. Harrs KPG, Lefkowith JB, Klahr S, et al. Essential fatty acid deficiency ameliorates acute renal dysfunction in the rat after the administration of the aminonucleoside of puromycin. *J Clin Invest* 1990;86:1115–1123.
161. de Jong G, van Dijk JP, van Eijk HG. The biology of transferrin. *Clin Chim Acta* 1990;190:1–46.
162. Ellis D. Anemia in the course of the nephrotic syndrome secondary to transferrin depletion. *J Pediatr* 1977;90:953–955.
163. Rifkind D, Kravetz HM, Knight V, et al. Urinary excretion of iron-binding protein in the nephrotic syndrome. *N Engl J Med* 1961;265:115–118.
164. Jensen H, Bro-Jorgensen K, Jarnum S, et al. Transferrin metabolism in the nephrotic syndrome and in protein-losing gastroenteropathy. *J Clin Lab Invest* 1968;21:293–304.
165. Vaziri ND, Kaupke CJ, Barton CH, et al. Plasma concentration and urinary excretion of erythropoietin in adult nephrotic syndrome. *Am J Med* 1992;92:35–40.
166. Zhou XJ, Vaziri ND. Erythropoietin metabolism and pharmacokinetics in experimental nephrosis. *Am J Physiol* 1992;263: F812–F815.
167. Vaziri ND. Erythropoietin and transferrin metabolism in nephrotic syndrome. *Am J Kidney Dis* 2001;38:1–8.
168. Cartwright GE, Gubler CJ, Wintrobe MM. Studies on copper metabolism: copper and iron metabolism in the nephrotic syndrome. *J Clin Invest* 1954;33:685–698.
169. Reichel M, Mauro TM, Ziboh VA, et al. Acrodermatitis enteropathica in a patient with the acquired immune deficiency syndrome. *Arch Derm* 1992;128:415–417.
170. Goldstein DA, Haldimann B, Sherman D, et al. Vitamin D metabolites and calcium metabolism in patients with nephrotic syndrome and normal renal function. *J Clin Endocrinol Metab* 1981;53:116–121.
171. Emerson K Jr, Beckman WW. Calcium metabolism in nephrosis. I. A description of an abnormality in calcium metabolism in children with nephrosis. *J Clin Invest* 1945;24:564–572.
172. Lim P, Jacob E, Chio LF, et al. Serum ionized calcium in nephrotic syndrome. *Q J Med* 1976;45:421–426.
173. Stickler GB, Hayles AB, Power MH, et al. Renal tubular dysfunction complicating the nephrotic syndrome. *Pediatrics* 1960; 26:75–85.
174. Goldstein DA, Oda Y, Kurokawa K, et al. Blood levels of 25-hydroxy-vitamin D in nephrotic syndrome. Studies in 26 patients. *Ann Intern Med* 1977;87:664–667.
175. Haddad JG Jr, Walgate J. Radioimmunoassay of the binding protein for vitamin D and its metabolites in human serum: Concentrations in normal subjects and patients with disorders of mineral homeostasis. *J Clin Invest* 1976;58:1217–1222.
176. Yoshioka T, Mitarai T, Kon V, et al. Role for angiotensin II in an overt functional proteinuria. *Kidney Int* 1986;30:538–545.
177. Stickler GB, Rosevear JW, Ulrich JA. Renal tubular dysfunction complicating the nephrotic syndrome: the disturbance in calcium and phosphorus metabolism. *Proc Mayo Clin* 1962;37: 376–387.
178. Kaysen GA, Myers BD, Couser WG, et al. Mechanisms and consequences of proteinuria. *Lab Invest* 1986;54:479–498.
179. Koomans HA, Kortlandt W, Geers AB, et al. Lowered protein content of tissue fluid in patients with the nephrotic syndrome: observations during disease and recovery. *Nephron* 1985;40: 391–395.
180. Koomans HA, Boer WH, Dorhout Mees EJ. Renal function during recovery from minimal lesions nephrotic syndrome. *Nephron* 1987;47:173–178.
181. Geers AB, Koomans HA, Roos JC, et al. Functional relationships in the nephrotic syndrome. *Kidney Int* 1984;26:324–330.
182. Perico N, Delaini F, Lupini C, et al. Blunted excretory response to atrial natriuretic peptide in experimental nephrosis. *Kidney Int* 1989;36:57–64.
183. Ichikawa I, Rennke HG, Hoyer JR, et al. Role for intrarenal mechanisms in the impaired salt excretion of experimental nephrotic syndrome. *J Clin Invest* 1983;71:91–104.
184. Valentin JP, Qiu C, Muldowney WP, et al. Cellular basis for blunted volume expansion natriuresis in experimental nephrotic syndrome. *J Clin Invest* 1992;90:1302–1312.
185. Feraille E, Vogt B, Rousselot M, et al. Mechanisms of enhanced Na-K-ATPase activity in cortical collecting duct from rats with nephrotic syndrome. *J Clin Invest* 1993;91:1295–1300.
186. Lewis EJ, Hunsicker LG, Bain RP, et al. The effect of angiotensin-converting enzyme inhibition on diabetic nephropathy. *N Engl J Med* 1993;329:1456–1462.
187. Maschio G, Albert D, Janin G, et al. Effect of the angiotensin-converting-enzyme inhibitor benazepril on the progression of chronic renal insufficiency. *N Engl J Med* 1996;334:939–945.
188. Parving H-H, Lehnert H, Brochner-Mortensen J, et al. The effect of irbesartan on the development of diabetic nephropathy in patients with type 2 diabetes. *N Engl J Med* 2001;345: 870–878.
189. Brenner BM, Cooper ME, DeZeeuw D, et al. Effects of losartan on renal and cardiovascular outcomes in patients with type 2 diabetes and nephropathy. *N Engl J Med* 2001;345:861–869.
190. Keilani T, Schleuter WA, Levin ML, et al. Improvement of lipid abnormalities associated with proteinuria using fosinopril, an angiotensin-converting enzyme inhibitor. *Ann Intern Med* 1993;118:246–354.
191. de Zeeuw D, Gansevoort RT, Dullaart RP, et al. Angiotensin II antagonism improves the lipoprotein profile in patients with nephrotic syndrome. *J Hypertens* 1995;13:(Suppl 1)S53.
192. Iida H, Izumino K, Asaka M, et al. Effect of probucol on hyperlipidemia in patients with nephrotic syndrome. *Nephron* 1987; 47:280–283.
193. Valeri A, Gelfand J, Blum C, et al. Treatment of the hyperlipidemia of the nephrotic syndrome a controlled trial. *Am J Kidney Dis* 1986;8:388–396.
194. Groggel GC, Cheung AK, Ellis-Benigni K, et al. Treatment of nephrotic hyperlipoproteinemia with gemfibrozil. *Kidney Int* 1989;36:266–271.
195. Rabelink AJ, Hené RJ, Erkelens DW, et al. Effects of simvastatin and cholestyramine on lipoprotein profile in hyperlipidaemia of nephrotic syndrome. *Lancet* 1988;11:1335–1338.
196. Kasiske BL, Velosa JA, Halstenson CE, et al. The effects of lovastatin in hyperlipidemic patients with the nephrotic syndrome. *Am J Kidney Dis* 1990;15:8–15.
197. Golper TA, Illingworth DR, Morris CD, et al. Lovastatin in the treatment of multifactorial hyperlipidemia associated with proteinuria. *Am J Kidney Dis* 1989;13:312–320.
198. Corpier CL, Jones PH, Suki WN, et al. Rhabdomyolysis and renal injury with lovastatin use. Report of two cases in cardiac transplant recipients. *JAMA* 1988;260:239–241.
199. Marais GE, Larson KK. Rhabdomyolysis and acute renal failure induced by combination lovastatin and gemfibrozil therapy. *Ann Intern Med* 1990;112:228–230.
200. Smith DE, Hyneck ML, Beradi RR, et al. Urinary protein binding kinetics and dynamics of furosemide in nephrotic patients. *J Pharm Sci* 1985;74:603–607.
201. Inoue M, Okajima K, Itoh K, et al. Mechanisms of furosemide resistance in analbuminemic rats and hypoalbuminemic patients. *Kidney Int* 1987;32:198–203.
202. Kirchner KA, Voelker JR, Brater DC. Binding inhibitors restore furosemide potency in tubule fluid containing albumin. *Kidney Int* 1991;40:418–424.

25

NUTRITIONAL MANAGEMENT OF PATIENTS UNDERGOING MAINTENANCE HEMODIALYSIS

KAMYAR KALANTAR-ZADEH
JOEL D. KOPPLE

Protein-energy malnutrition (PEM) is common in patients undergoing maintenance hemodialysis (MHD). Up to 40% or more of patients undergoing MHD are reported to suffer from PEM (1–6). As discussed in detail in Chapter 12, there is a strong association between PEM and greater risk of morbidity and mortality (4,7–9). In particular, low body weight-for-height or body mass index (BMI), reduced serum cholesterol, albumin and prealbumin (transthyretin), and decreased protein intake have been shown to occur frequently in patients undergoing MHD and also are associated with increased risk of morbidity and mortality (10, 11). Other measures of PEM that are common in patients undergoing MHD but had not yet been shown to correlate with poor outcome include energy intake, mid-arm muscle circumference, skeletal muscle alkali soluble protein, and total body fat, among others. The relationship between outcome and some of these measures, such as low body weight-for-height (11) or BMI (10), and reduced serum cholesterol (12,13) in patients undergoing MHD are to a substantial degree in opposition to the epidemiologic relationships between nutritional measures and outcome that have been observed repeatedly in the general population (14). This paradoxical reversal of risk factors in patients undergoing MHD (the so-called "reverse epidemiology") (10) might underscore the importance of nutrition as a predictor for outcome in these individuals because body weight or serum cholesterol can be increased with the appropriate type of nutritional intake. This thesis (i.e., increasing nutritional intake will reduce mortality risk) still needs to be tested in randomized prospective clinical trials.

Inflammation, which also is associated with increased morbidity and mortality in patients undergoing MHD, itself may promote malnutrition by engendering both anorexia and a catabolic state (4,15). It is also possible but not proven that PEM actually may predispose to inflammation as well (4). The findings that measures of inflammation as well as PEM, either independently or combined, predict mortality and that there may be an interaction between inflammation and PEM have given rise to the concept of the "malnutrition-inflammation complex syndrome" (MICS) (4,7,15,16). The fact that mortality of patients undergoing MHD still averages about 20% per year in the United States emphasizes the importance of examining the causes of this high mortality in these individuals (17). The recently completed HEMO study failed to show an improvement in morbidity or mortality in patients undergoing MHD who were treated with higher dialysis dose (average single-pool Kt/V of 1.71 ± 0.11) versus lower dose (average single-pool Kt/V of 1.32 ± 0.09) and/or high-flux dialyzer membranes (18). This suggests the possibility that other factors such as PEM and/or inflammatory diseases may play a more central causal role in the poor outcome of this group of patients.

PEM is not the only form of malnutrition in patients undergoing MHD. It has long been recognized that patients undergoing MHD may suffer from deficiency of micronutrients as well. Deficiencies have been particularly commonly reported for such vitamins as ascorbate, folate, pyridoxine (vitamin B_6), and calcitriol (1,25-dihydroxycholecalciferol) (19–23) and for such minerals as iron and zinc (24–26). Some deficiencies, such as for ascorbate, carotenoids, and folate, could play an important role in the development of atherosclerotic cardiovascular diseases (27–29). Indeed, studies using food-frequency questionnaires have found a higher intake of atherogenic diets in patients undergoing MHD in association with inadequate ingestion of these antioxidant vitamins (30,31). Moreover, management of such important conditions as end-stage renal disease (ESRD)–associated anemia and osteodystrophy cannot be achieved without special attention to nutritional intake of such elements as iron, calcium, and phosphorus. However, excessive intake of a number of nutrients also can be hazardous in renal failure. This perhaps more commonly is shown for sodium, water, potassium, phosphorus, magnesium, calcium, and protein. For instance, excessive intake of calcium-containing foods and particularly medications may play a crucial role in the development of coronary artery calcification and the consequent increased rate of cardiovascular events in patients undergoing MHD (32,33).

Many factors have been implicated as the cause for malnutrition in patients with chronic kidney disease (CKD) or ESRD; these are described in detail in Chapters 11 and 23. This chapter focuses on the evaluation and management of the nutritional state in patients undergoing MHD.

FACTORS ALTERING NUTRIENT INTAKE IN PATIENTS UNDERGOING MAINTENANCE HEMODIALYSIS

Appetite is considered to be the gateway to the nutritional state. A diminished appetite occurs commonly in patients undergoing MHD and decreases the patient's ability to ingest a sufficient diet (34–36). Dietary protein intake (DPI) often is decreased in patients undergoing MHD. More strikingly, in almost all studies of nutritional intake, energy intake of individual patients undergoing MHD is below that of normal rather sedentary individuals and also is reduced below that recommended for MHD (6) (Chapter 11). A recent cross-sectional study in 331 patients undergoing MHD showed that at least 38% of the patients undergoing MHD reported reduced appetite, which was associated with a statistically significant decrease in their protein equivalent of total nitrogen appearance (PNA), also referred to as protein catabolic rate (PCR) (34). In this study a diminished appetite also was associated with decreased serum levels of such nutritional markers as prealbumin, total cholesterol, and total iron-binding capacity (TIBC) and increased serum levels of the inflammatory markers, C-reactive protein (CRP), interleukin-6 (IL-6), and tumor necrosis factor α (TNF-α). Moreover, patients undergoing MHD with a reduced appetite required higher doses of human recombinant erythropoietin and reported a lower quality of life and higher prospective mortality (34).

In contrast to patients undergoing chronic peritoneal dialysis (CPD), who frequently are encouraged to ingest foods high in potassium content, patients undergoing MHD often suffer from hyperkalemia, hyperphosphatemia, and excess sodium and water gain and therefore almost invariably are asked to reduce intake of foods rich in the aforementioned components. Such prescribed limitations in the diet of patients undergoing MHD may impose additional restrictions on their nutritional intake even with an intact appetite (30). Furthermore, the current interest in advocating antiatherogenic diets in patients undergoing MHD who have a high incidence and prevalence of atherosclerotic diseases may constrain further the ability of patients undergoing MHD to eat adequate energy, protein, and other nutrients (30). Dietary treatment of diabetes mellitus, which in patients undergoing MHD is very common (up to 55% of patients undergoing MHD in some parts of the United States) (17) and increasing in prevalence, leads to further dietary restriction. Also, many multimorbid and/or debilitated patients undergoing MHD have difficulty in procuring and preparing foods because of insufficient funds to purchase foods or physical or mental disabilities that may impair their capacity to shop, cook, or even ingest food (e.g., emotional depression or lack of dentures). An increased prevalence of metabolic acidemia and other catabolic comorbid conditions also may induce anorexia in patients undergoing MHD (35). Therefore, nutrient intake in patients undergoing MHD may be the most important single factor in the development and maintenance of malnutrition.

LOSS OF NUTRIENTS DURING MAINTENANCE HEMODIALYSIS TREATMENT

Several studies have examined amino acid losses during hemodialysis (37–39). Kopple et al. showed that free amino acid losses ranged from 4.5 to 7.7 g per hemodialysis in fasting patients who were undergoing dialysis with a Kiil dialyzer for 11 hours (37); 3.7 g (range, 2.4 to 5.2 g) of bound amino acids (e.g., peptides) also were lost into the dialysate. When patients were fed during the hemodialysis procedure, the free amino acid losses increased to about 5 to 8 g per hemodialysis. These studies were conducted with glucose-free dialysate. When dialysis was carried out with glucose in dialysate, 450 mg/dL (405 mg/dL of anhydrous glucose), free amino acid losses diminished to 3.3 g and 6.0 g in the fasted and nonfasted state, respectively. Gutierrez et al. were unable to confirm that dialysate with glucose-suppressed amino acid losses (40); however, these authors used a standard glucose concentration of 180 mg/dL in the dialysate. These latter investigators used the Baxter cellulose acetate and Gambro GFS plus 20 dialyzers and found 8.3 ± 0.9 SEM (standard error of the mean) g and 7.9 ± 0.4 g of amino acid losses with glucose-containing and glucose-free dialysate, respectively.

Wolfson et al. (38) described losses of about 8.2 ± 3.1 g SD of free amino acids during a 5-hour hemodialysis using 1.5-m^2 hollow fiber or 1.0 or 1.5 mL parallel plate dialyzers. When patients were given intravenous infusions of 39.5 g of amino acids and 200 g of d-glucose monohydrate during the hemodialysis, losses increased only slightly, to 12.6 ± 3.6 g. The retention of about 89% of the infused amino acids (68% of the infused amino acids if the amino acid losses during fasting losses are not discounted) was predictable because the plasma amino acid concentrations at the end of the hemodialysis with the amino acid and glucose infusion had increased by only 70% over the plasma amino acid levels obtained at the end of a hemodialysis without the infusion of the nutrients. Thus, it was not anticipated that large amounts of the infused amino acids would be removed by hemodialysis.

Ikizler et al. examined amino acid and protein losses in patients undergoing hemodialysis with three different types of dialyzer membranes (39). The patients ingested a small meal about 1 hour prior to the hemodialysis procedure. Patients undergoing hemodialysis with high-flux polysulfone (HF-PS) membranes lost 8.0 ± 2.8 g of amino acid per dialysis session as compared to patients dialyzed with low-flux polymethylmethacrylate membranes, who lost 6.1 ± 1.5 g of amino acids, and those dialyzed with cellulose acetate membranes, who lost 7.1 ± 2.6 g. These small differences in amino acid losses may be the result of variations in the dialyzer surface area and blood flow rates and are probably biologically insignificant.

It should be noted that protein losses during hemodialysis are typically very small. However, several years ago, reuse of HF-PS dialyzers after reprocessing with bleach and formaldehyde resulted in a rather marked increase in protein losses as a result of increased permeability of these membranes (39,41). Ikizler et al. (39) found that albumin losses became apparent after the sixth reuse of the HF-PS membrane. These losses increased significantly, from 1.5 ± 1.3 SD g per dialysis session by the fifteenth reuse to 9.3 ± 5.5 g at the twentieth. Kaplan et al. observed similar results (41). The amino acid losses increased slightly, by 50%, after the sixth reuse in the HF-PS membranes. More recently, polysulfone membranes have been made more resistant to bleach that is used in the reuse process.

Blood sequestered in the hemodialyzer, clotted or leaking dialyzers, oozing of blood from the needle punctures of the vascular access site, and blood sampling for laboratory testing may contribute to protein losses. Approximately 5 to 10 mL of blood may be trapped in the dialyzer at the end of each dialysis. This could account for another 0.6 to 1.6 g of protein lost per dialysis session (42).

Several investigators have described a high prevalence of acidosis in patients undergoing MHD, as indicated by low predialysis serum bicarbonate concentrations (43–45). Metabolic acidemia has been shown to promote bone reabsorption and engender protein catabolism. It is, therefore, important to treat acidemia. The National Kidney Foundation Kidney Disease Outcomes Quality Initiative (NKF-K/DOQI) *Clinical Practice Guidelines for Nutrition in Chronic Renal Failure* recommends that the serum bicarbonate concentration should be maintained at or above 22 mEq/L (46). Some recent information suggests that the serum bicarbonate concentration should be maintained higher (47), possibly 24 mEq/L if not greater.

It has been argued that the hemodialysis procedure itself may be catabolic. Gutierrez et al. (48,49) demonstrated enhanced release of amino acids from the skeletal muscle of individuals who were sham-dialyzed with Cuprophan (Membrana, Wuppertal, Germany) dialyzers; no dialysate was used in these studies, and the investigators exclusively examined blood-membrane or blood-tubing interactions. This amino acid release could be abolished by pretreatment with indomethacin, suggesting that prostaglandins were involved in the genesis of the catabolic effects. The data of Borah et al. (50) also suggest that hemodialysis may induce catabolism, although the nitrogen balance studies were short term and the lack of time for equilibration after changing the DPI inadvertently may have prejudiced their findings.

It has been argued that the activation of complement and leukocytes by less biocompatible dialyzer membranes may lead to release of such proinflammatory cytokines as TNF-α, IL-1, IL-6, and granulocyte proteases (15,51–53). Oxidative stress also may play a central role in activation of the inflammatory cascade in patients undergoing MHD (54). The proinflammatory cytokines can induce catabolism (55–57). In recent years, increasing attention has been paid to the role of inflammation as a cause of the hypercatabolic state in patients undergoing MHD (4,15,58). Indeed, some investigators maintain that inflammation plays a primary role in the complex constellation of malnutrition-inflammation-atherosclerosis (the MIA syndrome) (59), whereas others suggest that anorexia, inadequate nutritional intake, and nutrient losses as well as inflammation may predispose to tissue wasting. Inflammation appears to promote anorexia, inadequate intake, and protein catabolism, whereas PEM also might predispose to inflammation (4), although evidence for this is still preliminary. Thus, the previously mentioned term "malnutrition-inflammation complex syndrome" (MICS) may be a more appropriate appellation (4, 10,60). Recent data also suggest the intriguing possibility that metabolic acidemia may predispose to inflammation (6).

Nutrient losses during MHD are not restricted to protein and amino acids; other macronutrients and micronutrients also may be lost. Gutierrez et al. (40) found that about 26 g of glucose were removed during a hemodialysis with glucose-free dialysate and about 30 g of glucose were absorbed by the patient when dialysate-containing glucose, 180 mg/dL, was used. Wathen et al. obtained similar results (61). The quantities of water-soluble vitamins lost during hemodialysis are not large because plasma concentrations of the water-soluble vitamins are not great and the molecular weights of these compounds are somewhat larger (i.e., greater than many amino acids). Losses are particularly prone to occur for vitamins B_1 (thiamin), B_2 (riboflavin), and B_6 (pyridoxine); ascorbic acid; and folic acid (19,22, 23,62–64). Although vitamin B_{12} is water soluble, its losses during hemodialysis are negligible because it is largely protein bound in plasma. The losses of these vitamins in dialysate are to some extent offset by the lack of urinary vitamin excretion in patients undergoing MHD. Thus, the removal of water-soluble vitamins by hemodialysis is easily replaceable by food intake and supplements of vitamins. The losses of vitamins during hemodialysis are discussed in more detail in Chapter 20.

IMPORTANCE OF PROTEIN-ENERGY MALNUTRITION AND DIET AS PATIENTS APPROACH END-STAGE RENAL DISEASE AND COMMENCE MAINTENANCE HEMODIALYSIS

Data suggest that the nutritional status of both pediatric and adult patients at the onset of maintenance dialysis is a predictor of their nutritional status 1 or 2 years later (6, 65–67), although nutritional status may undergo improvement with the advent of dialysis therapy. Thus, to prevent malnutrition in patients undergoing MHD, it would seem important to monitor the nutritional status and to endeavor to prevent malnutrition from occurring in patients before MHD is instituted (i.e., during progressive phases of CKD) (Chapter 23). In this regard, many patients become frankly anorectic, eat poorly, and sustain a deterioration in their nutritional and clinical status prior to the onset of dialysis therapy and particularly between the time when their glomerular filtration rate (GFR) decreases to about 5 to 10 mL/min (CKD stage 5) and the time when they are established on MHD therapy (68). It follows that steps should be taken to ensure a smooth transition to MHD when the patient has stage 4 or 5 of CKD (i.e., creatinine clearance less than 30 ml/min) (69).

Indeed, the NKF-K/DOQI Nutrition Work Group has recommended the following as a nutritional indication for commencing renal replacement therapy in individuals with advanced CKD: "In patients with chronic renal failure (e.g., GFR <15–20 mL/min) who are not undergoing maintenance dialysis, if protein-energy malnutrition develops or persists despite vigorous attempts to optimize protein and energy intake and there is no apparent cause for malnutrition other than low nutrient intake, initiation of maintenance dialysis or a renal transplant is recommended (70)."

ASSESSMENT OF NUTRITIONAL STATUS IN PATIENTS UNDERGOING MAINTENANCE HEMODIALYSIS

Because malnutrition can be insidious in patients undergoing MHD, their nutritional status should be assessed when they commence MHD and at monthly intervals thereafter (Chapter 15 and Tables 25.1 and 25.2). Moreover, because

TABLE 25.1. RECOMMENDED MEASURES FOR MONITORING NUTRITIONAL STATUS OF PATIENTS UNDERGOING MAINTENANCE HEMODIALYSIS BASED ON NATIONAL KIDNEY FOUNDATION KIDNEY/DIALYSIS OUTCOME QUALITY INITIATIVE GUIDELINES

Category	Measure	Minimum Frequency of Measurement
I. Measurements that should be performed routinely in all patients	Predialysis or stabilized serum albumin	Monthly
	% of usual postdialysis body weight, body mass index[a] and interdialytic weight gain[a]	Monthly
	% of standard (NHANES II) body weight	Every 4 months
	Subjective global assessment	Every 6 months
	Dietary interview and/or diary	Every 6 months
	nPNA (nPCR)	Monthly
II. Measures that can be useful to confirm or extend the data obtained from the measures in Category I	Predialysis or stabilized serum prealbumin (transthyretin)	As needed
	Skinfold thickness	As needed
	Midarm muscle area, circumference, or diameter	As needed
	Dual energy x-ray absorptiometry	As needed
III. Clinically useful measures, which, if low, might suggest the need for a more rigorous examination of protein-energy nutritional status	Predialysis or stabilized serum	
	—Creatinine	As needed
	—Urea nitrogen	As needed
	—Cholesterol	As needed
	Creatinine index	

NHANES, National Health and Nutrition Evaluation Survey; nPNA, normalized protein equivalent of total nitrogen appearance; nPCR, normalized protein catabolic rate.
From Clinical practice guidelines for nutrition in chronic renal failure. K/DOQI, National Kidney Foundation. *Am J Kidney Dis* 2000;35:S1–S140, with permission.

TABLE 25.2. ADDITIONAL RECOMMENDED MEASURES FOR MONITORING NUTRITIONAL STATUS OF PATIENTS UNDERGOING MAINTENANCE HEMODIALYSIS (SEE ALSO TABLE 25.1)

IV. Additional measures and tools	Serum calcium, phosphorus, and Ca-P product	Monthly
	Serum potassium	Monthly
	Serum bicarbonate, anion gap	Every 3 months
	Serum TIBC or transferrin, iron saturation ratio	Monthly
	Serum ferritin	Every 3 months
	Lipid panel: total cholesterol, triglyceride, LDL and HDL cholesterol	Every 6 months
	Serum C-reactive protein[a]	Every 3 to 6 months
	Plasma total homocysteine	Every 12 months

TIBC, total iron-binding capacity; LDL, low-density lipoprotein; HDL, high-density lipoprotein.
[a]Other inflammatory markers in serum that may be increased include interleukin-6 (IL-6), IL-1β, and tumor necrosis factor alpha (TNF-α).

of the strong association between the nutritional state and outcome in patients undergoing MHD and because of the high mortality and hospitalization rate in these individuals, many nutritional markers are outcome predictors. For example, serum albumin, serum creatinine, and body weight-for-height or BMI are independently associated with survival (71). Data from the United States Renal Data System confirm these findings, using the serum albumin and BMI (kg/m^2) (72). In the Canada-USA Study, both the serum albumin and Subjective Global Assessment (SGA) of nutrition were independent predictors of death or treatment failure (73). Chapter 12 includes an outcome-oriented approach to the nutritional assessment of patients with renal failure.

The NKF-K/DOQI guidelines include comprehensive recommendations pertaining to the nutritional and dietary assessment of patients undergoing MHD. According to these guidelines, nutritional status in patients undergoing MHD should be assessed with a combination of valid, complementary measures rather than any single measure alone because there is no single measure that provides a comprehensive indication of protein-energy nutritional status (Table 25.1). Moreover, measures of energy and protein intake, visceral protein pools, muscle mass, other dimensions of body composition, and functional status identify different aspects of protein-energy nutritional status, and malnutrition may be identified with greater sensitivity and specificity using a combination of factors. The NKF-K/DOQI guidelines recommend that nutritional status of patients undergoing MHD should be assessed routinely by predialysis or stabilized serum albumin, percent of usual body weight, percent of standard (National Health and Nutrition Evaluation Survey II) body weight, SGA, dietary interviews and diaries, and nPNA (69). Table 25.1 shows a list of parameters and tools to evaluate nutritional status and the assessment intervals as recommended by NKF-K/DOQI.

NKF-K/DOQI nutritional assessment guidelines include three categories. The first category includes those measurements that should be performed routinely on all patients undergoing MHD. Serum albumin should be assessed monthly as should the percentage of posthemodialysis body weight, but percentage of standard body weight may be evaluated every 4 months (see Table 25.1). There is no specific recommendation regarding the BMI, but because of the ease of its calculation based on posthemodialysis dry weight and height (weight in kg divided by height in meters squared) many health care workers in dialysis facilities calculate and evaluate the BMI routinely on a monthly to quarterly basis. For routine overall assessment, the conventional version of the SGA (74–78) (Chapter 15) and/or its newer derivatives such as the Malnutrition-Inflammation Score (MIS) (34,79) (Chapter 12) should be evaluated semiannually. The NKF-K/DOQI guidelines recommend calculating nPNA (also known as nPCR) every month.

The second category (Table 25.1) includes those measures that can be useful to confirm or extend data obtained from the measures in Category 1. Serum prealbumin (transthyretin) has a strong association with hospitalization and mortality and, like serum albumin, is a negative acute-phase reactant (80,81). Caliper anthropometry can be used to measure skinfold thicknesses, usually obtained in the biceps, triceps, and subscapular and suprailiac areas (an indicator of body fat mass). Midarm muscle circumference (an indicator of skeletal muscle mass) as well as its area and diameter can be measured simultaneously. Anthropometry should be carried out by personnel who have been trained specifically in these techniques and who have accurate and reliable equipment, which is not expensive. Although body-composition parameters, such as the percentage of body fat, can be assessed by such convenient methods as bioelectrical impedance analysis (BIA) (82,83) or near infrared interactance (NIR) (84), a more objective method of estimating body composition, dual energy X-ray absorptiometry

(DEXA), is the recommended technique according to the NKF-K/DOQI guidelines (85,86). Although the availability of these energy-beam based methods (DEXA, BIA, NIR) is increasing, their routine use is still largely limited to the research setting and a few health care center clinical treatment programs (4,86,87). There is not yet evidence that the use of these techniques improves the management or outcome of patients undergoing MHD over the generally simpler methods of nutritional assessment indicated in the Category I level of Table 25.1.

The third category includes several clinically useful measures, which, if low, might suggest the need for a more rigorous examination of protein-energy nutritional status. These consist of serum concentrations of creatinine, urea nitrogen, and cholesterol as well as the creatinine index (Table 25.1). The NKF-K/DOQI nutritional guidelines do not recommend serum TIBC, which is a reliable estimator of serum transferrin, because serum TIBC concentrations are influenced by inflammation and iron stores as well as by protein-energy nutritional status (69). However, recent studies in patients undergoing MHD have shown a strong association between serum TIBC and such nutritional markers as SGA and also between TIBC and outcome (77, 88,89). Many of the biochemical measurements are influenced by nonnutritional factors. For example, serum albumin is affected by the hydration status as well as by acute illness and inflammation (90,91). Serum albumin, prealbumin, and TIBC are negative acute-phase reactants (15,92). Serum creatinine and urea nitrogen also strongly reflect the dose of dialysis. Notwithstanding these factors, a number of epidemiologic studies have demonstrated clearly that these common laboratory measurements are strong predictors of hospitalization and death in patients undergoing MHD (13, 72,93,94). Dietary history also can provide a useful estimate of the patient's intake of protein, energy, and other nutrients. However, the services of a trained dietitian are almost always required to achieve acceptable accuracy. More convenient, self-administered food frequency questionnaires (FFQ) also been have used to compare dietary intake of patients undergoing MHD with other individuals; however, FFQs may not be sufficiently precise, and they tend to underestimate food intake (30). Their use essentially is limited to epidemiologic studies.

Because the foregoing recommendations are based on NKF-K/DOQI guidelines that focus mainly on protein and energy malnutrition (69), we propose an addendum (Table 25.2) for some important nutritional parameters that are not recommended for monitoring in the original NKF-K/DOQI panel. In many dialysis facilities, serum concentrations of potassium, calcium, and phosphorus are measured routinely on a monthly basis as are iron status indicators including serum ferritin, TIBC, and iron saturation ratio. At least biannual measurements of serum lipids including total serum cholesterol and low-density lipoprotein (LDL) are recommended because an increasing proportion of patients undergoing MHD, particularly those with diabetes mellitus, are hyperlipidemic. However, a low serum cholesterol is a strong predictor of poor outcome in patients undergoing dialysis (12,13). Although inflammatory markers currently are not measured routinely, we recommend that at least CRP be measured every several months, so that high-risk patients with inflammation can be identified (95). Finally, total plasma homocysteine is a cardiovascular risk factor and also a nutritional marker. Both high (96) and low (97,98) levels have been associated with poor outcome in patients undergoing MHD.

UREA KINETIC, ADEQUACY OF DIALYSIS, AND NUTRITIONAL STATUS

The urea nitrogen appearance (UNA) is used to estimate nitrogen losses and, hence, in the steady state, nitrogen intake. UNA is the quantity of nitrogen that appears in the urine, dialysate, and all other outputs plus the change in body urea nitrogen. The PNA (PCR) expresses total nitrogen appearance in terms of the equivalent amount of protein lost that is represented by the UNA (99,100). In patients undergoing MHD the UNA is calculated directly from urea kinetics by techniques that have been discussed extensively elsewhere (100,101). PNA can be calculated from the UNA by one of several formulas (99,101,102). Under steady-state conditions, the UNA also can be used to estimate the dietary nitrogen intake. Because of nitrogen losses through pathways that are difficult to measure (e.g., respiration, sweat, exfoliated skin, hair and nail growth, flatus, blood drawing), the UNA and PNA essentially always underestimate the dietary nitrogen or protein intake under metabolic steady-state conditions. Hence, a different regression equation must be used to estimate DPI, as compared to the PNA, from the UNA (99,100). A fuller discussion of these terms and the methods for calculating these processes in nondialyzed patients and patients undergoing MHD is given in Chapter 23 and elsewhere (103).

Several studies have shown a correlation between the prescribed dose of hemodialysis as defined by the Kt/V_{urea} and the DPI as estimated from the PNA (104–107). The direct relationship between Kt/V and PNA also has been observed in patients undergoing CPD (104,108,109), although the slope of the relationship is different in the patients undergoing CPD as compared to patients undergoing MHD (104). Some studies of patients undergoing MHD described a direct correlation between Kt/V and serum albumin levels (107). However, most of these studies correlating Kt/V and PNA or serum albumin were not prospective or randomized, and conclusions from these studies therefore must be considered tentative. Lindsay et al. (110) showed a direct relation between Kt/V and PNA in a prospective, randomized study in which Kt/V was increased from 0.82 ± 0.19 (SD) to 1.32 ± 0.21 for 3 months in one of the two groups of patients. The PNA rose in the experimental group from an initial value of 0.81 ± 0.08 g/kg/day to 1.02 ± 0.15 (p = 0.005), whereas it did not change in the control group. These studies suggest that increasing the dose of hemodialysis from a Kt/V of roughly 0.6 to a Kt/V_{sp} of which 1.5 to 1.6 will increase the DPI of patients undergoing MHD. Harty et al. have pointed out that in patients undergoing MHD the correlation between Kt/V_{urea} and PNA is partly a consequence of mathematic coupling because the two parameters are obtained from the same plasma predialysis and postdialysis measurements and also are normalized to body size (111). However, others have shown that a significant correlation exists between dialysis dose and DPI even when dialysis dose is not normalized for body size and when DPI is estimated by dietary histories (112, 113).

It should be emphasized that the correlation between Kt/V_{urea} and PNA, although significant, is not precise, and many patients with a relatively high Kt/V (i.e., = 1.5 for hemodialysis) have a very low PNA and, hence, a reduced DPI (105–107,110). This is not surprising because many patients undergoing MHD have comorbid conditions that may lead to a reduction in the DPI independent of their uremic status. Moreover, there are currently no data as to what extent the Kt/V_{urea} affects the dietary energy intake. A recent prospective study of 122 patients undergoing MHD who were dialyzed adequately (i.e., with a delivered average Kt/V >1.20 [single pool] over the first 3 months of the cohort) independent of their residual renal function, showed strong associations between normalized PNA (nPNA), measured for 3 months and the subsequent 12-month hospitalization and mortality rates (101). In this latter study, delivered Kt/V ranged from 1.23 to 2.71 (1.77 ± 0.34) and nPNA ranged from 0.5 to 2.15 (1.13 ± 0.29 g/kg/day). The nPNA and Kt/V did not correlate significantly (r = .09) except when analysis was limited to Kt/V values of less than 1.5 (r = .54) (Fig. 25.1). nPNA and albumin were the only variables with statistically significant correlations with three different measures of hospitalization and mortality (101). These data are consistent with the possibility that protein intake affects the clinical course of patients undergoing MHD even in the setting of an adequate to high dose of dialysis. Moreover, the so-called mathematic coupling between Kt/V and nPCR found in older studies does not appear to occur when Kt/V is greater than 1.50. Studies based on randomized assignments to different protein intakes will be necessary to confirm these conclusions. Current NKF-K/DOQI recommendations are to provide patients undergoing MHD with a Kt/V_{urea} dose of at least 1.20 (114); for many dialysis facilities, the Kt/V target is 1.40 or higher. However, the HEMO study failed to show any improvement in hospitalization or mortality with Kt/V (single pool) values of 1.71 ± 0.11 SE (standard error) as compared to 1.32 ± 0.09 (18), a result that is not consistent with many epidemiologic studies based on large sample sizes of 1,000 to 40,000 patients undergoing MHD (115–118).

ACIDOSIS AND PROTEIN WASTING

Experimental evidence suggests that acidemia may enhance protein catabolism (119–126). In rats, acidemia has been shown to increase the activity of branched-chain ketoacid dehydrogenase, which participates in the catabolism of branched-chain amino acids (119). Bergström et al. (125) found a linear correlation between predialysis plasma bicarbonate levels and muscle-free valine, suggesting that even

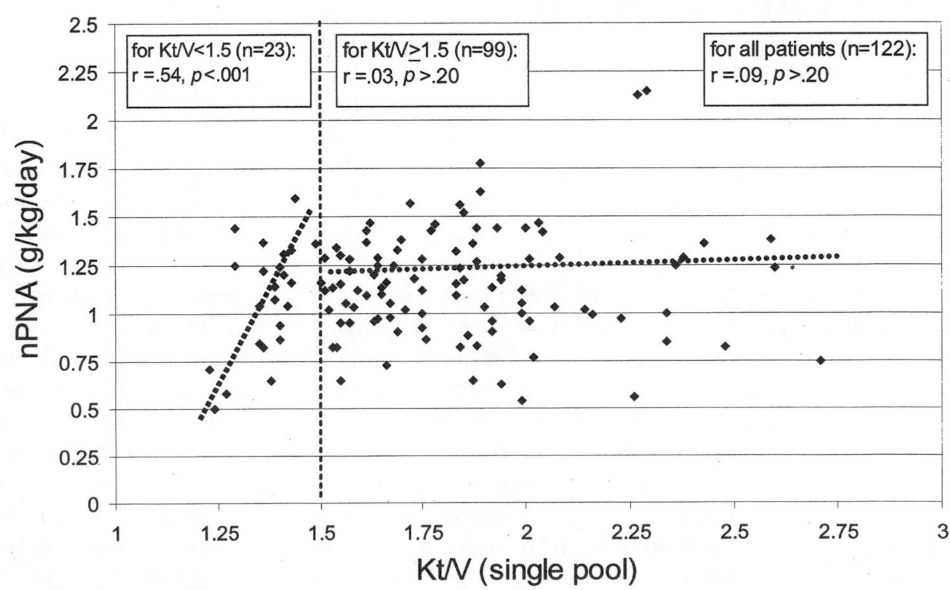

FIGURE 25.1. Exploring the association between normalized protein nitrogen appearance (nPNA) and Kt/V_{sp} in 122 patients undergoing maintenance hemodialysis with a Kt/V_{sp} value of more than 1.20. No significant correlation existed between these two urea kinetic indices despite their known mathematic association (r = .09, p >.20). However, by dividing the patients into two distinct subgroups based on a Kt/V_{sp} cutoff of 1.50, there was a strong, significant correlation between Kt/V and nPNA for the lower Kt/V_{sp} values less than 1.50 (r = .54, p <.001), whereas there was essentially no correlation at higher Kt/V_{sp} values (r = .03, p >.20). (From Kalantar-Zadeh K, Supasyndh O, Lehn RS, et al. Normalized protein nitrogen appearance is correlated with hospitalization and mortality in hemodialysis patients with Kt/V greater than 1.20. *J Ren Nutr* 2003; 13:15–25, with permission.)

transient acidemia may enhance amino acid degradation. Acidemia also increases protein catabolism in skeletal muscle of normal rats and rats with chronic renal failure (CRF) (121), increases total body protein catabolism, and induces negative nitrogen balance in humans with CRF (127). Normal individuals made acutely acidemic develop reduced albumin synthesis rates and negative nitrogen balance (128). The acidemia-induced increased proteolysis in skeletal muscle appears to be caused by enhanced activity of the ATP (adenosine triphosphate)-dependent ubiquitin–proteosome pathway (122,124).

Because patients undergoing MHD often have low predialysis serum bicarbonate concentrations (43–45,104), acidemia may be common in these patients, at least predialysis. However, low serum bicarbonate is not proof of acidemia; direct measurements of blood pH will provide more definitive information. Nonetheless, the evidence from the foregoing studies that acidemia is harmful appears to be so strong that we currently recommend that bicarbonate supplements be given, when needed, to maintain serum bicarbonate of 22 mEq/L or higher throughout the interdialytic interval unless the low serum bicarbonate levels are shown to be associated with a normal blood pH. This is consistent with the NKF-K/DOQI guidelines on nutrition (69).

GOALS OF NUTRITIONAL MANAGEMENT OF PATIENTS UNDERGOING MAINTENANCE HEMODIALYSIS

The goals of dietary therapy and nutritional interventions in patients undergoing MHD are the following: (a) to achieve and maintain good nutritional status; (b) to prevent or retard the development of cardiovascular, cerebrovascular, and peripheral vascular diseases; (b) to prevent or treat hyperparathyroidism and other forms of renal osteodystrophy; and (d) to prevent or ameliorate uremic toxicity and other nutritionally influenced metabolic disorders that occur in renal failure and that are not treated adequately by MHD. Compliance to special diets is often a challenging endeavor for patients undergoing MHD and their families. It may require a significant change in their dietary habits as well as their behavioral pattern. They often are required to limit the intake of favorite foods and ingest certain less desirable ones to avoid hyperkalemia or hyperphosphatemia. Patients undergoing MHD often ingest too little of a required nutrient rather than too much. To enable patients undergoing MHD to achieve the desired goals, it is important that they be educated in the principles of dietary therapy and its targets. Patients and their spouses or other close associates should be instructed in the nutritional content of various foods as well as the preparation of prescribed diets. Even patients who appear to have no interest in dietary management may benefit from nutritional therapy for several reasons. First, they may decide in the future to follow dietary therapy. Second, even if the patient adheres poorly to the diet, this is better than no adherence. Finally, nutrition, education, and encouragement may prevent nonadherent patients from deviating further from good nutrient intake, particularly as they age or are subjected to emotional or physical stress. Chapters 36 and 37 review methods for preparing patients for dietary therapy and maximizing compliance and indicate menu planning and some food preparations and supplements available for patients with CRF.

DIETARY NUTRIENT REQUIREMENTS

Protein Requirements

Table 25.3 includes dietary nutrient requirements for patients undergoing MHD. Surprisingly few studies have assessed the dietary protein requirements for these patients (1,50,129–131). Moreover, there is not a single randomized prospective clinical trial in which patients undergoing MHD were randomly assigned to different levels of DPI as the independent variable and the effect of protein intake on morbidity and mortality was examined. The publications that address protein requirements are of two types:

1. Several prospective studies compared the effects of different DPIs on the nutritional status of the patients; these studies used measures of nutritional status as the indication of a beneficial clinical response. Most of these studies were carried out in hospital research wards or clinical facilities modified for research activities, and the numbers of patients included in each study were small (130–132). It is noteworthy that most of these studies addressing protein requirements in patients undergoing hemodialysis were carried out several years ago and used dialyzers and dialyzer clearances that are no longer in use (131,132).
2. The other type of study involved retrospective analyses in larger numbers of patients of the relationships between DPI, assessed from the nPNA, and morbidity or mortality (1,133).

The NKF-K/DOQI guidelines on nutrition in CRF recommends a DPI for clinically stable patients undergoing MHD of 1.2 g/kg body weight/day; at least 50% of the dietary protein should be of high biologic value to ensure adequate intake of essential amino acids (70). These recommendations are based on the level of protein intake that, for the great majority of patients undergoing MHD, will maintain neutral or positive nitrogen balance and lead to maintenance or improvement in other such markers of nutritional status as serum albumin (70). Many patients undergoing MHD will maintain protein balance with lower DPIs (70). However, this protein intake is considered to be about the minimum level that will maintain neutral or positive nitrogen balance in the great majority, approximately 97%, of clinically stable patients undergoing MHD.

TABLE 25.3. RECOMMENDED DIETARY NUTRIENT INTAKE FOR ADULT PATIENTS UNDERGOING MAINTENANCE HEMODIALYSIS

Macronutrients and fiber	
Dietary protein intake (DPI)[a]	1.2 g/kg body weight/day for clinically stable patients undergoing MHD (at least 50% of the dietary protein should be of high biologic value) ≥ 1.2 to 1.3 g/kg/day for acutely ill patients
Dietary energy intake (DEI)[b]	35 kcal/kg body weight/day for those who are less than 60 years of age, and 30 to 35 kcal/kg body weight/day for individuals 60 years or older
Total fat intake[c,d]	30% of total energy intake
Saturated fat[c]	Up to 10% of total energy intake
Polyunsaturated fatty acids[c]	Up to 10% of total calories
Monounsaturated fatty acids[c]	Up to 20% of total calories
Carbohydrate[c,d,e]	Rest of nonprotein calories
Total fiber[f]	20–25 g/day
Minerals and water (range of intake)	
Sodium	750 to 2,000 mg/day
Potassium	Up to 70–80 mEq/day
Phosphorus[g]	10–17 mg/kg/day
Calcium[h]	≤ 1,000 mg/day
Magnesium	200–300 mg/day
Iron[i]	See text
Zinc	15 mg/day
Water	Usually 750–1,500 mL/day
Vitamins (including dietary supplements)	
Vitamin B_1 (thiamin)	1.1–1.2 mg/day
Vitamin B_2 (riboflavin)	1.1–1.3 mg/day
Pantothenic acid	5 mg/day
Biotin	30 μg/day
Niacin	14–16 mg/day
Vitamin B_6 (pyridoxine)	10 mg/day
Vitamin B_{12}	2.4 μg/day
Vitamin C	75–90 mg/day
Folic acid[j]	1–10 mg/day
Vitamin A	See text
Vitamin D	See text
Vitamin E[k]	400–800 IU (optional—see text)
Vitamin K[l]	See text

MHD, maintenance hemodialysis.
[a,b]According to Clinical practice guidelines for nutrition in chronic failure. K/DOQI, National Kidney Foundation. *Am J Kidney Dis* 2000;35:S1–S140, with permission.
[b]Refers to percent of total energy intake (diet plus dialysate).
[c]Although atherosclerotic vascular disease constitutes a common and serious problem for patients undergoing MHD, these recommendations often are hard to adhere to. Moreover, there is no prospective interventional study indicating these dietary modifications are beneficial for patients undergoing MHD, although, reasonably, the potential benefits of these modifications seem valuable. They are strongly recommended only if patients adhere closely to more critical aspects of the diet (e.g., sodium, water, potassium, phosphorus, protein, and energy intake) and have expressed a particular interest in these modifications or have a specific disorder that may respond to their medications.
[d]Refers to percent of total energy intake; if triglyceride levels are very high, the percentage of fat in the diet may be increased to about 35% of total calories; otherwise, 25% to 30% of total calories is preferable. Intake of fatty acids should be kept low because they raise low-density-lipoprotein cholesterol (see text).
[e]Should be primarily complex carbohydrates.
[f]Less critical to adhere to for the typical patient undergoing MHD.
[g]Phosphate binders (aluminum carbonate or hydroxide, or calcium carbonate or acetate) often are needed to maintain normal serum phosphorus levels.
[h]These calcium intakes commonly are ingested because of the use of calcium binders of phosphate. Excess calcium intake must be avoided (see text).
[i]Iron requirements vary according to the dose of administered erythropoietin.
[j]Folic acid 1 mg/day should be routine, but up to 10 mg/day may be given to reduce elevated plasma homocysteine levels.
[k]Vitamin E, 300 or 800 IU day, may be given to reduce oxidative stress and prevent cardiovascular disease, but the value of these supplements is controversial (see text and Chapter 20).
[l]Vitamin K supplements may be needed for patients who are not eating and who receive antibiotics.

These are the same nitrogen balance criteria used for determining the recommended dietary protein allowances for the general population by both the World Health Organization and the Food and Nutrition Board, National Research Council of the United States National Academy of Sciences (70,134). Because, *a priori*, it is generally impossible to ascertain which MHD may maintain protein balance on lower levels of protein intake, this quantity of dietary protein is recommended. The nitrogen balance data on which this recommended protein intake is based are surprisingly sparse, and more research clearly is indicated in this area. A brief review of the research to date is as follows.

Ginn et al. carried out nitrogen balance studies in four men who were undergoing MHD twice weekly (131). Two of these patients were fed 18 g protein/day and were in severely negative nitrogen balance. The two other patients, who were anephric, were fed higher protein diets. Their nitrogen balance was positive when they ingested 0.8 g/kg/day of primarily high biologic value protein. Nitrogen balance was sometimes negative with higher protein diets when the protein was of low biologic value. These patients almost certainly were malnourished, and this factor, as well as the reduced (by present standards) frequency of hemodialysis, might have accounted for their positive nitrogen balance with such low protein intakes. In an outpatient study of at least 6 months duration, Shinaberger and Ginn reported that 10 patients who ingested 0.75 g/kg/day showed improvement in nutritional status (135). Again many of these patients were malnourished at the onset of study. Also, provision of dialysis only twice weekly could have lowered amino acid and peptide losses into dialysate and reduced the catabolic stress of hemodialysis (see earlier in this chapter). These two factors may have increased the patient's ability to develop an anabolic response on this low protein intake. Also, the daily protein intake of these outpatients probably exceeded the prescribed 0.75 g/kg/day.

Kopple et al. carried out nitrogen balance studies on three patients who were living in a metabolic balance unit and were undergoing MHD for 11 hours twice weekly with a Kiil dialyzer (132). Each patient was fed two isocaloric diets that provided 0.75 or 1.25 g protein/kg/day for about 3 weeks with each diet. The two diets provided, respectively, 0.63 and 0.88 g/kg/day of high biologic value protein. Nitrogen balance, after equilibration and adjusted for unmeasured losses, was negative or neutral with the 0.75 g protein/kg/day diet and strongly positive with the diet providing 1.25 g protein/kg/day. Kopple et al. then carried out an outpatient study in 23 patients who were randomly assigned to receive either diet while they were treated twice weekly with hemodialysis for 10 to 12 hours with Kiil dialyzers. The patients prescribed the lower protein diet were estimated to have ingested closer to 0.8 to 0.9 g protein/kg/day, whereas the patients receiving the higher protein prescription ingested about 1.1 to 1.2 g/kg/day of protein. The lower protein diet group demonstrated a slight but statistically significant gain in serum albumin and body weight. In contrast, patients prescribed the higher protein diet demonstrated a statistically significant increase in both serum albumin and body weight. Borah et al. studied five patients undergoing hemodialysis given either 0.50 or 1.44 g protein/kg/day under metabolic balance conditions (50). Each diet was used for only 7 days. They concluded that the lower protein diet caused negative nitrogen balance, whereas the higher protein intake maintained neutral or positive nitrogen balance.

Slomowitz et al. carried out metabolic balance studies in six patients undergoing MHD who lived in a clinical research center for 63 to 65 days each and underwent hemodialysis for 4 hours three times weekly with Cuprophan or cellulose acetate dialyzers (136). This study was carried out to assess the dietary energy requirements of the patients (see later in this chapter), but some of the data obtained may be relevant to the dietary protein needs of patients undergoing MHD. These individuals were fed a constant protein diet throughout the study that provided 1.13 ± 0.02 SEM g protein/kg/day. All patients were fed, in random fashion, three different dietary energy intakes for 21 to 23 days each that provided 25, 35, or 45 kcal/kg/day. Of the six patients, the number that were in neutral or positive nitrogen balance with the 25, 35, and 45 kcal/kg/day intakes were, respectively, one (possibly), four, and six individuals. Because the usual energy intake of clinically stable patients undergoing MHD is less than 30 kcal/kg/day (137), these results suggest that for many of the patients undergoing MHD who ingest about 25 or even 35 kcal/kg/day, a DPI of 1.1 g/kg/day may not be sufficiently great to maintain protein balance. The nitrogen balance data with the energy intake of 35 kcal/kg/day and protein intake of 1.1 ± 0.02 SEM g/kg/day are shown in Table 25.4 (136).

Thus, these nitrogen balance studies suggest that some clinically stable MHD will not maintain protein balance with DPIs of 1.1 g protein/kg/day and adequate energy intakes (see later in this chapter). Therefore, the NKF-K/DOQI recommendation, following the general principles used for determining the RDA [(i.e., an intake that should satisfy the nutritional needs of about 97% of the general population (70,134)], proposed somewhat higher DPIs. The dietary protein level selected to be the recommended (i.e., safe) amount for stable patients undergoing MHD was 1.2 g protein/kg/day. According to this methodologic approach, many patients undergoing MHD will maintain protein balance with lower protein intakes. However, there is no way to identify prospectively who these patients are. Therefore, safety concerns suggest recommending this higher intake. Moreover, with the current doses of hemodialysis used, a protein intake of 1.20 g/kg/day will not induce uremic toxicity. Thus, we believe that, until more data are available, the current NKF-K/DOQI recommendations are safe and justifiable. Clearly more information concerning protein requirements is needed.

TABLE 25.4. NITROGEN BALANCE DATA IN SIX PATIENTS UNDERGOING MAINTENANCE HEMODIALYSIS[a] INGESTING A DIET PROVIDING ABOUT 1.13 G PROTEIN/KG/DAY AND ABOUT 35 KCAL/KG/DAY

Gender	Age (years)	Body Weight (kg)	Energy Intake per kg Actual Body Weight (kcal/kg/day)	Duration of Study (days)	Stable Period (days)[b]	Nitrogen Intake[c]	Urine Nitrogen	Fecal Nitrogen	Dialysate Nitrogen (g/day)	Total Nitrogen Output[d]	Adjusted Nitrogen Balance[e]
Female	61	60.6	35.8	21	14	11.0	0.78	0.68	7.40	8.86	+2.09
Female	64	73.6	31.3	21	7	11.4	0.20	1.15	9.15	10.50	+0.68
Male	46	73.3	35.6	21	14	13.4	0.84	0.99	10.52	12.35	+1.02
Male	43	58	45.4	21	7	14.0	0	1.60	12.07	13.67	+0.06
Male	24	51.4	41.2	21	14	11.2	0.12	1.14	8.80	10.06	+0.61
Male	42	70.5	34.5	21	7	12.8	0	1.70	11.90	13.75	−1.02
Mean	46.7	64.6	37.3	21	10.5	12.18	0.32	1.21	9.97	11.53	+0.57
SEM	59	3.8	2.1	0	1.6	0.53	0.16	0.16	0.75	0.83	0.42

[a] Balance data were obtained during the stable period, which is the time after patients had stabilized or equilibrated on each diet.
[b] Refers to the period in which nitrogen balance had equilibrated and was no longer changing.
[c] Refers to the measured nitrogen intake minus the nitrogen content of rejected or vomited food.
[d] Sum of urine, fecal, and dialysate nitrogen.
[e] Indicates nitrogen balance adjusted for changes in body urea nitrogen but not unmeasured losses from skin, nails or hair, growth, respiration, or blood drawing.
From Slomowitz LA, Monteon FJ, Grosvenor M, et al. Effect of energy intake on nutritional status in maintenance hemodialysis patients. *Kidney Int* 1989; 35:704–711, with permission.

The second type of studies, which are retrospective and observational, provides results that are consistent with these conclusions. Data from the National Cooperative Dialysis Study indicated that patients with a DPI of less than 0.80 g/kg/day, as estimated by the PNA, had increased morbidity (138). However, these patients were randomized to a specified midweek predialysis serum urea nitrogen (SUN) and a given range of time for hemodialysis treatment, and, hence, to a given range of dialysis doses. Thus, it could not be stated conclusively that the higher morbidity of these patients was the result of lower nutritional intake *per se* and not the result of a decreased Kt/V.

In a retrospective study, Acchiardo et al. examined the relationship in 98 nondiabetic patients between DPI, determined from the PNA, and frequency of hospitalizations, number of total days hospitalized, and mortality rate during a 12-month period (1). Patients were divided into four groups based on their mean PNA: 0.63, 0.93, 1.02, and 1.2 g/kg/day. Both the frequency of hospitalizations and the mortality rate were inversely correlated with DPI. The frequency and number of days of hospitalization and the mortality rate were particularly likely to be elevated in patients with a PNA of 0.63 g/kg/day. Because the group with the highest PNA averaged 1.2 g/kg/day, it is not known whether an increase in PNA above this level (or an increase in the equivalent DPI necessary to maintain this PNA) would result in any further reduction in morbidity or mortality. A study published in 2003 on 122 patients undergoing MHD whose Kt/V were greater than 1.20 (recommended NKF-K/DOQI target) did not show any correlation between nPNA and Kt/V, especially among those with a Kt/V of more than 1.50 (101) (Fig. 25.1).

Some investigators report that some patients undergoing MHD are in nitrogen balance even with a protein intake as low as 0.7 g/kg/day and contend that in stable patients undergoing dialysis a safe requirement for protein intake would not be greater than 1 g/kg/day. They suggest that attempts at increasing protein intake beyond this value are not warranted (139,140). However, given the findings that there is a high incidence of PEM in patients undergoing MHD and especially among those with a poor outcome (4, 7,141), that metabolic studies clearly indicate that 0.75 g protein/kg/day is nutritionally inadequate for many patients (129), and that 1.1 g protein/kg/day will maintain nitrogen balance in some but not all patients undergoing MHD who are ingesting 25 or 35 kcal/kg/day (136), a DPI of 1.20 g/kg/day has been recommended by NKF-K/DOQI guidelines (Table 25.3).

Energy Requirements

Epidemiologic studies in patients undergoing MHD suggest that low energy intakes are probably even more common and more severe than the protein intakes (5,133,137, 142–146). Virtually every survey of the energy intake of patients undergoing MHD indicates that it is frequently below the recommended energy intake for normal healthy adults engaged in mild physical activity and that it usually averages about 24 to 27 kcal/kg/day (146,147). Indeed, even in the HEMO study, in which patients were seen periodically by renal dietitians, the energy intake averaged 22.8 $\pm$ 8.8 SD kcal/kg adjusted body weight/day (137,148).

The low energy intakes of patients undergoing MHD do not reflect a decrease in energy requirements. Studies indicate that under basal metabolic conditions energy expenditure in patients undergoing MHD under resting, basal conditions is normal or slightly increased (149–151). Resting basal energy expenditure in 12 normal subjects and 16 patients undergoing MHD was 0.94 ± 0.24 SD and 0.97 ± 0.1 kcal/min/1.73 m^2, respectively; each group was composed of both men and women (149). Schneeweiss et al. (152) performed indirect calorimetry on 24 normal adults and 86 patients with various forms of CRF of whom 25 were undergoing chronic hemodialysis. The resting energy expenditure was 1.03 ± 0.04 SEM kcal/min/1.73 m^2 in patients undergoing MHD, which was slightly but not statistically increased over values for the control subjects, 0.96 ± 0.02. Neyra et al. (153) measured resting energy expenditure using a whole-room indirect calorimeter (metabolic chamber) after 12-hour fasting in 15 patients with advanced CRF, 15 patients undergoing MHD, and 10 patients undergoing peritoneal dialysis. Patients undergoing hemodialysis were assessed on a nondialysis day. Resting energy expenditure, adjusted for fat-free mass, was similar in patients undergoing hemodialysis or peritoneal dialysis but was significantly higher than in patients with CRF ($p < .05$). It was generally about 10% to 20% higher in the patient with CRF in comparison to the predicted value for normal individuals. Thus, the patients undergoing MHD displayed increased resting energy expenditure (153). Energy expenditure in patients undergoing MHD measured by indirect calorimetry, when sitting quietly, with physical activity (Fig. 25.2), and after a defined meal appears to be similar to that of normal individuals (149). Energy expenditure during a maintenance hemodialysis treatment also may be increased (153).

In the study by Slomowitz et al. (136), in which nitrogen balance studies were carried out on six clinically stable patients undergoing MHD and who were prescribed, in random order, constant protein diets providing 25, 35, or 45 kcal/kg/day (136), both change in body weight and nitrogen balance correlated directly with the dietary energy intake (Figs. 25.3 and 25.4). The grand mean of the nitrogen balances, after equilibration on each diet, was significantly negative with the 25-kcal/kg/day diet, neutral with the 35-kcal/kg/day diet, and significantly positive with the 45-kcal/kg/day intake. Changes in body weight, midarm muscle circumference, and estimated body fat also correlated directly and significantly with dietary energy intake, and these parameters tended to increase with the highest energy intake and decrease with the lowest intake. Indeed, one can assess from the regression equations of these outcome measures the level of energy intake at which nitrogen balance and anthropometric parameters were neither increasing nor decreasing. This value, which can be construed to indicate the level of energy intake at which patients neither are in positive nor negative energy balance, is about 32 to 38 kcal/kg/day, depending on the nitrogen balance or body composition parameter in question (136). For an unchanging nitrogen balance, adjusted for estimated unmeasured nitrogen losses (i.e., through respiration, skin and integumentary structures, flatus, and semen or menses), the energy intake value was 38 kcal/kg/day.

The findings of low body fat and decreased skinfold thicknesses in patients undergoing MHD, which have been noted in several studies (143,145,146), seem to support the thesis that the usual energy intakes of these individuals are inadequate for their needs. Moreover, according to the "reverse epidemiology" hypothesis based on a number of epidemiologic studies, those patients undergoing MHD who have larger body mass for a given height survive longer (10). Based on the foregoing studies, and particularly the energy

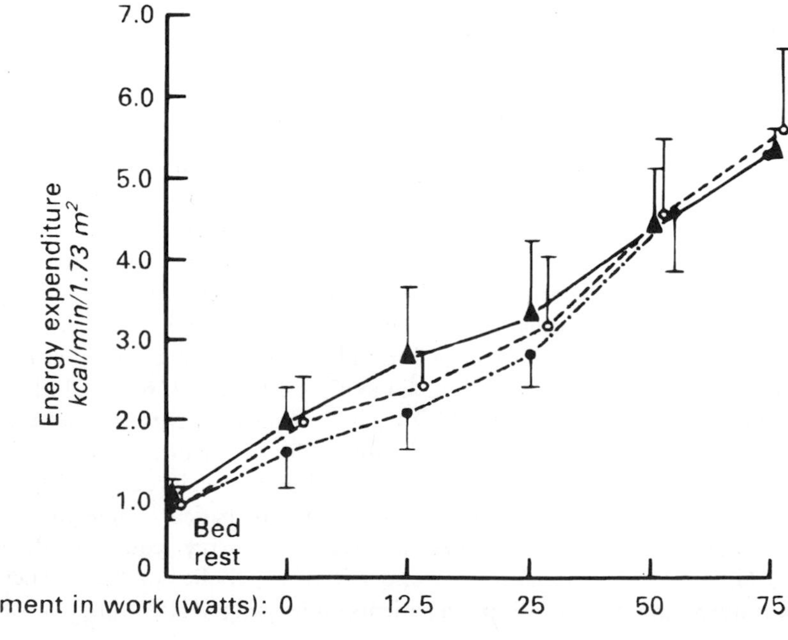

FIGURE 25.2. The direct correlation between the work of bicycle exercise and energy expenditure in normal subjects, nondialyzed patients with chronic renal failure, and patients undergoing maintenance hemodialysis. Symbols: (○) normal individual, $n = 12$; (•) patients with CRF, $n = 7$; (▲) patients undergoing hemodialysis, $n = 12$; (T), SD. (From Monteon FJ, Laidlaw SA, Shaib JK, et al. Energy expenditure in patients with chronic renal failure. *Kidney Int* 1986;30:741–747, with permission.)

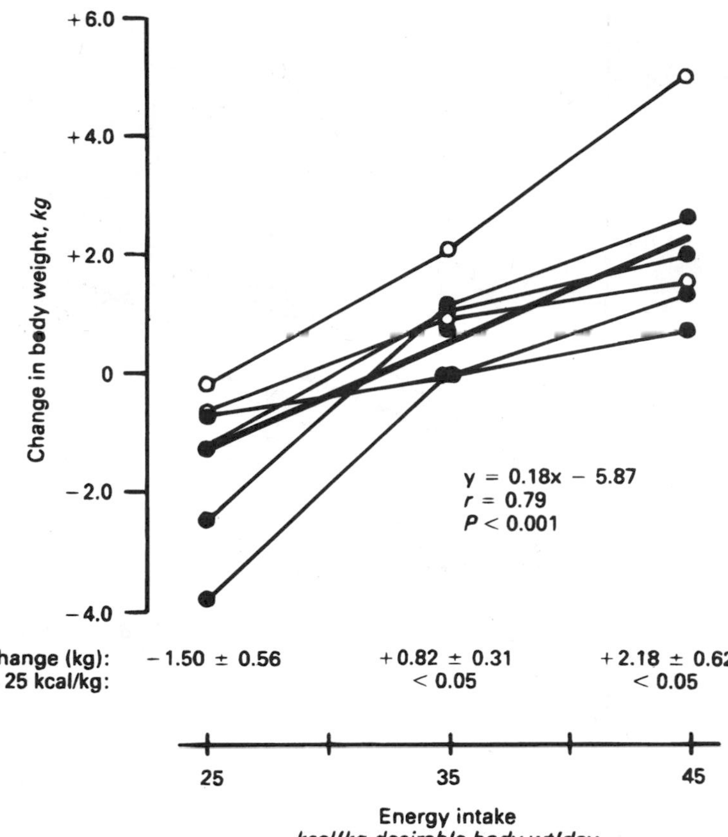

FIGURE 25.3. The direct correlation between the dietary energy intake and the change in body weight during each intake. Six patients undergoing maintenance hemodialysis were studied while they were living in a clinical research center and ingesting a constant protein diet. Energy intake was varied in random order between 25, 35, and 45 kcal/kg/day. Circles indicate values from an individual patient. Open circles indicate the two female patients. Thin lines connect data from the same individual. The heavy line indicates the least square regression line. (From Slomowitz LA, Monteon FJ, Grosvenor M, et al. Effect of energy intake on nutritional status in maintenance hemodialysis patients. *Kidney Int* 1989;35:704–711, with permission.)

expenditure measurements and nitrogen balance studies, the NKF-K/DOQI Nutrition Workgroup developed the following guideline: "the recommended daily energy intake for MHD or patients undergoing CPD is 35 kcal/kg body weight/day for those who are less than 60 years of age and 30 to 35 kcal/kg body weight/day for individuals 60 years or older" (70). This recommendation is based on the findings that: (a) energy expenditure of patients undergoing MHD is similar to or possibly slightly greater than that of normal, healthy individuals who are involved in mild physical activity (153); (b) metabolic balance studies of people undergoing MHD indicate that a total daily energy intake of about 35 kcal/kg/day induces neutral nitrogen balance and is adequate to maintain serum albumin and anthropometric indices (136); (c) because individuals 60 years of age or older tend to be more sedentary, a total energy intake of 30 to 35 kcal/kg is acceptable (70). Individuals involved in vigorous physical activity may require greater energy intakes. These recommendations are similar to the RDAs for sedentary healthy adults by the Food and Nutrition Board of the National Research Council (134).

The daily energy intake from the diet may be increased or decreased according to the net glucose balance across the hemodialyzer. However, the amount of glucose lost or taken up from hemodialysate generally is quite small. Gutierrez et al. (40) described average glucose losses of about 26 g per hemodialysis when glucose-free dialysate was used and a glucose uptake of about 30 g per hemodialysis when dialysate containing 180 mg/dL of glucose was used. The calorie balance across the dialyzer under these two conditions would be about −88 kcal and +102 kcal, respectively (i.e., based on a factor of 3.4 kcal/g of dextrose monohydrate). It should be remembered that these energy accruals or losses only occur three times per week for the typical patient undergoing MHD. Thus, under most conditions, and unlike the situation with CPD, the dietary energy intake for patients undergoing MHD usually does not have to be modified for a standard dialysis treatment. However, with the addition of larger glucose concentrations in hemodialysate, especially if hemodialysis treatments are conducted more frequently or for longer periods, the contribution of dialysis treatments to energy balance would be greater.

LIPIDS AND HEMODIALYSIS

The abnormalities in lipid metabolism and the causes for these disorders in patients with CRF are discussed in Chapter 3. Lipid disorders in this population constitute a highly significant problem because they are so prevalent, they involve so many of the traditional risk factors for vascular disease, and cardiovascular deaths account for one-half of

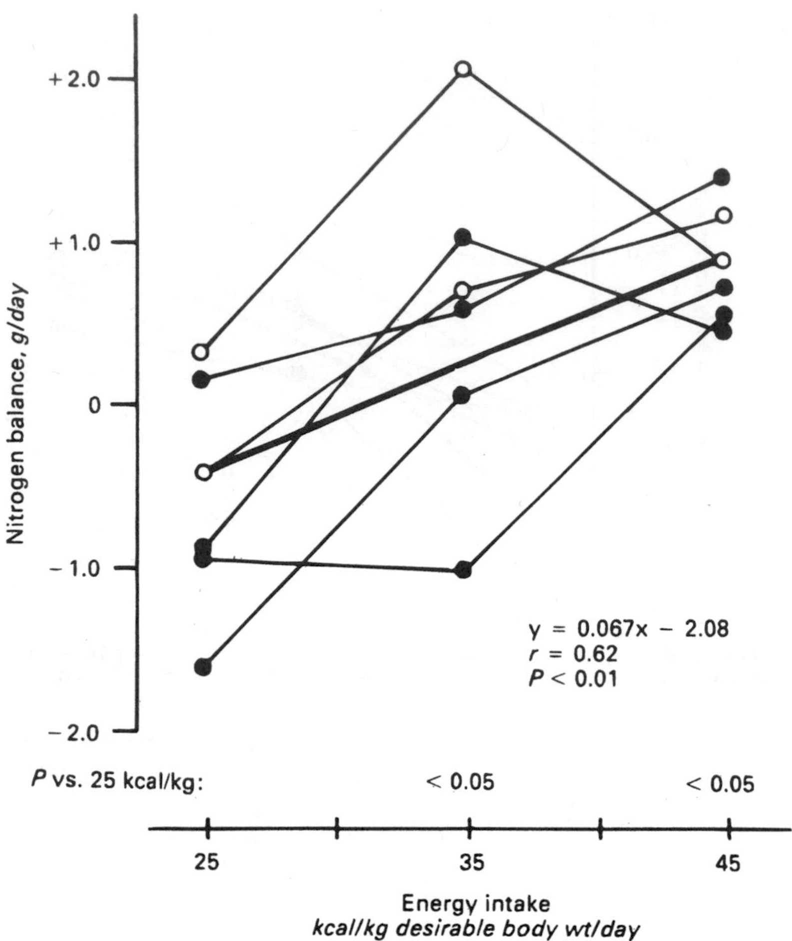

FIGURE 25.4. The direct correlation between dietary energy intake and nitrogen balance after equilibration on each diet. Six patients undergoing maintenance hemodialysis were studied while they lived in a clinical research center. Circles indicate values from an individual patient. Open circles indicate the two female patients. Thin lines connect data from the same individual. The heavy line indicates the least square regression line. (From Slomowitz LA, Monteon FJ, Grosvenor M, et al. Effect of energy intake on nutritional status in maintenance hemodialysis patients. *Kidney Int* 1989;35:704–711, with permission.)

the mortality of patients undergoing MHD (17,154). The growing number of patients with diabetes who develop ESRD; who are particularly likely to have lipid disorders; and who have an especially high incidence of cardiovascular, cerebrovascular, and peripheral vascular diseases have added to the severity of the problem. However, the paradoxical risk factor reversal that is observed in many epidemiologic studies in patients undergoing MHD with large sample sizes indicates that a low total serum cholesterol level poses at least as great a mortality risk as severe hypercholesterolemia (10,12) (Chapter 12). As serum total cholesterol decreases below roughly 200 to 250 mg/dL, the relative risk of death in patients undergoing MHD increases (12). Nevertheless, despite the association between a low serum cholesterol level and poor outcome in patients undergoing MHD, students of lipid metabolism in renal failure generally have concluded that until more data are available, it is still advantageous to create the same serum lipid pattern and dietary lipid intake that is recommended for the general population (Chapter 3).

Dyslipidemia is more prevalent in patients with ESRD than in the general population (155,156). In patients undergoing MHD, hypertriglyceridemia and low serum concentrations of high-density lipoprotein (HDL) frequently are observed (157–161). Moreover, very–low-density lipoprotein cholesterol usually is increased, but serum LDL and total cholesterol levels are usually within the normal range or even lower than that seen in the general population (162–164). Increased serum apolipoprotein B (apo B) containing triglyceride-rich lipoprotein particles containing C-III and (a) or lipoprotein(Bc) particles often are observed in patients undergoing MHD (165–167). A defect in postprandial chylomicron remnant clearance has been described (159,168). Moreover, there is a high incidence of type IV hyperlipidemia among patients with ESRD (165, 168). All serum HDL cholesterol fractions often are decreased, possibly secondary to reduced LCAT (lecithin:cholesterol/acyltransferase) activity; and HDL_3, which is not a major risk factor for reduced adverse cardiovascular events, is relatively spared. In contrast, there is a greater reduction in the larger HDL_2 fraction, which has a stronger association with a low incidence of cardiovascular morbidity and mortality. The antiatherogenic HDL-associated Apo A-I and Apo A-II also are diminished in sera. Lp(a) levels often are elevated. Lipoprotein lipase activities in serum and liver are decreased. The serum levels of oxidized lipids and thiobarbituric acid-reactive substances (TBARS) are elevated in patients with CKD and those undergoing MHD. There is some speculation as to whether the hemodialysis procedure increases lipid oxidation; the data of Schettler et al. suggest that this is not the case (169).

In contrast to the moderate prevalence of hypercholesterolemia, hypertriglyceridemia is more common in patients undergoing MHD (170) (Chapter 3). Patients undergoing MHD should be evaluated for systemic causes of hypertriglyceridemia, including diabetes mellitus and hypothyroidism. Dietary therapy, because of its greater safety, in general is used when the serum triglyceride concentrations are about 1.25 to 1.50 times the upper limit of normal values. Under these circumstances, patients should be urged to reduce ethanol intake to no more than one drink per day. Attempts should be made to lower the intake of purified sugars and saturated fat. If dietary therapy does not lower serum triglyceride concentrations sufficiently, and if serum triglycerides, after a 10-hour fast, remain higher than about 500 mg/dL, triglyceride-lowering medications generally are prescribed. Medical therapy can be given concurrently with a lipid-lowering to lower hypertriglyceridemia (171–173). Gemfibrozil and fibric acid derivatives such as clofibrate are effective agents for lowering serum triglyceride levels. However, there is a risk of myositis, cholelithiasis, and other disorders with these medicines, and the doses of these medicines should be decreased in patients undergoing hemodialysis (174–177).

There is currently no consensus as to the exact lipid composition of the diet for patients undergoing MHD. The National Cholesterol Education Program (NCEP) Expert Panel has recommended the Therapeutic Lifestyle Changes (TLC) diet in all individuals with LDL cholesterol of 100 to 129 mg/dL or triglycerides higher than 180 mg/dL (178). Table 25.5 shows the nutrient composition of the TLC diet. Its essential features are the following: (a) reduced intakes of saturated fats (<7% of total calories) and cholesterol (<200 mg/day); (b) sources of total calories in the diet should include up to 10% for polyunsaturated fats, up to 20% from monounsaturated fats, 25% to 35% from all fat sources, and the rest from protein and carbohydrate. Dietary protein should be modified from the TLC diet to provide 1.20 g protein/kg/day, and dietary carbohydrate should be modified accordingly so as to maintain desirable energy intake; (c) therapeutic options for enhancing LDL lowering such as plant stanols/sterols (2 g/day) and increased viscous (soluble) fiber (20 to 30 g/day); (d) attainment and maintenance of desirable body weight and physical activity to consume approximately 200 kcal/day (178) (Chapter 3).

These guidelines for the treatment of hypercholesterolemia are based on the same principles as for the general population. The TLC diet is a health-enhancing diet and, in general, all individuals in the population at large should be encouraged to adhere to it. Patients undergoing MHD are considered to be at high risk for coronary artery disease and stroke, and the target for their serum LDL cholesterol is to maintain it below 100 mg/dL. This sometimes can be attained by the TLC diet, but often pharmacologic therapy must be given in association with dietary therapy to attain target LDL cholesterol levels (see also Chapter 3) (178). Hydroxy-methyl-glutaryl coenzyme A reductase inhibitors, also known as statins, and fibric acid derivatives, such as clofibrate, have been used successfully to treat hypercholesterolemia. The recently described antiinflammatory characteristics of statins may play a major role in improving outcome in patients undergoing MHD (179–182). Some statins also have a modest HDL-cholesterol raising effect (183).

TABLE 25.5. NUTRIENT COMPOSITION OF THE THERAPEUTIC LIFESTYLE CHANGES (TLC) DIET

Nutrient	Recommended Intake
Saturated fat[a]	<7% of total calories
Polyunsaturated fat	Up to 10% of total calories
Monounsaturated fat	Up to 20% of total calories
Total fat	25%–35% of total calories
Carbohydrate[b,c]	50%–60% of total calories
Fiber	20–30 g/day
Protein[c]	Approximately 15% of total calories
Cholesterol	<200 mg/day
Total calories[d]	Balance energy intake and expenditure to maintain desirable body weight/prevent weight gain

[a] *Trans* fatty acids are another low-density-lipoprotein raising fat that should be kept at a low intake.
[b] Carbohydrates should be derived predominantly from foods rich in complex carbohydrates including grains, especially whole grains, fruits, and vegetables.
[c] Dietary content of protein and, hence carbohydrate, should be modified according to the specific needs of the patient undergoing maintenance hemodialysis (i.e., 1.20 g protein/kg/day). (See text.)
[d] Daily energy expenditure should include at least moderate physical activity (contributing approximately 200 kcal/day).
From Executive Summary of the Third Report of the National Cholesterol Education Program [NCEP] Expert Panel on Detection, Evaluation, and Treatment of High Blood Cholesterol in Adults [Adult Treatment Panel III]. *JAMA* 2001;285:2486–2497, with permission.

SODIUM AND WATER

Sodium and its most prevalent anion, chloride, are the most abundant extracellular solutes, and hence extracellular fluid volume and plasma volume are regulated largely by salt (sodium chloride) balance (184). Fecal sodium excretion usually amounts to 1 to 3 mmol/day, and in individuals who are not actively sweating, integumentary sodium losses are generally less than 3 to 4 mEq/day. Hence, in health, it is renal sodium excretion that maintains sodium balance across wide variations in sodium intake. As GFR falls, the fractional excretion of sodium (FeNa) increases so that sodium excretion usually remains equal to sodium intake (185–187). However, when the GFR falls below approximately 15 mL/min, the increase in FeNa often does not fully compensate for the fall in the GFR and filtered sodium load, and even a typical dietary sodium intake (e.g., 120 to 200 mmol/day) may lead to sodium retention. Within the first several weeks or months after MHD therapy is inaugurated, the GFR usually decreases to less than 1 or 2 mL/min, and by 12 months of MHD most patients are oliguric or anuric (188). Thus, sodium balance is dictated largely by the intake and removal by dialysis of sodium.

Patients must be counseled against ingesting high-sodium diets (Chapter 18). Excessive sodium intake may lead to a large interdialytic weight gain, hypertension, edema, and congestive heart failure (189). When patients gain large volumes of sodium and water during the interdialytic interval, the rapid removal of this fluid during the brief period of the hemodialysis treatment may cause sudden decreases in blood volume and hence engender hypotension, angina, arrhythmias, or muscle cramps. Shaldon (190), Krautzig et al. (191), and Tomson (192) emphasized the importance of restricted dietary sodium intake in patients undergoing MHD to achieve drug-free control of blood pressure and to limit interdialytic fluid gain. To that end, it has been contended that longer hours of MHD treatment achieve better blood pressure control by greater effectiveness in reducing total body sodium and water (193,194). However, excess intradialytic sodium gain is not always the result of dietary indiscretion because some medications can be major sources of sodium, such as some combined analgesics in effervescent form (e.g., co-codamol, a combination of codeine and paracetamol used especially in Europe) (195). This preparation is soluble because of 18 mmol sodium bicarbonate contained in each tablet. If a patient takes 6 to 8 tablets per day, the sodium intake from this medication can drive the intake of an extra 800 mL of water per day to maintain a normal extracellular sodium concentration.

It is not clear whether patients undergoing MHD with a high interdialytic weight gain have a higher risk of death (192). The largest study examining this issue showed the converse: Those patients undergoing MHD with low interdialytic weight gain are at highest risk of dying, although it is true that very high interdialytic weight gains also were associated with a modestly increased risk (192). The most likely explanation for this finding is that low interdialytic weight gain is associated with poor nutritional intake and therefore may be associated with serious comorbid disease. This explanation was supported by a study showing that low interdialytic weight gain was associated with poor nutritional status, which is an important predictor of poor outcome in patients undergoing MHD (196). In another smaller study, high interdialytic weight gain was associated with increased mortality in diabetic, but not in nondiabetic, patients undergoing MHD (197). A number of investigations indicate that high interdialytic weight gain may contribute to hypertension (198–201), but most studies show no such relationship (202–205) or show it only in a subset of "volume-responsive" patients (196,206). This lack of a relationship is less surprising than it may seem because it is the change in plasma volume, not in total extracellular volume or total body water, which is likely to result in acute changes in blood pressure during fluid removal (207). Nonetheless, given the high morbidity associated with excessive intake of sodium and water intake and interdialytic weight gain and the very high frequency of hypertension and need for antihypertensive medications in patients undergoing MHD, dietary salt and water restriction appear to be strongly indicated.

A sodium intake of 1,000 to 1,500 mg Na per day (43 to 64.5 mmol/day, or 2.54 to 3.82 g/day of sodium chloride or salt) is recommended for patients undergoing MHD (192,208). Precooked, processed, and canned foods usually have high sodium content, and the intake of these foods should be minimized. Salt substitutes prepared from herbs often can satisfy a patient's desire for sodium. Salt substitutes composed of potassium chloride generally contain 13 mEq of potassium per packet and may induce hyperkalemia in patients undergoing MHD.

Excessive water intake can contribute to these problems (208). Whereas sodium balance is a key regulator of extracellular fluid volume, the cell volume is regulated by plasma tonicity, which in turn is regulated by water balance. Thirst and the renal excretion of water are the two major regulators of water homeostasis (209,210). Although the ability of the kidney to excrete or retain large amounts of free water is reduced severely in patients with advanced stages of CKD, thirst and the consequent water ingested generally will maintain plasma sodium concentration within or slightly below the normal range. When sodium intake is restricted adequately and if patients are not hyperglycemic, individuals usually automatically will adjust their water intake to appropriate levels. However, perturbations of thirst may interfere with this homeostatic mechanism. Also, because patients undergoing MHD are usually oliguric or anuric, a separate prescription for water intake is usually necessary to prevent fluid overload, excessive interdialytic weight gain, and hyponatremia (192). In general, the water intake for patients undergoing MHD should not exceed 750 to 1,500 mL per day, including the water ingested in food, unless the patient has a urine output substantially above the oliguric range.

POTASSIUM

Normally, the kidney excretes at least 80% to 90% of the total daily potassium intake, which is usually between 50 to 150 mEq/day (about 2 to 6 g/day) but may vary even more widely. About 7 to 10 mEq per day of potassium normally are excreted in the feces; in patients with advanced CKD, fecal potassium excretion increases to about 14 to 25 mEq/day (211–215). Normally, in the nephron, almost all filtered potassium is reabsorbed and urinary potassium is largely derived from tubular secretion. As with sodium, when the GFR falls, the fractional excretion of potassium increases (214). This adaptive response increases the magnitude by which renal failure can progress before the urinary potassium excretion is no longer sufficient to prevent potassium retention and hyperkalemia. An early response to an increase in the extracellular potassium is to shift potassium inside the cell (216). Factors that inhibit this transcellular potassium shift or that promote movement of potassium extracellularly may exacerbate the tendency to hyperkalemia in patients undergoing MHD. These include insulin deficiency, metabolic acidemia, hypercatabolic states, and treatment with beta blockers or aldosterone antagonists; these conditions are not infrequently present in a typical multimorbid patient with CRF (120,217,218).

In general, a diet providing no more than 50 to 75 mmol/day (roughly 2 to 3 g/day) of potassium should be prescribed for patients undergoing MHD, although for patients with persistent hyperkalemia even lower amounts may be required (214). This restricted intake of potassium is well tolerated by most but not all patients undergoing MHD. Because severe hyperkalemia (e.g., greater than 7.0 mmol/L) may precipitate fatal arrhythmias, patients undergoing MHD should receive detailed instructions concerning the potassium content of various foods and should be instructed to avoid or strictly regulate the intake of potassium-rich foods. Constipation should be avoided or treated promptly because of the importance of fecal potassium losses to the body potassium economy in these individuals (212). In the past, patients with elevated serum potassium invariably were dialyzed with very–low-potassium dialysate containing 0 to 1.0 mmol/L. This practice has raised the question of a possible contribution of postdialysis hypokalemia to sudden cardiac death syndrome observed in patients undergoing MHD (219). Karnik et al. examined the records of 400 reported cardiac arrests over a 9-month period in a nationally representative cohort of 77,000 patients undergoing MHD dialyzed at outpatient facilities of a for-profit dialysis company in North America (220). They found that patients with cardiac arrest were nearly twice as likely to have been dialyzed with a dialysate containing 0 or 1.0 mEq/L potassium on the day of the cardiac arrest (17.1% versus 8.8%). Hence, the current trend is to avoid the use of very–low-potassium dialysate and to use longer dialysis hours, averaging 4 hours or more, using dialysate bath with potassium as high as 3.0 or 4.0 mmol/L, if possible. A possible alternative approach might be to ask these very–low-potassium–containing dialysates for only the first one-half of the dialysis treatment; the safety of this course of action would need to be tested. For noncompliant patients undergoing MHD or those who adhere poorly to their dietary potassium prescription, administration of ion-exchange resins, such as sodium polystyrene, by mouth or rectum, may be considered to enhance potassium excretion on off-dialysis days, especially during long intradialytic breaks and weekends. It should be noted that this ion-exchange resin exchanges sodium for potassium; hence, this procedure will increase sodium intake.

MAGNESIUM

As is the case for potassium, the kidney is the major excretory organ for magnesium (221–226). However, because in most foods the magnesium content is lower than the content of phosphorus or potassium and the net fractional absorption of magnesium by the intestine is less (roughly 50% of ingested magnesium) (223), hypermagnesemia is usually a less serious problem than hyperphosphatemia or hyperkalemia. Although mild hypermagnesemia is common in patients undergoing MHD, severe hypermagnesemia is rare unless patients ingest magnesium-containing antacids or laxatives, such as Maalox, Gelusil, milk of magnesia, or cascara sagrada, or receive large doses of intravenous magnesium (224). Patients with ESRD, most of whom were undergoing MHD, have been reported to have increased magnesium content of bone and some soft tissues (221, 226,227). In nondialyzed patients with chronic uremia, the magnesium requirement is about 2 to 4 mg/kg/day (i.e., about 200 mg/day) (223). Patients who are undergoing hemodialysis with 1.0 mEq/L of magnesium in the dialysate and whose dietary magnesium intakes range between 200 and 300 mg/day generally maintain normal or only slightly elevated serum magnesium levels.

CALCIUM

The normal dietary calcium requirement for nonpregnant, nonlactating adults is 800 to 1,200 mg per day (134). Vitamin D deficiency and resistance to the actions of vitamin D on bone and in the intestinal tract may increase the dietary calcium requirements of patients with CRF including those undergoing MHD (222,228) (Chapter 17). Foods rich in calcium are often rich in phosphorus; thus patients undergoing MHD usually should not ingest these foods in large amounts (223). With the widespread use of calcium-containing phosphate binders, oral calcium intake commonly has been 1.0 to 1.5 g/day or greater (229). Indeed, daily calcium intakes from calcium-containing phosphate binders and foods could be excessive, equaling or exceeding 3.0 g/day. Because the net intestinal absorption of calcium increases with high-calcium diets (223), these latter calcium intakes may engender continuing positive calcium balance and lead to hypercalcemia and calcium deposition in soft tissues (see later). Therefore, to avoid hypercalcemia and calcification, a hemodialysate bath containing 1.25 or 1.5 mmol/L (5.0 to 6.0 mg/dL) of calcium currently is used for most patients undergoing MHD if they are taking calcium-containing phosphate binders.

Concerns have been raised about the contributing role of ingested calcium to the development of coronary artery calcification and atherosclerotic plaques in patients undergoing MHD (33,230–234). A major source of excessive calcium intake in patients undergoing MHD is from calcium-containing phosphorus binders such as calcium carbonate or calcium gluconate (229). Several studies comparing patients undergoing MHD receiving the non-calcium–containing binder sevelamer hydrochloride with those taking calcium-containing binders showed significantly less progression of vascular and coronary calcification in the former patients (32,235,236), although concerns have been expressed regarding the increased incidence of metabolic acidosis as a result of ingestion of excessive amounts of sevelamer HCl usually required to treat hyperphosphatemia (237). These considerations suggest that control of serum phosphorous may be more safely achieved by using binders that do not contain calcium. If calcium-containing phosphate binders are not used, the recommended dietary calcium intake should be about 1,200 to 1,600 mg/day. If serum phosphorous cannot be controlled without the additional use of calcium-containing binders, then dietary calcium intake from foods should be reduced to below 1.0 g calcium/day, and hemodialysate using less than 3.5 mEq/L of calcium should be used.

Patients who are receiving calcium salts or 1,25-dihydroxyvitamin D should be monitored for hypercalcemia. Hypercalcemia can cause hypertension, pruritus, restlessness, and metastatic calcification, also known as calciphylaxis, particularly if the serum calcium–phosphorus product exceeds 70. Thus, the goal is to maintain the morning fasting serum calcium–phosphorus product well below this level and certainly below 60 (Chapter 17).

PHOSPHORUS

In general, hemodialysis is not a highly efficient method for removing excessive phosphorus. On average, approximately 250 mg of phosphorus are removed during each hemodialysis session depending on the predialysis serum phosphorus concentrations (238). The typical American diet provides about 1,500 to 1,700 mg/day of phosphorus (134). Roughly 60% of ingested phosphorus is absorbed from the gastrointestinal tract (134,211,216,222,223). Thus, the quantity of phosphorus removed by hemodialysis is less than that required to avoid severe hyperphosphatemia in most patients. Hence, patients undergoing MHD must decrease phosphorus intake and intestinal phosphorus absorption to prevent hyperphosphatemia.

It is recommended that patients undergoing MHD should be prescribed not more than 10 to 17 mg/kg/day of phosphorus (223,239,240). The dietary phosphorus content usually is directly related to the quantity of protein, dairy products, and certain cola drinks in the diet (223, 239). Very–low-phosphorus diets (e.g., less than 800 mg/day) are often unpalatable to the patient, particularly when the DPI is high (e.g., about 1.2 g/kg/day or greater). For these reasons, intestinal phosphorus binders almost invariably are required, in addition to dietary phosphorus restriction, to reduce intestinal phosphorus absorption and prevent severe hyperphosphatemia. Both hyperphosphatemia (241) and hypophosphatemia (13) have been reported to be associated with poor outcome in patients undergoing MHD.

Because aluminum-containing binders such as aluminum hydroxide or aluminum carbonate led to serious side effects (low-turnover bone disease, refractory anemia, and dementia) (242–246), calcium-containing binders frequently were used, including calcium carbonate (40% calcium), calcium acetate (25% calcium), and calcium citrate (21% calcium). More recently, calcium-free binders such as sevelamer hydrochloride frequently are prescribed (233). However, aluminum carbonate or hydroxide, because of its superior potency, still can be used on a short-term basis, especially when serum phosphorus levels are very high (>8 mg/dL) or when the product of the serum calcium and phosphorus approaches 70. This is recommended because calcium-based phosphorus binders may increase the risk of calcium–phosphate deposition, particularly when serum phosphorus is very high (241,247). Because citrate enhances the absorption of aluminum (248–250), calcium citrate should not be given with aluminum-containing phosphate binders. Calcium acetate is a more effective phosphate binder on a weight basis (presumably it is effective at a wider pH range than calcium carbonate) and may be associated less often with hypercalcemia (248,249). However, some research indicates that the incidence of hypercalcemia is similar to calcium acetate and calcium carbonate, and gastrointestinal symptoms such as nausea, bloating, or constipation may be more common with calcium acetate (251, 252). Moreover, calcium-containing binders are associated with a higher incidence of coronary artery calcification (33, 230). Large doses of calcium binders also have been implicated in adynamic bone disease (253,254).

Sevelamer hydrochloride and other calcium-free binders appear to be associated less often with such adverse effects. Indeed, some preliminary studies indicate a significantly lower incidence of hypercalcemia and coronary artery calcification (32). However, because of its hydrochloride content, sevelamer HCl can cause a hyperchloremic acidosis (237,255). This is especially likely to occur when sevelamer HCl is used in higher doses, up to 4 to 7 g given three times per day (237).

Lanthanum carbonate and trivalent iron-containing compounds are emerging non-calcium–containing phosphate binders that are almost as potent as calcium-containing binders (256–259). Lanthanum carbonate does not cause metabolic acidosis. Although individuals taking lanthanum carbonate may display an increase in serum or tissue lanthanum values, the increase appears to be small and, so far, has not been associated with adverse side effects (257–259).

VITAMIN D

Vitamin D is discussed in Chapter 17 and is addressed only briefly here. The enzyme, 1α-hydroxylase, which is present in the proximal tubule, converts 25-hydroxycholecalciferol to 1,25-dihydroxycholecalciferol (1,25-dihydroxyvitamin D), the most active form of vitamin D. Therefore, patients undergoing MHD are almost invariably deficient in this most active vitamin D analogue unless they take supplements of this compound or an analogue of this compound (260,261). 1,25-dihydroxycholecalciferol has pleiotropic actions. It facilitates calcium and phosphorus absorption from the gastrointestinal tract. It is a strong inhibitor of the production and secretion of parathyroid hormone (PTH). It inhibits PTH messenger RNA transcription (260) and also inhibits parathyroid cell hyperplasia (262,263). It also enhances the actions of PTH on bone and may act directly on bone as suggested by the presence of vitamin D receptors on osteoblasts and osteoclasts (264). Thus in CRF, vitamin D deficiency, coupled with the impaired ability to excrete phosphorus, results in low serum calcium levels and hyperparathyroidism.

Vitamin D supplements routinely are used in patients undergoing MHD to enhance calcium absorption, prevent or treat hyperparathyroidism, and improve bone metabolism. 1,25-dihydroxycholecalciferol (calcitriol) derivatives are commercially available in several oral and intravenous preparations (265–268). To replace low vitamin D levels, patients undergoing MHD may be given 0.25 to 1.0 μg/day of calcitriol as an oral dose or, as is a more common practice, intravenously with each hemodialysis session. To treat or prevent hyperparathyroidism, larger doses may be used, which may lead to hypercalcemia (Chapter 17). Some newer generations of vitamin D compounds such as paricalcitol are reported to cause less hypercalcemia and, hence, have a better safety profile as a suppressant of hyperparathyroidism (269). Occasionally, patients with refractory secondary (also known as tertiary) hyperparathyroidism may not respond to these medications and will require parathyroidectomy. After parathyroidectomy, many patients undergoing MHD may require high doses of calcium and vitamin D, especially during the first weeks to months postoperatively, as a result of the hungry bone syndrome (270, 271); after several months, this increased need for calcium and vitamin D tends to abate, presumably because bone has now become repleted with calcium.

For most patients undergoing MHD who do not have refractory hyperparathyroidism, 0.5 to 3.0 μg of calcitriol intravenously with each hemodialysis treatment or 0.25 to 3.0 μg by mouth every other day, three times per week, can be given (272,273). The equivalent dose for paricalcitol is higher and is in the range of 2 to 10 μg intravenously with each hemodialysis session (270,271). The relevant merits and disadvantages of oral and intravenous therapy for the treatment of hyperparathyroidism and a comparison among different forms of active vitamin D are discussed in detail in Chapter 17. Patients who are given supplemental 1,25-dihydroxycholecalciferol should be monitored routinely for hypercalcemia and hyperphosphatemia. As discussed earlier, an increasing number of reports indicate the possibility of an increased rate of coronary artery calcification with higher serum calcium concentrations (33,230, 236,247); hence, a more conservative approach to vitamin D and calcium therapy may be warranted with the possible utilization of lower dialysate calcium concentrations and with more reliance on medicines that are less potent at increasing serum calcium levels.

OTHER VITAMINS

Patients undergoing MHD are at increased risk for deficiencies of other vitamins (22,23,62,274–276), particularly folic acid and vitamins B and C. Vitamin metabolism and needs are described in more detail in Chapter 20. The causes for vitamin deficiencies in patients undergoing MHD include the following: (a) reduced overall food intake as a result of anorexia or MICS (see earlier and Chapter 12); (b) prescription of low-phosphorus, low-potassium diets that restrict intake of such nutritionally valuable foods as fresh fruits and vegetables, dairy products, and other items that are high in vitamins (30); (c) altered metabolism, as is the case for pyridoxine and possibly folate (276,277); (d) impaired synthesis (e.g., 1,25-dihydroxyvitamin D) (Chapter 17); (e) resistance to the actions of vitamins (e.g., vitamin D and possibly folate); (f) decreased intestinal absorption (e.g., decreased intestinal absorption of riboflavin, folate, and vitamin D have been described in rats with chronic renal insufficiency) (Chapter 23); and (g) dialysate losses of water-soluble vitamins (19,23,278).

In some studies, patients undergoing MHD who did not receive vitamin supplements did not develop signs of vitamin deficiency when followed for up to 1 year (278, 279). Based on these findings, some authors have questioned the need for vitamin supplementation for patients undergoing MHD (279). It is also true that many studies that suggest a need for vitamin supplements were carried out in the 1960s and early 1970s, when there was perhaps a higher incidence of malnutrition in patients undergoing MHD (278). Nevertheless, reports continue to show that many patients undergoing MHD ingest a vitamin intake that provides less than the RDA (19,30,280) and that there is a small but persistent prevalence of deficiencies for some water-soluble vitamins (as well as for 1,25-dihydroxyvitamin D) (19,63,281). At present, it does not seem feasible to identify, *a priori*, those patients who will develop vitamin deficiencies. Because the intake of water-soluble vitamins at the proposed levels appears to be safe, we propose that these vitamins be supplemented.

A 2002 study comparing food intake of 30 patients undergoing MHD with 30 normal individuals (matched for age, gender, and race) by means of a FFQ found that patients undergoing MHD consumed significantly lower amounts of potassium, vitamin C, and dietary fiber as well as lower amounts of some carotenoids including cryptoxanthin and lycopene (30). The lower vitamin C, fiber, and carotenoid intake of patients undergoing MHD may be atherogenic and also may be the result of the prescribed restrictions in potassium and phosphorus in patients undergoing MHD. These dietary restrictions may lead to reduced fruit, vegetable, and milk intake, leaving meat and fats as the main source of calories. The low energy intake of patients undergoing MHD often impels dietitians to recommend a higher fat diet. These factors could contribute to atherosclerosis and increased cardiovascular morbidity and mortality in these patients. This hypothesis needs to be evaluated in future studies.

Reports indicate that vitamin C supplementation may promote intestinal iron absorption and reduce the incidence of iron-deficiency anemia among patients undergoing MHD (Chapter 22) (282–286). Serum homocysteine concentration, a cardiovascular risk factor, is significantly increased in patients undergoing MHD and pharmacologic doses of folic acid can lower plasma total homocysteine levels. Generally, maximum homocysteine-lowering effects of folic acid occur with doses of 5 to 10 mg/day (29,287).

Erythrocyte or serum levels of riboflavin (vitamin B_2), thiamin (vitamin B_1), pantothenic acid, and biotin are usually normal in patients undergoing MHD. Case reports of Wernicke's encephalopathy in patients undergoing an MHD and CPD because of thiamin deficiency occasionally are described (288,289). Niacin levels are usually within the normal range in patients undergoing MHD (278,279,290, 291), although many years ago Lasker et al. reported low niacin levels (292). Pyridoxine (vitamin B_6) is removed by hemodialysis, and this factor, and possibly also altered vitamin B_6 metabolism, accounts for the increased daily requirement for this vitamin (293,294). Vitamin B_6 participates in the metabolism of homocysteine, although pyridoxine supplements have not been consistently shown to decrease plasma homocysteine in patients with CRF (Chapter 20).

The lipid-soluble vitamins are D, K, A, and E. Vitamin K levels are usually normal in patients undergoing MHD (278). Administration of a pharmacologic dose of vitamin K_2 (45 mg/day orally) for 1 year was found to prevent loss of bone mass in patients undergoing MHD with bone disease characterized by low bone turnover (295). Moreover, an inverse relationship between the frequency of bone fractures and plasma phylloquinone levels was reported in patients undergoing MHD (296). Also, in the same study, serum PTH was high (>300 ng/L) in patients with low plasma phylloquinone (vitamin K_1) concentrations who also had an abnormally high incidence of an apo E phenotype (297). However, several reports described a relationship between high plasma vitamin K levels and ectopic soft-tissue calcification in patients undergoing MHD (298–300). Because patients undergoing MHD generally do not have evidence for vitamin K deficiency, vitamin K supplements are not recommended for routine use (301). However, patients may be at increased risk for vitamin K deficiency if they are not eating, are not given vitamin K by parenteral administration, and are receiving antibiotics that suppress the intestinal bacteria that synthesize vitamin K. Under these conditions, vitamin K supplements should be given.

Serum vitamin A concentrations generally are increased in patients undergoing MHD, especially among long-term dialysis survivors of (302–304). Patients undergoing MHD who are binephrectomized are reported to have higher serum retinol levels than other patients undergoing MHD; this probably reflects the loss of the renal contribution to the degradation of retinal-binding protein (RBP), the carrier protein for vitamin A (305,306). Hemodialysis treatment does not change vitamin A levels (307,308); indeed, losses of vitamin A into dialysate would not be expected because of the relatively large size of the vitamin A-RBP-transthyretin (prealbumin) complex. However, beta carotene, ubiquinol, and lycopene have been found to be lower in patients undergoing MHD than in individuals without renal insufficiency, and beta carotene and ubiquinol decrease further after a single hemodialysis treatment (309). An individual's lipid metabolism also may affect serum vitamin A levels. In 72 patients undergoing MHD, Werb et al. (307) showed a positive correlation between plasma vitamin A levels and both serum total cholesterol and triglycerides. The hematocrit also has been found to correlate with the plasma vitamin A/RBP ratio in patients undergoing MHD, which is consistent with the evidence that vitamin A may promote erythropoiesis (Chapter 22) (310). Patients with advanced CRF appear to be particularly vulnerable to vitamin A toxicity. Hypercalcemia and elevated serum alkaline phosphatase levels have been described in patients undergoing MHD ingesting as little as 7,500 to 15,000 units/day of vitamin A (307,311). Therefore, it is recommended that the daily vitamin A intake from foods and supplements should not exceed the recommended dietary allowance of 800 to 1,000 μg/day (307–310).

Serum vitamin E (α-tocopherol) levels in patients undergoing MHD are reported to be low (312–314), normal (315), or increased (301). Significant amounts of α-tocopherol are not removed by the dialysis procedure (313, 314). In 10 long-term MHD survivors treated with MHD for an average of 274 ± 35 (SD) months, Chazot et al. found that serum vitamin E levels were abnormally high but not different from 10 age- and-gender-matched patients who were treated with MHD for 51 ± 29 months (316). There are contradictory results with regard to red blood cell (RBC) tocopherol concentrations in patients undergoing MHD (312,315). These findings may reflect either increased consumption of tocopherol, possibly as a result of oxidative stress, or a defect in the HDL-mediated transfer of tocopherol from plasma to the RBC membrane. Cohen et al. (317) showed that RBC tocopherol concentrations were low in patients undergoing MHD who had sustained hemolysis caused by a high chloramine concentration in the water and increased after the hemolytic condition was corrected by removal of the chloramine. Because patients undergoing MHD suffer not infrequently from oxidant stress (Chapter 5), several studies have examined the effects on oxidant stress of vitamin E supplementation given orally, during hemodialysis treatment using vitamin E-coated dialyzer membranes, or through dialysate (hemolipodialysis) (Chapter 20). In the SPACE (Secondary Prevention with Antioxidants of Cardiovascular disease in End-stage renal disease) study (a double-blind, prospective clinical trial of 196 patients undergoing MHD randomized to receive oral vitamin E, 800 IU/day, or placebo) patients undergoing MHD assigned to vitamin E treatment had a reduction in subsequent cardiovascular events (relative risk [RR] = 0.46) and myocardial infarction (RR = 0.30) (318). A number of other studies of vitamin E supplementation in patients undergoing MHD as well as in the general population have not always confirmed that such supplements reduce morbidity or mortality (319,320). Nonetheless, because CRF clearly is associated with increased oxidant stress and increased cardiovascular risk, and because vitamin E appears to be rather safe and may be beneficial, it is not unreasonable to consider prescribing a supplement of 400 to 800 IU/day of vitamin E.

Table 25.3 gives the dietary recommendations for various vitamins for maintenance hemodialysis patients. The recommended dietary allowances for patients undergoing maintenance hemodialysis are proposed for each of the water-soluble vitamins and for vitamin A except for higher doses of pyridoxine HCl (10 mg/day, 8.2 mg/day of pyridoxine) and folic acid (about 1 mg/day). Vitamin C is recommended only at the daily allowance levels (70 mg/day) because of the risk of increased oxalate formation at higher intakes (321,322). Vitamin E supplements appear safe; data concerning their effectiveness is equivocal so vitamin E supplements are considered optional.

TRACE ELEMENTS

Trace element nutrition in CRF is discussed in more detail in Chapter 19, and the nutritional requirements in patients undergoing MHD are reviewed briefly here. The advent of sophisticated analytic methodology allows for fairly accurate measurements of trace element levels. However, the blood and tissue levels of these elements may be affected by many factors, some of which are independent of the nutritional status for the trace elements. These factors include dietary intake, renal excretory function, environmental and occupational exposure, duration of renal failure, the concentrations in fresh dialysate, and possibly the mode of dialytic therapy (323–332). Also, many trace elements are highly protein bound. It is possible that uremia may be associated with altered serum-binding protein levels or increased serum concentrations of compounds that compete for binding sites on these proteins; such factors also may alter serum trace element concentrations independently of the body burden or nutritional needs for these elements. Malnutrition, or possibly inflammation leading to low serum proteins, may be one of the causes of low serum zinc, manganese, and nickel (333). In Chapter 19, Table 19.3 shows changes in the status of trace elements as renal failure progresses and in patients undergoing MHD.

Because many trace elements are present in trace amounts in the plasma and are protein bound, losses during hemodialysis may be minimal (334–336). Bromide and zinc, however, are removed during hemodialysis because a substantial proportion of the serum concentrations are not protein bound and because the levels in fresh dialysate are quite low (337). Conversely, the presence in the dialysate of even minute quantities of certain trace elements may lead to uptake by the body because of the avidity with which plasma-binding proteins bind to some trace elements. This phenomenon has been observed for lead, copper, and zinc (336,338).

Serum zinc levels are often low, but erythrocyte zinc is often high, normal, or elevated (24,221,339–343). Low serum zinc may be related to removal by dialysis (337) and inadequate dietary intake. Although serum zinc tends to increase at the end of dialysis, this can be attributed entirely to the increase in concentration of carrier proteins as a result of hemoconcentration (Chapter 19). Some reports indicate that dysgeusia, and impotence in males, may be ameliorated with zinc supplements (344–347); however, other studies have not confirmed these findings (348). Until more definitive studies are conducted concerning dietary zinc requirements, the current recommendation is that patients undergoing hemodialysis should receive the recommended dietary allowance for zinc, which is 15 mg/day. Intestinal zinc absorption is not affected by vitamin D metabolites (349).

Iron deficiency is common in patients undergoing MHD (Chapter 22). The causes include occult intestinal blood loss, sequestration of blood in the dialyzer at the termination of a hemodialysis procedure, binding of iron to the dialyzer membrane, and frequent blood drawing (284,350). Treatment with recombinant human erythropoietin (EPO) may reduce the non-hemoglobin–bound iron stores by enhancing erythropoiesis unless adequate iron supplementation is given. Malnutrition or inflammation, independently or in combination (i.e., MICS; see earlier), may lead to a state of refractory anemia and increase the dose of EPO (351) that is needed to attain the target range of hemoglobin of 11 to 12 g/dL according to the NKF-K/DOQI guidelines (352). Iron deficiency can be determined by measuring serum iron and TIBC; calculating their ratio, known as transferrin saturation; and assessing serum ferritin levels. However, serum TIBC is affected by nutritional status and inflammation (i.e., it is a negative acute-phase reactant), and its serum level generally is decreased in these conditions (77,353). Hence, in malnourished patients undergoing MHD, the transferrin saturation may be erroneously normal to high if the denominator (TIBC) is decreased (353). Serum ferritin is a positive acute-phase reactant and may increase as a result of non-iron–related factors, such as the MICS (89,354,355). Oral iron can be prescribed in the form of ferrous sulfate, fumarate, gluconate, or lactate. However, ingestion of oral iron compounds usually does not lead to sufficient uptake of iron for patients undergoing MHD, and they generally are given iron intravenously in the form of iron dextran, gluconate, and sucrose (saccharide) (284,356). Iron dextran seems to be associated more often with adverse reactions (356,357), and iron gluconate and iron sucrose are probably the safest compound because of their lower rate of generation of free radicals especially in iron gluconate (358).

Little is known concerning the nutritional requirements or tolerance for other trace elements in patients undergoing MHD. It is assumed that the trace quantities in foods and drinking water will satisfy the nutritional needs for these elements. However, the finding that serum selenium is low in patients undergoing dialysis has raised concerns that the dietary intake of selenium may not be adequate (359,360). This question is particularly relevant because selenium is an antioxidant and a component of the defense system against oxidative damage of tissues, which may be increased in renal failure (361–363). More research clearly is needed concerning the optimal intake for trace elements for patients undergoing chronic dialysis.

CARNITINE

Carnitine metabolism in renal failure is discussed in detail in Chapter 21. Carnitine is a naturally occurring compound that is essential for life and is ingested in foods as well as synthesized in the body by the liver and kidneys. Carnitine facilitates the transfer of long-chain (>10 carbon) fatty acids into skeletal muscle mitochondria (364). Because fatty acids are the major fuel source for muscle during both rest and mild to moderate exercise, carnitine is considered necessary for normal muscle function. In patients undergoing MHD, serum total carnitine levels are normal, free carnitine is below normal, and acylcarnitine (fatty acid–carnitine esters) levels are elevated (365,366). Free carnitine levels in skeletal muscle are often but not always low in patients undergoing MHD (70,367,368).

A number of studies have reported that carnitine supplementation in renal failure may increase blood hemoglobin levels, reduce erythropoietin requirements, reduce such intradialytic symptoms as hypotension and muscle cramps, decrease hyperlipidemia, increase skeletal muscle exercise capacity, improve sense of well-being, and reduce postdialysis asthenia and malaise (318,369–371). One randomized, double-blind prospective clinical trial reported that L-carnitine decreased predialysis serum urea, creatinine, and phosphorus concentrations and increased midarm muscle circumference. Interpretation of these data must be qualified because a number of the outcome measures that showed improvement are imprecise or difficult to quantitate. Also, although several studies showing benefits were randomized, prospective, and blinded (particularly the improvement in hemoglobin levels or reduction in erythropoietin needs, increase in exercise capacity, improvement in global well-being, and intradialytic and postdialytic symptoms), other studies showing benefits were not prospective, randomized, or blinded. Moreover, some randomized blinded studies did not confirm such benefits or did so only in *post hoc* analyses. The studies with regard to serum triglyceride levels are particularly conflicting. Some clinical trials show improvement in serum lipid profiles with L-carnitine treatment (372–374), whereas other clinical trials indicate no benefit (375,376) and some studies described an increase in serum triglycerides (366,377).

As a result of these outcomes, many nephrologists remain unconvinced of the therapeutic value of L-carnitine supplementation. However, a number of blinded prospective studies did show benefits, and L-carnitine appears to be quite a safe compound. The NKF-K/DOQI Nutrition Work Group concluded that there are insufficient data to support the routine use of L-carnitine for patients undergoing MHD (70). The NKF-K/DOQI guideline adds, "Although the administration of L-carnitine may improve subjective symptoms such as malaise, muscle weakness, intradialytic cramps and hypotension, and quality of life in selected patients undergoing MHD, the totality of evidence is insufficient to recommend its routine provision for any proposed clinical disorder without prior evaluation and attempts at standard therapy. The most promising of proposed applications is treatment of erythropoietin-resistant anemia" (70,371). Until more definitive data become available, one approach would be to use L-carnitine in the following clinical situations and only when all standard medical therapies have provided no benefit and when there is reason to believe that the medical condition is not irreversible (i.e., weakness associated with disseminated carcinomatosis).

1. Anemia resistant to erythropoietin, iron, and vitamin therapy

2. Intradialytic hypotension or muscle cramps
3. Impaired skeletal-muscle exercise capacity
4. Postdialysis asthenia or malaise

A thorough medical evaluation for other treatable causes should be conducted before instituting carnitine therapy. The optimal dosage and route of therapy for carnitine are unresolved. Gastrointestinal absorption of carnitine in patients undergoing MHD is not known and may be erratic. The United States Center for Medicare and Medicaid Services (CMS) has approved coverage for use of leucocarnitine for patients undergoing MHD if they have low plasma free carnitine (<40 micromoles/L) and either erythropoietin-resistant anemia or hypotension occurring during hemodialysis treatment (378,379). Continued coverage will not be given if improvement is not demonstrated within 6 months of starting treatment. L-carnitine, 10 to 20 mg/kg intravenously, three times per week after the end of each hemodialysis or 5 to 10 mg/kg/day orally, may be used.

MANAGEMENT OF PROTEIN-CALORIE MALNUTRITION

When patients undergoing MHD display evidence for PEM or appear to be at high risk for developing malnutrition, the following steps may be implemented to prevent or treat malnutrition:

1. Perform a medical and social history, physical examination, psychologic evaluation, and a nutritional assessment as indicated in Tables 25.1 and 25.2.
2. Identify the causes of the declining nutritional status. This assessment should include assessing dietary intake (e.g., UNA and dietary interviews and diaries) and the presence of acute illnesses, exacerbation of established comorbid illnesses or nonspecific inflammation (e.g., increased serum CRP). Also, the causes for acidemia or reduced food intake should be investigated (e.g., anorexia from inadequate dialysis, psychologic depression, poor dentition, poverty, inadequate social/family support).
3. Assess the patient's nutritional requirements.
4. Counsel the patient and spouse or significant others concerning the appropriate nutritional intake for the patient and strategies for attaining it.
5. If, despite dietary counseling, the nutrient intake remains inadequate for the patient's needs, the following maneuvers may be used.
   i. Oral supplements (Chapter 26)
   ii. Tube feeding
   iii. Intradialytic parenteral nutrition (Chapter 26)
   iv. Daily parenteral nutrition

Several studies have shown that nutritional supplements in association with dietary counseling can improve the nutritional status of patients undergoing MHD (151,380, 381). A 2002 study by Ikizler et al. showed a nutritional benefit from one can of supplement given three times weekly during each dialysis session (150). In the authors' experience, when malnourished patients undergoing MHD are given oral nutritional supplements, roughly, 20% to 40% of such individuals will take them on a continuing basis for several months or more. However, patients undergoing MHD commonly have modest financial resources, and when patients undergoing MHD must purchase the nutritional supplements, the long-term compliance rate is much lower. Tube feeding may be a more effective, less expensive method for nourishing malnourished adult dialysis patients, as it has been shown to be for the pediatric dialysis population (Chapter 29). There is a need for studies to examine the benefits and potential risks of tube feeding. Tube feeding may be particularly effective for patients with PEM who are anorexic or noncompliant or may have disorders of motility of the upper-gastrointestinal tract.

Several newer methods for the treatment of PEM in patients undergoing MHD have been investigated. These include appetite stimulants, particularly with megestrol acetate (36,382,383). This progestational agent has been shown to improve appetite and food intake and increase water-free body weight in patients with carcinomatosis or AIDS (384,385). However, some evidence suggests that the water-free weight gain is because of accrual of body fat rather than protein (386). There are currently no adequate experimental data as to whether megestrol acetate will improve appetite in patients undergoing MHD who are anorexic and malnourished.

The feasibility of administering amino acid supplements to the patient by hemodialysate was examined by Chazot et al. (387). Six clinically stable men underwent hemodialysis on three separate occasions with hemodialysate containing either no amino acids or one or three times the postabsorptive plasma amino acid concentrations. The patients lost 9.3 ± 2.7 g of amino acid when dialyzed with dialysate containing no amino acids. However, there was a net amino acid uptake of 1.5 ± 3.6 g and 37.1 ± 14.8 g when they used dialysate containing one or three times, respectively, the plasma concentrations of amino acids (387). Further studies will be necessary to demonstrate whether this treatment can be used to improve the nutritional or clinical status of patients undergoing MHD with inadequate nutritional intake or PEM.

Finally, a number of studies have examined the possible benefits of recombinant human growth hormone (rhGH) or recombinant human insulinlike growth factor-I (rhIGF-I) to improve nutritional status of malnourished patients undergoing MHD or CPD (Chapter 32) (388–393). Although patients with advanced CRF display resistance to both rhGH and rhIGF-I, pharmacologic doses of these agents still exert their effects on anabolism, growth, and hyperfiltration. rhGH may promote protein synthesis, decrease protein degradation and improve nitrogen balance in patients without renal failure with catabolic stress (393). It has been used to enhance growth in children with CRF and to maintain or increase the GFR in patients with stage 5 chronic kidney disease and kidney transplantation (394–398) (Chapter 32).

The rhGH also has been used to treat PEM in adult patients with CRF (Chapter 32). Several small, short-term trials have been carried out in patients with CRF to treat PEM with rhGH. Ziegler et al. (399) treated five outpatients undergoing MHD with rhGH for 2 weeks. The patients were prescribed a fixed protein and calorie diet. The SUN fell by 20% to 25% when patients received rhGH, 5 to 10 mg subcutaneously after each hemodialysis. Schulman et al. (400) treated seven malnourished patients undergoing MHD with intradialytic parenteral nutrition for 12 weeks. During the last 6 weeks, when patients also received rhGH, 5 mg subcutaneously, with each dialysis, there was a decrease in the PNA, from 0.81 ± 0.04 to 0.67 ± 0.03 g/kg/day and an increase in the serum albumin levels.

Kopple studied six patients undergoing MHD with PEM in a General Clinical Research Center for up to 35 days (401). After a baseline period of 14 to 21 days, patients were administered 0.05 mg rhGH/kg body weight/day for 17 ± SEM 2 days. During the study, patients 3 and 4 experienced acute illness with a reduction in protein and energy intake. Predialysis serum urea nitrogen fell markedly in patients 1, 2, 5, and 6 and less so in patients 3 and 4. Nitrogen balance was also markedly positive in patients 1, 2, 5, and 6 but much less so in patients 3 and 4 (401). Other studies on rhGH in patients with CKD who have not yet reached ESRD are reviewed in Chapter 23.

rhIGF-I also promotes positive nitrogen balance and decreases SUN in patients undergoing MHD or CPD (389). Side effects with rhGH injections include hyperglycemia and acromegaly (395,402). Treatment of critically ill patients in the intensive-care unit with rhIGF-I is reported to increase mortality (403) and should not be done. RhIGF-I, at doses currently used, may cause hypoglycemia and, uncommonly, cardiac arrhythmias and transient alterations in mental status. At present neither of these agents has been approved by the United States Food and Drug Administration for treatment of PEM or low GFR in patients with CRF or those undergoing MHD. rhGH has been approved for treatment of impaired growth in children with CRF.

TREATMENT OF ACUTE CATABOLIC ILLNESS

When patients undergoing MHD sustain superimposed catabolic illnesses, their intolerance for water, nitrogenous products, and many minerals and vitamins dictates that nutritional support must be modified extensively and controlled carefully. The high incidence of malnutrition in patients undergoing MHD and the close association between nutritional status and morbidity and mortality also suggest that it may be beneficial to provide nutritional support during acute illness if the patient's nutritional intake falls below his or her nutritional needs. The principles and techniques for nutritional support for patients undergoing MHD generally are similar to the methods for nutritional support for patients with acute renal failure and are discussed in Chapters 26 and 30. Nutritional management during treatment of the patient with renal failure with continuous renal replacement therapy is discussed in Chapter 31.

DAILY OR LONG-DURATION HEMODIALYSIS AND NUTRITIONAL STATUS

Several new approaches to standard hemodialysis therapy are currently either employed or are being examined in a small number of dialysis facilities. These include longer-duration and/or more frequent hemodialysis sessions (404–408). Long-duration hemodialysis is generally carried out for about 6 to 8 hours thrice weekly using lower blood flow rates of 200 to 250 mL/min (205). Short daily hemodialysis is characterized by 5 or 6 treatments per week, each lasting 1.5 to 2.5 hours, using conventional blood and dialysate flow rates (408,409). Nocturnal hemodialysis is performed 5 to 7 times per week; each treatment lasting 6 to 8 hours, with blood flow rates of about 200 to 300 mL/min and dialysate flows of approximately 200 to 300 mL/min (409,410). With each of these treatments, biocompatible hemodialysis membranes, often high flux, are generally employed. An increasing number of centers are experimenting with the latter two treatment schedules (411,412).

Preliminary data from the studies evaluating the effects of daily and nocturnal hemodialysis on nutritional status suggest a number of benefits. With both short daily hemodialysis and nocturnal hemodialysis the patient has less restrictions on dietary intake (404,405,413,414). Also, with long-duration, short daily and nocturnal dialyses, the patients' spontaneous dietary energy and protein intake appears to increase (316,404–407). This latter observation is supported by a rise in their dry weight, edema-free, fat-free body mass, or serum albumin levels (316,404,405,413, 414). There is often a striking lowering of the serum phosphorus concentrations that occurs with nocturnal hemodialysis (411). The reduced anorexia and nutritional improvement may be due to reduced uremia and also possibly the enhanced sense of well being, less dietetic constraints, and fewer drugs prescribed. These more intensive hemodialysis treatments are also reported to result in tighter blood pressure control, regression of left ventricular hypertrophy, correction of anemia, and improved quality of life (205,415). It is not clear whether these biological and clinical improvements are mainly the results of the greater frequency of dialysis treatments or higher weekly doses of dialysis. Prospective clinical trials are required to delineate the full potential of these therapies on nutritional status as well the differences between them.

There are little data on the nutritional needs of patients undergoing daily and/or longer duration hemodialyses. Energy, protein, mineral and vitamin needs are probably as described in Table 25.3. Exceptions to this may be the dietary potassium and phosphorus needs that may be increased (404,405,413,414). On the other hand, with more frequent or higher weekly doses of hemodialysis there is probably increased tolerance for higher intakes of protein, water, sodium, potassium, phosphorus, magnesium, and the potentially more hazardous of the water soluble (i.e., dialyzable) vitamins, such as ascorbic acid (316,404,405,413, 414). As in all MHD patients with more frequent and/or higher weekly doses of hemodialysis the nutrient intake, nutritional status, and serum mineral levels of the individual should be monitored closely.

REFERENCES

1. Acchiardo SR, Moore LW, Latour PA. Malnutrition as the main factor in morbidity and mortality of hemodialysis patients. *Kidney Int Suppl* 1983;16:S199–203.
2. Bergström J. Anorexia and malnutrition in hemodialysis patients. *Blood Purif* 1992;10:35–39.
3. Kopple JD. McCollum Award Lecture, 1996: Protein-energy malnutrition in maintenance dialysis patients. *Am J Clin Nutr* 1997;65:1544–1557.
4. Kalantar-Zadeh K, Kopple JD. Relative contributions of nutrition and inflammation to clinical outcome in dialysis patients. *Am J Kidney Dis* 2001;38:1343–1350.
5. Bilbrey GL, Cohen TL. Identification and treatment of protein calorie malnutrition in chronic hemodialysis patients. *Dial Transplant* 1989;18:669–677.
6. Mehrotra R, Kopple JD. Nutritional management of maintenance dialysis patients: Why aren't we doing better? In: McCormick DB, Bier DM, Cousins RJ, eds. *Annual review of nutrition* Vol. 21. Palo Alto, CA: Annual Reviews, 2001:343–380.
7. Kalantar-Zadeh K, Kopple JD, Block G, et al. A malnutrition-inflammation score is correlated with morbidity and mortality in maintenance hemodialysis patients. *Am J Kidney Dis* 2001; 38:1251–1263.
8. Ritz E, Vallance P, Nowicki M. The effect of malnutrition on cardiovascular mortality in dialysis patients: is L-arginine the answer? *Nephrol Dial Transplant* 1994;9:129–130.
9. Stenvinkel P, Heimburger O, Paultre F, et al. Strong association between malnutrition, inflammation, and atherosclerosis in chronic renal failure. *Kidney Int* 1999;55:1899–1911.
10. Kalantar-Zadeh K, Block G, Humphreys MH, et al. Reverse epidemiology of cardiovascular risk factors in maintenance dialysis patients. *Kidney Int* 2003;63:793–808.
11. Kopple JD, Zhu X, Lew NL, et al. Body weight-for-height relationships predict mortality in maintenance hemodialysis patients. *Kidney Int* 1999;56:1136–1148.
12. Iseki K, Yamazato M, Tozawa M, et al. Hypocholesterolemia is a significant predictor of death in a cohort of chronic hemodialysis patients. *Kidney Int* 2002;61:1887–1893.
13. Lowrie EG, Lew NL. Death risk in hemodialysis patients: the predictive value of commonly measured variables and an evaluation of death rate differences between facilities. *Am J Kidney Dis* 1990;15:458–482.
14. Calle EE, Thun MJ, Petrelli JM, et al. Body-mass index and mortality in a prospective cohort of U.S. adults. *N Engl J Med* 1999;341:1097–1105.
15. Kalantar-Zadeh K, Kopple J. Inflammation in renal failure. Up To Date 2003, Nephrology.
16. Stenvinkel P, Heimburger O, Paultre F, et al. Strong association between malnutrition, inflammation, and atherosclerosis in chronic renal failure. *Kidney Int* 1999;55:1899–1911.
17. U.S. Department of Public Health and Human Services, Public Health Service. United States Renal Data System. Bethesda: National Institutes of Health, 2002.
18. Eknoyan G, Beck GJ, Cheung AK, et al. Effect of dialysis dose and membrane flux in maintenance hemodialysis. *N Engl J Med* 2002;347:2010–2019.
19. Descombes E, Hanck AB, Fellay G. Water soluble vitamins in chronic hemodialysis patients and need for supplementation. *Kidney Int* 1993;43:1319–1328.
20. Moriwaki K, Kanno Y, Nakamoto H, et al. Vitamin B6 deficiency in elderly patients on chronic peritoneal dialysis. *Adv Perit Dial* 2000;16:308–312.
21. Yonemura K, Fujimoto T, Fujigaki Y, et al. Vitamin D deficiency is implicated in reduced serum albumin concentrations in patients with end-stage renal disease. *Am J Kidney Dis* 2000; 36:337–344.
22. Sullivan JF, Eisenstein AB. Ascorbic acid depletion during hemodialysis. *JAMA* 1972;220:1697–1699.
23. Sullivan JF, Eisenstein AB. Ascorbic acid depletion in patients undergoing chronic hemodialysis. *Am J Clin Nutr* 1970;23: 1339–1346.
24. Erten Y, Kayatas M, Sezer S, et al. Zinc deficiency: prevalence and causes in hemodialysis patients and effect on cellular immune response. *Transplant Proc* 1998;30:850–851.
25. Mahajan SK, Prasad AS, Rabbani P, et al. Zinc deficiency: a reversible complication of uremia. *Am J Clin Nutr* 1982;36: 1177–1183.
26. Blendis LM, Ampil M, Wilson DR, et al. The importance of dietary protein in the zinc deficiency of uremia. *Am J Clin Nutr* 1981;34:2658–2661.
27. Carr AC, Zhu BZ, Frei B. Potential antiatherogenic mechanisms of ascorbate (vitamin C) and alpha-tocopherol (vitamin E). *Circ Res* 2000;87:349–354.
28. Jialal I, Grundy SM. Effect of combined supplementation with alpha-tocopherol, ascorbate, and beta carotene on low-density lipoprotein oxidation. *Circulation* 1993;88:2780–2786.
29. Arnadottir M, Brattstrom L, Simonsen O, et al. The effect of high-dose pyridoxine and folic acid supplementation on serum lipid and plasma homocysteine concentrations in dialysis patients. *Clin Nephrol* 1993;40:236–240.
30. Kalantar-Zadeh K, Kopple JD, Deepak S, et al. Food intake characteristics of hemodialysis patients as obtained by food frequency questionnaire. *J Ren Nutr* 2002;12:17–31.
31. Facchini F, Schoenfeld P, Dixon B, et al. ESRD patients consume an atherogenic diet. *J Am Soc Neph* 1997;7:S133 (Abstract A1079).
32. Chertow GM, Burke SK, Raggi P. Sevelamer attenuates the progression of coronary and aortic calcification in hemodialysis patients. *Kidney Int* 2002;62:245–252.
33. Raggi P, Boulay A, Chasan-Taber S, et al. Cardiac calcification in adult hemodialysis patients. A link between end-stage renal disease and cardiovascular disease? *J Am Coll Cardiol* 2002;39: 695–701.
34. Kalantar-Zadeh K, Block G, McAllister C, et al. Association between self-reported appetite and markers of inflammation,

nutrition, anemia and quality of life in hemodialysis patients. 2003, *(in press).*

35. Bergström J. Regulation of appetite in chronic renal failure. *Miner Electrolyte Metab* 1999;25:291–297.
36. Yeh S, Wu SY, Levine DM, et al. Quality of life and stimulation of weight gain after treatment with megestrol acetate: correlation between cytokine levels and nutritional status, appetite in geriatric patients with wasting syndrome. *J Nutr Health Aging* 2000; 4:246–251.
37. Kopple JD, Swendseid ME, Shinaberger JH, et al. The free and bound amino acids removed by hemodialysis. *Trans Am Soc Artif Intern Organs* 1973;19:309–313.
38. Wolfson M, Jones MR, Kopple JD. Amino acid losses during hemodialysis with infusion of amino acids and glucose. *Kidney Int* 1982;21:500–506.
39. Ikizler TA, Flakoll PJ, Parker RA, et al. Amino acid and albumin losses during hemodialysis. *Kidney Int* 1994;46:830–837.
40. Gutierrez A, Bergström J, Alvestrand A. Hemodialysis-associated protein catabolism with and without glucose in the dialysis fluid. *Kidney Int* 1994;46:814–822.
41. Kaplan AA, Halley SE, Lapkin RA, et al. Dialysate protein losses with bleach processed polysulphone dialyzers. *Kidney Int* 1995; 47:573–578.
42. Vanherweghem JL, Drukker W, Schwarz A. Clinical significance of blood-device interaction in hemodialysis. A review. *Int J Artif Organs* 1987;10:219–232.
43. Oster JR, Lopez RA, Silverstein FJ, et al. The anion gap of patients receiving bicarbonate maintenance hemodialysis. *ASAIO Trans* 1989;35:800–804.
44. Tolchin N, Roberts JL, Hayashi J, et al. Metabolic consequences of high mass-transfer hemodialysis. *Kidney Int* 1977;11: 366–378.
45. Ward RA, Wathen RL, Williams TE, et al. Hemodialysate composition and intradialytic metabolic, acid-base and potassium changes. *Kidney Int* 1987;32:129–135.
46. (DOQI) NKFKDOQI. Clinical practice guidelines for nutrition in chronic renal failure. *Am J Kidney Dis* 2000;35:suppl 2.
47. Kovacic V, Roguljic L. Metabolic acidosis of chronically hemodialyzed patients. *Am J Nephrol* 2003;23:158–164.
48. Gutierrez A, Alvestrand A, Wahren J, et al. Effect of in vivo contact between blood and dialysis membranes on protein catabolism in humans. *Kidney Int* 1990;38:487–494.
49. Gutierrez A, Bergström J, Alvestrand A. Protein catabolism in sham-hemodialysis: the effect of different membranes. *Clin Nephrol* 1992;38:20–29.
50. Borah MF, Schonfeld PY, Gotch FA, et al. Nitrogen balance during intermittent dialysis therapy of uremia. *Kidney Int* 1978; 14:491–500.
51. Heidland A, Hörl WH, Heller N, et al. Proteolytic enzymes and catabolism: enhanced release of granulocyte proteinases in uremic intoxication and during hemodialysis. *Kidney Int Suppl* 1983;16:S27–36.
52. Baracos V, Rodemann HP, Dinarello CA, et al. Stimulation of muscle protein degradation and prostaglandin E2 release by leukocytic pyrogen (interleukin-1). A mechanism for the increased degradation of muscle proteins during fever. *N Engl J Med* 1983;308:553–558.
53. Stenvinkel P, Alvestrand A. Inflammation in end-stage renal disease: sources, consequences, and therapy. *Semin Dial* 2002; 15:329–337.
54. Himmelfarb J, Stenvinkel P, Ikizler TA, et al. The elephant in uremia: oxidant stress as a unifying concept of cardiovascular disease in uremia. *Kidney Int* 2002;62:1524–1538.
55. Nawabi MD, Block KP, Chakrabarti MC, et al. Administration of endotoxin, tumor necrosis factor, or interleukin 1 to rats activates skeletal muscle branched-chain alpha-keto acid dehydrogenase. *J Clin Invest* 1990;85:256–263.
56. Flores EA, Bistrian BR, Pomposelli JJ, et al. Infusion of tumor necrosis factor/cachectin promotes muscle catabolism in the rat. A synergistic effect with interleukin 1. *J Clin Invest* 1989;83: 1614–1622.
57. Perlmutter DH, Dinarello CA, Punsal PI, et al. Cachetin/tumor necrosis factor regulates hepatic acute-phase gene expression. *J Clin Invest* 1986;78:1349–1355.
58. Stenvinkel P. Malnutrition and chronic inflammation as risk factors for cardiovascular disease in chronic renal failure. *Blood Purif* 2001;19:143–151.
59. Stenvinkel P, Heimburger O, Lindholm B, et al. Are there two types of malnutrition in chronic renal failure? Evidence for relationships between malnutrition, inflammation and atherosclerosis (MIA syndrome). *Nephrol Dial Transplant* 2000;15: 953–960.
60. Ifudu O, Uribarri J, Rajwani I, et al. Low hematocrit may connote a malnutrition-inflammation syndrome in hemodialysis patients. *Dial Transplant* 2002;31:845–878.
61. Wathen RL, Keshaviah P, Hommeyer P, et al. The metabolic effects of hemodialysis with and without glucose in the dialysate. *Am J Clin Nutr* 1978;31:1870–1875.
62. Marumo F, Kamata K, Okubo M. Deranged concentrations of water-soluble vitamins in the blood of undialyzed and dialyzed patients with chronic renal failure. *Int J Artif Organs* 1986;9: 17–24.
63. Stone WJ, Warnock LG, Wagner C. Vitamin B6 deficiency in uremia. *Am J Clin Nutr* 1975;28:950–957.
64. Dobbelstein H, Korner WF, Mempel W, et al. Vitamin B6 deficiency in uremia and its implications for the depression of immune responses. *Kidney Int* 1974;5:233–239.
65. Jansen MAM, Korevaar JC, Dekker FW, et al. Renal function and nutritional status at the start of dialysis treatment. *J Am Soc Nephrol* 2001;12:157–163.
66. Kopple JD, Massry SG. Nutritional management of renal disease. In: Kopple JD, Massry SG, eds. *Nutritional management of nondialyzed patients with chronic renal failure.* Baltimore: William and Wilkins, 1996:479–531.
67. Mailloux LU, Napolitano B, Bellucci AG, et al. The impact of co-morbid risk factors at the start of dialysis upon the survival of ESRD patients. *ASAIO J* 1996;42:164–169.
68. Kopple JD. Nutrition in renal failure. Causes of catabolism and wasting in acute or chronic renal failure. In: Robinson RR, ed. *Nephrology. Proceedings of the IXth International Congress of Nephrology*, Vol. 2. New York: Springer-Verlag, 1984: 1498–1515.
69. K/DOQI clinical practice guidelines for chronic kidney disease: evaluation, classification, and stratification. Kidney Dialysis Outcome Quality Initiative. *Am J Kidney Dis* 2002;39:S1–246.
70. Clinical practice guidelines for nutrition in chronic renal failure. K/DOQI, National Kidney Foundation. *Am J Kidney Dis* 2000; 35:S1–S140.
71. Lowrie EG, Huang WH, Lew NL. Death risk predictors among peritoneal dialysis and hemodialysis patients. *Am J Kidney Dis* 1995;26:220–228.
72. Leavey SF, Strawderman RL, Jones CA, et al. Simple nutritional indicators as independent predictors of mortality in hemodialysis patients. *Am J Kidney Dis* 1998;31:997–1006.
73. Canada-USA Peritoneal Dialysis Study Group. Adequacy of dialysis and nutrition in continuous peritoneal dialysis: association with clinical outcomes. *J Am Soc Nephrol* 1996;7:198–207.
74. Enia G, Sicuso C, Alati G, et al. Subjective global assessment of nutrition in dialysis patients. *Nephrol Dial Transplant* 1993; 8:1094–1098.
75. Hirsch S, de Obaldia N, Petermann M, et al. Subjective global

assessment of nutritional status: further validation. *Nutrition* 1991;7:35–37; discussion 37–38.

76. Detsky AS, McLaughlin JR, Baker JP, et al. What is subjective global assessment of nutritional status? *JPEN J Parenter Enteral Nutr* 1987;11:8–13.
77. Kalantar-Zadeh K, Kleiner M, Dunne E, et al. Total iron-binding capacity-estimated transferrin correlates with the nutritional subjective global assessment in hemodialysis patients. *Am J Kidney Dis* 1998;31:263–272.
78. McCann L. Using subjective global assessment to identify malnutrition in the ESRD patient. *Nephrol News Issues* 1999;13: 18–19.
79. Kalantar-Zadeh K, Kleiner M, Dunne E, et al. A modified quantitative subjective global assessment of nutrition for dialysis patients. *Nephrol Dial Transplant* 1999;14:1732–1738.
80. Kopple JD, Mehrotra R, Suppasyndh O, et al. Observations with regard to the National Kidney Foundation K/DOQI clinical practice guidelines concerning serum transthyretin in chronic renal failure. *Clin Chem Lab Med* 2002;40:1308–1312.
81. Chertow GM, Ackert K, Lew NL, et al. Prealbumin is as important as albumin in the nutritional assessment of hemodialysis patients. *Kidney Int* 2000;58:2512–2517.
82. Chertow GM, Jacobs D, Lazarus J, et al. Phase angle predicts survival in hemodialysis patients. *J Renal Nutrition* 1997;7: 204–207.
83. Chertow GM, Lowrie EG, Wilmore DW, et al. Nutritional assessment with bioelectrical impedance analysis in maintenance hemodialysis patients. *J Am Soc Nephrol* 1995;6:75–81.
84. Kalantar-Zadeh K, Dunne E, Nixon K, et al. Near infra-red interactance for nutritional assessment of dialysis patients. *Nephrol Dial Transplant* 1999;14:169–175.
85. Chertow GM. Estimates of body composition as intermediate outcome variables: are DEXA and BIA ready for prime time? *J Ren Nutr* 1999;9:138–141.
86. Dumler F. Use of bioelectric impedance analysis and dual-energy X-ray absorptiometry for monitoring the nutritional status of dialysis patients. *Asaio J* 1997;43:256–260.
87. Woodrow G, Oldroyd B, Turney JH, et al. Whole body and regional body composition in patients with chronic renal failure. *Nephrol Dial Transplant* 1996;11:1613–1618.
88. Neyra NR, Hakim RM, Shyr Y, et al. Serum transferrin and serum prealbumin are early predictors of serum albumin in chronic hemodialysis patients. *J Ren Nutr* 2000;10:184–190.
89. Kalantar-Zadeh K, Don BR, Rodriguez RA, et al. Serum ferritin is a marker of morbidity and mortality in hemodialysis patients. *Am J Kidney Dis* 2001;37:564–572.
90. Kaysen GA, Rathore V, Shearer GC, et al. Mechanisms of hypoalbuminemia in hemodialysis patients. *Kidney Int* 1995;48: 510–516.
91. Kaysen GA, Chertow GM, Adhikarla R, et al. Inflammation and dietary protein intake exert competing effects on serum albumin and creatinine in hemodialysis patients. *Kidney Int* 2001;60:333–340.
92. Kaysen GA. The microinflammatory state in uremia: causes and potential consequences. *J Am Soc Nephrol* 2001;12:1549–1557.
93. Owen WF Jr, Lew NL, Liu Y, et al. The urea reduction ratio and serum albumin concentration as predictors of mortality in patients undergoing hemodialysis. *N Engl J Med* 1993;329: 1001–1006.
94. Leavey SF, McCullough K, Hecking E, et al. Body mass index and mortality in 'healthier' as compared with 'sicker' haemodialysis patients: results from the Dialysis Outcomes and Practice Patterns Study (DOPPS). *Nephrol Dial Transplant* 2001;16: 2386–2394.
95. Bergström J. Inflammation, malnutrition, cardiovascular disease and mortality in end-stage renal disease. *Pol Arch Med Wewn* 2000;104:641–643.
96. Wilcken DE, Dudman NP, Tyrrell PA, et al. Folic acid lowers elevated plasma homocysteine in chronic renal insufficiency: possible implications for prevention of vascular disease. *Metabolism* 1988;37:697–701.
97. Suliman ME, Lindholm B, Barany P, et al. Hyperhomocysteinemia in chronic renal failure patients: relation to nutritional status and cardiovascular disease. *Clin Chem Lab Med* 2001;39: 734–738.
98. Wrone EM, Zehnder JL, Hornberger JM, et al. An MTHFR variant, homocysteine, and cardiovascular comorbidity in renal disease. *Kidney Int* 2001;60:1106–1113.
99. Daugirdas JT. The post: pre dialysis plasma urea nitrogen ratio to estimate Kt/V and NPCR: validation. *Int J Artif Organs* 1989; 12:420–427.
100. Sargent J, Gotch F, Borah M, et al. Urea kinetics: a guide to nutritional management of renal failure. *Am J Clin Nutr* 1978; 31:1696–1702.
101. Kalantar-Zadeh K, Supasyndh O, Lehn RS, et al. Normalized protein nitrogen appearance is correlated with hospitalization and mortality in hemodialysis patients with Kt/V greater than 1.20. *J Ren Nutr* 2003;13:15–25.
102. Keshaviah PR, Emerson PF, Nolph KD. Timely initiation of dialysis: a urea kinetic approach. *Am J Kidney Dis* 1999;33: 344–348.
103. Kopple JD, Jones MR, Keshaviah PR, et al. A proposed glossary for dialysis kinetics. *Am J Kidney Dis* 1995;26:963–981.
104. Bergström J. Nutrition and adequacy of dialysis in hemodialysis patients. *Kidney Int Suppl* 1993;41:S261–267.
105. Lindsay RM, Spanner E. A hypothesis: the protein catabolic rate is dependent upon the type and amount of treatment in dialyzed uremic patients. *Am J Kidney Dis* 1989;13:382–389.
106. Hakim RM, Breyer J, Ismail N, et al. Effects of dose of dialysis on morbidity and mortality. *Am J Kidney Dis* 1994;23: 661–669.
107. Yang CS, Chen SW, Chiang CH, et al. Effects of increasing dialysis dose on serum albumin and mortality in hemodialysis patients. *Am J Kidney Dis* 1996;27:380–386.
108. Nolph KD. What's new in peritoneal dialysis—an overview. *Kidney Int Suppl* 1992;38:S148–152.
109. Lysaght MJ, Pollock CA, Hallet MD, et al. The relevance of urea kinetic modeling to CAPD. *ASAIO Trans* 1989;35:784–790.
110. Lindsay R, Spanner E, Heienheim P, et al. Which comes first, Kt/V or PCR—chicken or egg? *Kidney Int* 1992;42(Suppl 3): S32–S37.
111. Harty JC, Boulton H, Curwell J, et al. The normalized protein catabolic rate is a flawed marker of nutrition in CAPD patients. *Kidney Int* 1994;45:103–109.
112. Nolph KD, Moore HL, Prowant B, et al. Cross sectional assessment of weekly urea and creatinine clearances and indices of nutrition in continuous ambulatory peritoneal dialysis patients. *Perit Dial Int* 1993;13:178–183.
113. Bergström J, Furst P, Alvestrand A, et al. Protein and energy intake, nitrogen balance and nitrogen losses in patients treated with continuous ambulatory peritoneal dialysis. *Kidney Int* 1993;44:1048–1057.
114. National Kidney Foundation I, Kidney-Dialysis Outcome Quality Initiative: K/DOQI Clinical Practice Guidelines: Peritoneal Dialysis Adequacy. *Am J Kidney Dis* 2001;37(Suppl 1): S65–136.
115. Port FK, Wolfe RA. How will the results of the HEMO Study impact dialysis practice? *Semin Dial* 2003;16:13–16.
116. Rayner HC, Pisoni RL, Gillespie BW, et al. Creation, cannulation and survival of arteriovenous fistulae: Data from the Di-

alysis Outcomes and Practice Patterns Study. *Kidney Int* 2003; 63:323–330.
117. Konner K, Hulbert-Shearon TE, Roys EC, et al. Tailoring the initial vascular access for dialysis patients. *Kidney Int* 2002;62: 329–338.
118. Port FK, Ashby VB, Dhingra RK, et al. Dialysis dose and body mass index are strongly associated with survival in hemodialysis patients. *J Am Soc Nephrol* 2002;13:1061–1066.
119. Straumann E, Keller U, Kury D, et al. Effect of acute acidosis and alkalosis on leucine kinetics in man. *Clin Physiol* 1992;12: 39–51.
120. Papadoyannakis NJ, Stefanidis CJ, McGeown M. The effect of the correction of metabolic acidosis on nitrogen and potassium balance of patients with chronic renal failure. *Am J Clin Nutr* 1984;40:623–627.
121. May RC, Kelly RA, Mitch WE. Mechanisms for defects in muscle protein metabolism in rats with chronic uremia: the influence of metabolic acidosis. *J Clin Invest* 1987;79: 1099–1103.
122. Mitch WE, Medina R, Grieber S, et al. Metabolic acidosis stimulates muscle protein degradation by activating the adenosine triphosphate-dependent pathway involving ubiquitin and proteasomes. *J Clin Invest* 1994;93:2127–2133.
123. Bailey JL, Wang X, England BK, et al. The acidosis of chronic renal failure activates muscle proteolysis in rats by augmenting transcription of genes encoding proteins of the ATP-dependent ubiquitin-proteasome pathway. *J Clin Invest* 1996;97: 1447–1453.
124. Price SR, England BK, Bailey JL, et al. Acidosis and glucocorticoids concomitantly increase ubiquitin and proteasome subunit mRNAs in rat muscle. *Am J Physiol* 1994;267:C955–960.
125. Bergström J, Alvestrand A, Furst P. Plasma and muscle free amino acids in maintenance hemodialysis patients without protein malnutrition. *Kidney Int* 1990;38:108–114.
126. Williams AJ, Dittmer ID, McArley A, et al. High bicarbonate dialysate in haemodialysis patients: effects on acidosis and nutritional status. *Nephrol Dial Transplant* 1997;12:2633–2637.
127. Williams B, Hattersley J, Layward E, et al. Metabolic acidosis and skeletal muscle adaptation to low protein diets in chronic uremia. *Kidney Int* 1991;40:779–786.
128. Ballmer PE, McNurlan MA, Hulter HN, et al. Chronic metabolic acidosis decreases albumin synthesis and induces negative nitrogen balance in humans. *J Clin Invest* 1995;95:39–45.
129. Kopple JD, Shinaberger JH, Coburn JW, et al. Optimal dietary protein treatment during chronic hemodialysis. *Trans Am Soc Artif Int Org* 1969;15:302–308.
130. Kluthe R, Luttgren FM, Capetianu T, et al. Protein requirements in maintenance hemodialysis patients. *Am J Clin Nutr* 1978;31:1812–1820.
131. Ginn HE, Frost A, Lacy WW. Nitrogen balance in hemodialysis patients. *Am J Clin Nutr* 1968;21:385–393.
132. Kopple JD, Shinaberger JH, Coburn JW, et al. Optimal dietary protein treatment during chronic hemodialysis. *Trans Am Soc Artif Intern Organs* 1969;15:302–308.
133. Schoenfeld PY, Henry RR, Laird NM, et al. Assessment of nutritional status of the National Cooperative Dialysis Study population. *Kidney Int Suppl* 1983;23:S80–88.
134. Food and Nutrition Board. *Dietary Reference Intakes*. Washington, DC: National Academy Press, 2001.
135. Shinaberger JH, Ginn HE. Low protein, high essential amino acid diet for nitrogen equilibrium in chronic dialysis. *Am J Clin Nutr* 1968;21:618–625.
136. Slomowitz LA, Monteon FJ, Grosvenor M, et al. Effect of energy intake on nutritional status in maintenance hemodialysis patients. *Kidney Int* 1989;35:704–711.
137. Dwyer JT, Cunniff PJ, Maroni BJ, et al. The hemodialysis pilot study: nutrition program and participant characteristics at baseline. The HEMO Study Group. *J Ren Nutr* 1998;8:11–20.
138. Gotch FA, Sargent JA. A mechanistic analysis of the National Cooperative Dialysis Study (NCDS). *Kidney Int* 1985;28: 526–534.
139. Uribarri J. Doqi guidelines for nutrition in long-term peritoneal dialysis patients: a dissenting view. *Am J Kidney Dis* 2001;37: 1313–1318.
140. Lim VS, Flanigan MJ. Protein intake in patients with renal failure: comments on the current NKF-DOQI guidelines for nutrition in chronic renal failure. *Semin Dial* 2001;14: 150–152.
141. Kopple JD. Nutritional status as a predictor of morbidity and mortality in maintenance dialysis patients. *Asaio J* 1997;43: 246–250.
142. Bansal VK, Popli S, Pickering J, et al. Protein-calorie malnutrition and cutaneous anergy in hemodialysis maintained patients. *Am J Clin Nutr* 1980;33:1608–1611.
143. Blumenkrantz MJ, Kopple JD, Gutman RA, et al. Methods for assessing nutritional status of patients with renal failure. *Am J Clin Nutr* 1980;33:1567–1585.
144. Thunberg BJ, Swamy AP, Cestero RV. Cross-sectional and longitudinal nutritional measurements in maintenance hemodialysis patients. *Am J Clin Nutr* 1981;34:2005–2012.
145. Young GA, Swanepoel CR, Croft MR, et al. Anthropometery and plasma valine, amino acids and protein in the nutritional assessment of hemodialysis patients. *Kidney Int* 1982;21: 492–499.
146. Wolfson M, Strong CJ, Minturn D, et al. Nutritional status and lymphocyte function in maintenance hemodialysis patients. *Am J Clin Nutr* 1984;39:547–555.
147. Blumenkrantz MJ, Gahl GM, Kopple JD, et al. Protein losses during peritoneal dialysis. *Kidney Int* 1981;19:593–602.
148. Dwyer JT, Larive B, Leung J, et al. Nutritional status affects quality of life in Hemodialysis (HEMO) Study patients at baseline. *J Ren Nutr* 2002;12:213–223.
149. Monteon FJ, Laidlaw SA, Shaib JK, et al. Energy expenditure in patients with chronic renal failure. *Kidney Int* 1986;30: 741–747.
150. Ikizler TA, Pupim LB, Brouillette JR, et al. Hemodialysis stimulates muscle and whole body protein loss and alters substrate oxidation. *Am J Physiol Endocrinol Metab* 2002;282:E107–116.
151. Pupim LB, Flakoll PJ, Brouillette JR, et al. Intradialytic parenteral nutrition improves protein and energy homeostasis in chronic hemodialysis patients. *J Clin Invest* 2002;110:483–492.
152. Schneeweiss B, Graninger W, Stockenhuber F, et al. Energy metabolism in acute and chronic renal failure. *Am J Clin Nutr* 1990;52:596–601.
153. Neyra R, Chen KY, Sun M, et al. Increased resting energy expenditure in patients with end-stage renal disease. *JPEN J Parenter Enteral Nutr* 2003;27:36–42.
154. Keane WF, Collins AJ. Influence of co-morbidity on mortality and morbidity in patients treated with hemodialysis. *Am J Kidney Dis* 1994;24:1010–1018.
155. Kasiske B. Hyperlipidemia in patients with chronic renal disease. *Am J Kidney Dis* 1998;32:S142–S156.
156. Brunzell JD, Albers JJ, Haas LB, et al. Prevalence of serum lipid abnormalities in chronic hemodialysis. *Metabolism* 1977;26: 903–910.
157. Pedro-Botet J, Senti M, Rubies-Prat J, et al. When to treat dyslipidaemia of patients with chronic renal failure on haemodialysis? A need to define specific guidelines. *Nephrol Dial Transplant* 1996;11:308–313.
158. Lacour B, Roullet JB, Beyne P, et al. Comparison of several atherogenicity indices by the analysis of serum lipoprotein composition in patients with chronic renal failure with or without

haemodialysis, and in renal transplant patients. *J Clin Chem Clin Biochem* 1985;23:805–810.

159. Cheung AK, Wu LL, Kablitz C, et al. Atherogenic lipids and lipoproteins in hemodialysis patients. *Am J Kidney Dis* 1993; 22:271–276.

160. Brook JG, Chaimovitz C, Rapoport J, et al. High-density lipoprotein composition in chronic hemodialysis. *N Engl J Med* 1979;300:1056.

161. Rapoport J, Aviram M, Chaimovitz C, et al. Defective high-density lipoprotein composition in patients on chronic hemodialysis. A possible mechanism for accelerated atherosclerosis. *N Engl J Med* 1978;299:1326–1329.

162. Attman PO. Hyperlipoproteinaemia in renal failure: pathogenesis and perspectives for intervention. *Nephrol Dial Transplant* 1993;8:294–295.

163. Attman PO, Alaupovic P. Lipid and apolipoprotein profiles of uremic dyslipoproteinemia—relation to renal function and dialysis. *Nephron* 1991;57:401–410.

164. Oi K, Hirano T, Sakai S, et al. Role of hepatic lipase in intermediate-density lipoprotein and small, dense low-density lipoprotein formation in hemodialysis patients. *Kidney Int Suppl* 1999; 71:S227–228.

165. Senti M, Romero R, Pedro-Botet J, et al. Lipoprotein abnormalities in hyperlipidemic and normolipidemic men on hemodialysis with chronic renal failure. *Kidney Int* 1992;41: 1394–1399.

166. Parsy D, Dracon M, Cachera C, et al. Lipoprotein abnormalities in chronic haemodialysis patients. *Nephrol Dial Transplant* 1988;3:51–56.

167. Attman PO, Alaupovic P, Tavella M, et al. Abnormal lipid and apolipoprotein composition of major lipoprotein density classes in patients with chronic renal failure. *Nephrol Dial Transplant* 1996;11:63–69.

168. Weintraub M, Burstein A, Rassin T, et al. Severe defect in clearing postprandial chylomicron remnants in dialysis patients. *Kidney Int* 1992;42:1247–1252.

169. Schettler V, Wieland E, Verwiebe R, et al. Plasma lipids are not oxidized during hemodialysis. *Nephron* 1994;67:42–47.

170. Turgan C, Feehally J, Bennett S, et al. Accelerated hypertriglyceridemia in patients on continuous ambulatory peritoneal dialysis—a preventable abnormality. *Int J Artif Organs* 1981;4: 158–160.

171. Breuer HW. Hypertriglyceridemia: a review of clinical relevance and treatment options: focus on cerivastatin. *Curr Med Res Opin* 2001;17:60–73.

172. Rosenson RS. Hypertriglyceridemia and coronary heart disease risk. *Cardiol Rev* 1999;7:342–348.

173. Rapp RJ. Hypertriglyceridemia: a review beyond low-density lipoprotein. *Cardiol Rev* 2002;10:163–172.

174. Wanner C. Lipids in end-stage renal disease. *J Nephrol* 2002; 15:202–204.

175. Hendriks F, Kooman JP, van der Sande FM. Massive rhabdomyolysis and life threatening hyperkalaemia in a patient with the combination of cerivastatin and gemfibrozil. *Nephrol Dial Transplant* 2001;16:2418–2419.

176. Ozdemir O, Boran M, Gokce V, et al. A case with severe rhabdomyolysis and renal failure associated with cerivastatin-gemfibrozil combination therapy—a case report. *Angiology* 2000;51: 695–697.

177. Al Shohaib S. Simvastatin-induced rhabdomyolysis in a patient with chronic renal failure. *Am J Nephrol* 2000;20:212–213.

178. Executive Summary of the Third Report of The National Cholesterol Education Program (NCEP) Expert Panel on Detection, Evaluation, and Treatment of High Blood Cholesterol in Adults (Adult Treatment Panel III). *JAMA* 2001;285:2486–2497.

179. Chang JW, Yang WS, Min WK, et al. Effects of simvastatin on high-sensitivity C-reactive protein and serum albumin in hemodialysis patients. *Am J Kidney Dis* 2002;39:1213–1217.

180. Halkin A, Keren G. Potential indications for angiotensin-converting enzyme inhibitors in atherosclerotic vascular disease. *Am J Med* 2002;112:126–134.

181. Oda H, Keane WF. Recent advances in statins and the kidney. *Kidney Int Suppl* 1999;71:S2–5.

182. Bickel C, Rupprecht HJ, Blankenberg S, et al. Influence of HMG-CoA reductase inhibitors on markers of coagulation, systemic inflammation and soluble cell adhesion. *Int J Cardiol* 2002;82:25–31.

183. Ansell BJ, Watson KE, Weiss RE, et al. hsCRP and HDL Effects of Statins Trial (CHEST): Rapid Effect of Statin Therapy on C-Reactive Protein and High-Density Lipoprotein Levels A Clinical Investigation. *Heart Dis* 2003;5:2–7.

184. Alderman MH, Cohen HW. Impact of dietary sodium on cardiovascular disease morbidity and mortality. *Curr Hypertens Rep* 2002;4:453–457.

185. Pru C, Kjellstrand CM. On the clinical usefulness of the FENa test in acute renal failure: a critical analysis. *Proc Clin Dial Transplant Forum* 1980;10:240–247.

186. Espinel CH. The FENa test. Use in the differential diagnosis of acute renal failure. *JAMA* 1976;236:579–581.

187. Kahn T, Mohammad G, Stein RM. Alterations in renal tubular sodium and water reabsorption in chronic renal disease in man. *Kidney Int* 1972;2:164–174.

188. Jansen MA, Hart AA, Korevaar JC, et al. Predictors of the rate of decline of residual renal function in incident dialysis patients. *Kidney Int* 2002;62:1046–1053.

189. Maduell F, Navarro V. Dietary salt intake and blood pressure control in haemodialysis patients. *Nephrol Dial Transplant* 2000;15:2063.

190. Shaldon S. Dietary salt restriction and drug-free treatment of hypertension in ESRD patients: a largely abandoned therapy. *Nephrol Dial Transplant* 2002;17:1163–1165.

191. Krautzig S, Janssen U, Koch KM, et al. Dietary salt restriction and reduction of dialysate sodium to control hypertension in maintenance haemodialysis patients. *Nephrol Dial Transplant* 1998;13:552–553.

192. Tomson CR. Advising dialysis patients to restrict fluid intake without restricting sodium intake is not based on evidence and is a waste of time. *Nephrol Dial Transplant* 2001;16:1538–1542.

193. Charra B, Chazot C, Laurent G. Hypertension/hypotension in dialysis. *Kidney Int* 1999;55:1128.

194. Charra B, Calemard E, Cuche M, et al. Control of hypertension and prolonged survival on maintenance hemodialysis. *Nephron* 1983;33:96–99.

195. Strain WD, Lye M. Chronic pain, bereavement and overdose in a depressed elderly woman. *Age Ageing* 2002;31:218–219.

196. Sherman RA, Cody RP, Rogers ME, et al. Interdialytic weight gain and nutritional parameters in chronic hemodialysis patients. *Am J Kidney Dis* 1995;25:579–583.

197. Kimmel PL, Varela MP, Peterson RA, et al. Interdialytic weight gain and survival in hemodialysis patients: effects of duration of ESRD and diabetes mellitus. *Kidney Int* 2000;57:1141–1151.

198. Fishbane S, Youn S, Flaster E, et al. Ankle-arm blood pressure index as a predictor of mortality in hemodialysis patients. *Am J Kidney Dis* 1996;27:668–672.

199. Fishbane S, Youn S, Kowalski EJ, et al. Ankle-arm blood pressure index as a marker for atherosclerotic vascular diseases in hemodialysis patients. *Am J Kidney Dis* 1995;25:34–39.

200. Ventura JE, Sposito M. Volume sensitivity of blood pressure in end-stage renal disease. *Nephrol Dial Transplant* 1997;12: 485–491.

201. Rahman M, Dixit A, Donley V, et al. Factors associated with

inadequate blood pressure control in hypertensive hemodialysis patients. *Am J Kidney Dis* 1999;33:498–506.

202. Luik AJ, Gladziwa U, Kooman JP, et al. Blood pressure changes in relation to interdialytic weight gain. *Contrib Nephrol* 1994; 106:90–93.
203. Luik AJ, Gladziwa U, Kooman JP, et al. Influence of interdialytic weight gain on blood pressure in hemodialysis patients. *Blood Purif* 1994;12:259–266.
204. Kooman JP, Gladziwa U, Bocker G, et al. Blood pressure during the interdialytic period in haemodialysis patients: estimation of representative blood pressure values. *Nephrol Dial Transplant* 1992;7:917–923.
205. Chazot C, Charra B, Laurent G, et al. Interdialysis blood pressure control by long haemodialysis sessions. *Nephrol Dial Transplant* 1995;10:831–837.
206. Sherman RA, Daniel A, Cody RP. The effect of interdialytic weight gain on predialysis blood pressure. *Artif Organs* 1993; 17:770–774.
207. Lins LE, Hedenborg G, Jacobson SH, et al. Blood pressure reduction during hemodialysis correlates to intradialytic changes in plasma volume. *Clin Nephrol* 1992;37:308–313.
208. Geddes CC, Houston M, Pediani L, et al. Excess interdialytic sodium intake is not always dietary. *Nephrol Dial Transplant* 2003;18:223.
209. Dominic SC, Ramachandran S, Somiah S, et al. Quenching the thirst in dialysis patients. *Nephron* 1996;73:597–600.
210. Shen FH, Sherrard DJ, Scollard D, et al. Thirst, relative hypernatremia, and excessive weight gain in maintenance peritoneal dialysis. *Trans Am Soc Artif Intern Organs* 1978;24:142–145.
211. Blumenkrantz MJ, Kopple JD, Moran JK, et al. Metabolic balance studies and dietary protein requirements in patients undergoing continuous ambulatory peritoneal dialysis. *Kidney Int* 1982;21:849–861.
212. Martin RS, Panese S, Virginillo M, et al. Increased secretion of potassium in the rectum of humans with chronic renal failure. *Am J Kidney Dis* 1986;8:105–110.
213. Sandle GI, Gaiger E, Tapster S, et al. Evidence for large intestinal control of potassium homeostasis in uraemic patients undergoing long-term dialysis. *Clin Sci (Lond)* 1987;73: 247–252.
214. Kopple JD, Coburn JW. Metabolic studies of low protein diets in uremia. I. Nitrogen and potassium. *Medicine* 1973;52: 583–595.
215. Boddy K, King PC, Lindsay RM, et al. Total body potassium in non-dialysed and dialysed patients with chronic renal failure. *Br Med J* 1972;1:771–775.
216. Hsu CY, Chertow GM. Elevations of serum phosphorus and potassium in mild to moderate chronic renal insufficiency. *Nephrol Dial Transplant* 2002;17:1419–1425.
217. Abbott KC. Ace inhibitors and survival in dialysis patients: effects on serum potassium? *Am J Kidney Dis* 2003;41:520–521.
218. Allon M, Shanklin N. Effect of bicarbonate administration on plasma potassium in dialysis patients: interactions with insulin and albuterol. *Am J Kidney Dis* 1996;28:508–514.
219. Dolson GM. Do potassium deficient diets and K+ removal by dialysis contribute to the cardiovascular morbidity and mortality of patients with end stage renal disease? *Int J Artif Organs* 1997; 20:134–135.
220. Karnik JA, Young BS, Lew NL, et al. Cardiac arrest and sudden death in dialysis units. *Kidney Int* 2001;60:350–357.
221. Pietrzak I, Bladek K, Bulikowski W. Comparison of magnesium and zinc levels in blood in end stage renal disease patients treated by hemodialysis or peritoneal dialysis. *Magnes Res* 2002;15: 229–236.
222. Coburn JW, Hartenbower DL, Brickman AS, et al. Intestinal absorption of calcium, magnesium and phosphorus in chronic renal insufficiency. In: David DS, ed. *Perspectives in hypertension and nephrology-calcium metabolism in renal disease.* New York: Wiley, 1977:77–109.
223. Kopple JD, Coburn JW. Metabolic studies of low protein diets in uremia. II. Calcium, phosphorus and magnesium. *Medicine (Baltimore)* 1973;52:597–607.
224. Mansouri K, Halsted JA, Gombos EA. Zinc, copper, magnesium and calcium in dialyzed and nondialyzed uremic patients. *Arch Intern Med* 1970;125:88–93.
225. Wallach S. Effects of magnesium on skeletal metabolism. *Magnes Trace Elem* 1990;9:1–14.
226. Navarro-Gonzalez JF. Magnesium in dialysis patients: serum levels and clinical implications. *Clin Nephrol* 1998;49:373–378.
227. Contiguglia SR, Alfrey AC, Miller N, et al. Total-body magnesium excess in chronic renal failure. *Lancet* 1972;1:1300–1302.
228. Coburn JW, Hartenbower DL, Massry SG. Intestinal absorption of calcium and the effect of renal insufficiency. *Kidney Int* 1973;4:96–104.
229. Addison JF, Foulks CJ. Calcium carbonate: An effective phosphorus binder in patients with chronic renal failure. *Curr Ther Res* 1985;38:241.
230. Goodman WG, Goldin J, Kuizon BD, et al. Coronary-artery calcification in young adults with end-stage renal disease who are undergoing dialysis. *N Engl J Med* 2000;342:1478–1483.
231. Chertow GM, Burke SK, Dillon MA, et al. Long-term effects of sevelamer hydrochloride on the calcium x phosphate product and lipid profile of haemodialysis patients. *Nephrol Dial Transplant* 1999;14:2907–2914.
232. Chertow GM, Dillon M, Burke SK, et al. A randomized trial of sevelamer hydrochloride (RenaGel) with and without supplemental calcium. Strategies for the control of hyperphosphatemia and hyperparathyroidism in hemodialysis patients. *Clin Nephrol* 1999;51:18–26.
233. Chertow GM, Dillon MA, Amin N, et al. Sevelamer with and without calcium and vitamin D: observations from a long-term open-label clinical trial. *J Ren Nutr* 2000;10:125–132.
234. Chertow GM, Burke SK, Dillon MA, et al. Long-term effects of sevelamer hydrochloride on the calcium x phosphate product and lipid profile of haemodialysis patients. *Nephrol Dial Transplant* 2000;15:559.
235. Fournier A, Presne C, Oprisiu R, et al. Oral calcium, sevelamer and vascular calcification in uraemic patients. *Nephrol Dial Transplant* 2002;17:2276–2277.
236. Reslerova M, Moe SM. Vascular calcification in dialysis patients: pathogenesis and consequences. *Am J Kidney Dis* 2003; 41:S96–99.
237. Marco MP, Muray S, Betriu A, et al. Treatment with sevelamer decreases bicarbonate levels in hemodialysis patients. *Nephron* 2002;92:499–500.
238. Hou SH, Zhao J, Ellman CF, et al. Calcium and phosphorus fluxes during hemodialysis with low calcium dialysate. *Am J Kidney Dis* 1991;18:217–224.
239. Lorenzo V, Martin M, Rufino M, et al. Protein intake, control of serum phosphorus, and relatively low levels of parathyroid hormone in elderly hemodialysis patients. *Am J Kidney Dis* 2001;37:1260–1266.
240. Barsotti G, Morelli E, Giannoni A, et al. Restricted phosphorus and nitrogen intake to slow the progression of chronic renal failure: a controlled trial. *Kidney Int Suppl* 1983;16:S278–284.
241. Block GA, Port FK. Re-evaluation of risks associated with hyperphosphatemia and hyperparathyroidism in dialysis patients: recommendations for a change in management. *Am J Kidney Dis* 2000;35:1226–1237.
242. Chazan JA, Lew NL, Lowrie EG. Increased serum aluminum. An independent risk factor for mortality in patients undergoing long-term hemodialysis. *Arch Intern Med* 1991;151:319–322.

243. Hercz G, Pei Y, Greenwood C, et al. Aplastic osteodystrophy without aluminum: the role of "suppressed" parathyroid function. *Kidney Int* 1993;44:860–866.
244. Malluche HH, Faugere MC. Aluminum-related bone disease. *Blood Purif* 1988;6:1–15.
245. Norris KC, Crooks PW, Nebeker HG, et al. Clinical and laboratory features of aluminum-related bone disease: differences between sporadic and "epidemic" forms of the syndrome. *Am J Kidney Dis* 1985;6:342–347.
246. Ott SM, Maloney NA, Coburn JW, et al. The prevalence of bone aluminum deposition in renal osteodystrophy and its relation to the response to calcitriol therapy. *N Engl J Med* 1982; 307:709–713.
247. Ibels LS, Alfrey AC, Huffer WE, et al. Calcification in end-stage kidneys. *Am J Med* 1981;71:33–37.
248. Schiller LR, Santa Ana CA, Sheikh MS, et al. Effect of the time of administration of calcium acetate on phosphorus binding. *N Engl J Med* 1989;320:1110–1113.
249. Sheikh MS, Maguire JA, Emmett M, et al. Reduction of dietary phosphorus absorption by phosphorus binders. A theoretical, in vitro, and in vivo study. *J Clin Invest* 1989;83:66–73.
250. Mai ML, Emmett M, Sheikh MS, et al. Calcium acetate, an effective phosphorus binder in patients with renal failure. *Kidney Int* 1989;36:690–695.
251. Schaefer K, Scheer J, Asmus G, et al. The treatment of uraemic hyperphosphataemia with calcium acetate and calcium carbonate: a comparative study. *Nephrol Dial Transplant* 1991;6: 170–175.
252. Pflanz S, Henderson IS, McElduff N, et al. Calcium acetate versus calcium carbonate as phosphate-binding agents in chronic haemodialysis. *Nephrol Dial Transplant* 1994;9: 1121–1124.
253. Fournier A, Yverneau PH, Hue P, et al. Adynamic bone disease in patients with uremia. *Curr Opin Nephrol Hypertens* 1994;3: 396–410.
254. Malluche HH, Monier-Faugere MC. Risk of adynamic bone disease in dialyzed patients. *Kidney Int Suppl* 1992;38:S62–67.
255. Borras M, Marco MP, Fernandez E. Treatment with sevelamer decreases bicarbonate levels in peritoneal dialysis patients. *Perit Dial Int* 2002;22:737–738.
256. Hutchison AJ. Calcitriol, lanthanum carbonate, and other new phosphate binders in the management of renal osteodystrophy. *Perit Dial Int* 1999;19 Suppl 2:S408–412.
257. Cases A. Recent advances in nephrology: highlights from the 35th annual meeting of the American Society of Nephrology. *Drugs Today (Barc)* 2002;38:797–805.
258. Nelson R. Novel phosphate binder is effective in patients on haemodialysis. *Lancet* 2002;360:1483.
259. Hergesell O, Ritz E. Phosphate binders on iron basis: a new perspective? *Kidney Int Suppl* 1999;73:S42–45.
260. Gray RW, Weber HP, Dominguez JH, et al. The metabolism of vitamin D3 and 25-hydroxyvitamin D3 in normal and anephric humans. *J Clin Endocrinol Metab* 1974;39:1045–1056.
261. Vaziri ND, Hollander D, Hung EK, et al. Impaired intestinal absorption of vitamin D3 in azotemic rats. *Am J Clin Nutr* 1983;37:403–406.
262. Silver J, Russell J, Sherwood LM. Regulation by vitamin D metabolites of messenger ribonucleic acid for preproparathyroid hormone in isolated bovine parathyroid cells. *Proc Natl Acad Sci U S A* 1985;82:4270–4273.
263. Fukagawa M, Kitaoka M, Fukuda N, et al. Pathogenesis and management of parathyroid hyperplasia in chronic renal failure: role of calcitriol. *Miner Electrolyte Metab* 1995;21:97–100.
264. Bellido T, Girasole G, Passeri G, et al. Demonstration of estrogen and vitamin D receptors in bone marrow-derived stromal cells: up-regulation of the estrogen receptor by 1,25-dihydroxy-vitamin-D3. *Endocrinology* 1993;133:553–562.
265. Beckerman P, Silver J. Vitamin D and the parathyroid. *Am J Med Sci* 1999;317:363–369.
266. Roussanne MC, Duchambon P, Gogusev J, et al. Parathyroid hyperplasia in chronic renal failure: role of calcium, phosphate, and calcitriol. *Nephrol Dial Transplant* 1999;14 Suppl 1:68–69.
267. Dahl NV, Foote EF. Pulse dose oral calcitriol therapy for renal osteodystrophy: literature review and practice recommendations. *ANNA J* 1997;24:550–555.
268. Salusky IB, Goodman W. Skeletal response to intermittent calcitriol therapy in secondary hyperparathyroidism. *Kidney Int Suppl* 1996;53:S135–139.
269. Martin KJ, Gonzalez EA. Vitamin D analogues for the management of secondary hyperparathyroidism. *Am J Kidney Dis* 2001; 38:S34–40.
270. Kaye M. Hungry bone syndrome after surgical parathyroidectomy. *Am J Kidney Dis* 1997;30:730–731.
271. Slatopolsky E, Brown AJ. Vitamin D analogs for the treatment of secondary hyperparathyroidism. *Blood Purif* 2002;20: 109–112.
272. Slatopolsky E, Brown A, Dusso A. Pathogenesis of secondary hyperparathyroidism. *Kidney Int Suppl* 1999;73:S14–19.
273. Slatopolsky E, Weerts C, Thielan J, et al. Marked suppression of secondary hyperparathyroidism by intravenous administration of 1,25-dihydroxy-cholecalciferol in uremic patients. *J Clin Invest* 1984;74:2136–2143.
274. Hampers CL, Streiff R, Nathan DG, et al. Megaloblastic hematopoiesis in uremia and in patients on long-term hemodialysis. *N Engl J Med* 1967;276:551–554.
275. Whitehead VM, Comty CH, Posen GA, et al. Homeostasis of folic acid in patients undergoing maintenance hemodialysis. *N Engl J Med* 1968;279:970–974.
276. Jennette JC, Goldman ID. Inhibition of the membrane transport of folates by anions retained in uremia. *J Lab Clin Med* 1975;86:834–843.
277. Spannuth CL Jr, Warnock LG, Wagner C, et al. Increased plasma clearance of pyridoxal 5′-phosphate in vitamin B6-deficient uremic man. *J Lab Clin Med* 1977;90:632–637.
278. Kopple JD, Swendseid ME. Vitamin nutrition in patients undergoing maintenance hemodialysis. *Kidney Int Suppl* 1975: 79–84.
279. Ramirez G, Chen M, Boyce HW Jr, et al. Longitudinal follow-up of chronic hemodialysis patients without vitamin supplementation. *Kidney Int* 1986;30:99–106.
280. Sharman VL, Cunningham J, Goodwin FJ, et al. Do patients receiving regular haemodialysis need folic acid supplements? *Br Med J (Clin Res Ed)* 1982;285:96–97.
281. Porrini M, Simonetti P, Ciappellano S, et al. Thiamin, riboflavin and pyridoxine status in chronic renal insufficiency. *Int J Vitam Nutr Res* 1989;59:304–308.
282. Giancaspro V, Nuzziello M, Pallotta G, et al. Intravenous ascorbic acid in hemodialysis patients with functional iron deficiency: a clinical trial. *J Nephrol* 2000;13:444–449.
283. Sezer S, Ozdemir FN, Yakupoglu U, et al. Intravenous ascorbic acid administration for erythropoietin-hyporesponsive anemia in iron loaded hemodialysis patients. *Artif Organs* 2002;26: 366–370.
284. Van Wyck DB, Bailie G, Aronoff G. Just the FAQs: frequently asked questions about iron and anemia in patients with chronic kidney disease. *Am J Kidney Dis* 2002;39:426–432.
285. Tarng DC, Huang TP, Wei YH. Erythropoietin and iron: the role of ascorbic acid. *Nephrol Dial Transplant* 2001;16 Suppl 5:35–39.
286. Petrarulo F, Giancaspro V. Intravenous ascorbic acid in haemo-

dialysis patients with functional iron deficiency. *Nephrol Dial Transplant* 2000;15:1717–1718.

287. Lasseur C, Parrot F, Delmas Y, et al. Impact of high-flux/high-efficiency dialysis on folate and homocysteine metabolism. *J Nephrol* 2001;14:32–35.
288. Ihara M, Ito T, Yanagihara C, et al. Wernicke's encephalopathy associated with hemodialysis: report of two cases and review of the literature. *Clin Neurol Neurosurg* 1999;101:118–121.
289. Jagadha V, Deck JH, Halliday WC, et al. Wernicke's encephalopathy in patients on peritoneal dialysis or hemodialysis. *Ann Neurol* 1987;21:78–84.
290. Allman MA, Pang E, Yau DF, et al. Elevated plasma vitamers of vitamin B6 in patients with chronic renal failure on regular haemodialysis. *Eur J Clin Nutr* 1992;46:679–683.
291. Allman MA, Truswell AS, Tiller DJ, et al. Vitamin supplementation of patients receiving haemodialysis. *Med J Aust* 1989; 150:130–133.
292. Lasker N, Harvey A, Baker H. Vitamin levels in hemodialysis and intermittent peritoneal dialysis. *Trans Am Soc Artif Intern Organs* 1963;9:51.
293. Teehan BP, Smith LJ, Sigler MH, et al. Plasma pyridoxal-5′-phosphate levels and clinical correlations in chronic hemodialysis patients. *Am J Clin Nutr* 1978;31:1932–1936.
294. Lacour B, Parry C, Drueke T, et al. Pyridoxal 5′-phosphate deficiency in uremic undialyzed, hemodialyzed, and non-uremic kidney transplant patients. *Clin Chim Acta* 1983;127:205–215.
295. Akiba T, Kurihara S, Tachibana K, et al. Vitamin K increased bone mass in hemodialysis patients with low turn over bone disease. *J Am Soc Nephrol* 1991;2:608.
296. Kohlmeier M, Saupe J, Shearer MJ, et al. Bone health of adult hemodialysis patients is related to vitamin K status. *Kidney Int* 1997;51:1218–1221.
297. Kohlmeier M, Saupe J, Schaefer K, et al. Bone fracture history and prospective bone fracture risk of hemodialysis patients are related to apolipoprotein E genotype. *Calcif Tissue Int* 1998; 62:278–281.
298. Hodges SJ, Akesson K, Vergnaud P, et al. Circulating levels of vitamins K1 and K2 decreased in elderly women with hip fracture. *J Bone Miner Res* 1993;8:1241–1245.
299. Bitensky L, Hart JP, Catterall A, et al. Circulating vitamin K levels in patients with fractures. *J Bone Joint Surg Br* 1988;70: 663–664.
300. Soundararajan R, Leehey DJ, Yu AW, et al. Skin necrosis and protein C deficiency associated with vitamin K depletion in a patient with renal failure. *Am J Med* 1992;93:467–470.
301. Stein G, Sperschneider H, Koppe S. Vitamin levels in chronic renal failure and need for supplementation. *Blood Purif* 1985; 3:52–62.
302. Farrington K, Miller P, Varghese Z, et al. Vitamin A toxicity and hypercalcaemia in chronic renal failure. *Br Med J (Clin Res Ed)* 1981;282:1999–2002.
303. Smith FR, Goodman DS. The effects of diseases of the liver, thyroid, and kidneys on the transport of vitamin A in human plasma. *J Clin Invest* 1971;50:2426–2436.
304. Stein G, Schone S, Geinitz D, et al. No tissue level abnormality of vitamin A concentration despite elevated serum vitamin A of uremic patients. *Clin Nephrol* 1986;25:87–93.
305. Vahlquist A. Metabolism of the vitamin-A-transporting protein complex: turnover of retinol-binding protein, prealbumin and vitamin A in a primate (Macaca Irus). *Scand J Clin Lab Invest* 1972;30:349–360.
306. Vahlquist A, Peterson PA. Comparative studies on the vitamin A transporting protein complex in human and cynomolgus plasma. *Biochemistry* 1972;11:4526–4532.
307. Werb R, Clark WF, Lindsay RM, et al. Serum vitamin A levels and associated abnormalities in patients on regular dialysis treatment. *Clin Nephrol* 1979;12:63–68.
308. Werb R. Vitamin A toxicity in hemodialysis patients. *Int J Artif Organs* 1979;2:178–180.
309. Ha TK, Sattar N, Talwar D, et al. Abnormal antioxidant vitamin and carotenoid status in chronic renal failure. *QJM* 1996; 89:765–769.
310. Ono K, Waki Y, Takeda K. Hypervitaminosis A: a contributing factor to anemia in regular dialysis patients. *Nephron* 1984;38: 44–47.
311. Yatzidis H, Digenis P, Fountas P. Hypervitaminosis A accompanying advanced chronic renal failure. *Br Med J* 1975;3: 352–353.
312. Nenov D, Paskalev D, Yankova T, et al. Lipid peroxidation and vitamin E in red blood cells and plasma in hemodialysis patients under rhEPO treatment. *Artif Organs* 1995;19: 436–439.
313. Hultqvist M, Hegbrant J, Nilsson-Thorell C, et al. Plasma concentrations of vitamin C, vitamin E and/or malondialdehyde as markers of oxygen free radical production during hemodialysis. *Clin Nephrol* 1997;47:37–46.
314. De Bevere VO, Nelis HJ, De Leenheer AP, et al. Vitamin E levels in hemodialysis patients. *JAMA* 1982;247:2371.
315. Roob JM, Khoschsorur G, Tiran A, et al. Vitamin E attenuates oxidative stress induced by intravenous iron in patients on hemodialysis. *J Am Soc Nephrol* 2000;11:539–549.
316. Chazot C, Laurent G, Charra B, et al. Malnutrition in long-term haemodialysis survivors. *Nephrol Dial Transplant* 2001; 16:61–69.
317. Cohen JD, Viljoen M, Clifford D, et al. Plasma vitamin E levels in a chronically hemolyzing group of dialysis patients. *Clin Nephrol* 1986;25:42–47.
318. Ahmad S, Robertson HT, Golper TA, et al. Multicenter trial of L-carnitine in maintenance hemodialysis patients. II. Clinical and biochemical effects. *Kidney Int* 1990;38:912–918.
319. Lonn E, Yusuf S, Hoogwerf B, et al. Effects of vitamin E on cardiovascular and microvascular outcomes in high-risk patients with diabetes: results of the HOPE study and MICRO-HOPE substudy. *Diabetes Care* 2002;25:1919–1927.
320. Mann JF, Gerstein HC, Pogue J, et al. Renal insufficiency as a predictor of cardiovascular outcomes and the impact of ramipril: the HOPE randomized trial. *Ann Intern Med* 2001;134: 629–636.
321. Balcke P, Schmidt P, Zazgornik J, et al. Effect of vitamin B6 administration on elevated plasma oxalic acid levels in haemodialysed patients. *Eur J Clin Invest* 1982;12:481–483.
322. Balcke P, Schmidt P, Zazgornik J, et al. Ascorbic acid aggravates secondary hyperoxalemia in patients on chronic hemodialysis. *Ann Intern Med* 1984;101:344–345.
323. Zima T, Tesar V, Mestek O, et al. Trace elements in end-stage renal disease. 1. Methodological aspects and the influence of water treatment and dialysis equipment. *Blood Purif* 1999;17: 182–186.
324. Zima T, Mestek O, Nemecek K, et al. Trace elements in hemodialysis and continuous ambulatory peritoneal dialysis patients. *Blood Purif* 1998;16:253–260.
325. Surian M, Bonforte G, Scanziani R, et al. Trace elements and micropollutant anions in the dialysis and reinfusion fluid prepared on-line for haemodiafiltration. *Nephrol Dial Transplant* 1998;13 Suppl 5:24–28.
326. D'Haese PC, De Broe ME. Adequacy of dialysis: trace elements in dialysis fluids. *Nephrol Dial Transplant* 1996;11 Suppl 2: 92–97.
327. Hasanoglu E, Altan N, Sindel S, et al. The relationship between erythrocyte superoxide dismutase activity and plasma levels of

some trace elements (Al, Cu, Zn) of dialysis patients. *Gen Pharmacol* 1994;25:107–110.
328. Jervis RE, Kua BT, Hercz G. Hair trace elements in kidney dialysis patients by INAA. *Biol Trace Elem Res* 1994;43–45: 335–342.
329. Padovese P, Gallieni M, Brancaccio D, et al. Trace elements in dialysis fluids and assessment of the exposure of patients on regular hemodialysis, hemofiltration and continuous ambulatory peritoneal dialysis. *Nephron* 1992;61:442–448.
330. Berlyne GM, Diskin C, Gonick H, et al. Trace elements in dialysis patients. *ASAIO Trans* 1986;32:662–670.
331. Thomson NM, Stevens BJ, Humphery TJ, et al. Comparison of trace elements in peritoneal dialysis, hemodialysis, and uremia. *Kidney Int* 1983;23:9–14.
332. Sandstead HH. Trace elements in uremia and hemodialysis. *Am J Clin Nutr* 1980;33:1501–1508.
333. Hosokawa S, Oyamaguchi A, Yoshida O. Trace elements and complications in patients undergoing chronic hemodialysis. *Nephron* 1990;55:375–379.
334. Mahler DJ, Walsh JR, Haynie GD. Magnesium, zinc, and copper in dialysis patients. *Am J Clin Pathol* 1971;56:17–23.
335. Gallery ED, Blomfield J, Dixon SR. Acute zinc toxicity in haemodialysis. *Br Med J* 1972;4:331–333.
336. Blomfield J, McPherson J, George CR. Active uptake of copper and zinc during haemodialysis. *Br Med J* 1969;1:141–145.
337. Van Renterghem D, Cornelis R, Vanholder R. Behaviour of 12 trace elements in serum of uremic patients on hemodiafiltration. *J Trace Elem Electrolytes Health Dis* 1992;6:169–174.
338. Blomfield J. Dialysis and lead absorption. *Lancet* 1973;2: 666–667.
339. Chevalier CA, Liepa G, Murphy MD, et al. The effects of zinc supplementation on serum zinc and cholesterol concentrations in hemodialysis patients. *J Ren Nutr* 2002;12:183–189.
340. Jern NA, VanBeber AD, Gorman MA, et al. The effects of zinc supplementation on serum zinc concentration and protein catabolic rate in hemodialysis patients. *J Ren Nutr* 2000;10: 148–153.
341. Turk S, Bozfakioglu S, Ecder ST, et al. Effects of zinc supplementation on the immune system and on antibody response to multivalent influenza vaccine in hemodialysis patients. *Int J Artif Organs* 1998;21:274–278.
342. Schabowski J, Ksiazek A, Paprzycki P, et al. Ferrum, copper, zinc and manganese in tissues of patients treated with longstanding hemodialysis programme. *Ann Univ Mariae Curie Sklodowska (Med)* 1994;49:61–66.
343. Reid DJ, Barr SI, Leichter J. Effects of folate and zinc supplementation on patients undergoing chronic hemodialysis. *J Am Diet Assoc* 1992;92:574–579.
344. Mahajan SK, Abraham J, Hessburg T, et al. Zinc metabolism and taste acuity in renal transplant recipients. *Kidney Int Suppl* 1983;16:S310–314.
345. Mahajan SK, Bowersox EM, Rye DL, et al. Factors underlying abnormal zinc metabolism in uremia. *Kidney Int Suppl* 1989; 27:S269–273.
346. Mahajan SK, Prasad AS, Lambujon J, et al. Improvement of uremic hypogeusia by zinc: a double-blind study. *Am J Clin Nutr* 1980;33:1517–1521.
347. Sprenger KB, Bundschu D, Lewis K, et al. Improvement of uremic neuropathy and hypogeusia by dialysate zinc supplementation: a double-blind study. *Kidney Int Suppl* 1983;16: S315–318.
348. Rodger RS, Sheldon WL, Watson MJ, et al. Zinc deficiency and hyperprolactinaemia are not reversible causes of sexual dysfunction in uraemia. *Nephrol Dial Transplant* 1989;4:888–892.
349. Kiilerich S, Christiansen C, Christensen MS, et al. Zinc metabolism in patients with chronic renal failure during treatment with 1.25-dihydroxycholecalciferol: a controlled therapeutic trial. *Clin Nephrol* 1981;15:23–27.
350. Kalantar-Zadeh K, Hoffken B, Wunsch H, et al. Diagnosis of iron deficiency anemia in renal failure patients during the post-erythropoietin era. *Am J Kidney Dis* 1995;26:292–299.
351. Kalantar-Zadeh K, McAllister C, Lehn R, et al. Effect of malnutrition-inflammation complex syndrome on erythropoietin hyporesponsiveness in maintenance hemodialysis patients. *J Ren Nutr* 2003;13:15–25.
352. K/DOQI Clinical Practice Guidelines: Anemia of chronic kidney disease. Kidney Dialysis Outcome Quality Initiative. *Am J Kidney Dis* 2001;37(Suppl 1):S182–238.
353. Kalantar-Zadeh K, Luft FC. Diagnosis of iron deficiency in ESRD patients. *Am J Kidney Dis* 1997;30:455–456.
354. Kalantar-Zadeh K, Luft FC, Humphreys MH. Moderately high serum ferritin concentration is not a sign of iron overload in dialysis patients. *Kidney Int* 1999;56:758–759.
355. Barany P, Divino Filho JC, Bergström J. High C-reactive protein is a strong predictor of resistance to erythropoietin in hemodialysis patients. *Am J Kidney Dis* 1997;29:565–568.
356. Fishbane S, Maesaka JK. Iron management in end-stage renal disease. *Am J Kidney Dis* 1997;29:319–333.
357. Fishbane S, Ungureanu VD, Maesaka JK, et al. The safety of intravenous iron dextran in hemodialysis patients. *Am J Kidney Dis* 1996;28:529–534.
358. Coyne DW, Adkinson NF, Nissenson AR, et al. Sodium ferric gluconate complex in hemodialysis patients. II. Adverse reactions in iron dextran-sensitive and dextran-tolerant patients. *Kidney Int* 2003;63:217–224.
359. Kostakopoulos A, Kotsalos A, Alexopoulos J, et al. Serum selenium levels in healthy adults and its changes in chronic renal failure. *Int Urol Nephrol* 1990;22:397–401.
360. Sher L. Role of selenium depletion in the effects of dialysis on mood and behavior. *Med Hypotheses* 2002;59:89–91.
361. Dworkin B, Weseley S, Rosenthal WS, et al. Diminished blood selenium levels in renal failure patients on dialysis: correlations with nutritional status. *Am J Med Sci* 1987;293:6–12.
362. Hampel G, Schaller KH, Rosenmuller M, et al. Selenium-deficiency as contributing factor to anemia and thrombocytopenia in dialysis patients. *Life Support Syst* 1985;3 Suppl 1:36–40.
363. Turan B, Delilbasi E, Dalay N, et al. Serum selenium and glutathione-peroxidase activities and their interaction with toxic metals in dialysis and renal transplantation patients. *Biol Trace Elem Res* 1992;33:95–102.
364. Bremer J. Carnitine—metabolism and functions. *Physiol Rev* 1983;63:1420–1480.
365. Vacha GM, Corsi M, Giorcelli G, et al. Serum and muscle L-carnitine levels in hemodialyzed patients, during and after long-term L-carnitine treatment. *Curr Ther Res* 1985;37:505.
366. Wanner C, Forstner-Wanner S, Schaeffer G, et al. Serum free carnitine, carnitine esters and lipids in patients on peritoneal dialysis and hemodialysis. *Am J Nephrol* 1986;6:206–211.
367. Bellinghieri G, Santoro D, Calvani M, et al. Carnitine and hemodialysis. *Am J Kidney Dis* 2003;41:S116–122.
368. Chazot C, Blanc C, Hurot JM, et al. Nutritional effects of carnitine supplementation in hemodialysis patients. *Clin Nephrol* 2003;59:24–30.
369. Golper TA, Ahmad S. L-carnitine administration to hemodialysis patients: Has its time come? *Semin Dial* 1992;5:94–98.
370. Labonia WD. L-carnitine effects on anemia in hemodialyzed patients treated with erythropoietin. *Am J Kidney Dis* 1995;26: 757–764.
371. Hurot JM, Cucherat M, Haugh M, et al. Effects of L-carnitine supplementation in maintenance hemodialysis patients: a systematic review. *J Am Soc Nephrol* 2002;13:708–714.
372. Guarnieri G, Toigo G, Crapesi L, et al. Carnitine metabolism in chronic renal failure. *Kidney Int Suppl* 1987;22:S116–127.
373. Guarnieri GF, Ranieri F, Toigo G, et al. Lipid-lowering effect

of carnitine in chronically uremic patients treated with maintenance hemodialysis. *Am J Clin Nutr* 1980;33:1489–1492.
374. Lacour B, Di Giulio S, Chanard J, et al. Carnitine improves lipid anomalies in haemodialysis patients. *Lancet* 1980;2:763–764.
375. Bellinghieri G, Savica V, Mallamace A, et al. Correlation between increased serum and tissue L-carnitine levels and improved muscle symptoms in hemodialyzed patients. *Am J Clin Nutr* 1983;38:523–531.
376. Brass EP, Adler S, Sietsema KE, et al. Intravenous L-carnitine increases plasma carnitine, reduces fatigue, and may preserve exercise capacity in hemodialysis patients. *Am J Kidney Dis* 2001;37:1018–1028.
377. Weschler A, Aviram M, Levin M, et al. High dose of L-carnitine increases platelet aggregation and plasma triglyceride levels in uremic patients on hemodialysis. *Nephron* 1984;38:120–124.
378. Eknoyan G, Latos DL, Lindberg J. Practice recommendations for the use of L-carnitine in dialysis-related carnitine disorder National Kidney Foundation Carnitine Consensus Conference. *Am J Kidney Dis* 2003;41:868–876.
379. Ahmad S. L-carnitine in dialysis patients. *Semin Dial* 2001;14: 209–217.
380. Kuhlmann MK, Schmidt F, Kohler H. High protein/energy vs. standard protein/energy nutritional regimen in the treatment of malnourished hemodialysis patients. *Miner Electrolyte Metab* 1999;25:306–310.
381. Leon JB, Majerle AD, Soinski JA, et al. Can a nutrition intervention improve albumin levels among hemodialysis patients? A pilot study. *J Ren Nutr* 2001;11:9–15.
382. Boccanfuso JA, Hutton M, McAllister B. The effects of megestrol acetate on nutritional parameters in a dialysis population. *J Ren Nutr* 2000;10:36–43.
383. Kopple JD. Therapeutic approaches to malnutrition in chronic dialysis patients: the different modalities of nutritional support. *Am J Kidney Dis* 1999;33:180–185.
384. Timpone JG, Wright DJ, Li N, et al. The safety and pharmacokinetics of single-agent and combination therapy with megestrol acetate and dronabinol for the treatment of HIV wasting syndrome. The DATRI 004 Study Group. Division of AIDS Treatment Research Initiative. *AIDS Res Hum Retroviruses* 1997;13: 305–315.
385. Strang P. The effect of megestrol acetate on anorexia, weight loss and cachexia in cancer and AIDS patients (review). *Anticancer Res* 1997;17:657–662.
386. Engelson ES, FX PI-S, Kotler DP. Effects of megestrol acetate and testosterone on body composition in castrated male Sprague-Dawley rats. *Nutrition* 1999;15:465–473.
387. Chazot C, Shahmir E, Matias B, et al. Dialytic nutrition: provision of amino acids in dialysate during hemodialysis. *Kidney Int* 1997;52:1663–1670.
388. Fouque D, Peng SC, Kopple JD. Impaired metabolic response to recombinant insulin-like growth factor-1 in dialysis patients. *Kidney Int* 1995;47:876–883.
389. Fouque D, Peng SC, Shamir E, et al. Recombinant human insulin-like growth factor-1 induces an anabolic response in malnourished CAPD patients. *Kidney Int* 2000;57:646–654.
390. Fouque D, Peng SC, Kopple JD. Impaired metabolic response to recombinant insulin-like growth factor-1 in dialysis patients. *Kidney Int* 1995;47:876–883.
391. Fouque D, Peng SC, Kopple JD. Pharmacokinetics of recombinant human insulin-like growth factor-1 in dialysis patients. *Kidney Int* 1995;47:869–875.
392. Fouque D, Tayek JA, Kopple JD. Altered mental function during intravenous infusion of recombinant human insulin-like growth factor 1. *JPEN J Parenter Enteral Nutr* 1995;19: 231–233.
393. Kopple JD, Ding H, Qing DP. Physiology and potential use of insulin-like growth factor 1 in acute and chronic renal failure. *Nephrol Dial Transplant* 1998;13:34–39.
394. Fine RN, Stablein D, Cohen AH, et al. Recombinant human growth hormone post-renal transplantation in children: a randomized controlled study of the NAPRTCS. *Kidney Int* 2002; 62:688–696.
395. Fine RN, Sullivan EK, Tejani A. The impact of recombinant human growth hormone treatment on final adult height. *Pediatr Nephrol* 2000;14:679–681.
396. Fine RN, Sullivan EK, Kuntze J, et al. The impact of recombinant human growth hormone treatment during chronic renal insufficiency on renal transplant recipients. *J Pediatr* 2000;136: 376–382.
397. Ben-Atia I, Fine M, Tandler A, et al. Preparation of recombinant gilthead seabream (Sparus aurata) growth hormone and its use for stimulation of larvae growth by oral administration. *Gen Comp Endocrinol* 1999;113:155–164.
398. Fine RN. Growth hormone treatment of children with chronic renal insufficiency, end-stage renal disease and following renal transplantation—update 1997. *J Pediatr Endocrinol Metab* 1997;10:361–370.
399. Ziegler TR, Lazarus JM, Young LS, et al. Effects of recombinant human growth hormone in adults receiving maintenance hemodialysis. *J Am Soc Nephrol* 1991;2:1130–1135.
400. Schulman G, Wingard RL, Hutchison RL, et al. The effects of recombinant human growth hormone and intradialytic parenteral nutrition in malnourished hemodialysis patients. *Am J Kidney Dis* 1993;21:527–534.
401. Kopple JD. The rationale for the use of growth hormone or insulin-like growth factor I in adult patients with renal failure. *Miner Electrolyte Metab* 1992;18:269–275.
402. Saadeh E, Ikizler TA, Shyr Y, et al. Recombinant human growth hormone in patients with acute renal failure. *J Ren Nutr* 2001; 11:212–219.
403. Van den Berghe G. Endocrinology in intensive care medicine: new insights and therapeutic consequences. *Verh K Acad Geneeskd Belg* 2002;64:167–187; discussion 187–188.
404. McPhatter LL, Lockridge RS Jr. Nutritional advantages of nightly home hemodialysis. *Nephrol News Issues* 2002;16: 31,34–36.
405. McPhatter LL, Lockridge RS Jr, Albert J, et al. Nightly home hemodialysis: improvement in nutrition and quality of life. *Adv Ren Replace Ther* 1999;6:358–365.
406. Pierratos A. Daily hemodialysis: why the renewed interest? *Am J Kidney Dis* 1998;32:S76–82.
407. Pierratos A. Nocturnal home haemodialysis: an update on a 5-year experience. *Nephrol Dial Transplant* 1999;14:2835–2840.
408. Pierratos A. Daily hemodialysis. *Curr Opin Nephrol Hypertens* 2000;9:637–642.
409. Lindsay RM, Kortas C. Hemeral (daily) hemodialysis. *Adv Ren Replace Ther* 2001;8:236–249.
410. Lacson E Jr, Diaz-Buxo JA. Daily and nocturnal hemodialysis: how do they stack up? *Am J Kidney Dis* 2001;38:225–239.
411. Schulman G. Nutrition in daily hemodialysis. *Am J Kidney Dis* 2003;41:S112–115.
412. Goffin E, Pirard Y, Francart J, et al. Daily hemodialysis and nutritional status. *Kidney Int* 2002;61:1909–1910.
413. Galland R, Traeger J, Arkouche W, et al. Short daily hemodialysis rapidly improves nutritional status in hemodialysis patients. *Kidney Int* 2001;60:1555–1560.
414. Galland R, Traeger J, Arkouche W, et al. Short daily hemodialysis and nutritional status. *Am J Kidney Dis* 2001;37:S95–98.
415. Mohr PE, Neumann PJ, Franco SJ, et al. The quality of life and economic implications of daily dialysis. *Policy Anal Brief H Ser* 1999;1:1–4.

26

INTRADIALYTIC PARENTERAL NUTRITION

CHARLES J. FOULKS

The passage and implementation of Public Law 92-603 have permitted patients with chronic kidney disease to live and to be active members of society. As the age of patients undergoing dialysis has increased and the criteria for not offering dialysis or transplantation have become fewer, more patients with chronic kidney disease are malnourished as they begin dialysis. These malnourished patients undergoing maintenance hemodialysis (MHD) clearly have increased morbidity and mortality (1–5), but the causes for malnutrition are varied and may be difficult to treat (6). Decreased nutritional intake resulting from a variety of factors, loss of amino acids into dialysate, superimposed illnesses, and other factors that increase catabolism or decrease anabolism all may contribute to the malnutrition seen in patients undergoing MHD (7–10).

Nutritional intervention in these patients is difficult and expensive, and it has not been convincingly shown in prospective, randomized trials to be of clear benefit, although intuitively it should be beneficial (11–13). Recent nonrandomized trials in a large number of malnourished patients undergoing MHD have suggested that intervention with intradialytic parenteral nutrition (IDPN) may be associated with a decrease in hospitalization rate and mortality (12, 13). Although these reports are encouraging, they do not convincingly support the use of IDPN in all malnourished patients undergoing MHD.

A liberalization of the diet with increased dialysis and the use of oral supplements may be indicated in malnourished patients undergoing MHD (6,14). Unfortunately, data demonstrating success of these strategies are nonexistent, and the effectiveness of appetite stimulants in this population is unknown. Clinical nephrologists and renal dietitians also observe that supplements and diet liberalization are often not effective (6,12,13). For these reasons, a passive form of nutritional support, such as parenteral nutrition, becomes very appealing.

HISTORICAL PERSPECTIVE

In 1975 Heidland and Kult reported the first use of IDPN in patients undergoing MHD (15). Eighteen patients were studied during a 60-week period while they received an intravenous infusion during the last 90 minutes of MHD. The nutritive mixture contained D,L-malic acid, xylitol, sorbitol (about 100 kcal), and 2 g of nitrogen (N) as essential amino acids (EAA) including histidine. During the first 90 days, some patients received nonessential amino acids (NEAA) as well. The patients also were supplemented with 100 g of steak and curds during dialysis, but the amount that was ingested was not reported. Although the patients had some minor biochemical evidence of malnutrition, most patients were probably not severely malnourished. The patients tolerated the infusions well, and they experienced a significant increase in the serum albumin, total protein, transferrin, and complement concentrations after 16 weeks of therapy. An insignificant increase in body weight was noted, and the patients reported an increase in appetite. Therapy was discontinued for 6 weeks in 13 patients. During this later time, these 13 patients had a significant decrease in serum transferrin and complement ($p < 0.05$) and reported a subjective loss of strength.

Hecking et al. treated seven patients undergoing MHD with 17.25 g of EAA intravenously during the last 90 minutes of hemodialysis for 6 months; the patients also received oral EAA for 3 of these 6 months (16). The patients apparently were well nourished before IDPN, and no benefit from the therapy was noted.

A group of 18 stable patients undergoing were was treated with IDPN for 8 weeks by Guarnieri et al. (17). No clinical data were reported. The patients manifested a number of signs felt to be associated with malnutrition, including low serum albumin and complement concentrations, body weight, triceps skinfold thickness, midarm circumference, and midarm muscle circumference and depressed phytohemagglutination response. The 18 patients were divided into two groups. The first group received IDPN providing only 5% dextrose in water. The second group received an isocaloric quantity of IDPN with 5% dextrose and 3 g of nitrogen provided as EAA. The only variable that improved was the body weight in the EAA group. The average intake of calories and protein before the use of IDPN was 31 kcal/kg/day and 1.23 g/kg/ day, respectively, which was in excess of that reported in the National Cooperative Dialysis Study (2). Clinically significant malnutrition was probably not present in these patients.

Thunberg et al. reported the results in four patients undergoing MHD treated with IDPN for 6 months (18). The patients were presumed to be malnourished and received customized formulas consisting of amino acids, dextrose, and lipids. The patients developed positive nitrogen balance and had a significant increase in serum albumin. Other relevant clinical data, including adequacy of dialysis, were not presented.

Piraino et al. treated 21 patients undergoing MHD with IDPN over a 5-month period (19). Five patients who had lost more than 15% of their usual body weight were treated with a dextrose and EAA solution. The other 16 patients were treated with an EAA/NEAA (Travasol, Baxter International, Deerfield, IL) and dextrose solution. This group received 680 nonprotein calories and 42.5 g of EAA and NEAA during each dialysis session. The other group of five patients received 680 kcal and 21.6 g of EAA per dialysis. This latter group had been treated with MHD for a significantly shorter period than the group receiving EAA and NEAA. IDPN was not initiated during an acute illness, and patients with diabetes mellitus, malignancy, and intractable heart disease were excluded from the study. Eight patients in the EAA/NEAA group gained more than 10% of their starting body weight, whereas the other eight continued to lose weight. These patients differed from each other, with the responders (those who gained weight) having biochemical evidence of more severe secondary hyperparathyroidism. However, the clinical importance of this elevation in parathyroid hormone concentrations is questionable. The group of patients given EAA gained weight unless they were stressed by an acute illness.

Predialysis and postdialysis amino acid concentrations also were measured. Postdialysis concentrations of phenylalanine, methionine, leucine, and isoleucine were higher in the nonresponders (i.e., no weight gain) than in the responders. The group of patients receiving the EAA-based IDPN exhibited very low plasma NEAA concentrations. These findings led the investigators to recommend a reformulation of the amino acid (AA) solution for patients with end-stage renal disease (ESRD) to include increased proportions of valine, serine, arginine, and histidine; the addition of tyrosine; and decreased proportions of phenylalanine and methionine. The use of an IDPN solution containing EAA as the only protein source was not recommended. The authors also concluded that IDPN was safe, was effective if severe secondary hyperparathyroidism defined as an elevated parathyroid hormone concentration was not present, and would not prevent weight loss during an acute illness. Unfortunately, it is not clear that other factors that could have affected outcome were not operative. Morbidity was not reported, mortality apparently did not occur, and dialysis adequacy was not measured.

The report by Piraino et al. led Baxter International to reformulate Travasol to RenAmin (20). RenAmin contained an increase in the proportion (from 40% to 66%) of the nine EAA including histidine. Arginine, serine, and tyrosine also were included. Eighteen weight-losing patients undergoing MHD were selected for study with a RenAmin-based IDPN formula; three had been treated with MHD for less than 6 months. Thirteen of the other 15 patients had lost weight to less than their ideal body weight. Each patient received 250 mL of 50% dextrose and 250 mL of RenAmin, which delivered 65 g of amino acids per hemodialysis. Patients received from 45 to 165 infusions during MHD. Eleven of the 18 patients gained weight and were considered to be responders (12.6 + 4.9 lb), whereas seven did not ($-9.71 + 9.6$ lb, $p < 0.03$). Three of these latter seven patients stabilized their weight, and further weight loss was not seen. These two groups were considered to have not been different at baseline, although the data to support this contention were not presented. The group of responders had a significant increase in triceps skinfold, biceps skinfold, total fat folds, midarm circumference, and midarm muscle circumference, with no change in serum albumin concentration. The authors noted that the return of appetite was predictive of weight gain or response. Changes in plasma amino acid concentrations were not measured. Morbidity and dialysis adequacy were not reported, and there was no mortality during the study.

In 1982 Wolfson et al. treated eight patients undergoing MHD with an EAA and NEAA dextrose solution (21). Positive amino acid balance was demonstrated with about 90% of the infused AA being retained. Older dialyzers with a thick dialysis membrane and low blood flow were used, making the comparison to more modern, high-efficiency, thin-membrane dialyzers with high blood flow difficult. Nevertheless, the feasibility of IDPN-related retention of nutrients was established. More recent studies using high-flux dialyzers have shown similar or only slightly greater amino acid transfer rates across the dialyzer (22,23). Navarro et al. reported a greater loss of AA when these were infused during dialysis without accompanying glucose or lipid infusion (24).

Olshan et al. reported the use of an EAA and NEAA, lipid, and dextrose IDPN solution in 10 patients undergoing MHD who had lost more than 10% of their usual body weight (25). Only four of the patients had a low serum albumin concentration. An improved appetite was seen in eight patients who also gained weight (2 to 6 lb). Oral intake, comorbidities, or acute illnesses were not reported. No allowance was made for the effects of physician or dietitian intervention, selection bias, or adequacy of dialysis.

The first study to use a run-in observation period after selection for study was completed by Moore and Acchiardo (26). Patients undergoing MHD were chosen based on a low, midweek serum urea nitrogen (SUN); a decreased serum albumin; or a protein intake less than 0.8 g/kg/day. After 2 weeks of dietary counseling, the patients accepted for study were required to meet the inclusion criteria a second time. Those selected were treated for 3 months with a mixture of 500 mL of 50% dextrose and 500 mL of 8.5% EAA/NEAA infused during hemodialysis and were compared to an age-, sex-, and disease-matched control group of patients undergoing MHD. The study subjects were not randomized. The treatment group also received 240 mL of Ensure Plus (Ross Laboratories, Columbus, OH) on nondialysis days and 180 mL on dialysis days. A significant increase was noted in the serum albumin concentration in the treatment group, but no significant change was seen in the protein nitrogen appearance (PNA) (i.e., net protein catabolic rate) or SUN. The authors concluded that IDPN was an effective form of therapy for patients with hypoalbuminemia or those with an inadequate protein intake. However, the changes seen could have been the result of the supplementation with Ensure Plus, increased dietitian and physician effort or attention, or the motivation of the patient. The clinical outcome of these patients was not reported.

Bilbrey and Cohen (5) reported a series of 204 patients undergoing MHD of whom 21 were classified as having severe protein-calorie malnutrition and 42 were considered to be moderately malnourished. Twenty of the patients with moderate to severe protein-calorie malnutrition were treated with IDPN for at least 90 days. Criteria used to choose these 20 patients were not presented. The only nutritional marker to undergo improvement during this period was the midarm muscle circumference. No comparison with oral supplements was done, although the patients were considered to have failed other attempts to reverse their malnutrition. In 1993 Bilbrey further reported the findings of a group of 47 patients undergoing MHD with severe protein-calorie malnutrition who failed other therapeutic attempts aimed at reversing their malnutrition (27). The report was unclear as to whether some of these 47 patients had been included in his earlier study (5). These patients were treated with IDPN for at least 90 days; 29 survived (62%) and 18 died (38%). A significant increase in serum albumin was noted in the survivors: 3.30 ± 0.38 to 3.71 ± 0.30 g/dL (± standard deviation; $p < 0.001$) as well as an increase in serum transferrin (165 ± 37 to 200 ± 62, units of measurement not given; $p < 0.001$). No increase in serum albumin or transferrin was noted in the nonsurvivors. In addition, the prevalence of diabetes mellitus, average time undergoing dialysis, and time being treated with IDPN were not reported. The groups also could not be separated by dialysis dosage, comorbid conditions, or cause of death. IDPN was considered to be beneficial.

Twenty-six malnourished patients undergoing MHD were chosen by Cano et al. to receive or not receive IDPN (28). Each patient was given IDPN during MHD thrice weekly for 3 months. These patients undergoing MHD received 1.6 g/kg/hemodialysis as lipids (Intralipid, Kabi-Vitrum, Stockholm, Sweden) and 0.08 g N/kg/hemodialysis as EAA/NEAA and glycyl-tyrosine peptide. An increase in oral intake of about 9 kcal/kg/day and 0.25 g/kg/day of protein (0.04 g N/kg/day) was noted in these individuals ($p < 0.05$). The lipids were well tolerated, and no adverse effects on serum cholesterol, triglyceride, or phospholipid concentrations were observed.

Nine patients undergoing MHD with diabetes mellitus were treated with IDPN by Madigan et al. (29). After 2 months of therapy, three patients had gained weight, four lost weight, and two patients demonstrated no change. Four of the five patients manifested increased appetites. A similar small study by Snyder et al. demonstrated no effect of IDPN on serum chemistry values of five patients undergoing MHD treated with IDPN (30). An increase in dietary protein intake was noted. Few clinical outcomes were reported, and the patients' morbidity and mortality rates were not discussed.

Schulman et al. reported the results of treatment of eight malnourished patients undergoing hemodialysis with recombinant human growth hormone (rhGH) and IDPN (31). After 6 weeks of therapy with IDPN, a significant increase in the serum transferrin concentration was noted, whereas there was no significant change in PNA, serum albumin, or insulinlike growth factor-1 (IGF-1). IDPN was continued for another 6 weeks, along with the addition of 5 mg of rhGH administered at each hemodialysis session. This resulted in a significant increase in serum albumin and IGF-1 concentrations at the end of therapy. No significant change in anthropometric measurements was noted. The sample size was small, and although the results are encouraging, interpretation must be qualified. The beneficial response seen may have been secondary to the continuation of the IDPN for a longer period—a phenomenon reported by other investigators (12,13).

In 1991 Foulks reported the results of a large group of patients undergoing MHD treated with IDPN (12). All patients who were treated with MHD and IDPN from July 1, 1989 through March 15, 1991 or who died during this period were evaluated. All patients met at least one criterion for malnutrition (weight loss >10% of the usual body weight over 30 days or a serum albumin <3.5 g/dL). Patients were not started on IDPN until a 2-week course of intensive dietary counseling and a trial use of nutritional supplements (in 64% of patients) were completed. Additionally, IDPN was not started within 180 days of commencing MHD therapy, within 14 days of hospitalization, or in patients with a protein intake higher than 0.75 g/kg/day.

Patients were described as either responders (>10% weight gain or an increase in serum albumin >0.5 g/dL or serum total protein >0.5 g/dL) or nonresponders (absence of defined increases in weight, serum albumin, or serum total protein). The only difference between the groups at the start of the study was that the responders had significantly lower serum albumin (2.2 + 0.7 versus 3.0 + 0.8 g/dL, $p < 0.0001$) and total protein (5.3 + 1.0 versus 6.2 + 1.3 g/dL, $p < 0.0001$). A significant increase in weight gain, serum albumin, and total protein in the responders was observed, whereas weight loss and a decrease in serum albumin and total protein were observed in the nonresponders ($p < 0.0001$).

Hospitalization rates were also significantly different: the prestudy hospitalization rate (hospitalizations/patient per month) was greater in the responders than in the nonresponders (0.36 ± 0.23 versus 0.25 + 0.20, $p < 0.0001$). No change was noted in the hospitalization rate during the study in the nonresponders (0.25 ± 0.20, $p = 1.0$), and a significant decrease was seen in the hospitalization rate of the responders (0.12 ± 0.20, $p < 0.0001$). During IDPN therapy 52% of the responders were hospitalized at least once, as compared to 76% of the nonresponders ($p < 0.001$). Additionally, a marked difference was observed in mortality between the responders and nonresponders (9/52 versus 13/20, $p < 0.0001$). Half of the responders were able to discontinue IDPN because of an increase in dietary protein intake to more than 0.90 g/kg/day. Of the responders who were able to discontinue therapy, 88% did so within 9 months (four patients in <3 months, 16 patients in 3 to 6 months, and three patients in 6 to 9 months).

Although this study avoided many of the flaws of previous investigations, its findings must be interpreted with caution. The study was not randomized; not all patients received oral supplements; dialysis adequacy was not measured but was assessed clinically; and there was no untreated control group. No differences of great importance were noted between the responders and nonresponders prior to the study, and although the groups seem equally matched, there can be no firm conclusion that the two groups were at the same risk for hospitalization or death before treatment.

Capelli et al. studied 81 malnourished patients undergoing MHD treated with IDPN (13). Malnutrition was defined as a serum albumin of less than 3.5 g/dL and either a body weight less than 90% of desirable body weight or a loss of body weight of more than 10% over 2 consecutive months. Fifty-one patients who did not show a response to dietary counseling or oral supplements (Ensure or Ensure Plus, Ross Laboratories, Columbus, OH) were treated with IDPN. The remaining 30 patients demonstrated a serum albumin less than 3.5 g/dL, and they were within 10% of desirable body weight or had a weight loss less than 10% of the usual body weight. The dietary supplements were continued in these 30 patients, although most patients discontinued the supplements after 3 months of therapy. The supplements were not continued in the IDPN group. Urea kinetic modeling was used to maintain Kt/V at 1.0 to 1.2 and normalized PNA (nPNA or nPCR) between 0.9 and 1.1 g/kg/day.

All patients being treated with IDPN received 50 g of AA during each dialysis session. Nondiabetic patients received 270 to 450 kcal/hemodialysis as dextrose and 200 to 500 kcal/hemodialysis as lipid. Patients with diabetes received 102 to 170 kcal/hemodialysis as dextrose and 200 to 500 kcal/hemodialysis as lipid. Total nonprotein calories delivered to nondiabetic patients ranged from 470 to 950 kcal/hemodialysis, whereas diabetics received 302 to 670 nonprotein kcal/hemodialysis. It is impossible to determine the amounts of nonprotein calories or the proportions of dextrose and lipid used in the IDPN formulas delivered to each patient group.

Baseline demographics were not different between treated and untreated patients with the exception that patients with diabetes had been undergoing dialysis for a shorter period than nondiabetic patients. Significant weight gains were seen in the treated patients who survived but not in the survivors who were not treated. Neither treated nor untreated nonsurvivors experienced weight gain. It is noteworthy that survivors had a higher body weight at the start of the study as compared to nonsurvivors (143.8 ± 35 lb versus 115.9 ± 25 lb, $p = 0.02$). An insignificant improvement in serum albumin was observed in the treated survivors comparing baseline to the 12-month values. The nonsurvivors also demonstrated an increase in the serum albumin in the first 6 months of therapy (p = ns) with values declining by the twelfth month. Upwards of 8 months of therapy were required before the serum albumin normalized in some treated patients, and 6 months of IDPN were needed before changes in weight or serum albumin were noted.

Thirty-two of the 50 treated patients survived, as compared to 16 of the 31 untreated patients (64% versus 52%, p = ns). Untreated nonsurvivors lived a shorter time than did treated nonsurvivors (7.5 ± 4.2 versus 16.9 ± 7.9 months, $p < 0.01$). Age, length of time on dialysis, sex, race, diabetic status, body weight at 1 month, and Kt/V and serum albumin at 1 month did not correlate with survival (Cox Proportional Hazards Regression Model). Treatment with IDPN was significantly related to survival ($p = 0.01$), and the change in the nPNA at 1 month approached significance ($p = 0.077$). Although the study was retrospective and nonrandomized, and the statistical analysis plan was developed after the data were accumulated, the authors concluded that IDPN was an effective form of therapy that could improve survival, presumably by improving protein-calorie malnutrition.

The experience of National Medical Care with IDPN-treated patients undergoing MHD has been reported (32, 33). The initial analysis compared data between 2,363 patients undergoing MHD treated with IDPN by National Medical Care and 53,663 patients undergoing MHD not treated with IDPN in the time period of January 1, 1989 through December 31, 1992 (32). Data were compiled from the central National Medical Care laboratory data files and reimbursement files from National Medical Care Home-care, Inc. Only patients with complete data were selected for analysis. Logistic regression techniques were used; odds of death and probability of death were computed. Variables examined were age, sex, race, diabetic status, serum albumin, and serum creatinine concentrations. Patients treated with IDPN were more likely to be older, white, and diabetic and to have lower serum albumin and creatinine concentrations, higher urea reduction ratios (URR) and SUN, lower cholesterol and iron concentrations, and a higher serum bicarbonate concentration (all significant at $p < 0.002$ to $p < 0.0001$). The primary predictors of death in the untreated patients were age, sex, presence of diabetes, and serum albumin. Observed and expected death from a risk of death of 0.0 to 1.0 resulted in a line of identity for non-IDPN–treated patients undergoing MHD. However, at a risk of death above 0.4, the observed deaths in the patients treated with IDPN were decreased and differed significantly from the line of identity. Serum albumin and creatinine concentrations trended slowly upward in the IDPN-treated group over 6 months of therapy. The authors suggested that IDPN might be associated with decreased death rate in patients undergoing MHD who have a risk of death above 0.4. However, they cautioned that the putative benefits from IDPN might be related to physician bias and selection, use of other therapies not measured, or convalescence from acute illnesses.

A second analysis of National Medical Care patients who were undergoing hemodialysis and treated with IDPN was reported in 1994 (33). Patients undergoing MHD at their dialysis units who were alive and receiving MHD on January 1, 1991 and who either lived until December 3l, 1991 or died between these two dates were selected for analysis. All of these patients who received IDPN during the year were evaluated as the treatment group (n = 1,679), and the remaining patients served as a control group (n = 22,517).

Patients were stratified by serum albumin and creatinine concentrations and were adjusted for case mix and URR. The risk of death then was calculated following this stratification. Patients with a low serum creatinine (<8.0 g/dL) and low serum albumin (<3.3 g/dL) had a significant decrease in mortality if they were treated with IDPN. Those patients treated with IDPN with serum albumin higher than 4.0 g/dL did not benefit from therapy with IDPN but demonstrated an increase in death risk when compared to similar patients not treated with IDPN. Likewise IDPN-treated patients with creatinine above 8.0 and serum albumin above 3.5 did not benefit from therapy and had an increase in death risk associated with IDPN. Again, these data suggest benefit from IDPN therapy for malnourished patients undergoing hemodialysis. However, the same caveats to the earlier evaluation of National Medical Care patients are still operative. These data also suggest that the increase in death risk seen with IDPN-treated patients without malnutrition (defined as an serum albumin >3.5 and creatinine >8.0) is not related to any nutritional disorder but perhaps to another illness not affected by nutrition. Clearly, no definitive statement concerning efficacy of IDPN can be made based on these observations.

Ruggian et al. reported the results of IDPN therapy in 31 patients undergoing MHD (34). Patients who had received IDPN for at least 3 consecutive months and who were without hospitalization or illness in the 3 months prior to or during IDPN therapy were analyzed. A significant increase in serum albumin was noted (2.67 ± 0.14 versus 3.13 ± 0.10 g/dL (mean ± standard error of the mean); $p < 0.05$). No changes in SUN, creatinine, total protein, or body weight were observed. Of the 10 patients who were able to discontinue IDPN, no change in these variables was noted after 6 months of follow-up. The data have been reported only in abstract form (29), and conclusions from this study must be considered tentative.

Although the data from National Medical Care indicate that 6.9% of their patients undergoing hemodialysis received IDPN (33), data concerning the incidence of IDPN use in all patients undergoing hemodialysis in the United States are scanty. The Medical Review Board of End Stage Renal Disease Network 14 (Texas) conducted a survey of the dialysis unit practices concerning the use of IDPN (35). The response rate from the dialysis units in Network 14 was 100% (n = 143). The dialysis unit medical directors and the renal dietitian completed the surveys. The most widely used criteria for selection of patients for IDPN were serum albumin less than 3.5 g/dL, enteral supplement intolerance, malabsorption, and weight loss. Patient progress and the decision to discontinue IDPN were suggested by increased oral intake; weight change; improvement in serum albumin; and subjective reports of well-being, improved serum cholesterol concentration, and food records.

Between 4.5% and 7.5% of all patients undergoing MHD in Texas were treated with IDPN. The use of IDPN at these facilities was quite variable: 0% use in 44 units, 1% to 5% in 51, 5% to 10% in 36, 10% to 20% in 10, and greater than 20% in two. Of even greater interest was the finding that the decision to initiate IDPN was not solely a physician decision. Physicians were involved in the decision to use IDPN in 98% of cases, dietitians in 92%, nurses in 63%, proprietary infusion providers in 30%, and insurers in 15%. Of physicians, 44% used a standard one-size-fits-all formula, whereas 56% customized the IDPN prescription. An EAA/NEAA solution was used in 73% of prescriptions, whereas EAA was used in 27%. An average of 57 g of amino acids were delivered per hemodialysis, with 36% of calories from lipids; lipids were included in 92% of the formulas. The use of IDPN in Network 14 was not uniform, and criteria to select, monitor, and deselect patients were nonexistent. The use of EAA cannot be justified from these data, especially considering the expense and previous reports (19,20). Adequacy of dialysis prior to initiation of IDPN therapy was not noted, and oral supplements and diet liberalization generally were not used or commented on. The survey indicated that an unproved therapy often was used for unclear and possibly unsound reasons. It was also not clear that any investigation of other deleterious factors, including emotional depression or the presence of an acute illness or a serious non-nutrition–related illness, had been performed. The finding that therapy providers and insurers participated in patient selection is cause for concern.

CRITIQUE OF PUBLISHED STUDIES

An evidence-based review of the published IDPN studies has been published and will be briefly summarized (36). An extensive search of Medline and an extensive hand search of journals and published articles concerning IDPN were completed. All articles were categorized according to (a) strength of evidence, (b) size of treatment effect, (c) magnitude of risk of nontreatment, and (d) the precision of the estimate of treatment effect. The characteristics of each study that was examined are noted in Table 26.1.

Each study specifically was evaluated for evidence that could be used to validate the following statement: "Is there reliable evidence that proves that IDPN therapy in clearly malnourished HD patients causes a decrease in mortality, decrease in morbidity, an improved quality of life, or the successful treatment and reversal of malnutrition?"

Of all of the studies reviewed only one was a randomized, double-blinded, controlled trial (16). Unfortunately, apparently well-nourished patients were studied. Three studies were randomized (17,21,28). One was a feasibility study (21), one used an IDPN formulation not available today (17), and the other was not blinded and the randomization schema was not described; therefore, a causal relationship cannot be described (28). This study also used a form of IDPN that currently is not used. Their definition of malnutrition is suspect, and clinically important changes were not seen. The intent of this study was to evaluate the safety of lipid as a calorie source in patients undergoing MHD, not to study the effects of IDPN on morbidity and mortality.

There were 20 nonrandomized, observational studies of IDPN that described 362 patients (5,11,13,15,18–20, 25–30,33,37–41). None of these studies can be used to support the use of IDPN. The weaknesses of these studies are listed in Table 26.2.

TABLE 26.1. STUDY CHARACTERISTICS USED FOR ARTICLE CATEGORIZATION

Strength of evidence
Significance of treatment effect
Sources/significance of bias
Applicability of results
Trade-offs
Size of treatment effect
Clear causal relationship
Sources/magnitude of variation
Variance in risk
Evidence supporting inferences

TABLE 26.2. STUDY WEAKNESSES

Poor criteria to diagnose malnutrition
Use of nonmalnourished patients
Poor or undescribed selection criteria
Poorly standardized or described dialysis regimens
Nonexclusion of confounding factors (e.g., intercurrent illness, recent hospitalization, inadequate dialysis)
Disparate baseline risks
Differing intradialytic parenteral nutrition formulas

Only two studies indicated an IDPN-related effect in malnourished patients (12,13). In the study by Foulks, patients treated with IDPN who had a biochemical response (increase in serum albumin or total protein) or weight gain had a significant decrease in mortality and hospitalization rate (12). However, this study was not randomized and it is not clear that baseline risk for mortality or morbidity were the same in the responders and the nonresponders. The report of Capelli et al. indicated that IDPN treatment of malnourished HD patients led to a prolonged survival in nonsurvivors when compared to the nonsurvivors not treated with IDPN (13). There was a significant correlation of IDPN use with survival, although there was no significant difference in the survival rates of the IDPN-treated patients undergoing MHD compared to those not treated with IDPN. Multiple confounding factors keep this study from providing conclusive evidence that IDPN prolongs survival, decreases morbidity, or reverses malnutrition. It is interesting that several studies suggest that merely being selected to receive IDPN results in an improved outcome (12,13, 31) with the exception that patients with a serum albumin of more than 3.4 g/dL or a serum creatinine of more than 8.0 mg/dL had an increase in mortality over that expected had they not received IDPN (33). No good studies concerning the effect of IDPN therapy on quality of life exist (37).

Three studies (12,13,33) allow the calculation of the number needed to treat, or NNT (i.e., the number of patients who must be treated before one patient is likely to show benefit from the therapy). When calculating the NNT mortality, one has to perform the calculation based on a range of assumptions of mortality rate. However, in the Foulks study (12), the risk of death in the responders was 0.17 and 0.65 in the nonresponders, leading to an NNT of 2. The NNT from the Capelli study was 8.3. Using the United States Renal Data System mortality rate of 24%, the Chertow et al. study had an NNT of 17 (33). Although these studies do not possess the power of well-done, randomized, blinded trials, they at least offer the clinician a basis for comparison of therapies. If the NNT is 2, the cost of 1 year of IDPN therapy is about $60,000 to provide benefit to one patient. If the NNT is 17, the cost of 1 year of therapy to benefit one patient is about \$510,000. As a comparison, 1 quality-of-life–adjusted year of life improvement from erythropoietin therapy is at least \$130,000.

A recent study of IDPN by Pupim et al. has offered new insights into the possible contribution of IDPN to improved outcomes in patients undergoing dialysis (42). Seven stable patients undergoing hemodialysis without history of signs, symptoms, or biochemical evidence of malnutrition or inflammation were studied during dialysis. All patients had a Kt/V 1.4 and all had protein intake of more than 0.97 g/kg body weight. Patients were studied with and without the administration of IDPN, and constant infusions of L-(1-^{13}C) leucine and L-(ring-$^{2}H_5$) phenylalanine were used in all dialysis periods to measure whole-body protein synthesis and proteolysis and forearm muscle protein synthesis. They found that IDPN promoted a significant increase in whole-body protein synthesis and a decrease in whole-body proteolysis. There was a significant increase in forearm muscle protein synthesis. IDPN usage caused the hemodialysis session to convert from a catabolic state to one of positive protein balance. Unfortunately, these effects did not carry over into the interdialytic period. Nevertheless, for the first time, there has been a mechanistic evaluation that suggests that IDPN might be useful in reversing the protein catabolism of dialysis. Clearly, this area needs to be investigated more fully.

In summary, the data that IDPN is an effective therapy are not definitive. The cost and reimbursement problems are formidable, and it is unlikely under current funding mechanisms that IDPN will become a widely used therapy.

INDICATIONS FOR INTRADIALYTIC PARENTERAL NUTRITION

Several years ago, the National Kidney Foundation appointed a group of professional renal nutrition experts who drafted a position paper on these reimbursement issues in response to the proposed changes. The recommendations of this position paper represent reasonable guidelines for the practitioner to follow in responding to the need for nutritional support of the patient undergoing MHD (38). Chan et al., representing a group of professional renal nutrition experts from ESRD Network 14, also have published an algorithm for the team management of the malnourished patient undergoing MHD (39). Both of these articles strongly recommend that all remedial causes of malnutrition and poor nutritional intake be identified and an attempt at reversal be made prior to considering invasive nutritional support.

Those patients who have a functional gastrointestinal tract, and for whom enteral nutrition is not contraindicated, should be offered enteral feedings (38,39). IDPN represents a next logical step for those patients who cannot tolerate or cannot be treated successfully with enteral feedings. However, if the patient cannot consume sufficient calories and protein to adequately supplement the IDPN, total parenteral nutrition should be considered. It is clear that IDPN by itself does not represent full nutritional support and cannot meet total nutritional requirements. However, in the patient undergoing MHD, daily intravenous feeding may lead to multiple complications including line sepsis, subclavian or internal jugular stenosis or thrombosis, volume overload, electrolyte and mineral imbalance, and the need for extra MHD sessions. It is likely that these adverse events will occur less commonly or will be nonexistent with IDPN.

Currently it is extremely difficult if not almost impossible for one to receive reimbursement for IDPN therapy from Medicare without demonstrating a severe gastrointestinal dysfunction. The therapy is not reimbursed by state Medicaid, and only some private, commercial insurers will cover the cost of IDPN. Most of the large IDPN providers (i.e., Fresenius) do not cover the cost or supply IDPN unless there is a funding source available.

INTRADIALYTIC PARENTERAL NUTRITION ADMINISTRATION

Before IDPN is used, the nursing staff should be thoroughly acquainted with the rationale and the use and monitoring of IDPN. Proprietary companies that provide IDPN services already have prepared protocols for the use and monitoring of IDPN. These companies will offer in-service teaching for the nursing and medical staff. However, one must be careful when using these services, especially in light of the observation of Network 14 that providers often were involved in the decision to use IDPN (35). Such involvement represents a serious conflict of interest and should be avoided.

The original Heidland and Kult article on IDPN used a peripheral vein for IDPN administration (15). Wolfson et al. used the venous drip chamber of the dialysis blood lines for IDPN administration (21), and this has been the practice in the United States. This is the preferred delivery site because it does not involve another percutaneous venous access and avoids predialyzer delivery of the nutrients that would be expected to increase the amount of amino acids lost into the dialysate.

Several formulations have been used for IDPN (5,12,13, 15–22,26). These have ranged from those with minimal provision of nutrients (15,17), to those that deliver significant amounts of calories and amino acids (12,13,19–21, 27,28). Until the report of Cano et al. (28), lipid administration was thought to be contraindicated; however, experience as well as the Cano report suggest otherwise, and lipids are used routinely. Table 26.3 lists several representative formulas; Goldstein and Strom also offer other formulations (40). Although a lipid-based IDPN formula is well tolerated, as reported by Cano et al. (28), there are anecdotal reports of lipid intolerance in patients undergoing MHD

TABLE 26.3. IDPN FORMULATIONS[a]

	Standard Amount	Nutrient Delivery
Lipids (20%)	250 mL	500 kcal
Amino acids (10%)	500 mL	50 g
Dextrose (g)	175 g	595 kcal
Lipid-free IDPN[a]		
Amino acids (10%)	500 mL	50 g
Dextrose (g)	250 g	850 kcal

IDPN, intradialytic parenteral nutrition.
[a]To be given during a single hemodialysis treatment.

(40). If this occurs, the lipid-free IDPN formulation may be used. It may be wise to only use half of the standard formula for the first two or three treatments until the glycemic response of the patient can be determined. Following this, the formula may be increased to full strength. The amount of amino acids delivered by these formulas is greater than that studied by Wolfson et al. (21); however, clinical experience has not suggested any harm from this.

MONITORING INTRADIALYTIC PARENTERAL NUTRITION ADMINISTRATION

IDPN treatment monitoring has been well reviewed by Goldstein and Strom (40). In brief, disorders of glucose metabolism, lipid intolerance, and mineral and electrolyte imbalance may occur. The administration rate of the first IDPN solution should be 1 mL/min for 30 minutes while the patient is observed closely for signs of lipid intolerance. Also, the use of IDPN requires a readjustment of the calculated fluid removal or ultrafiltration needed over the dialysis period. Initial and routine monitoring recommendations for IDPN are listed in Table 26.4.

If the patient develops hyperglycemia (>300 mg/dL) during the hemodialysis procedure, intravenous human regular insulin should be given; 2 to 6 units are generally adequate. The posthemodialysis goal for glycemic control is 200 to 300 mg/dL. Either intravenous regular insulin may be used to attain this goal or insulin may be added to the IDPN solution. Some authors recommend that patients receive an oral intake of a carbohydrate at the end of the hemodialysis session, but it is the author's viewpoint that rebound hypoglycemia is seen only in those patients who are treated with a lipid-free formula (12,40).

TABLE 26.4. RECOMMENDED MONITORING OF IDPN

Pre-HD	1 Hour	Post-HD	2 Weeks	Monthly
Glucose	X[a]	X[a]	X[a]	X
Sodium			X[a]	X
Potassium	X[a]		X[a]	X
Phosphorus				X
Cholesterol				X
Triglycerides				X
Liver function				X
KT/V (or URR)			X	X

IDPN, intradialytic parenteral nutrition; HD, hemodialysis; KT/V, a measure of dialysis adequacy; URR, urea reduction ratio.
[a]These tests should be done until the patient has had 3 days of full-strength IDPN and then may be deleted if the values are acceptable.

If hypokalemia is noted, either potassium may be added to the IDPN solution or the potassium concentration of the dialysate may be increased. It is important to monitor the patient's oral intake because as the patient improves, oral intake also improves and there is the risk that hyperkalemia may occur. Hypophosphatemia may occur, especially if the patient has become severely malnourished and a high efficiency dialyzer is used. Phosphorus may be added to the IDPN solution as either potassium phosphate or sodium phosphate. Generally, 10 to 20 mM per 1,000 kcal administered are adequate. Again, as oral intake improves, hyperphosphatemia may occur.

Occasionally intradialytic skeletal muscle cramping is noted in patients treated with IDPN. This may be treated by adding sodium chloride, 75 to 150 mEq, to the IDPN formula. The cramping may be secondary to osmolar changes or to too rapid ultrafiltration. Quinine sulfate may be a useful therapy if given prior to hemodialysis. Sodium profiling also may be of benefit.

Elevated hepatic transaminases secondary to the use of IDPN have not been reported but theoretically could be induced by the rapid administration of 125 to 250 g of dextrose over 3 or 4 hours. Additionally, elevations of lipids have not been reported and were not seen by Cano et al. (28). It is important to monitor serum cholesterol and triglyceride concentrations because as the oral intake of a patient improves, an increase in these chemistries will signal to the clinician that improvement has occurred.

Most patients undergoing MHD will respond to IDPN after 90 to 180 days of therapy, and the continuation of IDPN beyond this is not generally recommended (12). Response to therapy is indicated by an increase in appetite, nonfluid weight gain, and improvement of the serum albumin concentration (12). In general, when patients can consume more than 90% of their prescribed diet, IDPN can be discontinued. It is important to monitor the adequacy of dialysis carefully because dialysis requirements will increase as the patient's appetite improves. It is the author's practice to increase the dose of dialysis by 25% to 30% when IDPN is initiated, although the pre-IDPN dialysis adequacy has been acceptable. It is also unwise to use IDPN during hemodialysis sessions less than 3 hours long. IDPN usually is tolerated better and dialysis runs are smoother with fewer hypotensive episodes when the dialysis time is 3½ to 4 hours.

CONCLUSIONS

IDPN has not yet been established conclusively as being responsible for the salutary benefits accredited to its use. As newer technologies and advances in diagnosis and therapy abound and compete for scarce health care dollars, it will be hard to justify such monies for an unproved therapy such as IDPN. A randomized prospective trial of IDPN versus oral supplements in a group of malnourished patients undergoing hemodialysis with a study group large enough to lend adequate power to the study should be undertaken.

Until the efficacy of IDPN is demonstrated definitively, it should be reserved for those malnourished patients undergoing hemodialysis who have failed conventional measures to improve protein-calorie malnutrition and for whom other treatment options are neither available nor appropriate (39). Such patients first should undergo an evaluation for treatable causes of malnutrition and anorexia. Dialysis adequacy must be assured, and psychiatric disorders must be diagnosed and treated. Zinc deficiency should be excluded, as should be hormonal disorders such as hypothyroidism and hypoadrenalism, both of which are often difficult to diagnose in the patient undergoing MHD. A liberalization of diet and use of supplements should be undertaken (39). Appetite stimulants such as megestrol acetate or cyproheptadine should be considered, although their efficacy in patients undergoing MHD is unknown. Enteral feedings using a nocturnal patient-placed feeding tube should be considered, although it is the author's experience that patients usually refuse this form of therapy. Continuous enteral feeding with nasoenteric or percutaneous gastrostomy/jejunostomy tubes is also a therapeutic option. Finally, barring all else, daily total parenteral nutrition might be considered if American Society of Parenteral and Enteral Nutrition criteria are met (41). Before using such invasive therapy as tube feedings or parenteral nutrition, the physician must be satisfied that the patient is not so ill (e.g., from disseminated cancer) that benefits are very unlikely to be attained.

REFERENCES

1. Kelly MP, Gottel S, Gee C, et al. Nutritional and demographic data related to the hospitalization of hemodialysis patients. *CRN Q* 1987;11:16–22.
2. Schoenfeld P, Henry R, Kaurd N, et al. Assessment of nutritional status of the National Cooperative Dialysis Study population. *Kidney Int* 1983;23(Suppl 13):S80–S88.
3. Acchiardo S, Moore L, Latour P. Malnutrition as the main factor in morbidity and mortality of hemodialysis patients. *Kidney Int* 1983;24(Suppl 16):S19–S203.
4. Mattern W, Hak L, Lamanna R, et al. Malnutrition altered immune function and the risk of infection in maintenance hemodialysis patients. *Am J Kidney Dis* 1982;1:206–218.
5. Bilbrey GL, Cohen T. Identification and treatment of protein calorie malnutrition in chronic hemodialysis patients. *Dial Transplant* 1989;8:669–677.
6. Foulks CJ. Nutritional evaluation and management of patients on chronic hemodialysis therapy. *CRN Q* 1989;13:10–13.
7. Lazarus JM. Nutrition in hemodialysis patients. *Am J Kidney Dis* 1993;21:99–105.
8. Fouque D. Causes and interventions for malnutrition in patients undergoing maintenance dialysis. *Blood Purification* 1997;15(2): 112–120.
9. Mitch WE, Maroni BJ. Factors causing malnutrition in patients with chronic uremia. *Am J Kidney Dis* 1999;33(1):176–179.
10. Kaysen GA. C-reactive protein: A story half told. *Semin Dial* 2000;13:143–146.
11. Foulks CJ, Goldstein DJ, Kelly MP, et al. Indications for the use of intradialytic parenteral nutrition in the malnourished hemodialysis patient. *J Renal Nutr* 1991;1:23–33.
12. Foulks CJ. The effect of intradialytic parenteral nutrition on hospitalization rate and mortality in malnourished hemodialysis patients. *J Renal Nutr* 1991;4:5–10.
13. Capelli JP, Kushner H, Camiscioli TC, et al. Effect of intradialytic parenteral nutrition on mortality rates in end-stage renal disease care. *Am J Kidney Dis* 1994;23:808–816.
14. Kopple J. Therapeutic approaches to malnutrition in chronic dialysis patients: the different modalities of nutritional support. *Am J Kidney Dis* 1999;33(1):180–185.
15. Heidland A, Kult J. Long-term effects of essential amino acids supplementation inpatients on regular dialysis treatment. *Clin Nephrol* 1975;3:234–239.
16. Hecking E, Post F, Brehym R, et al. A controlled study on the value of amino acid supplementation with essential amino acids and ketoanalogues in chronic hemodialysis. *Proc Eur Dial Transplant Forum* 1977;7:157–161.
17. Guarnieri B, Faccini L, Lipartiti, et al. Simple methods for nutritional assessment in hemodialyzed patients. *Am J Clin Nutr* 1980; 33:1598–1607.
18. Thunberg B, Jain V, Patterson P, et al. Nutritional measurements and urea kinetics to guide intradialytic hyperalimentation. *Proc Eur Dial Transplant Forum* 1980;10:22–28.
19. Piraino A, Tirpo J, Powers D. Prolonged hyperalimentation in catabolic chronic dialysis therapy patients. *JPEN J Parenter Enteral Nutr* 1981;5:463–477.
20. Powers DV, Jackson A, Piraino AJ. Prolonged intradialysis hyperalimentation in chronic hemodialysis patients with an amino acid solution RenAmin® (Amino Acid Injection) formulated for renal failure. In: Kinney JM, Brown PR, eds. *Perspectives in clinical nutrition.* Baltimore-Munich: Urban & Schwarzenberg, 1989: 191–205.
21. Wolfson M, Jones M, Kopple J. Amino acids losses during hemodialysis with infusion of amino acids and glucose. *Kidney Int* 1982;21:500–506.
22. Chazot C, Smair E, Matias B, et al. Provision of amino acids by dialysis during maintenance hemodialysis (MHD). *J Am Soc Nephrol* 1995;6:574.
23. Berneis K, Iseli-Schaub J, Garbani E, et al. Effects of intradialytic parenteral nutrition in chronic hemodialysis patients with malnutrition. A pilot study. *Wien Klin Wochenschr* 1999;111:876–881.
24. Navarro JF, Mora C, León C, et al. Amino acid losses during hemodialysis with polyacrylonitrile membranes: effect of intradialytic amino acid supplementation on plasma amino acid concentrations and nutritional variables in nondiabetic patients. *Am J Clin Nutr* 2000;71:765–773.
25. Olshan A, Bruce J, Schwartz A. Intradialytic parenteral nutrition administration during outpatient hemodialysis. *Dial Transplant* 1987;16:495–496.
26. Moore L, Acchiardo S. Aggressive nutritional supplementation in chronic hemodialysis patients. *CRN Q* 1987;11:14–17.
27. Bilbrey GL. Is intradialytic parenteral nutrition of benefit in he-

modialysis patients? In Lazarus JM, ed. *Semin Dial* 1993;6(3): 168–170.
28. Cano N, Labastie-Coeyrehourq J, Lacombe P, et al. Perdialytic parenteral nutrition with lipids and amino acids in malnourished hemodialysis patients. *Am J Clin Nutr* 1990;52:726–730.
29. Madigan KM, Olshan A, Yingling DJ. Effectiveness of intradialytic parenteral nutrition in diabetic patients with end-stage renal disease. *J Am Diet Assoc* 1990;90:861–863.
30. Snyder S, Bergen C, Sigler MH, et al. Intradialytic parenteral nutrition in chronic hemodialysis patients. *ASAIO Trans* 1991; 37:M373–M375.
31. Schulman G, Wingard RL, Hutchison RL, et al. The effects of recombinant human growth hormone and intradialytic parenteral nutrition in malnourished hemodialysis patients. *Am J Kidney Dis* 1993;21:527–534.
32. Lowrie EG, Ling J, Lew NL. The effect of IDPN on patient survival: A retrospective examination of existing data. National Medical Care, July 1993, personal communication.
33. Chertow GM, Ling J, Lew NL, et al. The association of intradialytic parenteral nutrition administration with survival in hemodialysis patients. *Am J Kidney Dis* 1994;24:912–920.
34. Ruggian JC, Fishbane S, Frei GL. Effect of intradialytic parenteral nutrition (IDPN) on hypoalbuminemic hemodialysis (HD) patients [Abstract]. *J Am Soc Nephrol* 1994;5:502.
35. Chan A, Cochran C, Harbert G, et al. Use of intradialytic parenteral nutrition: An end-stage renal disease network perspective. *J Renal Nutr* 1994;4:11–14.
36. Foulks CJ. An evidence-based evaluation of intradialytic parenteral nutrition. *Am J Kidney Dis* 1999;33(1):186–192.
37. United States Renal Data System (USRDS): Patient mortality and survival. *Am J Kidney Dis* 1997;30(Suppl 1):S86–S106.
38. Kopple JD, Foulks CJ, Piraino B, et al. Proposed health care financing administration guidelines for reimbursement of enteral and parenteral nutrition. *Am J Kidney Dis* 1995;26:995–997.
39. Chan A, Cochran C, Harbert G, et al. Management of hypoalbuminemia: A challenge for the health care team. *J Renal Nutr* 1996;6(1)38–44.
40. Goldstein DJ, Strom JA. Intradialytic parenteral nutrition: Evolution and current concepts. *J Renal Nutr* 1991;1:9–22.
41. Guidelines for the use of parenteral and enteral nutrition in adult and pediatric patients. *JPEN J Parenter Enteral Nutr* 1993; 17(Suppl):1SA–52SA.
42. Pupim LB, Flakoll PJ, Brouillette JR, et al. Intradialytic parenteral nutrition improves protein and energy homeostasis in chronic hemodialysis patients. *J Clin Invest* 2002;110:483–492.

27

NUTRITIONAL EFFECTS AND NUTRITIONAL MANAGEMENT OF CHRONIC PERITONEAL DIALYSIS

OLOF HEIMBÜRGER
PETER STENVINKEL
BENGT LINDHOLM

Patients with chronic renal failure display a variety of metabolic and nutritional abnormalities, and a large proportion of the patients demonstrate signs of protein-energy malnutrition. This may be a consequence of multiple factors related to uremia, including disturbances in protein and energy metabolism; hormonal derangements; and poor food intake because of anorexia, nausea, and vomiting caused by uremic toxicity (1,2). With peritoneal dialysis (PD) some—but not all—of these factors can be partly or fully corrected.

However, additional metabolic and nutritional problems may be induced by the dialysis procedure, including dialytic losses of proteins, amino acids, water-soluble vitamins, and other essential small molecular solutes. Suppression of appetite by glucose absorption from dialysate and abdominal discomfort induced by the dialysate also may occur.

When evaluating the nutritional effects of dialysis therapies it should be kept in mind that the patient starting dialysis often is suffering from malnutrition and wasting (3–6). During the period before the institution of dialysis therapy the patients usually are anorectic and spontaneously decrease their protein intake (7). In addition, the patients may be treated with low-protein diets and a variety of drugs that may worsen anorexia. In addition, underlying or intercurrent diseases (such as diabetes mellitus, cardiovascular disease, and inflammation), complications of therapy, and certain medications (in particular, corticosteroid therapy) may worsen malnutrition and wasting in these patients (8).

Once dialysis therapy begins, accompanied by reduction of uremic symptoms and liberalization of the diet, some patients may show improved nutritional status (5,9). However, many of the indicators of malnutrition that are present at the onset of therapy remain abnormal and some aspects of malnutrition may become even more severe.

INTERMITTENT PERITONEAL DIALYSIS

Although the first clinical application of PD was reported as early as 1923 by Ganter (10), it was not until the early 1960s, following the work of several investigators, that PD became accepted as a long-term treatment for chronic uremia (11–14). Although capable of transiently improving uremic symptoms, long-term intermittent PD frequently was associated with progressive tissue wasting and malnutrition. Insufficient dialysis as the residual renal function declines and inadequate nutrient intake are considered to be the two major factors contributing to the frequently observed development of malnutrition and wasting in patients treated with long-term intermittent PD.

CONTINUOUS AMBULATORY PERITONEAL DIALYSIS

The number of patients treated with PD grew very slowly, and by the end of 1975 only 1.5% of the patients undergoing dialysis in Europe were treated with PD (15), despite several improvements in the PD technique. It was not until 1976, when Popovich and Moncrief first described "a novel portable/wearable equilibrium PD technique" (16), that the number of patients undergoing PD started to grow. The concept of this technique, which later was called continuous ambulatory PD (CAPD), was that the patient is dialyzed continuously with 2 to 3 L of dialysis fluid in the peritoneal cavity, interrupted only by short periods to exchange the fluid four to five times a day (16). Following the preliminary experiences with CAPD in the late 1970s, it soon was reported that CAPD had several advantages over intermittent PD, such as increased hematocrit levels, improved fluid and blood pressure and biochemical control, and improved physical and psychosocial well-being (17–21). The patients

TABLE 27.1. NUTRITIONAL ADVANTAGE OF CAPD COMPARED TO INTERMITTENT DIALYSIS THERAPIES

Stable metabolite levels and fluid status as a result of continuous removal
Increased clearance of middle molecules
Improved control of metabolic acidosis
Prevention of severe electrolyte disturbances such as hyperkalemia (before dialysis)
Continuous energy supply

CAPD, continuous ambulatory peritoneal dialysis.

TABLE 27.2. CATABOLIC FACTORS IN PATIENTS UNDERGOING PERITONEAL DIALYSIS

Factors resulting from uremia
- Poor food intake because of anorexia caused by uremic toxicity (underdialysis)
- Increased circulating levels of anorexins like cholecystokinin, leptin, tumor necrosis factor-α, interleukin-6, and other cytokines
- Abnormal protein and amino acid metabolism
- Acidosis
- Decreased biologic activity of anabolic hormones such as insulin and insulinlike growth factors (somatomedins) and increased circulating levels of catabolic hormones such as glucagon, parathyroid hormone, leptin, and proinflammatory cytokines
- Abnormal cell energy metabolism, carbohydrate intolerance, and impaired lipid metabolism, contributing to negative energy balance
- Inflammation

Factors related to the dialysis procedure
- Dialytic losses of amino acids, water-soluble vitamins, and other essential small molecular solutes
- Protein losses in dialysate
- Suppression of appetite by glucose absorption from dialysate and abdominal discomfort induced by the dialysate
- Infectious complications such as peritonitis and exit-site infection

Other catabolic factors
- Comorbidity such as cardiovascular disease and chronic obstructive pulmonary disease
- Gastrointestinal problems
- Low physical activity
- Frequent blood sampling

starting treatment with CAPD appeared to thrive—their body weight increased and the control of serum biochemistries, acid-base equilibrium, and fluid balance was reported to be comparable to, or better than, patients undergoing other forms of dialysis therapy. These effects, which suggested an anabolic state, were attributed to the continuous dialytic process and to an effective removal of uremic middle molecules (Table 27.1).

However, CAPD also involves several catabolic factors, such as loss of appetite, insufficient removal of small solutes, dialysate loss of proteins and amino acids, and recurrent peritonitis (1,22,23). In addition, the continuous supply of glucose (100 to 200 g/24 hr) and lactate from the dialysate represents a sizable and perhaps undesirable energy load that may induce or accentuate hyperglycemia, hyperinsulinemia, hypertriglyceridemia, and other metabolic abnormalities (24,25). These factors, in addition to the already deranged metabolism and nutritional state of patients with chronic renal failure, may have serious consequences in the form of aggravated malnutrition and wasting, susceptibility to infection, anemia, progressive neuropathy, hyperlipidemia, failure of rehabilitation, and increased morbidity and mortality.

PROTEIN-ENERGY MALNUTRITION IN PATIENTS UNDERGOING CHRONIC PERITONEAL DIALYSIS

Several reports have documented that protein-energy malnutrition and wasting frequently are present in nondialyzed patients with chronic renal failure as well as in patients undergoing maintenance dialysis therapy. It may occur even in those patients who appear to be normal and who have had a successful clinical course (1,3–6,26).

Causes of Protein-Energy Malnutrition in Patients Treated with Peritoneal Dialysis

A variety of causes contribute to impaired nutritional status in patients with chronic renal failure (see Chapter 11). When dialysis therapy begins, the uremic symptoms are reduced, the diet is less restricted, and most patients may show improved nutritional status. However, anorexia may persist in patients undergoing PD and many of the catabolic factors found at the onset of therapy remain abnormal (Table 27.2). Furthermore, the dialytic procedure induces additional catabolic factors (Table 27.2), in particular dialytic losses of proteins (5 to 15 g/24 hr), and hence increases the protein requirements above those for nondialyzed patients with uremia.

Despite the increased nutritional requirements, patients undergoing PD often have a low nutritional intake because of anorexia and nausea and vomiting, which may be caused by uremic toxicity (because of underdialysis), medications, unpalatable diets, infections, and other complicating illnesses. In addition, PD may aggravate anorexia as a result of absorption of glucose or amino acids from the dialysate as well as abdominal discomfort induced by the dialysate (Table 27.3).

Signs of Protein-Energy Malnutrition

To prevent and treat malnutrition in patients undergoing dialysis, it is important to assess the nutritional status appro-

TABLE 27.3. ANORECTIC FACTORS IN PATIENTS UNDERGOING PERITONEAL DIALYSIS

Effects induced by peritoneal dialysis
- Abdominal discomfort induced by the dialysate
- Absorption of glucose from the dialysate
- Peritonitis

Other factors
- Uremic toxicity (underdialysis)
- Increased circulating levels of anorexins such as cholecystokinin, leptin, tumor necrosis factor α, and other cytokines
- Reduced circulating levels of orexigens such as neuropeptide Y
- Unpalatable or inadequate diets
- Gastropathy (particularly in diabetics)
- Medications
- Psychosocial factors such as poverty, loneliness, and depression

priately and to identify patients at risk (1,22,23,27). Validation of nutritional status may be based on clinical evaluation, anthropometric measurements, and various biophysical and biochemical methods. Based on the complex nature of nutrition involving several different components, such as fat mass (FM), lean body mass (LBM), and plasma proteins, we do not believe that there is a single best nutritional marker, but that several nutritional markers should be evaluated together in patients undergoing PD as well as in other patients with chronic renal failure (CRF).

Common signs of malnutrition in patients undergoing PD (Table 27.4) are reduced muscle mass as assessed by anthropometric methods; low serum concentrations of albumin, transferrin, prealbumin (transthyretin), and other liver-derived proteins; and low alkali-soluble protein in muscle in relation to dry fat-free weight and DNA. Today, the serum albumin and the method of subjective global assessment (SGA) of nutritional status (5,26,28–32) are the most commonly used methods to identify malnutrition in patients undergoing CAPD.

TABLE 27.4. EVIDENCE OF MALNUTRITION IN PATIENTS UNDERGOING PERITONEAL DIALYSIS

- Subjective global assessment of nutritional status indicates a high prevalence of malnutrition.
- Body weight (% relative body weight, % preuremic body weight) is low.
- Skinfold thicknesses (triceps and other) are low.
- Midarm muscle circumference is low.
- Total body nitrogen and total body potassium are low.
- Lean body mass (estimated with DEXA, bioimpedance, and creatinine kinetics) is low.
- Visceral proteins (total serum protein, albumin, prealbumin, transferrin, immunoglobulins, C_3, C_4) are low.
- Essential amino acids (plasma and muscle) are low.
- Nonessential amino acids (plasma and muscle) are high.
- Muscle intracellular alkali-soluble protein to DNA ratio (ASP/DNA) is low.

DEXA, dual-energy X-ray absorptiometry.

Subjective Global Assessment of Nutritional Status

Although SGA has not been fully validated as a gold standard for the assessment of nutritional status in patients undergoing PD, SGA has been used widely in patients undergoing hemodialysis or PD (26,31,33) as well as in patients with CRF at the start of dialysis therapy (3,5,32). These studies have shown a high prevalence of malnutrition already at the start of dialysis therapy (3,5,32), and SGA has been demonstrated to have good correlations to other nutritional markers in patients undergoing PD (5,26,31) and to have a high predictive value for mortality in patients starting PD therapy (5,32,34). However, one potential problem with SGA is the subjective nature of SGA, which may reduce its reproducibility, and small differences in SGA scores must be interpreted with great caution.

Serum Albumin as a Marker of Nutritional Status in Patients Undergoing Peritoneal Dialysis

Although several methods are available for the assessment of nutritional status, serum albumin by far has been the most commonly used marker of nutritional status in patients undergoing PD (35). Furthermore, serum albumin has been shown to be a powerful predictor of mortality as well as morbidity in patients undergoing CAPD. Previously, it generally was assumed that the reason why a low serum albumin predicted outcome was that albumin is a key index of nutritional status and reflects visceral protein stores. However, the serum albumin levels also are influenced by several other factors (Table 27.5) (35–42). Today it generally is accepted that a low serum albumin level mainly represents the acute-phase response and albumin losses in dialysate and urine and that albumin levels only to a lesser extent reflect a poor nutritional status of the patient (35,40,42).

Methods of Albumin Determination

The routine methods applied in most previous studies for determination of serum or plasma albumin concentration

TABLE 27.5. FACTORS AFFECTING THE MEASURED SERUM ALBUMIN LEVEL IN PATIENTS UNDERGOING PERITONEAL DIALYSIS

Factor	Effect
• Method of albumin determination	
• Abnormal distribution of albumin between extravascular and intravascular spaces	⇓
• Fluid status (increased plasma volume)	⇓
• Increased albumin synthesis rate	⇑
• Peritoneal transport characteristics (albumin losses in dialysate)	⇓
• Protein intake	⇑
• Nutritional status	⇑
• Inflammation (acute-phase response)	⇓
• Systemic disease	⇓

are the two dye-binding methods with bromcresol green or bromcresol purple. The *bromcresol green method* is still the most commonly used method, although it has been shown to markedly overestimate the plasma albumin concentration compared to nephelometry (the gold standard) (43,44) because the bromcresol green dye is not specific for albumin but also binds to globulins (45). This overestimation is more marked in patients undergoing dialysis and includes systematic constant and proportional errors (43,44). The *bromcresol purple method*, however, yields serum albumin values that have a close correlation to the values determined with nephelometry (43,44), although it may underestimate serum albumin slightly (by about 1 to 2 g/L) in patients undergoing CAPD (43). Thus, the method of albumin determination is of crucial importance for the interpretation of serum albumin levels in individual patients as well as the serum albumin levels associated with increased risk of complication in different studies of patients undergoing dialysis.

Albumin Metabolism in Patients Undergoing Peritoneal Dialysis

The serum albumin level is the net result of four dynamic processes: albumin synthesis in the liver; body distribution of albumin; albumin catabolism; and albumin losses in dialysate and, in patients with remaining residual renal function, in urine (36,42,46,47). In healthy individuals, the albumin synthesis rate is considered to be driven by dietary protein intake (47), and a correlation between protein intake (as assessed from dietary history or urea kinetics) and serum albumin also has been demonstrated in several studies of patients undergoing CAPD (36,48–54), although a few studies have failed to demonstrate any correlation (42, 55–59). In conclusion, taking all these studies together, it seems likely that there is a correlation between protein intake and serum albumin in patients undergoing CAPD, although this correlation may be weak. Also, addition of high-protein nutrients to the diet has been reported to result in increased serum albumin levels in patients with hypoalbuminemia undergoing CAPD (60).

Hypoalbuminemia is an almost universal finding during severe acute illness because albumin synthesis is reduced during the acute-phase response (38,39,41,61). In a study of 27 patients undergoing CAPD, Yeun and Kaysen elegantly demonstrated that the acute-phase response and transperitoneal albumin losses are the major causes of hypoalbuminemia in patients undergoing PD (42), and similar findings also have been seen in predialysis patients (3) and patients undergoing hemodialysis (41,62,63). Inflammatory markers have been shown to be strong predictors of mortality in patients undergoing PD, and it is likely that the close relation between hypoalbuminemia and mortality in patients undergoing dialysis to a large extent results from the relation between inflammation and outcome. Several studies have found that, whereas serum albumin and C-reactive protein (CRP) predict mortality in univariate analysis, only CRP is a predictor in multivariate analysis (64–66).

Albumin synthesis also is known to be influenced by the plasma colloid osmotic pressure (40,46,47,67). It has been suggested that albumin synthesis is regulated by an oncotically sensitive compartment in the abdomen (67). Furthermore, it also has been suggested that PD might directly deplete this interstitial pool of albumin in the liver and hence stimulate the albumin synthesis rate (36). However, many regulatory mechanisms involved in albumin metabolism remain unknown at present (40).

The plasma albumin concentration is equal to plasma albumin mass divided by the plasma volume. Thus, the fluctuating fluid balance status in patients undergoing dialysis may result in various degrees of dilution with differences in the serum/plasma concentration, although this effect is less marked in patients undergoing CAPD than in patients undergoing intermittent hemodialysis therapy (68). In a study of albumin turnover in nine patients undergoing CAPD, Kaysen and Schoenfeld (36) found that, although the serum albumin level was decreased (by 9 g/L) in patients undergoing CAPD compared to a group of healthy controls, this was partly because of an increased plasma volume, and the plasma albumin mass did not differ between the patients undergoing CAPD and healthy controls (36). The normal plasma albumin mass in the patients undergoing CAPD was found to be an effect of both decreased catabolism of albumin and increased albumin synthesis (gram for gram) with increasing albumin loss (36). However, the serum albumin concentration still exhibited an inverse correlation to the peritoneal albumin loss (36), and this also has been demonstrated by several other investigators (42,49,69–71). Thus, although albumin loss in dialysate may induce increased albumin synthesis, this may not always be enough to prevent a decrease in serum albumin levels.

Note that about 50% to 70% of the total albumin mass in patients undergoing CAPD (36) (similar to that in healthy controls) (39,46,47) is found in the extravascular storage sites in the body (mainly skin and muscle). Thus, it must be kept in mind that decreased serum albumin levels in many clinical conditions may be related to disturbances in the distribution of albumin between intravascular and extravascular compartments (37,39,40).

Other factors such as systemic disease and old age also have been reported to have an impact on the serum albumin level in patients undergoing CAPD (50,71,72), and it is not established if or to what extent the low serum albumin levels in these patient groups are related to the nutritional status of the patients. Because these patient groups in general are known to have higher CRP levels, it is likely that the hypoalbuminemia in these patient groups to a large extent results from inflammation.

Relationship Between Serum Albumin and Other Estimates of Nutritional Status in Patients Undergoing Peritoneal Dialysis

Although the serum albumin level is used widely as a marker of nutritional status, it is obvious from the various factors that affect the serum albumin level (*vide supra*) that the serum albumin levels do not only reflect the nutritional status of the patient. Thus, serum albumin levels do not always directly correlate to other measures of nutritional status in patients undergoing CAPD.

In a large cross-sectional study of 224 patients undergoing CAPD from six centers, plasma albumin, midarm muscle circumference, and weight loss were the objective variables that showed the best correlation to a subjective nutritional assessment (based on 21 variables derived from history, clinical examination, anthropometry, and biochemistry), although this correlation was significant in females only (26). In a study of 134 patients Pollock et al. (49) found that serum albumin correlated significantly with anthropometric measurements (apart from percentage body fat) as well as with total body nitrogen in a subgroup of 29 patients. Similarly, serum albumin levels have been found to correlate to midthigh muscle area (as assessed using computed tomography) (73) in patients undergoing CAPD and to SGA and bioelectrical impedance (BIA) in a combined group of patients undergoing CAPD and hemodialysis (31). Significant correlations also have been reported in patients undergoing CAPD between changes in serum albumin concentration versus nitrogen balance (as estimated from monthly 24-h collections of dialysate, urine, and feces and dietary interview) (74) and versus changes in total body potassium (75). In contrast, other authors have failed to find any correlation between serum albumin levels in patients undergoing CAPD and LBM (as assessed by single-frequency body electrical impedance [76] or dual energy x-ray absorptiometry [DEXA]) (77).

Goodship et al. found that although serum albumin (measured using the bromcresol green method) decreased from 37.9 ± 1.5 g/L (SEM, or standard error of the mean) before the start of CAPD to 33.9 ± 1.2 g/L 3 months later in 10 patients undergoing CAPD, total body potassium did not change during the 3-month period and, furthermore, was normal, indicating a normal nutritional status (78). Protein turnover (which was measured using whole-body leucine turnover in the same study) was lower in the patients undergoing CAPD than in normal subjects, but the balance between synthesis and breakdown was significantly higher and was maintained after 3 months of treatment with CAPD (78). These results indicate that the decrease in serum albumin with the start of CAPD treatment (possibly as a result of peritoneal albumin losses) may not abate the nutritional status of the patients undergoing CAPD in other respects. The serum albumin level is therefore not a good estimate of nutritional status when comparing patients undergoing CAPD to other patient groups such as patients undergoing hemodialysis, as demonstrated by de Fijter et al. (76), who reported that although serum albumin levels were reduced in patients undergoing CAPD compared to patients undergoing hemodialysis, LBM (as assessed by single-frequency BIA) was higher in patients undergoing CAPD compared to the patients undergoing hemodialysis.

Other Plasma Proteins and Amino Acids as Markers of Nutritional Status

Because the value of serum albumin as a nutritional marker has been questioned, other visceral proteins have been used for nutritional assessment in patients undergoing PD, including prealbumin, transferrin, and retinol-binding protein (79). For these proteins in general, there is considerable overlap between malnourished and well-nourished patients (3). Prealbumin has a shorter half-life than albumin, has a close relation to nutritional status, and is a good predictor of clinical outcome (79,80). However, prealbumin is also a negative acute-phase protein (3).

In addition, abnormal plasma amino acid and intracellular amino acid profiles similar to those found in untreated uremia have been reported in patients undergoing PD, indicating that PD does not reverse these abnormalities (81). However, the intracellular free amino acid pattern in muscle is less abnormal in patients undergoing CAPD than in patients with uremia undergoing other forms of therapy (82). In contrast, the plasma levels of most of the essential and several nonessential amino acids appear to be lower in patients undergoing CAPD than in other categories of patients with uremia. Note that the abnormal plasma amino acid pattern in the patients undergoing CAPD may not necessarily be a consequence of amino acid depletion; instead, it may reflect an increased transport of amino acids across the cell membrane, possibly because of the sustained hyperinsulinemia during CAPD treatment, resulting in an increased intracellular uptake of amino acids into the cells (82).

Assessment of Body Composition

Because protein malnutrition with loss of muscle mass is particularly common in patients undergoing PD, various methods have been applied for objective monitoring of muscle mass or LBM (e.g., anthropometrics, creatinine kinetics, bioimpedance, DEXA, total body potassium and neutron activation) (83). In general, bearing the high prevalence of malnutrition in mind, it is not surprising that several studies have demonstrated a decreased LBM at the start of dialysis therapy and after the start of PD therapy using these methods (5,6,84,85). Of these methods, total body potassium and neutron activation are accurate research methods that need very expensive devices, but they are not widely available. Of the other methods, DEXA seems to be the most reliable (86,87).

With DEXA, bone mineral, fat, and LBM distribution are estimated directly without making assumptions about the two-compartment model (88). DEXA is considered to be superior to the other easily available methods for determining body composition in renal failure (83,89) and has been applied widely for studies of body composition in patients undergoing dialysis (83). However, it must be kept in mind that, although the state of hydration does not affect the estimate of FM with DEXA, it does affect that of LBM, and, ideally, for assessment of body cell mass, it should be combined with the estimation of the extracellular fluid volume with the tracer dilution technique. With anthropometric methods, the sum of skinfolds at the four sites can be used to calculate body density (e.g., using the equations of Durnin and Womersley [90]), and FM and LBM then can be obtained from body density and body weight. Although the use of anthropometrics is an indirect and rather insensitive method, with several errors (including sensitivity to hydration status), the estimation of LBM and FM agree reasonably well with results from DEXA (3). Because anthropometrics is easy and cheap to apply, it can be recommended for routine assessment of nutritional status, bearing the limitations in mind.

Creatinine kinetics (CK) also has been used to calculate LBM in patients undergoing PD from creatinine excretion in the urine and dialysate (91). However, the estimated LBM from CK is usually markedly lower than with other methods such as total body potassium (92), anthropometry (86,93), bioimpedance (86,94), or DEXA (89,94,95). Furthermore, LBM estimated from CK is dependent on the creatinine content in the diet (mainly related to the meat content) and the metabolic degradation of creatinine, which is poorly understood in uremia (92,96,97). Finally, the variation in LBM with repeated measures of LBM using CK is unacceptably high (92). Therefore, CK is not a good method for monitoring LBM in patients undergoing PD.

Single-frequency and multifrequency BIA recently has been used in many studies of nutritional status of patients undergoing dialysis. However, it is not clear to what extent the measured impedance really contributes to the results because it has been suggested that height and body weight are the major sources of the variance in the BIA prediction models (98). Furthermore, the technique is not well validated against more specific methods, and bioimpedance does not measure FM and LBM accurately in patients with a body composition that differs from young healthy adults with a normal body mass index (BMI) (98,99). In patients undergoing PD, bioimpedance does not agree well with neutron activation and total body potassium (83,89). Therefore, the different BIA methods need further validation.

Prevalence of Protein-Energy Malnutrition in Patients Undergoing Peritoneal Dialysis

Several reports have shown a high prevalence of protein-energy malnutrition in patients undergoing CAPD, with 18% to 56% of patients undergoing CAPD showing anthropometric and biochemical evidence of malnutrition (4–6,9,26,32,48,78,82,100–107).

An extensive evaluation of nutritional status in patients undergoing CAPD included patients from six centers in Europe and North America (26). A total of 224 patients, 132 males and 92 females, ranging in age from 14 to 87 years, were selected. All patients had been maintained on CAPD for more than 3 months and had remained free from peritonitis for at least 1 month before the study. The patients had a mean ($\pm$SD) age of 53, $\pm$15 years, and had on average been maintained on CAPD for 32 $\pm$ 27 months. Their residual renal function (estimated as the average of creatinine and urea clearance) was 1.3 $\pm$ 2.0 mL/min (26).

A "subjective nutritional assessment" was made, using 21 variables derived from history, clinical examination, anthropometry, and biochemistry. Eighteen patients (8%) were judged to be severely malnourished, 73 (32.6%) were mildly to moderately malnourished, and 133 (59.4%) did not show evidence for malnutrition.

There was a higher incidence of mild to moderate malnutrition among diabetics (47%) than among nondiabetics (29%), but there was no difference in the prevalence of severe malnutrition between diabetics (4%) and nondiabetics (9%). The variables that most frequently were correlated with subjective nutritional assessment and with one another included plasma albumin, midarm muscle circumference, weight loss, and the clinical judgment of muscle wasting and loss of subcutaneous fat. Loss of residual renal function correlated with muscle wasting and months on CAPD. Variables that did *not* correlate with other estimates of nutritional status included peritonitis rate, patient age, serum transferrin, dialysate protein loss, and serum cholesterol and triglycerides (26).

Patients with severe malnutrition (8%) had minimal or no residual renal function and were either older or had been treated with CAPD longer than other patients. Of the patients with severe malnutrition, 94% were anuric (26). Compared with well-nourished patients with no residual renal function, severely malnourished patients were prescribed a lower total volume of dialysate (108). From this study (26,108) one may conclude that progression of malnutrition may occur in patients undergoing CAPD as a result of the synergistic effects of loss of residual renal function, anorexia, and inadequate dietary intake. In some patients, especially patients with minimal or no residual renal function, more efficient dialysis may be required before nitrogen depletion can be reversed by either dietary supplementation or alternative therapies.

Comparison of the Prevalence of Protein-Energy Malnutrition in Patients Undergoing Peritoneal Dialysis and Hemodialysis

A few studies have compared the prevalence of malnutrition in patients undergoing CAPD and hemodialysis. Marckmann (104) studied 32 patients undergoing hemodialysis and 16 patients being treated with CAPD, using a nutritional score (including relative body weight, anthropometrics and s-transferrin), and found an equally high prevalence of malnutrition in both groups (54% and 52%, respectively). In a multicenter study comparing 609 patients undergoing hemodialysis and 138 patients undergoing CAPD, Nelson et al. (109) noted no difference in nutritional status between the two groups. However, a large study of 224 patients undergoing CAPD and 263 patients undergoing hemodialysis from eight centers in Italy reported on a greater prevalence of malnutrition among patients undergoing CAPD (42%) compared to patients undergoing hemodialysis (31%) using SGA of nutritional status (110). The patients undergoing CAPD were slightly older, had a higher prevalence of cardiovascular disease, tended to have greater muscle wasting, and had markedly lower serum albumin levels compared to the patients undergoing hemodialysis (110). In contrast, among the patients undergoing CAPD body weight was higher, and body fat (as assessed from anthropometrics) was higher than among the patients undergoing hemodialysis. Protein intake (as estimated from urea kinetics) did not differ between the two groups. The lower serum albumin levels among patients undergoing CAPD is in agreement with the observation by Maiorca et al. (111) that patients undergoing CAPD, in contrast to patients undergoing hemodialysis, failed to correct the slight hypoalbuminemia present at the start of dialysis treatment, possibly as a result of the protein losses in dialysate. In contrast, the results from the prospective nutritional follow-up for 24 months of 132 patients starting hemodialysis and 118 patients starting PD from the Netherlands Cooperative Study on the Adequacy of Dialysis (NECOSAD) was reported in 2001 (9). Although the initial (after 3 months of dialysis) serum albumin levels were slightly lower among the patients undergoing PD, the serum albumin increased among the patients undergoing PD and was in fact higher than among the patients undergoing hemodialysis after 24 months of treatment (9). They also reported on a larger gain in body fat in women starting on PD compared to the other patient groups (9). However, it should be noted the women starting PD initially had lower body fat and BMI (9).

In conclusion, the prevalence of protein-energy malnutrition is high in patients undergoing hemodialysis or PD. No definite conclusions can be drawn from the data available in the literature as to which method is superior regarding adequacy of nutrition, especially because the patient populations in the various studies differed with regard to modality selection, age, time on dialysis, incidence of complicating diseases, socioeconomic conditions, residual renal function, dialysis dose, and dietary recommendations. In summary, there does not seem to be any clear nutritional advantage for either PD or hemodialysis.

MALNUTRITION AND CLINICAL OUTCOME IN PATIENTS UNDERGOING PERITONEAL DIALYSIS

Several studies suggest that malnutrition is an important risk factor for morbidity and mortality in patients undergoing CAPD (6,32,34,112–115). Similar results also have been reported in patients undergoing hemodialysis (64,113, 116–119).

Patients undergoing CAPD that were judged to be malnourished at the start of CAPD (using SGA) have been shown to have increased mortality compared to well-nourished patients undergoing CAPD (6,32,34). In a study of 35 patients undergoing CAPD (studied at the start of CAPD and reassessed 17.5 ± 4.4 months later), Pollock et al. (112) found that total body nitrogen (determined by neutron activation) was significantly lower in patients who died or suffered serious morbidity requiring transfer from CAPD to hemodialysis (n = 10) than in those patients that remained on CAPD or underwent successful renal transplantation (n = 25), indicating that low total body nitrogen may be associated with a poor clinical outcome. Also, cachexia has been reported to be a major cause of death in patients undergoing CAPD (120,121) as well as in patients undergoing hemodialysis (121).

Furthermore, low serum albumin levels in patients undergoing CAPD have been shown to be associated with increased mortality and morbidity (35,48,49,53,54,58,71, 72,122–127). Unfortunately, the method of albumin determination is not reported in several studies of patients undergoing CAPD (48,49,53,58,71,123,124).

Patients with a serum albumin level equal to or greater than 35 g/L demonstrated survival of more than 50 months, whereas those with lower values were all likely to die within 40 months in a 5-year study of 51 patients undergoing CAPD (58,122). In a study of 61 patients undergoing CAPD followed for 2 years, Struijk et al. reported that the mortality was increased in the group of patients undergoing CAPD with a serum albumin level below 30.9 g/L (measured with immunoturbidometry) (72). This is similar to a report from the U.S. Renal Data System showing that the relative risk of mortality (in 666 patients undergoing CAPD entering treatment from 1986 to 1987) started to increase in patients with a serum albumin below 30 g/L (128). This may seem not to be entirely in agreement with a study by Fine and Cox (129), who found that a moderately decreased serum albumin level of 25 to 33 g/L was persistent for 12 months in 19 patients undergoing CAPD and had no obvious clinical consequence. Note, however, that serum albumin in this study (129) was measured using the bromcresol purple method, which, in patients undergoing dialysis, yields serum albumin levels that are about 5 to 8 g lower than the bromcresol green method (43,44), which is the most commonly used method in the United States (44) and thus possibly the most commonly used method in the patients reported to the U.S. Renal Data System. Because the bromcresol purple method may yield serum albumin values in patients undergoing CAPD that are about 2 g lower than values obtained with immunoturbidometry or nephelometry (43), the finding by Fine and Cox is in good agreement with the study by Struijk et al. (72).

The relation between nutritional status and outcome was studied in detail in the CANUSA study (5,34,114). The CANUSA study was a prospective cohort study of nutrition and adequacy in CAPD involving 698 patients undergoing PD from 14 centers in Canada and the United States. Significant demographic risk factors for death included age, presence of insulin-dependent diabetes, a history of cardiovascular disease, and country of residence (United States versus Canada), and low serum albumin levels, low SGA, and low normalized protein intake (as assessed from urea kinetics as the normalized protein equivalent of nitrogen appearance rate, or nPNA; see page 496) were significant nutritional risk factors for death (114). When serum albumin and SGA were included in the Cox proportional hazards model together with the demographic risk factors, the predictive power of the model increased, whereas the additional inclusion of nPNA did not result in any additional increase in the predictive power of the model (34). This is similar to the study by Genestier et al. of 201 patients undergoing CAPD from one unit in France where low nPNA and serum albumin were nutritional risk factors for mortality in univariate analysis but not in multivariate analysis (130). However, low nPNA was a rather strong predictor of technique failure in this study.

It should be kept in mind that the relationship between malnutrition and mortality and increased morbidity (usu-

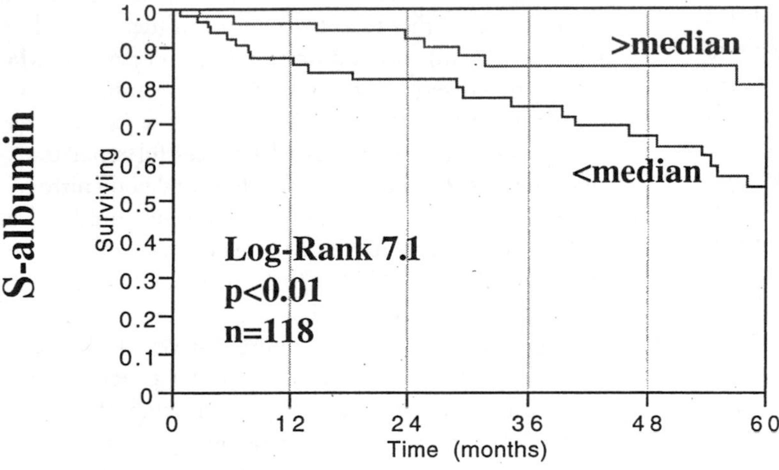

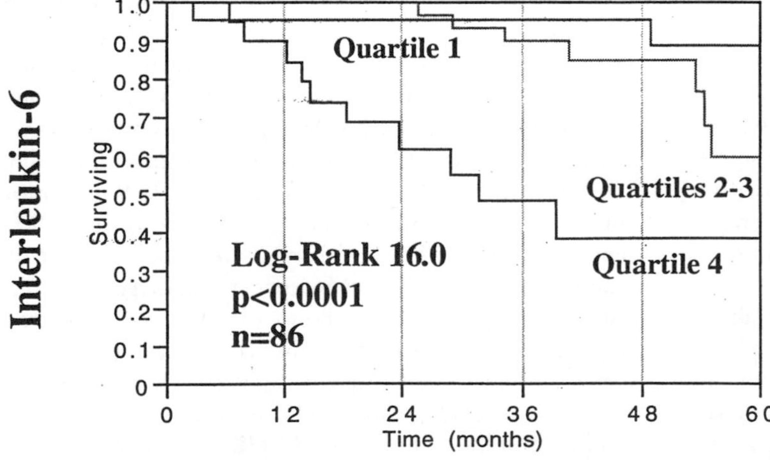

FIGURE 27.1. Low serum albumin and elevated level of interleukin-6 (IL-6) are both strong predictors of mortality in a cohort of patients undergoing peritoneal dialysis from our unit in univariate analysis, as illustrated here. The upper panel shows survival in patients with a serum albumin level above and below the median value, and the lower panel shows survival in patients in quartile 1, 2, 3, and 4 of plasma IL-6 levels. When multivariate analysis was performed using the Cox proportional hazards model, IL-6 was still a strong predictor of mortality (chi-square 11.2, $p < 0.001$), whereas serum albumin lost its significance (chi-square 0.26, $p = 0.61$), indicating that low serum albumin is more a marker of inflammation than an independent nutritional marker. (Unpublished observation.)

ally assessed as hospitalization rate) is not necessarily a cause-and-effect one. In addition to uremia, a large proportion of patients undergoing dialysis have complicating illnesses such as diabetic vascular complications, severe cardiovascular disease, and other systemic diseases with unfavorable prognosis. Such sick patients may be anorexic and malnourished; thus, malnutrition may be a marker of illness (8,35, 41,50,54,71,72) but not the direct cause of death. Furthermore, one has to be very cautious in drawing conclusions regarding the role of malnutrition for dialysis-associated morbidity and mortality based only on serum albumin data, considering that comorbid conditions (the severity of which are reflected in low serum albumin levels, rather than malnutrition) may be instrumental in causing complications, including death of the patient.

Hypoalbuminemia may be more a marker of illness, and it is crucial to look not only for other signs of malnutrition but also for comorbid conditions in patients with hypoalbuminemia. Because recent evidence suggests that S-albumin is very vulnerable to the effects of inflammation (3,42, 63) it could be hypothesized that the association between low S-albumin levels and outcome is caused by chronic inflammation rather than poor nutritional intake. Strong associations between malnutrition, inflammation, and atherosclerosis (MIA syndrome) have been found in patients with CRF, a syndrome associated with poor outcome and elevated levels of proinflammatory cytokines (8,131). The prevalence of elevated CRP levels is high in patients with CRF (33,65,131,132) and reflects the generation of proinflammatory cytokines such as interleukin-1 (IL-1), IL-6, and tumor necrosis factor α (TNF-α), which also have been reported to be increased in patients with CRF (133,134). CRP has been shown to be a strong predictor of mortality in patients undergoing PD (135,136), and it is likely that the close relationship between hypoalbuminemia and mortality in patients undergoing dialysis to a large extent is the result of the relationship between inflammation and outcome. Several studies have found that whereas serum albumin and CRP predict mortality in patients undergoing hemodialysis in univariate analysis, only CRP is a predictor in multivariate analysis (64–66). In Fig. 27.1, we show the relation between albumin and IL-6 versus patient survival in patients undergoing PD from our hospital. Furthermore, recent studies have documented that elevated levels of proinflammatory cytokines, such as IL-6, not only predict outcome (133,137,138) but also the development of malnutrition (139) and atherosclerosis (140). The impact of inflammation on the development of malnutrition and atherosclerosis are discussed further in Chapter 13.

NUTRITIONAL REQUIREMENTS IN PATIENTS UNDERGOING PERITONEAL DIALYSIS

For an individual to thrive, nutrients must be ingested and used in sufficient amounts to serve as metabolic fuel, to serve as a substrate for tissue growth and maintenance, and to regulate the cellular and metabolic processes. If a macronutrient (protein, energy) or an essential nutrient (e.g., essential amino and fatty acids, vitamins, and trace minerals) are provided in insufficient amounts, this will eventually have serious consequences for the individual. However, a nutritional deficiency may be subclinical for some time before it will result in more overt clinical signs and symptoms, which may develop into morbidity and, as a final consequence, the death of the subject (141). It thus may be a long time before a nutritional deficiency is reflected in vital statistics. However, less severe deficiencies may have a negative effect indirectly by sensitizing the individual to other morbid factors (e.g., protein malnutrition may impair the immune response, resulting in an increased risk of severe infections) (142).

Protein Requirement in Patients Undergoing Continuous Ambulatory Peritoneal Dialysis

To maintain a satisfactory nutritional status, it is mandatory that the nutritional intake of protein and energy meet the requirements. A low protein intake is especially detrimental if the protein requirements are increased, which seems to be the case in patients undergoing CAPD.

In normal adults, the average minimum requirements for protein are about 0.6 g/kg body weight/day, which, after correction for 25% variability to include 97.5% of the population of young adults, increases the safe level of intake to about 0.75 g/kg body weight/day (143). This variability is the result of genetic differences, age, sex, physical activity, environmental factors, the chemical form of the nutrients, and the effect of other dietary constituents (143).

The protein requirements in patients undergoing maintenance dialysis are not well defined. It may be assumed that the variation in protein requirements is much larger among patients undergoing dialysis than in healthy subjects because of additional sources of variability, such as endocrine and biochemical abnormalities, anemia, drugs, physical inactivity, and comorbid conditions (e.g., cardiovascular disease, diabetes, and infections). In addition, specific effects of the dialytic process may increase the protein requirements, especially in patients treated with hemodialysis (23).

In patients undergoing CAPD the daily protein intake is recommended to be at least 1.2 g/kg body weight/24 h (Table 27.6) (144,145). This recommendation mainly is based on the nitrogen balance studies performed by Blumenkrantz et al. (146), showing that patients undergoing CAPD were at high risk of a negative nitrogen balance when the protein intake was less than 1.1 g/kg body weight. However, in another study (in which nitrogen balance was measured in patients undergoing CAPD receiving an individualized diet composed to resemble the patients' spontaneously chosen diets regarding daily intake of protein and energy)

TABLE 27.6. RECOMMENDED NUTRITIONAL INTAKES PER DAY FOR PATIENTS TREATED WITH PERITONEAL DIALYSIS

Protein	= 1.2 g/kg body weight (= 50% of high biologic value)
Energy	= 35 kcal/kg (including glucose absorption from the dialysate)
Fat	30% of total energy supply (high content of unsaturated lipids)
Water and sodium	As tolerated by fluid balance
Potassium	40–80 mmol
Calcium	Individualized, usually not <1,000 mg (supplements may be required)
Phosphorous	8–17 mg/kg (phosphate binders often are needed)
Magnesium	200–300 mg
Iron	10–15 mg (supplements often are needed)
Zinc	15 mg (supplements may be required)
Vitamins (recommended supplementation)	
Pyridoxine (B_6)	10 mg
Ascorbic acid	60–100 mg
Thiamin	1–5 mg
Folic acid	1 mg
Vitamin A, E, and K	Not routinely (vitamin E may be indicated in some patients)
Vitamin D	Individual supplementation

some of the patients were in neutral or positive nitrogen balance with a protein intake as low as 0.7 g/kg body weight/day (147). Moreover, most comparative studies show comparable survival in patients undergoing hemodialysis or CAPD despite a lower protein intake as calculated from urea appearance rate among the patients undergoing CAPD (148). However, it is important to distinguish between the average dietary protein intake that will maintain nitrogen balance in some individuals and the safe protein intake that will maintain nitrogen balance in almost all (97.5%) individuals (145). It should be noted that patients undergoing PD have a significant loss of nonurea nitrogen in dialysate (147,149) and the daily protein intake in patients undergoing CAPD may be underestimated if the commonly applied equations (which were not based on nitrogen balance studies in patients undergoing CAPD) (150) are used to estimate protein intake in patients undergoing CAPD (149). Several studies have shown that protein intake as measured in nitrogen balance studies (147) or estimated from dietary recall (49,105,149) is markedly higher in patients undergoing CAPD than protein intake estimated from urea generation rate using the Randerson equation (150) in the same patients.

An equation published in 1998 (151) (based on the pooled data from 36 nitrogen balance studies in patients undergoing CAPD) (146,147) provides a higher and more correct estimate of protein intake in patients undergoing CAPD (151). However, many patients undergoing CAPD still have a protein intake lower than 1.2 g/kg body weight. Moreover, although a positive nitrogen balance has been reported in a few patients undergoing CAPD with a protein intake as low as 0.7 g/kg body weight/day (147), a much higher protein intake must be recommended because currently it is not possible to identify which patients will manage on such a low protein intake; the majority of patients undergoing CAPD will need a much higher protein intake to avoid negative nitrogen balance. Also, note that the nitrogen balance in patients undergoing CAPD has been shown to be closely related to the energy intake (147) and that a sufficient energy intake is needed to avoid protein being used as an energy source through gluconeogenesis.

Energy Intake in Patients Undergoing Continuous Ambulatory Peritoneal Dialysis

The energy requirements are dependent on the level of physical activity. In healthy individuals an energy intake of 35 to 40 kcal/kg body weight/day is recommended to individuals not performing heavy physical exercise.

There is no evidence that the energy requirements of chronic dialysis patients are systematically different from those of normal subjects. Monteon et al. (152) measured energy expenditure in normal subjects, nondialyzed patients with chronic renal failure, and patients undergoing maintenance hemodialysis and found no differences between the three groups with the subjects sitting, exercising, or in the postprandial state. This suggests that the energy expenditure of chronic hemodialysis patients does not differ from that in normal subjects during a given physical activity. There also are no data indicating that the energy requirements of patients undergoing CAPD differ from normal subjects. In a recent study, Harty et al. (153) found no difference in resting energy expenditure measured with indirect calorimetry in 12 patients undergoing CAPD compared to 11 healthy controls. Thus, patients undergoing CAPD are recommended an energy intake of at least 35 kcal/kg body weight (147 kJoule/kg body weight), which is similar to recommendations for healthy individuals (1) (Table 27.6). In addition to the oral energy intake, patients undergoing

CAPD with normal peritoneal transport capacity absorb about 60% of the daily dialysate glucose load, resulting in a glucose absorption of about 100- to 200-g glucose/24 h (25). However, the total energy intake in patients undergoing CAPD has been reported to be low in many patients undergoing CAPD despite the additional supply of energy provided from the glucose absorbed from the dialysate (1, 22,147,154).

It generally is recommended that 35% of the energy should be given as fat, of which a substantial part should be unsaturated (1). Obese patients, however, for body weight reduction should be recommended a low energy intake and restrictions in the use of hypertonic dialysis fluid; this also may have salutary effects regarding glucose intolerance and lipid abnormalities.

Vitamin and Trace Mineral Requirements of Patients Undergoing Continuous Ambulatory Peritoneal Dialysis

The vitamin and trace mineral requirements of patients undergoing CAPD have been reviewed in detail (155,156) (Table 27.6). Inadequate dietary intake, altered metabolism in uremia, and vitamin loss into dialysate may lead to vitamin deficiencies (in particular, deficiencies of water-soluble vitamins) in a few patients treated with PD (155–161). The serum levels of ascorbic acid, thiamin (B_1), pyridoxine (B_6), and folic acid have been reported to be low in some studies of patients undergoing dialysis (155). Vitamin B_1 deficiency with encephalopathy has been described in patients undergoing dialysis (162) and may be confounded with other neurologic diseases. A common dietary intake of 0.5 to 1.5 mg/day can be supplemented with a daily dose of 1 to 5 mg of thiamin hydrochloride. Vitamin B_6 coenzymes play a vital role in several aspects of amino acid utilization, and the need for vitamin B_6 is particularly critical if protein and amino acid intake is limited (156,163). Changes in fasting plasma amino acid and serum high-density lipoprotein (HDL) levels after correction of the vitamin B_6 deficiency in patients undergoing dialysis indicates its role in the pathogenesis of the abnormal amino acid and lipid metabolism (164). There are data suggesting that the daily requirement of pyridoxine may be higher in patients undergoing dialysis than in normal subjects and that patients undergoing dialysis should be supplemented with a minimum of 10 mg of vitamin B_6 per day (159,160,163). Folate is lost in dialysate, and because folate levels have been reported to be reduced in serum, it is recommended to give 1 mg of folic acid daily. High doses of folic acid (5 to 10 mg/day) have been shown to reduce the markedly elevated plasma homocysteine by about two-thirds; however, this does not fully correct it to normal levels (165). The question of whether these high doses of folate should be prescribed to decrease plasma homocysteine levels and improve cardiovascular morbidity and mortality is still unanswered, and prospective studies are needed in this area.

Supplementation with vitamin C also has been recommended (158–161). However, high intake of vitamin C may aggravate hyperoxalemia in patients undergoing dialysis.

Supplementation of the fat-soluble vitamins A, D, E, and K have not been not recommended on a routine basis (155). Vitamin A tends to accumulate in patients undergoing PD as well as in other patients with renal failure, and supplementation should be avoided because vitamin A may have potentially harmful effects. Vitamin D and its active forms should not be prescribed as a routine but should be given on the basis of an evaluation of the bone metabolic status and taking the risks of hyperphosphatemia and hypercalcemia into consideration. Blood levels of vitamin E has been found to be normal or high in most studies in patients with uremia, and vitamin K deficiency has not been reported in patients with renal failure (155). However, because vitamin E (tocopherol) is a strong antioxidant compound it may be worthwhile to consider treating selected patients undergoing dialysis at high cardiovascular risk with vitamin E. A recent randomized controlled high-dose vitamin E (800 IU α-tocopherol/day) supplementation in patients undergoing hemodialysis at high cardiovascular risk showed a significant (50%) decrease in a cardiovascular composite index as compared with the placebo group (166). However, other studies in nonrenal patient groups have not shown results as good, possibly partly because different doses and forms of vitamin E were used.

Dietary requirements for trace elements are not well defined in patients undergoing PD. Trace element metabolism frequently is altered in patients with chronic renal failure (155,157). High levels of trace elements have been attributed to impaired renal elimination or contamination of dialysis fluids, and low levels of trace elements may occur as a result of inadequate dietary intake or loss of protein-bound trace elements into the dialysate. Several groups have reported on decreased levels of zinc in serum, leukocytes, and muscle of patients undergoing CAPD (155). Zinc deficiency has been reported to be associated with anorexia, hypogeusia, hyperprolactinemia, and impotence, which have been alleviated by zinc administration. However, these results generally have not been confirmed, and the role of zinc deficiency and requirements for extra supply of zinc in the diet of patients undergoing CAPD remains controversial (155,157), although supplementation with zinc has been suggested in patients with hypogeusia, anorexia, and muscle weakness.

Carnitine Depletion

The myocardial and skeletal muscle exhibit the highest concentrations of L-carnitine (L-3-hydroxy-4-N-trimethylaminobutyrate), which is an amino acid that transfers long-chain fatty acids from the cytoplasm through the inner mitochondrial membrane. A deficiency of L-carnitine may lead to impaired oxidation of long-chain fatty acids, inefficient energy production, and derangements of intermediary metabolism.

Low and normal plasma and muscle concentrations of carnitine and carnitine esters have been reported in patients undergoing CAPD (167,168). Although only a minor portion of patients undergoing hemodialysis seem to exhibit severe carnitine deficiency (169), several positive clinical effects of L-carnitine administration on patients undergoing hemodialysis have been reported, including improved nutritional status and muscle strength, increased well-being, and reduction of cardiac arrhythmias and angina, suggesting that carnitine depletion may be a pathogenic factor in skeletal muscle weakness and uremic heart disease (169). However, a metaanalysis of all randomized controlled clinical trials of L-carnitine supplementation did not show any effect of L-carnitine supplementation on cholesterol and triglyceride profiles in patients undergoing hemodialysis (170). The effects of L-carnitine supplementation on muscle weakness, asthenia, and cardiovascular symptoms could not be assessed reliably because of insufficient number or quality of the trials (170).

It is not established if patients undergoing CAPD will benefit from L-carnitine supplementation. Patients eating well will probably have well-maintained carnitine stores as a result of an adequate intake of both carnitine and the carnitine precursors, lysine and methionine, in the food. However, patients undergoing CAPD with a poor nutritional intake may be at risk of developing a carnitine deficiency.

PROTEIN CATABOLIC FACTORS IN PATIENTS UNDERGOING PERITONEAL DIALYSIS

The observation that patients undergoing CAPD seem to have a decreased use of ingested protein and increased protein requirements compared to healthy subjects indicates that several metabolic factors that are not fully corrected by the treatment, as well as effects of the treatment itself, may enhance net protein catabolism and impair the utilization of dietary protein (*vide infra*). Furthermore, many patients undergoing PD are physically inactive because of several factors such as fatigue, anemia, and intercurrent diseases. Physical inactivity may result in muscle wasting and a negative nitrogen balance (171).

Anorexia and Low Nutritional Intake

Considering all evidence that the requirements for protein are increased in patients undergoing CAPD and that an adequate energy supply is crucial for optimizing utilization of ingested protein, low protein and energy intakes must be especially harmful in such patients. However, it may be difficult to fulfill the nutritional requirements because some patients undergoing CAPD lose their appetite (172) and reduce their protein and energy intakes spontaneously.

Low Protein and Energy Intake

A large proportion of patients undergoing CAPD ingest a considerably lower amount of protein than the recommended intake of 1.2 g/kg body weight/day (6,49,105–107, 173–178). This may be especially harmful because energy intake also has been reported to be low despite the additional supply of energy from the amount of glucose absorbed from the dialysate (23,154,179). Metabolic studies indicate that the utilization of protein is greatly dependent on the energy intake, so a low energy intake reduces utilization, whereas a high energy intake has a protein-saving effect (180). In patients undergoing CAPD, the nitrogen balance is strongly correlated to the total energy intake (23). About 60% of the 24-h peritoneal glucose load is absorbed from dialysate in patients undergoing CAPD with normal peritoneal transport characteristics (25). Thus, 100 to 200 g of glucose will be absorbed per day, averaging about 8 kcal/kg body weight/day (varying between 5 and 20 kcal/kg body weight/day), which should be advantageous regarding the utilization of protein (25). However, despite glucose uptake, many patients undergoing CAPD have a total energy intake of less than 35 kcal/kg body weight/day (1,23,154,179,181–183). Considering that many patients undergoing PD ingest less than 35 kcal/kg body weight/day, energy deficiency may be an important factor contributing to poor utilization of dietary protein (147).

Underdialysis and Uremic Toxicity

Anorexia, nausea, and vomiting are signs of severe uremic intoxication. It is a common clinical experience that patients with uremia who are anorexic regain appetite after the initiation of maintenance dialysis. This suggests that uremic toxins causing anorexia have been removed by dialysis. Assuming that dialyzable uremic toxins accumulate in severe renal failure and causes anorexia, it is conceivable that underdialysis may affect the appetite, and insufficient removal of appetite-reducing uremic toxins resulting from underdialysis is considered to be the most important anorectic factor in patients undergoing CAPD (184). There are studies in patients undergoing CAPD and hemodialysis that report a correlation between the dose of dialysis for small solute removal (Kt/V urea) and protein intake (as assessed by urea kinetics), especially in the lowest dose intervals (23,50,147, 174,185–187), although there is no consensus if this relationship is a physiologic one (188) or a mathematic artifact (105,189,190). It has been argued that the relationship between Kt/V urea and protein intake (urea appearance) reflects a mathematic coupling rather than a biologic relationship because the two variables are to some extent dependent (both are normalized to body size and both are dependent on urea excretion in dialysate and urine) (105,189). However, protein intake as assessed by dietary recall also shows similar relationships to Kt/V urea (147), and prospective studies in small groups of patients have indicated that increasing the dose of PD results in an increased protein intake (191–193). However, these studies were confounded by the concomitant decline in residual renal function. A preliminary study of 100 Chinese patients with anuria undergoing CAPD has been reported (194), showing that in half of the patients that had their dialysis prescription increased, protein intake increased in parallel with increased Kt/V when the prescription was increased from three to four exchanges per day, whereas an increase from four to five exchanges per day did not increase protein intake (194).

A few studies also have demonstrated a decrease of protein and energy intake with length of time being treated with CAPD, which is paralleled by a decrease in nitrogen balance (103,195,196). The reduced nutritional intake with time undergoing CAPD seems to be caused by anorexia, with a reduced nutritional intake as a consequence, probably because patients undergoing CAPD become underdialyzed as the total solute clearance falls as a result of a decrease in residual renal function.

Abdominal Distension and Absorption of the Osmotic Agent

In CAPD, the presence of dialysate in the peritoneal cavity may suppress appetite because of an interference with gastric emptying and abdominal discomfort as a result of low pH and high osmolarity of the solution. Furthermore, absorption of the osmotic agent from the dialysate also may contribute to a reduced appetite in patients undergoing CAPD.

Upper gastrointestinal symptoms are common among patients undergoing CAPD (197), and a high frequency of gastroesophageal reflux (198) and retarded gastric emptying for solid foods also has been reported in patients treated with CAPD (199–201) especially in diabetics (201). It is, however, not established how much of these changes may be related to PD because diabetes is known to cause delayed gastric emptying as a result of autonomic neuropathy, and delayed gastric emptying also has been reported in patients undergoing hemodialysis (202,203). Furthermore, the presence of fluid in the peritoneal cavity did not affect intragastric or lower esophageal sphincter pressure in a study of 11 patients undergoing CAPD (204).

Hylander et al. (205) investigated hunger, "fullness," and food preferences in healthy controls, patients undergoing hemodialysis, and patients undergoing CAPD by serving a test meal placed on a hidden scale with a computer registering the eating process on-line. The patients undergoing CAPD had a significantly lower food intake than the patients undergoing hemodialysis, whereas the patients undergoing hemodialysis and CAPD had a reduced food intake and eating velocity compared to the healthy controls (205). The patients undergoing CAPD were studied twice, once with dialysate in the abdomen and once without to evaluate the effect of the presence of dialysate in the peritoneal cavity. No differences in food intake or eating velocity were observed among the patients undergoing CAPD with a full compared to empty abdomen, indicating that the higher sugar load contributes to the feeling of fullness and is more important than the discomfort caused by the dialysate (205). In a separate study, patients undergoing CAPD were studied before the start of CAPD, during CAPD treatment, and after renal transplantation in some patients (206). The feeling of fullness before meals was higher in patients undergoing CAPD than during the predialytic phase, and food intake was similar. After renal transplantation, the feeling of fullness decreased markedly and food intake increased (206). These findings are supported by a study of food consumption in 10 patients undergoing CAPD with persistent hypoalbuminemia (207). The patients recorded food intake for 2 weeks; during one of the weeks the patients were eating after draining out the fluid, and in the other week, meals were consumed with the dialysate in the peritoneal cavity. No significant differences were found in protein, carbohydrate, fat, or energy intakes, irrespective of the presence of dialysate in the peritoneal cavity (207). In contrast, Brown-Cartwright et al. reported that the presence of dialysate in the peritoneal cavity retarded gastric emptying of solid foods in a study of 10 patients without diabetes undergoing CAPD (200).

Balaskas et al. (208) studied the effect on food intake in rabbits after intraperitoneal infusion of different volumes and concentrations of glucose and amino acid solutions. They reported that high-osmolality solutions and large filling volumes suppressed the appetite. They found no difference in suppression of appetite between glucose and amino acid solutions and concluded that the absorption of these nutrients from the dialysate had no specific appetite-suppressing effect (208). These results are in agreement with the results of a crossover study in 16 patients undergoing CAPD that did not show any difference in subjective appetite and food intake during a 4-week period with one daily exchange with amino acid–based dialysis fluid compared to a control period with glucose–based dialysis fluid (209). Our group has introduced a highly reproducible experimental model for the study of ingestive behavior in unstressed, free-moving, male Wistar rats with catheters channeled from the top of the skull to the oral cavity (210,211). The ingestion behavior is tested with registration of the time (volume) of ingestion when nutritional solutions are infused intraorally (1 mL/min) through this catheter. By using solutions with different compositions (e.g., high content of protein or carbohydrates) it is possible to test the effect of various factors on ingestion of protein and carbohydrates independently of each other. Intraperitoneal injection of up to 30 mL 0.9% NaCl solution did not affect protein or carbohydrate ingestion (211). Intraperitoneal injection of PD solutions containing 13.6%, 22.7%, and 38.6% of glucose induced a dose-dependent inhibition of sucrose intake but had no effect on protein intake, whereas intraperitoneal injection of amino acid solutions reduced the ingestion of both sucrose and protein in a dose-dependent manner (211). These results indicate that the inhibition of appetite caused by solutions containing glucose or amino acids is specific to each nutritional constituent and is not simply an effect of hyperosmolarity of large filling volumes. Zheng et al. found that lactate solutions may inhibit appetite more than bicarbonate solutions (212) and that the degree of appetite inhibition was higher with a higher concentration of glucose (213). However, Davies et al. reported that calories derived from the dialysate in patients undergoing CAPD do not suppress appetite; instead they found that they provide a useful and significant proportion of the total energy intake that does not necessarily cause excessive obesity or have a negative effect on patient survival (214).

Patients with chronic renal failure also have an impaired taste acuity that is not fully corrected by CAPD or hemodialysis, which may contribute to low nutritional intake (215, 216). The plasma levels of several anorectic factors such as cholecystokinin, leptin, TNF-α, and IL-6 are markedly increased among patients undergoing PD (138,217–219). Whereas leptin and cholecystokinin (217) have not been demonstrated to correlate to nutritional status, malnourished patients have been reported to have higher TNF-α (217) and IL-6 (138) compared to well-nourished patients. Recently, orexins, a family of hypothalamic peptides that stimulate appetite, was identified (220), but no studies of orexins in patients undergoing PD have been reported so far. However, the plasma level of neuropeptide Y—another peptide that stimulates appetite—has been reported to be low in patients undergoing PD (217). In addition, several other factors, such as medications, unpalatable diets, and psychosocial problems (e.g., poverty, loneliness, social isolation, and depression), also may contribute to a reduced appetite in patients undergoing CAPD.

Protein and Amino Acid Losses in Dialysate

The average dialysate losses of free amino acids into the dialysate during CAPD are reported to vary between 1.2 and 3.4 g/24 h in different studies (1). About 30% of the amino acids lost into the dialysate are essential amino acids. The weekly losses of amino acids into the dialysate are of the same order of magnitude as in patients undergoing hemodialysis (1).

Substantial loss of protein into dialysate is a major drawback with PD; this is not present in hemodialysis. The reported average loss of protein into the dialysate varies between 5 and 15 g/24 h in different studies with large interindividual differences (1,221–223). Albumin is the main constituent comprising 50% to 65% of the total protein loss, but several other proteins also are present in the dialysate (221–223) in amounts depending on the serum concentrations and peritoneal clearances of the different proteins. The peritoneal clearances of proteins of different molecular weight show a bimodal pattern (69,224,225). The clearances of proteins up to the size of albumin is related to the ultrafiltration rate and is inversely related to the molecular weight of the protein, whereas the larger proteins show a much smaller decrease in clearance with increasing molecular weight, and the clearances of large proteins are, furthermore, independent of the ultrafiltration rate (69,224, 225).

It should be noted that protein losses indirectly may contribute to various nutritional and metabolic disturbances in patients undergoing CAPD (e.g., low HDL-cholesterol levels as a result of losses of apolipoproteins in the dialysate (226), hypercholesterolemia, increased lipoprotein(a) levels (227), altered amino acid metabolism, and metabolic bone disease as a result of losses of vitamin D–binding protein) (1). Furthermore, the decreased serum albumin concentration in patients undergoing CAPD shows an inverse correlation to peritoneal albumin loss in several studies (36,49,54, 69–71). Thus, although albumin loss seems to stimulate the albumin synthesis rate (36), this may not always be enough to prevent a decrease in serum albumin levels.

Impact of Peritoneal Transport Rate on Nutritional Status

Because there is a close relationship between the peritoneal transport characteristics of solutes of different molecular weight up to the size of albumin (225,228) it is not surprising that patients undergoing CAPD with relatively high transport rates of small solutes as assessed by the dialysate to plasma concentration ratios (D/P) during the peritoneal equilibration test (PET) also exhibit increased protein losses. It also comes as no surprise that these patients have more severe hypoalbuminemia than patients with lower D/P ratios (70,71,125,229–234). Furthermore, a large influx of glucose absorbed from the dialysate may suppress appetite (229,230). Hypophagia induced by PD solutions because of the utilization of absorbed nutrients from the solutions has been emphasized by our group (211,213) and other authors (208), using an animal appetite model. More recently, Zheng et al. found that the degree of appetite inhibition was higher with a higher concentration of glucose (213), which may be needed in high transporters. However, Davies et al. reported that calories derived from the dialysate in patients undergoing CAPD did seem to reduce appetite (214).

The patients with high transport rates have in a few studies been reported to have lower nPNA and lower daily creatinine production (indicating lower muscular mass) compared to patients with lower D/P values during the PET (229,230). Furthermore, the morbidity has been reported to be increased among the patients with high transport rates (230,235–237), although this has not been seen in all studies (125,238). Also, Kang et al. reported on a correlation between a nutritional index and peritoneal transport characteristics (239). However, serum albumin was included in the nutritional index used in this study (239). In contrast, Churchill et al. found no difference in nutritional status at the start of treatment (except for serum albumin) between patients in different peritoneal transport groups in the CANUSA study (236). Harty et al. found no difference in anthropometrics (midarm circumference and arm-muscle area) between patients undergoing CAPD with high peritoneal transport rates versus patients with low peritoneal transport rates in a cross-sectional study of 147 patients undergoing CAPD (231). Cueto-Manzano et al. found no relation between nutritional status (except serum albumin) and peritoneal transport rate in a cross-sectional study of 42 patients undergoing CAPD (234). Selgas et al. found no difference in nPNA between different transport groups in a prospective study, and although they reported on a higher hospitalization rate among patients with high transport rates, they found no impact of peritoneal transport rates on long-term morbidity and mortality (125). Furthermore, in a study of 235 patients undergoing CAPD Szeto et al. found that there were weak inverse correlations between 4-hour dialysate to plasma concentration (D/P) of creatinine versus baseline serum albumin, percentage LBM (estimated using creatinine kinetics), and nPNA, which only were higher in the lowest transport group (240). However, during a prospective follow up of 24 months, there were no signs of change in any nutritional parameter, and they concluded that transport status is not associated with longitudinal change of nutritional parameters (240).

In conclusion, there is poor evidence that peritoneal transport characteristics will influence nutritional status (other than the influence of serum protein levels) in patients undergoing CAPD. A possible link between high peritoneal transport status and the poor outcome seen in several studies is the risk of fluid overload in high transporters (237,241). We also have seen that there is a relation between high peritoneal transport rate, inflammation, and cardiovascular disease (242,243). It is striking that the relation between peritoneal transport rate and serum albumin (236) and some other nutritional markers was seen already at the start of CAPD (240). Therefore, it is likely that the relation between peritoneal transport and some nutritional parameters seen in some of the studies discussed earlier, in fact, are the result of a relation between peritoneal transport and the MIA syndrome (244). High peritoneal membrane transport characteristics merely may be another feature of the MIA syndrome (244).

Metabolic Acidosis

It has become increasingly evident that metabolic acidosis is an important stimulus for net protein catabolism. A study of leucine kinetics in normal subjects during acute acidosis and alkalosis showed that total body protein breakdown and apparent leucine oxidation increase more during acidosis than during alkalosis (245). In nondialyzed chronic uremic patients the correction of metabolic acidosis improves nitrogen balance (246). Acidosis, rather than uremia, appears to enhance protein catabolism in rats with chronic renal failure (247). This effect seems to be mediated by the stimulation of skeletal muscle branched-chain keto acid decarboxylation, resulting in increased catabolism of the branched-chain amino acids (valine, leucine, and isoleucine), which mainly are metabolized in muscle tissue (248,249). Mitch et al. have shown that metabolic acidosis elicits the transcription of genes for proteolytic enzymes in muscle (249). Our group previously has reported that low intracellular valine concentration in muscle correlated with the predialysis blood standard bicarbonate level (which varied between 18 and 24 mmol/L) in a group of patients undergoing hemodialysis (250). This finding indicates that even slight, and intermittent, acidosis may have stimulated the catabolism of valine in muscle, resulting in valine depletion that may be a limiting factor for protein synthesis. In patients undergoing CAPD, Kang et al. reported that patients with metabolic acidosis seemed to be more malnourished compared to the other patients using a composite nutritional score including clinical, biochemical, and anthropometric parameters (177).

Note that acidosis is today the only identified uremic "toxic" factor that induces catabolism and impairs nitrogen utilization. Lim et al. reported that correction of acidosis in seven patients with CRF studied with L-(1-13C) leucine kinetics resulted in decreased protein degradation, although protein synthesis capacity was preserved and the patients adapted successfully to lower dietary protein intake (251). After initiation of dialysis, all components of protein flux were accelerated, in particular protein synthesis (251). Also, correction of acidosis (from a HCO_3 level of 19 to 26 mmol/L) with oral sodium bicarbonate in seven patients undergoing CAPD resulted in an improvement in protein turnover with a decrease of whole-body protein degradation as determined from L-(1-13C) leucine kinetics (252). Furthermore, a short-term study of correction of acidosis with oral sodium bicarbonate for 2 weeks in 11 patients undergoing PD showed that urea appearance decreased significantly, whereas there was no significant change in protein intake (as assessed by a 1-week dietary record), indicating that the bicarbonate supplementation may have induced net anabolism (253). In addition, oral treatment with sodium bicarbonate in patients with acidosis undergoing hemodialysis resulted in increased plasma levels of branched-chain amino acids (254). Thus, full correction of acidosis is an obvious goal for treatment in patients undergoing CAPD, and oral bicarbonate should be prescribed even when the blood standard bicarbonate level only marginally is decreased.

In general, patients undergoing CAPD are less acidotic than patients undergoing hemodialysis (23), and many patients undergoing CAPD using standard lactate-buffered dialysis solutions have a normal blood standard bicarbonate level without any additional oral bicarbonate supplementation (23). Because hydrogen ions are produced from the catabolism of proteins, it is not surprising that the bicarbonate levels (in arterialized capillary blood) have been reported to correlate to protein intake as assessed from urea kinetics (nPNA) in patients undergoing CAPD (255). The absorption of lactate from dialysate is related to the peritoneal transport characteristics, and the buffer absorption from dialysate is more efficient in patients with a high peritoneal transport rate (256). However, the previous most commonly applied lactate concentration of 35 mmol/L may not be enough to provide full correction of acidosis in all patients (23,257). Therefore, the lactate concentration was increased to 40 mmol/L in PD solutions, which still may not always be enough to correct acidosis in all patients undergoing CAPD (258). However, a detailed study of acid-base balance in 19 stable patients undergoing CAPD using a solution with a lactate concentration of 40 mmol/L showed that all of these patients had a normal or high serum bicarbonate concentration without oral bicarbonate supplementation. Furthermore, a detailed analysis showed that these patients were in steady state with a neutral acid-base balance (259). Stein et al. performed a large prospective controlled trial of 200 consecutive new patients undergoing CAPD who were randomized to a lactate 40 mmol/L ($n = 100$) versus 35 mmol/L ($n = 100$) PD solution (178). After 1 year of treatment, the venous serum bicarbonate (27.2 ± 0.3 versus 23.0 ± 0.3 mmol/L, $p < 0.001$) and arterial pH (7.44 ± 0.004 versus 7.40 ± 0.004, $p < 0.001$) levels were significantly higher in the 40 mmol/L lactate solution group. The patients in the 40 mmol/L lactate solution group also had a higher increase in body weight (6.1 versus 3.7 kg, $p < 0.05$), a higher increase in midarm circumference, and less hospitalization, whereas the serum albumin and protein intake did not differ between the groups (178). However, no specific method was applied for estimation of fluid status in this study. Recently, a new bicarbonate 25 mmol/L and lactate 15 mmol/L PD solution has been introduced. It seems to give similar correction of acidosis as compared to a lactate 40 mmol/L solution (260). Also, a 34 mmol bicarbonate-based PD solution has been tested and gives similar arterial acid-base status as a 35 mmol lactate-based solution, which, however, may not be enough for correction of acidosis in all patients (261). Therefore, a 39 mmol/L bicarbonate-based solution was tested and resulted in improved acid-base status compared to the 34 mmol/L bicarbonate-based solutions (262).

Loss of Residual Renal Function and Metabolizing Renal Tissue

The normal kidneys actively take part in the metabolism of amino acids, and loss of metabolizing renal tissue may be one important pathogenic factor for the amino acid abnormalities frequently observed in patients with uremia (1, 184). In the normal kidneys, among other processes, phenylalanine hydroxylation to tyrosine (263,264) and glycine conversion to serine take place (265). Low plasma and intracellular concentrations of tyrosine and a reduced ratio of tyrosine to phenylalanine persist in patients undergoing dialysis, and serine depletion appears to become more severe than in nondialyzed patients because not only the plasma concentration but also the muscle concentration of serine is low (23). A possible explanation for these findings is that the patients undergoing dialysis have less metabolizing renal tissue left compared to nondialyzed patients with uremia. It is conceivable that under conditions of low protein intake or increased catabolic stress, depletion of valine, tyrosine, and serine may become limiting for protein synthesis in patients undergoing maintenance dialysis. This partly may explain why loss of the residual renal function was the factor that was connected most closely to severe malnutrition in the large cross-sectional study of nutritional status (involving 224 patients undergoing CAPD from six centers (26); see page 482). Poor residual renal function also has been shown to correlate to malnutrition in several other studies (108,175,234,266) and Wang et al. reported in 2001 that residual renal function has an independent and better effect than peritoneal clearance on protein intake, energy intake, and other nutrient intake in patients undergoing CAPD (267).

The residual renal function may be better preserved in patients undergoing CAPD than in patients treated with hemodialysis (268,269), and patients undergoing CAPD often have some residual renal function several years after the start of dialysis therapy (268), which may, at least in part, explain why the intracellular free amino acid pattern in muscle seems to be less abnormal in patients undergoing CAPD than in patients undergoing hemodialysis (82). However, there seems to be close relation between inflammation (as assessed by increase CRP levels) and more rapid decline of residual renal function in patients undergoing PD (242). In Chapter 13, the relation between inflammation and residual renal function is discussed in detail.

Recurrent Peritonitis and Other Infections

Uremia leads to disturbances in the immune response, with cutaneous anergy and impaired granulocyte function, thus increasing the susceptibility to infections. Although marked improvement of cell-mediated immunity (as assessed by hypersensitivity skin testing) has been reported during the first year of CAPD treatment (48), several patients undergoing CAPD still show relative anergy (48).

In patients undergoing CAPD with mild peritonitis the dialysate protein losses increased by 50% to 100% to an average of 15 ± 3.6 g/24 h (270) and also have been reported to remain elevated for several weeks (100,271). In addition, the spontaneous energy and protein intake has been shown to be extremely low during peritonitis (272, 273). Furthermore, the inflammatory response may be a strong catabolic stimulus superimposed on the enhanced protein losses. Nitrogen balance studies during CAPD peritonitis demonstrated a markedly negative nitrogen balance (272,273). Adverse effects of recurrent peritonitis on nutritional status were reported by Rubin et al. (75,274), who observed that changes in total body potassium correlated negatively with the number of episodes of peritonitis per month and, furthermore, that patients with a high incidence of peritonitis had lower arm-muscle circumference and lower plasma protein compared to patients with lower incidence of peritonitis. Note, however, that this study was performed during the early days of CAPD when the peritonitis incidence was much higher than today—on average 0.6 peritonitis episodes/months (75).

Dialysis Procedure, Biocompatibility, and Protein Catabolism in Hemodialysis Versus Continuous Ambulatory Peritoneal Dialysis

A major difference between CAPD and hemodialysis is that the blood-membrane contact during the hemodialysis procedure may give rise to an inflammatory reaction, the intensity of which depends on the membrane material that is used (275–277). *In vivo* blood-membrane interaction in a dialyzer without dialysate during sham hemodialysis also has been shown to stimulate net protein catabolism in normal individuals, especially when membranes of low biocompatibility were used, demonstrating that the effect is the result of the interaction between blood and the membrane (278, 279). IL-1 and TNF-α may act in concert and induce *inter alia* lysosomal catabolism of muscle protein (280), an effect that is mediated by the release of prostaglandin E2 (281). Furthermore, IL-1, TNF-α, and endotoxin may induce net catabolism of muscle protein by stimulating branched-chain keto acid dehydrogenase, which leads to an enhanced oxidation of branched-chain amino acids (282).

Compared to the hemodialysis procedure, the PD procedure is apparently not such a strong catabolic stimulus, provided that the patient is free from peritonitis. However, there is a possibility that in PD the dialytic procedure elicits a low-grade inflammatory response, induced by substances other than live bacteria, thereby stimulating protein catabolism (283). These substances could be microbial products (endotoxins), plastics, silicon, glucose breakdown products (284), or other products from the system that elute into the peritoneal cavity.

EFFECTS OF PERITONEAL DIALYSIS ON NUTRITIONAL STATUS

Early Effects of Peritoneal Dialysis on Nutritional Status

During the first year of CAPD, there is improvement of nutritional status with weight gain (285,286), improvement in anthropometric parameters (9,32,49), and an increase in plasma proteins (9,32,100,286–288), indicating that there is an increased net anabolism during the first years of CAPD. Detailed prospective studies of body composition during the first year of PD, using bioimpedance (289), anthropometrics (9,49), DEXA (219,290,291), and the combination of total body potassium and tritium dilution (84), show that whereas LBM seems to be rather stable, body FM increases considerably. Fernström reported that the body fat distribution changed with a marked increase in intraperitoneal fat (as estimated using computed tomography) (292). In addition, part of the weight gain may be the result of increased body water.

Nitrogen balance studies from our unit performed in patients undergoing CAPD during the first year of CAPD (prescribed an individualized diet composed to resemble the patients' spontaneously chosen diets regarding dietary protein and energy intake) show that most of these patients were in a positive nitrogen balance during the first year of CAPD (147). These results are in agreement with the results from a study of protein turnover (using whole-body leucine turnover) showing that the balance between synthesis and breakdown was significantly higher in 10 patients undergoing CAPD (after 3 months of CAPD treatment as well as before the start of CAPD) compared to healthy controls, indicating net anabolism among the patients undergoing CAPD. Furthermore, total body potassium was normal in these 10 patients, indicating a normal nutritional status (78).

An increase in total body nitrogen (which was low at the start of CAPD, indicating protein malnutrition) also has been reported during the first year of CAPD in a prospective study (49,112). In contrast, a few old prospective studies of total body nitrogen indicate that a gradual deterioration in nutritional status is common after the start of CAPD, especially in male patients, with large protein stores at the beginning of treatment (100,103,293). Although diverging results have been reported concerning the changes in total body nitrogen in patients undergoing CAPD, they all show that patients undergoing CAPD in general have decreased total body nitrogen during the first year of treatment, indicating that protein malnutrition is common among patients undergoing CAPD despite normal anthropometric measurements (49,100,103,112,293).

Long-Term Effects of Peritoneal Dialysis on Nutritional Status

Most long-term studies of nutrition in patients undergoing CAPD have used rather indirect measures of nutritional status. In general, protein intake (49,56,294), energy intake (295), serum albumin and total protein levels (49,56,111, 294,296), body weight (49,286,289,294,296,297), and anthropometrics (9,49,294) seem to be maintained on stable levels without further decrease in patients undergoing long-term CAPD. Prospective studies of body composition using bioimpedance (289) and anthropometrics (294) show a tendency toward a further increase in FM in patients undergoing long-term CAPD.

However, a progressive decrease in serum albumin has been reported in patients undergoing CAPD after 3 years or more (286,289,297), and Davies et al. reported on decreased protein intake with time on CAPD (295). Furthermore, the patients with severe malnutrition in the international cross-sectional study of nutritional status in 224 patients undergoing CAPD were either older or had been on CAPD longer than other patients (26). Also, because there is a high mortality rate among patients undergoing CAPD (286,295,298) and a high transfer rate of patients undergoing CAPD to hemodialysis (286,295,298) because of various complications, few patients are maintained on CAPD for 5 years or more. The patients that were treated with CAPD for longer time periods consequently will represent a positive selection of patients undergoing CAPD that have a more favorable clinical course, and these patients also may have a more favorable evolution of nutritional status compared to patients that die or are transferred to hemodialysis (295). The relative stability of nutritional status in patients undergoing long-term CAPD therefore may not necessarily be typical for the general evolution of nutritional status in most patients treated with CAPD.

Decline in Lean Body Mass During Long-Term Peritoneal Dialysis

Davies et al. (295) have reported that following an initial improvement of nutritional status, a decline may occur after about 2 years of PD treatment. Recently, several studies suggest that during long-term PD a gradual deterioration in nutritional status may occur with a decrease in LBM (84, 85,291,293).

The reasons for the tendency toward a decrease in LBM during long-term PD are not evident but are probably multifactorial. At first, residual renal function declines with time on dialysis treatment and many patients are anuric after 2 to 3 years of PD. This results in decreased solute clearances, which may result in inadequate dialysis. Secondly, it is likely that the continuous loss of protein into the dialysate may contribute to a negative protein balance. Furthermore, a low eating drive has been demonstrated in patients undergoing PD despite an increased need for protein (205). Finally, in 2000 we reported that a high level of the anorexic hormone serum leptin relative to the body fat mass was associated with weight loss in patients undergoing PD (290). However, because others have found no association between the leptin concentration and recent weight change or nutritional status in patients with end-stage renal disease (299, 300) more prospective studies are needed to investigate the role of hypoleptinemia in the loss of LBM in PD. The cause(s) of hypoleptinemia in PD may be multifactorial, but because a significant positive correlation between initial CRP and the increase in serum leptin levels has been demonstrated in patients undergoing PD (290), this could suggest that inflammation may be one contributor. Indeed, in recent years malnutrition has been linked to inflammation (8,244), and it has been postulated that proinflammatory cytokines may be an important cause of muscle wasting and hypoalbuminemia (138,139). It should be noted that an increase in leptin was associated with increased CRP in our patients, and the role of leptin compared to other inflammatory mediators for the decrease in LBM is not clear. Indeed, elevated levels of proinflammatory cytokines do predict outcome in patients undergoing dialysis (133,137,138). Thus, more research is needed to investigate whether elevated levels of proinflammatory cytokines may be a significant mediator of wasting in patients undergoing long-term PD and if selective anticytokine treatment may be one way to improve nutritional status and outcome.

Total Body Water in Patients Treated with Peritoneal Dialysis

The estimation of total body water in patients undergoing PD is important for the assessment of nutritional status as well as for the calculation of Kt/V urea as a marker of dialysis adequacy. The Watson equation has been adopted widely for the latter purpose (301), and for this the Watson equation gives a reasonable good estimate in most patients undergoing PD, although it has been shown to slightly overestimate total body water in obese subjects and to underestimate total body water in lean subjects (302,303). However, for the assessment of nutritional status, better methods for determination of total body water are needed. At present, indicator dilution methods (e.g., using tritium, deuterium, or ethanol) are the gold standards for assessment of fluid status in patients undergoing PD (302,303). Bioelectrical impedance has been used more for this purpose, but still this method is not well validated for patients undergoing PD.

In a study of 82 patients undergoing PD studied at the start of treatment and followed for an average of 26 months (range 11 to 80 months) Johansson showed that with time of PD, there was an increase in extracellular water with time on PD (calculated from the four-compartment model using measured values of total body potassium and total body water from tritium dilution) (85). This is well in agreement with the recent study by Enia et al. showing that patients undergoing CAPD had more antihypertensive treatment, higher plasma levels of atrial natriuretic factor, and higher left atrial volume and left ventricular hypertrophy compared to patients undergoing hemodialysis, indicating volume overload (304). It also has been reported that after an initial improvement after initiation of dialysis, there is an increase in hypertension with time on PD (305,306), which is associated with declining residual renal function (306) and may be related to fluid overload. Thus, patients undergoing PD are at risk to become volume overloaded with time on PD, in particular as residual renal function and ultrafiltration capacity declines with time (295,306,307).

Increase in Fat Mass and Obesity in Patients Undergoing Peritoneal Dialysis

As mentioned earlier, weight gain and accumulation of fat tissue are seen after the start of PD (9,49,84,219,289,290). However, this is not seen in all patients starting PD treatment.

Glucose is absorbed to a large extent from the dialysate, and conventional PD results in an almost unique metabolic situation involving continuous 24-hour absorption of glucose. It has been estimated that during conventional PD about 100 to 200 g of glucose are absorbed during 24 hours (25) and glucose uptake from the dialysis fluid represents a significant portion of the energy intake (24,182,183). It generally is assumed that the accumulation of adipose tissue is related to the glucose absorption from the dialysate. However, there is no clear relation between the gain in weight and the amount absorbed, and marked variations exist between patients. It is notable that patients with diabetes (9, 290) and obese females in particular tend to gain fat mass during PD (9,290).

The reason(s) why only some PD patients accumulate fat mass during PD are not clear. However, because it has been shown that genetic factors may contribute to about 70% of the variations in BMI in nonrenal patient groups (308) it could be speculated that genetic factors also are of importance in patients undergoing PD. Obviously, there is no way to accumulate excess adipose tissue without disequilibrium between the intake and expenditure of calories. It has been found that small reductions in energy expenditure increase the risk for developing obesity (309) and that genetic factors may influence the resting metabolic rate (310, 311). One reason for increased energy expenditure appears to entail an increased thermogenesis in adipose tissue. A key element in adipose tissue is the unique expression of a mitochondrial inner-membrane protein called uncoupling protein (UCP), which is a transporter of free fatty acid anions, allowing free fatty acids to function as proton carriers. Whereas UCP3 expression has been found only in skeletal muscle, UCP2 has a wide tissue distribution, and it has been speculated that UCP2 may play a role in fat-tissue accumulation (312,313). Indeed, because it has been demonstrated that a considerable contribution of the exon 8 UCP2 polymorphism contributes to variations in body composition in patients undergoing PD, this suggests that genetic factors may be important factors contributing to fat-tissue accumulation in these patients (314).

In nonuremic patient populations, a marked accumulation of abdominal fat tissue has been regarded as an important risk factor for cardiovascular disease. However, to the best of our knowledge, no studies have demonstrated that obesity and fat tissue accumulation are risk factors for cardiovascular disease and death in patients undergoing dialysis. In fact, in 1999 Fleischmann et al. (315) showed that patients undergoing hemodialysis with a high BMI had a better survival than patients with a normal BMI, suggesting that obesity actually may reduce the risk of death in patients undergoing dialysis. In this respect, it is noteworthy that it has been demonstrated that patients undergoing PD who do not accumulate fat tend to lose more LBM (i.e., muscle mass) during PD (314). This finding agrees with other studies demonstrating that some patients may be at risk of losing LBM during long-term PD treatment (84,290,293,295). Indeed, a recent study concluded that patients with low energy stores might benefit to a larger extent from PD and that the nutritional status at the start of dialysis is an important factor to consider when a choice for the dialysis modality is made (9).

PREVENTION AND TREATMENT OF MALNUTRITION IN PATIENTS UNDERGOING PERITONEAL DIALYSIS

To prevent and treat malnutrition among patients undergoing PD it is important to monitor nutritional status. Various methods are available for follow-up of nutritional status (see Chapter 15).

It is obvious that a sufficient intake of energy and protein is necessary for the maintenance of nutritional status and the prevention of malnutrition in patients undergoing CAPD. Furthermore, even slight acidosis should be corrected by oral supplementation with sodium bicarbonate (or altered dialysate buffer concentration). Physical exercise should be encouraged, and intercurrent diseases should be treated actively. The prevention of peritonitis and other infectious complications is also crucial for the maintenance of adequate nutrition in patients undergoing CAPD, but this lies outside the scope of the present review. Optimal treatment of comorbidity is an obvious goal; in particular, if there are signs of inflammation, such as increased CRP levels, it is important to look for the cause.

Monitoring and Maintenance of Adequate Protein and Energy Intakes

To ensure a safe supply of protein to the majority of patients undergoing CAPD it is recommended that patients undergoing CAPD should have a protein intake of at least 1.2 g/kg body weight/day of which a large part should be of high biologic value (i.e., the protein should have a high content of essential amino acids, usually animal proteins from milk, eggs and meat). It is likely that some patients may require less than this to maintain nitrogen equilibrium (147,316); however, it is difficult to identify such patients by simple methods. The patients who are initially malnourished or later develop signs of protein-energy malnutrition may require higher amounts of protein (and energy) for repleting the protein and energy stores. Some patients may benefit by eating as much as 1.4 to 2.1 g protein/kg/day, especially during the initial months of PD treatment (147).

The protein intake can be estimated from dietary recall or from urea kinetics (assuming that the patient is in nitrogen balance). A prospective dietary history is not always possible to obtain and is highly dependent on the cooperation of the patient and the skill of the dietitian (317). However, the PNA can be calculated easily from urea appearance rate (147). Note that PNA previously often has been denoted protein catabolic rate (PCR). PNA has been suggested as a more accurate term because the true protein catabolic rate is about six times higher than PNA estimated from urea appearance rate—most of the catabolized protein is not catabolized to urea but is used for protein synthesis again (147,318).

It is strongly advisable to monitor the estimated protein intake as assessed by urea kinetics on a regular basis for all patients undergoing CAPD to identify patients with a suboptimal protein intake. Repeated values below 1.0 g/kg body weight/day should arouse the suspicion that the protein intake is too low, and the patient should be advised to increase the intake of dietary protein. However, in patients with even slight variations in body weight or in the serum urea levels (which may suggest net protein catabolism or anabolism) the estimation of protein intake based on urea kinetic modeling should be interpreted with great caution (147,149). In addition, the active cooperation of the patient is needed because it is crucial that the dialysate and urine collections be complete. Note that the previously applied equations for the estimation of PNA from urea appearance rate (150) yield values of protein intake lower than the values obtained from diet history (49,105,147,149). However, our group established a new equation (which was based on 36 complete nitrogen balance studies in patients undergoing CAPD [146,147]) that will yield a more accurate, and higher, estimate of dietary protein intake in patients undergoing CAPD (151).

Thus, when urea appearance (UA) or urea nitrogen appearance (UNA) (151) and protein losses have been calculated from routine determinations of urea and protein concentrations and volumes of 24-h collections of urine and drained dialysate, PNA simply can be calculated, using the following equation derived from Bergström et al. (151):

$$\text{PNA (g/24 h)} = 15.1 + 0.195\ \text{UA (mmol/24-h)} + \text{protein losses (g/24 h)}$$

$$[\text{PNA (g/24 h)} = 15.1 + 6.95\ \text{UNA (g/24-h)} + \text{protein losses (g/24 h)}]$$

In the absence of excessive protein losses, PNA can be calculated even more simply, without determination of protein losses in dialysate and urine (151):

$$\text{PNA (g/24 h)} = 20.1 + 0.209\ \text{UA (mmol/24 h)}$$

$$[\text{PNA (g/24 h)} = 20.1 + 7.50\ \text{UNA (g/24 h)}]$$

The recommended and the estimated nutritional intakes of various nutrients usually are normalized for body size. Several different ways of normalization have been applied, although there is no general agreement on which way is the best. When PNA has been calculated, it is usually normalized to g/kg body weight/day (*normalized* PNA, or nPNA). However, this normalization has been performed using several different weight standards (105,108,319). The easiest, and most common, way to normalize PNA is simply to divide it by the patient's *actual* dry body weight. This method is applied often, although it does not take into account that the protein requirements per kg body weight possibly are lower in obese subjects. Furthermore, this method will yield high values of nPNA in malnourished patients with a low body weight (105,108). Other possibilities are to normalize PNA to normal body weight (from the National Health Examination Survey, NHANES) (320), to desirable body weight (from the Metropolitan Life Insurance Company) (321), to other weight standards (319), or to the patient's preuremic weight (if it is known).

An alternative method to normalize PNA that is commonly applied is to first calculate total body water (V, liter) from the Watson nomogram (301), for example, and then normalize PNA to "idealized body weight" using the equation: nPNA = PNA/(V/0.58) (105). This method, however, is perhaps not appropriate because it assumes that the absolute value of total body water should not differ from the absolute value of the total body water at "idealized body weight," an assumption that can be questioned. Note that the calculated total body water using the Watson nomogram is directly proportional to the actual body weight (301) and that the "idealized body weight" thus will be directly proportional to the actual body weight of the patients. Harty et al. (105) reported from a cross-sectional study of 147 patients undergoing CAPD that nPNA normalized using V/0.58 did not differ between a group of severely malnourished patients undergoing CAPD (n = 25) compared to well-nourished patients undergoing CAPD (n = 46).

In the study by Harty et al. (105) nPNA normalized to normal body weight, calculated from the 50th percentile for weight obtained from the NHANES tables (320), showed a significant correlation to nutritional status. However, the correlation with nutritional status was even better when PNA was not normalized to body weight (105). However, it is obvious that PNA and other nutritional intakes should, at least to some extent, take body size into account, especially for interpatient comparisons. Prospective studies are needed to clarify which normalization factor should be used for various nutritional intakes. At present, it seems to be most reasonable to normalize PNA to desirable body weight, normal body weight, or some other weight standard. Until a single uniform way of normalization has been established, it is important to be aware of the problems involved in normalization, and, furthermore, to state *how* nPNA is normalized when it is reported.

The addition of oral essential amino acids to the diet may increase the biologic value and the total intake of ingested protein and may improve the nutritional status. Special amino acid formulas with a modified amino acid composition (high valine, addition of tyrosine and serine) have been designed to compensate for amino acid deficiencies present in uremia (322,323).

As pointed out previously, energy depletion may be as common, and as important, as protein depletion in patients undergoing CAPD. An energy intake of 35 kcal (145 kJoule)/kg body weight/day generally is recommended, and even higher intakes may be necessary if the patient is energy depleted or is regularly doing physical exercise. The energy intake presently can be assessed only by dietary recall, which requires a high level of patient skill and cooperation. In addition, patients with a high energy intake tend to underestimate their true intake, whereas patients with a low intake tend to overestimate the nutritional intake. In a review it was concluded that "in order to gain a representative assessment of energy, protein, fat and carbohydrate intakes, dietary intake should be measured for a minimum of one week in free-living individuals" (317). Thus, it may be difficult to monitor dietary energy intake with precision on a regular basis.

The glucose absorption from dialysate can be calculated easily from the volume and glucose concentration of a 24-h collection of dialysate (25). According to our experience a rough, but for the clinical setting accurate, estimate of the amount of glucose absorbed from the dialysate (in patients undergoing CAPD with normal peritoneal transport characteristics) can be made by multiplication of the 24-h glucose load with 0.6. A patient using, for example, four exchanges of (anhydrous) glucose 2.27% (usually denoted 2.5% in the United States) will absorb about 110 g of glucose (corresponding to about 440 kcal) per 24 h (25).

If the dietary energy supply is considered insufficient, oral liquid or powder mixtures of glucose polymers may be used as energy supplement. For a more complete supplementation of both protein and energy several liquid formulas containing large amounts of protein of high biologic value, lipids, and carbohydrates in a small amount of fluid are available, which are suitable for the supplementary nutrition of patients undergoing dialysis (because they have a low content of phosphate, potassium, and sodium) (60). However, Heaf et al. reported that oral protein supplements (two times 20 g/day for 10 weeks) were unable to improve nutritional status in 14 malnourished patients undergoing CAPD (324). Part of the reason was that half of the patients were unable to drink the prescribed nutritional supplement because of nausea, but the results also were unimpressive among the compliant patients. However, these patients were old and had a high prevalence of comorbidity (79%) and high transporters (46%), suggesting that factors other than poor nutritional intake possibly were causing the malnutrition among these patients (324).

If severe malnutrition develops in patients undergoing CAPD despite adequate dialysis, measures to eliminate anorectic and catabolic factors and food supplements, such as enteral or parenteral nutritional supplementation with energy and amino acids, may be necessary. Severely malnourished patients may have to be hospitalized temporarily for such treatment. Enteral nutrition through a thin nasogastric tube is preferable whenever possible because it is less expensive than parenteral nutrition and does not carry the risk of catheter sepsis. In patients who need parenteral nutrition with amino acids, a mixture of essential and nonessential amino acids seems better than a solution with only essential amino acids (1). Energy should be provided simultaneously as hypertonic glucose or a mixture of glucose and lipid emulsion. Parenteral nutrition may be needed especially during peritonitis because the spontaneous nutritional intake may be extremely low during peritonitis, which in combination with the catabolic stimuli of the peritonitis results in markedly negative nitrogen balance (272,273). Early intravenous hyperalimentation has been shown to be effective to maintain a positive nitrogen balance during peritonitis in five of seven patients undergoing CAPD that received intravenous hyperalimentation during peritonitis (325).

Dialysis Dose, Anorexia, and Nutritional Intake

To maintain an adequate nutritional intake, it is obvious that the patients should receive an adequate amount of dialysis, and increased dialysis dose always should be considered in patients with nutritional intakes that are too low. The residual renal function has been shown to be a major determinant of the total small solute clearance in patients undergoing CAPD (326,327). Because the residual renal function declines with time in most patients undergoing PD, it is important to monitor residual renal function (in addition to dialysis efficiency) and to increase the dialysis dose as residual renal function declines. However, several recent studies have demonstrated that residual renal, but not peritoneal, clearances are related to clinical outcome in patients undergoing PD (328,329), and an increase in peritoneal urea and creatinine clearance by increased dialysate volume may not be enough to compensate for the loss of residual renal function, as regards mortality (329). Therefore, patients with anuria undergoing PD need special attention and careful follow-up. However, it seems that increased dialysate volume still may improve nutritional status (see later in this chapter).

As pointed out previously (see page 488), there are several cross-sectional studies in patients undergoing CAPD or hemodialysis that report a correlation between the dose of dialysis (as assessed by Kt/V urea) and PNA, although there is no consensus regarding whether this is mainly the result of a physiologic relationship (188) or a mathematic artifact (105,189,190). Lindsay and Spanner (185) have shown in a prospective study that nPNA increased when Kt/V urea was increased in patients undergoing hemodialysis. Several cross-sectional studies among patients undergoing CAPD also have demonstrated a similar correlation, and the regression line seems to be steeper, perhaps indicating a more marked favorable effect on PNA per unit of increase in Kt/V among patients undergoing CAPD (50,55,147,330).

A few prospective studies of increased dialysis dose have been reported in patients undergoing CAPD (191,192). We have reported that when the dialysate volume was increased in 19 patients undergoing CAPD, there was a significant correlation between the changes in Kt/V urea and nPNA 3 months later (191). There was also a tendency toward increased serum albumin levels (from 29.1 g/L to 30.5 g/L 3 months later), although there was no correlation between the changes in Kt/V or nPNA versus the changes in serum albumin (191). Burkart et al. (192) reported on an increase in serum albumin (from 35.1 g/L to 36.9 g/L) 1 month after an increase of the dialysate volume in a group of 17 patients undergoing CAPD. However, the observed increase in serum albumin may not necessarily be the result of an increase in the plasma albumin mass because the increase in dialysate volume among the patients undergoing CAPD may provide improved ultrafiltration, which, in turn, may result in a concentration effect as a result of a decrease in plasma volume. In a similar study, Williams et al. studied 10 patients with increased CAPD and a smaller group of five patients with anuria undergoing CAPD that were switched to continuous cycling peritoneal dialysis (331). They found a tendency toward an increase in nPNA that was not significant in any of the two groups of patients. Furthermore, the serum albumin levels were not influenced by the increase in dialysis dose (331). Recently, a randomized prospective study (n = 82) showed that increasing the number of exchanges from three to four per day in patients undergoing CAPD improved protein intake (nPNA) in the treatment group (n = 30) from 1.10 to 1.24 g/kg/day after 1 year (193). However, there was no change in serum albumin levels. Also, a preliminary study of 100 Chinese patients with anuria undergoing CAPD was reported (194). Fifty of the patients had their dialysate volume increased, and 50 patients had their dialysis prescription unchanged. This study showed that protein intake increased in parallel with increased Kt/V when the prescription was increased from three to four exchanges per day, whereas an increase from four to five exchanges per day did not increase protein intake (194). These results need to be interpreted with some caution because Chinese patients tend to have a small body size and excellent compliance and clinical outcome (332). In addition, Davies et al. have reported that when dialysis volume was increased by 25% in 48 malnourished patients undergoing PD who had evidence of declining nutrition over the past 12 months (333) nutritional status stabilized, in general, but clear signs of improvement (increased nPNA and plasma albumin) were significant only in patients without comorbidity.

In conclusion, the prospective studies of increased dialysis dose (as assessed by Kt/V urea) among patients undergoing CAPD tend to show a less steep relationship (or even no relationship) between Kt/V urea and nPNA than the cross-sectional studies among patients undergoing CAPD. Furthermore, the increase in dialysate volume often is counterbalanced by a spontaneous gradual decrease in residual renal function resulting in no change of solute removal as assessed by small solute clearances (327,331,334, 335). An increased dialysis dose seems to be efficient in some patient groups undergoing CAPD, although it may not always be enough to treat and prevent malnutrition among other patient groups, in particular among patients with comorbidity (333).

Clinical Use of Amino Acid–Based Dialysis Fluids

Short-term studies have shown that PD solutions containing amino acids may supplement in excess the daily losses of amino acids during dialysis with glucose-based solutions (336,337). The amino acid solutions produce ultrafiltration and solute transport patterns that are similar to those with the standard glucose solutions, although the period of effective ultrafiltration, for the same concentration of the osmotic agent, is slightly shorter (336,338).

During the early 1980s several investigators developed and tested different amino acid solutions for PD (336,339). The initial clinical experience with amino acid solutions containing large amounts of nonessential amino acids were discouraging, in general (340–343). The patients, who were not always malnourished and tended to have a low energy intake, developed increased blood urea nitrogen (BUN) levels; acidosis (because the amount of buffer was too low); and, in some cases, anorexia and had no improvement in nutritional status or amino acid abnormalities (340–343).

In 1985 a new 1% amino acid solution, containing an

increased buffer amount (lactate 35 mmol/L) and mainly essential amino acids in proportions that take the amino acid abnormalities in patients with uremia into account, became available (316,137,344–347). The use of this amino acid solution resulted in some improvement in the plasma amino acid pattern and nutritional parameters, but acidosis and increased BUN levels still remained problems (316,344–347). The experiences from these and previous studies showed that (a) the altered amino acid composition of this solutions was beneficial, (b) patients included should have signs of protein malnutrition combined with low dietary protein intake to benefit from the use of intraperitoneal amino acid supply, (c) a further increase of the buffer amount was needed, and (d) it is important for the energy intake to be sufficient to prevent amino acids ending up as an energy source (316,336,344–347). A study of protein synthesis estimated with leucine kinetics during intraperitoneal use of this solution demonstrated that the absorbed amino acids are used efficiently for protein synthesis, whereas protein breakdown is unaffected (348). The simultaneous infusion of energy from a carbohydrate-lipid meal inhibits protein breakdown and reinforces a positive effect of the amino acid solution on protein breakdown (348).

For this purpose, a new improved 1.1% amino acid solution was developed, containing a further increase of some essential amino acids and an increased amount of lactate (40 mmol/L). This solution was tested in a nitrogen balance study of 19 malnourished patients undergoing CAPD eating 0.8 g protein/kg/day and 25 to 30 kcal/kg/day. The patients lived in the hospital for 35 days while they ate a constant diet. The first 15 days served as a baseline phase, and the patients used their usual glucose-based dialysis solution. Then, for the last 20 days, one or two of the patients' usual exchanges with glucose-based solution per day was replaced with amino acid–based dialysis solution (316). During the baseline phase the patients were in neutral nitrogen balance and net protein anabolism was positive (as determined from total body protein turnover studies with 15N-glycine). The treatment with intraperitoneal amino acid solution resulted in a markedly positive nitrogen balance, a significant increase in net protein anabolism, a more normal fasting plasma amino acid pattern, and significant increases in serum total protein and transferrin (316). A marked improvement of nitrogen balance with this amino acid solution also was reported in all patients in a small study of three patients undergoing CAPD (349). It also has been demonstrated that the absorption of amino acids from the dialysate during one exchange of amino acid solution resulted in amino acid absorption (on average 17.6 g/day) that was twice as large as the dialysate losses of amino acids and protein (on average 9.2 g/day) (337).

A prospective study of the use of this solution for 3 months in 15 patients undergoing CAPD resulted in significant increases in serum albumin (from 32.7 ± 2.3 to 35.1 ± 2.2, $p < 0.01$) and transferrin (2.21 ± 0.25 to 2.39 ± 0.27, $p < 0.05$) (350). Also, a large randomized study with this solution was reported in 1998 (351). In this study, 134 malnourished patients undergoing PD were randomized to either use one or two exchanges of this amino acid solution per day (n = 71) or to continue with their usual glucose-based dialysis solution for 3 months (351). At 1 month of study, there were (by analysis of covariance) significant increases in albumin, prealbumin, transferrin, and total proteins compared to baseline values in the amino acid group. Midarm muscular circumference also increased significantly in the amino acid group. At 3 months of the study, 70% of the patients in the amino acid group had improved in two or more nutritional variables versus only 45% among the patients that were randomized to the control group. Furthermore, there was a significant difference between the two groups in insulinlike growth factor-1, or IGF-1 (which is considered to be a good marker of nutritional status; see later in this chapter) compared to baseline values: IGF-1 increased with 38 ± 89 ng/L in the amino acid group versus a decrease in the control group of 12 ± 83 ng/mL (p = 0.001) between the two groups (351). One exchange per day of amino acid solution also has been tested as nutritional support during peritonitis (352). The patients treated with amino acid solution (n = 13) returned to preperitonitis levels of serum total protein and albumin more rapidly than the patients in the control group (n = 11) (352). The amino acid solution also has been shown to improve the serum amino acid profile without change of other nutritional parameters in relatively well-nourished patients undergoing PD (353).

In conclusion, the possibility to use amino acid solutions should be of value in malnourished patients, in particular in those patients with low nutritional intake and in whom attempts to increase the dose of dialysis and measures to increase the dietary intake have failed. However, amino acid solution may not be as efficient in patients with malnutrition arising from causes other than a low protein intake, intercurrent illnesses, and inflammation (MIA syndrome) (354). Nevertheless, PD supplemented with amino acid solutions is an important component of CAPD therapy to reduce the high prevalence of malnutrition among these patients.

Hormonal Treatment of Malnutrition in Patients Undergoing Peritoneal Dialysis

The dramatic evolution of molecular biology and new biotechnologic tools have resulted in the possibility to produce recombinant human hormones that may be used to treat disease. In nephrology, the use of erythropoietin has dramatically changed the ability to treat renal anemia. Furthermore, the possibility to treat malnutrition among patients undergoing dialysis with recombinant human growth stimulating hormones seems to be a promising perspective in the future.

Correction of Anemia and Erythropoietin Treatment

Anemia is present in most patients undergoing dialysis and may be severe, especially in anephric patients with and in patients who are dialyzed inadequately. Anemia leads to fatigue, which diminishes exercise capacity, and physical inactivity, which may contribute to muscle wasting and malnutrition. Correction of anemia with recombinant human erythropoietin (rHu-EPO) has been reported to improve nutritional status to a moderate degree in patients undergoing hemodialysis (355), which is presumably a secondary effect of anemia correction on physical work capacity, general well-being, and appetite, rather than a specific anabolic effect of rHu-EPO. Although anemia is often less severe in patients undergoing CAPD than in patients undergoing hemodialysis, correction of anemia with rHu-EPO in patients undergoing CAPD possibly may contribute to improved nutritional status among patients undergoing CAPD. Positive effects (i.e., increased body weight, serum albumin, and total protein, as well as improvement in appetite, sleep, and well-being, by patients' self-assessments) were reported in a small retrospective study of 17 patients undergoing CAPD that started treatment with rHu-EPO (356).

The use of rHu-EPO for correction of renal anemia should be accompanied by an increased supply of iron to nonoverloaded patients as the hemoglobin mass increases. Therefore the use of rHu-EPO in patients undergoing CAPD requires assessment of iron stores because iron depletion will impair the response to rHu-EPO and rHu-EPO can cause iron deficiency. The increased iron requirements should be met if possible by oral substitution with iron (155),although parenteral iron supplementation may be needed in many cases.

Anabolic Steroids

Anabolic steroids frequently were used during the 1960s and 1970s in attempts to improve nutritional status among malnourished patients undergoing dialysis. In 1980, a review concluded that androgens are of no value in the management of nitrogen retention in chronic renal failure, and, at best, they induce a transient improvement in nitrogen balance that is of doubtful significance (357). In contrast, a recent review of the same literature concluded that anabolic steroids exert a beneficial effect on the malnutrition of renal failure (358). One retrospective study of 13 patients undergoing CAPD showed increasing serum albumin and creatinine levels (interpreted as improved nutritional status) among nine patients who received small doses of nandrolone decanoate intramuscularly for 3 months, whereas no beneficial effect was observed among four patients who received both nandrolone decanoate and one daily exchange of a 1% amino acid solution (359). The lack of anabolic effect among the four patients who received both nandrolone decanoate and amino acids was attributed to the low dose of nandrolone decanoate, the increased acidosis with the amino acid solution, the severity of malnutrition, and the advanced age of these four patients (359). These retrospective data may indicate that anabolic steroids may have a beneficial effect in some malnourished patients undergoing CAPD and that larger prospective studies are needed to clarify the role of treatment with anabolic steroids among these patients as well as the severity of possible adverse effects.

Growth Hormone and Insulinlike Growth Factor-1

Recombinant human growth hormone (rhGH) administration enhances the growth velocity of children undergoing CAPD (360) and may reduce urea generation and improve the efficiency of dietary protein utilization in stable adult patients undergoing hemodialysis (361). Furthermore, the combination of intradialytic parenteral nutrition and rhGH treatment in seven malnourished patients undergoing hemodialysis resulted in improved nutritional parameters (increased serum albumin, transferrin, and IGF-1) as well as in a decreased intradialytic urea appearance, indicating that the treatment promoted net anabolism (362). Similarly, Sinobe et al. reported on decreased urea appearance, improved nitrogen balance, and increased levels of IGF-1 and albumin in 26 patients with hypoalbuminemia undergoing hemodialysis who received rhGH (363). In addition, rhGH treatment has been shown to enhance growth, food efficiency, plasma IGF-1 levels, and the *in vivo* fractional muscle protein synthesis rate (as assessed by 3H-phenylalanine incorporation) in uremic rats (364). Note, however, that the presence of chronic metabolic acidosis resulted in a complete resistance to rhGH for all studied parameters among the uremic rats (364).

A short-term study of rhGH treatment in 10 patients undergoing CAPD was reported in 1994 (365). Treatment with rhGH for 1 week resulted in a decrease in serum urea, PNA, and dialysate urea appearance consistent with a decrease in urea appearance as well as a marked increase in IGF-1 levels, indicating that rhGH treatment had a net anabolic effect (365). Furthermore, administration of rhGH resulted in a decline of essential amino acids, both in plasma and in dialysate, simultaneous with a decrease in serum urea nitrogen, strongly suggesting an increased utilization of essential amino acids for protein anabolism (366). In addition, a randomized study in a small group of 17 malnourished patients undergoing dialysis (hemodialysis and CAPD) showed, after 1 month of rhGH treatment, decreased serum urea levels, increased serum IGF-1 levels, increased body weight and midarm muscular circumference, and reduced triceps skinfold among the patients treated with rhGH ($n = 8$), whereas no differences were found among the controls (n = 9), indicating a protein anabolic affect of the rhGH treatment (367).

Many of the effects of growth hormone are mediated via the IGFs (previously denoted somatomedins) (368). The IGFs are a group of serum proteins that are produced in the liver and have insulinlike metabolic effects (368). The circulating IGFs are bound almost completely to IGF-binding proteins (of which at least six have been identified) (369), and the IGF-binding proteins interact with the biologic activity of the IGFs (370,371). A low serum level of IGF-1 has been reported to be good marker of malnutrition in patients undergoing dialysis (351,372–374) (although this was not confirmed in one study) (375).

Because some individual may become resistant to the anabolic affects of rhGH as a result of malnutrition or uremia (376–379), and this resistance seems to be partly associated with a low IGF-1 response to growth hormone as well as a reduced bioactivity of IGF-1 in uremic serum (371), treatment with IGF-1 was applied in a small study of six patients undergoing CAPD (380). These six patients exhibited a marked anabolic effect within hours after commencing the rhIGF-1 treatment, with a strongly positive nitrogen balance (+2.0 g/day) that was sustained over the 20 days of the study without any sign of attenuation (380). Data from normal humans indicate that the positive nitrogen balance with IGF-1 treatment mainly may be an effect of decreased catabolism rather than net stimulation of anabolism (381).

In the future growth hormone and IGF-1 may turn out to be useful adjunctive therapy to diminish body protein catabolism in patients undergoing CAPD, and one may speculate that the combination of rhGH or IGF-1 treatment with use of dialysis solutions containing amino acids one day may be the treatment of choice for the malnutrition of patients undergoing CAPD. However, larger long-term studies are needed to clarify if the positive effects rhGH and IGF-1 treatment can be sustained for longer time periods, to determine which patients may benefit from the different treatments, and to assess the potential side effects of these hormones.

SUMMARY AND CONCLUSIONS

A large proportion of patients undergoing PD demonstrate signs of protein-energy malnutrition as a result of various factors, including disturbances in protein and energy metabolism, hormonal derangements, infections and other superimposed illnesses, and poor food intake because of anorexia and nausea. Signs of malnutrition have been found to correlate to the MIA syndrome and clinical outcome among patients being treated with PD.

The safe protein requirement in patients undergoing CAPD appears to be increased to about 1.2 g protein/kg/day, which is twice that of normal individuals, although some patients are in neutral balance with a protein intake as low as 0.7 g/kg/day. The nitrogen balance is strongly dependent on the energy intake, which often is lower than the recommended 35 kcal/kg/day in patients undergoing CAPD.

It is important to monitor protein intake (preferably by urea kinetics) and nutritional status (preferably by SGA, body weight, serum albumin, and an estimation of LBM) in patients undergoing PD. Note, however, that a low serum albumin level does not always reflect a poor nutritional status of the patient and that, in the medical decisionmaking process, it is important to consider the multiple factors, other that poor nutrition, that may contribute to low serum albumin concentrations in patients undergoing PD, in particular inflammation and losses of albumin in the dialysate. If the patients have signs of inflammation, such as increased CRP levels, it is important to look for and treat the cause.

Anorexia with low protein and energy intake results from a variety of factors of which underdialysis with insufficient control of uremic toxicity seems to be a major one. Malnourished patients undergoing CAPD should be recommended to increase the protein and energy intake; acidosis also should be corrected, and the dialysis dose should be increased, if possible. Amino acid–based dialysis fluids may provide new opportunities to improve the nutritional status in malnourished patients undergoing CAPD, and treatment with hormones promoting net anabolism may turn out to be a useful adjunctive therapy to diminish body protein catabolism in patients undergoing CAPD in the future.

ACKNOWLEDGMENTS

We acknowledge gratefully the important contributions of our friend, colleague, and mentor Dr. Jonas Bergström for this chapter and for stimulating the authors to participate in and continue his lifelong work in the field of nutrition in renal disease.

REFERENCES

1. Lindholm B, Bergström J. Nutritional requirements of peritoneal dialysis. In: Gokal R, Nolph KD, eds. *Textbook of peritoneal dialysis.* Dordrecht: Kluwer Academic Publishers, 1994; 443–472.
2. May RC. Effects of renal insufficiency on nutrient metabolism and endocrine function. In: Mitch WE, Klahr S, eds. *Nutrition and the kidney.* Boston: Little, Brown and Co, 1993;35–59.
3. Heimbürger O, Qureshi AR, Blanner B, et al. Hand-grip muscle strength, lean body mass and plasma proteins as markers of nutritional status in patients with advanced renal failure. *Am J Kidney Dis* 2000;36:1213–1225.
4. Jansen MAM, Korevaar JC, Dekker FW, et al. Renal function and nutritional status at the start of chronic dialysis treatment. *J Am Soc Nephrol* 2001;12:157–163.
5. McCusker FX, Teehan BP, Thorpe KE, et al. How much perito-

neal dialysis is required for the maintenance of a good nutritional state? *Kidney Int* 1996;50(Suppl 56):S56–S61.
6. Chung SH, Lindholm B, Lee HB. Influence of initial nutritional status on continuous ambulatory peritoneal dialysis patient survival. *Perit Dial Int* 2000;20:19–26.
7. Ikizler TA, Greene J, Wingard RL, et al. Spontaneous dietary protein intake during progression of chronic renal failure. *J Am Soc Nephrol* 1995;6:1386–1391.
8. Stenvinkel P, Heimbürger O, Lindholm B, et al. Are there two types of malnutrition in chronic renal failure? *Nephrol Dial Transplant* 2000;15:953–960.
9. Jager KJ, Merkus MP, Huisman RM, et al. Nutritional status over time in haemodialysis and peritoneal dialysis. *J Am Soc Nephrol* 2001;12:1272–1279.
10. Ganter G. Über die Beseitigung giftiger Stoffe aus dem Blute durch Dialyse. *Münch Med Wochenshcr* 1923;70:1478–1480.
11. Fine J, Frank HA, Seligman AM. The treatment of acute renal failure by peritoneal irrigation. *Ann Surg* 1946;124:857–875.
12. Grollman A, Turner LB, McLean JA. Intermittent peritoneal lavage in nephrectomized dogs and its application to the human being. *Arch Intern Med* 1951;87:379–390.
13. Maxwell MH, Rockney RE, Kleeman CR, et al. Peritoneal dialysis, techniques and applications. *JAMA* 1959;170:917–924.
14. Boen ST, Mion CM, Curtis FK, et al. Periodic peritoneal dialysis using the repeated puncture technique and an automatic cycling machine. *ASAIO Trans* 1964;10:409–413.
15. Gurland HJ, Brunner FP, Chantler C, et al. Combined report on regular dialysis and transplantation in Europe, VI, 1975. In: Robinson BHB, Vereestraeten P, Hawkins JB, eds. *Dialysis, transplantation, nephrology. Proceedings of the 13th Congress of the EDTA, held in Hamburg, Germany, 1976.* London: Pitman Medical, 1976;2–58.
16. Popovich RP, Moncrief JW, Decherd JF, et al. The definition of a novel portable/wearable equilibrium peritoneal dialysis technique. *Abstracts ASAIO* 1976;5:64.
17. Popovich RP, Moncrief JW, Nolph KD, et al. Continuous ambulatory peritoneal dialysis. *Ann Intern Med* 1978;88:449–456.
18. Oreopoulos DG, Khanna R, Williams P, et al. A simple and safe technique for continuous ambulatory peritoneal dialysis (CAPD). *ASAIO Trans* 1978;24:484–489.
19. Nolph KD, Popovich RP, Moncrief JW. Theoretical and practical implications of continuous ambulatory peritoneal dialysis. *Nephron* 1978;21:117–122.
20. Madden MA, Zimmerman SW, Simpson DP. Longitudinal comparison of intermittent versus continuous ambulatory peritoneal dialysis, in the same patients. *Clin Nephrol* 1981;16: 293–299.
21. Lacke C, Senekjian HO, Knight TF, et al. Twelve months' experience with continuous ambulatory and intermittent peritoneal dialysis. *Arch Intern Med* 1981;141:187–190.
22. Lindholm B, Bergström J. Nutritional management of patients undergoing peritoneal dialysis. In: Nolph KD, ed. *Peritoneal dialysis.* Dordrecht: Kluwer Academic Publishers, 1989; 230–260.
23. Bergström J, Lindholm B. Nutrition and adequacy of dialysis. How do hemodialysis and CAPD compare? *Kidney Int* 1993; 43 (Suppl 40):S39–S50.
24. DeSanto NG, Capodicasa G, Senatore R, et al. Glucose utilization from dialysate in patients on CAPD. *Int J Artif Organs* 1979;2:119–125.
25. Heimbürger O, Waniewski J, Werynski A, et al. A quantitative description of solute and fluid transport during peritoneal dialysis. *Kidney Int* 1992;41:1320–1332.
26. Young GA, Kopple JD, Lindholm B, et al. Nutritional assessment of continuous ambulatory peritoneal dialysis patients: an international study. *Am J Kidney Dis* 1991;17:462–471.
27. Bergström J. Protein catabolic factors in patients on renal replacement therapy. In-depth review. *Blood Purif* 1985;3: 215–236.
28. Detsky AS, McLaughlin JR, Baker JP, et al. What is subjective global assessment? *J Parenteral Enteral Nutr* 1987;11:8–13.
29. Baker JP, Detsky AS, Wesson DE, et al. Nutritional assessment: a comparison of clinical judgement and objective measurements. *N Engl J Med* 1982;16:969–972.
30. Jeejeebhoy KN, Detsky AS, Baker JP. Assessment of nutritional status. *J Parenteral Enteral Nutr* 1990;14:193S–196S.
31. Enia G, Sicuso C, Alati G, et al. Subjective global assessment of nutrition in dialysis patients. *Nephrol Dial Transplant* 1993; 8:1094–1098.
32. Fenton SSA, Johnston N, Delmore T, et al. Nutritional assessment of continuous ambulatory peritoneal dialysis patients. *ASAIO Trans* 1987;33:650–653.
33. Qureshi AR, Alvestrand A, Danielsson A, et al. Factors predicting malnutrition in hemodialysis patients: a cross-sectional study. *Kidney Int* 1998;53:773–782.
34. CANADA-USA (CANUSA) Peritoneal Dialysis Study Group. Adequacy of dialysis and nutrition in continuous ambulatory peritoneal dialysis: Association with clinical outcomes. *J Am Soc Nephrol* 1996;7:198–207.
35. Heimbürger O, Bergström J, Lindholm B. Is serum albumin an indication of nutritional status in CAPD patients? *Perit Dial Int* 1994;14:108–114.
36. Kaysen GA, Schoenfeld PY. Albumin homeostasis in patients undergoing continuous ambulatory peritoneal dialysis. *Kidney Int* 1984;25:107–114.
37. Fleck A, Raines G, Hawker F, et al. Increased vascular permeability: a major cause of hypoalbuminemia in disease and injury. *Lancet* 1985;I:781–784.
38. Klein S. The myth of serum albumin as a measure of nutritional status. *Gastroenterology* 1990;99:1845–1846.
39. Marik PE. The treatment of hypoalbuminemia in the critically ill patient. *Heart Lung* 1993;22:166–170.
40. Schoenfeld PY. Albumin is an unreliable marker of nutritional status. *Semin Dial* 1992;5:218–223.
41. Kaysen GA, Rathore V, Shearer GC, et al. Mechanisms of hypoalbuminemia in hemodialysis patients. *Kidney Int* 1995;48: 510–516.
42. Yeun JY, Kaysen GA. Acute phase proteins and peritoneal dialysate albumin loss are the main determinants of serum albumin in peritoneal dialysis patients. *Am J Kidney Dis* 1997;30:923–927.
43. Koomen GCM, van Straalen JP, Boeschoten EW, et al. Comparison between dye binding methods and nephelometry for the measurement of albumin in plasma of peritoneal dialysis (abstract). *Perit Dial Int* 1992;12(Suppl 1):S133.
44. Blagg CR, Liedtke RJ, Batjer JD, et al. Serum albumin concentration-related health care financing administration quality assurance criterion is method-dependent: revision is necessary. *Am J Kidney Dis* 1993;21:138–144.
45. Leerink CB, Winckers EK. Multilayer-film bromcresol green method for albumin measurement significantly inaccurate when albumin/globulin ratio is less than 0.8. *Clin Chem* 1991;223: 626–633.
46. Rothschild MA, Oratz M, Schreiber SS. Albumin synthesis (first of two parts). *N Engl J Med* 1972;286:748–757.
47. Rothschild MA, Oratz M, Schreiber SS. Albumin metabolism. *Gastroenterology* 1973;64:324–337.
48. Young GA, Young JB, Young SM, et al. Nutrition and delayed hypersensitivity during continuous ambulatory peritoneal dialysis in relation to peritonitis. *Nephron* 1986;43:177–186.
49. Pollock CA, Ibels LS, Caterson RJ, et al. Continuous ambulatory peritoneal dialysis, eight years of experience at a single center. *Medicine* 1989;68:293–308.

50. Nolph KD, Moore HL, Prowant B, et al. Cross-sectional assessment of weekly urea and creatinine clearance and indices of nutrition in continuous ambulatory peritoneal dialysis patients. *Perit Dial Int* 1993;13:178–183.
51. Spinowitz BS, Gupta BK, Kulogowski J, et al. Dialysis adequacy in hypoalbuminemic continuous ambulatory peritoneal dialysis patients. *Perit Dial Int* 1993;13(Suppl 2):S221–S223.
52. Lindsay RM, Spanner E. The lower serum albumin does reflect nutritional status. *Semin Dial* 1992;5:215–218.
53. Germain M, Harlow P, Mulhern J, et al. Low protein catabolic rate and serum albumin correlate with increased mortality and abdominal complications in peritoneal dialysis patients. In: Khanna R, Nolph KD, Prowant BF, et al., eds. *Advances in peritoneal dialysis 1992.* Toronto: Peritoneal Publications, Inc., 1992;113–115.
54. Heimbürger O, Bergström J, Lindholm B. Albumin and amino acids as markers of adequacy in CAPD. *Perit Dial Int* 1994; 14(Suppl 3):S123–S132.
55. Blake PG, Sombolos K, Abraham G, et al. Lack of correlation between urea kinetic indices and clinical outcome in CAPD patients. *Kidney Int* 1991;39:700–706.
56. Cancarini G, Constantino E, Brunori G, et al. Nutritional status in long-term CAPD patients. In: Khanna R, Nolph KD, Prowant BF, et al., eds. *Advances in peritoneal dialysis 1992.* Toronto: Peritoneal Publications, Inc., 1992;84–87.
57. Kumano K, Takagi Y, Yokata S, et al. Urea kinetics and clinical features of long-term continuous ambulatory peritoneal dialysis patients. *Perit Dial Int* 1993;13(Suppl 2):S180–S182.
58. Teehan BP, Schleifer CR, Brown JM, et al. Urea kinetic analysis and clinical outcome on CAPD. A five year longitudinal study. In: Khanna R, Nolph KD, Prowant BF, et al., eds. *Advances in peritoneal dialysis 1990.* Toronto: University of Toronto Press, 1990;181–185.
59. Abdo F, Clemente L, Davy J, et al. Nutritional status and efficiency of dialysis in CAPD and CCPD patients. In: Khanna R, Nolph KD, Prowant BF, et al., eds. *Advances in peritoneal dialysis 1993.* Toronto: Peritoneal Publications, Inc., 1993; 76–79.
60. Shimomura A, Tahara D, Azekura H. Nutritional improvement in elderly CAPD patients with additional high protein foods. In: Khanna R, Nolph KD, Prowant BF, et al., eds. *Advances in peritoneal dialysis 1993.* Toronto: Peritoneal Publications, Inc., 1993;80–86.
61. Moshage HJ, Janssen JAM, Franssen JH, et al. Study of the molecular mechanisms of decreased liver synthesis of albumin in inflammation. *J Clin Invest* 1987;79:1635–1641.
62. Kaysen GA. Hypoalbuminemia in dialysis patients. *Semin Dial* 1996;9:249–256.
63. Kaysen GA. Biological bases of hypoalbuminemia in ESRD. *J Am Soc Nephrol* 1998;9:2368–2376.
64. Qureshi AR, Alvestrand A, Divino-Filho JC, et al. Inflammation, malnutrition and cardiac disease as predictors of mortality in hemodialysis patients. *J Am Soc Nephrol* 2002;13(Suppl 1): S28–S36.
65. Zimmermann J, Herrlinger S, Pruy A, et al. Inflammation enhances cardiovascular risk and mortality in hemodialysis patients. *Kidney Int* 1999;55:648–658.
66. Yeun JY, Levine RA, Mantadilok V, et al. C-reactive protein predicts all-cause and cardiovascular mortality in hemodialysis patients. *Am J Kidney Dis* 2000;35:469–476.
67. Rothschild MA, Oratz M, Evans CD, et al. Role of hepatic interstitial albumin in regulating albumin synthesis. *Am J Physiol* 1966;210:57–68.
68. Jones CH, Smye SW, Newstead CG, et al. Extracellular fluid volume determined by bioelectric impedance and serum albumin in CAPD patients. *Nephrol Dial Transplant* 1998;13: 393–397.
69. Kagan A, Bar-Khayim Y, Schafer Z, et al. Kinetics of peritoneal protein loss during CAPD: I. Different characteristics for low and high molecular weight proteins. *Kidney Int* 1990;37: 971–979.
70. Lamb E, Buhler R, Cattell WR, et al. Albumin transport during the peritoneal equilibration test (PET): relationship to solute transport and effect of diabetes (abstract). *J Am Soc Nephrol* 1991;2:364.
71. Blake PG, Flowerdew G, Blake RM, et al. Serum albumin in patients on continuous ambulatory peritoneal dialysis—Predictors and correlations with outcomes. *J Am Soc Nephrol* 1993; 3:1501–1507.
72. Struijk DG, Krediet RT, Koomen GCM, et al. The effect of serum albumin at the start of CAPD treatment on patient survival. *Perit Dial Int* 1994;14:121–126.
73. Saxenhofer H, Scheidegger J, Descoeudres C, et al. Impact of dialysis modality on body composition in patients with end-stage renal disease. *Clin Nephrol* 1992;38:219–223.
74. Buchwald R, Peña JC. Evaluation of nutritional status in patients on continuous ambulatory peritoneal dialysis (CAPD). *Perit Dial Int* 1989;9:295–301.
75. Rubin J, Flynn MA, Nolph KD. Total body potassium—a guide to nutritional health in patients undergoing continuous ambulatory peritoneal dialysis. *Am J Clin Nutr* 1981;34:94–98.
76. de Fijter CWH, Oe LP, de Fijter MW, et al. Is serum albumin a marker for nutritional status in dialysis patients? (abstract). *J Am Soc Nephrol* 1993;4:402.
77. Saxenhofer H, Horber FF, Jaeger P. Predictors of nutritional status in CAPD patients (abstract). *J Am Soc Nephrol* 1993;4: 416.
78. Goodship THJ, Lloyd S, Clague MB, et al. Whole body leucine turnover and nutritional status in continuous ambulatory peritoneal dialysis. *Clin Sci* 1987;73:463–469.
79. Sreedhara R, Avram MM, Blanco M, et al. Prealbumin is the best nutritional predictor of survival in hemodialysis and peritoneal dialysis. *Am J Kidney Dis* 1996;28:937–942.
80. Avram MM, Sreedhara R, Fein P, et al. Survival in hemodialysis and peritoneal dialysis over 12 years with emphasis of nutritional parameters. *Am J Kidney Dis* 2001;37(Suppl 2):S77–S88.
81. Qureshi ART. *Malnutrition in patients with chronic renal failure.* PhD Thesis. Stockholm: Karolinska Institutet, 2000.
82. Lindholm B, Alvestrand A, Fürst P, et al. Plasma and muscle free amino acids during continuous ambulatory peritoneal dialysis. *Kidney Int* 1989;35:1219–1226.
83. Kerr PG, Strauss BJG, Atkins RC. Assessment of the nutritional state of dialysis patients. *Blood Purif* 1996;14:382–387.
84. Johansson A-C, Samuelsson O, Haraldsson B, et al. Body composition in patients treated with peritoneal dialysis. *Nephrol Dial Transpl* 1998;13:1511–1517.
85. Johansson A-C, Haraldsson B. Body composition and comorbidity in long term peritoneal dialysis (abstract). *J Am Soc Nephrol* 2000;11:210A.
86. Jones CH, Newstead CG, Will EJ, et al. Assessment of nutritional status in CAPD patients: serum albumin is not a useful measure. *Nephrol Dial Transplant* 1997;12:1406–1413.
87. Abrahamsen B, Hansen TB, Høgsberg IM, et al. Impact of hemodialysis on dual energy X-ray absorptiometry, bioelectrical impedance measurements, and anthropometry. *Am J Clin Nutr* 1996;63:80–86.
88. Jebb SA, Elia M. Techniques for the measurement of body composition: a practical guide. *Int J Obes Relat Metab Disord* 1993;17:611–621.
89. Borovnicar DJ, Wong KC, Kerr PG, et al. Total body protein

status assessed by different estimates of fat-free mass in adult peritoneal dialysis patients. *Eur J Clin Nutr* 1996;50:607–616.
90. Durnin JVGA, Womersley J. Body fat assessed from total body density and its estimation from skinfolds thickness: measurements on 481 men and women aged from 16 to 72 years. *Br J Nutr* 1974;32:77–79.
91. Keshaviah P, Nolph KD, Moore HL, et al. Lean body mass estimation by creatinine kinetics. *J Am Soc Nephrol* 1994;4: 1475–1485.
92. Johansson A-C, Attman P-O, Haraldsson B. Creatinine generation rate and lean body mass: a critical analysis in peritoneal dialysis patients. *Kidney Int* 1997;51:855–859.
93. Szeto CC, Kong J, Wu AKL, et al. The role of lean body mass as a nutritional index in Chinese peritoneal dialysis patients—comparison of creatinine kinetics method and anthropometric method. *Perit Dial Int* 2000;20:708–714.
94. Bhatla B, Moore H, Emerson P, et al. Lean body mass estimation by creatinine kinetics, bioimpedance, and dual energy X-ray absorptiometry in patients on continuous ambulatory peritoneal dialysis. *ASAIO J* 1995;41:M442–M446.
95. Nielsen PK, Ladefoged J, Olgaard K. Lean body mass by dual energy x-ray absorptiometry (DEXA) and by urine and dialysate creatinine recovery in CAPD and pre-dialysis patients compared to normal subjects. *Adv Perit Dial* 1994;10:99–103.
96. Forbes GB, Bruining GJ. Urinary creatinine excretion and lean body mass. *Am J Clin Nutr* 1976;29:1359–1366.
97. Blake PG, Chu KH. Creatinine production and excretion in end-stage renal disease. *Am J Kidney Dis* 2001;38:1119–1121.
98. Jackson AS, Pollock ML, Graves JE, et al. Reliability and validity of bioelectrical impedance in determining body composition. *J Appl Physiol* 1988;64(2):529–534.
99. Deurenberg P, van der Kooij K, Evers P, et al. Assessment of body composition by bioelectrical impedance in a population aged greater than 60 y. *Am J Clin Nutr* 1990;51:3–6.
100. Williams P, Kay R, Harrison J, et al. Nutritional and anthropometric assessment of patients on CAPD over one year: Contrasting changes in total body nitrogen and potassium. *Perit Dial Bull* 1981;1:82–87.
101. Dombros N, Oren A, Marliss EB, et al. Plasma amino acid profiles and amino acid losses in patients undergoing CAPD. *Perit Dial Bull* 1982;2:27–32.
102. Kopple JD, Blumenkrantz MJ, Jones MR, et al. Plasma amino acid levels and amino acid losses during continuous ambulatory peritoneal dialysis. *Am J Clin Nutr* 1982;36:395–402.
103. Heide B, Pierratos A, Khanna R, et al. Nutritional status of patients undergoing continuous ambulatory peritoneal dialysis (CAPD). *Perit Dial Bull* 1983;3:138–141.
104. Marckmann P. Nutritional status of patients on hemodialysis and peritoneal dialysis. *Clin Nephrol* 1988;29:75–78.
105. Harty JC, Boulton H, Curwell J, et al. The normalized protein catabolic rate is a flawed marker of nutrition in CAPD patients. *Kidney Int* 1994;45:103–109.
106. Flanigan MJ, Bailie GR, Frankenfield DL, et al. 1996 peritoneal dialysis core indicators study: report on nutritional indicators. *Perit Dial Int* 1998;18:489–496.
107. Kumano K, Kawaguchi Y, and the group for Water and Electrolyte Balance Study in CAPD. Multicenter cross-sectional study for dialysis dose and physician's subjective judgement in Japanese peritoneal dialysis patients. *Am J Kidney Dis* 2000;35: 515–525.
108. Jones MR. Etiology of severe malnutrition: results of an international cross-sectional study in continuous ambulatory peritoneal dialysis patients. *Am J Kidney Dis* 1994;23:412–420.
109. Nelson EE, Hong CD, Pesce AL, et al. Anthropometric norms for the dialysis population. *Am J Kidney Dis* 1990;16:32–37.
110. Cianciaruso B, Brunori G, Kopple JD, et al. Cross-sectional comparison of malnutrition in continuous ambulatory peritoneal dialysis and hemodialysis patients. *Am J Kidney Dis* 1995; 26:475–486.
111. Maiorca R, Cancarini GC, Camerini C, et al. Is CAPD competitive with hemodialysis for long-term treatment of uremic patients? *Nephrol Dial Transplant* 1989;4:244–253.
112. Pollock CA, Allen BJ, Warden RA, et al. Total body nitrogen by neutron activation in maintenance dialysis. *Am J Kidney Dis* 1990;16:38–45.
113. Marckmann P. Nutritional status and mortality of patients in regular dialysis therapy. *J Int Med* 1989;226:429–432.
114. Keshaviah P, Churchill DN, Thorpe K, et al. Impact of nutrition on CAPD mortality (abstract). *J Am Soc Nephrol* 1994.
115. Jager KJ, Merkus MP, Dekker FW, et al. Mortality and technique failure in patients starting chronic peritoneal dialysis: results of the Netherlands Cooperative Study on the Adequacy of Dialysis. *Kidney Int* 1999;55:1476–1485.
116. Lowrie EG, Lew NL. Death risk in hemodialysis patients: the predictive value of commonly measured variables and an evaluation of death rate differences between facilities. *Am J Kidney Dis* 1990;15:458–482.
117. Oksa H, Ahonen K, Pasternack A, et al. Malnutrition in hemodialysis patients. *Scand J Urol Nephrol* 1991;25:157–161.
118. Degoulet P, Legrain M, Réach I, et al. Mortality risk factors in patients treated by chronic hemodialysis. *Nephron* 1982;31: 103–110.
119. Bilbrey GL, Cohen TL. Identification and treatment of protein calorie malnutrition in chronic hemodialysis patients. *Dial Transplant* 1989;18:669–677.
120. Maiorca R, Vonesh E, Cancarini GC, et al. A six year comparison of patient and technique survivals in CAPD and HD. *Kidney Int* 1988;34:518–524.
121. Maiorca R, Vonesh EF, Cavalli PL, et al. A multicenter, selection-adjusted comparison of patient and technique survivals on CAPD and hemodialysis. *Perit Dial Int* 1991;114:118–127.
122. Teehan BP, Schleifer CR, Brown J. Urea kinetic modelling is an appropriate assessment of adequacy. *Semin Dial* 1992;5: 189–192.
123. Gamba G, Mejía JL, Saldívar S, et al. Death risk in CAPD patients. *Nephron* 1993;65:23–27.
124. Spiegel DM, Andersson M, Campbell U, et al. Serum albumin: a marker for morbidity in peritoneal dialysis patients. *Am J Kidney Dis* 1993;21:26–30.
125. Selgas R, Bajo MA, Fernandez-Reyes MJ, et al. An analysis of adequacy of dialysis in a selected population on CAPD for over three years: the influence of urea and creatinine kinetics. *Nephrol Dial Transplant* 1993;8:1244–1253.
126. Spiegel DM, Breyer JA. Serum albumin: a predictor of long-term outcome in peritoneal dialysis patients. *Am J Kidney Dis* 1994;23:283–285.
127. Avram MM, Goldwasser P, Erroa M, et al. Predictors of survival in continuous ambulatory peritoneal dialysis patients: The importance of prealbumin and other nutritional and metabolic markers. *Am J Kidney Dis* 1994;23:91–98.
128. Winchester J. The albumin dilemma. *Am J Kidney Dis* 1992; 20:76–77.
129. Fine A, Cox D. Modest reduction of serum albumin in continuous ambulatory peritoneal dialysis patients is common and of no apparent clinical consequence. *Am J Kidney Dis* 1992;20: 50–54.
130. Genestier S, Hedelin G, Schaffer P, et al. Prognostic factors in CAPD patients: a retrospective study of a 10-year period. *Nephrol Dial Transpl* 1995;10:1905–1911.
131. Stenvinkel P, Heimbürger O, Paultre F, et al. Strong association between malnutrition, inflammation, and atherosclerosis in chronic renal failure. *Kidney Int* 1999;55:1899–1911.

132. Haubitz M, Brunkhorst R, Wrenger E, et al. Chronic induction of C-reactive protein by hemodialysis, but not by peritoneal dialysis therapy. *Perit Dial Int* 1996;16:158–162.
133. Kimmel PL, Phillips TM, Simmens SJ, et al. Immunologic function and survival in hemodialysis patients. *Kidney Int* 1998;54: 236–244.
134. Pereira BJG, Shapiro L, King AJ, et al. Plasma levels of IL-1b, TNF-a and their specific inhibitors in undialyzed chronic renal failure, CAPD and hemodialysis patients. *Kidney Int* 1994;45: 890–896.
135. Herzig KA, Purdie DM, Chang W, et al. Is C-reactive protein a useful predictor of outcome in peritoneal dialysis patients? *J Am Soc Nephrol* 2001;12:814–821.
136. Noh H, Lee SW, Kang SW, et al. Serum C-reactive protein: a predictor of mortality in continuous ambulatory peritoneal dialysis. *Perit Dial Int* 1998;18:387–394.
137. Bologa RM, Levine DM, Parker TS, et al. Interleukin-6 predicts hypoalbuminemia, hypocholesterolemia, and mortality in hemodialysis patients. *Am J Kidney Dis* 1998;32:107–114.
138. Pecoits-Filho R, Bárány P, Lindholm B, et al. Interleukin-6 is in an independent predictor of mortality in patients starting dialysis treatment. *Nephrol Dial Transplant* 2002;17: 1684–1688.
139. Kaizu Y, Kimura M, Yoneyama T, et al. Interleukin-6 may mediate malnutrition in chronic hemodialysis patients. *Am J Kidney Disease* 1998;31:93–100.
140. Stenvinkel P, Heimbürger O, Jogestrand T. Elevated interleukin-6 predicts progressive carotid artery atherosclerosis in dialysis patients: association to chlamydia pneumoniae seropositivity. *Am J Kidney Dis* 2002;39:274–282.
141. Young VR. Nutritional requirements in normal adults. In: Mitch WE, Klahr S, eds. *Nutrition and the kidney.* Boston: Little, Brown and Company, 1993;1–34.
142. Chandra RK. Nutrition, immunity, and infection: present knowledge and future direction. *Lancet* 1983;i:688–691.
143. FAO/WHO. *Energy and protein requirements, Report of a joint FAO/WHO ad hoc Expert Committee. Tech Rep Ser No 522.* Geneva: World Health Organization; 1973.
144. National Kidney Foundation. K/DOQI clinical practice guidelines for nutrition in chronic renal failure. *Am J Kidney Dis* 2000;35(Suppl 2):S1–S140.
145. Kopple JD. The national kidney foundation K/DOQI clinical practice guidelines for dietary protein intake for chronic dialysis patients. *Am J Kidney Dis* 2001;38(Suppl 1):S68–S73.
146. Blumenkrantz MJ, Kopple JD, Moran JK, et al. Metabolic balance studies and dietary protein requirements in patients undergoing continuous ambulatory peritoneal dialysis. *Kidney Int* 1982;21:849–861.
147. Bergström J, Fürst P, Alvestrand A, et al. Protein and energy intake, nitrogen balance and nitrogen losses in patients treated with continuous ambulatory peritoneal dialysis. *Kidney Int* 1993;44:1048–1057.
148. Blake PG. Urea kinetic modelling is of no proven benefit. *Semin Dial* 1992;5:193–196.
149. Lindholm B, Heimbürger O, Ahlberg M, et al. Urea kinetic modelling in peritoneal dialysis. In: Lopot F, ed. *Urea kinetic modelling.* Ruddervoorde: EDTNA-ERCA, 1990;134–146.
150. Randerson DH, Chapman GV, Farrell PC. Amino acids and dietary status in CAPD patients. In: Atkins RC, Thomson NM, Farrell PC, eds. *Peritoneal dialysis.* Edinburgh: Churchill Livingstone, 1981;179–191.
151. Bergström J, Heimbürger O, Lindholm B. Calculation of the protein equivalent of total nitrogen appearance from urea appearance. Which formulas should be used? *Perit Dial Int* 1998; 18:467–473.
152. Monteon FJ, Laidlaw SA, Shaib JK, et al. Energy expenditure in patients with chronic renal failure. *Kidney Int* 1986;30: 741–747.
153. Harty J, Conway L, Keegan M, et al. Energy metabolism during CAPD—a controlled study. *Adv Perit Dial* 1995;11:229–233.
154. Marckmann. Dialyse patienters kost bestemt ved 7 dages kostregistrering. *Ugeskr Laeger* 1990;152:317–320.
155. Gilmour ER, Hartley GH, Goodship THJ. Trace elements and vitamins in renal disease. In: Mitch WE, Klahr S, eds. *Nutrition and the kidney.* Boston: Little, Brown and Co, 1993;114–131.
156. Chazot C, Kopple JD. Vitamin metabolism and requirements in renal disease and renal failure. In: Kopple JD, Massry SG, eds. *Nutritional management of renal disease.* Baltimore: Williams & Wilkins, 1997;415–477.
157. Kopple JD, Hirschberg R. Nutrition and peritoneal dialysis. In: Mitch WE, Klahr S, eds. *Nutrition and the kidney.* Boston: Little, Brown and Co, 1993;114–131.
158. Blumberg A, Hanck A, Sander G. Vitamin nutrition in patients on continuous ambulatory peritoneal dialysis (CAPD). *Clin Nephrol* 1983;20:244–250.
159. Henderson IS, Leung ACT, Shenkin A. Vitamin status in continuous ambulatory peritoneal dialysis. *Perit Dial Bull* 1984;4: 143–145.
160. Boeshoten EW, Schriever J, Krediet RT, et al. Vitamin deficiencies in CAPD patients. *Perit Dial Bull* 1984;4(Suppl):S7.
161. Boeshoten EW, Schriever J, Krediet RT, et al. Deficiencies of vitamins in CAPD patients: the effect of supplementation. *Nephrol Dial Transpl* 1988;2:187–193.
162. Hung SC, Hung SH, Tarng DC, et al. Thiamine deficiency and unexplained encephalopathy in hemodialysis and peritoneal dialysis patients. *Am J Kidney Dis* 2001;38:941–947.
163. Kopple JD, Mercurio K, Blumenkrantz MJ, et al. Daily requirement for pyridoxine supplements in chronic renal failure. *Kidney Int* 1981;19:694–704.
164. Kleiner MJ, Tate SS, Sullivan JF, et al. Vitamin B6 deficiency in maintenance dialysis patients: metabolic effects of repletion. *Am J Clin Nutr* 1980;33:1612–1619.
165. Arnadottir M, Brattström L, Simonsen O, et al. The effect of high dose pyridoxine and folic acid supplementation on serum lipid and plasma homocysteine concentrations in dialysis patients. *Clin Nephrol* 1993;40:236–240.
166. Boaz M, Smetana S, Weinstein T, et al. Secondary prevention with antioxidants of cardiovascular disease in endstage renal disease (SPACE): randomised placebo-controlled trial. *Lancet* 2000;356:1213–1218.
167. Moorthy AV, Rosenbaum M, Rajaram R, et al. A comparison of plasma and muscle carnitine levels in patients on peritoneal and hemodialysis for chronic renal failure. *Am J Nephrol* 1983; 3:205–208.
168. Amair P, Gregordiadis A, Rodela H, et al. Serum carnitine in patients on continuous ambulatory peritoneal dialysis (CAPD). *Perit Dial Bull* 1982;2:11–12.
169. Wanner C, Hörl WH. Carnitine abnormalities in patients with renal insufficiency. *Nephron* 1988;50:89–102.
170. Hurot JM, Cucherat M, Haugh M, et al. Effects of L-carnitine supplementation in maintenance hemodialysis patients: a systematic review. *J Am Soc Nephrol* 2002;13:708–714.
171. Schoenheyder F, Heilskov NSC, Olsen K. Isotopic studies on the mechanism of negative nitrogen balance produced by immobilization. *Scand J Clin Bal Invest* 1954;6:178–188.
172. Dobell E, Chan M, Williams P, et al. Food preferences and food habits of patients with chronic renal failure undergoing dialysis. *J Am Diet Assoc* 1993;93:1129–1135.
173. Guarnieri G, Toigo G, Situlin R, et al. Muscle biopsy studies in chronically uremic patients: evidence for malnutrition. *Kidney Int* 1983;24(Suppl 16):S187–S193.

174. Lysaght MJ, Pollock CA, Hallet MD, et al. The relevance of urea kinetic modeling to CAPD. *ASAIO Trans* 1989;35:784–790.
175. Szeto CC, Lai KN, Wong TYH, et al. Independent effect of residual renal function and dialysis adequacy on nutritional status and patient outcome in continuous ambulatory peritoneal dialysis. *Am J Kidney Dis* 1999;34:1056–1064.
176. Cho DK. Nutritional status in long-term peritoneal dialysis. *Perit Dial Int* 1999;19(Suppl 2):S337–S340.
177. Kang DH, Lee R, Lee HY, et al. Metabolic acidosis and composite nutritional index (CNI) in CAPD patients. *Clin Nephrol* 2000;53:124–131.
178. Stein A, Moorhouse J, Iles-Smith H, et al. Role of an improvement in acid-base status and nutrition in CAPD patients. *Kidney Int* 1997;52:1089–1095.
179. von Bayer H, Gahl GM, Riedinger H, et al. Adaptation of CAPD patients to the continuous peritoneal energy uptake. *Kidney Int* 1983;23:29–34.
180. Kishi K, Miytani K, Inoue G. Requirement and utilization of egg protein by Japanese young men with marginal intakes of energy. *J Nutr* 1978;198:658–669.
181. Lindholm B, Berström J. Nutritional aspects on peritoneal dialysis. *Kidney Int* 1993;42(Suppl 38):165–171.
182. Fernström A, Hylander B, Rössner S. Energy intake in patients on continuous ambulatory peritoneal dialysis and hemodialysis. *J Intern Med* 1996;240:211–218.
183. Uribarri J, Leibowitz J, Dimaano F. Caloric intake in a group of peritoneal dialysis patients. *Am J Kidney Dis* 1998;32: 1019–1022.
184. Bergström J. Malnutrition in patients on renal replacement therapy. In: Andreucci VE, Fine LG, eds. *International yearbook of nephrology 1993.* London: Springer-Verlag, 1993;245–265.
185. Lindsay RM, Spanner E. A hypothesis: the protein catabolic rate is dependent on the type and amount of treatment in dialyzed uremic patients. *Am J Kidney Dis* 1989;13:382–389.
186. Goodship THJ, Passlick-Deetjen J, Ward MK, et al. Adequacy of dialysis and nutritional status in CAPD. *Nephrol Dial Transplant* 1993;8:1366–1371.
187. Ronco C, Conz P, Agostini F, et al. The concept of adequacy in peritoneal dialysis. *Perit Dial Int* 1994;14(Suppl 3):S93–S98.
188. Gotch FA. Dependence of normalized protein catabolic rate on Kt/V in continuous ambulatory peritoneal dialysis: Not a mathematical artifact. *Perit Dial Int* 1993;13:173–175.
189. Stein A, Walls J. The correlation between Kt/V and protein catabolic rate—a self-fulfilling prophecy. *Nephrol Dial Transplant* 1994;9:743–745.
190. Harty J, Venning M, Gokal R. Does CAPD guarantee adequate dialysis delivery and nutrition. *Nephrol Dial Transplant* 1994; 9:1721–1723.
191. Heimbürger O, Tranæus A, Bergström J, et al. The effect of increased PD on Kt/V, protein catabolic rate (PCR) and serum albumin (abstract). *Perit Dial Int* 1992;12(Suppl 2):S19.
192. Burkart J, Jordan J, Garchow S, et al. Using a computer kinetic modelling program to prescribe PD (abstract). *Perit Dial Int* 1993;13(Suppl 1):S77.
193. Mak SK, Wong PN, Lo KY, et al. Randomized prospective trial study of the effect of increased dialytic dose on nutritional and clinical outcome in continuous ambulatory peritoneal dialysis patients. *Am J Kidney Dis* 2000;36:105–114.
194. Szeto CC, Wong TY, Chow KM, et al. The impact of increasing daytime dialysis exchange frequency on the peritoneal dialysis adequacy and dietary protein intake in anuric Chinese patients (abstract). *J Am Soc Nephrol* 2001;12:457A.
195. Lindholm B, Alvestrand A, Fürst P, et al. Efficacy and clinical experience of CAPD—Stockholm, Sweden. In: Atkins R, Thomson N, Farrell PC, eds. *Peritoneal Dialysis.* Edinburgh: Churchill Livingstone, 1981;147–161.
196. Oreopoulos DG, Marliss E, Anderson GH, et al. Nutritional aspects of CAPD and the potential use of amino acid containing dialysis solutions. *Perit Dial Bull* 1983;3(Suppl 3):S10–S15.
197. Björvell H, Hylander B. Functional status and personality in patients on chronic dialysis. *J Intern Med* 1990;226:319–324.
198. Anderson JE, Yim KB, Crowell MD. Prevalence of gastroesophageal reflux in peritoneal dialysis and hemodialysis patients. *Adv Perit Dial* 1999;75–78.
199. Fernström A, Hylander B, Grytbäck P, et al. Gastric emptying and electrogastrography in patients on CAPD. *Perit Dial Int* 1999;19:429–437.
200. Brown-Cartwright D, Smith HJ, Feldman G. Gastric emptying of indigestible solid??? in patients with end-stage renal disease on continuous ambulatory peritoneal dialysis. *Gastroenterology* 1988;95:49–51.
201. Bird NJ, Streather CP, O'Dohery MJ, et al. Gastric emptying in patients with chronic renal failure on continuous ambulatory peritoneal dialysis. *Nephrol Dial Transplant* 1993;9:287–290.
202. Grodstein PA, Harrison A, Roberts C, et al. Impaired gastric emptying in hemodialysis patients (abstract). *Kidney Int* 1979; 16:952A.
203. Van Vlem B, Schoonjans R, Vanholder R, et al. Delayed gastric emptying in dyspeptic chronic hemodialysis patients. *Am J Kidney Dis* 2000;36:962–968.
204. Hylander BI, Dalton CB, Castell DO, et al. Effect of intraperitoneal fluid volume changes on esophageal pressure: studies in patients on continuous ambulatory peritoneal dialysis. *Am J Kidney Dis* 1991;17:307–310.
205. Hylander BI, Barkeling B, Rössner S. Eating behavior in continuous ambulatory peritoneal dialysis and hemodialysis patients. *Am J Kidney Dis* 1992;20:592–597.
206. Hylander BI, Barkeling B, Rössner S. Changes in patients' eating behavior: in uremic state, on continuous ambulatory peritoneal dialysis treatment and after transplantation. *Am J Kidney Dis* 1997;29:691–698.
207. Torrington J, Jenkins JH, Coles GA. The effect of the dialysate on food consumption by continuous ambulatory peritoneal dialysis patients. *J Renal Nutr* 1992;2:113–116.
208. Balaskas EV, Rodela H, Oreopoulos DG. Effect of intraperitoneal infusion of dextrose and amino acids on the appetite of rabbits. *Perit Dial Int* 1993;13(Suppl 2):S490–S498.
209. Musk M, Anderson H, Oreopoulos D, et al. Effects of amino acid dialysate on appetite in CAPD patients. In: Khanna R, Nolph KD, Prowant BF, et al., eds. *Advances in peritoneal dialysis 1992.* Toronto: Peritoneal Dialysis Bulletin, Inc., 1992; 153–156.
210. Anderstam B, Mamoun A-H, Södersten P, et al. Middle-sized molecule fractions isolated from uremic ultrafiltrate and normal urine inhibit ingestive behavior in the rat. *J Am Soc Nephrol* 1996;7:2453–2460.
211. Mamoun AH, Anderstam B, Södersten P, et al. Influence of peritoneal dialysis solutions with glucose and amino acids on ingestive behavior in rats. *Kidney Int* 1996;49:1276–1282.
212. Zheng ZH, Anderstam B, Sederholm F, et al. Less inhibition of appetite with IP bicarbonate—than with lactate-based electrolyte solution (abstract). *Perit Dial Int* 2000;20:155.
213. Zheng ZH, Sederholm F, Qureshi AR, et al. Peritoneal dialysis solutions affect ingestive behavior in rats appetite model (abstract). *Perit Dial Int* 2000;20(Suppl 1):S45.
214. Davies SJ, Russel L, Bryan J, et al. Impact of peritoneal absorption of glucose on appetite, protein catabolism and survival in CAPD patients. *Clin Nephrol* 1996;45:194–198.
215. Fernström A, Hylander B, Rössner S. Taste acuity in patients with chronic renal failure. *Clin Nephrol* 1996;45:169–174.
216. Middleton RA, Allman-Farinelli MA. Taste sensitivity is altered

in patients with chronic renal failure receiving continuous ambulatory peritoneal dialysis. *J Nutr* 1999;129:122–125.
217. Aguilera A, Codoceo R, Selgas R, et al. Anorexigen (TNF-a, cholecystokinin) and orexigen (neuropeptide Y) plasma levels in peritoneal dialysis (PD) patients: their relationship with nutritional parameters. *Nephrol Dial Transplant* 1998;13: 1476–1483.
218. Espinoza M, Aguilera A, Bajo MA, et al. Tumor necrosis factor alpha as a uremic toxin: correlation with neuropathy, left ventricular hypertrophy, anemia, and hypertriglyceridemia in peritoneal dialysis patients. *Adv Perit Dial* 1999;15:82–86.
219. Heimbürger O, Lönnqvist F, Danielsson A, et al. Serum immunoreactive leptin concentration and its relation to body fat content in chronic renal failure. *J Am Soc Nephrol* 1997;8: 1423–1430.
220. Wolf G. Orexins: a newly discovered family of hypothalamic regulators of food intake. *Nutr Rev* 1998;56:172–173.
221. Blumenkrantz MJ, Gahl GM, Kopple JD, et al. Protein losses during peritoneal dialysis. *Kidney Int* 1981;19:593–602.
222. Young GA, Brownjohn AM, Parsons FM. Protein losses in patients receiving continuous ambulatory peritoneal dialysis. *Nephron* 1987;45:196–201.
223. Dulaney JT, Hatch FE. Peritoneal dialysis and loss of proteins: A review. *Kidney Int* 1984;26:253–262.
224. Rippe B, Haraldsson B. How are macromolecules transported across the capillary wall. *N I P S* 1987;2(August):135–138.
225. Rippe B, Stelin G. Simulations of peritoneal solute transport during CAPD. Applications of two-pore formalism. *Kidney Int* 1989;35:1234–1244.
226. Kagan A, Bar-Khayim Y, Schafer Z, et al. Kinetics of peritoneal protein loss during CAPD: II. Lipoprotein leakage and its impact on plasma lipid levels. *Kidney Int* 1990;37:980–990.
227. Heimbürger O, Stenvinkel P, Berglund L, et al. Increased plasma lipoprotein(a) in CAPD is related to peritoneal transport of proteins and glucose. *Nephron* 1995;72:135–144.
228. Heimbürger O. *Peritoneal transport in patients treated with continuous peritoneal dialysis.* [Ph.D. Thesis]: Karolinska Institute, Stockholm; 1994.
229. Nolph KD, Moore HL, Prowant B, et al. Continuous ambulatory peritoneal dialysis with a high flux membrane. *ASAIO J* 1993;39:904–909.
230. Heaf J. CAPD adequacy and dialysis morbidity: detrimental effect of a high peritoneal equilibration rate. *Renal Failure* 1995; 17:575–587.
231. Harty J, Boulton H, Venning M, et al. Is peritoneal permeability an adverse risk factor for malnutrition in CAPD patients? *Miner Electrolyte Metab* 1996;22:97–101.
232. Kagan A, Bar-Khayim Y, Schafer Z, et al. Heterogeneity in peritoneal transport during continuous ambulatory peritoneal dialysis and its impact on ultrafiltration, loss of macromolecules and plasma levels of proteins, lipids and lipoproteins. *Nephron* 1993;63:32–42.
233. Diaz-Alvarenga A, Abasta-Jimenez M, Bravo B, et al. Serum albumin and body surface area are the strongest predictors of the peritoneal transport type. *Adv Perit Dial* 1994;10:47–51.
234. Cueto-Manzano AM, Espinosa A, Hernández A, et al. Peritoneal transport kinetics correlate with serum albumin but not with the overall nutritional status in CAPD patients. *Am J Kidney Dis* 1997;30:229–236.
235. Davies SJ, Phillips L, Russell GI. Peritoneal solute transport predicts survival on CAPD independently of residual renal function. *Nephrol Dial Transpl* 1998;13:962–968.
236. Churchill DN, Thorpe KE, Nolph KD, et al. Increased peritoneal membrane transport is associated with decreased patient and technique survival for continuous peritoneal dialysis patients. *J Am Soc Nephrol* 1998;9:1285–1292.
237. Wang T, Heimbürger O, Waniewski J, et al. Increased peritoneal permeability is associated with decreased fluid and small-solute removal and higher mortality in CAPD patients. *Nephrol Dial Transplant* 1998;13:1242–1249.
238. Cueto-Manzano AM, Correa-Rotter R. Is high peritoneal transport rate an independent risk factor for CAPD mortality? *Kidney Int* 2000;57:314–320.
239. Kang DH, Yoon KI, Choi KB, et al. Relationship of peritoneal membrane transport characteristics to the nutritional status in CAPD patients. *Nephrol Dial Transplant* 1999;14:1715–1722.
240. Szeto CC, Law MC, Wong TYH, et al. Peritoneal transport status correlates with morbidity but not longitudinal change of nutritional status of continuous ambulatory peritoneal dialysis patients: a 2-year prospective study. *Am J Kidney Dis* 2001;37: 329–336.
241. Tzamaloukas AH, Saddler MC, Murata GH, et al. Symptomatic fluid retention in patients on continuous peritoneal dialysis. *J Am Soc Nephrol* 1995;6:198–206.
242. Chung SH, Heimbürger O, Stenvinkel P, et al. Association between inflammation and changes in residual renal function and peritoneal transport rate during the first year of dialysis. *Nephrol Dial Transplant* 2001;16:2240–2245.
243. Heimbürger O, Wang T, Chung SH, et al. Increased peritoneal transport rate from an early peritoneal equilibration test (PET) is related to inflammation, cardiovascular disease and mortality (abstract). *J Am Soc Nephrol* 1999;10:315A.
244. Stenvinkel P, Chung SH, Heimbürger O, et al. Malnutrition, inflammation and atherosclerosis in peritoneal dialysis patients. *Perit Dial Int* 2001;21(Suppl 3):S157–S162.
245. Straumann E, Keller U, Küry D, et al. Effect of acute acidosis and alkalosis on leucine kinetics in man. *Clin Physiol* 1992;12: 39–51.
246. Papadoyannakis NJ, Stefanidis CJ, McGeown M. The effect of the correction of metabolic acidosis on nitrogen and potassium balance of patients with chronic renal failure. *Am J Clin Nutr* 1984;40:623–627.
247. Hara Y, May RC, Kelly RC, et al. Acidosis, not azotemia, stimulates branched-chain, amino acid catabolism in uremic rats. *Kidney Int* 1987;32:808–814.
248. May RC, Hara Y, Kelly RA, et al. Branched-chain amino acid metabolism in rat muscle: Abnormal regulation in acidosis. *Am J Physiol* 1987;252:E712–E718.
249. Mitch WE, Jurkovic C, England BK. Mechanisms that cause protein and amino acid catabolism in uremia. *Am J Kidney Dis* 1993;21:91–95.
250. Bergström J, Alvestrand A, Fürst P. Plasma and muscle free amino acids in maintenance hemodialysis patients without protein malnutrition. *Kidney Int* 1990;38:108–114.
251. Lim VS, Yarasheski KE, Flanigan MJ. The effect of uremia, acidosis, and dialysis treatment on protein metabolism: a longitudinal leucine kinetic study. *Nephrol Dial Transplant* 1998;13: 1723–1730.
252. Graham KA, Reaich D, Channon SM, et al. Correction of acidosis in CAPD decreases whole body protein degradation. *Kidney Int* 1996;49:1396–1400.
253. Stein A, Baker F, Larratt C, et al. Correction of metabolic acidosis and the protein catabolic rate in PD patients. *Perit Dial Int* 1994;14:187–189.
254. Kooman JP, Deutz NEP, Zijlmans P, et al. The influence of bicarbonate supplementation on plasma levels of branched-chain amino acids in haemodialysis patients with metabolic acidosis. *Nephrol Dial Transplant* 1997;12:2397–2401.
255. Marcinkowski K, Grzegorzewska A. Protein catabolic rate (PCR), dietary protein intake (DPI) and metabolic acidosis (letter). *Nephrol Dial Transpl* 1999;14:2266–2267.
256. Kang DH, Yoon KI, Lee HY, et al. Impact of peritoneal mem-

brane transport characteristics on acid-base status in CAPD patients. *Perit Dial Int* 1998;18:294–302.

257. Gokal R. Continuous ambulatory peritoneal dialysis. In: Maher JF, ed. *Replacement of renal function by dialysis.* Dordrecht: Kluwer Academic Publisher, 1989;590–615.
258. Feriani M. Adequacy of acid base correction in continuous ambulatory peritoneal dialysis patients. *Perit Dial Int* 1994; 14(Suppl 3):S133–S138.
259. Uribarri J, Buquing J, Oh MS. Acid-base balance in chronic peritoneal dialysis patients. *Kidney Int* 1995;47:269–273.
260. Tranæus A, for The Bicarbonate/Lactate study group. A long-term study of a bicarbonate/lactate based peritoneal dialysis solution—clinical benefits. *Perit Dial Int* 2000;20:516–523.
261. Feriani M, Kirchgessner J, La Greca G, et al. Randomized long-term evaluation of bicarbonate-buffered CAPD solution. *Kidney Int* 1998;54:1731–1738.
262. Feriani M, Carobi C, La Greca G, et al. Clinical experience with a 39 mmol/L bicarbonate-buffered peritoneal dialysis solution. *Perit Dial Int* 1997;17:9–10.
263. Fukuda S, Kopple JD. Uptake and release of amino acids by the kidney of dogs made chronically uremic with uranyl nitrate. *Min Electr Metab* 1980;3:248–260.
264. Tizianello A, Deferrari G, Garibotto G, et al. Renal metabolism of amino acids and ammonia in subjects with normal renal function and in patients with chronic renal insufficiency. *J Clin Invest* 1980;65:1162–1173.
265. Pitts RF, Macleod MB. Synthesis of serine by the dog kidney in vivo. *Am J Physiol* 1972;222:394–398.
266. Lopez-Menchero R, Miguel A, Garcia-Ramon R, et al. Importance of residual renal function in continuous ambulatory peritoneal dialysis: its influence of different parameters of renal replacement treatment. *Nephron* 1999;83:219–225.
267. Wang AYM, Sea MMM, Ip R, et al. Independent effect of residual renal function and dialysis adequacy on actual dietary protein intake, calorie, and other nutrient intake in patients on continuous ambulatory peritoneal dialysis. *J Am Soc Nephrol* 2001;12:2450–2457.
268. Rottembourg J. Residual renal function and recovery of renal function in patients treated by CAPD. *Kidney Int* 1993; 43(Suppl 40):S106–S110.
269. Lysaght MJ, Vonesh EF, Gotch F, et al. The influence of dialysis treatment modality on the decline of remaining renal function. *ASAIO Trans* 1991;37:598–604.
270. Bannister DK, Acchiardo SR, Moore LW, et al. Nutritional effects of peritonitis in continuous ambulatory peritoneal dialysis. *J Am Diet Ass* 1987;87:53–56.
271. Verger C, Larpent L, Dumontet M. Prognostic value of peritoneal equilibration curves (EC) in CAPD patients. In: Maher JF, Winchester JF, eds. *Frontiers in peritoneal dialysis.* New York: Field, Rich and Assoc., Inc., 1986;88–93.
272. Gahl G, Hain H. Nutrition and metabolism in continuous ambulatory peritoneal dialysis. In: Scarpione LL, Ballocchi S, eds. *Evolution and trends in peritoneal dialysis.* Basel: Karger, 1990;36–44.
273. Gahl G, Gebler H, Becker H, et al. Dietary intake, peritoneal glucose absorption and nitrogen balance during continuous ambulatory peritoneal dialysis-associated peritonitis (abstract). *Nephrol Dial Transplant* 1987;2:453.
274. Rubin J, Kirchner K, Barnes T, et al. Evaluation of continuous ambulatory peritoneal dialysis. *Am J Kidney Dis* 1983;3: 199–204.
275. Cheung AK. Biocompatibility of hemodialysis membranes. *J Am Soc Nephrol* 1990;1:150–161.
276. Betz M, Haenisch GM, Rauterberg EW, et al. Cuprammonium membranes stimulates interleukin-1 release and archidonic acid metabolism in monocytes in the absence of complement. *Kidney Int* 1988;34:67–73.
277. Lonnemann G, Bingel M, Floege J, et al. Detection of endotoxin-like interleukin-1-inducing activity during in vitro dialysis. *Kidney Int* 1988;33:29–35.
278. Gutierrez A, Alvestrand A, Wahren J, et al. Effect of in vivo contact between blood and dialysis membranes on protein catabolism in humans. *Kidney Int* 1990;38:487–494.
279. Gutierrez A, Bergström J, Alvestrand A. Protein catabolism in sham-hemodialysis: the effect of different membranes. *Clin Nephrol* 1992;38:20–29.
280. Flores EA, Bistrian BR, Pomposelli JJ, et al. Infusion of tumor necrosis factor. Cachectin promotes muscle catabolism in the rat. *J Clin Invest* 1989;83:1614–1622.
281. Baracos V, Rodeman HP, Dinarello CA, et al. Stimulation of muscle protein degradation and prostaglandin E2 release by leukocytic pyrogen (interleukin-1). *N Engl J Med* 1983;308: 553–558.
282. Nawabi MD, Block KP, Chakrabarti MC, et al. Administration of endotoxin, tumor necrosis factor, or interleukin-1 to rats activates skeletal muscle branched-chain alpha-keto acid dehydrogenase. *J Clin Invest* 1990;85:256–263.
283. Shaldon S, Koch KM, Quellhorst E, et al. CAPD is a second-class treatment. *Contr Nephrol* 1985;44:163–172.
284. Nilsson-Thorell CB, Muscalu N, Andrén AHG, et al. Heat sterilization of fluids for peritoneal dialysis gives rise to aldehydes. *Perit Dial Int* 1993;13:208–213.
285. Boeshoten EW, Zuyderhoudt FMJ, Krediet RT, et al. Changes in weight and lipid concentrations during CAPD treatment. *Perit Dial Int* 1988;8:19–24.
286. Tranæus A, Heimbürger O, Lindholm B, et al. Six years' experience of CAPD at one centre: A survey of major findings. *Perit Dial Int* 1988;8:31–41.
287. Nolph KD, Sorkin MN, Rubin J, et al. Continuous ambulatory peritoneal dialysis: Three-year experience at one center. *Ann Intern Med* 1980;92:609–613.
288. Kurtz SB, Wong VH, Anderson CF, et al. Continuous ambulatory peritoneal dialysis. Three years' experience at the Mayo Clinic. *Mayo Clin Proc* 1983;58:633–639.
289. Bazzato G, Scanferla F, Landini S, et al. Bioimpedance: a new tool to assess nutritional status. Longitudinal study in peritoneal vs. hemodialysis patients. In: Ota K, Maher JF, Winchester JF, et al., eds. *Current concepts in peritoneal dialysis. Proceedings of the Fifth Congress of the International Society of Peritoneal Dialysis, Kyoto, July 21–24, 1990.* Amsterdam: Excerpta Medica, 1992; 516–522.
290. Stenvinkel P, Lindholm B, Lönnqvist F, et al. Increases in serum leptin during peritoneal dialysis are associated with inflammation and a decrease in lean body mass. *J Am Soc Nephrol* 2000; 11:1303–1309.
291. Numata M, Yamamoto H, Kawaguchi Y, et al. A study of association between lean body mass and serum insulin-like growth factor-1 in continuous ambulatory peritoneal dialysis patients. *Nippon Jinzo Gakkai Shi* 1999;41:8–13.
292. Fernström A, Hylander B, Moritz Å, et al. Increase of intra-abdominal fat in patients treated with continuous ambulatory peritoneal dialysis. *Perit Dial Int* 1998;18:166–171.
293. Schilling H, Wu G, Petit J, et al. Nutritional status of patients on long-term CAPD. *Perit Dial Bull* 1985;5:12–18.
294. Viglino G, Gallo M, Cottino R, et al. Assessment of nutritional status of CAPD patients during five-year follow-up. In: Ota K, Maher JF, Winchester JF, et al., eds. *Current concepts in peritoneal dialysis. Proceedings of the Fifth Congress of the International Society of Peritoneal Dialysis, Kyoto, July 21–24, 1990.* Amsterdam: Excerpta Medica, 1992;497–505.
295. Davies SJ, Phillips L, Griffiths AM, et al. What really happens

to people on long-term peritoneal dialysis? *Kidney Int* 1998;54: 2207–2217.

296. Boeschoten EW. Nutritional deficiencies during long-term CAPD. In: Ota K, Maher JF, Winchester JF, et al., eds. *Current concepts in peritoneal dialysis. Proceedings of the Fifth Congress of the International Society of Peritoneal Dialysis, Kyoto, July 21–24, 1990.* Amsterdam: Excerpta Medica, 1992;506–515.
297. Faller B, Lameire N. Evolution of clinical parameters and peritoneal function in a cohort of CAPD patients followed over 7 years. *Nephrol Dial Transplant* 1994;9:280–286.
298. Gokal R, King J, Bogle S, et al. Outcome in patients on continuous ambulatory peritoneal dialysis and haemodialysis: 4-year analysis of a prospective multicentre study. *Lancet* 1987;ii: 1105–1109.
299. Dagogo-Jack S, Ovalle F, Geary B, et al. Hyperleptinaemia in patients with end-stage renal disease treated by peritoneal dialysis. *Perit Dial Int* 1998;18:34–40.
300. Merabet E, Dagogo-Jack S, Coyne DW, et al. Increased plasma leptin concentrations in end-stage renal disease. *J Clin Endocrinol Metab* 1997;82:847–850.
301. Watson PE, Watson ID, Batt RD. Total body water volumes for adult males and females estimated from simple anthropometric measurements. *Am J Clin Nutr* 1980;33:27–39.
302. Johansson A-C, Samuelsson O, Attman P-O, et al. Limitations in anthropometric calculations of total body water in patients on peritoneal dialysis. *J Am Soc Nephrol* 2001;12:568–573.
303. Arkouche W, Fouque D, Pachiaudi C, et al. Total body water and body composition in chronic peritoneal dialysis patients. *J Am Soc Nephrol* 1997;8:1906–1914.
304. Enia G, Mallamaci F, Benedetto FA, et al. Long-term CAPD patients are volume expanded and display more severe left ventricular hypertrophy than haemodialysis patients. *Nephrol Dial Transplant* 2001;16:1459–1464.
305. Lameire N. Cardiovascular risk factors and blood pressure control in continuous ambulatory peritoneal dialysis. *Perit Dial Int* 1993;13:S394–S395.
306. Menon MK, Naimark DM, Bargman JM, et al. Long-term blood pressure control in a cohort of peritoneal dialysis patients and its association with residual renal function. *Nephrol Dial Transpl* 2001;16:2207–2213.
307. Heimbürger O, Wang T, Lindholm B. Alterations in water and solute transport with time on peritoneal dialysis. *Perit Dial Int* 1999;19 (suppl 2):S83–S90.
308. Stunkard AJ, Harris JR, Pederson NL, et al. The body-mass index in twins who have been reared apart. *N Engl J Med* 1990; 322:1483–1487.
309. Ravussin E, Lillioja S, Knowler WC, et al. Reduced rate of energy expenditure as a risk factor for body-weight gain. *N Engl J Med* 1988;318:467–472.
310. Bogardus C, Lillioja S, Ravussin E, et al. Familial dependence of the resting metabolic rate. *N Engl J Med* 1986;315:96–100.
311. Walder K, Norman RA, Hanson RL, et al. Association between uncoupling protein polymorphism (UCP2-UCP3) and energy expenditure/obesity in Pima indians. *Hum Mol Gen* 1998;7: 1431–1435.
312. Nordfors L, Hoffstedt J, Nyberg B, et al. Reduced gene expression of UCP2 but not UCP3 in skeletal muscle of human obese subjects. *Diabetologia* 1998;41:935–939.
313. Schrauwen P, Walder K, Ravussin E. Human uncoupling proteins and obesity. *Obesity Research* 1999;7:97–105.
314. Nordfors L, Heimbürger O, Lönnqvist F, et al. Fat tissue accumulation during peritoneal dialysis is associated with a polymorphism in uncoupling protein 2. *Kidney Int* 2000;57: 1713–1719.
315. Fleischmann E, Teal N, Dudley J, et al. Influence of excess weight on mortality and hospital stay in 1346 hemodialysis patients. *Kidney Int* 1999;55:1560–1567.
316. Kopple JD, Bernard D, Messana J, et al. Treatment of malnourished CAPD patients with an amino acid based dialysate. *Kidney Int* 1995;47:1148–1157.
317. Levine JA, Morgan MY. Assessment of dietary intake in man: a review of available methods. *J Nutr Med* 1991;2:65–81.
318. Kopple JD, Jones MR, Keshaviah PR, et al. A proposed glossary for dialysis kinetics. *Am J Kidney Dis* 1995;26:963–981.
319. Dwyer J, Kenler SR. Assessment of nutritional status in renal disease. In: Mitch WE, Klahr S, eds. *Nutrition and the kidney.* Boston: Little, Brown and Co, 1993;61–95.
320. Frisancho AR. New standards of weight and body composition by frame size and height for assessment of nutritional state of adults and the elderly. *Am J Clin Nutr* 1984;40:808–819.
321. 1983 Metropolitan height and weight tables. *Stat Bull Metrop Life Insur Co* 1983;64:3.
322. Alvestrand A, Ahlberg M, Fürst P, et al. Clinical results of long-term treatment with a low protein diet and a new amino acid preparation in patients with chronic uremia. *Clin Nephrol* 1983; 19:67–73.
323. Garibotto G, Defarrari G, Robaudo C, et al. Effects of a new amino acid supplement on blood AA pools in patients with chronic renal failure. *Amino Acids* 1991;1:319–329.
324. Heaf JG, Honoré K, Valeur D, et al. The effect of oral protein supplements on the nutritional status of malnourished CAPD patients. *Perit Dial Int* 1999;19:78–81.
325. Rubin J. Nutritional support during peritoneal dialysis-related peritonitis. *Am J Kidney Dis* 1990;15:551–555.
326. Heimbürger O, Tranæus A, Park MS, et al. Relationships between peritoneal equilibration test (PET) and 24 h clearances in CAPD (abstract). *Perit Dial Int* 1992;12 (suppl 2):S12.
327. Tattersall JE, Doyle S, Greenwood RN, et al. Kinetic modelling and underdialysis in CAPD patients. *Nephrol Dial Transplant* 1993;8:535–538.
328. Bargman J, Thorpe KE, Churchill DN, et al. Relative contributions of residual renal function and peritoneal clearance to adequacy of dialysis: A reanalysis of the CANUSA study. *J Am Soc Nephrol* 2001;12:2158–2162.
329. Paniagua R, Amato D, Ramos A, et al. Summary results from the Mexican adequacy (ADEMEX) clinical trial on mortality and morbidity in peritoneal dialysis (abstract). *J Am Soc Nephrol* 2001;12:235A.
330. Bergström J, Alvestrand A, Lindholm B, et al. Relationship between Kt/V and protein catabolic rate (PCR) is different in continuous peritoneal dialysis (CPD) and hemodialysis (HD) patients (abstract). *J Am Soc Nephrol* 1991;2:358.
331. Williams P, Jones J, Marriott J. Do increases in dialysis dose in CAPD patients lead to nutritional improvements? *Nephrol Dial Transplant* 1994;9.
332. Szeto CC, Wong TYH, Leung CB, et al. Importance of dialysis adequacy in mortality and morbidity of Chinese CAPD patients. *Kidney Int* 2000;58:400–407.
333. Davies SJ, Phillips L, Griffiths AM, et al. Analysis of the effects of increasing delivered dialysis treatment to malnourished peritoneal dialysis patients. *Kidney Int* 2000;57:1743–1754.
334. Harty JC, Boulton H, Uttley L, et al. Limitations of modelling dialysis therapy in CAPD: the impact of increasing dialysis prescription (abstract). *Perit Dial Int* 1995;15(Suppl 1):S40.
335. Tattersall JE, Doyle S, Greenwood RN, et al. Maintaining adequacy in CAPD by individualizing the dialysis prescription. *Nephrol Dial Transplant* 1994;9:749–752.
336. Lindholm B, Park MS, Bergström J. Supplemented dialysis: Amino acid-based solutions in peritoneal dialysis. In: Bonomini

V, ed. *Evolution in dialysis adequacy.* Basel: Karger, 1992; 168–182.

337. Jones M, Gehr T, Burkart J, et al. Replacement of amino acid and protein losses with 1.1% amino acid peritoneal dialysis solution. *Perit Dial Int* 1998;18:210–216.
338. Park MS, Heimbürger O, Bergström J, et al. Peritoneal transport during dialysis with amino acid-based solution. *Perit Dial Int* 1993;13:280–288.
339. Paniagua R, Amato D, Vonesh E, et al. Effects of increased peritoneal clearances on mortality rates in peritoneal dialysis: ADEMEX, a prospective, randomized, controlled trial. *J Am Soc Nephrol* 2002;13(5):1307–1320.
340. Oren A, Wu G, Anderson E, et al. Effective use of amino acid dialysate over four weeks in CAPD patients. *Trans Am Soc Artif Intern Organs* 1983;29:604–610.
341. Schilling H, Wu G, Petit J, et al. Use of amino acid containing solutions in continuous ambulatory peritoneal dialysis patients after peritonitis: Result of a prospective controlled trial. *Proc EDTA-ERA* 1985;22:421–425.
342. Dombros N, Prutis K, Tong M, et al. Six-month overnight intraperitoneal amino-acid infusion in continuous ambulatory dialysis (CAPD) patients: no effect on nutritional status. *Perit Dial Intern* 1990;10:79–84.
343. Schilling H, Wu G, Petit J, et al. Effect of prolonged CAPD with amino acid-containing solutions in three patients. In: Khanna R, Nolph KD, Prownar B, et al., eds. *Advances in continuous ambulatory peritoneal dialysis.* Toronto: Peritoneal Dialysis Bulletin, Inc., 1985;49–55.
344. Dibble JB, Young GA, Hobson SM, et al. Amino-acid-based continuous ambulatory peritoneal dialysis (CAPD) fluid over twelve weeks: Effects on carbohydrate and lipid metabolism. *Perit Dial Int* 1990;10:71–77.
345. Bruno M, Bagnis C, Marangella M, et al. CAPD with an amino acid dialysis solution: A long-term, cross-over study. *Kidney Int* 1989;35:1189–1194.
346. Arfeen A, Goodship THJ, Kirkwood A, et al. The nutrition/metabolic and hormonal effects of 8 weeks continuous ambulatory peritoneal dialysis with a 1% amino acid solution. *Clin Nephrol* 1990;33:192–199.
347. Young GA, Dibble JB, Hobson SM, et al. The use of an amino-acid-based CAPD fluid over 12 weeks. *Nephrol Dial Transplant* 1989;4:285–292.
348. Delarue J, Maingourd C, Objois M, et al. Effects of an amino acid dialysate on leucine metabolism in continuous ambulatory peritoneal dialysis. *Kidney Int* 1999;56:1934–1943.
349. Rubin J, Garner T. Positive nitrogen balance after intraperitoneal administration of amino acids in three patients. *Perit Dial Int* 1994;14:223–226.
350. Faller B, Aparicio M, Faict D, et al. Clinical evaluation of an optimized 1.1% amino-acid solution for peritoneal dialysis. *Perit Dial Int* 1995;10(8):1432–1437.
351. Jones M, Hagen T, Boyle CA, et al. Treatment of malnutrition with 1.1% amino-acid peritoneal dialysis solution: results of a multicenter outpatient study. *Am J Kidney Dis* 1998;32: 761–769.
352. Dratwa M, Vladutiu D, Keller J. Nutritional support with Nutrineal[R] (N) for CAPD peritonitis (abstract). *Perit Dial Int* 1995;15(Suppl 1):S39.
353. Grzegorzewska AE, Mariak I, Dobrowolska-Zachwieja A, et al. Effects of amino acid dialysis solution on the nutrition of continuous ambulatory peritoneal dialysis patients. *Perit Dial Int* 1999;19:462–470.
354. Bruno M, Gabella P, Ramello A. Use of amino acids in peritoneal dialysis solutions. *Perit Dial Int* 2000;20(Suppl 2): S166–S171.
355. Bárány P, Pettersson E, Ahlberg M, et al. Nutritional assessment in anemic hemodialysis patients treated with recombinant human erythropoietin. *Clin Nephrol* 1991;35:270–279.
356. Balaskas EV, Melamed IR, Gupta A, et al. Effect of erythropoietin treatment on nutritional status of continuous ambulatory peritoneal dialysis patients. *Perit Dial Int* 1993;13(Suppl 2): S544–S549.
357. Wilson JD, Griffin JE. The use and misuse of androgens. *Metabolism* 1980;29:1278–1295.
358. Soliman G, Oreopoulos DG. Anabolic steroids and malnutrition in chronic renal failure. *Perit Dial Int* 1994;14:362–365.
359. Dombros N, Digenis GE, Soliman G, et al. Anabolic steroids in the treatment of malnourished CAPD patients: a retrospective study. *Perit Dial Int* 1994;14:344–347.
360. Fine RN. Growth in children undergoing CAPD/CCPD/APD. *Perit Dial Int* 1993;13(Suppl 2):S247–S250.
361. Ziegler TR, Lazarus JM, Young LS, et al. Effects of recombinant human growth hormone in adults receiving maintenance hemodialysis. *J Am Soc Nephrol* 1991;2:1130–1135.
362. Schulman G, Wingard RL, Hutchinson RL, et al. The effects of recombinant human growth hormone and intradialytic parenteral nutrition in malnourished hemodialysis patients. *Am J Kidney Dis* 1993;21:527–534.
363. Sinobe M, Sanaka T, Higuchi C, et al. The improvement of catabolic state in hemodialysis patients by recombinant human growth hormone (r-hGH) (abstract). *J Am Soc Nephrol* 1993; 4:431.
364. Kleinknecht C, Maniar S, Zhou X, et al. Acidosis prevents growth hormone-induced growth in experimental uremia. *Pediatr Nephrol* 1996;10:256–260.
365. Ikizler TA, Wingard RL, Breyer JA, et al. Short-term effects of recombinant human growth hormone in CAPD patients. *Kidney Int* 1994;46:1178–1183.
366. Ikizler TA, Wingard RL, Flakoll PJ, et al. Effects of recombinant human growth hormone on plasma and dialysate amino acid profiles in CAPD patients. *Kidney Int* 1996;50:229–234.
367. Iglesias P, Díez JJ, Fernández-Reyes MJ, et al. Recombinant human growth hormone therapy in malnourished patients: a randomized controlled study. *Am J Kidney Dis* 1998;32: 454–463.
368. Hammerman MR. The growth hormone-insulin-like growth factor axis in kidney. *Am J Physiol* 1989;26:F503–F514.
369. Allander SV, Bjalica S, Larsson C, et al. Structure and chromosomal localization of human insulin-like growth factor binding genes. *Growth Regul* 1993;3:3–5.
370. Blum WF, Ranke MB, Kietzman K, et al. Growth hormone resistance and inhibition of somatomedin activity by excess of insulin-like growth factor binding protein in uremia. *Pediatr Nephrol* 1991;5:539–544.
371. Blum WF. Insulin-like growth factors (IGFs) and IGF binding proteins in chronic renal failure: Evidence for reduced secretion of IGFs. *Acta Paediatr Scand* 1991;379(Suppl):24–31.
372. Jacob V, Le Carpentier JE, Salzano S, et al. IGF-1, a marker of undernutrition in hemodialysis patients. *Am J Clin Nutr* 1990;52:39–44.
373. Sanaka T, Shinobe M, Ando M, et al. IGF-1 as an early indicator of malnutrition in patients with end-stage renal disease. *Nephron* 1994;67:73–81.
374. Kagan A, Altman Y, Zadik Z, et al. Insulin-like growth factor-a in patients on CAPD and hemodialysis: relationship to body weight and albumin level. *Adv Perit Dial* 1995;11:47–52.
375. Himmelfarb J, Holbrook D, McMonagle E, et al. Kt/V, nutritional parameters, serum cortisol, and insulin growth factor-1 and patient outcome in hemodialysis. *Am J Kidney Dis* 1994; 24:473–479.
376. Ramirez G, O'Neill WM, Bloomer A, et al. Abnormalities in

the regulation of growth hormone in chronic renal failure. *Arch Intern Med* 1978;138:267–271.

377. Tönshoff B, Schäfer F, Mehls O. Disturbance of growth hormone-insulin-like growth factor axis in uremia. *Pediatr Nephrol* 1990;4:654–662.
378. Kopple JD. The rationale for the use of growth hormone or insulin-like growth factor 1 in adult patients with renal failure. *Miner Electrolyte Metab* 1992;18:269–275.
379. Tönshoff B, Edén S, Weiser E, et al. Reduced hepatic growth hormone (GH) receptor gene expression and increased plasma GH binding protein in experimental uremia. *Kidney Int* 1994; 45:1085–1092.
380. Fouque D, Peng S, Shamir E, et al. Recombinant human insulin-like growth factor-1 induces an anabolic response in malnourished CAPD patients. *Kidney Int* 2000;57:646–654.
381. Giordano M, DeFronzo RA. Acute effects of insulin-like growth factor 1 (IGF-1) on protein metabolism in humans (abstract). In: *Abstract book, 7th International Congress of Nutrition and Metabolism in Renal Disease, Stockholm 1994.* Stockholm, 1994; 26.

28

NUTRITIONAL MANAGEMENT OF RENAL TRANSPLANTATION

BERTRAM L. KASISKE
MAGDALENA ADEVA-ANDANY

Cardiovascular disease is a leading cause of morbidity and mortality in renal transplant recipients (1). Pharmacologic treatment of hyperlipidemia, hypertension, and other cardiovascular risk factors is generally safe and effective; however, dietary management continues to be an important adjunctive measure. Specifically, diet is important in managing obesity, insulin resistance, diabetes, hyperlipidemia, and hypertension. Other posttransplant conditions for which diet and/or nutritional supplements also may be beneficial include hypomagnesemia, hypophosphatemia, hyperuricemia, hyperkalemia, hyperhomocysteinemia, chronic renal allograft failure, and osteoporosis.

NUTRITIONAL ASSESSMENT IN RENAL TRANSPLANT RECIPIENTS

Nutritional assessment includes the evaluation of net energy balance and body composition. Body mass index (BMI) (weight in kg divided by height in m^2) is one estimate of energy balance. Obesity is defined by the World Health Organization as BMI of 27.3 mg/m^2 or more (women) and 27.8 kg/m^2 or more (men). The waist-to-hip ratio or the waist circumference, measured at the umbilicus with the patient standing, helps to define central (abdominal, visceral) obesity (2). A waist-to-hip ratio greater than 1.0 for men or 0.9 for women or a waist circumference greater than 1.0 m for men or 0.9 m for women indicates central obesity.

The assessment of body composition may be performed by various procedures, including anthropometric measurements, laboratory analysis, and other more complex techniques (3). Anthropometric measures include estimation of the fat mass by caliper evaluation of triceps or subscapular skinfold thickness and assessment of the protein mass in the body through the estimation of muscle mass by the midarm circumference, taking into account the amount of fat. Useful laboratory parameters include serum protein levels and urine creatinine excretion. So-called visceral proteins, such as albumin, transferrin, and prealbumin, can be influenced by many factors, rendering their interpretation as nutritional parameters problematic. In addition, they are negative acute-phase reactants, and their levels decrease in a variety of acute and chronic inflammatory conditions (4). Serum transferrin concentration may be influenced by iron and erythropoietin therapy. Serum prealbumin concentration is closely associated with the level of renal function. Serum insulinlike growth factor 1 (IGF-1) concentration has been described as another index of nutritional status. Serum IGF-1 level is influenced by dietary protein and energy intake, and it can change with modifications in nutrient intake (5). Furthermore, IGF-1 is a negative acute-phase protein (4), and its serum concentrations may decline in acute and chronic inflammatory situations. Urinary creatinine excretion in renal transplant recipients is determined primarily by muscle mass (6). The lean body mass can be estimated by the 24-hour urinary creatinine or by the ratio of urinary creatinine to height.

There are also more complex techniques for evaluating body composition. Isotope dilution allows the assessment of total body water. Because the proportion of fat-free body mass to water is 0.732, this technique predicts the fat-free body mass and the fat mass (body weight–fat-free body mass) (3). Bioimpedance analysis is a method of estimating total, extracellular, and intracellular body water, and it can be used for estimating body fat and fat-free mass. It also has been used in renal transplant recipients (7). Dual-energy X-ray absorptiometry (DEXA) is a method to quantify bone-mineral mass, total and regional fat mass, and muscle mass. Whole-body counting/*in vivo* neutron activation analysis encompasses a group of techniques for estimating elements such as potassium, nitrogen (which can be used to measure total body protein), calcium and phosphorus (useful to estimate bone-mineral mass), hydrogen, oxygen, carbon, sodium, and chlorine. Computerized axial tomography and magnetic resonance imaging can be used to measure muscle mass and fat mass (3).

NUTRITIONAL STATUS OF RENAL TRANSPLANT RECIPIENTS

Patients with chronic renal failure may develop protein-energy malnutrition and negative nitrogen balance, with loss of lean body mass and fat deposits. Approximately one-third of patients undergoing maintenance dialysis have mild to moderate protein-energy malnutrition, and about 6% to 8% have severe malnutrition (8). However, patients undergoing maintenance dialysis often come to renal transplantation with a BMI higher than normal.

Information on nutritional status and body composition in renal transplant recipients is limited. There are several small observational studies, most performed early after transplantation (9–16). In 45 renal transplant recipients, both diabetic and nondiabetic, there was significant improvement of weight posttransplant. Of patients, 42% with diabetes and 29% without diabetes had a midarm muscle circumference less than the 5th percentile, indicating protein-calorie malnutrition (9). Weight was greater posttransplant, with an increase in body fat, in a study using *in vivo* neutron activation analysis and tritium dilution in five patients before transplant and 4.4 months posttransplant. Total body protein was similar pretransplant and posttransplant and slightly decreased compared with the predicted value in normals. Body water and minerals were also similar before and after transplant (10). Body weight increased in both patients with diabetes and in control patients in another retrospective study. Subcutaneous fat thickness (measured from computed tomography scans of the calf) increased in patients with diabetes, but the cross-sectional area of triceps and calf muscles did not increase, suggesting that the increase in body weight was the result of an increase in fat (11).

The effects of renal transplantation on the nutritional status, muscle composition, and plasma and muscle free amino acid pattern were analyzed in 30 renal transplant recipients several times after transplantation. Conventional anthropometric measurements were normal in renal transplant recipients. There was an elevated percentage of body fat 13 months after transplant. The muscle intracellular content of alkaline-soluble protein (ASP) relative to DNA, which is a sensitive index of protein depletion on the cellular level, was decreased in patients 45 days after transplant (12). However, it was normal in the longer follow-up, suggesting that cellular protein malnutrition may persist for a short period after kidney transplantation, but it subsequently normalizes in patients with functioning renal graft (12). In 11 children who had received kidney transplants, height was reduced, but the skinfold thickness, arm-muscle circumference, and serum proteins were normal. The muscle contents of ASP, DNA, and the ASP/DNA ratio were similar in patients and controls (13). Body composition, resting energy expenditure, and substrate oxidation were similar in three groups of 77 renal transplant recipients (a) without steroids, (b) taking 5 mg/day prednisolone, and (c) taking 10 mg/day of prednisolone (14). Physical activity was positively related with lean mass and inversely related with fat mass, especially in females (14). A prospective study of 15 patients analyzed changes in body composition after renal transplantation, using the DEXA technique. Thirteen patients (87%) showed an increase in the amount of fat (15). Body composition was prospectively assessed by DEXA 1, 3, and 6 months posttransplant in a study of 11 renal transplant recipients without acute rejection or severe disease (16). There was weight gain after transplantation because of an increase in fat mass, which is evident within 3 months after transplantation (16).

In a retrospective analysis of 115 adult renal transplant recipients, 21% were overweight before transplant (17). During the first posttransplant year, patients 18 to 29 years old and African-American recipients experienced greater weight gains than patients older than 50 years and white recipients. Men and women experienced comparable weight gains during the first year, but women continued to gain weight throughout the 5 years follow-up. Men remained stable after the first year. Weight gain did not correlate with cumulative steroid dose, donor source, rejections, preexisting obesity, or renal function (17).

In summary, most studies observed an increase in body weight after successful kidney transplantation, indicating an improvement of the overall energy balance (9–11,16). This weight gain occurs with an increase in the amount of fat mass (10,12,15,16). Most patients were protein deficient prior to transplant (10), and this state persisted to some degree in the first few weeks to months after transplantation (9–12,15). However, protein malnutrition normalized in patients with a functioning renal graft in the long term (12). The major long-term nutritional problem after kidney transplantation is obesity.

IMPACT OF PRETRANSPLANT OBESITY ON POSTTRANSPLANT OUTCOMES

The effect of pretransplant obesity on long-term patient and graft survival is controversial. In a case-control study of 46 obese (BMI >30 kg/m^2) and 50 control renal transplant recipients, postoperative mortality was increased in the obese recipients, but patient survival over a 2-year follow-up period was similar in the two groups. Graft survival at 1 year was reduced in obese recipients (66% versus 84%, $p < 0.05$). Delayed graft function, duration of surgery, wound complications, and posttransplant diabetes mellitus (PTDM, 12% versus 0%, $p < 0.02$) were more frequent in the obese group (18). In a retrospective study, 15% of 263 renal transplant recipients were obese (weight $>120\%$ of ideal body weight) before transplant (19). Patient survival, graft survival, and the incidence of acute rejection were similar for obese and nonobese recipients. Wound infections were more frequent in obese recipients (17.5% versus 6.3%, $p = 0.036$) (19). In another case-control study, 85 obese

TABLE 28.1. RECIPIENT BODY MASS INDEX AT TRANSPLANTATION

Reference	Body Mass Index	Patients (%)
Johnson (17)	<26–27	79
	≥26–27	21
Pirsch (21)	<27.5	80
	27.5–30	10
	>30	10
Drafts (22)	<30	81
	30–40	17
	>40	2
Meier-Kriesche (24)	≤25	59
	>25	41
Bumgardner (25)	≤27	88
	>27	12

(BMI >30 kg/m^2) and 85 controls (BMI <27 kg/m^2) renal transplant recipients were compared (20). Patient survival at 5 years in the obese group was reduced (55% versus 90%, $p = 0.0003$), and, as a result, graft survival was also lower. Wound complications (25% versus 8%, $p = 0.006$) and PTDM (14% versus 1%, $p = 0.002$) were more common in obese renal transplant recipients than in controls (20). In a retrospective analysis of 584 renal transplant recipients, delayed graft function was more common in obese compared with nonobese recipients (80%) and mildly obese (BMI 27.5–30 kg/m^2, 10%) patients (27% versus 9%, $p = 0.001$) (21). There were no differences in the incidence of acute rejection or graft survival among the groups, but wound complications were more frequent in both obese groups (21).

In 408 renal transplant recipients, categorized as either nonobese (BMI <30 mg/m^2, 81%), moderately obese (BMI 30–40 mg/m^2, 17%) or morbidly obese (BMI >40 mg/m^2, 2%), wound infections, delayed graft function, and PTDM were significantly more common in moderately and morbidly obese patients (22). Graft survival was not different, whether calculated for all graft losses or for graft losses resulting from immunologic causes, including acute and chronic rejection. Similarly, patient survival was not different between groups (22). In another retrospective case-control study, 127 renal transplant recipients with a BMI >30 mg/m^2 were compared with 127 nonobese recipients over a mean follow-up of 5 years (23). Obese patients were significantly older (43.8 versus 39.8 years, $p = 0.01$). More obese patients had a pretransplant history of angina or myocardial infarction. Nonobese recipients had a significantly greater patient survival (89.2% versus 67.1%, $p = 0.0002$) at 5 years. There was no difference in death-censored graft failure between obese and lean renal transplant recipients. Similarly, there were no significant differences in delayed graft function, acute rejection, chronic rejection, length of hospital stay, or mean serum creatinine during the first 5 years. Obese patients experienced a greater incidence of posttransplant diabetes (12% versus 2%, $p = 0.0003$) (23). In a retrospective study of 405 renal transplant recipients, a BMI of more than 25 mg/m^2 was an independent risk factor for both decreased graft and patient survival (24). Graft survival at 7 years was better in lean than in obese recipients (88% versus 72%, $p = 0.002$). Patient survival at 7 years was also better in nonobese patients (92% versus 81%, $p = 0.01$). Acute tubular necrosis was more common in obese than in nonobese recipients (24% versus 13%, $p < 0.01$). There were no differences in the incidences of acute or chronic rejection between the two groups (24). In a retrospective study of 240 pancreas-kidney recipients, 12% had a BMI of more than 27 kg/m^2 at transplant. Actuarial patient survival was comparable between obese and nonobese recipients. Actuarial graft survival, both renal and pancreas, was decreased significantly in patients with a BMI of more than 27 mg/m^2. There was no difference in the frequency of acute rejection episodes, and the type and frequency of posttransplant complications were not significantly different (25). Cyclosporine A (CsA) pharmacokinetics appears to be similar in obese and nonobese candidates for renal transplantation (26). The BMI detected at the time of the transplant and the results of different studies about obesity in renal transplant recipients are summarized in Tables 28.1 and 28.2, respectively.

TABLE 28.2. EFFECT OF OBESITY ON OUTCOMES AFTER RENAL TRANSPLANTATION

	Patient Survival	Graft Survival	Acute Rejection	DGF	Wound Complications	PTDM	N
Holley (18)	=	↓		↑	↑	↑	96
Merion (19)	=	=	=		↑		263
Gill (20)	↓	=			↑	↑	170
Pirsch (21)		=	=	↑	↑		584
Drafts (22)	=	=		↑	↑	↑	408
Modlin (23)	↓	=	=	=		↑	304
Meier-Kriesche (24)	↓	↓	=	↑			405
Bumgardner (25)	=	↓	=				240

DGF, delayed graft function; PTDM, posttransplant diabetes mellitus. Results indicated by arrows and equals sign are significant at $p < 0.05$.

In summary, obesity is associated with wound complications (18–22), delayed graft function (18,21,22,24), and PTDM (18,20,22,23). The incidence of acute rejection is not altered by obesity in most studies (19,21,23–25). The effects of obesity on long-term patient and graft survival remain controversial (18–25). The effects of pretransplant obesity on long-term graft and patient survival, although poorly defined, do not seem to be great enough to exclude most obese patients from transplantation. However, obesity increases morbidity after kidney transplantation and obese individuals should be encouraged to lose weight prior to transplant. Unfortunately, there are no controlled studies examining the efficacy of pretransplant weight loss on outcomes.

INSULIN RESISTANCE AFTER RENAL TRANSPLANTATION

In renal transplant recipients there is a high incidence of impaired glucose tolerance and insulin resistance, excluding patients who were already diabetic at the time of transplantation. In a prospective study examining the incidence and risk factors of posttransplant glucose intolerance, 173 consecutive renal transplant recipients underwent either an oral glucose tolerance test (n = 167) or were treated for diabetes mellitus (n = 6) at 10 weeks after transplantation. Of these 173 renal transplant recipients, 18% had PTDM and 31% showed impaired glucose tolerance. All patients received prednisolone, 97% received CsA, 87% received azathioprine, and 86% were undergoing triple therapy (27). Age, prednisolone dose, and the use of beta blockers were associated with impaired glucose tolerance in a multivariate analysis.

In another study, an oral glucose tolerance test was used to categorize 46 renal transplant recipients as having either normal glucose tolerance (54%), impaired glucose tolerance (33%), or PTDM (13%) (28). Insulin sensitivity was measured using a hyperinsulinemic, euglycemic clamp technique. Insulin response was estimated by the increase in serum insulin levels during the oral glucose tolerance test. Those with impaired glucose tolerance or PTDM had the same degree of insulin resistance, and they had a reduction in insulin-stimulated glucose disposal rate compared to the normal glucose tolerance group (4.6 ± 1.6 and 3.4 ± 1.3, respectively, versus 7.1 ± 2.4, $p < 0.05$). The insulin response was reduced in the PTDM group compared to the other two groups (170 ± 128 versus 448 ± 310 and 450 ± 291, $p < 0.05$). All recipients received CsA, azathioprine, and prednisolone, and there were no other major differences between the groups (28).

Insulin resistance is common after renal transplantation (31% to 33% versus 20% to 25% in the nondiabetic general population). Renal transplant recipients often have predisposing conditions for insulin resistance, including obesity; mild or moderate renal failure; and medication use such as glucocorticoids, diuretics, and beta blockers (29). Whatever the cause, it is likely that insulin resistance contributes to the high incidence of cardiovascular disease in renal transplant recipients.

Obesity is common among renal transplant recipients, and insulin resistance is a uniform feature of obesity. Insulin resistance also is related to the severity and type of obesity. Abdominal (visceral) obesity predisposes to insulin resistance much more than peripheral (gluteal or subcutaneous) obesity. The amount of intraabdominal fat may be an important determinant of the effect of obesity on glucose metabolism (2). The relationship between obesity, insulin resistance, leptin, and neuropeptide Y in renal transplant recipients is poorly defined. Leptin is a protein produced by adipose tissue that has an anorectic effect. Neuropeptide Y is produced in the arcuate nucleus and acts in the hypothalamus to stimulate eating. The kidney contributes to the clearance of leptin from the circulation (30). However, both decreased (31,32) and increased (33,34) leptin levels have been reported after renal transplantation. Neuropeptide Y also has been reported to be increased (34).

Mild or moderate renal insufficiency frequently is present in renal transplant recipients and may predispose to insulin resistance. Insulin resistance is common in severe chronic renal failure (29,35) and may be present in earlier stages of renal dysfunction. In a cross-sectional study, insulin sensitivity was diminished in mild renal insufficiency, irrespective of the type of renal disease (29). In another study of 52 patients with mild or moderate renal failure, almost half had insulin resistance. However, in this study, patients with insulin resistance were also significantly more obese (35). Finally, in a study of 18 patients with chronic glomerulonephritis but only mild renal insufficiency, the glomerular filtration rate (estimated by creatinine clearance) was lower in the insulin-resistant group than in the insulin-sensitive group. BMI and family history of non–insulin-dependent diabetes mellitus tended to be greater, however, in the insulin-resistant group (36).

Insulin resistance is associated with a group of conditions that together are known as the "metabolic syndrome" or "syndrome X." This syndrome includes hyperinsulinemia, abdominal (visceral) obesity, hypertension, dyslipidemia, glucose intolerance, abnormalities of blood coagulation (elevated plasminogen-activator inhibitor type 1 and fibrinogen), hyperuricemia, and microalbuminuria. Insulin resistance also is associated with an increased risk of cardiovascular events, and this risk may be attributable to some individual components of the syndrome, such as dyslipidemia and hypertension, or to hyperinsulinemia itself (2,37).

Insulin promotes uptake and transportation of glucose into cells, mainly muscle and fat, and inhibits hepatic glucose production (gluconeogenesis). In addition, insulin stimulates the synthesis and storage of triglycerides in adipocytes (lipogenesis) and inhibits the release of free fatty acids from adipose tissue (lipolysis). Insulin also stimulates the synthesis and secretion of lipoprotein lipase (LPL). LPL is formed in fat and muscle and binds to proteoglycans on the luminal surfaces in the adjacent capillary beds. LPL induces the hydrolysis of triglycerides in chylomicrons and very–low-density lipoprotein (VLDL) to produce free fatty acids and glycerol. The free fatty acids are oxidized to produce energy or are stored as fat.

In insulin resistance there is increased hydrolysis of triglycerides in adipocytes, resulting in the release of free fatty acids into the blood. These free fatty acids constitute the substrate for increased hepatic synthesis of VLDL, leading to hypertriglyceridemia. In addition, LPL activity is reduced in insulin resistance, and this may contribute to reduced VLDL clearance and hypertriglyceridemia (2). Also, when the uptake of free fatty acids by the liver is increased, gluconeogenesis is promoted, resulting in higher production of glucose by the liver (2,37).

In plasma, VLDL transfers triglycerides to high-density lipoprotein (HDL), in exchange for cholesterol esters from HDL, through the action of cholesterol ester transfer protein (CETP). The triglyceride-enriched HDL that results is a substrate for hepatic lipase, which hydrolyzes the triglycerides, and renders a smaller HDL that subsequently is cleared from the circulation. VLDL also can transfer triglycerides to low-density lipoprotein (LDL), in exchange for cholesterol esters, again under the action of CEPT. This results in triglyceride-enriched LDL that generates small, dense particles after hydrolysis of their triglycerides (37). These small, dense LDL are more susceptible to oxidation and are felt to be more atherogenic than regular LDL (2,37–39). Small, dense LDL particles are typically found in the insulin-resistance syndrome (2).

Dyslipidemia of insulin resistance is characterized by increased triglycerides (and VLDL); low HDL-c (HDL-associated cholesterol) concentration; and small, dense LDL. Low HDL-c and the increase in small, dense LDL are an indirect consequence of elevated triglyceride-rich VLDL by means of CETP and hepatic lipase activity. Small, dense LDL is common after renal transplantation. In one study small, dense LDL was more frequent in 47 renal transplant recipients compared to 44 controls (38). In another study LDL size was significantly less in 19 renal transplant recipients than in 19 controls (39). The LDL size was inversely correlated with plasma triglyceride levels (39). It is likely that small, dense LDL results from insulin resistance and other factors after renal transplantation.

When insulin resistance is treated with thiazolidinedione derivatives (troglitazone, rosiglitazone), the dyslipidemia usually improves but does not resolve (2). Triglycerides and free fatty acids tend to decrease, but HDL-c and LDL-c levels do not change significantly (2). Likewise, weight loss can improve insulin resistance and glycemic control in obese non–insulin-dependent diabetes mellitus, but weight loss usually does not correct the dyslipidemia (40).

Diet, exercise, and lifestyle modification have an important role in the prevention and treatment of insulin resistance. Insulin sensitivity is enhanced by reducing weight and visceral adiposity. Regular physical activity ameliorates insulin sensitivity and improves HDL-c and triglyceride levels. Mild alcohol consumption also has been reported to enhance insulin sensitivity and improve HDL-c concentration. However, smoking aggravates insulin resistance and may contribute to decrease HDL-c (41).

Specific dietary components, especially the amount and composition of fatty acids, also may modify insulin sensitivity. For example, in a study of 162 healthy individuals from the general population, dietary monounsaturated fatty acids improved insulin sensitivity compared to saturated fat. However, the beneficial effect of monounsaturated fat is lost when total fat intake is greater than 38% of total calories (42).

The role of dietary carbohydrates in insulin resistance is controversial (43). The glycemic index is a measure of the rate of carbohydrate absorption. Dietary carbohydrates with a high glycemic index produce an elevated postprandial glucose and subsequent insulin response and are associated with reduced insulin sensitivity. In a cross-sectional study of 1,420 adults, there was an inverse relationship between HDL-c levels and the glycemic index of dietary carbohydrates for men and women. The glycemic index was the only dietary variable that correlated with the HDL-c concentration, suggesting that the glycemic index is a better predictor than dietary fat intake for HDL-c levels (44). Interventional studies are needed to assess the role of dietary carbohydrates on insulin resistance and lipid levels.

The CARDIA (Coronary Artery Risk Development in Young Adults) study is a multicenter population-based cohort study of cardiovascular risk factor evolution in 2,909 healthy adults between 18 and 30 years followed for more than 10 years. This study was designed to assess the effect of dietary fiber on weight gain, insulin levels, and other cardiovascular risk factors. Dietary fiber consumption was inversely associated with weight gain, waist-to-hip ratio, and fasting and 2-hour postglucose insulin levels adjusted for BMI in young adults. Intake of fat, protein, and carbohydrate were not associated with insulin levels or cardiovascular risk factors (43).

The amount of dietary fiber in foods contributes to their glycemic index. Fiber has been shown to account for 40% of the variance in glycemic index in foods, and it exerts influence on the insulinemic response to carbohydrates in meals. Low-fiber diets have a higher glycemic index and subsequently tend to stimulate more insulin secretion than high-fiber diets (43). However, randomized, controlled trials are needed to determine the role of fiber on insulin resistance and cardiovascular risk.

In summary, nutritional advice targeting the prevention

and treatment of insulin resistance should be focused on weight loss, and the diet should be rich in fiber, should contain low-glycemic index carbohydrates (pasta, oats, whole grain, vegetables, whole fruit), and should be limited in total and saturated fat. Dietary counseling should be combined with regular exercise and lifestyle modifications, especially smoking cessation.

POSTTRANSPLANT DIABETES MELLITUS

Glucocorticoids are associated with the development of PTDM, probably as a result of insulin resistance and a relative deficiency in insulin production (45). Calcineurin inhibitors, CsA and tacrolimus, also have been implicated in the development of PTDM. In a multicenter, randomized trial comparing tacrolimus and CsA over 1 year of follow-up, 25.4% of patients treated with tacrolimus developed PTDM (requiring insulin) compared to 5% treated with CsA (p = 0.06) (46). In another multicenter, randomized trial, 12% of patients treated with tacrolimus developed PTDM compared to 2.1% receiving CsA (p = 0.001). Altogether, these results suggest that tacrolimus may be more diabetogenic than CsA.

In a prospective, randomized, multicenter study the incidences of PTDM were similar in patients treated with sirolimus (rapamycin) versus CsA (48). In another prospective, randomized, single-center study the incidence of PTDM was similar in patients treated with sirolimus + CsA + prednisone compared to patients treated with CsA + prednisone (49). Thus, sirolimus does not appear to cause PTDM.

DYSLIPIDEMIA AFTER KIDNEY TRANSPLANTATION

Dyslipidemia is a major complication of kidney transplantation that usually requires both diet and pharmacologic management. The prevalence of lipid abnormalities after kidney transplantation is very high (50). The lipid profile in renal transplant recipients is variable, possibly because a number of different factors influence posttransplant lipid metabolism to a greater or lesser degree in individual renal transplant recipients. These include genetic predisposition, immunosuppressive drugs (sirolimus, CsA, tacrolimus, glucocorticoids), other medications (diuretics, beta blockers), obesity, insulin resistance, proteinuria, and impairment of renal function. Sometimes other illnesses promoting lipid abnormalities also are present, such as diabetes, hepatic dysfunction, or infections (51).

The most common dyslipidemias in renal transplant recipients are elevated total cholesterol (about 60% of renal transplant recipients have greater than 240 mg/dL of total cholesterol) and LDL-c (60% have LDL-c greater than 130 mg/dL). However, hypertriglyceridemia is present in 35% of renal transplant recipients. The prevalence of decreased HDL-c is similar in renal transplant recipients and the general population (15%) (50). As discussed earlier, small, dense LDL particles also have been found in renal transplant recipients (38,39,52).

Although lipid-lowering diets have been found to be less effective in renal transplant recipients than in the general population (53,54), they are still an important adjunct in the treatment of dyslipidemia in these patients. In one study, the step-one diet of the American Heart Association (55) was modified by increasing monounsaturated fats and alimentary fiber (56). Patients received a diet with carbohydrates 54% ± 2% (complex carbohydrates 49% ± 2%), proteins 13% ± 1%, lipids 25% ± 2% (saturated fats 9% ± 1%, polyunsaturated fats 2.5% ± 0.5%, monounsaturated fats 14% ± 1%) of total calories, cholesterol 202 ± 10 mg/day and fiber 23 ± 3 g/day. This diet reduced total cholesterol and LDL cholesterol by 10%, and triglycerides by 6.5%, without altering HDL-c in renal transplant recipients (56).

In renal transplant recipients there appears to be an increased susceptibility of LDL to oxidation. This may be the result, in part, of calcineurin inhibitors (39,52). It has been suggested that vitamin C and E supplementation could reduce the risk of cardiovascular disease in renal transplant recipients (52,57). However, there have been no controlled trials examining whether antioxidant vitamins reduce cardiovascular disease after transplantation. Indeed, several large, randomized controlled trials in the general population failed to find any benefit of antioxidant vitamins on cardiovascular disease events. It also has been suggested that vitamin E supplementation may ameliorate chronic renal allograft nephropathy. However, randomized, controlled trials are needed to test this hypothesis as well (58).

DIETARY MANAGEMENT IN HYPERTENSION

Dietary salt restriction is considered to be important in the treatment of hypertension. However, the relationship between sodium intake and blood pressure control is still controversial, possibly because the individual response of blood pressure to variations in sodium intake differs widely (59). Nevertheless, the nutritional recommendations in the sixth report of the Joint National Committee on the Prevention, Detection, Evaluation, and Treatment of High Blood Pressure include dietary sodium restriction (no more than 100 mmol/day) as well as maintenance of adequate dietary potassium (90 mmol/day), calcium, and magnesium. Other nutritional measures recommended include losing weight, if necessary; avoiding excessive alcohol intake, increasing physical activity, abstaining from smoking, and reducing dietary saturated fat and cholesterol intake (59).

Hypertension is common after kidney transplantation, occurring in 50% to 80% of patients. Several factors have been implicated in the pathogenesis of posttransplant hypertension. These include immunosuppressive agents (corticosteroids, CsA, and to a lesser extent tacrolimus), renal allograft dysfunction, hypertension associated with the native kidneys, essential hypertension, and allograft renal artery stenosis (1,60). CsA causes afferent arteriolar vasoconstriction that may lead to a reduced glomerular filtration rate and enhanced tubular sodium reabsorption, both of which may contribute to volume-dependent hypertension (59, 61).

The effect of dietary salt restriction on high blood pressure has not been investigated thoroughly in renal transplant recipients. In an observational study examining the relationship between dietary salt intake and the prevalence of hypertension in 129 renal transplant recipients, there was no significant difference in the frequency of antihypertensive medication between recipients with low, medium, or high urinary sodium excretion (as a measure of salt intake). There was no correlation between sodium excretion and systolic or diastolic blood pressure (61). Prospective controlled trials are needed to better define the role of dietary salt on high blood pressure after kidney transplantation.

In the absence of data from randomized, controlled trials in renal transplant recipients it is reasonable to treat blood pressure using recommendations for the general population. However, some fluid and electrolyte problems that are common in renal transplant recipients occasionally may alter the approach to hypertension. Hyperkalemia, for example, is more common in renal transplant recipients than in the general population, and recommendations regarding potassium intake also may differ.

HYPERURICEMIA

Hyperuricemia is common after kidney transplantation and is probably a consequence of immunosuppressive medications (CsA, tacrolimus), diuretics, and impaired renal function (62,63). A number of epidemiologic studies in the general population have reported an association between hyperuricemia and cardiovascular disease. However, the causal relationship between hyperuricemia and atherosclerotic cardiovascular disease remains unproven, and there are no data from randomized trials demonstrating that reducing uric acid lowers the risk of cardiovascular disease (64). Indeed, it is not clear whether uric acid has a damaging or protective role on cardiovascular system (65). Hyperuricemia also could be a manifestation of insulin resistance (66). In a retrospective study of 375 kidney transplant cases, hyperuricemia was found to be a significant risk factor for graft survival (67). However, there are no randomized trials examining the effects of lowering uric acid on cardiovascular disease in renal transplant recipients.

Gout is more common in renal transplant recipients than in the general population. Nevertheless, most hyperuricemia in renal transplant recipients is mild, is asymptomatic, and does not require treatment with diet or medication (62). Pharmacologic management of hyperuricemia in patients with symptomatic gout is problematic in renal transplant recipients. Allopurinol interferes with azathioprine metabolism; nonsteroidal antiinflammatory agents can reduce glomerular filtration rate and colchicine can cause myopathy (68–70). Dietary management of gout has been largely displaced by drug therapy, but diet continues to be important, especially in renal transplant recipients whose pharmacologic management options are limited. Patients should be advised to avoid excessive alcohol intake and purine-rich foods, such as liver, kidney, sardines, anchovies, fish roe, and sweetbreads.

HYPOMAGNESEMIA

In renal transplant recipients, the calcineurin inhibitors CsA and tacrolimus may cause renal magnesium wasting and hypomagnesemia. Hypomagnesemia has been reported to occur in 7.1% of renal transplant recipients treated with either CsA or tacrolimus (71). Hypomagnesemia has been linked to increased calcineurin-inhibitor toxicity, including neurotoxicity, in renal transplant recipients (62,72–74). Magnesium supplementation also has been reported to reduce total and LDL-c in renal transplant recipients with hypomagnesemia (71). However, others have failed to confirm this (75). In a controlled study of 43 patients in the general population, magnesium lowered apolipoprotein B (76).

Magnesium deficiency has been linked to coronary heart disease, insulin resistance, and type 2 diabetes mellitus in the general population, but the causal nature of these associations remain very much in doubt. The Atherosclerosis Risk in Communities (ARIC) study prospectively investigated the possible influence of serum and dietary magnesium on coronary heart disease in 13,992 adults (77). In this study, there was an inverse relationship between serum magnesium and cardiovascular disease; however, this relationship was no longer statistically significant once LDL-c, diabetes, and systolic blood pressure were taken into account (77). In addition, dietary magnesium was not associated with serum magnesium levels (77). The ARIC study also failed to find convincing evidence for a relationship between either serum or dietary magnesium and the risk for type 2 diabetes mellitus (78). Magnesium deficiency has been suggested to promote insulin resistance (79), but hypomagnesemia also could be a result rather than a cause of insulin resistance (78). Clearly, controlled trials of magnesium supplementation are needed to better understand the relationship between magnesium, coronary heart disease, insulin resistance, and diabetes.

HYPERHOMOCYSTEINEMIA

Hyperhomocysteinemia is associated with cardiovascular disease in the general population, but the pathogenic role of hyperhomocysteinemia in cardiovascular disease is controversial (80). Renal transplant recipients are at increased risk of cardiovascular disease and have a high prevalence of elevated homocysteine (81,82). However, there are no controlled trials in renal transplant recipients or in the general population examining whether lowering homocysteine reduces cardiovascular disease.

Homocysteine is an amino acid created during the metabolism of methionine, an essential amino acid obtained in the diet. Homocysteine can be metabolized through two pathways, remethylation and transsulfuration. The remethylation pathway produces back methionine and requires vitamin B_{12} (cobalamin) and folate. The transsulfuration pathway produces cysteine and glutathione and requires vitamin B_6 (pyridoxine). When cysteine synthesis is required or when there is an excess of methionine, homocysteine is metabolized by the transsulfuration pathway. Enzymes in the transsulfuration pathway are responsible for reversing transient postprandial increases in homocysteine concentration, and their activity can be evaluated by a methionine-challenge test (83).

Depending on the specific vitamin deficiency, increased homocysteine levels may occur after either fasting or methionine loading. If there is a deficit of vitamin B_{12} or folate, the remethylation pathway is inhibited, homocysteine cannot be converted to methionine, and fasting hyperhomocysteinemia results. When there is a deficiency of vitamin B_6, the transsulfuration pathway is impaired. In this case, fasting homocysteine levels are normal or only slightly elevated, but they increase after methionine loading (84).

Nutritional deficiencies in folate, vitamin B_{12}, and vitamin B_6 may promote hyperhomocysteinemia. It also may be caused by other conditions, including several genetic defects, renal insufficiency, hypothyroidism, smoking, some carcinomas, and some medications (83). Albumin and creatinine are independent determinants of homocysteine levels, unrelated to B-vitamin status (85).

In 1998, the U.S. Food and Drug Administration mandated the fortification of cereal grains with folic acid. This folic acid supplementation resulted in an increase in plasma folate in the general population (86). In 86 renal transplant recipients studied after the dietary folic acid fortification policy was instituted, mild fasting hyperhomocysteinemia was still evident (82). In renal transplant recipients renal function is probably the major determinant of elevated plasma homocysteine levels, with vitamins playing a lesser role (82).

In people with normal renal function, vitamin B is very effective in normalizing homocysteine levels. However, the dose needed to decrease homocysteine levels in patients with renal failure has not been determined. In a study comparing the response to hyperhomocysteinemia treatment in renal transplant recipients and patients undergoing hemodialysis, it was found that hyperhomocysteinemia of patients undergoing hemodialysis was more refractory to vitamin B therapy (81).

In summary, vitamin supplementation with folate, B_6, and B_{12} reduces homocysteine level, but the effects on cardiovascular disease currently are being tested in randomized controlled trials in the general population. In renal transplant recipients, the prevalence of hyperhomocysteinemia is high, but its effect on cardiovascular disease is unclear. There is currently insufficient evidence to recommend vitamin supplementation for lowering homocysteine in renal transplant recipients.

THE ROLE OF A LOW-PROTEIN DIET IN THE TREATMENT OF CHRONIC ALLOGRAFT NEPHROPATHY

The efficacy and safety of dietary protein restriction to slow the progression of renal insufficiency in native kidneys remains controversial. The balance of evidence from randomized controlled trials suggests that a low-protein diet indeed slows the rate of decline (87,88). However, the magnitude of the effect is relatively small (89). Indeed, the largest and best-designed randomized trial failed to demonstrate a significant effect on the rate of decline in renal function (90). There are very few studies addressing the role of a low-protein diet in the progression of renal graft dysfunction (91–93), and there are no adequately powered, randomized trials. Additional controlled trials are necessary to determine the role, if any, of dietary protein restriction in the treatment of chronic allograft nephropathy.

CALCIUM, PHOSPHORUS, AND METABOLIC BONE DISEASE

The metabolic bone disease that is common in patients undergoing dialysis usually improves after successful kidney transplantation. Nevertheless, some bone abnormalities persist in renal transplant recipients and other metabolic abnormalities that threaten bone integrity first may appear after renal transplantation. Hyperparathyroidism, which is common among patients undergoing hemodialysis, may persist posttransplant and contribute to both hypophosphatemia and occasionally hypercalcemia. Hypophosphatemia is very common in the first few weeks after kidney transplantation, even in the absence of hyperparathyroidism.

Hypophosphatemia is most often a consequence of renal tubular phosphate wasting. The causes of the renal phosphate wasting are probably multiple. In some patients elevated parathyroid hormone contributes. Glucocorticoids also promote urinary phosphate loss. Reduced dietary intake or inadequate intestinal absorption from medications that bind phosphate or vitamin D deficiency also may play a role. Hypophosphatemia contributes to hypercalcemia by stimulating 1α hydroxylase in the proximal tubule (94). Hypophosphatemia, if severe, can have other adverse metabolic consequences including bone-marrow suppression, insulin resistance, and muscle weakness. Hypophosphatemia from urinary phosphate wasting in the absence of hyperparathyroidism generally can be treated successfully with oral phosphate supplements (62,94). The typical American diet is rich in phosphorus because of the addition of phosphates to foods in processing, especially fast foods, snacks, and soft drinks, the consumption of which is increasing (95). Nevertheless, supplemental phosphate often is required in the early posttransplant period.

Bone loss is a significant complication in renal transplant recipients and is attributable to several factors, including persistent hyperparathyroidism, renal dysfunction, acidosis, and glucocorticoids. The effect of CsA on bone metabolism remains controversial. In renal transplant recipients with normal renal function and normal parathyroid hormone levels, glucocorticoids are the major cause of osteoporosis. Glucocorticoid-induced osteoporosis occurs early after initiation of the therapy, and most posttransplant bone loss occurs during the first 6 to 12 months, when glucocorticoid doses are relatively high. Glucocorticoids inhibit osteoblastic bone formation. They also impair the intestinal absorption of calcium and enhance renal calcium wasting. The resultant negative calcium balance causes parathyroid hormone–mediated bone resorption. In addition, glucocorticoids decrease sex hormone levels and cause muscle weakness, which predisposes to fractures from falling. Preventive measures, when necessary, should be implemented early, if possible, and should include smoking cessation, exercise, nutritional management (see later in this chapter), hormone replacement therapy, thiazide diuretics for hypercalciuria (96), and antiresorptive agents such as calcitonin and bisphosphonates (97).

The effectiveness of diet in preventing glucocorticoid-induced osteoporosis has not been established. Malnutrition has been associated with an increased risk of fractures, but the amount and type of dietary protein and other constituents that are needed to avoid osteoporosis has not been established (98). Certainly, calcium and vitamin D supplementation have been used to prevent osteoporosis in the general population. Milk is the major source of both nutrients, and milk is also rich in high biologic value protein and vitamin A (95). However, at least one observational study in the general population has linked an increased intake of vitamin A to reduced bone mineral density and an increased risk for hip fractures (99). Plasma levels of vitamin A (retinol) and retinol-binding protein have been reported to be increased in renal transplant recipients (100,101). However, the consequences of this increase in vitamin A are unclear (101). Nevertheless, it may be prudent to avoid unnecessary vitamin A supplementation in renal transplant recipients.

HYPOALBUMINEMIA

Hypoalbuminemia is a predictor of all-cause mortality in observational studies from the general population (102), patients undergoing dialysis (103), and renal transplant recipients (104). In addition, hypoalbuminemia has been associated with graft loss in renal transplant recipients (105) and in kidney-pancreas transplant recipients (106). In renal transplant recipients, hypoalbuminemia was present in 31%, 12%, 14%, 20%, and 29% of patients at 3 months, 1 year, 4 years, 8 years, and 12 years, respectively, and it was an independent risk factor for both cardiac and noncardiac mortality (104).

Albumin is synthesized exclusively in the liver and has a half-life of 14 to 20 days. Although the mechanisms that regulate albumin synthesis are not well known, albumin production is increased in response to a reduced plasma oncotic pressure (107). However, the synthesis of albumin decreases when there is extensive hepatocellular injury. Albumin synthesis also is influenced by the availability of amino acid precursors, especially tryptophan. Thus, serum albumin can decline when nutritional status is poor. Serum albumin also can decrease when there are losses related to extensive injury to skin (burns), nephrotic syndrome, blood loss, or protein-losing enteropathy. Serum albumin levels also are affected by shifts between intravascular and extravascular spaces and by changes in intravascular volume. Dehydration causes an increase in serum albumin, whereas overhydration can cause a decline.

Albumin is a negative acute-phase protein, and its synthesis declines during acute and chronic systemic inflammatory states, including infections, trauma, surgery, tissue infarction, cancer, and immunologically mediated conditions (4). The response to inflammation involves changes in the concentrations of several proteins. Positive acute-phase reactants increase and negative acute-phase reactants decrease in response to acute and chronic inflammatory disorders. Positive acute-phase proteins include C-reactive protein (CRP), serum amyloid A, ferritin, sialic acid, and fibrinogen. Negative acute-phase reactants include albumin, transthyretin (prealbumin), transferrin, and IGF-1. The major stimuli for acute-phase protein synthesis are inflammation-associated cytokines (e.g., interleukin-6). Glucocorticoids seem to enhance the stimulatory effect of cytokines on the production of acute-phase reactants (4,108).

Why hypoalbuminemia is a predictor of graft loss and all-cause mortality is uncertain. Low oncotic pressure associated with hypoalbuminemia might lead to a hypercoagulable state, as in nephrotic syndrome (103). Hypoalbuminemia could decrease the antioxidant potential in plasma(109), or it could be associated with impaired endothelial-dependent vasodilatation (110,111). Low serum albumin levels could have a detrimental effect in the free fatty acid transport (102). Serum albumin levels also correlate with HDL-c (112) and homocysteine levels (85). However, the effect of low serum albumin is so strong and pervasive that it is likely that other, more fundamental mechanisms explain the association between hypoalbuminemia and mortality. For example, it recently has been reported that acute-phase reactants, which are associated with hypoalbuminemia, are independent risk factors for cardiovascular disease in both the general population and in patients with chronic renal failure.

In a nested case-control analysis of the Physicians' Health Study, baseline plasma CRP predicted myocardial infarction and stroke, but not venous thrombosis, in apparently healthy men (113). The reduction in the risk of a first myocardial infarction associated with the use of aspirin seemed to be related with the level of CRP (113). CRP was an independent predictor of cardiovascular death in 280 stable patients undergoing hemodialysis (108). CRP and age, but not serum albumin, were significant independent predictors of cardiovascular death in the multivariate Cox regression analysis (108). In another prospective study with 6 years of follow-up, CRP also was reported to be a significant predictor of death in 163 patients undergoing dialysis (114). In both of these studies, there was an inverse correlation between serum albumin and CRP levels, indicating that hypoalbuminemia in patients undergoing dialysis indeed may be an acute-phase reactant.

In renal transplant recipients, CRP and other acute-phase reactants, such as serum amyloid A protein, may be markers of acute rejection (115,116). In a retrospective analysis of 97 patients, with mean follow-up of 564 days, pretransplant CRP levels were higher in recipients who had an acute rejection episode after transplant compared to those without rejection (116). In the Cox regression analysis, pretransplant CRP level was the only independent risk factor for subsequent acute rejection (116).

In summary, hypoalbuminemia is common in renal transplant recipients. It is associated with cardiovascular disease, mortality, and chronic allograft nephropathy. It is likely that hypoalbuminemia reflects an underlying relationship between systemic inflammation and the synthesis and degradation of acute-phase reactants. Thus, it is unlikely that diet or other measures designed to increase albumin synthesis will be effective in improving outcomes after renal transplantation.

POSSIBLE EFFECTS OF DIET ON DRUGS IMPORTANT IN TRANSPLANTATION

There is a potential for interactions between various medications and some dietary components and herbs (e.g., grapefruit juice, St. John's wort). These interactions occasionally have deleterious consequences, and it is conceivable that reported interactions underestimate the full extent of the problem.

Bioavailability of calcineurin inhibitors, CsA and tacrolimus, is highly variable. Both drugs are metabolized primarily by cytochrome P450 isoenzymes in the liver and small intestine, mainly isoenzymes 3A4 (CYP3A4). There are numerous substrates of CYP3A4, including rapamycin, verapamil, diltiazem, nifedipine, felodipine, colchicine, and lovastatin. Inhibitors of these isoenzymes comprise itraconazole, ketoconazole, and erythromycin, whereas inducers of CYP3A4 include phenobarbital, phenytoin, and rifampin (117). Administration of CsA and tacrolimus with these and other medications may cause potentially serious interactions.

P-glycoprotein is a versatile carrier protein located in the enterocyte cellular membrane, which actively transports some substances back into the intestinal lumen, including CsA. P-glycoprotein also is expressed in other tissues, such as liver and kidney. P-glycoprotein first was described as responsible for resistance of tumoral cells to chemotherapy, and it has been recognized as a determinant for drug availability. CYP3A4 and P-glycoprotein share a broad range of substrates, including CsA, tacrolimus, rapamycin, diltiazem, verapamil, nicardipine, colchicine, and cortisol (117,118). CsA availability appears to be determined by CYP3A4 in the liver and small intestine and by P-glycoprotein (117, 118).

The ingestion of grapefruit juice increases the oral availability and concentrations of many CYP3A4 substrates, including CsA, felodipine, and nicardipine. The compounds and mechanisms responsible for this effect of grapefruit juice are being investigated. Grapefruit juice does not modify the availability of intravenous CsA and does not alter hepatic CYP3A4 activity, as measured by the erythromycin breath test (119). Grapefruit juice seems to be an inhibitor of intestinal CYP3A4 and P-glycoprotein (119,120). Some compounds in orange juice also have been reported to be P-glycoprotein inhibitors without having an effect on CYP3A4. The ingestion of orange juice also could have the potential for drug interactions (121). There are studies showing an effect of St. John's wort, a popular herb commonly used for treating depression, inducing intestinal and hepatic CYP3A4 enzymes and intestinal P-glycoprotein (122). Serious clinical consequences have been reported after interaction of CsA with St. John's wort, including acute rejection related to low CsA levels (123,124).

REFERENCES

1. Kasiske BL. Cardiovascular disease after renal transplantation. *Semin Nephrol* 2000;20:176–187.
2. Timar O, Sestier F, Levy E. Metabolic syndrome X: A review. *Can J Cardiol* 2000;16:779–789.
3. Jeejeebhoy KN. Nutritional assessment. *Nutrition* 2000;16: 585–589.

4. Gabay C, Kushner I. Acute-phase proteins and other systemic responses to inflammation. *N Engl J Med* 1999;340:448–454.
5. Ikizler TA, Hakim RM. Nutrition in end-stage renal disease. *Kidney Int* 1996;50:343–357.
6. Kasiske BL. Creatinine excretion after renal transplantation. *Transplantation* 1989;48:424–428.
7. Van den Ham ECH, Kooman JP, Christiaans MHL, et al. Body composition in renal transplant patient: bioimpedance analysis compared to isotope dilution, dual energy x-ray absorptiometry, and anthropometry. *J Am Soc Nephrol* 1999;10:1067–1079.
8. Kopple JD. Pathophysiology of protein-energy wasting in chronic renal failure. *J Nutr* 1999;129(1S):247S–251S.
9. Miller DG, Levine SE, D'Elia JA, et al. Nutritional status of diabetic and nondiabetic patients after renal transplantation. *Am J Clin Nutr* 1986;44:66–69.
10. Verran D, Munn S, Collins J, et al. Impact of renal allograft implantation and immunosuppression on body composition using in vivo neutron activation analysis. *Transplant Proc* 1992; 24:173–174.
11. Ekstrand A, Groop L, Pettersson E, et al. Metabolic control and progression of complications in insulin-dependent diabetic patients after kidney transplantation. *J Intern Med* 1992;232: 253–261.
12. Qureshi AR, Lindholm B, Alvestrand A, et al. Nutritional status, muscle composition and plasma and muscle free amino acids in renal transplant patients. *Clin Nephrol* 1994;42:237–245.
13. Perfumo F, Canepa A, Divino Filho JC, et al. Muscle and plasma amino acids and nutritional status in kidney-transplanted children. *Nephrol Dial Transplant* 1994;1778–1785.
14. van den Ham E, Kooman JP, Christiaans MHL, et al. Relation between steroid dose, body composition and physical activity in renal transplant patients. *Transplantation* 2000;69:1591–1598.
15. Isiklar I, Akin O, Demirag A, et al. Effect of renal transplantation on body composition. *Transplant Proc* 1998;30:831–832.
16. van den Ham E, Kooman JP, Christiaans MHL, et al. Posttransplantation weight gain is predominantly due to an increase in body fat mass. *Transplantation* 2000;70:241–243.
17. Johnson CP, Gallagher-Lepak S, Zhu Y, et al. Factors influencing weight gain after renal transplantation. *Transplantation* 1993;56:822–827.
18. Holley JL, Shapiro R, Lopatin WB, et al. Obesity as a risk factor following cadaveric renal transplantation. *Transplantation* 1990; 49:387–389.
19. Merion RM, Twork AM, Rosenberg L, et al. Obesity and renal transplantation. *Surg Gynecol Obstet* 1991;172:367–376.
20. Gill IS, Hodge EE, Novick AC, et al. Impact of obesity on renal transplantation. *Transplant Proc* 1993;25:1047–1048.
21. Pirsch JD, Armbrust MJ, Knechtle SJ, et al. Obesity as a risk factor following renal transplantation. *Transplantation* 1995;59: 631–647.
22. Drafts HH, Anjum MR, Wynn JJ, et al. The impact of pre-transplant obesity on renal transplant outcomes. *Clin Transplantation* 1997;11:493–496.
23. Modlin CS, Flechner SM, Goormastic M, et al. Should obese patients lose weight before receiving a kidney transplant? *Transplantation* 1997;64:599–604.
24. Meier-Kriesche HU, Vaghela M, Thambuganipalle R, et al. The effect of body mass index on long-term renal allograft survival. *Transplantation* 1999;68:1294–1297.
25. Bumgardner GL, Henry ML, Elkhammas E, et al. Obesity as a risk factor after combined pancreas/kidney transplantation. *Transplantation* 1995;60:1426–1430.
26. Flechner EM, Kolbeinsson ME, Tam J, et al. The impact of body weight on cyclosporine pharmacokinetics in renal transplant recipients. *Transplantation* 1989;47:806–810.
27. Hjelmesætj J, Hartmann A, Kofstad J, et al. Glucose intolerance after renal transplantation depends upon prednisolone dose and recipient age. *Transplantation* 1997;64:979–983.
28. Midtvedt K, Hartmann A, Hjelmesætj J, et al. Insulin resistance is a common denominator of post-transplant diabetes mellitus and impaired glucose tolerance in renal transplant recipients. *Nephrol Dial Transplant* 1998;13:427–431.
29. Fliser D, Pacini G, Engelleiter R, et al. Insulin resistance and hyperinsulinemia are already present in patients with incipient renal disease. *Kidney Int* 1998;53:1343–1347.
30. Sharma K, Considine RV, Michael B, et al. Plasma leptin is partly cleared by the kidney and is elevated in hemodialysis patients. *Kidney Int* 1997;51:1980–1985.
31. Landt M, Brennan DC, Parvis CA, et al. Hyperleptinemia of end-stage renal disease is corrected by renal transplantation. *Nephrol Dial Transplant* 1998;13:2271–2275.
32. Kotok F, Adamczak M, Więcek A. Plasma leptin concentration in kidney transplant patients during the early post-transplant period. *Nephrol Dial Transplant* 1998;13:2276–2280.
33. Kagan A, Haran N, Leschinsky L, et al. Leptin in CAPD patients: serum concentrations and peritoneal loss. *Nephrol Dial Transplant* 1999;14:400–405.
34. Kotok F, Adamczak M, Więcek A, et al. Plasma immunoreactive leptin and neuropeptide Y levels in kidney transplant patients. *Am J Nephrol* 1999;19:28–33.
35. Dzúrik R, Spustová V, Janeková K. The prevalence of insulin resistance in kidney disease patients before the development of renal failure. *Nephron* 1995;69:281–285.
36. Kato Y, Hayashi M, Ohno Y, et al. Mild renal dysfunction is associated with insulin resistance in chronic glomerulonephritis. *Clin Nephrol* 2000;54:366–373.
37. Ginsberg HN. Insulin resistance and cardiovascular disease. *J Clin Invest* 2000;106:453–458.
38. Rajman I, Harper L, McPake D, et al. Low-density lipoprotein subfraction profiles in chronic renal failure. *Nephrol Dial Transplant* 1998;13:2281–2287.
39. Ghanem H, van den Dorpel MA, Weimar W, et al. Increased low density lipoprotein oxidation in stable kidney transplant recipients. *Kidney Int* 1996;49:488–493.
40. Carruthers SG. Diet and hypertension. In: Carroll KK, ed. *Current perspectives on nutrition and health.* Canada: McGill-Queen's University Press, 1998.
41. Gordon DJ. Factors affecting high-density lipoproteins. *Endocrinol Metab Clin North Am* 1998;27:699–709.
42. Ricardi G, Rivellese AA. Dietary treatment of the metabolic syndrome—the optimal diet. *Br J Nutr* 2000;83(Suppl 1): S143–S148.
43. Ludwig DS, Pereira MA, Kroenke CH, et al. Dietary fiber, weight gain, and cardiovascular disease risk factors in young adults. *JAMA* 1999;282:1539–1546.
44. Frost G, Leeds AA, Doré CJ, et al. Glycaemic index as a determinant of HDL-cholesterol concentration. *Lancet* 1999;353: 1045–1048.
45. Weir MR, Fink JC. Risk for posttransplant diabetes mellitus with current immunosuppressive medications. *Am J Kidney Dis* 1999;34:1–13.
46. Vincenti F, Laskow DA, Neylan JF, et al. One-year follow-up of an open-label trial of FK506 for primary kidney transplantation. *Transplantation* 1996;61:1576–1581.
47. Mayer AD, Dmitrewski J, Squifflet JP, et al. Multicenter randomized trial comparing tacrolimus (FK506) and cyclosporine in the prevention of renal allograft rejection. *Transplantation* 1997;64:436–443.
48. Groth CG, Bäckman L, Morales JM, et al. Sirolimus (rapamycin)-based therapy in human renal transplantation. *Transplantation* 1999;67:1036–1042.
49. Kahan BD, Podbielski J, Napoli KL, et al. Immunosuppressive

effects and safety of a sirolimus/cyclosporine combination regimen for renal transplantation. *Transplantation* 1998;66: 1040–1046.

50. Kasiske BL. Hyperlipidemia in patients with chronic renal disease. *Am J Kidney Dis* 1998;5(Suppl 3):S142–S156.
51. Khovidhunkit W, Memon RA, Feingold KR, et al. Infection and inflammation-induced proatherogenic changes of lipoproteins. *J Infect Dis* 2000;181(Suppl 3):S462–S472.
52. Varguese Z, Fernando RL, Turakhia G, et al. Calcineurin inhibitors enhance low-density lipoprotein oxidation in transplant patients. *Kidney Int* 1999;56(Suppl 71):S134–S140.
53. Bastani B, Robinson S, Heisler T, et al. Post-transplant hyperlipidemia: Risk factors and response to dietary modification and gemfibrozil therapy. *Clin Transplantation* 1995;9:340–348.
54. Tonstad S, Holdaas H, Gørbitz C, et al. Is dietary intervention effective in post-transplant hyperlipidemia? *Nephrol Dial Transplant* 1995;10:82–85.
55. National Cholesterol Education Program. Second Report of the Expert Panel on Detection, Evaluation, and Treatment of High Blood Cholesterol in Adults (Adult Treatment Panel II). *Circulation* 1994;89:1329–1445.
56. Barbagallo CM, Cefalù AB, Gallo S, et al. Effects of Mediterranean diet on lipid levels and cardiovascular risk in renal transplant recipients. *Nephron* 1999;82:199–204.
57. Juskowa J, Paczek L, Laskowska-Klita T, et al. Antioxidant potential in renal allograft recipients with stable graft function. *Transplant Proc* 2000;32:1353–1357.
58. Vela C, Cristol JP, Ribstein J, et al. Antioxidant supplementation and chronic renal transplant dysfunction. *Transplant Proc* 2000;32:427–428.
59. The Sixth Report of the Joint National Committee on Prevention, Detection, Evaluation, and Treatment of High Blood Pressure. *Arch Intern Med* 1997;157:2413–2446.
60. Kasiske BL. Risk factors for accelerated atherosclerosis in renal transplant recipients. *Am J Med* 1988;84:985–992.
61. Moeller T, Buhl M, Schorr U, et al. Salt intake and hypertension in renal transplant patients. *Clin Nephrol* 2000;53:159–163.
62. Kasiske BL, Vazquez MA, Harmon WE, et al. Recommendations for the Outpatient Surveillance of Renal Transplant Recipients. *J Am Soc Nephrol* 2000;11:S1–S86.
63. Clive DM. Renal transplant-associated hyperuricemia and gout. *J Am Soc Nephrol* 2000;11:974–979.
64. Rich MW. Uric acid: is it a risk factor for cardiovascular disease? *Am J Cardiol* 2000;85:1018–1021.
65. Waring WS, Webb DJ, Maxwell SRJ. Uric acid as a risk factor for cardiovascular disease. *Q J Med* 2000;93:707–713.
66. Reaven GM. The kidney: an unwilling accomplice in syndrome X. *Am J Kidney Dis* 1997;30:928–931.
67. Gerhardt U, Hüttmann MG, Hohage H. Influence of hyperglycemia and hyperuricemia on long-term transplant survival in kidney transplant recipients. *Clin Transplantation* 1999;13: 375–379.
68. Jonsson J, Gelpi JR, Light JA, et al. Colchicine-induced myoneuropathy in a renal transplant patient. *Transplantation* 1992; 53:1369–1371.
69. Cook M, Ramos E, Peterson J, et al. Colchicine neuromyopathy in a renal transplant patient with normal muscle enzyme levels (letter). *Clin Nephrol* 1994;42:67–68.
70. Kuncl RW, Duncan G, Watson D, et al. Colchicine myopathy and neuropathy. *N Engl J Med* 1987;316:1562–1568.
71. Gupta BK, Glicklick D, Tellis VA. Magnesium repletion therapy improves lipid metabolism in hypomagnesemic renal transplant recipients. *Transplantation* 1999;69:1485–1487.
72. Niederstadt C, Steinhojj J, Erbslöh-Möller B, et al. Effect of FK506 on magnesium homeostasis after renal transplantation. *Transplant Proc* 1997;29:3161–3162.
73. Ramos EL, Barri YM, Kubilis P, et al. Hypomagnesemia in renal transplant patients: improvement over time and association with hypertension and CsA levels. *Clin Transplantation* 1995;9: 185–189.
74. Vannini SD, Mazzola BL, Rodoni L, et al. Permanently reduced plasma ionized magnesium among renal transplant recipients on cyclosporine. *Transpl Int* 1999;12:244–249.
75. Nguyen T, Steiner RW. A trial of oral magnesium supplementation in renal transplant recipients receiving cyclosporine. *Transplant Proc* 1998;30:4317–4319.
76. Rasmussen HS, Aurup P, Goldstein K, et al. Influence of magnesium substitution therapy on blood lipid composition in patients with ischemic heart disease: a double-blind, placebo controlled study. *Arch Intern Med* 1989;149:1050–1053.
77. Liao F, Folsom AR, Brancati FL. Is low magnesium concentration a risk factor for coronary heart disease? The Atherosclerosis Risk in Communities (ARIC) Study. *Am Heart J* 1998;136: 480–490.
78. Orchard TJ. Magnesium and type 2 diabetes mellitus. *Arch Intern Med* 1999;159:2119–2120.
79. Nadler JL, Buchanan T, Natarajan R, et al. Magnesium deficiency produces insulin resistance and increased thromboxane synthesis. *Hypertension* 1993;21:1024–1029.
80. Brattström L, Wilcken DEL. Homocysteine and cardiovascular disease: cause or effect? *Am J Clin Nutr* 2000;72:315–323.
81. Bostom AG, Shemin D, Gohh RY, et al. Treatment of hyperhomocysteinemia in hemodialysis and renal transplant recipients. *Kidney Int* 2001;59(Suppl 78):S246–S252.
82. Bostom AG, Gohh RY, Beaulieu AJ, et al. Determinants of fasting plasma total homocysteine levels among chronic stable renal transplant recipients. *Transplantation* 1999;68:257–261.
83. Welch GN, Loscalzo J. Homocysteine and atherothrombosis. *N Engl J Med* 1998;338:1042–1050.
84. Selhub J, Miller JW. The pathogenesis of homocysteinemia: interruption of the coordinate regulation by S-adenosylmethionine of the remethylation and transsulfuration of homocysteine. *Am J Clin Nutr* 1992;55:131–138.
85. Bostom AG, Lathrop L. Hyperhomocysteinemia in end-stage renal disease: prevalence, etiology, and potential relationship to arteriosclerotic outcomes. *Kidney Int* 1997;52:10–20.
86. Jacques PF, Selhub J, Bostom AG, et al. The effect of folic fortification on plasma folate and total homocysteine concentrations. *N Engl J Med* 1999;340:1449–1454.
87. Fouque D, Laville M, Boissel JP, et al. Controlled low protein diets in chronic renal insufficiency: meta-analysis. *Br Med J* 1992;304:216–220.
88. Pedrini MT, Levey AS, Lau J, et al. The effect of dietary protein restriction on the progression of diabetic and nondiabetic renal diseases: a meta-analysis. *Ann Med Intern* 1996;124:627–632.
89. Kasiske BL, Lakatua JDA, Ma JZ, et al. A meta-analysis of the effects of dietary protein restriction on the rate of decline in renal function. *Am J Kidney Dis* 1998;31:954–961.
90. Klahr S, Levey AS, Greene T, et al. The effects of dietary protein restriction and blood-pressure control on the progression of chronic renal disease. *N Engl J Med* 1994;330:877–884.
91. Bernardi A, Biasia F, Piva M, et al. Dietary protein intake and nutritional status in patients with renal transplant. *Clin Nephrol* 2000;53:3–5.
92. Rosenberg ME, Salahudeen AK, Hostetter TH. Dietary protein and the renin-angiotensin system in chronic renal allograft rejection. *Kidney Int* 1995;48(Suppl 52):S102–S106.
93. Remuzzi G, Perico N. Protecting single-kidney allografts from long-term functional deterioration. *J Am Soc Nephrol* 1998;9: 1321–1332.
94. Heering P, Degenhardt S, Grabensee B. Tubular dysfunction following kidney transplantation. *Nephron* 1996;74:501–511.

95. Calvo MS. Dietary considerations to prevent loss of bone and renal function. *Nutrition* 2000;16:564–566.
96. LaCroix AZ, Ott SM, Ichikawa L, et al. Low-dose hydrochlorothiazide and preservation of bone mineral density in older adults. a randomized, double-blind, placebo-controlled trial. *Ann Intern Med* 2000;133:516–526.
97. Lane NE, Lukert B. The science and therapy of glucocorticoid-induced bone loss. *Endocrinol Metab Clin North Am* 1998;27: 465–483.
98. Munger RG, Cerhan JR, Chiu BCH. Prospective study of dietary protein intake and risk of hip fracture in postmenopausal women. *Am J Clin Nutr* 1999;69:147–152.
99. Melhus H, Michaëlsson K, Kindmark A, et al. Excessive dietary intake of vitamin A is associated with reduced bone mineral density and increased risk for hip fracture. *Ann Intern Med* 1998; 129:770–778.
100. Kelly GE, Yow D, Meikle W, et al. The retinoid status of kidney transplant recipients. *Nephron* 1988;50:68–69.
101. Kelleher J, Humphrey CS, Homer D, et al. Vitamin A and its transport proteins in patients with chronic renal failure receiving maintenance haemodialysis and after renal transplantation. *Clin Sci* 1983;65:619–623.
102. Gillum RF, Makuc DM. Serum albumin, coronary heart disease, and death. *Am Heart J* 1992;123:507–513.
103. Foley RN, Parfrey PS, Harnett JD, et al. Hypoalbuminemia, cardiac morbidity, and mortality in end-stage renal disease. *J Am Soc Nephrol* 1996;7:728–736.
104. Guijarro C, Massy ZA, Wiederkehr MR, et al. Serum albumin and mortality after renal transplantation. *Am J Kidney Dis* 1996; 27:117–123.
105. Massy ZA, Guijarro C, Wiederkehr MR, et al. Chronic renal allograft rejection: Immunologic and nonimmunologic risk factors. *Kidney Int* 1996;49:518–524.
106. Becker BN, Becker YT, Heisey DM, et al. The impact of hypoalbuminemia in kidney-pancreas transplant recipients. *Transplantation* 1999;68:72–75.
107. Kaysen GA. Biological basis of hypoalbuminemia in ESRD. *J Am Soc Nephrol* 1998;9:2368–2376.
108. Zimmerman J, Herrlinger S, Pruy A, et al. Inflammation enhances cardiovascular risk and mortality in hemodialysis patients. *Kidney Int* 1999;55:648–658.
109. Cha MK, Kim IH. Glutathione-linked thiol peroxidase activity of human serum albumin's possible antioxidant role of serum albumin in blood plasma. *Biochem Biophys Res Commun* 1996; 222:619–625.
110. Keaney JF Jr, Simon DL, Stamler JS, et al. NO forms an adduct with serum albumin that has endothelium-derived relaxing factor-like properties. *J Clin Invest* 1993;91:1582–1589.
111. Minamiyama Y, Takemura S, Inove M. Albumin is an important vascular tonus regulator as a reservoir of nitric oxide. *Biochem Biophys Res Commun* 1996;225:112–115.
112. Nanji AA, Reddy S. Use of total cholesterol/albumin ratio as an alternative to high density lipoprotein cholesterol measurement. *J Clin Pathol* 1983;36:716–718.
113. Ridker PM, Cushman M, Stampfer MJ, et al. Inflammation, aspirin, and the risk of cardiovascular disease in apparently healthy men. *N Engl J Med* 1997;336:973–979.
114. Iseki K, Tozawa M, Yoshi S, et al. Serum C-reactive protein (CRP) and risk of death in chronic dialysis patients. *Nephrol Dial Transplant* 1999;14:1956–1960.
115. Harris KR, Digard NJ, Lee HA. Serum C-reactive protein. A useful and economical marker of immune activation in renal transplantation. *Transplantation* 1996;61:1593–1600.
116. Perez RV, Brown DJ, Katznelson SA, et al. Pretransplant systemic inflammation and acute rejection after renal transplantation. *Transplantation* 2000;69:869–874.
117. Wacher VJ, Silverman JA, Zhang Y, et al. Role of P-glycoprotein and cytochrome P450 3A in limiting oral absorption of peptides and peptidomimetics. *J Pharm Sci* 1998;87:1322–1330.
118. Lown KS, Mayo RR, Leichtman AB, et al. Role of intestinal P-glycoprotein (mdr1) in interpatient variation in the oral bioavailability of cyclosporine. *Clin Pharmacol Ther* 1997;62: 248–260.
119. Edwards DJ, Fitzsimmons ME, Schuetz EG, et al. 6′,7′-Dihydroxybergamottin in grapefruit juice and Seville orange juice: effects on cyclosporine disposition, enterocyte CYP3A4, and P-glycoprotein. *Clin Pharmacol Ther* 1999;65:237–244.
120. Bailey DG, Malcolm J, Arnold O, et al. Grapefruit juice-drug interactions. *Br J Clin Pharmacol* 1998;46:101–110.
121. Takanaga H, Ohnishi A, Yamada S, et al. Polymethoxylated flavones in orange juice are inhibitors of P-glycoprotein but not cytochrome P450 3A4. *J Pharmacol Exp Ther* 2000;293: 230–236.
122. Dürr D, Steiger B, Kullak-Ublick GA, et al. St. John's Wort induces intestinal P-glycoprotein/MDR1 and intestinal and hepatic CYP3A4. *Clin Pharmacol Ther* 2000;68:598–604.
123. Barone GW, Gurley BJ, Ketel BL, et al. Herbal supplements: a potential for drug interactions in transplant recipients. *Transplantation* 2001;71:239–241.
124. Cheng TO. Comment: drug-herb interaction (letter). *Ann Pharmacother* 2001;35:124–125.

29

NUTRITIONAL MANAGEMENT OF THE CHILD WITH KIDNEY DISEASE

VIMAL CHADHA
BRADLEY A. WARADY

ETIOLOGY AND IMPACT OF MALNUTRITION

Protein-energy malnutrition (PEM) is a common problem in patients with chronic kidney disease (CKD) and those undergoing maintenance dialysis therapy. Although the exact prevalence of PEM in children is not known, an indirect estimate of the problem can be gauged from the prevalence of growth failure in these patients because growth retardation is a major consequence of PEM in children. Although several factors such as acidemia, calcitriol deficiency, renal osteodystrophy, and most importantly tissue resistance to the actions of growth hormone (GH) and insulinlike growth factor-1 (IGF-1) contribute to the impaired skeletal growth of pediatric patients with CKD, malnutrition plays a critical role, especially during the first few years of life. Clinical experience also suggests that suboptimal nutrition may contribute to an impaired neurodevelopmental outcome in the youngest patients with renal insufficiency (1–4).

Malnutrition in children with CKD and end-stage renal disease (ESRD) is multifactorial in origin (Table 29.1). However, inadequate voluntary nutritional intake is a major contributing factor, especially in infants (5). A number of studies in infants and children undergoing peritoneal dialysis (PD) have documented mean energy intakes of less than 75% of recommended levels (6–8). In a large, prospective study of growth failure in children with CKD, calorie intakes were less than 80% of the recommended dietary allowance (RDA) for age in more than one-half of food records obtained (9). In contrast, protein intake normally exceeded the RDA (6,8,10).

The taste sensation of patients with renal disease frequently is altered and probably also influences the voluntary nutrient intake. Although zinc depletion has been linked to anorexia and a low dietary intake of zinc and low serum zinc concentration have been reported in children with decreased taste acuity undergoing maintenance dialysis (11,12), it has not clearly been demonstrated that zinc supplementation improves taste acuity and appetite. Serum levels of a recently identified small peptide hormone "leptin" have been shown to be elevated in patients with CKD and those undergoing maintenance dialysis. Produced mainly in the adipose tissue and primarily cleared by the kidney, it is speculated that hyperleptinemia also might contribute to uremic anorexia and malnutrition (13–15). Finally, patients with CKD usually receive multiple medications, and drugs such as angiotensin converting enzyme (ACE) inhibitors or antihistamines may adversely influence taste perception and, in turn, nutrient intake (16,17).

Nausea and vomiting are common in infants and children with CKD/ESRD and contribute to feeding dysfunction and a poor nutritional status. Delayed gastric emptying and gastroesophageal reflux have been detected in as many as 70% of patients with these problems (18). Although the etiology of these gastrointestinal abnormalities is unclear, factors such as autonomic dysfunction and the actions of uremic toxins on gastric smooth muscle activity have been implicated (19).

The diagnosis of CKD also results in substantial emotional distress in many patients and their families, which may affect nutritional intake adversely. The social and financial situation of the family also might prevent, on occasion, the patient and family from procuring or preparing appropriate food items.

The provision of adequate nutrition and the prevention of PEM are necessary to promote optimal growth and development in children with impaired kidney function while minimizing the physiologic and biochemical consequences of uremia. The goal of this chapter is to provide a comprehensive review of the many factors that impact the nutritional status of infants, children, and adolescents with CKD or receiving maintenance dialysis and to provide treatment recommendations. Since the initial publication of this chapter in 1997, a European committee has published guidelines for the assessment of growth and nutritional status in children undergoing chronic PD (20) and the National Kidney Foundation Kidney/Disease Outcome Quality Initiative

TABLE 29.1. CAUSES OF PROTEIN-ENERGY MALNUTRITION IN CHILDREN WITH CHRONIC KIDNEY DISEASE

Inadequate food intake secondary to
Anorexia
Altered taste sensation
Nausea/vomiting
Emotional distress
Intercurrent illness
Unpalatable prescribed diets
Impaired ability to procure food because of socioeconomic situation
Chronic inflammatory state
Catabolic response to superimposed illnesses
Possible accumulation of endogenously formed uremic toxins and/or the ingestion of exogenous toxins
Removal of nutrients during dialysis procedure
Endocrine causes such as
Resistance to the actions of insulin, growth hormone, and insulinlike growth factor-1
Hyperglucagonemia
Hyperparathyroidism

(NKF-K/DOQI) (21) has published clinical practice guidelines addressing the nutritional status of children with renal insufficiency following a review of the pertinent medical/nutrition literature and the collection of expert clinical opinion. Where appropriate, the latter guidelines will be incorporated into this text.

ASSESSMENT OF NUTRITIONAL STATUS

There is no single measure available that alone can assess a patient's nutritional status accurately. Multiple indices, therefore, are measured concurrently and evaluated collectively to provide an overall impression (Table 29.2).

Evaluation of Nutrient Intake

Dietary recall and food intake records kept in a diary are the two most common methods used for estimating the nutrient intake (22). The dietary recall (usually obtained for the previous 24 hours) is a simple and rapid method of obtaining a crude assessment of dietary intake. Because it relies on the patient's (or their parents') memory, the responses may not always be valid. However, the advantages to the recall method are that respondents usually will not be able to modify their eating behavior in anticipation of this dietary evaluation, and they do not have to be literate to provide the information. A trained dietitian can obtain useful information from patients by using various models of foods and measuring devices to estimate food portion sizes.

Dietary diaries are written reports of foods eaten during a specified length of time, characteristically 3 to 4 days,

TABLE 29.2. INDICES USED FOR NUTRITIONAL ASSESSMENT

Nutrient intake estimation
Dietary recall
Dietary diary
Physical measurements
Weight
Length/height
Head circumference
Skinfold thickness
Body mass index
Midarm circumference
Midarm muscle circumference
Midarm muscle area
Biochemical determinations
Serum albumin
Serum prealbumin
Serum retinol-binding protein
Serum transferrin
Serum complement fractions
Serum insulinlike growth factor-1
Special studies
Protein equivalent of total nitrogen appearance
Bioelectrical impedance analysis
Dual-energy X-ray absorptiometry
Subjective global assessment
Nutritional physical examination

including a weekend day. A 3-day food intake diary provides a more reliable estimate of an individual's nutrient intake than do single-day records. The actual number of days chosen to collect food records should depend on the degree of accuracy needed, the day-to-day variability in the intake of the nutrient being measured, and the cooperation of the patient. Records kept for more than 3 days increase the likelihood of inaccurate reporting because an individual's motivation typically will decrease with an increasing number of days of dietary data collection, especially if the days are consecutive (23).

The validity and reliability of the dietary interviews and diaries are dependent on the patient's ability to provide accurate data and the ability of the dietitian to conduct detailed, probing interviews. Food records must be maintained meticulously to maximize the accuracy of the diary. Food intake should be recorded at the time the food is eaten to minimize any reliance on memory. Recording errors can be minimized if proper directions on how to approximate portion sizes and servings of fluid are provided. The dietitian should review carefully the food record with the patient for accuracy and completeness shortly after it is completed. In most cases the intake of nutrients is then calculated using computer-based programs.

Physical Measurements (Anthropometry)

The evaluation of anthropometric parameters is a fundamental component of the nutritional assessment in pediatrics. Measurement must be done according to standardized protocols with accurate and consistent equipment and, ideally, by the same person on each occasion (21,24,25). Recumbent length, height, weight, head circumference, midarm circumference (MAC), and skinfold thickness are measured directly, whereas body mass index (BMI), midarm muscle circumference (MAMC), and midarm muscle area (MAMA) are calculated from the primary measurements. It is important to note that serial measurements are necessary for the assessment of growth because one-time measurements reflect only a patient's size.

Once measured, weight, length/height, head circumference, and BMI should be plotted on the appropriate Centers for Disease Control and Prevention (CDC) growth chart specific for the patient's age and sex (26). For premature infants until 2 years of age, the growth chart should be corrected for gestational age. The year 2000 CDC growth charts are revised versions of the 1977 National Center for Health Statistics (NCHS) growth charts (27). The data used to construct the revised CDC charts were derived from the National Health and Nutrition Examination Survey. Most of the differences between the revised and old charts pertain to data for infants; the revised charts include a better mix of both breastfed and formula-fed infants in the U.S. population.

All anthropometric measurements should be expressed as a Standard Deviation Score (SDS), also known as z score. The SDS is calculated using the patient's actual measurement compared with control values of the same chronologic age and sex, according to the following equation:

$$\text{SDS} = \frac{[\text{Patient's actual value}] - [\text{value at 50th percentile for controls}]}{\text{Standard deviation of the control subject}}$$

The tables of 50th percentile and standard deviation values used for calculating SDS still are based on the 1977 NCHS data (27) and are available in the NKF-K/DOQI guidelines (21). An SDS within two standard deviations of the mean encompasses 95% of healthy children; an SDS greater than +2.0 or more negative than −2.0 is abnormal and mandates further evaluation. For children who are growth stunted, recommendations on whether their anthropometric measurements should be compared to children of the same chronologic age or height age are inconsistent.

Recumbent length is measured in children up to approximately 24 months of age or in older children who are unable to stand without assistance. The measurement is performed by laying the child supine on an infant stature board with a fixed headboard and a moveable footboard positioned perpendicular to the table surface with a measuring scale on one side. The head of the infant should be held in contact with the headboard and a second person should grasp one or both feet at the ankle, moving the footboard close to the infant's feet as the legs are gently straightened. The footboard should rest firmly against the infant's heels, making sure the toes point straight upward and the knees are pressed down on the table. The length is read to the nearest 0.1 cm.

Height is measured when the child is able to stand unassisted. The child is made to stand barefooted with his back toward the stadiometer fixed on a wall. The heels, buttocks, shoulders, and head all should touch the stadiometer. The headboard is brought down until it touches the head firmly and is perpendicular to the measuring scale. The height is measured to the nearest 0.1 cm. Usually, three measurements within 0.2 cm of each other are performed, and the average of the three is used for the final value. The timing of when the length measurement is changed to height measurement should be noted on the growth chart because of the discrepancy between the two measurements that commonly exists.

Weight is measured to the nearest 0.1 kg and should be measured while the child is nude (young infants) or wearing very light clothing. The infant scale or the standing machine scale should be calibrated to zero before a measurement is made. Special attention should be devoted to patients with edema or who are undergoing maintenance dialysis because changes in weight are more reflective of shifts in fluid balance than of true weight gain or loss of solid matter. It is important to determine the patient's "dry weight," which can be challenging because growing children are expected to gain weight. Five parameters are helpful for this estimate: measured weight, presence of edema, blood pressure, laboratory data, and the dietary interview. The midweek, postdialysis weight is used for evaluation purposes in the patient undergoing hemodialysis, and the weight at a monthly visit (minus dialysis fluid in the peritoneal cavity) is used for the child undergoing PD. A careful physical examination should be conducted to look for edema in the periorbital, pedal, and other regions of the body. Hypertension that resolves with dialysis can be indicative of excess fluid weight. Decreased serum sodium and albumin levels may be markers of overhydration. Likewise, a rapid weight gain in the absence of a significant increase in reported energy intake or decrease in physical activity must be evaluated critically before it is assumed to be dry weight gain.

The head circumference is measured in children up to 36 months of age with a firm nonstretchable tape. The tape is placed just above the supraorbital ridges and over the most prominent point on the occiput as the maximum head circumference to the nearest 0.1 cm is recorded.

Skinfold thickness measurement is a well-established clinical method for measuring body fat (28). The subcutaneous fat measurement is a reliable estimate of total body fat in nutritionally stable individuals because one-half of the body's fat content is located in the subcutaneous layer (29). Ideally, the skinfold thickness should be measured at four sites (triceps, biceps, subscapular, and iliac crest) that quantify subcutaneous adipose tissue thickness on the limbs and trunk to make an accurate assessment of body fat (30). However, the most common skinfold thickness measured in children is the triceps skinfold (TSF) because of the availability of normal values and the ease of measurement (31). Skinfold measurements only should be made when patients treated with maintenance dialysis are at their dry weight because fluid retention may falsely increase the skinfold thickness.

The MAC is measured to the nearest 0.1 cm using a nonstretchable flexible steel tape measure at the midpoint between the acromion and the olecranon process. The MAC is used for calculating the MAMC and the MAMA by the following formulas:

$$\text{MAMC (cm)} = \text{MAC (cm)} - (3.14 \times \text{TSF in cm})$$

$$\text{MAMA (for males): } [(\text{MAC} - 3.14 \times \text{TSF})^2/4 \times 3.14] - 10$$

$$\text{MAMA (for females): } [(\text{MAC} - 3.14 \times \text{TSF})^2/4 \times 3.14] - 6.5$$

Anthropometric measures of skeletal muscle mass (MAMC and MAMA) are an indirect assessment of skeletal muscle mass, and muscle and somatic protein as approximately 60% of total body protein are located in the skeletal muscle (29). The MAC, MAMC, MAMA, and TSF are evaluated according to tables of normal values for children of the same age and sex (32). The tables are available in the NKF-K/DOQI guidelines (21).

BMI has proved to be another useful and practical method for assessing the level of body fatness (33). It is calculated by dividing weight (in kilograms) by height (in meters) squared; reference values are available for children older than 1 year of age (31,34). Although BMI is a good measure of obesity, it does not provide information regarding the distribution of lean body mass and fat mass, and it also will be influenced by altered states of hydration in patients undergoing dialysis.

Biochemical Determinations

Serum total protein, albumin, prealbumin, retinol-binding protein, transferrin, and complement fractions are measurements of visceral protein stores. Serum albumin levels have been used extensively to assess the nutritional status of individuals with and without CKD (35). Many studies have shown that hypoalbuminemia present at the time of initiation of chronic dialysis as well as during the course of dialysis is a strong independent predictor of patient morbidity and mortality (36–49). In a recent pediatric study by Gulati et al. (49), hypoalbuminemia was associated with an increased incidence of technique failure in patients undergoing PD. Despite its clinical utility, serum albumin levels may be insensitive to changes in nutritional status, do not necessarily correlate with changes in other nutritional parameters, and can be influenced by nonnutritional factors, such as infection/inflammation, hydration status, peritoneal or urinary albumin losses, and acidemia (50–57). In addition, because of its long half-life (20 days) and large body pool size, serum albumin can be a relatively insensitive index of protein nutritional status. Mak et al. found that serum albumin levels remained unchanged in association with an increasing dose of dialysis, despite documentation of an increased normalized protein equivalent of total nitrogen appearance (nPNA) (*vide infra*) and the absence of increased peritoneal losses (58). Serum albumin concentrations are also inversely correlated with the serum levels of acute-phase proteins such as C-reactive protein (57,59). Therefore, the patient's clinical status (e.g., comorbid conditions, dialysis modality, acid-base status, and degree of proteinuria) must be taken into consideration when evaluating the changes in the serum albumin level.

Serum prealbumin and retinol-binding protein are very sensitive to acute changes in protein nutrition because of their short half-lives (1 day and 12 hours, respectively) and small body pool size. Prealbumin has also been found to correlate strongly with mortality risk in adult patients treated with hemodialysis and PD (60). However, serum concentrations of both proteins are elevated in patients with CKD because of impaired degradation by the kidney and the value of prealbumin is limited by many of the same factors that affect albumin.

Although infrequently used to assess a patient's nutritional status, serum C_3 may be decreased in association with chronic renal failure and is considered to be a very sensitive index of protein-calorie malnutrition (61). Similarly, serum transferrin may be a sensitive indicator of the nutritional status because of its relatively short half-life (8 to 9 days) and smaller body pool size. However, its usefulness is limited by the substantial influence that iron stores have on its level. Finally, the creatinine-height index is reflective of body muscle mass and dietary muscle protein intake. It is directly related to nPNA (62), and the index has been used in adults to calculate the edema-free lean body mass. However, reference data are not available for use in the pediatric population.

Special Studies

Protein Equivalent of Total Nitrogen Appearance

Protein equivalent of total nitrogen appearance (PNA) is a useful tool for the indirect estimation of dietary protein intake. It is based on the simple principle that during steady-state conditions, total nitrogen losses are equal to or slightly less than the total nitrogen intake (63). The majority of nitrogen losses (approximately 65% or greater) occur as urea excretion in urine and/or dialysate (64). Nitrogen is also lost as nonurea nitrogen in creatinine, uric acid, feces, skin, and hair. Protein loss in urine and/or dialysate is an additional source of nitrogen loss. The total nitrogen losses from the body are represented as total nitrogen appearance (TNA). The PNA, in turn, can be estimated by multiplying the TNA by 6.25 based on the fact that the nitrogen content of protein is relatively constant at 16%. Recognizing the practical difficulties associated with the measurement of all sources of nitrogen loss, in addition to the fact that a portion of these losses (e.g., hair and skin) are small and fixed, several researchers have attempted to derive quantitative relationships between TNA and the easily measurable and most abundant source of nitrogen loss, urea nitrogen (64–68).

The most commonly used formula to estimate dietary protein intake by urinary urea-nitrogen excretion in adults, published by Maroni et al. (65), is as follows:

$$\text{Total nitrogen intake (g/kg/day)} = [\text{urea-N excretion (g/kg/day)} + 0.031 \text{ g/kg/day}] \times 6.25$$

Maroni et al. proposed that the nonurea-N excretion (0.031 g/kg/day) was constant. In fact, this later formulation more closely reflects measured total nitrogen output than nitrogen intake because it does not adjust for unmeasured nitrogen losses (67). Wingen et al. (66) documented that in children (2 to 18 years of age) the nonurea-N excretion was higher (0.085 ± 0.061 g/kg/day) and was highly correlated to dietary protein intake ($r = 0.839$). This relationship did not appear to be influenced by the age of the patient. They derived the following formula:

$$\text{Protein intake (g/kg/day)} = [\text{urea-N excretion (g/kg/day)} \times 15.39] - 0.8$$

Mendley and Majkowski (64) initially defined the relationship between urea-N and TNA in children undergoing PD as follows:

$$\text{TNA (g/day)} = 1.26 \text{ (urea-N appearance)} + 0.83$$

Their data suggested that the nonurea nitrogen appearance in children was greater than that reported by Maroni et al. (65) and supported the observations of Wingen et al. (66). However, in contrast to Wingen et al.'s observation in children with CKD, the nonurea nitrogen excretion in patients undergoing PD varied by age, being significantly greater in the youngest patients. This is likely a result of the relatively greater dialysate protein losses that occur in younger patients. The authors' formula subsequently was revised to reflect the impact of age as follows:

$$\text{TNA} = 1.03 \text{ (urea-N appearance)} + 0.02 \text{ (weight in kg)} + 0.56 \text{ (for subjects age 0 to 5 years) or } 0.98 \text{ (for subjects age 6 to 15 years)}$$

Edefonti et al. (68) later reported that incorporating the dialysate protein-nitrogen and body surface area (BSA) in the formula could make the best prediction of TNA in children undergoing PD. They recommended that the TNA be calculated in the following manner:

$$\text{TNA (g/day)} = 0.03 + 1.138 \text{ urea-N}_{\text{urine}} + 0.99 \text{ urea-N}_{\text{dialysate}} + 1.18 \text{ BSA} + 0.965 \text{ protein-N}_{\text{dialysate}}$$

In patients undergoing maintenance hemodialysis, the estimation of PNA is dependent on the urea generation rate (G) during the interdialytic period. The PNA can be calculated simultaneously during Kt/V estimations by urea kinetic modeling. A simple formula for the calculation of nPNA (69) in pediatric patients undergoing hemodialysis is as follows:

$$\text{nPNA} = 5.43 \times {}_{est}G/V_1 + 0.17; \quad {}_{est}G = [(C_2 \times V_2) - (C_1 \times V_1)]/t$$

where C_1 and V_1 are postdialysis serum urea nitrogen (SUN) and total body water (TBW), respectively, from the previous hemodialysis treatment; C_2 and V_2 are predialysis SUN and TBW, respectively, from the current hemodialysis treatment; and t is time (minutes) from the end of one dialysis treatment to the beginning of the next treatment. Currently, the formulas of Mellits and Cheek (70) commonly are used to estimate TBW in children, as per the recommendation of NKF-K/DOQI (21).

Because protein requirements are determined primarily from fat-free, edema-free body mass, PNA usually is normalized (nPNA) to some function of body weight. The usual weight used to normalize PNA is derived from the urea distribution space (approximate weight × 0.58) because this idealized weight does not include the body fat weight.

Several important limitations of PNA should be recognized. PNA is known to approximate protein intake only when the patient is in nitrogen equilibrium. However, because of growth, children are in an anabolic state and the PNA therefore typically will underestimate the actual dietary protein intake. In addition, it has been demonstrated that children treated with recombinant human growth hormone may have a significantly increased dietary protein intake without exhibiting greater nitrogen excretion, reflective of an anabolic state (64). However, in the catabolic patient, PNA will exceed protein intake to the extent that there is net degradation and metabolism of endogenous protein pools to form urea. It also should be noted that urea nitrogen appearance (and hence PNA) changes rapidly following variations in protein intake. Therefore, PNA can fluctuate from day-to-day as a function of dietary protein intake, and a single measurement of PNA may not reflect the usual protein intake. Additionally, PNA estimates have been found to be inaccurate at extremes of protein intake (71, 72).

Bioelectrical Impedance Analysis

Bioelectrical impedance analysis (BIA) is an attractive tool for the nutritional assessment of individuals undergoing dialysis because it is noninvasive, painless, and relatively inexpensive to perform and requires minimal operator training. Whereas BIA allows for an accurate assessment of fat-free mass in healthy children (73), the estimate of fat-free mass of patients undergoing dialysis may be confounded by variations in hydration.

Dual-Energy X-Ray Absorptiometry

Whole-body dual-energy x-ray absorptiometry (DEXA) is a reliable, noninvasive method to assess the three main components of body composition: fat mass, fat-free mass, and bone mineral mass/density. The accuracy of DEXA is influenced minimally by the variations in hydration that commonly occur in patients receiving dialysis, and studies of DEXA in this patient population have demonstrated its superior precision and accuracy when compared to anthropometry, total body potassium counting, creatinine index, and BIA (74–77). The main limitations of DEXA in pediatrics are its substantial cost and the lack of reliable normal values in children undergoing dialysis.

Subjective Global Assessment

The subjective global assessment (SGA) is a useful tool that assesses a patient's nutritional status based on features of the history and physical examination (78). The history focuses on gastrointestinal symptoms (anorexia, nausea, vomiting, diarrhea) and weight loss over the preceding 6 months. The physical examination focuses on the loss of subcutaneous fat, muscle wasting, and the presence of edema. The SGA is easy to perform, has low interobserver and intraobserver variability, and does not require sophisticated equipment. It has been used successfully as part of the nutritional assessment of adult patients undergoing maintenance dialysis (79). However, this inexpensive and attractive tool has not yet been validated in the pediatric population.

Nutritional Physical Examination

Finally, the so-called nutritional physical examination can be used as an adjunct to other nutritional assessment and monitoring techniques. The nutritional physical examination involves the assessment of a patient for the presence or absence of physical signs suggestive of nutrient deficiency or excess. A careful examination of the tongue, skin, teeth, breath, and hair may provide important clues to the nutritional status (80).

Nutritional Requirements

The nutritional requirements for children with CKD and those undergoing maintenance dialysis generally are based on the published RDA for healthy children (81). However, it is important to recognize that the RDAs are estimates of the average needs of the normal population, are meant to be applied to children as a group, and do not take into account the specific requirements of an individual patient. The American Academy of Pediatrics' Committee on Nutrition states that RDAs cannot be used as a measure of nutritional adequacy in children (82).

The basis for the RDA values vary for different nutrients. Whereas the RDA for energy reflects the average energy intake needed to maintain body weight and activity of well-nourished normal-sized individuals (with an additional provision for infants and children to ensure normal growth), the RDAs for protein are based on protein nitrogen loss (mean + 2 SD) and are further adjusted to account for poor protein quality and individual variability (83). Whereas most of the RDAs are based on the patient's weight, Grupe et al. (84) proposed using an RDA for length in pediatric patients with renal failure because many patients have low body weight for length and the latter is not affected by fluid balance and body fat. Unfortunately, sufficient normative data are not available to support the use of a height-standardized RDA.

The RDAs for a number of nutrients have been replaced by dietary reference intakes (DRIs) (85). The DRIs are comprised of a set of four reference values: *Estimated Average Requirement* (EAR), *RDA*, *Adequate Intake* (AI), *and Tolerable Upper Intake Level* (UL). The EAR is the median usual intake value that is estimated to meet the requirements of half of the healthy individuals in a specific age and gender group, whereas the other half of individuals are at risk for nutritional deficiency and/or chronic disease. EARs are used to assess the prevalence of nutrient inadequacy in a group of individuals. RDAs are intake levels that, according to the available scientific evidence, meet the nutrient requirement of almost all (>97%) healthy individuals in a specific age and gender group. AI values are used when the scientific evidence is lacking to establish an EAR or an RDA. AIs are derived from experimental data or are approximated from the observed mean nutrient intakes of apparently healthy people. The UL is the highest level of daily nutrient intake that is likely to pose no risk of adverse health effects in almost all individuals in a specified group. The UL is not intended to be a recommended intake level, and the potential risk for adverse effects increases if the intake exceeds the UL.

Energy Requirements

A variety of studies have shown that the majority of pediatric patients with CKD exhibit an inadequate dietary energy intake (10,86–89). Furthermore, the energy intake progressively decreases with worsening renal failure (89). Betts and Magrath (90) demonstrated decreased growth velocity in children when the energy intake was less than 80% of the RDA, and they were unable to increase their patient's growth velocity with caloric supplementation (91). Maximizing caloric intake has been noted to be particularly effective in improving height velocity only in infants with CKD or undergoing dialysis (92,93). Because children older than 2 years of age with CKD do not generally experience catch-up growth (94), the provision of adequate energy intake early in life is crucial.

Energy intakes for children with CKD should be at least equal to the RDA for normal children of the same chronologic age (21,95) (Table 29.3). Rizzoni et al. (5) demonstrated that the growth of infants with CKD receiving ≤100% of the RDA averaged 53% (range 10% to 72%) of expected, whereas it averaged 97% (range 61% to 130%) of expected during periods when the energy intake was ≤100% of the RDA. When chronologic and height ages are widely discrepant, the treatment goals should be individualized. Height age may be used to estimate the energy requirements if the patient fails to gain appropriate weight with a consistent energy intake at the RDA based on chronologic age.

Energy requirements for patients treated with maintenance hemodialysis or PD are similar to those of predialysis patients and may be achieved best in those children whose dialysate clearance is enhanced. Unique to patients treated with PD, the calculation of total caloric intake should include calories derived from the absorption of dialysate glucose. The glucose absorption will increase the total caloric intake by 7 to 10 kcal/kg per day or 7% to 15% of the total daily caloric intake (6,10,96).

Dietary therapy should provide 50% of total calories from primary complex carbohydrates, and the remainder of the nonprotein calories should be fat, with a polyunsaturated/saturated ratio of 2:1. Carbohydrate intake should be decreased to 35% of total calories in patients with very elevated serum triglyceride levels. An adequate amount of nonprotein calories should be provided for protein-sparing effects. However, it should be noted that during the advanced stages of uremia, the protein-sparing effect of added fat calories may be inferior to the effect of added concentrated carbohydrate calories (24).

Finally, although energy supplementation resulting in a total energy intake exceeding the RDA for age has been administered to children treated with long-term dialysis, there are no data that demonstrate a resultant and consistent improvement in growth velocity. In fact, in the absence of malnutrition, there are no outcome data that have been documented to correlate with energy supplementation in the pediatric patient.

TABLE 29.3. ESTIMATED ENERGY ALLOWANCES FOR INFANTS AND CHILDREN

	Age (years)	kcal/kg/day
Infants	0.0–0.5	108
	0.5–1.0	98
Children	1–3	102
	4–6	90
	7–10	70
Males	11–14	55
	15–18	45
	18–21	40[a]
Females	11–14	47
	15–18	40
	18–21	38[a]

[a]Based on recommended dietary allowances and increased physical activity.
From Food and Nutrition Board, Commission on Life Sciences, National Research Council. *Recommended dietary allowances*, ed 10. Washington, DC: National Academies Press, 1989, with permission.

Protein Requirements

Chronic Kidney Disease

Low-protein diets reduce the generation of nitrogenous wastes and inorganic ions that might be responsible for many of the clinical and metabolic disturbances characteristic of uremia. Moreover, low-protein diets can modify the development of hyperphosphatemia, metabolic acidosis, hyperkalemia, and other electrolyte disorders and possibly delay the progression of renal failure. A large number of clinical trials and experimental studies have examined the effect of dietary protein restriction on the rate of progression to ESRD in adults (97–103). Although the initial analysis of the most prominent study, "Modification of Diet in Renal Disease," provided equivocal results (100), a secondary analysis of the data and three separate metaanalyses each indicated that low-protein diets could retard the progression of renal failure or delay the onset of maintenance dialysis therapy (104–108). Accordingly, it is recommended that a low-protein (0.6 g/kg/day) diet be considered in adults with renal failure who are not yet undergoing dialysis.

Experimental studies in young animals have shown that a decrease in dietary protein intake, sufficient to slow the deterioration of renal function, has a resultant adverse effect on growth (98,109). In turn, concerns regarding the potential for harmful effects of protein deficiency on the growth of infants and young children have resulted in very few studies on protein restriction being conducted in the pediatric population (110–113). Moreover, in contrast to the adult studies, the investigators of pediatric studies typically have compared a very modest decrease in protein intake with a higher protein intake.

In a randomized, multicenter prospective study (111) involving 56 children (aged 2 to 18 years) with CKD (glomerular filtration rate [GFR]: 15 to 60 mL/min/1.73 m^2), the "study group" received the protein intake recommended by the World Health Organization (0.8 to 1.1 g/kg/day) (114) and the control group was advised to eat 1.5 to 2.0 times the WHO recommendation, which equates to the intake of normal healthy children. Energy intake was adequate (>80% of the recommended amount) and similar in both groups. The researchers did not observe any beneficial effect of the low-protein diet on the progression of renal failure or any adverse effect of the diet on growth parameters.

However, Uauy et al. reported a negative impact of a modest protein restriction on the growth of infants with CKD during the feasibility phase of a multicenter trial (112). These investigators compared the rate of progression of renal insufficiency and the height velocity of 24 infants with a GFR less than 55 mL/min/1.73 m^2 who were randomly assigned to two different protein intakes (study group, 1.4 g/kg/day and control group, 2.4 g/kg/day) for 10 months. Overall, energy intakes were 92% of RDA and similar in both groups. Although the change in GFR did not differ between the two groups, the height velocity decreased in the study group. The height SDS in the study group worsened from -2.2 ± 1.4 to -2.6 ± 1.2, whereas it remained the same in the control group (-1.7 ± 1.4).

In 1997, the European Study Group for Nutritional Treatment of Chronic Renal Failure in Childhood reported the final results of a project designed to evaluate the impact of a low-protein diet on the progression of CKD in children (113). In this study, 191 patients (aged 2 to 18 years) completed 2 years of follow-up and 112 patients completed 3 years of follow-up. After a run-in period of at least 6 months, patients were stratified into either a progressive or nonprogressive category based on the change in creatinine clearance during this period. The patients were also stratified into three renal-disease categories and then randomly assigned to a control or diet group. Patients in the diet group were advised to decrease their protein intake to the "safe amounts" recommended by the WHO (0.8 to 1.1 g/kg ideal body weight/day) (114). The advised energy intake was 80% of the RDA of the Natural Academy of Science (81). Patients in the control group were instructed to consume a similar amount of calories but with no restriction on protein intake. The study concluded that a reduction in dietary protein intake to "safe amounts" for 3 years did not interfere with the children's growth, but it also did not influence the progression of renal insufficiency.

In conclusion, current data suggest that in children with CKD, moderate dietary protein restriction has no beneficial effect in preventing the progression of renal insufficiency. On the contrary, such interventions may be associated with a loss of growth velocity, particularly in infants. Thus, it does not appear advisable to reduce dietary protein intake below the safe levels recommended by the WHO for protein intake of children in the process of growth. Current recommendations are to provide 100% of the RDA (81) for healthy children of the same gender and chronologic age (Table 29.4). It is advised that at least 50% of the total protein intake should be from proteins of high biologic value such as from milk, egg, meat, fish, and poultry. Suggested protein intake levels have been extrapolated from energy requirements for a given age and the ratio of protein to energy contained in the diet of adults. Because the calorie requirement is higher in children, the extrapolated recommendations for protein intake are also higher. Note that the suggested RDA for protein intake is 15% to 50% higher in comparison to WHO recommendations because the latter are based on protein of high biologic value, whereas RDA recommendations are adjusted for proteins of mixed biologic value found in a typical American diet of animal and plant proteins.

TABLE 29.4. RECOMMENDED DIETARY PROTEIN (GM/KG/DAY) FOR CHILDREN WITH CHRONIC KIDNEY DISEASE AND THOSE UNDERGOING MAINTENANCE DIALYSIS

		Protein Intake (g/kg/day)		
	Age (years)	CKD	HD	PD
Infants	0.0–0.5	2.2	2.6	2.9–3.0
	0.5–1.0	1.6	2.0	2.3–2.4
Children	1–3	1.2	1.6	1.9–2.0
	4–6	1.2	1.6	1.9–2.0
	7–10	1.0	1.4	1.7–1.8
Males	11–14	1.0	1.4	1.7–1.8
	15–18	0.9	1.3	1.4–1.5[a]
	19–21	0.8	1.2	1.3[a]
Females	11–14	1.0	1.4	1.7–1.8
	15–18	0.8	1.2	1.4–1.5[a]
	19–21	0.8	1.2	1.3[a]

CKD, chronic kidney disease; HD, hemodialysis; PD, peritoneal dialysis.
[a]Based on growth potential.
From Clinical practice guidelines for nutrition in chronic renal failure. K/DOQI, National Kidney Foundation. *Am J Kidney Dis* 2000; 35:S1–S140, with permission.

Maintenance Dialysis

The optimal protein intake for pediatric patients on maintenance dialysis has not yet been well defined. Most of the recommendations are based on expert opinion or derived from data extrapolated from adult studies. Currently, it has been suggested that patients undergoing hemodialysis should be prescribed the RDA for chronologic age plus an increment of 0.4 g/kg/day to consistently achieve a positive nitrogen balance (21). This recommendation is based on studies performed in adult patients undergoing hemodialysis who demonstrated evidence of malnutrition when they received a protein intake of only 0.75 g/kg/day and in whom the ingestion of 1.1 g/kg/day of protein, which was much of high biologic value, was not adequate enough to maintain nitrogen balance routinely (21,115). Moreover, the use of dietary protein restriction has led to poor growth in children undergoing hemodialysis (116). There are no data, however, that demonstrate any advantage of protein supplemented at a level above the combination of the RDA and the assumed dialysate losses with regard to growth rate or other measures of nutritional status in children.

The protein requirements for children treated with PD are higher than for those receiving hemodialysis because of the constant loss of protein and amino acids across the peritoneal membrane (6,10,117–119). The dialysate protein losses usually range from 100 to 300 mg/kg/day and are similar for chronic ambulatory peritoneal dialysis and chronic cycling peritoneal dialysis, but they show interindividual variation (117). The peritoneal protein loss is inversely related to age and size, so that smaller and, therefore, younger children have proportionately the greatest losses. The recommendations for daily protein intake in children undergoing PD therefore are based on the RDA, dialysate protein losses, and the results of nitrogen balance studies. Edefonti et al. (118) calculated the dietary protein requirements from equations of correlation obtained from 42 nitrogen balance studies conducted on 31 children undergoing PD. They demonstrated that a dietary protein intake of 144% of RDA and a total energy intake of 89% of RDA is required to obtain an estimated positive nitrogen balance of more than 50 mg/kg per day. A value of 50 mg of nitrogen/kg per day is considered adequate to guarantee metabolic and growth requirements in children undergoing PD. This value was derived from nitrogen balance studies in normal children where a value of 40 mg/kg per day is considered adequate (120–121). The additional 10 mg/kg per day accounts for the nitrogen losses experienced by children with uremia.

Typically, the initial diet prescription advocates a protein intake at the higher end of the recommended levels for infants and toddlers and the lower end for older children and adolescents. Subsequent adjustments in the recommended intake are based on follow-up evaluations and routine measures of nutritional status. Although protein intakes that meet the standard recommendations are advocated by some, the advisability of this approach has been challenged because of concern regarding the associated daily load of phosphorus and the risk of hyperphosphatemia (122).

LIPIDS

Lipid profiles characterized by hypertriglyceridemia, elevated cholesterol and low-density lipoprotein, decreased high-density lipoprotein, and abnormal apolipoprotein values commonly are seen in children with ESRD (96, 123–127). Moreover, the composition of these lipoproteins is atherogenic (128). Dyslipidemia increases the risk of cardiovascular disease among individuals with renal disease—a growing concern in children (129,130). There is also a body of evidence that an abnormal lipid status hastens the progression of renal disease itself (131). The etiology of the lipid disorders is likely multifactorial, resulting from a combination of decreased lipoprotein catabolism resulting from reduced activity of the enzymes lipoprotein lipase, lecithin–cholesterol acyltransferase, and hepatic triglyceride lipase and increased very–low-density lipoprotein synthesis as a result of glucose uptake from dialysis fluid in those patients receiving PD. In one study of children undergoing PD, hyperlipidemia was shown to be inversely related to the patient's age (132). In a more recently published study, the hypertriglyceridemia seen in young children undergoing PD was shown to be related directly to dietary energy intake but with no significant relationship to protein loss in the dialysate or to serum albumin levels (133).

Accordingly, in patients with substantially elevated serum triglycerides levels, the carbohydrate intake should be decreased from 50% to 35% of the total caloric intake. The remainder of the nonprotein calories should be supplied as fat with a polyunsaturated to saturated ratio of >2:1. The child should be encouraged to ingest complex carbohydrates in lieu of simple sugars and concentrated sweets and to use unsaturated fats such as oils and margarines from corn, safflower, and soy in an effort to control the hyperlipidemia. The pharmacologic treatment of dyslipidemia with medications such as hepatic 3 methylglutaryl coenzyme A reductase inhibitors (statins) is controversial because conclusive data regarding the risks and benefits of such therapy in children are lacking (128,131).

CALCIUM, PHOSPHORUS, AND VITAMIN D

It is well recognized that phosphorus retention in patients with advanced CKD plays a central role in the development and maintenance of secondary hyperparathyroidism (HPT) by causing hypocalcemia and reducing the rate of conversion of 25-hydroxyvitamin D3 to 1,25-dihydroxyvitamin D3 (134). A deficit of calcitriol synthesis has also been shown to be a major factor in the development of HPT (135,136). In fact, a study involving a large number of adult patients with CKD revealed that HPT developed at a time when the serum calcium and phosphorus were still normal (137). Thus, the current belief is that calcium, phosphorus, and calcitriol play an integrated role and all are important in the pathogenesis of HPT.

Although dietary phosphorus restriction is the usual firstline approach to the management of HPT, phosphorus restriction alone may not be very effective in suppressing parathyroid hormone (PTH) if the calcium intake is inadequate (137). Apart from having an independent effect on parathyroid gland activity (137), dietary calcium also may be a signal to upregulate the vitamin D receptor density in the parathyroid glands (138,139). Thus, the appropriate dietary intakes of calcium, phosphorus, and vitamin D are crucial for the management of HPT in patients with CKD.

Adequate dietary calcium intake during childhood is necessary for the development of optimal peak bone mass (140). In addition and as mentioned earlier, inadequate calcium intake in patients with CKD or ESRD is an important factor contributing to the development of HPT. The current rec-

TABLE 29.5. RECOMMENDED CALCIUM INTAKE FOR CHILDREN WITH CHRONIC KIDNEY DISEASE

Age (years)	Dietary Reference Intake (mg/day)	Recommended Maximum Intake (mg/day)
0.0–0.5	210	420
0.5–1.0	270	520
1–3	500	1,000
4–8	800	1,600
9–18	1,300	2,500[a]

Tolerable upper intake level (UL); DRI and UL
[a]Recommended maximum intake—recommendation by a pediatric workgroup developing guidelines for "the management of dietary calcium intake in children with CKD."
From Baker SS, Cochran WJ, Flores CA, et al. American Academy of Pediatrics, Committee on Nutrition. Calcium requirements of infants, children, and adolescents. *Pediatrics* 1999;104:1152–1157, with permission.

ommendation is that patients with CKD should achieve a calcium intake of 100% of the DRI (141) (Table 29.5). Infants and young children usually meet the DRI for calcium with the consumption of adequate volumes of breast milk/formula. Unfortunately, the largest source of dietary calcium for most people are dairy products that are also rich in phosphorus; in turn, phosphorus restriction universally leads to a decreased calcium intake. In these situations, calcium supplementation may be required because low-phosphorus, high-calcium foods such as collards, dandelion greens, kale, rhubarb, and spinach usually do not make up a substantial part of a child's diet and are rich in potassium as well. Several products fortified with calcium such as fruit juices and breakfast foods are commercially available, and limited studies have suggested that the bioavailability of calcium from these products is at least comparable to that of milk (142). Calcium also can be supplemented in medicinal forms such as carbonate, acetate, and gluconate salts of calcium that are used commonly as phosphate binders. When used for calcium supplementation alone, ingesting these products between meals maximizes calcium absorption (143). Chloride and citrate salts of calcium should be avoided; the former may lead to acidosis in patients with CKD or ESRD, and the latter may enhance aluminum absorption.

However, excessive calcium intake in conjunction with activated vitamin D analogues can lead to (a) hypercalcemia, (b) adynamic bone disease, and (c) systemic calcification. Accordingly, in the absence of definitive pediatric studies, a pediatric workgroup developing guidelines for "the management of dietary calcium intake in children with CKD" is likely to recommend a maximal intake of two times the DRI for age, except for ages 9 to 18 years (both genders), in which two times the DRI (2,600 mg) exceeds the UL of 2,500 mg (141). The serum calcium and phosphorus product probably should be kept below 60 in all but possibly the youngest (<3 years) children, although this important issue clearly is unsettled and in need of data.

The calcium balance in patients undergoing maintenance dialysis is also affected by the dialysate calcium concentration. The calcium balance during PD is usually negative with use of a 2.5 mEq/L calcium dialysate and positive with a calcium concentration of 3.0 to 3.5 mEq/L (144). As a result, it may be wise to use a low calcium dialysate (2.5 mEq/L) in children undergoing dialysis who are receiving calcium-containing phosphate binders along with activated vitamin D sterols. On the contrary, a 3.0 to 3.5 mEq/L calcium dialysate should be used if hypocalcemia is present in a child with an elevated PTH (>300 pg/mL) as part of the treatment of HPT and may be needed in children restricted to non-calcium–containing phosphate binders only.

The dietary phosphorus intake in children with CKD/ESRD should be restricted to less than 800 mg/day with recognition that dairy products and high-protein foods are the main sources of dietary phosphorus (24). However, strict dietary phosphorus restriction is often impractical and ill advised because it may lead to an inadvertent poor protein intake. In addition, extremely low phosphorus diets are typically unpalatable. Although young infants may be managed effectively by a low-phosphorus–containing milk formula such as Similac PM 60/40 (Ross Laboratories, OH), and Nestle Good Start Supreme (Nestle USA, Glendale, CA), most other patients require oral intestinal phosphate binders to control hyperphosphatemia. Phosphorus control is particularly difficult in vegetarians because for the same total quantity of dietary protein delivered, the phosphorus content is greater in protein derived from vegetable sources versus animal protein. Although food labels rarely state the phosphorus content, chocolates, nuts, dried beans, and cola drinks are rich in phosphorus and should be avoided; nondairy creamers and certain frozen nondairy desserts may be used in place of milk and ice cream.

Aluminum hydroxide and carbonate were used widely as phosphate binders in the past, but their use was markedly reduced once they were found to be associated with severe toxicity in adults and children with renal insufficiency (145, 146). Currently, calcium-containing salts such as calcium carbonate and calcium acetate are commonly used as phosphate binders, with the latter often reported to be a more effective binder than the former (147). To be maximally effective, their intake should coincide with that of meals or snacks. The optimal timing for the administration of binders with tube feedings has not been clearly defined. As noted earlier, calcium-containing phosphate binders also serve as an important source of supplemental calcium. More recently, excessive calcium intake in the form of phosphate binders has been implicated as one of the factors responsible for the development of coronary artery calcification in young adults who started dialysis as young children (148–150). These findings have focused attention on calcium and aluminum free phosphate binders such as sevelamer hydrochloride (RenaGel, GelTex Pharmaceuticals, Waltham, MA) (151,152), although no calcium-free phosphate binder is currently approved by the FDA for use in children. On rare occasions, a closely monitored low-dose (<30 mg/kg per day) of aluminum-containing phosphate binders may be tried as a last resort for those patients in whom hyperphosphatemia remains uncontrolled despite the previously recommended medical/dietary management. Finally, in contrast to the successful pretreatment of milk with ion-exchange resins to decrease potassium content, studies on the pretreatment of milk with calcium acetate to reduce the phosphate content found the procedure ineffective (153).

It should be noted that the serum phosphorus levels are normally higher (4.8 to 8.2 mg/dL) in young infants presumably because of the need for rapid mineralization of growing cartilage and bone in this age group. Roodhooft et al. (154) reported hypophosphatemia in three infants undergoing PD and receiving a low-phosphorus–containing formula; one of them had osteomalacic osteodystrophic changes on bone biopsy. Accordingly, dietary phosphorus restriction and the use of phosphate binders should be applied with caution in infants undergoing PD, and serum phosphate levels should be monitored regularly.

In the absence of 1α-hydroxylation of vitamin D, synthetic 1,25-dihydroxyvitamin D (the active metabolite) or dihydrotachysterol (requires only hepatic hydroxylation for activation) are used in pediatric patients with CKD. These preparations are often started early in the course of CKD on the basis of an elevation of serum PTH and alkaline phosphatase levels. As suggested previously, one of the serious complications associated with the use of these activated vitamin D metabolites is the development of hypercalcemia. Several newer noncalcemic vitamin D analogues, such as paricalcitol (19-nor-1,25-dihydroxyvitamin D_2) (155) and doxercalciferol (1α-hydroxyvitamin D_2) (156), selectively depress the parathyroid gland with a lower incidence of hypercalcemia when compared to current agents. Pediatric studies with these medications are under way.

SODIUM

Sodium is the major determinant of the body's extracellular volume status, and its balance is usually maintained by appropriate alterations in urinary sodium excretion in patients with normal kidney function. In children with CKD, sodium requirements are dependent on the underlying kidney disease and the GFR. Children with CKD as a result of obstructive uropathy or renal dysplasia are often polyuric and demonstrate increased urinary sodium losses. The growth of these children is hampered if ongoing sodium and water losses are not corrected. In 2001 Parekh et al. (157) reported the beneficial effect of a dilute, sodium-supplemented (2 to 4 mEq sodium per 100 mL formula), high-volume (180 to 240 mL/kg per 24 hours, depending on urine output) feeding regimen on the linear growth of 24 young children with severe polyuric CKD. The treated group of patients was able to maintain a nearly normal height SDS despite the presence of significant renal insufficiency.

In contrast, children with CKD resulting from primary glomerular disease, or those who are oliguric or anuric, typically require sodium and fluid restriction to minimize fluid gain, edema formation, and hypertension. These patients should be advised to avoid processed foods (e.g., meat and cheese) and snacks from fast-food restaurants, which typically are high in sodium content. The sodium content of other food items should be checked carefully on food labels. In addition, the sodium content of the medications may need to be monitored. While undergoing maintenance dialysis, the restrictions on fluid and sodium allowances are more stringent for children receiving hemodialysis than for those undergoing PD because of the continuous nature of the latter therapy. In fact, sodium losses associated with PD in infants can be substantial, necessitating aggressive sodium supplementation.

POTASSIUM

Children with CKD are usually able to maintain potassium homeostasis with a mild reduction in intake because hyperkalemia generally does not occur until the GFR falls to less than 10% of normal. However, children with renal dysplasia, postobstructive renal damage, severe reflux nephropathy, and renal insufficiency secondary to interstitial nephritis who are recognized to be salt losers often demonstrate renal tubular resistance to aldosterone action and manifest hyperkalemia even when their creatinine clearance is relatively well preserved (158). The hyperkalemia experienced by these children is exacerbated by volume contraction, and the majority of the patients respond to salt and water repletion. For patients who are persistently hyperkalemic, dietary potassium intake should be limited. Because potassium is listed infrequently on food labels and cannot be tasted, a list of foods rich in potassium such as chocolates, french fries, potato chips, bananas, green leafy vegetables, dried fruits, and orange juice should be provided to patients and their families. Altering the methods of food preparation, such as soaking vegetables before cooking, help decrease potassium content. For infants and young children being fed milk formula, the potassium content of the formula can be reduced by incorporating the potassium exchange resin sodium polystyrene sulfonate (Kayexalate, Sanofi-Synthelabo, Markham, Ontario, Canada) (159). Attention also should be paid to such medications as potassium-sparing diuretics, cyclosporine, and ACE inhibitors that may cause or exacerbate hyperkalemia. If constipated, the patient should be treated aggressively because significant quantities of potassium are eliminated through the intestinal tract in patients with CKD. Finally, in children undergoing PD, hyperkalemia is usually not a problem; this is in contrast to patients undergoing hemodialysis, in whom dietary potassium intake should be distributed throughout the day because high serum concentrations of potassium can develop when a large quantity of potassium is ingested at one time, regardless of the total daily dietary potassium content.

ACID-BASE STATUS

Bicarbonate reabsorption, hydrogen ion excretion, or both may be disturbed in children with CKD. Infants and children normally have a relatively larger endogenous hydrogen ion load per kg body weight than adults do, and persistent metabolic acidosis frequently is associated with a child's failure to thrive. Studies performed in adult patients also have shown that chronic acidosis is associated with increased oxidation of branched-chain amino acids (160), increased protein degradation (161), and decreased albumin synthesis (162). In addition, persistent acidosis has detrimental effects on bone because it alters the normal accretion of hydroxyapatite into bone matrix and causes bone demineralization as the bone buffers increasingly are used to bind with the excess hydrogen ions. Thus, the serum bicarbonate level of children should be maintained at or above 22 mmol/L by supplementing with oral bicarbonate, altering the base content of dialysate, or both when deemed necessary.

Vitamins and Micronutrients

Vitamins and minerals are essential for normal growth and development, and their deficiency or excess can be harmful. Unfortunately, the vitamin and mineral needs of pediatric patients with CKD and those undergoing maintenance dialysis are not clearly defined. Indeed, there are virtually no data on the vitamin status of children with CKD, whereas a limited amount of data exists for those undergoing maintenance dialysis. This is of particular concern because children are prone to develop vitamin deficiencies as a result of anorexia, dietary restrictions, and the needs for growth; however, they can develop toxic levels of vitamins because of impaired renal clearance. In addition, their vitamin needs may be increased because of altered metabolism of the vitamins by medications or uremia itself.

All of the water-soluble vitamins except pyridoxine are eliminated by the kidneys, and their clearance in patients with CKD is not known. However, most water-soluble vitamins are lost during maintenance dialysis and, in turn, routinely are supplemented by special vitamin formulations that do not contain vitamins A and D. Studies conducted in the adult dialysis population have provided evidence of low blood concentrations of water-soluble vitamins and minerals because of inadequate intake, increased losses, and, in some cases, increased needs (163,164). Deficiency of vitamin B6 can result from poor dietary intake as well as inhibition of activity and/or increased clearance of pyridoxal phosphate in the dialysis fluid (165). Vitamin B12 and folic acid, both of which are important for effective erythropoiesis, differ in their peritoneal clearance; whereas there can be significant losses of folic acid, only small quantities of vitamin B12 are lost by this route (166). Accordingly, supplementation with 0.8 to 1.0 mg folic acid routinely is recommended; the necessity of vitamin B12 supplementation remains unsettled. More recently, a higher dose of folic acid (2.5 mg per day) has been suggested for children with CKD because supplemental folic acid has been shown to decrease the elevated homocysteine level that commonly is seen in patients with renal failure and is a potential risk factor for cardiovascular morbidity and mortality (167,168). In contrast, serum thiamin and riboflavin levels have been reported to be normal in patients undergoing PD, with or without supplementation, in association with negligible losses during dialysis (169).

Supplementation with vitamin C is occasionally recommended because of the significant quantity that can be lost during PD (170). It is important to recognize, however, that although adequate levels of vitamin C are necessary for the formation of collagen, an excessive intake of vitamin C in the dialysis population may result in elevated oxalate levels as an end-product of vitamin C metabolism and lead to the development of significant vascular complications (171). Accordingly, vitamin C intake should not exceed 100 mg/day. Vitamin K deficiency may occur in patients who receive antibiotics and do not eat; this deficiency has been reported in a small number of adults (172). Vitamin A levels usually are elevated in patients undergoing PD despite the lack of vitamin A in the vitamin-supplement formulation. The elevated levels are a result of the loss of the kidney's normal ability to degrade or excrete retinol-binding protein or excrete vitamin A metabolites (173). Because elevated levels of vitamin A can be associated with the development of hypercalcemia and complications related to a high calcium–phosphorus product, it is critically important to avoid the use of vitamin supplements that include much vitamin A.

In children older than 6 years of age undergoing PD, vitamin supplementation has been associated with normal or greater than normal serum levels of the water-soluble vitamins (170). However, no published studies have assessed the blood vitamin levels of children undergoing maintenance dialysis in the absence of the use of a vitamin supplement. Because most infant milk formulas are fortified with both water-soluble and fat-soluble vitamins, most infants with CKD/ESRD receive the DRI/RDA for all vitamins (including vitamin A) by dietary intake alone. Warady et al. (174) reported on the vitamin status of a group of seven infants undergoing PD; their main nutrient intake was infant milk formula (Similac PM 60/40) and they received a water-soluble vitamin supplement (Iberet, Abbott Laboratories, Abbott Park, IL). The combined dietary and supple-

TABLE 29.6. DIETARY REFERENCE INTAKES (PER DAY) OF VITAMINS AND TRACE ELEMENTS FOR NORMAL CHILDREN AND ADOLESCENTS

Age Group	Thiamin (mg)	Riboflavin (mg)	Vitamin B_6[a] (mg)	Niacin[b] (mg)	Folate (μg)	Vitamin B_{12} (μg)	Vitamin C (mg)	Vitamin A[c] (μg)	Vitamin E[d] (mg)	Vitamin K (μg)	Zinc (mg)	Copper (μg)
Infants												
0–6 mo	0.2	0.3	0.1	2	65	0.4	40	400	4	2	2	200
7–12 mo	0.3	0.4	0.3	4	80	0.5	50	500	5	2.5	3	220
Children												
1–3 yr	0.5	0.5	0.5	6	150	0.9	15	300	6	30	3	340
4–8 yr	0.6	0.6	0.6	8	200	1.2	25	400	7	55	5	440
Males												
9–13 yr	0.9	0.9	1.0	12	300	1.8	45	600	11	60	8	700
14–18 yr	1.2	1.3	1.3	16	400	2.4	70	900	15	75	11	890
Females												
9–13 yr	0.9	0.9	1.0	12	300	1.8	45	600	11	60	8	700
14–18 yr	1.0	1.0	1.2	14	400	2.4	65	700	15	75	11	890

[a]Vitamin B_6 comprises a group of six related compounds—pyridoxal, pyridoxine, pyridoxamine, and 5′-phosphates (PLP, PNP, PMP).
[b]Includes nicotinic acid amide, nicotinic acid (pyridine 3-carboxylic acid), and derivatives that exhibit the biologic activity of nicotinamide.
[c]Includes provitamin A carotenoids that are dietary precursors of retinol. Given as retinol activity equivalents (RAEs). 1 RAE = 1 μg retinol, 12 μg β-carotene, 24 μg α-carotene.
[d]Also known as α-tocopherol.
From Food and Nutrition Board, Institute of Medicine. Dietary reference intakes for thiamine, riboflavin, niacin, vitamin B_6, folate, vitamin B_{12}, pantothenic acid, biotin, and choline. Washington, DC: National Academies Press, 2000, with permission; Food and Nutrition Board, Institute of Medicine. Dietary reference intakes for vitamin A, vitamin K, arsenic, boron, chromium, copper, iodine, iron, manganese, molybdenum, nickel, silicon, vanadium, and zinc. Washington, DC: National Academies Press, 2002, with permission; and Food and Nutrition Board, Institute of Medicine. Dietary reference intakes for vitamin C, vitamin E, selenium, and carotenoids. Washington, DC: National Academies Press, 2000, with permission.

ment intake exceeded the RDA for the water-soluble vitamins in all but one patient, who received only 79% of the RDA for vitamin B_6 because of inadequate formula intake. In all cases, the patient's serum concentrations of the water-soluble vitamins were comparable to or greater than the values reported in normal infants. In addition, the serum vitamin A levels were significantly greater than normal values, despite the lack of supplemental vitamin A. Accordingly, the current NKF-K/DOQI guidelines recommend an intake of 100% of the DRI for water-soluble vitamins (Table 29.6) as a reasonable starting point for children undergoing maintenance dialysis therapy. Supplementation should be considered if the dietary intake alone does not meet or exceed the DRI, if measured blood vitamin levels are below normal values, if clinical evidence of deficiency is present (21), or if the vitamin need exceeds normal (e.g., folic acid and pyridoxine) (see earlier in this chapter).

Aluminum, copper, chromium, lead, strontium, tin, and silicon levels have all been noted to be elevated in patients with CKD, reflecting the fact that their clearance is dependent on an adequate GFR (175,176) (Chapter 19). As mentioned previously, aluminum salts were commonly used in the 1970s and early 1980s as phosphate binders and were found to cause severe toxicity manifested by encephalopathy with seizures, osteomalacia, and microcytic anemia, even in children with mild renal insufficiency (145,146). Subsequently, the use of aluminum-containing phosphate binders was discontinued. Aluminum absorption is enhanced by citrate, but it is uncertain whether citrate alone can cause aluminum toxicity by enhancing the absorption of environmental aluminum. The Growth Failure in Renal Disease Study (177) showed that serum aluminum levels were elevated only in children taking antacids containing aluminum, which provides 1,000 times more aluminum than environmental exposure (approximately 3 to 5 mg/day). Other trace elements have not been well studied in children; however, blood zinc levels have been shown to be low in malnourished children and should be monitored and supplemented as necessary (175).

CARNITINE

Carnitine, a low–molecular-weight substance, plays a critical role in the oxidation of long-chain fatty acids (178), and the kidney is a major site for its synthesis in humans (179) (Chapter 21). Although patients undergoing prolonged dialysis are potentially at risk for carnitine deficiency as carnitine is removed both by hemodialysis and PD (180,181), there is little information on the carnitine status of children with CKD and those undergoing dialysis (182,183). Carnitine has been proposed as a treatment for a variety of metabolic abnormalities in patients with ESRD, including hypertriglyceridemia, hypercholesterolemia, and anemia. It has also been proposed as a treatment for several symptoms or complications of dialysis, including intradialytic arrhythmias and hypotension, low cardiac output, interdialytic and postdialytic symptoms of malaise or asthenia, general weakness or fatigue, skeletal muscle cramps, and decreased exercise capacity or low peak oxygen consumption. Unfortunately, there is currently insufficient evidence to support the routine use of carnitine for these conditions in patients undergoing dialysis; however, in selected patients receiving maintenance dialysis who manifest these symptoms or disorders and who have not responded adequately to standard therapies, a trial of carnitine may be considered (21).

NUTRITION MANAGEMENT

A registered dietitian with experience in pediatric renal diseases should play the central role in the dietary management of children with CKD/ESRD. In addition to possessing knowledge related to nutritional requirements, this person should also be skilled in the evaluation of physical growth, developmental assessment, and the educational and social needs of this special population. The dietitian must be able to establish a positive rapport with both the child and the primary caretakers to enhance compliance with the recommended nutritional regimen. The focus of the dietitian's treatment plan is determined by the patient's age. In the case of infants, the parents or primary caretaker who is responsible for feeding the child has the greatest interaction with the dietitian; in contrast, adolescents must receive the majority of information directly because they often eat independently. For children between these two extremes, both the parents and the child typically are involved in different aspects of the dietary management. It is noteworthy that the two most vulnerable groups for malnutrition are infants and adolescents. Whereas infants are at special risk because of the frequent occurrence of anorexia and emesis, many adolescents have poor eating habits. They skip meals, favor fast foods, and, in the presence of imposed dietary restrictions, find it difficult to meet the nutritional requirements of normal pubertal growth and development.

An individualized nutrition plan taking into account a variety of factors (Table 29.7) should be developed for each patient by the dietitian in consultation with the physician, patient (when appropriate) and family, with clearly defined short-term and long-term objectives. Because cultural food preferences play an important role in the family's ability to adhere to dietary changes, dietary instructions should be tailored to help families modify, but not eliminate, cultural food preferences. Background information on cultural diets and translated versions of renal diets and food lists are available for reference (184). The plan should be modified as necessary according to changes in the child's nutritional status, renal function, dialytic therapy, medication regimen, and psychosocial situation. Routinely, the specific recommendations of the plan are updated and/or reinforced at least every 3 to 4 months. However, certain conditions (Table 29.8) may dictate a more frequent reevaluation of the plan of care. It is important for any changes to be shared with all members of the multidisciplinary team.

Dietary restrictions should be limited as much as possible with a goal of enhancing nutrient intake. Restrictions of nutrients should ideally be imposed only when there is a clear indication, rather than an anticipated need. It is also important to find substitutes for restricted foods so as to maintain an adequate caloric intake. A simple explanation of the role of the nutrient in the body, the rationale for the diet modification, and the desired outcomes to be achieved (e.g., normalization of biochemical parameter, specific amount of weight gain) is helpful in obtaining cooperation of the patient and caretakers, thereby increasing the likelihood of success. Adopting and maintaining changes in eating habits is also easier for a child if family members make similar changes, or at least avoid eating restricted foods in the child's presence. In addition, caregivers outside of the immediate family (e.g., grandparents, school staff, baby sitters) should be aware of the diet restrictions and should be asked to provide consistency of care in helping the child follow his/her diet. Although the ideal goal is full compliance with the prescribed regimen, it is not always a realistic

TABLE 29.7. ASSESSMENTS CONDUCTED IN THE DEVELOPMENT OF AN INDIVIDUALIZED NUTRITION PLAN OF CARE

Medical history and medications
Dietary interview
Cultural preferences
Comparison of actual intake with estimated needs
Estimates of actual nutrient intake for macronutrients (such as energy and protein) from oral and/or enteral feeds
Assessment and evaluation of growth parameters
Laboratory values associated with nutrient intake
Review of fluid balance and blood pressure
Assessment of physical eating skills
Estimation of urine, stool, emesis, and ostomy output
Signs of specific vitamin deficiencies
Psychosocial status
Questions regarding consumption of unusual nonfood substances such as mud, paper, paint (e.g., pica)

TABLE 29.8. CONDITIONS DICTATING A MORE FREQUENT EVALUATION OF THE NUTRITION PLAN OF CARE

Dry-weight loss
Decrease in oral intake
Change in gastrointestinal function
Significant change in standard deviation scores (e.g., 0.5 standard deviation decrease in height SDS)
Abnormal laboratory values related to nutrients
Repeated excess interdialytic weight gain
Concern for compliance with recommendations
Change in psychosocial situation
Placement of a feeding tube

expectation, and "partial compliance" is often acceptable. Rigidity with the dietary prescription adds to parental stress and increases the risk for behavioral eating problems in the young child, such as food refusal, gagging, and vomiting.

ORAL SUPPLEMENTATION

Infants with CKD requiring fluid restriction or those who have a poor oral intake may require a greater caloric density of their milk formula than the standard 20 kcal/oz. The increase in caloric density should not be achieved by concentrating the milk formula because this approach also will increase the protein and mineral content. The provision of extra calories can be achieved by adding carbohydrate and/or fat modules to the formula. A glucose polymer such as Polycose (Ross Laboratories, Columbus, OH) has a low osmolality and is generally the initial supplement added to infant formulas. Additional calories can be added in the form of corn oil. Oils containing medium chain triglycerides are generally not necessary unless there is coexistent malabsorption. Older infants may tolerate the addition of corn syrup or sugar, which is readily available and inexpensive. The quantity of both carbohydrate and fat modules can be increased gradually to raise the calorie density to as much as 60 kcal/oz (185). It is important to wait at least 24 hours following each 2- to 4-kcal/oz incremental increase in concentration to enhance patient tolerance of the formula. To facilitate digestion of the formula, efforts should be made to keep the total fat to carbohydrate ratio close to that contained in the base formula (24). If, however, the patient is intolerant of the formula as manifested by persistent vomiting or diarrhea, the composition of the formula may need to be altered (24).

Children beyond infancy characteristically refuse the high-calorie carbohydrate supplements. For them, it is often easier to encourage common foods that have a high caloric content but a relatively low mineral and protein content. Powdered fruit drinks, frozen fruit-flavored desserts, candy, jelly, honey, and other concentrated sweets can be used for this purpose. However, the altered taste acuity associated with uremia may limit the acceptability of these foods. In addition, one may need to avoid high carbohydrate foods in the presence of hypertriglyceridemia. Under these circumstances, unsaturated fats may be the preferred choice of high-calorie food sources. Children and adolescents also should be encouraged to use margarine on popcorn, bread, vegetables, rice, and noodles for added calories. It, however, should be noted that during advanced stages of uremia, the protein-sparing effect of added fat calories may be inferior to the effect of concentrated carbohydrate calories (24).

A variety of calorie-dense (2 calorie/cc) preparations, such as Nepro and Suplena (Ross Laboratories) and Magnacal Renal (Mead Johnson, Evansville, IN), have been formulated specifically for renal patients and are commercially available. Suplena has a lower protein content than Nepro (30 g/L versus 70 g/L). These preparations are characterized by a low renal osmolar load and have a low vitamin A and D content. Although initially produced for patients older than 10 years, they have been used successfully in younger children.

In contrast to energy intake, the protein requirements of children with CKD usually are met by voluntary, unsupplemented consumption. If the protein intake is insufficient because of concomitant phosphorus restriction in the patient with significantly impaired renal function, the protein module, Promod (Ross Laboratories), which is a whey protein concentrate, can be added to the formula to increase the protein content. As much as 1 gm of Promod, which is equivalent to 0.76 gm protein, can be added to each ounce of formula. Semisynthetic diets supplemented with either amino or keto forms of essential amino acid (EAA) also have been tried to ensure an adequate protein intake. The ketoanalogues are nitrogen free and allow nitrogen sparing by using nonessential nitrogen when they are converted to the corresponding EAA in the body through reversible transamination. Ketoacid analogues generally are provided in a mixture that contains some EAA. In experimental studies in rats, the diets based on EAA did not improve growth rates above those achieved with the casein diets, despite much lower plasma levels of urea. The lack of sufficient data in children precludes making any firm recommendation regarding its possible clinical application.

ENTERAL NUTRITIONAL SUPPORT

Aggressive enteral feeding should be considered if the nutritional intake by the oral route is suboptimal despite all attempts at oral supplementation. The use of enteral support has resulted in maintenance or improvement of SD scores for weight and/or height in infants and young children with moderate to severe CKD and those undergoing maintenance dialysis (4,5,21,186–189). In fact, several investigators, including Kari et al. (190), have advocated early enteral feeding at the first sign of growth failure in infants.

Nasogastric (NG) tubes (187,189,191,192), gastrostomy catheters (193), gastrostomy buttons (194,195), and gastrojejunostomy (196) have been used to provide supplemental enteral feeding to children with renal disease with encouraging results. The feeding can be given as an intermittent bolus or more commonly by continuous infusion during the night. Continuous overnight feeds generally are preferred to allow time during the day for regular oral intake. The NG tube has been used most frequently in infants and young children, is easily inserted, and is generally well tolerated (189,197). In a recent study conducted by the North American Pediatric Renal Transplant Cooperative Study (NAPRTCS) of children who received tube feeding, the NG tube was used by 78% and 68% of children who initiated dialysis at less than 3 months and 3 to 20 months of age, respectively (198). However, this route of therapy often is complicated by recurrent emesis, the need for frequent tube replacement, the risk of pulmonary aspiration, nasoseptal erosion, and psychologic distress of the caretaker because of the cosmetic appearance. Persistent emesis can be addressed by slowing the rate of formula delivery and by the addition of antiemetic agents such as metoclopramide or domperidol. Additionally, whey predominant formulas can be used because they have been shown to stimulate gastric emptying (199,200).

The gastrostomy tube or button has the advantage of being hidden beneath clothing. Once placed, it can be used within several days. Most, but not all, clinicians recommend that the patient should be investigated for gastroesophageal reflux before undertaking gastrostomy placement so that a Nissen fundoplication can be created at the same sitting, if required. The reported complications of gastrostomy tubes/buttons include exit-site infection, leakage, obstruction, gastrocutaneous fistula, and peritonitis (201,202). Peritonitis is potentially the most serious complication and is a factor inhibiting the more widespread adoption of gastrostomy as opposed to NG feeding in the PD population (203). A recent review of the NAPRTCS data revealed that 11 (24%) of 45 episodes of fungal peritonitis were associated with the presence of a gastrostomy tube or button, but there was no statistically significant correlation between the presence of a gastrostomy and the development of fungal peritonitis (204). Nonetheless, it may be better to avoid combining gastrostomy placement and PD catheter placement in a malnourished patient until the nutritional status and general immunity of the patient can be improved by other means, such as NG tube feeds (202). Gastrojejunostomy feedings usually are considered for those children who have associated severe gastroesophageal reflux that is not amenable to medical therapy and have failed surgical repair (202).

A common and serious complication of using any form of enteral tube feeding is a prolonged and potentially difficult transition from tube to oral feeding (205,206). Regular nonnutritive sucking and repetitive oral stimulation are recommended for all tube-fed infants. A multidisciplinary feeding team consisting of a dietitian, occupational therapist, and behavioral psychologist can help facilitate the transition from tube to oral feeding.

ALTERNATIVE ROUTES OF NUTRITIONAL SUPPORT

The substitution of amino acids for dextrose in the PD fluid and the provision of parenteral nutrition during hemodialysis sessions (intradialytic parenteral nutrition, or IDPN) are two additional aggressive approaches to nutritional supplementation that have had limited pediatric application. Intraperitoneal nutrition has been evaluated in only a small number of children receiving PD and for a limited time (207–210). The quantity of amino acids absorbed from the dialysate routinely exceeded the protein lost in the dialysate. Very little experience with IDPN has been reported in the pediatric population. A short-term study of 10 chronic hemodialysis patients, ages 10 to 18 years, conducted in the Netherlands documented weight gain in nine patients with no significant change in plasma amino acid profile (211). Similarly, Goldstein et al. (212) demonstrated reversal of weight loss and initiation of weight gain within 6 weeks of IDPN initiation in three malnourished adolescents undergoing hemodialysis. Future studies may prove these routes of nutritional supplementation to be valuable adjuncts to the oral and enteral routes of therapy.

REFERENCES

1. Warady BA, Kriley M, Lovell H, et al. Growth and development of infants with end-stage renal disease receiving long-term peritoneal dialysis. *J Pediatr* 1988;112:714–719.
2. Geary DF, Haka Ikse K. Neurodevelopmental progress in young children with chronic renal disease. *Pediatrics* 1989;84:68–72.
3. Geary DF, Haka Ikse K, Coulter P, et al. The role of nutrition in neurology health and development of infants with chronic renal failure. *Adv Perit Dial* 1990;6:252–254.
4. Claris-Appiani A, Arissino GL, Dacco V, et al. Catch-up growth in children with chronic renal failure treated with long-term enteral nutrition. *JPEN J Parenter Enteral Nutr* 1995;19:175–178.
5. Rizzoni G, Basso T, Setari M. Growth in children with chronic renal failure on conservative treatment. *Kidney Int* 1984;26:52–58.
6. Broyer M, Niaudet P, Champion G, et al. Nutritional and metabolic studies in children on continuous ambulatory peritoneal dialysis. *Kidney Int (Suppl)* 1983;15/24:S106–S110.
7. Macdonald A. The practical problems of nutritional support for children on continuous ambulatory peritoneal dialysis. *Hum Nutr Appl Nutr* 1986;40A:253–261.
8. Canepa A, Divino Filho JC, Forsberg AM, et al. Children on continuous ambulatory peritoneal dialysis: muscle and plasma proteins, amino acids and nutritional status. *Clin Nephrol* 1996;46:125–131.
9. Foreman JW, Abitol CL, Trachtman H, et al. Nutritional intake in children with renal insufficiency: A report of the Growth Failure in Children with Renal Diseases Study. *J Am Coll Nutr* 1996;15:579–585.
10. Salusky IB, Fine RN, Nelson P, et al. Nutritional status of children undergoing continuous ambulatory peritoneal dialysis. *Am J Clin Nutr* 1983;38:599–611.
11. Tamaru T, Vaughn WH, Waldo FB, et al. Zinc and copper balance in children on continuous ambulatory peritoneal dialysis. *Pediatr Nephrol* 1989;3:309–313.
12. Coleman JE, Watson AR. Micronutrient supplementation in children on continuous cycling peritoneal dialysis (CCPD). *Adv Perit Dial* 1992;8:396–401.
13. Daschner M, Tonshoff B, Blum WF, et al. Inappropriate elevation of serum leptin levels in children with chronic renal failure. European Study Group for Nutritional Treatment of Chronic Renal Failure in Childhood. *J Am Soc Nephrol* 1998;9:1074–1079.
14. Stenvinkel P. Leptin and its clinical implications in chronic renal failure. *Miner Electrolyte Metab* 1999;25:298–302.

15. Wolf G, Chen S, Han DC, et al. Leptin and renal disease. *Am J Kidney Dis* 2002;39:1–11.
16. Shiffman S. Changes in taste and smell: drug interactions and food preferences. *Nutr Rev* 1994;52:S11–S14.
17. van der Ejik I, Allman Farinelli MA. Taste testing in renal patients. *J Renal Nutr* 1997;7:3–9.
18. Ravelli AM, Ledermann SE, Bisset WM, et al. Foregut motor function in chronic renal failure. *Arch Dis Child* 1992;67: 1343–1347.
19. Bird NJ, Strather CP, O'Doherty MJ, et al. Gastric emptying in patients with chronic renal failure on continuous ambulatory peritoneal dialysis. *Nephrol Dial Transplant* 1993;9:287–290.
20. Coleman JE, Edefonti A, Watson AR. Guidelines by an ad hoc European Committee on the assessment of growth and nutrition status in children on chronic peritoneal dialysis. *Perit Dial Int* 2001;21(3):E-article.
21. Clinical practice guidelines for nutrition in chronic renal failure. K/DOQI, National Kidney Foundation. *Am J Kidney Dis* 2000; 35:S1–S140.
22. Buzzard M. 24-hour dietary recall and food record methods. In: Willett W, ed. *Nutritional epidemiology.* New York: Oxford, 1998:50–73.
23. Gersovitz M, Madden JP, Smiciklas-Wright H. Validity of the 24-hr. dietary recall and seven-day record for group comparisons. *J Am Diet Assoc* 1978;73:48–55.
24. Nelson P, Stover J. Nutrition recommendations for infants, children, and adolescents with end-stage renal disease. In: Gillit D, Stover J, eds. *A clinical guide to nutrition care in end-stage renal disease.* Chicago: American Dietetic Association, 1994: 79–97.
25. Centers for Disease Control and Prevention. Using the CDC growth charts: Accurately weighing and measuring: technique, equipment, training modules. Atlanta: CDC, 2001.
26. Centers for Disease Control and Prevention. CDC growth charts: United States. Atlanta: CDC, 2000.
27. National Center for Health Statistics. Growth curves for children 0–18 years. United States Vital and Health Statistics. Series II, No. 165. Washington, DC: Health Resources Administration, U.S. Government Printing Office, 1977.
28. Durnin JV, Womersley J. Body fat assessed from total body density and its estimation from skinfold thickness: Measurements on 481 men and women aged from 16 to 72 years. *Br J Nutr* 1974;32:77–97.
29. Heymsfield SB, Tighe A, Wang ZM. Nutritional assessment by anthropometric and biochemical methods. In: Shils ME, Olson JA, Shike M, eds. *Modern nutrition in health and disease.* Philadelphia: Lea and Febiger, 1984:812–841.
30. Oe B, De Fijter CWH, Oe PL, et al. Four-site skinfold anthropometry (FSA) versus body impedance analysis (BIA) in assessing nutritional status of patients on maintenance hemodialysis: Which method is to be preferred in routine patient care. *Clin Nephrol* 1998;49:180–185.
31. Must A, Dallal GE, Dietz WH. Reference data for obesity: 85th and 95th percentiles of body mass index (wt/ht^2) and triceps skin fold thickness. *Am J Clin Nutr* 1991;53:839–846.
32. Frisancho AR. New norms of upper limb fat and muscle areas for assessment of nutritional status. *Am J Clin Nutr* 1981;34: 2540–2545.
33. Malina RM, Katzmarzyk PT. Validity of the body mass index as an indicator of the risk and presence of overweight in adolescents. *Am J Clin Nutr* 1999;70:S131–S136.
34. Hammer LD, Kraemer HC, Wilson DM, et al. Standardized percentile curves of body-mass index for children and adolescents. *AJDC* 1991;145:259–263.
35. Blumenkrantz MJ, Kopple JD, Gutman RA, et al. Methods for assessing nutritional status of patients with renal failure. *Am J Clin Nutr* 1980;33:1567–1585.
36. Owen WF Jr, Lew NL, Liu Y, et al. The urea reduction ratio and serum albumin concentration as predictors of mortality in patients undergoing hemodialysis. *N Engl J Med* 1993;329: 1001–1006.
37. Goldwasser P, Mittman N, Antignani A, et al. Predictors of mortality in hemodialysis patients. *J Am Soc Nephrol* 1993;3: 1613–1622.
38. Spiegel DM, Breyer JA. Serum albumin: A predictor of long-term outcome in peritoneal dialysis patients. *Am J Kidney Dis* 1994;23:283–285.
39. Avram MM, Mittman N, Bonomini L, et al. Markers for survival in dialysis: A seven year prospective study. *Am J Kidney Dis* 1995;26:209–219.
40. Lowrie EG, Huang WH, Lew NL. Death risk predictors among peritoneal dialysis and hemodialysis patients: A preliminary comparison. *Am J Kidney Dis* 1995;26:220–228.
41. Churchill DN, Taylor DW, Keshaviah PR. Adequacy of dialysis and nutrition in continuous peritoneal dialysis: association with clinical outcomes. Canada-USA Peritoneal Dialysis Study Group. *J Am Soc Nephrol* 1996;7:198–207.
42. Foley RN, Pafrey PS, Harnett JD, et al. Hypoalbuminemia, cardiac morbidity, and mortality in end-stage renal disease. *J Am Soc Nephrol* 1996;7:728–736.
43. Fung L, Pollock CA, Caterson RJ, et al. Dialysis adequacy and nutrition determine prognosis in continuous ambulatory peritoneal dialysis patients. *J Am Soc Nephrol* 1996;7:737–744.
44. Iseki K, Uehara H, Nishime K, et al. Impact of the initial levels of laboratory variables on survival in chronic dialysis patients. *Am J Kidney Dis* 1996;28:541–548.
45. Soucie JM, McClellan WM. Early death in dialysis patients. Risk factors and impact on incidence and mortality rates. *J Am Soc Nephrol* 1996;7:2169–2175.
46. Barrett BJ, Parfrey PS, Morgan J, et al. Prediction of early death in end-stage renal disease patients starting dialysis. *Am J Kidney Dis* 1997;29:214–222.
47. Marcen R, Teruel JL, de la Cal MA, et al. The impact of malnutrition in morbidity and mortality in stable hemodialysis patients. Spanish Cooperative Study of Nutrition in Hemodialysis. *Nephrol Dial Transplant* 1997;12:2324–2331.
48. Wong CS, Hingorani S, Gillen DL, et al. Hypoalbuminemia and risk of death in the U.S. Pediatric ESRD population. *J Am Soc Nephrol* 2000;11:171A (Abstr).
49. Gulati S, Stephens D, Balfe JA, et al. Children with hypoalbuminemia on continuous peritoneal dialysis are at risk for technique failure. *Kidney Int* 2001;59:2361–2367.
50. Oksa H, Ahonen K, Pasternack A, et al. Malnutrition in hemodialysis patients. *Scan J Urol Nephrol* 1991;25:157–161.
51. Harty JC, Boulton H, Curwell J, et al. The normalized protein catabolic rate is a flawed marker of nutrition in CAPD patients. *Kidney Int* 1994;45:103–109.
52. Jacob V, Marchant PR, Wild G, et al. Nutritional profile of continuous ambulatory peritoneal dialysis patients. *Nephron* 1995;71:16–22.
53. Jones CH, Newstead CG, Will EJ, et al. Assessment of nutritional status in CAPD patients: Serum albumin is not a useful measure. *Nephrol Dial Transplant* 1997;12:1406–1413.
54. Yeun JY, Kaysen JA. Factors influencing serum albumin in dialysis patients. *Am J Kidney Dis* 1998;32:S118–S125.
55. Ballmer PE, McNurlan MA, Hulter HN, et al. Chronic metabolic acidosis decreases albumin synthesis and induces negative nitrogen balance in humans. *J Clin Invest* 1995;95:39–45.
56. Kaysen GA, Rathore V, Shearer GC, et al. Mechanisms of hypoalbuminemia in hemodialysis patients. *Kidney Int* 1995;48: 510–516.

57. Han DS, Lee SW, Kang SW, et al. Factors affecting low values of serum albumin in CAPD patients. *Adv Perit Dial* 1996;12: 288–292.
58. Mak SK, Wong PN, Lo KY et al. Randomized prospective study of the effect of increased dialytic dose on nutritional and clinical outcome in continuous ambulatory peritoneal dialysis patients. *Am J Kidney Dis* 2000;36:105–114.
59. Docci D, Bilancioni R, Baldrati L, et al. Elevated acute phase reactants in hemodialysis patients. *Clin Nephrol* 1990;34: 88–91.
60. Avram MM, Goldwasser P, Erroa M, et al. Predictors of survival in continuous ambulatory peritoneal dialysis patients: The importance of prealbumin and other nutritional and metabolic markers. *Am J Kidney Dis* 1994;23:91–98.
61. Olusi SO, McFarlane H, Osunkoya O, et al. Specific protein assays in protein-calorie malnutrition. *Clin Chem Acta* 1975; 62:107.
62. Canaud B, Garred IJ, Argiles A, et al. Creatinine kinetic modelling: A simple and reliable tool for the assessment of protein nutritional status in hemodialysis patients. *Nephrol Dial Transplant* 1995;10:1405–1410.
63. Kopple JD, Jones MR, Keshaviah PR, et al. A proposed glossary for dialysis kinetics. *Am J Kidney Dis* 1995;26:963–981.
64. Mendley SR, Majkowski NL. Urea and nitrogen excretion in pediatric peritoneal dialysis patients. *Kidney Int* 2000;58: 2564–2570.
65. Maroni BJ, Steinman TI, Mitch WE. A method for estimating nitrogen intake of patients with chronic renal failure. *Kidney Int* 1985;27:58–65.
66. Wingen AM, Fabian-Bach C, Mehls O. European Study Group for Nutritional Treatment of Chronic Renal Failure in Childhood. Evaluation of protein intake by dietary diaries and urea-N excretion in children with chronic renal failure. *Clin Nephrol* 1993;40:208–215.
67. Kopple JD, Gao XL, Qing DP. Dietary protein, urea nitrogen appearance and total nitrogen appearance in chronic renal failure and CAPD patients. *Kidney Int* 1997;52:486–494.
68. Edefonti A, Picca M, Damiani B, et al. Models to assess nitrogen losses in pediatric patients on chronic peritoneal dialysis. *Pediatr Nephrol* 2000;15:25–30.
69. Goldstein SL. Hemodialysis in the pediatric patient: State of the art. *Adv Renal Rep Ther* 2001;8:173–179.
70. Mellits ED, Cheek DB. The assessment of body water and fatness from infancy to adulthood. *Monogr Soc Res Child Dev Serial* 1970;35:12–26.
71. Kopple JD. Uses and limitations of the balance technique. *JPEN J Parenter Enteral Nutr* 1987;11:S79–S85.
72. Panzetta G, Tessitore N, Faccini G, et al. The protein catabolic rate as a measure of protein intake in dialysis patients: Usefulness and limits. *Nephrol Dial Transplant* 1990;5:S125–S127.
73. Schaefer F, Georgi M, Zieger A, et al. Usefulness of bioelectric impedance and skinfold measurements in predicting fat-free mass derived from total body potassium in children. *Pediatr Res* 1994;35:617–624.
74. Formica C, Atkinson MG, Nyulasi I, et al. Body composition following hemodialysis: Studies using dual-energy X-ray absorptiometry and bioelectrical impedance analysis. *Osteoporosis Int* 1993;3:192–197.
75. Stenver DI, Gotfredsen A, Hilsted J, et al. Body composition in hemodialysis patients measured by dual-energy X-ray absorptiometry. *Am J Nephrol* 1995;15:105–110.
76. Borovnicar DJ, Wong KC, Kerr PG, et al. Total body protein status assessed by different estimates of fat-free mass in adult peritoneal dialysis patients. *Eur J Clin Nutr* 1996;50:607–616.
77. Woodrow G, Oldroyd B, Smith MA, et al. Measurement of body composition in chronic renal failure: Comparison of skinfold anthropometry and bioelectrical impedance with dual energy X-ray absorptiometry. *Eur J Clin Nutr* 1996;50:295–301.
78. Detsky AS, McLaughlin JR, Baker JP, et al. What is subjective global assessment of nutritional status? *JPEN J Parenter Enteral Nutr* 1987;11:8–13.
79. Enia G, Sicuso C, Alati G, et al. Subjective global assessment of nutrition in dialysis patients. *Nephrol Dial Transplant* 1993; 8:1094–1098.
80. Kight MA, Kelly MP. Conducting physical examination round for manifestations of nutrient deficiency or excess: an essential component of JCAHO assessment performance. *Diagn Nutr Network* 1995;4:2–6.
81. Food and Nutrition Board, Commission on Life Sciences, National Research Council: Recommended Dietary Allowances, ed 10. Washington, DC: National Academies Press, 1989.
82. Kleinman RE. *Pediatric nutrition handbook*, 4th ed. Elk Grove Village, IL: American Academy of Pediatrics, 1998:126, 489, 648–649.
83. Holliday MA. Nutrition therapy in renal disease. *Kidney Int* 1986;30:S3–S6.
84. Grupe WE, Harmon WE, Spinozzi NS. Protein and energy requirements in children receiving chronic hemodialysis. *Kidney Int* 1983;24:S6–S10.
85. Food and Nutrition Boards. Institute of Medicine. Dietary reference intakes. Applications in dietary assessment. A report of the subcommittees on interpretation and uses of dietary reference intakes and upper reference levels of nutrients, and the Standing Committee on the Scientific Evaluation of Dietary Reference Intakes. Washington, DC: National Academies Press, 2001.
86. Holliday MA. Calorie deficiency in children with uremia: Effect upon growth. *Pediatrics* 1972;50:590–597.
87. Ratsch IM, Catassi C, Verrina E, et al. Energy and nutrient intake of patients with mild to moderate chronic renal failure compared with healthy children: An Italian multicenter study. *Eur J Pediatr* 1992;151:701–705.
88. Kuizon BD, Salusky IB. Growth retardation in children with chronic renal failure. *J Bone Miner Res* 1999;14:1680–1690.
89. Norman LJ, Coleman JE, Macdonald IA, et al. Nutrition and growth in relation to severity of renal disease in children. *Pediatr Nephrol* 2000;15:259–265.
90. Betts PR, Magrath G. Growth pattern and dietary intake of children with chronic renal insufficiency. *Br Med J* 1974;2: 189–193.
91. Betts PR, Magrath G, White RH. Role of dietary energy supplementation in growth of children with chronic renal insufficiency. *Br Med J* 1977;1:416–418.
92. Mehls O, Blum WF, Schaefer F, et al. Growth failure in renal disease. *Baillieres Clin Endocrinol Metab* 1992;6:665–685.
93. Sedman A, Friedman A, Boineau F, et al. Nutritional management of the child with mild to moderate chronic renal failure. *J Pediatr* 1996;129:S13–S18.
94. Foreman JW, Chan JCM. Chronic renal failure in infants and children. *J Pediatr* 1988;113:793–800.
95. Kurtin PS, Shapiro AC. Effect of defined caloric supplementation on growth of children with renal disease. *J Renal Nutr* 1992;2:13.
96. Querfeld U, Salusky IB, Nelson P, et al. Hyperlipidemia in pediatric patients undergoing peritoneal dialysis. *Pediatr Nephrol* 1988;2:447–452.
97. Kleinknecht C, Salusky IB, Broyer M, et al. Effect of various protein diets on growth, renal function, and survival of uremic rats. *Kidney Int* 1979;15:534–542.
98. Salusky IB, Kleinknecht C, Broyer M, et al. Prolonged renal survival and stunting, with protein-deficient diets in experimental uremia. *J Lab Clin Med* 1981;21–30.

99. Brenner BM, Meyer TW, Hostetter TH. Dietary protein intake and the progressive nature of kidney disease: The role of hemodynamically mediated glomerular injury in the pathogenesis of progressive glomerular sclerosis in aging, renal ablation and intrinsic renal disease. *N Engl J Med* 1982;652–659.
100. Klahr S, Levey AS, Beck GJ, et al. The effects of dietary protein restriction and blood-pressure control on the progression of chronic renal disease. Modification of Diet in Renal Disease Study Group. *N Engl J Med* 1994;330:877–884.
101. Walser M, Hill S. Can renal replacement be deferred by a supplemented very low protein diet? *J Am Soc Nephrol* 1999;10: 110–116.
102. Aparicio M, Chauveau P, Precigout VD, et al. Nutrition and outcome on renal replacement therapy of patients with chronic renal failure treated by a supplemented very low protein diet. *J Am Soc Nephrol* 2000;11:708–716.
103. Bernhard J, Beaufrere B, Laville M, et al. Adaptive response to a low-protein diet in predialysis chronic renal failure patients. *J Am Soc Nephrol* 2001;12:1249–1254.
104. Fouque D, Laville M, Boissel JP, et al. Controlled low protein diets in chronic renal insufficiency: meta-analysis. *Br Med J* 1992;304:216–220.
105. Levey AS, Adler S, Caggiula AW, et al. Effects of dietary protein restriction on the progression of advanced renal disease in the Modification of Diet in Renal Disease Study. *Am J Kidney Dis* 1996;27:652–663.
106. Pedrini MT, Levey AS, Lau J, et al. The effect of dietary protein restriction on the progression of diabetic and non-diabetic renal diseases: A meta-analysis. *Ann Intern Med* 1996;124:627–632.
107. Kasiske BL, Lakatua JD, Ma JZ, et al. A meta-analysis of the effects of dietary protein restriction on the rate of decline in renal function. *Am J Kidney Dis* 1998;31:954–961.
108. Levey AS, Greene T, Beck GJ, et al., for the MDRD Study Group. Dietary protein restriction and the progression of chronic renal disease: What have all the results of the MDRD study shown? *J Am Soc Nephrol* 1999;10:2426–2439.
109. Friedman AL, Pityer R. Benefit of moderate dietary protein restriction on growth in the young animal with experimental chronic renal insufficiency: importance of early growth. *Pediatr Res* 1989;25:509–513.
110. Wingen AM, Fabian-Bach, Mehls O. European Study Group for Nutritional Treatment of Chronic Renal Failure in Childhood. Multicenter randomized study on the effect of a low-protein diet on the progression of renal failure in childhood: One-year results. *Miner Electrolyte Metab* 1992;18:303–308.
111. Kist-van Holthe tot Echten JE, Nauta J, de Jong MCJW, et al. Protein restriction in chronic renal failure. *Arch Dis Child* 1993; 68:371–375.
112. Uauy RD, Hogg RJ, Brewer ED, et al. Dietary protein and growth in infants with chronic renal insufficiency: a report from the Southwest Pediatric Nephrology Study Group and the University of California, San Francisco. *Pediatr Nephrol* 1994;8: 45–50.
113. Wingen AM, Fabian-Bach C, Schaefer F, et al. for the European Study Group for Nutritional Treatment of Chronic Renal Failure in Childhood. Randomized multicenter study of a low-protein diet on the progression of chronic renal failure in children. *Lancet* 1997;349:1117–1123.
114. Food and Agriculture Organization/World Health Organization. Energy and protein requirements. In: Technical Report Series No 724, Report of a joint FAO/WHO Expert Committee. Geneva: WHO, 1985.
115. Slomowitz LA, Monteon FJ, Grosvenor M, et al. Effect of energy intake on nutritional status in maintenance hemodialysis patients. *Kidney Int* 1989;35:704–711.
116. Simmons JM, Wilson CJ, Potter DE, et al. Relation of caloric deficiency to growth failure in children on hemodialysis and the growth response to caloric supplementation. *N Engl J Med* 1971;285:653–656.
117. Quan A, Baum M. Protein losses in children on continuous cycler peritoneal dialysis. *Pediatr Nephrol* 1996;10:728–731.
118. Edefonti A, Picca M, Damiani B, et al. Dietary prescription based on estimated nitrogen balance during peritoneal dialysis. *Pediatr Nephrol* 1999;13:253–258.
119. Brem AS, Lambert C, Hill C, et al. Prevalence of protein malnutrition in children maintained on peritoneal dialysis. *Pediatr Nephrol* 2002;17:527–530.
120. Ziegler EE, O'Donnel AM, Stearns G, et al. Nitrogen balance studies in normal children. *Am J Clin Nutr* 1977;7:939–946.
121. Iyengar AK, Narasing Rao BS, Reddy V. Effect of varying protein and energy intakes on N balance in Indian pre-school children. *Br J Nutr* 1979;42:417–423.
122. Uribarri J. DOQI guidelines for nutrition in long-term peritoneal dialysis patients: a dissenting view. *Am J Kidney Dis* 2001; 37:1313–1318.
123. Pennisi AJ, Heuser ET, Mickey MR, et al. Hyperlipidemia in pediatric hemodialysis and renal transplant patients. Association with coronary artery disease. *Am J Dis Child* 1976;130: 957–961.
124. Querfeld U, LeBouef RC, Salusky IB, et al. Lipoproteins in children treated with continuous peritoneal dialysis. *Pediatr Res* 1991;29:155–159.
125. Attman PO, Alaupovic P. Lipid abnormalities in chronic renal insufficiency. *Kidney Int* 1991;31:516S.
126. Querfeld U. Disturbances of lipid metabolism in children with chronic renal failure. *Pediatr Nephrol* 1993;7:749–757.
127. Scolink D, Balfe JW. Initial hypoalbuminemia and hyperlipidemia persist during chronic peritoneal dialysis in children. *Perit Dial Int* 1993;13:136–139.
128. Querfeld U. Under treatment of cardiac risk factors in adolescents with renal failure. *Perit Dial Int* 2001;21:S285–S289.
129. Chavers BM, Li S, Collins AJ, et al. Cardiovascular disease in pediatric chronic dialysis patients. *Kidney Int* 2002;62: 648–653.
130. Parekh RS, Carroll CE, Wolfe RA, et al. Cardiovascular mortality in children and young adults with end-stage kidney disease. *J Pediatr* 2002;141:162–164.
131. Saland JM, Ginsberg H, Fisher EA. Dyslipidemia in pediatric renal disease: epidemiology, pathophysiology, and management. *Curr Opin Pediatr* 2002;14:197–204.
132. Matsuyama T, Honda M, Ito H. Lipoprotein and apoprotein abnormalities in children undergoing CAPD. In: Ota K, Maher J, Winchester J, et al., eds. *Current concepts in peritoneal dialysis.* Tokyo: Excerpta Medica 1992;555–559.
133. Tanaka Y, Hataya H, Araki Y, et al. Hyperlipidemia in children on peritoneal dialysis: Effect of energy intake on serum triglyceride. *Perit Dial Int* 2002;22:426–428.
134. Slatopolsky E, Caglar S, Gradowska L, et al. On the prevention of secondary hyperparathyroidism in experimental chronic renal disease using "proportional reduction" of dietary phosphorus intake. *Kidney Int* 1972;2:147.
135. Portale AA, Booth BE, Tsai HC, et al. Reduced plasma concentration of 1,25 dihydroxyvitamin D in children with moderate renal insufficiency. *Kidney Int* 1982;21:627–632.
136. Wilson I, Felsenfeld A, Drezner MK, et al. Altered divalent ion metabolism in early renal failure: Role of 1,25$(OH)_2D_3$. *Kidney Int* 1985;7:565–573.
137. Martinez I, Saracho R, Montenegro J, et al. The importance of dietary calcium and phosphorus in the secondary hyperparathyroidism of patients with early renal failure. *Am J Kidney Dis* 1997;29:496–502.
138. Russel J, Bar A, Sherwood LM, et al. Interaction between cal-

cium and 1,25-dihydroxyvitamin D3 in the regulation of pre-proparathyroid hormone and vitamin D receptor messenger ribonucleic acid in avian parathyroids. *Endocrinology* 1993;132: 2639–2644.

139. Denda M, Finch J, Brown Alex J, et al. 1,25-Dihydroxyvitamin D3 and 22-oxacalcitriol prevent the decrease in vitamin D receptor content in the parathyroid glands of uremic rats. *Kidney Int* 1996;50:344–349.
140. Baker SS, Cochran WJ, Flores CA, et al. American Academy of Pediatrics. Committee on Nutrition. Calcium requirements of infants, children and adolescents (RE 9904). *Pediatrics* 1999; 104:1152–1157.
141. Food and Nutrition Board, Institute of Medicine. Dietary reference intakes for calcium, phosphorus, magnesium, vitamin D, and fluoride. Washington, DC: National Academies Press, 1997.
142. Andon MB, Peacock M, Kanerva RL, et al. Calcium absorption from apple and orange juice fortified with calcium citrate malate (CCM). *J Am Coll Nutr* 1996;15:313–316.
143. Coburn W, Kopple MH, Brickman AS, et al. Study of intestinal absorption of calcium in patients with renal failure. *Kidney Int* 1973;3:264–272.
144. Sieniawska M, Roszkowska-Blaim M, Wojciechowska B. The influence of dialysate calcium concentration on the PTH level in children undergoing CAPD. *Perit Dial Int* 1996;16: S567–S569.
145. Andreoli SP, Bergstein JF, Sherrard DJ, et al. Aluminium-containing phosphate binders in children with azotemia not undergoing dialysis. *N Engl J Med* 1984;310:1079–1084.
146. Sedman A. Aluminium toxicity in childhood. *Pediatr Nephrol* 1992;6:383–393.
147. Mai ML, Emmett M, Sheikh MS, et al. Calcium acetate, an effective phosphorus binder in patients with renal failure. *Kidney Int* 1989;36:690–695.
148. Goodman WG, Goldin J, Kuizon BD, et al. Coronary-artery calcification in young adults with end-stage renal disease who are undergoing dialysis. *N Engl J Med* 2000;342:1478–1483.
149. Salusky IB, Goodman WG. Cardiovascular calcification in end-stage renal disease. *Nephrol Dial Transplant* 2002;17:336–339.
150. Oh J, Wunsch R, Turzer M, et al. Advanced coronary and carotid arteriopathy in young adults with childhood-onset chronic renal failure. *Circulation* 2002;106:100–105.
151. Bleyer AJ, Burke SK, Dillon M, et al. A comparison of the calcium-free phosphate binder sevelamer hydrochloride with calcium acetate in the treatment of hyperphosphatemia in hemodialysis patients. *Am J Kidney Dis* 1999;33:694–701.
152. Goldberg DI, Dillon MA, Slatopolsky EA, et al. Effect of RenaGel, a non-absorbed, calcium- and aluminum-free phosphate binder, on serum phosphorus, calcium, and intact parathyroid hormone in end-stage renal disease patients. *Nephrol Dial Transplant* 1998;13:2303–2310.
153. Schroder CH, Swinkels DW, Verschuur R, et al. Studies with pre-treatment of milk with calcium acetate to reduce the phosphate content. *Eur J Pediatr* 1995;154:689.
154. Roodhooft AM, Van Hoeck KJ, Van Acker KJ. Hypophosphatemia in infants on continuous ambulatory peritoneal dialysis. *Clin Nephrol* 1990;34:131–135.
155. Slatopolsky E, Finch J, Ritter C, et al. A new analog of calcitriol, 19-nor-1,25$(OH)_2D_2$ suppresses parathyroid hormone secretion in uremic rats in the absence of hypercalcemia. *Am J Kidney Dis* 1995;25:852–860.
156. Tan AU Jr, Levine BS, Mazess RB, et al. Effective suppression of parathyroid hormone by 1 α-hydroxyvitamin D_2 in hemodialysis patients with moderate to severe secondary hyperparathyroidism. *Kidney Int* 1997;51:317–323.
157. Parekh RS, Flynn JT, Smoyer WE, et al. Improved growth in young children with severe chronic renal insufficiency who use specified nutritional therapy. *J Am Soc Nephrol* 2001;12: 2418–2426.
158. Schrier RN, Regal EM. Influence of aldosterone on sodium, water, and potassium metabolism in chronic renal disease. *Kidney Int* 1972;1:156–168.
159. Bunchman TE, Wood EG, Schenck MH, et al. Pretreatment of formula with sodium polystyrene sulfonate to reduce dietary potassium intake. *Pediatr Nephrol* 1991;5:29–32.
160. Mitch WE, Clark AS. Specificity of the effects of leucine and its metabolites on protein degradation in skeletal muscle. *Biochem J* 1984;222:579–586.
161. Movilli E, Bossini N, Viola BF, et al. Evidence for an independent role of metabolic acidosis on nutritional status in hemodialysis patients. *Nephrol Dial Transplant* 1998;13:674–678.
162. Uribarri J. Moderate metabolic acidosis and its effects on nutritional parameters in hemodialysis patients. *Clin Nephrol* 1997; 48:238–240.
163. Makoff R. Water-soluble vitamin status in patients with renal disease treated with hemodialysis or peritoneal dialysis. *J Renal Nutr* 1991;1:56–73.
164. Makoff R, Dwyer J, Rocco MV. Folic acid, pyridoxine, cobalamin, and homocysteine and their relationship to cardiovascular disease in end-stage renal disease. *J Renal Nutr* 1996;6:2–11.
165. Stockberger RA, Parott KA, Lexander SR, et al. Vitamin B6 status of children undergoing continuous ambulatory peritoneal dialysis. *Nutr Res* 1987;7:1021–1030.
166. Blumberg A, Hanck A, Sander G. Vitamin nutrition in patients on continuous ambulatory peritoneal dialysis (CAPD). *Clin Nephrol* 1983;20:244–250.
167. Schroder CH, de Boer AW, Giesen AM, et al. Treatment of hyperhomocysteinemia in children on dialysis by folic acid. *Pediatr Nephrol* 1999;13:583–585.
168. Merouani A, Lambert M, Delvin EE, et al. Plasma homocysteine concentration in children with chronic renal failure. *Pediatr Nephrol* 2001;16:805–811.
169. Makoff R. Vitamin supplement in patients with renal disease. *Dial Transplant* 1992;21:18–24.
170. Kriley M, Warady BA. Vitamin status of pediatric patients receiving long-term peritoneal dialysis. *Am J Clin Nutr* 1991;53: 1476–1479.
171. Shah GM, Ross EA, Sabo A, et al. Effects of ascorbic acid and pyridoxine supplementation on oxalate metabolism in peritoneal dialysis patients. *Am J Kidney Dis* 1992;20:42–49.
172. Reddy J, Bailey RR. Vitamin K deficiency developing in patients with renal failure treated with cephalosporin antibiotics. *N Z Med J* 1980;92:378–379.
173. Werb R, Clark WF, Lindsay RM, et al. Serum vitamin A levels and associated abnormalities in patients on regular dialysis treatment. *Clin Nephrol* 1979;12:63–68.
174. Warady BA, Kriley M, Alon U, et al. Vitamin status of infants receiving long-term peritoneal dialysis. *Pediatr Nephrol* 1994; 8:354–356.
175. Smythe WR, Alfrey AC, Craswell PW, et al. Trace element abnormalities in chronic uremia. *Ann Intern Med* 1982;96: 302–310.
176. Thomson NM, Stevens BJ, Humphrey TJ, et al. Comparison of trace elements in peritoneal dialysis, hemodialysis, and uremia. *Kidney Int* 1983;23:9–14.
177. Chan JCM, McEnery PT, Chinchilli VM, et al. A prospective, double-blind study of growth failure in children with chronic renal insufficiency and the effectiveness of treatment with calcitriol vs dihydrotachysterol. *J Pediatr* 1994;124:520–528.
178. Fritz IB. Action of carnitine on long-chain fatty acid oxidation by liver. *Am J Physiol* 1959;197:297–304.
179. Englard S, Carnicero HH. a-Butyro betaine hydroxylation to

carnitine in mammalian kidney. *Arch Biochem Biophys* 1978; 190:361–364.
180. Bartel LL, Hussey JL, Shrago E. Perturbation of serum carnitine levels in human adults by chronic renal disease and dialysis therapy. *Am J Clin Nutr* 1981;34:1314–1320.
181. Moorthy A, Rosenblum M, Rajaram R, et al. A comparison of plasma and muscle carnitine levels in patients on peritoneal or hemodialysis for chronic renal failure. *Am J Nephrol* 1983;3: 205–208.
182. Warady BA, Borum P, Stall C, et al. Carnitine status of pediatric patients on continuous ambulatory peritoneal dialysis. *Am J Nephrol* 1990;10:109–114.
183. Gusmano R, Oleggini R, Perfumo F. Plasma carnitine concentrations and dyslipidemia in children on maintenance hemodialysis. *J Pediatr* 1981;99:429–432.
184. Patel C, Denny M. *Cultural foods and renal diets. A multilingual guide for renal patients.* Sections I and II. Reno, NV/San Mateo, CA: Council on Renal Nutrition, National Kidney Foundation of Northern California.
185. Yiu VW, Harmon WE, Spinozzi NS, et al. High calorie nutrition for infants with chronic renal disease. *J Renal Nutr* 1996; 6:203–206.
186. Balfe JW, Secker DJ, Coulter PE, et al. Tube feeding in children on chronic peritoneal dialysis. *Adv Perit Dial* 1990;6:257–261.
187. Brewer ED. Growth of small children managed with chronic peritoneal dialysis and nasogastric tube feedings: 203-month experience in 14 patients. *Adv Perit Dial* 1990;6:269–272.
188. Fine RN. Growth in children undergoing continuous ambulatory peritoneal dialysis/continuing cycling peritoneal dialysis/ automated peritoneal dialysis. *Perit Dial Int* 13:S247–S250, 1992.
189. Warady BA, Weis L, Johnson L. Nasogastric tube feeding in infants on peritoneal dialysis. *Perit Dial Int* 1996;16: S521–S525.
190. Kari JA, Gonzalez C, Ledermann SE, et al. Outcome and growth of infants with severe chronic renal failure. *Kidney Int* 2000;57: 1681–1687.
191. Warren S, Conley SB. Nutritional considerations in infants on peritoneal dialysis (CPD). *Dial Transplant* 1983;12:263–266.
192. Conley SB. Supplemental (NG) feedings of infants undergoing continuous peritoneal dialysis. In: Fine RN, ed. *Chronic ambulatory peritoneal dialysis (CAPD) and chronic cycling peritoneal dialysis (CCPD) in children.* Boston, Martinus Nijhoff, 1987: 263–269.
193. Watson AR, Taylor J, Balfe JW. Growth in children on CAPD: a reappraisal. In: Khanna R, et al., eds. *Adv Perit Dial.* Conference. 1985;171–177.
194. Watson AR, Coleman JE, Taylor EA. Gastrostomy buttons for feeding children on continuous cycling peritoneal dialysis. In: Khanna R et al., eds. *Adv Perit Dial* 1992:391–395.
195. Coleman JE, Watson AR, Rance CH, et al. Gastrostomy buttons for nutritional support on chronic dialysis. *Nephrol Dial Transplant* 1998;13:2041–2046.
196. O'Regan S, Garel L. Percutaneous gastrojejunostomy for caloric supplementation in children on peritoneal dialysis. In: Khanna R, et al., eds. *Adv Perit Dial* 1990:273–275.
197. Kohaut ED, Whelchel J, Waldo FB, et al. Aggressive therapy of infants with renal failure. *Pediatr Nephrol* 1987;1:150–153.
198. Ellis EN, Yiu V, Harley F, et al. The impact of supplemental feeding in young children on dialysis: a report of the North American Pediatric Renal Transplant Cooperative Study (NAPRTCS). *Pediatr Nephrol* 2001;16:404–408
199. Fried MD, Khoshoo V, Secker DJ, et al. Decrease in gastric emptying time and episodes of regurgitation in children with spastic quadriplegia fed a whey-based formula. *J Pediatr* 1992; 120:569–572.
200. Tolia V, Lin CH, Kuhns LP. Gastric emptying using three different formulas in infants with gastroesophageal reflux. *J Pediatr Gastroenterol Nutr* 1992;15:297–301.
201. Wood EG, Bunchman TE, Khurana R, et al. Complications of nasogastric and gastrostomy tube feedings in children with end-stage renal disease. *Adv Perit Dial* 1990;6:262–264.
202. Watson AR, Coleman JE, Warady BA. When and how to use nasogastric and gastrostomy feeding for nutritional support in infants and children on CAPD/CCPD. In: Fine RN, Alexander SR, Warady BA, eds. *CAPD/CCPD in children.* Boston: Kluwer Academic, 1998:281–300.
203. Murugaru B, Conley SB, Lemire JM, Portman RJ. Fungal peritonitis in children treated with peritoneal dialysis and gastrostomy feeding. *Pediatr Nephrol* 1991;5:620–621.
204. Warady BA, Bashir M, Donaldson LA. Fungal peritonitis in children receiving peritoneal dialysis: a report of the NAPRTCS. *Kidney Int* 2000;58:384–389.
205. Kamen RS. Impaired development of oral-motor functions required for normal oral feeding as a consequence of tube feeding during infancy. *Adv Perit Dial* 1990;6:276–278.
206. Strologo LD, Principato F, Sinibaldi D, et al. Feeding dysfunction in infants with severe chronic renal failure after long-term nasogastric tube feeding. *Pediatr Nephrol* 1997;11:84–86.
207. Hanning RM, Balfe JW, Zlotkin SH. Effect of amino acid containing dialysis solutions on plasma amino acid profiles in children with chronic renal failure. *J Pediatr Gastroenterol Nutr* 1987;6:942–947.
208. Hanning RM, Balfe JW, Zlotkin SH. Effectiveness and nutritional consequences of amino acid based vs glucose based dialysis solutions in infants and children receiving CAPD. *Am J Clin Nutr* 1987;46:22–30.
209. Canepa A, Perfumo F, Carrea A, et al. Long-term effect of amino-acid dialysis solution in children on continuous ambulatory peritoneal dialysis. *Pediatr Nephrol* 1991;5:215–219.
210. Qamar IU, Levin N, Balfe JW, et al. Effects of 3-month aminoacid dialysis compared to dextrose dialysis in children on continuous ambulatory peritoneal dialysis. *Perit Dial Int* 1994; 14:34–41.
211. Zachwieja J, Duran M, Joles JA, et al. Amino acid and carnitine supplementation in hemodialysed children. *Pediatr Nephrol* 1994;8:739–743.
212. Goldstein SL, Baronette S, Gambrell V, et al. nPCR assessment and IDPN treatment of malnutrition in pediatric hemodialysis patients. *Pediatr Nephrol* 2002;17:531–534.
213. Food and Nutrition Board, Institute of Medicine. Dietary reference intakes for thiamine, riboflavin, niacin, vitamin B6, folate, vitamin B12, pantothenic acid, biotin, and choline. Washington, DC: National Academies Press, 2000.
214. Food and Nutrition Board, Institute of Medicine. Dietary reference intakes for vitamin A, vitamin K, arsenic, boron, chromium, copper, iodine, iron, manganese, molybdenum, nickel, silicon, vanadium, and zinc. Washington, DC: National Academies Press, 2002.
215. Food and Nutrition Board, Institute of Medicine. Dietary reference intakes for vitamin C, vitamin E, selenium, and carotenoids. Washington, DC: National Academies Press, 2000.

30

NUTRITIONAL MANAGEMENT OF ACUTE RENAL FAILURE

JOEL D. KOPPLE

METABOLIC AND NUTRITIONAL DERANGEMENTS ASSOCIATED WITH ACUTE RENAL FAILURE

The patient with acute renal failure (ARF), particularly when sufficiently ill to require intensive care, constitutes one of the most challenging therapeutic dilemmas for the health care team. The overall mortality rate of individuals with ARF is 40% to 60% (1,2). However, patients with severe underlying illnesses have higher morbidity and mortality (3). This is particularly the case for patients with high APACHE II (Acute Physiology And Chronic Health Evaluation) or APACHE III scores and for patients who have multiorgan system failure syndrome (4). In our experience, patients with shock or sepsis as the cause of ARF who are unable to be nourished by oral or enteral feeding because of gastrointestinal dysfunction have a mortality rate of 80% to 90% (5,6). These latter groups of patients frequently display profound metabolic and nutritional disorders. There is often excess total body water, azotemia, hyperkalemia, hyperphosphatemia, hypocalcemia, hyperuricemia, and metabolic acidemia.

Net protein degradation in ARF can be massive. Protein losses as high as 200 to 250 g/day have been observed (5–7). Over a several day period, the cumulative protein losses can constitute a sizable proportion of total body protein; for comparison, the total noncollagen protein mass of a 70-kg man is about 6 kg (8). Patients are more likely to be catabolic when the ARF is caused by shock, sepsis, or rhabdomyolysis. Feinstein et al. reported an average urea nitrogen appearance (UNA) of 12.0 ± (standard deviation [SD]) 7.9 g/day (5); for patients with rhabdomyolysis, the mean UNA was 12.3 ± 7.9 g/day. These UNA rates were each significantly greater ($p < 0.05$, respectively) than in patients with ARF from other causes (3.8 ± 2.4 g/day) (5).

Marked net protein degradation may accelerate the rate of increase in plasma concentrations of potassium, phosphorus, nitrogenous metabolites, and hydrogen ion in patients with ARF. In patients without renal failure, severe protein or calorie malnutrition can impair normal wound healing and immune function (9,10) and enhance morbidity and mortality. Therefore, it is likely that the profound catabolic response of many patients with ARF may increase the risk of delayed wound healing, infection, prolonged convalescence, and mortality.

However, some patients with ARF maintain nitrogen balance and have normal or near normal total body water, plasma mineral concentrations, and acid–base status. Usually, these patients do not have severely catabolic underlying illnesses. They are generally not oliguric, and the cause of their ARF is typically an isolated, noncatabolic event, such as administration of radiocontrast media or antibiotic nephrotoxicity. However, most patients with ARF have some degree of net protein breakdown (i.e., protein synthesis minus degradation) and disordered fluid, electrolyte, or acid–base status.

Studies in animals suggest that acute uremia itself may cause disorders in amino acid and protein metabolism and promote wasting. UNA is increased in rats with ARF as compared to sham-operated controls. In acutely uremic rats there is enhanced hepatic uptake of several amino acids and increased hepatic release of glucose, urea, and the branched-chain amino acids valine, leucine, and isoleucine (11,12). When a mixture of amino acids was added to the perfusate in concentrations that were approximately similar to those found in plasma, the increment in hepatic glucose and urea formation in the rats with ARF was significantly greater than in control rats (12). These observations suggest that in rats, acute uremia stimulates both gluconeogenesis and protein degradation in the liver. There is increased protein degradation, impaired protein synthesis, and insulin resistance of rats made acutely uremic by bilateral nephrectomy (13,14). The hypercatabolic state appears to be more pronounced when the ARF is created by bilateral nephrectomy rather than other, less traumatic techniques.

Acute uremia seems to engender only a mild increase in catabolism (13,14). It is when sepsis, inflammation, trauma, or hypoxia is superimposed that catabolism often increases markedly (5–7,15).

Much evidence has accumulated concerning the mechanisms responsible for increased gluconeogenesis and net protein degradation in ARF. In acutely uremic rats, there is increased hepatic activity of two urea cycle enzymes, ornithine transaminase, which catalyzes the conversion of glutamate to ornithine, and arginase, which catalyzes formation of urea and ornithine from arginine (16). Increased activity of serine dehydratase, which oxidizes the gluconeogenic amino acid serine, is described. In addition, in rats with ARF, normal hepatic activity of phenylalanine hydroxylase and increased activity of tyrosine aminotransferase, key enzymes in the degradation of phenylalanine and tyrosine, are observed (16,17).

Reduced muscle glycogen is described in rats with bilateral nephrectomy (18). Increased activity of phosphorylase-a, which catalyzes glycogenolysis, and decreased activity of glycogen synthetase 1, which catalyzes glycogen synthesis, have been observed in muscle of these rats. Supplementing a low-protein diet with the amino acid serine led to increased glycogen synthetase 1 activity in these animals (18).

ARF frequently is associated with hyperglycemia, which primarily is the result of insulin resistance and increased hepatic gluconeogenesis (19). Infusion of exogenous glucose does not suppress hepatic glucose production normally (20). Plasma triglycerides (20) are increased and total cholesterol and high-density lipoprotein cholesterol are decreased (21). Decreased lipolysis appears to be a major contributory factor to these disorders (22). There is increased protein catabolism with enhanced release of amino acids from skeletal muscle (13). Despite this, plasma amino acid concentrations are reduced and the plasma clearance of most amino acids is increased in ARF (23). Also, intracellular pools of various amino acids are decreased. The combination of low plasma amino acid concentrations and accelerated protein degradation in skeletal muscle with increased release of amino acids suggests that there is enhanced hepatic removal of amino acids from the circulation, which is responsible for the low plasma and intracellular amino acid pools. Indeed, increased hepatic amino acid consumption and glucose production in dogs with ARF support this possibility (20). The end result of these processes is net protein degradation, negative nitrogen balance that often is profound, protein depletion, enhanced gluconeogenesis, glucose intolerance, and increased generation of urea and other potentially toxic metabolites.

There are many causes for the hypercatabolic state in ARF. First, there are many metabolic products, particularly those proteins, peptides, amino acids, and nucleic acids that normally are excreted in the urine or degraded by the kidney and that accumulate in ARF. Some of these compounds may induce negative protein balance. Indeed hydrogen ion is one such product (24–26). Second, acidemia activates the adenosine triphosphate (ATP)-dependent ubiquitin–proteosome system and increases protein degradation in skeletal muscle (26). Third, underlying catabolic conditions, such as sepsis, hypotension, surgery, polytrauma, or rhabdomyolysis, may cause increased plasma concentrations of counterregulatory hormones including epinephrine, norepinephrine, cortisone, and glucagon. These hormones, which can induce a catabolic state, often are elevated in patients with ARF (27,28). Fourth, underlying catabolic illnesses may stimulate the elaboration of endotoxin and other toxic compounds and the secretion of toxic acute-phase proteins, such as C-reactive protein, and such cytokines as tumor necrosis factor and interleukin-1 (IL-1) and IL-6; these compounds may induce inflammation and catabolism (29–32). Hemodialysis may engender catabolism by stimulating the release of cytokines (e.g., IL-1), which may induce the complement cascade, activate proteolytic enzymes, and increase net protein degradation (33–35). This is particularly likely to occur when hemodialysis is performed with bioincompatible membranes (36,37). Fifth, ARF itself can increase serum levels of certain catabolic hormones, including glucagon and parathyroid hormone (38–41).

Sixth, many patients are unable to eat adequately because they are anorexic, nauseated, or vomiting. These symptoms may be caused by uremia itself, underlying illnesses, or the anorectic effects of dialysis treatment. Other causes of poor food intake are medical or surgical disorders that alter cognitive performance or impair gastrointestinal function and the frequent diagnostic studies that require the patient to fast for several hours. Seventh, losses of nutrients in draining fistulas and during dialysis therapy (i.e., amino acids; peptides; proteins; water-soluble vitamins; and, with glucose-free dialysate, glucose) may contribute to malnutrition (42–45) (see Chapters 11, 25, and 31). Eighth, blood drawing; gastrointestinal bleeding, which may be occult; and blood trapped in the hemodialyzer also may contribute to protein depletion (46,47).

Severely ill patients with multiorgan failure and ARF may have a reduction in plasma concentrations of a number of antioxidants, including ascorbic acid, beta carotene, and selenium; an increase in plasma malondialdehyde, a marker of lipid peroxidation; and elevated hydrogen peroxide production from neutrophils (48). Some of these findings of oxidant stress were more pronounced in those patients with multiorgan failure and ARF as compared to those without ARF.

EFFECT OF NUTRITIONAL THERAPY ON METABOLIC STATUS AND MORTALITY RATE

From the 1940s to the mid-1960s, many clinicians recommended marked restriction or total avoidance of protein intake for patients with ARF (49–51). Small amounts of energy (e.g., 400 to 800 kcal/day) were provided from candy, butterballs, or intravenous infusions of hypertonic glucose to diminish protein degradation. The rationale for this approach was based on Gamble's studies of lifeboat rations for healthy young men. Gamble observed that administration of about 100 g/day of sugar could reduce substantially net protein breakdown in these starving but otherwise healthy volunteers (52).

In the 1950s, an era before most ARF patients could be readily treated with dialysis or hemofiltration, some investigators administered low-nitrogen diets and anabolic steroids to patients with ARF to reduce uremic toxicity and maintain life until renal function recovered. The maintenance of good nutrition was a secondary aim. Anabolic steroids may decrease transiently the UNA and slow the rate of increase in the serum urea nitrogen (SUN) or nonprotein nitrogen and the development of acidemia (53,54). In the 1960s, the Giordano–Giovannetti diet was developed for patients with advanced chronic renal failure (55,56). This diet, which provided about 20 g/day of protein, most of which usually was supplied by two eggs, provided the recommended dietary allowances for essential amino acids for young healthy adults. Some clinicians advocated this diet for patients with ARF who were able to eat with the anticipation that this diet would be used efficiently and would minimize the degree of protein wasting, reduce the UNA, and suppress the rate of the accumulation of nitrogenous metabolites (57).

When dialysis first became available, it usually was used only for specific sequelae of renal failure, such as uremic symptoms, fluid overload, heart failure, or hyperkalemia, and efforts often were made to avoid dialysis therapy. As modern techniques developed for the routine use of dialysis therapy and for parenteral and enteral nutrition, the focus of nutritional therapy gradually evolved so that the maintenance of good nutrition became a primary goal, and dialysis (58) and eventually continuous filtration and dialysis procedures (59) (see Chapter 31 and later in this chapter) were used as needed to control fluid and electrolyte balance and remove metabolic waste.

In 1967 Lee et al. administered solutions containing casein hydrolysate, fructose, ethanol, and lipid emulsions by peripheral vein to several patients with acute or chronic renal failure who were in need of nutritional support (60). Although the patients were often severely ill, these investigators reported that marked loss of weight did not occur, and convalescence was shortened. Dudrick et al. treated patients who had acute or chronic renal failure with infusions of essential amino acids and hypertonic glucose into the subclavian vein (61,62). The investigators reported weight gain, improved wound healing, and stabilization or reduction of SUN levels. Decreased serum potassium and phosphorus and positive nitrogen balance often were observed. Anephric beagles were given intravenous infusions of a solution of essential amino acids and 57% glucose and demonstrated a lower increase in SUN and a longer survival than similar animals that were given food or infusions of glucose (5% or 57%) alone without amino acids (63).

Abel et al. carried out a series of studies in patients with ARF who were treated with hypertonic glucose and eight essential amino acids but no histidine (64–68). Serum potassium, phosphorus, and magnesium concentrations fell, and SUN often stabilized or decreased. Baek et al. compared the outcome in 63 patients treated with total parenteral nutrition (TPN) that provided a fibrin hydrolysate and hypertonic glucose to 66 subjects who received varying quantities of glucose (69). The patients who were given the hydrolysate had lower morbidity and mortality. However, this did not appear to be a randomly assigned, concurrently controlled clinical trial.

McMurray et al. (70) and Milligan et al. (71) gave patients with acute tubular necrosis intravenous infusions of either hypertonic glucose alone (200 to 400 kcal/day) or a mixture of essential and nonessential amino acids and hypertonic glucose that provided 12 g nitrogen/day and more than 2,000 kcal/day. In the patients who had no complications, there was no difference in survival between the two intravenous treatments. However, among patients who had three or more clinical complications or who had peritonitis, those who received 12 g/day of amino acid nitrogen with hypertonic glucose had significantly greater survival as compared with patients receiving low quantities of glucose alone. This study was carried out retrospectively, and the patients who received amino acids and glucose were treated at a later time than those who received glucose alone.

There have been few prospective, randomized clinical trials of parenteral nutrition in patients with ARF, and these were conducted many years ago. No randomized clinical trials of enteral nutrition have been carried out in such patients. In the former studies essentially only three types of solutions have been used: glucose alone, glucose and about 13 to 26 g/day of essential amino acids, and glucose and approximately equal quantities of essential and nonessential amino acids. Vitamins and minerals also were supplied. Abel et al. carried out a prospective double-blind study in 53 patients with ARF who were randomly assigned to receive infusions of either a mean of 16 g/day of essential amino acids with hypertonic glucose or hypertonic glucose alone (66). The total energy intake with the two preparations averaged 1,426 and 1,641 kcal/day, respectively. Food intake may not have been strictly controlled during the study. The survival rate until renal function recovered was significantly higher in the patients receiving the essential amino acids and hypertonic glucose as compared to hypertonic glucose alone. However, although overall hospital mortality tended to be lower with the former treatment, it was not significantly different between the two treatment groups. Patients with more severe renal failure, as indicated by their need to receive dialysis treatments, and those with serious complications, such as pneumonia and generalized sepsis, displayed significantly greater hospital survival when essential amino acids and glucose were given than when glucose alone was infused.

Several studies have indicated that animals or patients with ARF often have increased nutritional needs for protein or amino acids and energy and that nitrogen balance is difficult to attain, particularly during the first few days of ARF (5–7,72–76). There have been a few studies that have examined, in a prospective fashion, nitrogen balance and requirements in severely ill patients with acute renal failure. Leonard et al. randomly assigned patients with ARF to receive intravenous infusions of 1.75% essential L-amino acids and 47% dextrose or 47% dextrose alone (7). Patients who were able to eat or tolerate tube feeding were excluded from the study. Hence, many of the patients were severely ill. Most patients required frequent dialysis treatments. The rate of increase in SUN was significantly less in the group that received the essential amino acids. However, the mean nitrogen balance was approximately 10 g/day negative in both groups, and there was no difference in the rate of survival or recovery of renal function in the two groups.

Feinstein et al. performed a prospective, double-blind study in 30 patients with ARF who were unable to eat adequately. Patients were randomly assigned to receive parenteral nutrition with glucose alone, glucose and 21 g/day of essential amino acids, or glucose and 21 g/day of essential amino acids and 21 g/day of nonessential amino acids (5). Mean energy intake varied from 2,300 to 2,700 kcal/day and did not differ significantly among the groups. Small supplements of glucose and, in the latter two treatment groups, essential amino acids or essential and nonessential amino acids, respectively, were given during hemodialysis treatments. The duration of the study in the three groups was 9.0 ± (SD) 7.7 days.

Many of the patients were in a markedly catabolic state, as indicated by the negative nitrogen balances, high UNA, low serum protein levels, and altered plasma amino acid concentrations. Mean nitrogen balance, estimated from the difference between nitrogen intake and UNA, which underestimates nitrogen losses by approximately 2 g/day, was −10.4 ± 5.7 g/day with glucose alone, −4.4 ± 7.3 g/day with glucose and essential amino acids, and −8.5 ± 7.9 g/day with glucose and essential and nonessential amino acids (5). Although the nitrogen balances were not different with three infusates, a few patients who received essential amino acids or essential and nonessential amino acids displayed only slightly negative nitrogen balance. In one patient receiving essential amino acids, the nitrogen balance was probably neutral or positive. Serum potassium, phosphorus, and urea often stabilized or decreased in patients in all three treatment groups; these changes in serum levels probably were influenced by dialysis therapy, recovering renal function, the natural history of the underlying metabolic disorders, and the patients' nutrient intakes. There was no difference in the rapidity or incidence of recovery of renal function or in the rate of survival among the three treatment groups, although recovery of renal function and survival tended to be greater in the patients receiving the essential amino acids.

Because these observations suggested that higher nitrogen intakes might be more effective at maintaining nitrogen balance in catabolic patients with ARF, Feinstein et al. conducted another randomized prospective clinical trial in a smaller number of patients (6). Patients received TPN providing 21 g/day of essential amino acids or TPN with essential and nonessential amino acids provided in a 1.0:1.0 ratio. With the latter treatment, attempts were made to infuse a quantity of amino acid nitrogen that was equal to the UNA. Thirteen patients with ARF were randomly assigned to one of the two treatment groups. The results indicated that although nitrogen intake was about five times greater and the essential amino acid intake was more than twice as great with the nonessential and essential amino acid regimen, the nitrogen balance, calculated from the difference between nitrogen intake and UNA, was not different between the two treatment groups. Moreover, the UNA fell significantly only in patients receiving essential amino acids. As would be expected in such a small clinical trial, there was no difference in the incidence of recovery of renal function or mortality rate between the two treatment groups.

These latter two studies, taken together, suggest that, at least for short periods, high-calorie solutions providing about 21 g/day of essential amino acids may be used more efficiently than isocaloric preparations containing larger quantities of essential and nonessential amino acids (e.g., 40 to 70 g/day provided in an essential to nonessential amino acid ratio of 1.0:1.0) (Figs. 30.1 and 30.2) (77). The essential amino acid solutions seem to reduce the UNA and total nitrogen output more than solutions containing both essential and nonessential amino acids. Consequently, nitrogen balance, although negative with both regimens, was no more negative with the low quantities of essential amino acids, but the accumulation of nitrogenous metabolites was less with this latter regimen. These findings are consistent with the thesis that a TPN regimen that provides larger quantities of essential and nonessential amino acids but that contains a larger proportion of essential amino acids may be used more effectively, especially if the solutions are enriched with the branched-chain amino acids (see later in this chapter). Clinical research trials will be necessary to test this hypothesis.

Lopez Martinez et al. treated 35 septic patients with ARF by parenteral nutrition for 12 days (74). The patients were in the polyuric phase of ARF, were not very uremic, and had not received dialysis therapy. Patients were given 4.4 g nitrogen/day from essential amino acids and 2,000 kcal/day (group 1) or 15 g nitrogen/day from essential and nonessential amino acids and 3,000 kcal/day, provided either by glucose (group 2) or by glucose and fat (group 3). Nitrogen balance, apparently estimated from the difference between nitrogen intake and UNA, was initially negative in all three

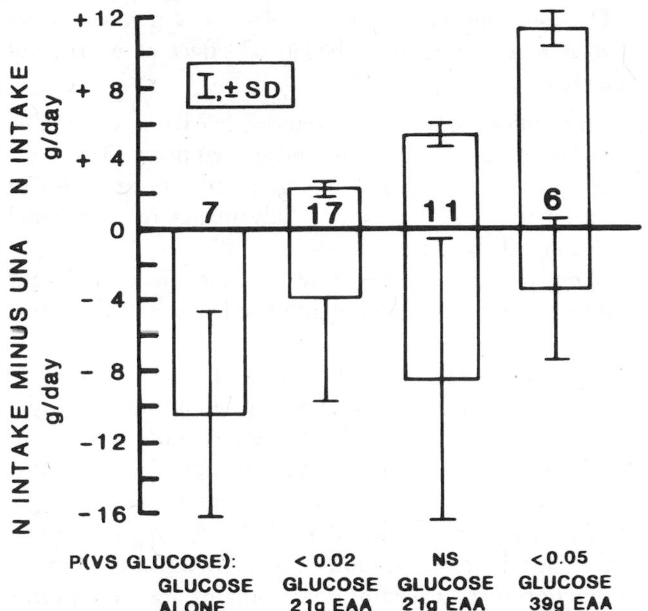

FIGURE 30.1. Mean nitrogen intake and approximate nitrogen balance in four groups of patients with acute renal failure who were receiving parenteral nutrition. Individuals were treated with glucose alone, glucose and 21 g/day of essential amino acids (EAA), glucose and 21 g/day of EAA and 21 g/day nonessential amino acids (NEAA), and glucose and approximately 39 g/day of EAA and 39 g/day of NEAA. Nitrogen intake was calculated from the measured nitrogen content of the infused parenteral nutrition solutions and is plotted above the horizontal line. The nitrogen balance, estimated as the difference between the nitrogen intake and nitrogen output, calculated as the urea nitrogen appearance (UNA), is plotted below the horizontal line. Data for patients who received a given parenteral nutrition formulation represent the mean values of the average daily intake and balance data obtained from each of the patients during the parenteral nutrition treatment. The calculated nitrogen intake was not adjusted for the nitrogen received from transfusions of blood or blood products that contain proteins and small amounts of peptides, free amino acids, and other nitrogen-containing compounds. Nitrogen balance was not adjusted for nonurea nitrogen in urine, fecal nitrogen, and other unmeasured nitrogen losses (e.g., from respiration, wound drainage, nasogastric tube or fistula drainage, flatus, sweat, skin desquamation and replacement, and hair and nail growth). The numbers in the vertical bars indicate the sample size of each group. Data from two separate studies (5,6) are combined in this figure. (From Kopple JD. The nutrition management of the patient with acute renal failure. *J Parenter Enteral Nutr* 1996;20:3–12, with permission.)

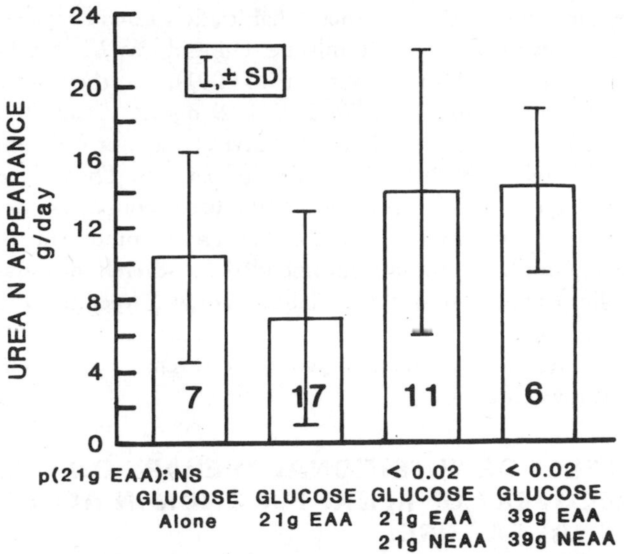

FIGURE 30.2. Urea nitrogen appearance (UNA) in four groups of patients with acute renal failure who were receiving parenteral nutrition (5,6). Data for patients who received a given parenteral nutrition formulation represent the mean values of the daily average UNA for the patients in that treatment group. Symbols are explained in the legend to Fig. 30.1 and in the text. (From Kopple JD. The nutrition management of the patient with acute renal failure. *J Parenter Enteral Nutr* 1996;20:3–12, with permission.)

groups and became more positive with time, particularly in groups 2 and 3. Over the 12-day period of the study, mean nitrogen balances were significantly more positive in both groups 2 and 3 than in group 1.

Hasik et al. fed diets varying in protein content to nine patients with ARF when they were polyuric (78). The authors concluded that these patients, who were probably not severely ill at the time of the study, required 0.97 g protein/kg/day to maintain nitrogen balance. Mirtallo et al. gave small amounts of either essential amino acids or essential and nonessential amino acids to patients with mild ARF (79). The patients had substantial renal function, and no patient received dialysis in this study. There were no differences in UNA, recovery of renal function, or mortality in the two groups. Because the patients in these last three studies were neither very uremic nor very ill, the results may be more applicable to the patient who is not very catabolic and either has mild ARF or is recovering from ARF.

Bellomo et al. carried out a sequential, nonrandomized study in two groups of critically ill patients with ARF (80). Patients were receiving continuous arteriovenous hemodiafiltration (CAVHDF) or continuous venovenous hemodiafiltration (CVVHDF). All patients were given the same amount of calories (30 to 35 kcal/kg/day) from intravenous nutrition and uptake of glucose from dialysate, with similar percentages of calories derived from carbohydrates and lipids. The protein source was provided as a mixture of essential and nonessential amino acids given intravenously. The quantity of amino acids received by the first group (24 patients) was determined by their attending physician and averaged 1.2 g/kg/day. The second group (16 patients) received a fixed amount of amino acids—2.5 g/kg/day. Patients were followed for a mean of 6.8 days.

Nitrogen balance was -5.50 ± 10.5 (SD) g/day with 1.2 g amino acids kg/day and tended to be less negative (-1.92 ± 15 g/day) with 2.5 g/kg/day of amino acids (p = NS). Patients receiving the higher amino acid intake were more likely to be in neutral or positive nitrogen balance (53.6% of patients) versus those given less amino acids (36.7% of subjects, $p < 0.05$). The former patients also required more aggressive hemodiafiltration to control uremia (mean volume of ultrafiltrate removed was 2,145 mL/hour versus 1,658 mL/hour, $p < 0.0001$), and they had a higher serum urea level (74.5 ± 19.9 mg/dL versus 50.4 ± 25.2 mg/dL, $p < 0.0001$). Survival was not different in this relatively small population of patients. These data, although obtained from a nonrandomized, nonparallel designed study, provide evidence that larger amino acid intakes, similar to those recommended for severely ill, catabolic patients without renal failure, are well tolerated and might engender less negative nitrogen balance in patients with ARF who are receiving continuous renal replacement therapy (CRRT).

EFFECT OF NUTRITIONAL THERAPY ON THE RECOVERY OF RENAL FUNCTION IN ACUTE RENAL FAILURE

Some reports have suggested that TPN in humans with ARF or parenteral administration of amino acids to rats with ARF may accelerate the rate of recovery of renal function (66,81–83). It has been argued that injured proximal tubular cells have increased requirements for amino acids and other nutrients and are likely to undergo more rapid recovery in response to nutritional support (81,84). Not all studies in rats with ARF confirmed these effects (85). Abel et al. reported that recovery from ARF was more rapid in patients with ARF given TPN providing an average of 16 g/day of essential amino acids as compared to glucose alone (66). Other clinical trials in humans with ARF have not shown that infusions of amino acids and glucose, as compared with glucose alone, accelerate the rate of recovery of renal failure (5,6,74,78,79). These latter studies had relatively small sample sizes, and in some of these studies the mortality rate was very high. It is reasonable to conclude that the question of whether nutritional support may accelerate the rate of recovery of renal function in humans has not been tested adequately.

WHY NUTRITIONAL THERAPY HAS NOT BEEN CLEARLY DEMONSTRATED TO BE BENEFICIAL

The foregoing studies, taken together, do not clearly demonstrate that nutritional therapy improves the rate or incidence of recovery of renal function, the nutritional or overall clinical status, or the survival of patients with ARF. However, intuitively, it seems reasonable to believe that nutritional therapy will benefit patients with ARF. This would seem particularly likely for patients who have ARF for extended periods (i.e., for 2 to 3 weeks or longer) or for patients who are convalescing from ARF but are still unable to eat. For these individuals, clinical experience more strongly suggests that oral or parenteral nutrition will improve nutritional status.

The following factors may explain why it has been so difficult to demonstrate a beneficial effect of nutritional therapy:

1. The clinical course of patients with ARF is so variable and often so complex that randomized prospective studies must be carried out in large numbers of patients to show statistically significant advantages to nutritional therapy, if these benefits exist.
2. Many previous studies were retrospective or not randomly controlled. This may have led to unintentional biases in the results.
3. The optimal nutrient composition of the TPN solutions has not been defined, and the use of suboptimal formulations of nutrients may have made it more difficult to demonstrate the clinical benefits of nutritional therapy. For example, recent studies suggest that critically ill patients may display reduced morbidity when given enteral feeding with a preparation designed to enhance immune function (e.g., a feeding that contains arginine, purine nucleotides given as yeast RNA, and omega-3 polyunsaturated fatty acids [86] or glutamine [87–90]) (see later in this chapter).
4. The previous studies in patients with ARF did not examine whether parenteral nutrition is beneficial. These studies only compared the response to different formulations of parenteral nutrition. There has been no prospective, randomized controlled study of the clinical course of patients with ARF who received nutritional therapy as compared to those who received no nutritional support. In each of the previously randomized studies, the control groups received some intravenous nutrition.
5. The route of nutritional support (i.e., total enteral nutrition [TEN] versus eating or intravenous nutrition) may be of substantial importance (see later in this chapter).
6. It is not unlikely that catabolic patients with ARF may need both good nutritional intake and metabolic intervention to suppress catabolic processes and promote anabolism in liver and other tissues (see later in this chapter).

Because patients with ARF who need nutritional therapy often have underlying catabolic illnesses, they have undergone a metabolic reorganization so that they are more prone to degrade administered amino acids and energy substrates. Thus, the provision of nutrients without altering these metabolic processes may be less likely to benefit their nutritional status or clinical outcome. This may be particularly true during the initial days after the onset of ARF.

ROLE OF CONTINUOUS OR LONG-DURATION RENAL REPLACEMENT THERAPY IN NUTRITIONAL MANAGEMENT OF PATIENTS WITH ACUTE RENAL FAILURE

Continuous renal replacement therapy (CRRT) is reviewed in detail in Chapter 31. There are several forms of CRRT:

CVVH (continuous venovenous hemofiltration) and CVVHD (CVVH with concurrent hemodialysis) commonly are used for the management of severely ill patients with ARF or other conditions associated with fluid or nonprotein nitrogen retention (e.g., severe liver or congestive heart failure). At present, CVVH/CVVHD generally are preferred to CAVH (continuous arteriovenous hemofiltration) or CAVHD (CAVH with concurrent hemodialysis) because of complications that arise from arterial catheter placement. CVVH and CAVH can be combined with hemodiafiltration (CVVHDF/CAVHDF).

Variants of CRRT are also in use. These include more frequent or even daily dialysis or slow, low-efficiency dialysis (SLED, which provides somewhat more intensive dialysis than CVVHD) (91,92). Occasionally peritoneal dialysis is used to treat patients with ARF (93). Because many of the same principles of nutritional support apply to all of these longer or more frequent dialysis or ultrafiltration therapies, and because CVVH/CVVHD are the most commonly used of these therapies, this discussion will emphasize more the interaction of nutrition with CVVHD (or CVVH) or standard hemodialysis (i.e., about 4 hours of duration three times per week).

CVVH/CVVHD/CVVHDF or SLED offer the following advantages to the patient (94–104):

1. Large quantities of water, electrolytes, and metabolites may be removed each day.
2. The rate of removal of water and electrolytes and metabolites is slow and therefore is less likely to cause or worsen hypotension.
3. Because of the high daily clearances of water and other small molecules, including metabolic waste products, one may safely administer greater amounts of amino acids and other nutrients to the patient. Also, the ability to ultrafilter more fluid from the patient with ARF each day actually may improve survival (105).
4. The high daily clearances by CVVH/CVVHD may enable patients to be treated with hemodialysis less frequently or, in many cases, to avoid it altogether.
5. CVVH/CVVHD/CVVHDF may be administered by nurses who are not specifically trained in hemodialysis (although special training of nursing personnel is required). Thus, CVVH/CVVHD/CVVHDF may be more convenient to use, and the cost for this therapy may be no more or possibly even less expensive than for intermittent hemodialysis.

Several studies have examined the mortality rate of patients with multiorgan failure treated with CVVH or CVVHD as compared to intermittent hemodialysis (106–107). In some studies, there was a trend toward greater survival with CRRT. It is surprising that a randomized prospective clinical trial comparing CAVHDF or CVVHDF to intermittent hemodialysis in patients with ARF in the intensive care unit (ICU) showed significant increases in ICU and in-hospital mortality with CAVHDF/CVVHDF (108). The authors of this paper suggested that the cause for the increased mortality with CAVHDF/CVVHDF treatment might be the result of the chance assignment of slightly higher-risk patients to this latter group. Prospective randomized comparisons of SLED with CVVHD/CVVHDF on morbidity and mortality have not yet been conducted. Recently, a randomized prospective clinical trial reported that in patients with severe ARF, daily hemodialysis, as compared to alternate-day hemodialysis, was associated with lower SUN and creatinine levels and reduced morbidity and mortality (109). These encouraging data need to be confirmed.

Glucose absorption from slow-flow dialysis in patients undergoing CVVHD/CAVHD or SLED may provide a substantial proportion of daily energy needs. Several investigators report that 36.7% to 70% of the dextrose in the dialysate is absorbed during CAVHD; the dialysate solutions contained dextrose (i.e., dextrose monohydrate) concentrations of 0.5% to 4.25% (94–96). The daily energy intake from the dialysate solutions, estimated from the measured dextrose absorption, varies from 123 to 2,388 kcal; the values depend on the dialysate and arterial plasma glucose concentrations and the flow rates of dialysate, blood, and ultrafiltrate. Monson and Mehta suggest that for clinical purposes one can assume a dextrose monohydrate absorption rate of 43% and 45% when dialysate solutions containing 1.5% and 2.5% dextrose monohydrate concentrations (1.34% and 2.25% anhydrous dextrose) are used (97). Some dialysate solutions used for CVVHD have lower glucose concentrations, and essentially no glucose (or calorie) uptake or loss occurs during treatment.

Lipids are not lost with CVVH/CVVHD. Infusion into blood of salts containing citrate, for anticoagulation, or lactate also may provide some calories.

Amino acid losses during CVVH/CVVHD are influenced by the permeability characteristics of the filter membrane; the ultrafiltration and dialysis flow rates; and the rate of amino acid infusion, which will influence the plasma amino acid concentrations (100–102). Approximately 4 to 7 g/day of amino acids are removed with CVVH (100). In one study, amino acid losses were about 8.9% ± 1.2% (standard error of the mean, or SEM) and 12.2% ± 2.2% of the daily quantity of amino acids infused in patients with renal failure undergoing CAVHD with a dialysate flow rate of 1 and 2 L/hour, respectively (101). For comparison, in patients with ARF receiving TPN, amino acid losses are reported to be 5.2 ± 0.6 g with hemodialysis using a conventional cuprophane membrane (45); 7.3 ± 1.8 g with hemodialysis using a high-flux, polysulphane membrane (45); and 6.2 ± SEM 0.6 g with 10 hours of slow diurnal hemodialysis (blood flow, 80 mL/min; dialysate flow, 30 mL/min) (110). Thus, the 24-hour amino acid losses with CVVH/CVVHD are similar to the losses during a single hemodialysis treatment or during slow diurnal hemodialysis (see Chapter 25).

CRRT usually clears minerals, including potassium, phosphorus, and magnesium, efficiently, and elevated concentrations of these minerals are uncommon once patients are established on treatment (103). Indeed, episodes of hypokalemia or hypophosphatemia may occur and may be the result of both efficient membrane clearance and the promotion of intracellular shifts by the glucose load (103, 104).

RECOMMENDED NUTRITIONAL MANAGEMENT OF PATIENTS WITH ACUTE RENAL FAILURE

As indicated earlier, no nutritional treatment has been shown definitively in randomized, prospective clinical trials to enhance the rate of recovery of renal function, reduce morbidity, or improve survival in patients with ARF. Thus, it is not possible to develop definitive protocols for the nutritional therapy of this condition. However, the body of research studies concerning the often severely hypercatabolic state, increased nutritional losses, and altered immunologic and organ function of acutely ill individuals with or without ARF suggests that there should be clinical value in providing nutritional support for physically stressed patients (111, 112). This research, combined with clinical experience, provides the basis for the therapeutic approach, which is summarized in Tables 30.1 and 30.2. In general, the policy is to administer sufficient quantities of nutrients to prevent or minimize the development of malnutrition and to provide sufficient dialysis or ultrafiltration to remove excess water, minerals, and metabolites.

Clinical trials indicate that TEN is preferable to TPN because the former is associated with a lower rate of morbid events (see later in this chapter) (111–114). This may be the consequence of better preservation of gut mass and host resistance in the intestinal tract and other organs with TEN as compared to TPN (115–121). Certain components in nutritional support solutions, such as arginine, RNA, and omega-3 fatty acids (122,123), or glutamine (88–90) appear to maintain more normal gut anatomy, enhance immune function, and possibly increase survival. The gut hormone, bombesin, also may improve intestinal structure and the immune function of the gut mucosa and upper-respiratory tract (124–126).

Because the clinical status of patients with ARF is so diverse, the prescribed nutrient intake will vary greatly and should depend on the patient's nutritional status, catabolic rate, residual glomerular filtration rate (GFR), and the indications for initiating intermittent or CRRT. A patient who is malnourished or hypercatabolic might receive a surfeit of nutrients and may be given dialysis or CVVH/CVVHD/CVVHDF as needed. Patients with a high residual GFR also may be given large quantities of nutrients because there is less risk of developing fluid and electrolyte disorders or accumulating metabolic waste products. For a patient who

TABLE 30.1. AMINO ACID COMPOSITION OF SOLUTIONS FOR TOTAL PARENTERAL NUTRITION FOR PATIENTS WITH ACUTE RENAL FAILURE[a,b,c]

	No Dialysis or Ultrafiltration	Intermittent Hemodialysis	CVVH/CVVHD/ CVVHDF/SLED
Volume	About 1.2–1.7 L	About 1.7–2.0 L	Standard TPN volumes
Essential amino acids (g/kg/day) (usually 5% solutions)	0.30–0.50[d]	Not applicable	Not applicable
Essential and nonessential amino acids (g/kg/day) (usually 8.5%–10% solutions)	0.60	1.0–1.2	1.5–2.5

CVVH, continuous venovenous hemofiltration; CVVHD, continuous venovenous hemofiltration with concurrent dialysis; CVVHDF, continuous venovenous hemodiafiltration; SLED, slow, low-efficiency dialysis.

[a]For patients who are more catabolic (e.g., urea nitrogen appearance ≥ 5 g/day), who are undergoing regular dialysis treatments (particularly for 2 or more weeks), or who are very wasted, essential and nonessential amino acids may be infused; about 1.0 to 1.2 g/kg/day for hemodialysis patients and 1.0 to 1.3 g/kg/day for patients undergoing intermittent peritoneal dialysis, continuous ambulatory peritoneal dialysis, or continuous cycling peritoneal dialysis. 1.5 to 2.5 g/kg/day of essential and nonessential amino acids may be given to patients undergoing CVVH, CVVHD, CVVHDF, or SLED. For patients who are not very wasted, who are less catabolic, who are not undergoing regular dialysis therapy, and who will not be receiving total parenteral nutrition for more than 2 or 3 weeks, 21 to 40 g/day of the nine purified essential amino acids may be infused. See text for discussion of the formulations of amino acids.

[b]Normally, formulations containing both essential and nonessential amino acids are constituted in about a 1.0 to 1.0 ratio. With administration of small quantities of amino acids, higher proportions of essential to nonessential amino acids sometimes have been advocated.

[c]Some authorities have recommended immune-enhancing nutritional formulations containing glutamine or the combination of arginine, RNA, and omega-3 fatty acids.

[d]No more than 30–40 g/day of essential amino acids if nonessential amino acids are not administered concomitantly (see text).

TABLE 30.2. COMPOSITION OF SOLUTIONS FOR TOTAL PARENTERAL NUTRITION FOR PATIENTS WITH ACUTE RENAL FAILURE[a]

Dextrose (D-glucose)[b]	350	g/L	Vitamin A[g]	See text
Lipid emulsion[c]	10% or 20%	in 500 mL	Vitamin D	See text
Energy (approximately)[b]	1,140	kcal/L	Vitamin K[h]	7.5 mg/week
Electrolytes[d]			Vitamin E[i]	10 IU/day
Sodium[e]	40–50	mmol/L	Niacin	20 mg/day
Chloride[e]	25–35	mmol/L	Thiamin HCl (B_1)	2 mg/day
Potassium[f]	≤35	mmol/day	Riboflavin (B_2)	2 mg/day
Acetate	35–40	mmol/day	Pantothenic acid	10 mg/day
Calcium	5	mmol/day	Pyridoxine HCl (B_6)	10 mg/day
Phosphorus	8	mmol/day	Ascorbic acid (C)	60 mg/day
Magnesium	4	mmol/day	Biotin	200 mg/day
Iron	2	mg/day	Folic acid[h]	1 mg/day
Other trace elements	See text		Vitamin B_{12}[h]	3 μg/day

CVVH, continuous venovenous hemofiltration; CVVHD, continuous venovenous hemofiltration with concurrent dialysis; CVVHDF, continuous venovenous hemodiafiltration; SLED, slow, low-efficiency dialysis; TPN, total parenteral nutrition.

[a]The nutrients listed are present in each bottle containing 500 mL of 8.5% to 10% crystalline amino acids or 250 to 500 mL of 5% essential amino acids and 500 mL of 70% D-glucose. The vitamins and trace elements are an exception because they are added to only one bottle per day. For those doses of nutrients that are expressed as concentrations rather than as quantities per day, the dose refers to the quantity present in each liter of dextrose and amino acids, with or without lipids. The patient's fluid status and serum electrolyte and glucose values must be monitored closely. The composition and volume of the infusate may be modified according to the nutritional status of the patient (see text).

[b]70% D-glucose is added as necessary to obtain an energy intake of 30 to 35 kcal/kg/day (see text); lower energy intakes may be used in very obese patients. For the higher levels of energy intake (i.e., 35 kcal/kg/day), additional 70% D-glucose may be added to the solutions. Patients who have greater tolerance to water loads (e.g., those with large volumes of water removed by CVVH/CVVHD/CVVHDF or SLED) may receive solutions with lower glucose concentrations (e.g., 50% D-glucose).

[c]Generally lipids are infused each day to provide 20% to 30% of total calories to balance the sources of calories and to prevent essential fatty acid deficiency. For patients who are septic or at high risk for sepsis, about 10% to 20% of calories may be given as lipids. The lipids probably should be infused for 12 to 24 hours to reduce the hyperlipidemia that occurs with intravenous infusion of lipid emulsions and to avoid impairment of the reticuloendothelial system. The lipids may be infused through a separate line or mixed with the amino acid and dextrose solutions and infused soon after mixing (see text). A 20% lipid emulsion (250 mL) often is used to reduce the water load. The approximate calorie values are dextrose monohydrate (the usual form of dextrose), 3.4 kcal per g; amino acids, 3.5 kcal per g.

[d]When adding electrolytes, the amounts intrinsically present in the amino acid solution should be taken into account.

[e]Refers to the final concentrations of electrolytes after any additional 70% dextrose or other solutions have been added.

[f]Larger amounts may be necessary with CVVH/CVVHD/CVVHDH or SLED.

[g]Vitamin A is best avoided unless TPN is continued for more than 2 or 3 weeks (see text).

[h]Should be given orally or parenterally and not in the TPN solution because of antagonisms.

[i]May need to be increased with use of lipid emulsions.

has little or no urine flow and is not very catabolic or uremic, a reduced intake of water, minerals, and amino acids, often given exclusively as essential amino acids, may decrease the need for dialysis; this may be particularly beneficial if the patient does not tolerate dialysis well because of underlying illnesses.

Similarly, a patient who is beginning to recover from ARF may be given small quantities of water, electrolytes, and amino acids to postpone the need for dialysis until renal function becomes adequate. In these latter patients, high-calorie diets and enteral feeding or intravenous infusates with small amounts of essential amino acids and little or no protein may be used for limited amounts of time. As indicated earlier, such nutritional therapy may maintain near-neutral nitrogen balance for short periods. Fluid and mineral balance should be monitored carefully in patients with ARF to avoid overhydration or electrolyte disorders. In general, the intake of water (including the water content from wet foods) should equal the output from urine and all other measured sources (e.g., nasogastric aspirate, fistula drainage) plus about 400 mL/day. This regimen takes into account the contributions to water balance of endogenous water production from metabolism and of insensible water losses (e.g., from respiration and skin). However, if the patient is catabolic and in negative energy and nitrogen balance, it may be advantageous to allow weight to decrease by about 0.2 to 0.5 kg/day to avoid excessive accumulation of fluid.

The intake of sodium, potassium, phosphorus, magnesium, calcium, and trace elements should be restricted to prevent accumulation of these minerals. Sodium intake should equal output but also should be coordinated with the water balance to prevent hyponatremia or hypernatremia. Potassium and phosphorus intake should be designed to prevent abnormally high or low serum levels. By controlling the water and electrolyte intake and lowering the rate of accumulation of urea and other nitrogenous metabolites, it may be possible to reduce the need for dialysis treatments.

The following discussion of specific nutrient intakes for patients with ARF can be applied to individuals receiving oral, enteral, or intravenous nutrition. TPN has been emphasized because this is frequently the route of choice for nutritional therapy in the sicker, more catabolic patients with ARF, and it is usually the most complicated of the techniques. However, as indicated earlier, there is a rationale for inaugurating TEN within 72 hours of the loss of the ability to eat adequately (86,127).

When the recommended nutrient intake is given in terms of body weight, the latter refers to the normal or standard body weight as determined from the National Health and Nutrition Evaluation Survey II (NHANES II) data (128, 129). An exception is when the patient is obese (e.g., greater than 115% of standard body weight) or very underweight (e.g., less than 90% of standard body weight). Under these latter conditions the patient's adjusted actual body weight (aBW) may be used for the body weight term (130). The use of the adjusted edema-free aBW, which is gaining in popularity but has not yet been validated by experimental studies, is calculated as follows:

$$\text{Adjusted aBW} = \text{edema-free aBW} + [(\text{standard normal BW} - \text{estimated edema-free aBW}) \times 0.25]$$

Amino Acid and Protein Intake

As discussed previously, the patient's metabolic and clinical status is most likely to be benefited if the amino acid or protein intake is tailored to the clinical condition of the patient. A low amino acid or protein intake, provided orally, enterally, or intravenously, may be prescribed for patients who have a small UNA (i.e., equal to or less than 4 to 5 g nitrogen/day), who have no evidence of severe protein malnutrition, and who probably will recover renal function within 1 to 2 weeks. A severely reduced GFR and the desire to avoid or reduce the frequency of dialysis therapy are other indications for low nitrogen intakes. One may give 0.30 to 0.50 g/kg standard body weight/day of essential amino acids with or without arginine. More than about 40 g/day of the nine essential amino acids are not prescribed because larger quantities may cause hazardous amino acid imbalances (see later in this chapter) (77,131,132). For patients who can eat, diets providing 0.10 to 0.30 g/kg/day of miscellaneous protein and 10 to 20 g/day of essential amino acids also may be used. These treatment protocols should promote a low rate of accumulation of nitrogenous metabolites, and unless the patient is very catabolic, they usually will maintain neutral or only mildly negative nitrogen balance. Hence, the need for dialysis therapy may be minimized or avoided. In the author's experience, only about 5% to 15% of patients with ARF who are unable to eat adequately will qualify for this type of therapy.

If the patient has a substantial residual renal function (e.g., GFR of 5 to 20 mL/min), is not very catabolic, and can eat well, he may be treated as a nondialyzed patient with chronic renal failure, receiving 0.55 to 0.60 g/kg body weight per day (128,130) of primarily high biologic value protein or about 0.28 g protein/kg/day supplemented with 6 to 10 g/day of essential amino acids. If such a patient cannot be fed orally or enterally, he may be given 0.55 to 0.60 g/kg/day of essential and nonessential amino acids intravenously. For patients who are more catabolic and have a higher UNA (greater than 5 g nitrogen/day), are severely wasted, and either have or are expected to have ARF for more than 2 weeks, a higher protein or amino acid intake usually is prescribed. This prescribed intake is generally 1.1 to 1.2 g/kg/day for patients undergoing regular hemodialysis; however, it is greater, approximately 1.5 to 2.5 g/kg/day, for individuals receiving CVVH/CVVHD/CVVHDF or SLED (133,134). It is anticipated that most acutely ill patients with ARF in the ICU will merit CVVH/CVVHD/CVVHDF or SLED in association with TEN or TPN providing 1.5 to 2.5 g of protein or peptides (for TEN) or essential and nonessential amino acids (for TEN or TPN).

In comparison with small quantities of essential amino acids, these larger nitrogen intakes may improve nitrogen balance, particularly after the first 1 or 2 weeks of dialysis treatments. However, the UNA almost invariably will rise, and the increased azotemia and water load (in patients treated with TEN or TPN) may increase the need for dialysis. Patients undergoing CVVH/CVVHD/CVVHDF or SLED appear to tolerate increased amino acid and water loads more effectively because of their greater weekly clearances. Peak SUN levels tend to be lower with CVVH/CVVHD or SLED, and if blood levels of metabolites become excessive, these patients can be treated with intermittent hemodialysis or SLED for longer periods as well.

As indicated earlier, large doses (i.e., more than about 0.50 g/kg/day) of essential amino acids alone may be hazardous. Several reports describe patients with ARF who were infused with, for their body weight, relatively large quantities of essential amino acids (77,131,132). Their plasma amino acid concentrations were bizarre; many plasma amino acids were markedly increased. Blood ammonia levels were high, and a metabolic acidosis occurred. Some patients became comatose, and death has been observed. The plasma amino acid pattern improved markedly when patients were given an infusion of essential and nonessential amino acids provided in a 1.0:1.0 ratio. We observed this phenomenon in a 72-year-old man given parenteral nutrition providing progressively larger amounts of eight essential amino acids (excluding histidine). The patient became progressively more obtunded, and we were asked to evaluate this individual. His plasma amino acid pattern was found to be profoundly deranged (Figs. 30.3 and 30.4). Most plasma essential and nonessential amino acids were markedly increased. Most striking were the plasma methionine concentrations, which were about 55 times normal fasting levels, and the plasma phenylalanine levels, which were approximately 17 times normal concentrations.

These findings underscore the critical importance of nonessential amino acids for normal protein and amino acid metabolism (135–137). Nonessential amino acids are necessary for the synthesis of proteins and other biologically valuable compounds. A deficiency of a nonessential amino acid inside the cell may disrupt protein synthesis (138). What defines an amino acid as nonessential is that it can be synthesized by the organism. However, the rate of synthesis may be inadequate for the body's needs, particularly in disease states and when there is malfunction of organs important in the synthesis or metabolism of amino acids (e.g., liver failure) or when artificial nutrient formulations lacking in some nonessential amino acids are given to the patient. This may be particularly likely to occur if the organism is flooded with large quantities of some amino acids (e.g., the essential amino acids) to the exclusion of others. Under these conditions an increase in protein synthesis may cause a selective depletion of certain nonessential amino acids not provided in the infusion, particularly for those nonessential amino acids that are not as readily synthesized in the body.

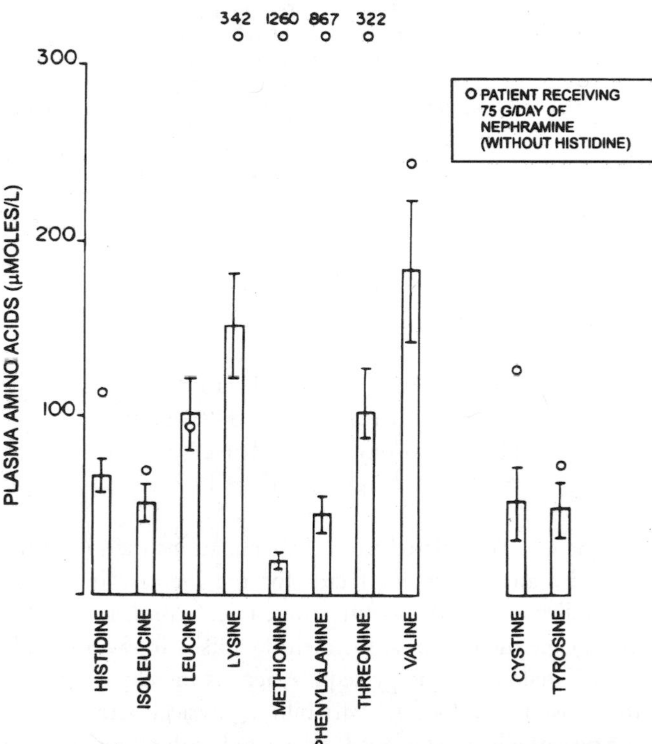

FIGURE 30.3. Plasma essential and semiessential amino acid concentrations (*open circles*) in a 72-year-old man with acute renal failure who received parenteral nutrition providing eight essential amino acids, but not histidine, and no nonessential amino acids. Amino acid intake was increased progressively to 75 g/day, and the patient lapsed into coma. For the plasma concentrations that are off scale, the actual amino acid concentration is indicated next to the circle. The normal mean plasma amino acid concentrations ± one standard deviation (*bars and brackets*) were obtained from healthy adults who had fasted overnight. They are shown for comparison. (From Kopple JD. The nutrition management of the patient with acute renal failure. *J Parenter Enteral Nutr* 1996; 20:3–12, with permission.)

During administration of preparations containing selected amino acids, competition between amino acids that share the same transport carriers into the cell may accentuate the amino acid imbalances and promote further increases in plasma concentrations of certain amino acids. However, because solutions with a high ratio of essential to nonessential amino acids may stimulate more anabolism than preparations with a 1.0:1.0 ratio (see earlier) and may be safer than high doses (greater than about 0.50 g/kg/day or approximately 30 to 40 g/day) of essential amino acids alone, the use of such formulations for patients with ARF should be investigated.

Branched-chain amino acids, particularly leucine, may promote anabolism (139,140). Studies in catabolic patients without renal failure suggest that the intravenous infusion of amino acid solutions containing a large proportion of branched-chain amino acids (i.e., isoleucine, leucine, and valine) may have a modest anabolic effect (141,142); not all reports confirm these findings. The fact that today the branched-chain amino acid content of standard amino acid solutions is high may explain why it is difficult to demonstrate greater anabolic effects of preparations with larger amounts of branched-chain amino acids.

Ketoacid analogues of the branched-chain amino acids also have been shown to enhance anabolism in *in vitro* tissue preparations and in clinical studies carried out in nonuremic individuals who are not hypercatabolic (140,143). In postoperative patients who were receiving TPN, intravenous infusion of the salt complex of α-ketoglutarate and ornithine was reported to decrease UNA and improve nitrogen balance (144). Further investigation into the anabolic properties and potential clinical usefulness of these preparations for patients with ARF would be helpful.

Energy and d-Glucose

The energy expenditure and requirements of patients with ARF primarily are determined by the same factors that affect nonuremic individuals and include weight, age, sex, associated diseases, and physical activity (if any). In nonuremic individuals, the energy intake necessary to obtain neutral or positive nitrogen balance increases when nitrogen intake is low. Because patients with ARF often are given low quan-

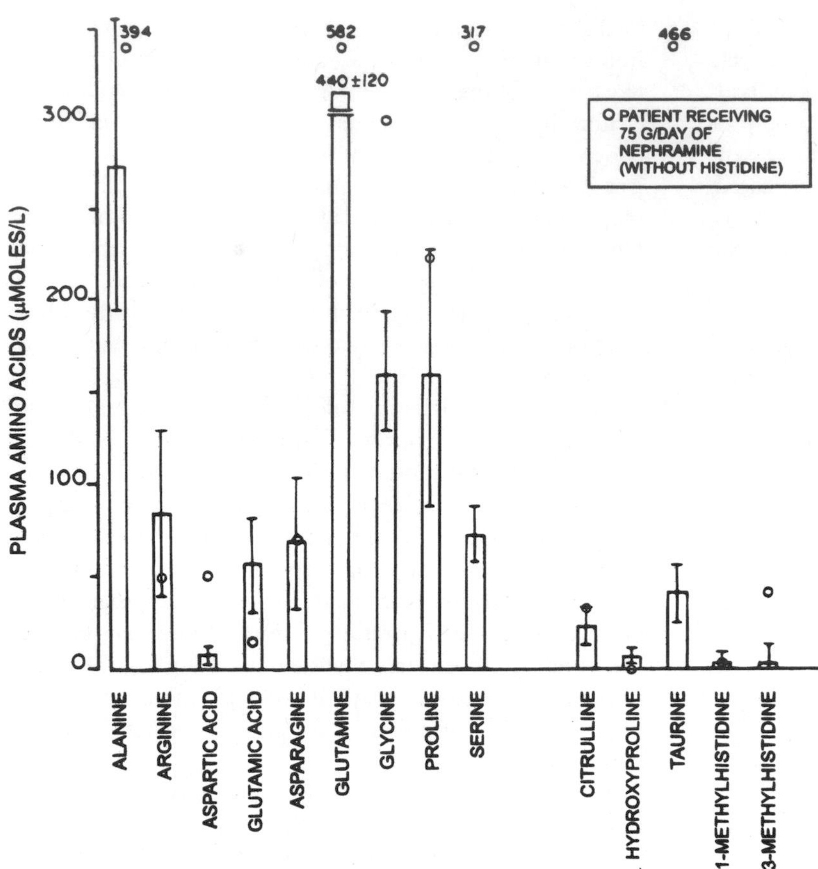

FIGURE 30.4. Plasma nonessential amino acid concentrations (*open circles*) in a 72-year-old man with acute renal failure given parenteral nutrition providing eight essential amino acids, without histidine. The amino acid intake was increased progressively to 75 g/day. Bars and brackets indicate mean values ± one standard deviation from normal adults. Symbols are described in detail in the legend to Fig. 30.3. (From Kopple JD. The nutrition management of the patient with acute renal failure. *J Parenter Enteral Nutr* 1996;20:3–12, with permission.)

tities of nitrogen, this may indicate a need for greater energy intake. Resting energy expenditure is reported to be normal or increased, by roughly 30%, in patients with ARF (76, 145,146). Elevated energy expenditure appears to be largely but not entirely the result of sepsis or other catabolic illnesses (76,145,146).

In a nonrandomized comparison, Mault et al. found that patients with ARF who died had a more negative energy balance than those who survived (76). We also have observed that patients with ARF given higher energy intakes had a greater survival (5). Although this might reflect a clinical benefit of high energy intakes, it is also possible that the patients who had more negative energy balance were sicker and had medical disorders that made them more difficult to nourish (e.g., shock, pulmonary edema). The fact that patients with ARF are often fluid intolerant sometimes influences the quantity of energy that may be safely given intravenously. CVVH/CVVHD may reduce energy expenditure in patients with ARF (98,99), presumably because of the cooling effect on the patient caused by the heat loss from the blood circulating through the apparatus. It is unclear whether this reduction in body temperature in severely ill patients is hazardous.

One standard method for assessing energy needs is based on the Harris–Benedict equations, which estimate basal energy expenditure (BEE) from age, sex, body weight, and height. The Harris–Benedict equations are as follows (147):

$$\text{For men: BEE (kcal/day)} = 66.5 + [13.8 \times \text{weight (kg)}] + [5.0 \times \text{height (cm)}] - [6.8 \times \text{age (years)}]$$

$$\text{For women: BEE (kcal/day)} = 655.1 + [9.6 \times \text{weight (kg)}] + [1.8 \times \text{height (cm)}] - [4.7 \times \text{age (years)}]$$

The value calculated from these equations then is multiplied by an adjustment factor for the increase in energy expenditure caused by different clinical conditions (148, 149). One such set of adjustment factors is shown in Table 30.3. Finally, the energy requirement is increased by 25% to adjust for individual variability, physical activity, and the potentially greater needs associated with a low nitrogen intake and ARF. Thus, the calculation of energy requirements in ARF is as follows:

$$\text{Energy requirements} = \text{estimated BEE} \times \text{adjustment for illness} \times 1.25$$

In recent years, the Harris–Benedict equation has been reported to overestimate the resting metabolic rate by about 10% to 15% (150). This overestimate may be greater in patients with low resting metabolic rates (150). The World

TABLE 30.3. PROPOSED ADJUSTMENT FACTORS FOR ESTIMATING ENERGY EXPENDITURE DURING ILLNESS

Type of Stress	Fraction of Normal Basal Energy Expenditure[a]
Malnutrition (chronic, severe)	0.70
Nondialyzed chronic renal failure	1.00
Maintenance hemodialysis	1.00–1.05
Elective surgery	
Early (1–4 days)[b]	1.00
Late (18–21 days)	0.95
Peritonitis	1.15
Soft-tissue trauma	1.15
Fractures	1.20–1.25
Infections	
Mild	1.00
Moderate	1.20–1.40
Severe	1.40–1.60
Burns (percent of body surface)	
0%–20%	1.00–1.50
21%–40%	1.50–1.85
41%–100%	1.85–2.05

[a]The basal energy expenditure values during the normal healthy state may be multiplied by these approximate factors to estimate resting energy expenditure during acute illness.
[b]Associated with early starvation.
Adapted from Wilmore DW. *The metabolic management of the critically ill.* New York: Plenum, 1977:34; and Monteon FJ, Laidlaw SA, Shaib JK, et al. Energy expenditure in patients with chronic renal failure. *Kidney Int* 1986;30(5):741–747.

Health Organization (WHO) equations appear to give more accurate estimates of resting metabolic rates, at least in normal men and women (150). These equations, compiled from about 11,000 measurements of individuals of both genders, all ages, and a wide variety of ethnic groups and body mass indices, are as follows (151):

Age (years)	Resting Metabolic Rate (RMR, kcal/day)
Men: 18 to 30:	RMR = 15.4 × weight (kg) − 27.0 × height (m) + 717
30 to 60:	RMR = 4.6 × weight (kg) + 16.0 × height (m) + 901
Women: 18 to 30:	RMR = 13.3 × weight (kg) + 334.0 × height (m) + 35
30 to 60:	RMR = 8.7 × weight (kg) − 25.0 × height (m) + 865

Another method used to estimate energy requirements is to measure energy expenditure by indirect calorimetry and multiply this value by 1.25. In some acutely ill patients, the calculated and measured rates of energy expenditure may vary widely. The use of indirect calorimetry will decrease these errors and reduce the risks of excessive (see later in this chapter) or insufficient energy intakes. For patients receiving CVVHD, SLED, or peritoneal dialysis, the energy intake from the glucose absorbed from dialysate should be considered as part of the patient's total daily energy load. In the author's experience, the estimated energy requirements for patients with ARF requiring nutritional support usually fall between 30 and 35 kcal/kg normal (standard) body weight/day.

The higher energy intakes (i.e., 35 kcal/kg/day) generally are prescribed for patients who have a higher UNA, who are severely ill, and who are not very obese. For example, if nitrogen balance, estimated from the difference between the patient's nitrogen intake and the nitrogen output calculated from the UNA (see earlier), is negative, despite an appropriate protein or amino acid intake, one may try to provide an energy intake even closer to 40 kcal/kg/day.

Larger energy intakes generally are not used because obesity and fatty liver may occur, there is little or no further increase in protein accrual or retardation of negative protein balance, and the large volume of fluids in the intravenous solutions will increase the water load to the patient (152). Also, because high energy intakes generate more carbon dioxide from the infused carbohydrates and fat, they can promote hypercapnia if pulmonary function is impaired (153). Carbon dioxide retention is particularly likely to occur with very high carbohydrate loads because, in comparison to fat, more carbon atoms from carbohydrates are necessary to provide the same quantity of energy.

Because most patients with ARF do not tolerate large water intakes, glucose usually is administered in a 70% solution. Glucose is added to intravenous solutions as d-glucose monohydrate, which is 90% anhydrous d-glucose. The energy available from glucose monohydrate is 3.4 kcal/g or, for 70% dextrose, about 2.38 kcal/mL. Patients receiving CVVH/CVVHD/CVVHDF or SLED usually tolerate larger water intakes and can receive glucose in lower concentrations (e.g., 50% dextrose). Amino acids provide about 3.5 kcal/g. The glucose and amino acid solutions are mixed so that the amino acids and calories are provided simultaneously (see Tables 30.1 and 30.2).

Lipids

Lipids generally will be given to all patients with ARF receiving TEN or TPN. However, patients receiving TPN for more than about 5 days must receive lipid emulsions to prevent essential fatty acid deficiency. The optimal amount of fat for TPN is somewhat controversial, especially because lipid clearance may be impaired in ARF (154). Taking 25 g/day of a lipid emulsion will prevent essential fatty acid deficiency. Some investigators recommend infusing up to 30% of calories as lipid emulsions to provide more normal amounts of fatty acids to organs that use lipids for energy and to more closely approximate the normal Western dietary intake. However, several studies suggest that infusion of lipid emulsions may lower host resistance. Infusions of large amounts of fat emulsions (e.g., 50 g for an 8-hour period) may impair reticuloendothelial system function

(155), presumably by overwhelming the phagocytic capacity of this system. Neonates receiving TPN with lipid emulsions are reported to have a higher incidence of bacteremia than similar infants given TPN without lipids (156).

A prudent approach may be to infuse lipid emulsions for 12 to 24 hours to minimize increases in plasma lipids and to avoid overwhelming the reticuloendothelial system. Patients who are not septic and not at high risk for infection may be given 20% to 30% of calories as lipid emulsions. Patients who are severely septic or at high risk for severe sepsis probably should not receive intravenous lipid emulsions for several days. Patients with less severe infection should not receive more than 10% to 20% of total calories from fat. Lipids are available as 10% and 20% fat emulsions that provide 1.1 and 2.0 kcal/mL, respectively. With careful attention to aseptic techniques, the lipid emulsions may be mixed with glucose and amino acids and infused shortly after preparation (157).

Minerals

Minerals should be added to parenteral nutrition solutions for ARF as shown in Table 30.2. Recommended intakes of minerals should be considered tentative and must be modified according to the clinical status of the patient. The patient must be monitored closely because the hormonal and metabolic changes that often occur in ARF may cause serum electrolytes to rise or fall dramatically. If the serum concentrations of an electrolyte are increased, it may be advisable to reduce the quantity infused or to refrain from administering it at the onset of parenteral nutrition. However, parenteral nutrition may rapidly lower certain serum electrolytes, particularly potassium and phosphorus, and a low serum concentration of a mineral may indicate that there is a need for a greater than usual intake of that element. Again, metabolic changes and the impaired GFR can lead to a rapid increase in the serum concentrations of electrolytes or glucose. As indicated earlier, removal of minerals is generally more efficient with CVVH/CVVHD/CVVHDF or SLED. Hypokalemia and hypophosphatemia may be particularly likely to occur and should be watched for in patients receiving these renal replacement therapies.

With the exception of iron and possibly zinc and selenium, there is no compelling evidence that addition of trace elements to parenteral nutrition solutions is helpful to patients with ARF unless this is the sole source of nutritional support for at least 2 to 3 weeks. Plasma selenium levels are reported to be low in patients with the multiple organ dysfunction syndrome (158). This might be related to reduced plasma concentrations or binding characteristics of the carrier protein. However, in a prospective open label trial, patients with the severe systemic inflammatory response syndrome were randomized to receive, intravenously, either replacement doses of sodium selenite for 9 days (535, 285, and 155 μg/day for 3 days each, in order of descending dosage) followed by sodium selenite, 35 μg/day, or else sodium selenite, 35 μg/day, throughout the treatment period (159). The patients given the larger doses of selenium displayed significantly reduced morbidity and need for CVVHD.

Many trace elements are added routinely to standard TEN preparations. The nutritional requirements for trace elements have not been established for patients with renal failure receiving TEN or TPN.

Vitamins

Vitamin requirements have not been well defined for patients with ARF, and there is a clear need for more research on this subject. Tentative recommendations for vitamin intake for patients receiving parenteral nutrition are shown in Table 30.2 (also see Chapters 20 and 31). The recommended intake is based largely on information obtained from studies in patients with chronic renal failure, normal individuals, or acutely ill patients not selected for renal failure. Patients with ARF need water-soluble vitamin supplements because their intake of these vitamins is often inadequate, they lose vitamins in dialysate, their vitamin needs may be increased, and they are given medicines that may antagonize the actions of certain vitamins (160–162) (see Chapter 33). A daily multivitamin supplement, as indicated in Table 30.2, should provide sufficient vitamins to replete and maintain adequate vitamin stores.

Vitamin A probably should be avoided or, at most, given in only the recommended dietary allowance. In patients with chronic renal failure serum vitamin A levels are elevated, and rather small supplements of vitamin A are reported to cause toxicity in individuals with advanced chronic renal failure (163,164). Gleghorn et al. reported biochemical and clinical evidence of vitamin A toxicity in three patients with acute or chronic renal failure who were receiving TPN (165). Each individual had been infused with a multivitamin additive that provided 1,500 μg of vitamin A (retinol).

The nutritional requirements for vitamin D in patients with ARF have not been well defined. Although vitamin D is fat soluble and vitamin D stores should not become depleted during the few days to weeks that most patients with ARF receive parenteral nutrition, the turnover of its most active analogue—1,25-dihydroxycholecalciferol—is much faster and it is synthesized in the kidney (166). Hence, patients with ARF may need supplements of this analogue. In patients undergoing maintenance hemodialysis, intravenous 1,25-dihydroxycholecalciferol can suppress parathyroid hormone secretion (167). The finding that hyperparathyroidism may occur in ARF and have adverse effects (38) suggests a possible therapeutic role for this vitamin D compound or possibly for one of its analogues that may have less calcemic effects (168). Deficiency of 1,25-dihydroxycholecalciferol has been reported in the oliguric phase of ARF caused by rhabdomyolysis (169).

Vitamin K deficiency may occur in nonuremic patients who are not eating and are receiving antibiotics that may suppress intestinal bacteria that synthesize vitamin K (170). Vitamin K therefore should be given routinely to patients receiving parenteral nutrition and also to those given enteral nutrition if the feeding does not contain vitamin K (Table 30.2). The recommendation of 10 mg/day of pyridoxine hydrochloride (8.2 mg/day of pyridoxine) is based on evidence for an increased need for pyridoxine hydrochloride in patients with chronic renal failure not receiving dialysis therapy. Also, studies in clinically stable individuals or acutely ill patients undergoing maintenance hemodialysis indicate that this quantity may be necessary to prevent or correct vitamin B_6 deficiency (171). Patients probably should not receive more than 60 to 100 mg/day of ascorbic acid because of the risk of increased serum oxalate concentrations (172,173). Indeed, there is one report of a child with ARF caused by the hemolytic uremic syndrome who received parenteral nutrition providing 500 mg/day of ascorbic acid (174). The patient was found to have deposits of calcium oxalate in the kidneys and pancreas.

Vitamin E supplements, alone or in combination with selenium or pentoxifylline, are often but not always reported to protect against or enhance recovery of experimentally induced ARF in rodents, presumably because of the antioxidant properties of this vitamin (175,176). There have been no large-scale clinical trials of vitamin E supplementation in humans with ARF. It should be emphasized that the nutrient needs of patients with ARF must be reevaluated carefully each day and sometimes more frequently. This is particularly important in the early stages of ARF because the clinical and metabolic condition of these patients may undergo rapid changes.

SPECIAL METHODS FOR MANAGING HYPERCATABOLISM OR PROVIDING NUTRITIONAL PHARMACOLOGY FOR PATIENTS WITH ACUTE RENAL FAILURE

Growth or Anabolic Factors

In the last several years, a number of reports have indicated the potential value of using growth factors to improve protein balance. Experience with these agents in individuals or animal models with or without kidney disease suggests that they may be useful for patients with acute or chronic renal failure and superimposed catabolic stress (177–181). Anabolic steroids were used more than 30 years ago to treat patients with ARF to suppress the accumulation of nitrogenous compounds (53,54). Evidence indicates that IGF-1 may suppress negative nitrogen balance in rats with ARF (179), but it does not appear to improve recovery of renal function or survival in humans (182).

Recombinant human growth hormone (rhGH) also may promote nitrogen balance in patients with acute catabolic stress or chronic illness, including chronic renal failure (177, 178). However, individuals who are acutely stressed from infection or physical trauma or who receive low quantities of nutrients sometimes become refractory to rhGH (183, 184), possibly because of downregulation of growth hormone receptors with reduced ability to express IGF-1. A more important concern is that a recent randomized clinical trial in critically ill adults has shown that growth hormone therapy doubles the mortality rate, and this increase in mortality was largely the result of multiple organ failure and infection but also of cardiovascular disorders (185). Thus, growth hormone therapy should not be given to critically ill patients with ARF.

Glucose intolerance is very common in patients with ARF. With the large glucose loads frequently administered to hypercatabolic patients with ARF, hyperglycemia is a common occurrence (5). Insulin can maintain normal glucose concentrations, and it also is an anabolic hormone. In nonuremic patients who have catabolic illnesses, insulin may reduce nitrogen output and improve negative nitrogen and protein balance (186,187).

More importantly, a recent prospective randomized clinical trial in 1,548 critically ill patients in the ICU, not selected for ARF, indicated that intensive insulin therapy to maintain blood glucose from 80 to 110 mg/dL reduced mortality from 8% with conventional insulin treatment to 4.6% ($p < 0.04$) (188). Conventional insulin treatment involved starting a continuous insulin infusion if the blood glucose exceeded 215 mg/dL and trying to maintain the blood glucose between 180 and 200 mg/dL. The decreased mortality with intensive insulin therapy was the result of the reduced fatality rate in patients who remained in the ICU for more than 5 days (mortality rates: 10.6% with intensive insulin treatment versus 20.2% with conventional therapy, $p < 0.005$). The greatest reduction in mortality was in patients with multiple organ failure with a known focus of sepsis. Also of pertinence, a lower percentage of patients receiving intensive insulin therapy as compared to conventional insulin therapy sustained a plasma creatinine higher than 2.5 mg/dL (9% versus 12.3%, $p = 0.04$) or plasma urea nitrogen higher than 54 mg/dL (7.7% versus 11.2%, $p = 0.02$) or received dialysis or CVVH (4.8% versus 8.2%, $p = 0.007$). Intensive insulin therapy also reduced the frequency or severity of other morbidity outcomes.

The authors of this study point out that hyperglycemia is reported to impair macrophage or neutrophil function (189–191), and possibly these factors or the potential trophic effects of insulin on mucosal or skin barriers may account for the lower morbidity and mortality with intensive insulin therapy (188). The authors also suggest that the higher mortality rate with growth hormone therapy in critically ill patients might be because growth hormone may increase insulin resistance and blood glucose levels (185, 188).

Nutrients Enhancing Immune Function

Administration of glutamine, arginine, RNA, or omega-3 fatty acids to acutely ill humans or animals is reported to improve immune function, reduce risk of infection, improve intestinal or extraintestinal mucosal structure and physiology and host resistance, and decrease the risk of bacterial translocation (86–90,127,192–197). Glutamine also may restore intracellular glutamine pools, which fall early in acute stress, and improve protein balance. Arginine may enhance T-lymphocyte proliferative responses to mitogens or cytokines (198). Nucleotides promote normal maturation of leukocytes and in animal models appear necessary for normal immune function (199,200). Several studies suggest that omega-3 fatty acids may enhance immune function and host resistance possibly by altering the pattern of cytokines elaborated by inflammatory cells (201–203).

The results of several clinical trials in surgical patients or critically ill or septic individuals living in an ICU in which they received enteral liquid diets enriched with arginine, nucleotides, omega-3 fatty acids, and structured lipids suggest that immune function, the incidence of infections, the duration of hospitalization, or mortality may be improved with these formulations (86,122,123,127). The provision of these potentially immune-enhancing agents by TEN may be particularly beneficial (see later in this chapter) (86,127). Further studies are needed to define the role, if any, for these compounds in critically ill patients with ARF. There are currently no data as to whether these nutrients may be beneficial for patients with ARF. Because metabolites of these nutrients could accumulate in renal failure, caution should be used concerning their use in this condition.

Peptides

Peptides in TPN solutions have been used to effectively provide unstable or poorly soluble amino acids to the patient (i.e., dipeptides of glutamine, cysteine, and tyrosine) (193). Peptides also can provide equal quantities of amino acids at lower osmolalities.

EFFECTS OF OTHER NUTRITIONAL INTERVENTIONS TO ENHANCE RECOVERY OF RENAL FUNCTION

Growth factors have been used in experimental models of ARF, both to accelerate recovery of renal function and to enhance anabolism (see earlier). Research suggests that epidermal growth factor (204), hepatocyte growth factor (205), and IGF-1 and IGF-1 analogues (179,206,207) may enhance the rate of recovery of renal function in rats with ARF. However, in humans, studies have shown no beneficial effects of recombinant human IGF-1 (rhIGF-1) on recovery of renal function or mortality rates in patients with ARF in the ICU (see earlier) (182).

It is possible rhIGF-1 acts differently on the injured kidney of rats as compared to humans or that the renal injuries associated with ARF in rats and humans have major dissimilarities. Alternatively, and more likely, the severity of the systemic illnesses; the heterogeneity of the causes of ARF in humans; or the fact that, because of the study protocol requirements, the rhIGF-1 treatment was delayed for 1 to 6 days after the onset of ARF may have contributed to the negative results of this latter study (182). It is hoped that further research will be carried out on the potential value of earlier onset of treatment with growth factors on the use of combinations of growth factors on the recovery of ARF or the reduction in morbidity or mortality in humans with ARF.

In rats with ischemic ARF, administration of L-arginine, 300 mg/kg for 60 minutes, is reported to increase GFR acutely, probably by increasing nitric oxide production (208). Other potential effects of arginine and arginine derivatives on nitric oxide production, and protection of the kidney from injury or enhancement of recovery from ARF are reviewed elsewhere (209). Other types of nutrition-related interventions have shown varying degrees of promise for preventing or ameliorating the severity of ARF or enhancing recovery from renal failure in experimental animal models. These interventions include treatment with calcium channel blockers to inhibit calcium flux into the cell, a preterminal event leading to cell death (210). Several studies have examined the benefits of maintaining or repleting the cellular energy supply in the acutely injured kidney in animals (211,212). A number of investigators have examined the role of oxidative stress and oxidant-free radicals in renal injury and the potential for antioxidants to ameliorate the injury (213,214). Other investigators have examined the role of certain amino acids, perhaps most notably glycine, but also alanine, in reducing renal injury from various insults (215,216).

Recent data indicate that hypoxia may induce an increase in cytosolic calcium $(Ca^{2+})_I$ in rat proximal tubular cells (217). This increase in cytosolic calcium often is followed by proximal tubular cell membrane damage. These factors may be one of the reasons why calcium channel blockers may reduce the propensity toward acute tubular necrosis in humans exposed to ischemic injury. These observations have been shown particularly well for kidney transplantation (218). The calcium channel blocker diltiazem also may lead to an amelioration of cyclosporine nephrotoxicity and better allograft survival (219).

Also, calpain, a cytosolic calcium-dependent cysteine protease, has been associated with ischemic injury (220, 221). Newly developed calpain inhibitors are being investigated for their ability to protect against development of acute renal injury (222,223).

METHODS OF NUTRIENT ADMINISTRATION FOR PATIENTS WITH ACUTE RENAL FAILURE

Enteral Versus Parenteral Nutrition

It generally is accepted that acutely or critically ill patients should be given oral or enteral nutrition whenever feasible (224). It would seem reasonable that patients with ARF should be treated in the same way. If the patient will not eat adequately, he may be offered liquid formula diets, elemental diets, or tube or enterostomy feeding. Often enteral tube or gastrostomy feeding is the only possible method of nourishment through the alimentary tract in critically ill patients (225). For patients who must be fed by an enteral tube or gastrostomy, there are many liquid protein or defined-formula (elemental) diets that may be prescribed.

Some evidence suggests that TEN may be more beneficial than TPN and that immune-enhancing components of the nutritional preparations may be advantageous. Metaanalysis of the results of TPN in critically ill patients not selected for ARF indicates no effect of TPN on mortality or the rate of complications (113). TPN in malnourished patients only showed a significant reduction in the complication rate (relative risk, 0.52; 95% confidence interval, 0.30–0.91) but, again, not in mortality (113). However, randomized clinical trials of critically ill patients given enteral nutrition, particularly when started no later than about the first 8 to 72 hours postoperatively or following admission to an ICU, show that enteral nutrition has been associated with reduction in permeability of the gastrointestinal mucosa (226), decreased rates of infection (86,111,112,127,227), and improved healing of wounds (228). The rationale for TEN as compared to TPN is that the former treatment promotes healthier gastrointestinal mucosal structure and function (229–232).

There are currently no large-scale, randomized, prospective clinical trials of enteral nutrition in patients with ARF. Mortality rates are not reduced by enteral feeding with immune-enhancing preparations containing such compounds as arginine, purine nucleotides (e.g., given as yeast RNA), and omega-3 fatty acids or glutamine. However, these individuals appear to have reduced infection rates, other medical complications, and lengths of stay in the ICU and/or hospital (127). Early commencement of TEN with immune-enhancing preparations (i.e., within the first 72 hours of admission to the ICU) may be important to attain some of these benefits (86,127).

Some liquid oral supplements or enteral feeding preparations have an electrolyte and protein content that is designed specifically patients with renal failure. Dietitians usually can provide information concerning the composition of these preparations. There are a number of reviews of the techniques and complications associated with the use of the chemically defined diets and tube feeding (225,233). Most of the principles are applicable to the patient with renal failure. Although tube feeding has been used extensively in pediatric patients, and particularly infants, with chronic renal failure (234,235), there has been a reluctance to use these techniques for adult patients with renal failure.

Many patients with ARF do not have well-functioning gastrointestinal tracts, and parenteral nutrition is the only technique that will provide adequate nutrient intake. This is particularly common in the more catabolic patients with ARF. Parenteral nutrition provides greater fluid loads and is more costly. Techniques for enteral and parenteral nutrition and the potential complications of this treatment have been reviewed elsewhere (236–239).

Peripheral parenteral nutrition has been suggested as an alternative to TPN (240). The solutions are infused into a peripheral vein, and the risks of inserting a central catheter are avoided. A limitation of peripheral parenteral nutrition is that the osmolality of the infusate must be restricted to about 600 mOsm or lower to prevent thrombophlebitis; even then, the needles or catheters must be changed frequently, usually every 18 to 48 hours. Thus, to provide adequate calories and amino acids, the patient must receive large fluid loads, which are not tolerated by most individuals with ARF who require parenteral nutrition. Moreover, the pharmaceutical costs of peripheral parenteral nutrition are usually similar to those of TPN because with the former technique, larger amounts of expensive lipid emulsions must be given to provide calories with a lower osmotic load.

Peripheral partial parenteral nutrition may be useful for patients with ARF who are able to receive only part of their daily nutritional requirements by oral or enteric feeding. The peripheral infusions may allow these patients to receive adequate nutrition without resorting to TPN through a large-flow vein. In these individuals it often is preferable to infuse an 8.5% to 10% amino acid solution or a 20% lipid emulsion into a peripheral vein and administer as much as possible of the other essential nutrients through the enteral tract, including carbohydrates, which provide most of the osmotic load when given intravenously.

To avoid the risk of central vein catheterization, a peripheral vascular fistula or graft that is used for hemodialysis or hemofiltration therapy also may be used for TPN (241). Because the blood flow through the vascular access is large, hypertonic solutions can be infused and the water load to the patient can be reduced. However, in our experience, this technique increases the risk of local infection, and it should not be used in patients who will need a hemodialysis access for extended periods.

NUTRIENTS THAT MAY PREDISPOSE TO ACUTE RENAL FAILURE

Amino Acids

Several studies in rats suggest that a high amino acid or protein intake may increase the susceptibility to ARF caused by ischemia or nephrotoxicity (242–246). The nutrients seem to increase both the incidence and the severity of ARF induced by these mechanisms. This effect is probably at least partly a result of the increased GFR induced by high amino acid or protein intakes. The increased GFR increases the quantity of solutes that are filtered and, hence, reabsorbed by the renal tubules. This, in turn, increases renal oxygen consumption and the susceptibility to ischemic and possibly toxic injury. Several individual amino acids, particularly D-serine, DL-ethionine, and L-lysine, appear to be nephrotoxic (244,247). In contrast, as indicated earlier, glycine and alanine may protect against ischemic- or toxic-induced renal tubular cell damage (215,216,246), at least in *in vitro* preparations.

If high amino acid or protein intakes predispose to renal failure in humans, then patients who receive nephrotoxic medicines or who are at high risk for renal ischemia might benefit from transiently lowering the amino acid or protein intake. However, if glycine and alanine are protective *in vivo*, it is possible that administration of these amino acids could reduce the likelihood of ARF in high-risk patients. Clearly, more research is needed in this area.

Vitamins and Minerals

Hypercalcemia caused by such disorders in nutrient intake as vitamin D intoxication (248) or milk alkali syndrome (249) can cause ARF. Renal oxalosis complicating ARF was reported in a patient receiving TPN providing 1 g/day of ascorbic acid (250).

REFERENCES

1. Kjellstrand CM, Ebben J, Davin T. Time of death, recovery of renal function, development of chronic renal failure and need for chronic hemodialysis in patients with acute tubular necrosis. *Trans Am Soc Artif Intern Organs* 1981;27:45–50.
2. Butkus DE. Persistent high mortality in acute renal failure. Are we asking the right questions? *Arch Intern Med* 1983;143(2): 209–212.
3. Mehta RL, Pascual MT, Gruta CG, et al. Refining predictive models in critically ill patients with acute renal failure. *J Am Soc Nephrol* 2002;13(5):1350–1357.
4. Mehta R, Farkas A, Pascual M, et al. Effect of serial APACHE and organ failure scores on prediction of mortality in acute renal failure (ARF). *J Am Soc Nephrol* 1995;550.
5. Feinstein EI, Blumenkrantz MJ, Healy M, et al. Clinical and metabolic responses to parenteral nutrition in acute renal failure. A controlled double-blind study. *Medicine (Baltimore)* 1981; 60(2):124–137.
6. Feinstein EI, Kopple JD, Silberman H, et al. Total parenteral nutrition with high or low nitrogen intakes in patients with acute renal failure. *Kidney Int Suppl* 1983;16:S319–S323.
7. Leonard CD, Luke RG, Siegel RR. Parenteral essential amino acids in acute renal failure. *Urology* 1975;6(2):154–157.
8. Cahill GF Jr. Starvation in man. *N Engl J Med* 1970;282(12): 668–675.
9. Law DK, Dudrick SJ, Abdou NI. Immunocompetence of patients with protein-calorie malnutrition. The effects of nutritional repletion. *Ann Intern Med* 1973;79:545.
10. Bozzetti F, Terno G, Longoni C. Parenteral hyperalimentation and wound healing. *Surg Gynecol Obstet* 1975;141(5):712–714.
11. Lacy WW. Effect of acute uremia on amino acid uptake and urea production by perfused rat liver. *Am J Physiol* 1969;216(6): 1300–1305.
12. Frohlich J, Scholmerich J, Hoppe-Seyler G, et al. The effect of acute uraemia on gluconeogenesis in isolated perfused rat livers. *Eur J Clin Invest* 1974;4(6):453–458.
13. Flugel-Link RM, Salusky IB, Jones MR, et al. Enhanced muscle protein degradation and urea nitrogen appearance (UNA) in rats with acute renal failure. *Am J Physiol* 1983;244:E615.
14. Clark AS, Mitch WE. Muscle protein turnover and glucose uptake in acutely uremic rats. Effects of insulin and the duration of renal insufficiency. *J Clin Invest* 1983;72(3):836–845.
15. Kuhlmann MK, Shahmir E, Maasarani E, et al. New experimental model of acute renal failure and sepsis in rats. *JPEN J Parenter Enteral Nutr* 1994;18(6):477–485.
16. Shear L, Sapico V, Litwack G. Induction of hepatic enzymes and translocation of cytosol tyrosine amino transaminase (TAT) in uremic rats. *Clin Res* 1973;21:707A.
17. Sapico V, Shear L, Litwack G. Translocation of inducible tyrosine aminotransferase to the mitochondrial fraction. Facilitation by acute uremia and other conditions. *J Biol Chem* 1974;249(7): 2122–2129.
18. Hörl WH, Heidland A. Glycogen metabolism in muscle in uremia. *Am J Clin Nutr* 1980;33(7):1461–1467.
19. May RC, Clark AS, Goheer MA, et al. Specific defects in insulin-mediated muscle metabolism in acute uremia. *Kidney Int* 1985;28(3):490–497.
20. Cianciaruso B, Bellizzi V, Napoli R, et al. Hepatic uptake and release of glucose, lactate, and amino acids in acutely uremic dogs. *Metabolism* 1991;40(3):261–269.
21. Druml W, Fischer M, Sertl S, et al. Fat elimination in acute renal failure: long-chain vs. medium-chain triglycerides. *Am J Clin Nutr* 1992;55(2):468–472.
22. Druml W, Zechner R, Magometschnigg D, et al. Post-heparin lipolytic activity in acute renal failure. *Clin Nephrol* 1985;23(6): 289–293.
23. Druml W, Fischer M, Liebisch B, et al. Elimination of amino acids in renal failure. *Am J Clin Nutr* 1994;60(3):418–423.
24. May RC, Kelly RA, Mitch WE. Metabolic acidosis stimulates protein degradation in rat muscle by a glucocorticoid-dependent mechanism. *J Clin Invest* 1986;77(2):614–621.
25. Ballmer PE, McNurlan MA, Hulter HN, et al. Chronic metabolic acidosis decreases albumin synthesis and induces negative nitrogen balance in humans. *J Clin Invest* 1995;95(1):39–45.
26. Mitch WE, Medina R, Grieber S, et al. Metabolic acidosis stimulates muscle protein degradation by activating the adenosine triphosphate-dependent pathway involving ubiquitin and proteasomes. *J Clin Invest* 1994;93(5):2127–2133.
27. Eigler N, Sacca L, Sherwin RS. Synergistic interactions of physiologic increments of glucagon, epinephrine, and cortisol in the dog: a model for stress-induced hyperglycemia. *J Clin Invest* 1979;63(1):114–123.
28. Bessey PQ, Watters JM, Aoki TT, et al. Combined hormonal infusion simulates the metabolic response to injury. *Ann Surg* 1984;200(3):264–281.
29. Pettipher ER, Higgs GA, Henderson B. Interleukin 1 induces leukocyte infiltration and cartilage proteoglycan degradation in the synovial joint. *Proc Natl Acad Sci U S A* 1986;83(22): 8749–8753.
30. Ito A, Itoh Y, Sasaguri Y, et al. Effects of interleukin-6 on the metabolism of connective tissue components in rheumatoid synovial fibroblasts. *Arthritis Rheum* 1992;35:1197–1201.

31. Souba WW. Cytokine control of nutrition and metabolism in critical illness. *Curr Probl Surg* 1994;31(7):577–643.
32. Pasceri V, Willerson JT, Yeh ET. Direct proinflammatory effect of C-reactive protein on human endothelial cells. *Circulation* 2000;102(18):2165–2168.
33. Baracos V, Rodemann HP, Dinarello CA, et al. Stimulation of muscle protein degradation and prostaglandin E2 release by leukocytic pyrogen (interleukin-1). A mechanism for the increased degradation of muscle proteins during fever. *N Engl J Med* 1983;308(10):553–558.
34. Horl WH, Jochum M, Heidland A, et al. Release of granulocyte proteinases during hemodialysis. *Am J Nephrol* 1983;3(4): 213–217.
35. Gutierrez A, Alvestrand A, Wahren J, et al. Effect of in vivo contact between blood and dialysis membranes on protein catabolism in humans. *Kidney Int* 1990;38(3):487–494.
36. Gutierrez A, Bergstrom J, Alvestrand A. Protein catabolism in sham-hemodialysis: the effect of different membranes. *Clin Nephrol* 1992;38(1):20–29.
37. Lindsay RM, Bergstrom J. Membrane biocompatibility and nutrition in maintenance haemodialysis patients. *Nephrol Dial Transplant* 1994;9(Suppl 2):150–155.
38. Massry SG, Arieff AI, Coburn JW, et al. Divalent ion metabolism in patients with acute renal failure: studies on the mechanism of hypocalcemia. *Kidney Int* 1974;5(6):437–445.
39. Pietrek J, Kokot F, Kuska J. Serum 25-hydroxyvitamin D and parathyroid hormone in patients with acute renal failure. *Kidney Int* 1978;13(2):178–185.
40. Moxley MA, Bell NH, Wagle SR, et al. Parathyroid hormone stimulation of glucose and urea production in isolated liver cells. *Am J Physiol* 1974;227(5):1058–1061.
41. Kopple JD, Cianciaruso B, Massry SG. Does parathyroid hormone cause protein wasting? *Contrib Nephrol* 1980;20: 138–148.
42. Wolfson M, Jones MR, Kopple JD. Amino acid losses during hemodialysis with infusion of amino acids and glucose. *Kidney Int* 1982;21(3):500–506.
43. Ikizler TA, Flakoll PJ, Parker RA, et al. Amino acid and albumin losses during hemodialysis. *Kidney Int* 1994;46(3):830–837.
44. Sullivan JF, Eisenstein AB, Mottola OM, et al. The effect of dialysis on plasma and tissue levels of vitamin C. *Trans Am Soc Artif Intern Organs* 1972;18:277–282.
45. Hynote ED, McCamish MA, Depner TA, et al. Amino acid losses during hemodialysis: effects of high-solute flux and parenteral nutrition in acute renal failure. *JPEN J Parenter Enteral Nutr* 1995;19(1):15–21.
46. Linton AL, Clark WF, Driedger AA, et al. Correctable factors contributing to the anemia of dialysis patients. *Nephron* 1977; 19(2):95–98.
47. Rosenblatt SG, Drake S, Fadem S, et al. Gastrointestinal blood loss in patients with chronic renal failure. *Am J Kidney Dis* 1982; 1(4):232–236.
48. Metnitz GH, Fischer M, Bartens C, et al. Impact of acute renal failure on antioxidant status in multiple organ failure. *Acta Anaesthesiol Scand* 2000;44(3):236–240.
49. Borst JGG. Protein metabolism in uraemia; effects of protein-free diet, infections and blood-transfusions. *Lancet* 1948;1:824.
50. Bull GM, Joekes AM, Lowe KG. Conservative treatment of anuric uremia. *Lancet* 1949;2:229.
51. Blagg CR, Parsons FM, Young BA. Effects of dietary glucose and protein in acute renal failure. *Lancet* 1962;1:608.
52. Gamble JL. The Harvey Lectures, Series XLIII 1946–1947: Physiological information gained from studies on the life raft ration. *Nutr Rev* 1989;47(7):199–201.
53. McCracken BH, Parsons FM. Nilevar (17-ethyl-19-nor-testosterone) to suppress protein catabolism in acute renal failure. *Lancet* 1958;2:885.
54. Gjorup S, Thavsen JH. The effect of anabolic steroid (Durabolin) in the conservative management of acute renal failure. *Acta Med Scand* 1960;167:227.
55. Giordano C. Use of exogenous and endogenous urea for protein synthesis in normal and uremic subjects. *J Lab Clin Med* 1963; 62:231.
56. Giovannetti S, Maggiore Q. A low nitrogen diet with proteins of high biological value for severe chronic uraemia. *Lancet* 1964; 1:1000.
57. Berlyne GM, Bazzard FJ, Booth EM. The dietary treatment of acute renal failure. *Q. J. Med* 1967;141:59.
58. Teschan PE, Baxter CR, O'Brien TF, et al. Prophylactic hemodialysis in the treatment of acute renal failure. *Ann Intern Med* 1960;53:992–1016.
59. Mehta RL. Symposium on practical issues in the use of continuous renal replacement therapies. *Semin Dial* 1996;9:79–221.
60. Lee HA, Sharpstone P, Ames AC. Parenteral nutrition in renal failure. *Postgrad Med J* 1967;43(496):81–91.
61. Wilmore DW, Dudrick SJ. Treatment of acute renal failure with intravenous essential L-amino acids. *Arch Surg* 1969;99(5): 669–673.
62. Dudrick SJ, Steiger E, Long JM. Renal failure in surgical patients. Treatment with intravenous essential amino acids and hypertonic glucose. *Surgery* 1970;68(1):180–185; discussion 185–186.
63. Van Buren CT, Dudrick SJ, Dworkin L. Effects of intravenous essential L-amino acids and hypertonic dextrose on anephric beagles. *Surg Forum* 1972;23:83.
64. Abbott WM, Abel RM, Fischer JE. Treatment of acute renal insufficiency after aortoiliac surgery. *Arch Surg* 1971;103(5): 590–594.
65. Abel RM, Abbott WM, Fischer JE. Intravenous essential L-amino acids and hypertonic dextrose in patients with acute renal failure. Effects on serum potassium, phosphate, and magnesium. *Am J Surg* 1972;123(6):632–638.
66. Abel RM, Beck CH Jr, Abbott WM, et al. Improved survival from acute renal failure after treatment with intravenous essential L-amino acids and glucose. Results of a prospective, double-blind study. *N Engl J Med* 1973;288(14):695–699.
67. Abel RM, Abbott WM, Beck CH Jr, et al. Essential L-amino acids for hyperalimentation in patients with disordered nitrogen metabolism. *Am J Surg* 1974;128(3):317–323.
68. Abel RM, Shih VE, Abbott WM, et al. Amino acid metabolism in acute renal failure: influence of intravenous essential L-amino acid hyperalimentation therapy. *Ann Surg* 1974;180(3): 350–355.
69. Baek SM, Makabali GG, Bryan-Brown CW, et al. The influence of parenteral nutrition on the course of acute renal failure. *Surg Gynecol Obstet* 1975;141(3):405–408.
70. McMurray SD, Luft FC, Maxwell DR, et al. Prevailing patterns and predictor variables in patients with acute tubular necrosis. *Arch Intern Med* 1978;138(6):950–955.
71. Milligan SL, Luft FC, McMurray SD, et al. Intra-abdominal infection and acute renal failure. *Arch Surg* 1978;113(4): 467–472.
72. Abitbol CL, Holliday MA. Total parenteral nutrition in anuric children. *Clin Nephrol* 1976;5(4):153–158.
73. Blackburn GL, Etter G, Mackenzie T. Criteria for choosing amino acid therapy in acute renal failure. *Am J Clin Nutr* 1978; 31(10):1841–1853.
74. Lopez Martinez J, Caparros T, Perez Picouto F, et al. Parenteral nutrition in septic patients with acute renal failure in polyuric phase. *Rev Clin Esp* 1980;157(3):171–177.
75. Spreiter SC, Myers BD, Swenson RS. Protein-energy require-

ments in subjects with acute renal failure receiving intermittent hemodialysis. *Am J Clin Nutr* 1980;33(7):1433–1437.
76. Mault JR, Bartlett RH, Dechert RE, et al. Starvation: a major contribution to mortality in acute renal failure? *Trans Am Soc Artif Intern Organs* 1983;29:390–395.
77. Kopple JD. The nutritional management of the patient with acute renal failure. *JPEN J Parenter Enteral Nutr* 1996;20(1): 3–12.
78. Hasik J, Hryniewiecki L, Baczyk K, et al. (Minimal protein requirements in patients with acute kidney failure). *Pol Arch Med Wewn* 1979;61(1):29–36.
79. Mirtallo JM, Schneider PJ, Mavko K, et al. A comparison of essential and general amino acid infusions in the nutritional support of patients with compromised renal function. *JPEN J Parenter Enteral Nutr* 1982;6(2):109–113.
80. Bellomo R, Seacombe J, Daskalakis M, et al. A prospective comparative study of moderate versus high protein intake for critically ill patients with acute renal failure. *Ren Fail* 1997; 19(1):111–120.
81. Toback FG, Dodd RC, Maier ER, et al. Amino acid enhancement of renal protein synthesis during regeneration after acute tubular necrosis. *Clin Res* 1979;27:432A.
82. Toback FG. Amino acid enhancement of renal regeneration after acute tubular necrosis. *Kidney Int* 1977;12(3):193–198.
83. Toback FG, Teegarden DE, Havener LJ. Amino acid-mediated stimulation of renal phospholipid biosynthesis after acute tubular necrosis. *Kidney Int* 1979;15(5):542–547.
84. Toback FG. Amino acid treatment of acute renal failure. In Stein JH, ed. *Acute renal failure.* Churchill Livingstone: London, 1980:202–228.
85. Oken DE, Sprinkel FM, Kirschbaum BB, et al. Amino acid therapy in the treatment of experimental acute renal failure in the rat. *Kidney Int* 1980;17(1):14–23.
86. Atkinson S, Sieffert E, Bihari D. A prospective, randomized, double-blind, controlled clinical trial of enteral immunonutrition in the critically ill. Guy's Hospital Intensive Care Group. *Crit Care Med* 1998;26(7):1164–1172.
87. Schloerb PR, Amare M. Total parenteral nutrition with glutamine in bone marrow transplantation and other clinical applications (a randomized, double-blind study). *JPEN J Parenter Enteral Nutr* 1993;17(5):407–413.
88. Li J, Kudsk KA, Janu P, et al. Effect of glutamine-enriched total parenteral nutrition on small intestinal gut-associated lymphoid tissue and upper respiratory tract immunity. *Surgery* 1997; 121(5):542–549.
89. DeWitt RC, Wu Y, Renegar KB, et al. Glutamine-enriched total parenteral nutrition preserves respiratory immunity and improves survival to a Pseudomonas Pneumonia. *J Surg Res* 1999;84(1):13–18.
90. Ziegler TR, Young LS, Benfell K, et al. Clinical and metabolic efficacy of glutamine-supplemented parenteral nutrition after bone marrow transplantation. A randomized, double-blind, controlled study. *Ann Intern Med* 1992;116(10):821–828.
91. Marshall MR, Golper TA, Shaver MJ, et al. Sustained low-efficiency dialysis for critically ill patients requiring renal replacement therapy. *Kidney Int* 2001;60(2):777–785.
92. Duggan KA, Macdonald GJ, Charlesworth JA, et al. Verapamil prevents post-transplant oliguric renal failure. *Clin Nephrol* 1985;24(6):289–291.
93. Chitalia VC, Almeida AF, Rai H, et al. Is peritoneal dialysis adequate for hypercatabolic acute renal failure in developing countries? *Kidney Int* 2002;61(2):747–757.
94. Bellomo R, Martin H, Parkin G, et al. Continuous arteriovenous haemodiafiltration in the critically ill: influence on major nutrient balances. *Intensive Care Med* 1991;17(7):399–402.
95. Bonnardeaux A, Pichette V, Ouimet D, et al. Solute clearances with high dialysate flow rates and glucose absorption from the dialysate in continuous arteriovenous hemodialysis. *Am J Kidney Dis* 1992;19(1):31–38.
96. Sigler MH, Teehan BP. Solute transport in continuous hemodialysis: a new treatment for acute renal failure. *Kidney Int* 1987; 32(4):562–571.
97. Monson P, Mehta RL. Nutritional considerations in continuous renal replacement therapies. *Semin Dial* 1996;9:152–160.
98. Bellomo R, Parkin G, Love J, et al. Use of continuous haemodiafiltration: an approach to the management of acute renal failure in the critically ill. *Am J Nephrol* 1992;12(4):240–245.
99. Matamis D, Tsagourias M, Koletsos K, et al. Influence of continuous haemofiltration-related hypothermia on haemodynamic variables and gas exchange in septic patients. *Intensive Care Med* 1994;20(6):431–436.
100. Davenport A, Roberts NB. Amino acid losses during continuous high-flux hemofiltration in the critically ill patient. *Crit Care Med* 1989;17(10):1010–1014.
101. Davies SP, Reaveley DA, Brown EA, et al. Amino acid clearances and daily losses in patients with acute renal failure treated by continuous arteriovenous hemodialysis. *Crit Care Med* 1991; 19(12):1510–1515.
102. Mehta R. Therapeutic alternatives to renal replacement for critically ill patients in acute renal failure. *Seminars in Nephrol* 1994; 14:64–82.
103. Weiss L, Danielson BG, Wikstrom B, et al. Continuous arteriovenous hemofiltration in the treatment of 100 critically ill patients with acute renal failure: report on clinical outcome and nutritional aspects. *Clin Nephrol* 1989;31(4):184–189.
104. Cottrell AC, Mehta RL. Phosphate kinetics in continuous renal replacement therapy (CRRT). *J Am Soc Nephrol* (abs) 1992;3: 360.
105. Ronco C, Bellomo R, Homel P, et al. Effects of different doses in continuous veno-venous haemofiltration on outcomes of acute renal failure: a prospective randomised trial. *Lancet* 2000; 356(9223):26–30.
106. Bartlett RH, Mault JR, Dechert RE, et al. Continuous arteriovenous hemofiltration: improved survival in surgical acute renal failure? *Surgery* 1986;100(2):400–408.
107. Bellomo R, Boyce N. Continuous venovenous hemodiafiltration compared with conventional dialysis in critically ill patients with acute renal failure. *ASAIO J* 1993;39(3):M794–M797.
108. Mehta RL, McDonald B, Gabbai FB, et al. A randomized clinical trial of continuous versus intermittent dialysis for acute renal failure. *Kidney Int* 2001;60(3):1154–1163.
109. Schiffl H, Lang SM, Fischer R. Daily hemodialysis and the outcome of acute renal failure. *N Engl J Med* 2002;346(5): 305–310.
110. Kihara M, Ikeda Y, Fujita H, et al. Amino acid losses and nitrogen balance during slow diurnal hemodialysis in critically ill patients with renal failure. *Intensive Care Med* 1997;23(1): 110–113.
111. Kudsk KA, Croce MA, Fabian TC, et al. Enteral versus parenteral feeding. Effects on septic morbidity after blunt and penetrating abdominal trauma. *Ann Surg* 1992;215(5):503–511, discussion 511–513.
112. Moore FA, Moore EE, Jones TN, et al. TEN versus TPN following major abdominal trauma—reduced septic morbidity. *J Trauma* 1989;29(7):916–922, discussion 922–923.
113. Heyland DK, MacDonald S, Keefe L, et al. Total parenteral nutrition in the critically ill patient: a meta-analysis. *JAMA* 1998;280(23):2013–2019.
114. Taylor SJ, Fettes SB, Jewkes C, et al. Prospective, randomized, controlled trial to determine the effect of early enhanced enteral nutrition on clinical outcome in mechanically ventilated pa-

tients suffering head injury. *Crit Care Med* 1999;27(11): 2525–2531.
115. Janu P, Li J, Renegar KB, et al. Recovery of gut-associated lymphoid tissue and upper respiratory tract immunity after parenteral nutrition. *Ann Surg* 1997;225(6):707–715, discussion 715–717.
116. Abraham E. Intranasal immunization with bacterial polysaccharide containing liposomes enhances antigen-specific pulmonary secretory response. *Vaccine* 1992;10:461–468.
117. Deitch EA, Winterton J, Li M, et al. The gut as a portal of entry for bacteremia. Role of protein malnutrition. *Ann Surg* 1987;205(6):681–692.
118. Purandare S, Offenbartl K, Westrom B, et al. Increased gut permeability to fluorescein isothiocyanate-dextran after total parenteral nutrition in the rat. *Scand J Gastroenterol* 1989;24(6): 678–682.
119. Wu Y, Kudsk KA, DeWitt RC, et al. Route and type of nutrition influence IgA-mediated intestinal cytokines. *Ann Surg* 1999; 229(5):662–667, discussion 667–668.
120. Alverdy JC, Aoys E, Moss GS. Total parenteral nutrition promotes bacterial translocation from the gut. *Surgery* 1988;104(2): 185–190.
121. King BK, Kudsk KA, Li J, et al. Route and type of nutrition influence mucosal immunity to bacterial pneumonia. *Ann Surg* 1999;229(2):272–278.
122. Daly JM, Lieberman MD, Goldfine J, et al. Enteral nutrition with supplemental arginine, RNA, and omega-3 fatty acids in patients after operation: immunologic, metabolic, and clinical outcome. *Surgery* 1992;112(1):56–67.
123. Bower RH, Cerra FB, Bershadsky B, et al. Early enteral administration of a formula (Impact) supplemented with arginine, nucleotides, and fish oil in intensive care unit patients: results of a multicenter, prospective, randomized, clinical trial. *Crit Care Med* 1995;23(3):436–449.
124. Li J, Kudsk KA, Hamidian M, et al. Bombesin affects mucosal immunity and gut-associated lymphoid tissue in intravenously fed mice. *Arch Surg* 1995;130(11):1164–1169, discussion 1169–1170.
125. DeWitt RC, Wu Y, Renegar KB, et al. Bombesin recovers gut-associated lymphoid tissue and preserves immunity to bacterial pneumonia in mice receiving total parenteral nutrition. *Ann Surg* 2000;231(1):1–8.
126. Janu PG, Kudsk KA, Li J, et al. Effect of bombesin on impairment of upper respiratory tract immunity induced by total parenteral nutrition. *Arch Surg* 1997;132(1):89–93.
127. Zaloga GP. Immune-enhancing enteral diets: where's the beef? *Crit Care Med* 1998;26(7):1143–1146.
128. Frisancho AR. New standards of weight and body composition by frame size and height for assessment of nutritional status of adults and the elderly. *Am J Clin Nutr* 1984;40(4):808–819.
129. Najjar MF, Rowland M. Anthropometric reference data and prevalence of overweight, United States, 1976–80. *Vital Health Stat 11* 1987(238):1–73.
130. Kopple JD, Jones MR, Keshaviah PR, et al. A proposed glossary for dialysis kinetics. *Am J Kidney Dis* 1995;26(6):963–981.
131. Motil KJ, Harmon WE, Grupe WE. Complications of essential amino acid hyperalimentation in children with acute renal failure. *JPEN J Parenter Enteral Nutr* 1980;4(1):32–35.
132. Nakasaki H, Katayama T, Yokoyama S, et al. Complication of parenteral nutrition composed of essential amino acids and histidine in adults with renal failure. *JPEN J Parenter Enteral Nutr* 1993;17(1):86–90.
133. Chima CS, Meyer L, Hummell AC, et al. Protein catabolic rate in patients with acute renal failure on continuous arteriovenous hemofiltration and total parenteral nutrition. *J Am Soc Nephrol* 1993;3(8):1516–1521.
134. Bellomo R, Mansfield D, Rumble S, et al. A comparison of conventional dialytic therapy and acute continuous hemodiafiltration in the management of acute renal failure in the critically ill. *Ren Fail* 1993;15(5):595–602.
135. Swendseid ME, Harris CL, Tuttle SG. The effect of sources of nonessential nitrogen on nitrogen balance in young adults. *J Nutr* 1960;71:105–108.
136. Anderson HL, Heindel MB, Linkswiler H. Effect on nitrogen balance of adult man of varying source of nitrogen and level of calorie intake. *J Nutr* 1969;99(1):82–90.
137. Laidlaw SA, Kopple JD. Newer concepts of the indispensable amino acids. *Am J Clin Nutr* 1987;46(4):593–605.
138. van Venrooij WJ, Henshaw EC, Hirsch CA. Effects of deprival of glucose or individual amino acids on polyribosome distribution and rate of protein synthesis in cultured mammalian cells. *Biochim Biophys Acta* 1972;259(1):127–137.
139. Buse MG, Reid SS. Leucine. A possible regulator of protein turnover in muscle. *J Clin Invest* 1975;56(5):1250–1261.
140. Mitch WE, Walser M, Sapir DG. Nitrogen sparing induced by leucine compared with that induced by its keto analogue, alpha-ketoisocaproate, in fasting obese man. *J Clin Invest* 1981;67(2): 553–562.
141. Cerra FB, Upson D, Angelico R, et al. Branched chains support postoperative protein synthesis. *Surgery* 1982;92(2):192–199.
142. Daly JM, Mihranian MH, Kehoe JE, et al. Effects of postoperative infusion of branched chain amino acids on nitrogen balance and forearm muscle substrate flux. *Surgery* 1983;94(2): 151–158.
143. Tischler ME, Desautels M, Goldberg AL. Does leucine, leucyl-tRNA, or some metabolite of leucine regulate protein synthesis and degradation in skeletal and cardiac muscle? *J Biol Chem* 1982;257(4):1613–1621.
144. Leander U, Furst P, Vesterberg K, et al. Nitrogen sparing effect of Ornicetil in the immediate postoperative state. Clinical biochemistry and nitrogen balance. *Clin Nutr* 1985;4:43.
145. Bouffard Y, Viale JP, Annat G, et al. Energy expenditure in the acute renal failure patient mechanically ventilated. *Intensive Care Med* 1987;13(6):401–404.
146. Schneeweiss B, Graninger W, Stockenhuber F, et al. Energy metabolism in acute and chronic renal failure. *Am J Clin Nutr* 1990;52:596–601.
147. Harris JA, Benedict FG. *A biometric study of basal metabolism in man.* Publ. No. 279. Washington, DC: Carnegie Institute, 1919.
148. Wilmore DW. *The metabolic management of the critically ill.* New York: Plenum, 1977:34.
149. Monteon FJ, Laidlaw SA, Shaib JK, et al. Energy expenditure in patients with chronic renal failure. *Kidney Int* 1986;30(5): 741–747.
150. Garrel DR, Jobin N, de Jonge LH. Should we still use the Harris and Benedict equations? *Nutr Clin Pract* 1996;11(3): 99–103.
151. WHO. *Energy and protein requirements.* WHO Tech. Rep. Ser. No. 724. Geneva: WHO, 1985.
152. Jeejeebhoy KN, Langer B, Tsallas G, et al. Total parenteral nutrition at home: studies in patients surviving 4 months to 5 years. *Gastroenterology* 1976;71(6):943–953.
153. Askanazi J, Rosenbaum SH, Hyman AI, et al. Respiratory changes induced by the large glucose loads of total parenteral nutrition. *JAMA* 1980;243(14):1444–1447.
154. Druml W, Laggner A, Widhalm K, et al. Lipid metabolism in acute renal failure. *Kidney Int Suppl* 1983;16:S139–S142.
155. Seidner DL, Mascioli EA, Istfan NW, et al. Effects of long-chain triglyceride emulsions on reticuloendothelial system function in humans. *JPEN J Parenter Enteral Nutr* 1989;13(6):614–619.
156. Freeman J, Goldmann DA, Smith NE, et al. Association of

intravenous lipid emulsion and coagulase-negative staphylococcal bacteremia in neonatal intensive care units. *N Engl J Med* 1990;323(5):301–308.

157. Driscoll DF, Baptista RJ, Bistrian BR, et al. Practical considerations regarding the use of total nutrient admixtures. *Am J Hosp Pharm* 1986;43(2):416–419.
158. Makropoulos W, Heintz B, Stefanidis I. Selenium deficiency and thyroid function in acute renal failure. *Ren Fail* 1997;19(1): 129–136.
159. Angstwurm MW, Schottdorf J, Schopohl J, et al. Selenium replacement in patients with severe systemic inflammatory response syndrome improves clinical outcome. *Crit Care Med* 1999;27(9):1807–1813.
160. Druml W, Schwarzenhofer M, Apsner R, et al. Fat-soluble vitamins in patients with acute renal failure. *Miner Electrolyte Metab* 1998;24(4):220–226.
161. Fortin MC, Amyot SL, Geadah D, et al. Serum concentrations and clearances of folic acid and pyridoxal-5-phosphate during venovenous continuous renal replacement therapy. *Intensive Care Med* 1999;25(6):594–598.
162. Story DA, Ronco C, Bellomo R. Trace element and vitamin concentrations and losses in critically ill patients treated with continuous venovenous hemofiltration. *Crit Care Med* 1999; 27(1):220–223.
163. Yatzidis H, Digenis P, Fountas P. Hypervitaminosis A accompanying advanced chronic renal failure. *Br Med J* 1975;3(5979): 352–353.
164. Farrington K, Miller P, Varghese Z, et al. Vitamin A toxicity and hypercalcaemia in chronic renal failure. *Br Med J (Clin Res Ed)* 1981;282(6281):1999–2002.
165. Gleghorn EE, Eisenberg LD, Hack S, et al. Observations of vitamin A toxicity in three patients with renal failure receiving parenteral alimentation. *Am J Clin Nutr* 1986;44(1):107–112.
166. Audran M, Kumar R. The physiology and pathophysiology of vitamin D. *Mayo Clin Proc* 1985;60(12):851–866.
167. Slatopolsky E, Weerts C, Thielan J, et al. Marked suppression of secondary hyperparathyroidism by intravenous administration of 1,25-dihydroxy-cholecalciferol in uremic patients. *J Clin Invest* 1984;74(6):2136–2143.
168. Sprague SM, Llach F, Amdahl M, et al. Paricalcitol versus calcitriol in the treatment of secondary hyperparathyroidism. *Kidney Int* 2003;63(4):1483–1490.
169. Massry SG, Smogorzewski M. Metabolic and endocrine abnormalities in acute renal failure. In: Massry SG, Glassock RJ. *Massry & Glassock's textbook of nephrology.* Baltimore: Williams & Wilkins, 1995;1004–1013.
170. Udall JA. Human sources and absorption of vitamin K in relation to anticoagulation stability. *JAMA* 1965;194(2):127–129.
171. Kopple JD, Mercurio K, Blumenkrantz MJ, et al. Daily requirement for pyridoxine supplements in chronic renal failure. *Kidney Int* 1981;19(5):694–704.
172. Balcke P, Schmidt P, Zazgornik J, et al. Ascorbic acid aggravates secondary hyperoxalemia in patients on chronic hemodialysis. *Ann Intern Med* 1984;101(3):344–345.
173. Pru C, Eaton J, Kjellstrand C. Vitamin C intoxication and hyperoxalemia in chronic hemodialysis patients. *Nephron* 1985; 39(2):112–116.
174. Friedman AL, Chesney RW, Gilbert EF, et al. Secondary oxalosis as a complication of parenteral alimentation in acute renal failure. *Am J Nephrol* 1983;3(5):248–252.
175. Fryer MJ. Treatment of acute renal failure with antioxidant vitamin E. *Ren Fail* 1999;21(2):231–233.
176. Akpolat T, Akpolat I, Ozturk H, et al. Effect of vitamin E and pentoxifylline on glycerol-induced acute renal failure. *Nephron* 2000;84(3):243–247.
177. Ponting GA, Halliday D, Teale JD, et al. Postoperative positive nitrogen balance with intravenous hyponutrition and growth hormone. *Lancet* 1988;1(8583):438–440.
178. Wilmore DW. Catabolic illness. Strategies for enhancing recovery. *N Engl J Med* 1991;325:695–702.
179. Ding H, Kopple JD, Cohen A, et al. Recombinant human insulin-like growth factor-I accelerates recovery and reduces catabolism in rats with ischemic acute renal failure. *J Clin Invest* 1993;91(5):2281–2287.
180. Kopple JD. Uses and limitations of growth factors in renal failure. *Perit Dial Int* 1997;17(Suppl 3):S63–S66.
181. Fouque D, Peng SC, Shamir E, et al. Recombinant human insulin-like growth factor-1 induces an anabolic response in malnourished CAPD patients. *Kidney Int* 2000;57(2):646–654.
182. Hirschberg R, Kopple J, Lipsett P, et al. Multicenter clinical trial of recombinant human insulin-like growth factor I in patients with acute renal failure. *Kidney Int* 1999;55(6): 2423–2432.
183. Dahn MS, Lange MP, Jacobs LA. Insulinlike growth factor 1 production is inhibited in human sepsis. *Arch Surg* 1988; 123(11):1409–1414.
184. Kopple JD. The rationale for the use of growth hormone or insulin-like growth factor I in adult patients with renal failure. *Miner Electrolyte Metab* 1992;18(2–5):269–275.
185. Takala J, Ruokonen E, Webster NR, et al. Increased mortality associated with growth hormone treatment in critically ill adults. *N Engl J Med* 1999;341(11):785–792.
186. Hinton P, Allison SP, Littlejohn S, et al. Insulin and glucose to reduce catabolic response to injury in burned patients. *Lancet* 1971;1(7703):767–769.
187. Woolfson AM, Heatley RV, Allison SP. Insulin to inhibit protein catabolism after injury. *N Engl J Med* 1979;300(1):14–17.
188. van den Berghe G, Wouters P, Weekers F, et al. Intensive insulin therapy in the critically ill patients. *N Engl J Med* 2001;345(19): 1359–1367.
189. Rayfield EJ, Ault MJ, Keusch GT, et al. Infection and diabetes: the case for glucose control. *Am J Med* 1982;72:439–450.
190. Rassias AJ, Marrin CA, Arruda J, et al. Insulin infusion improves neutrophil function in diabetic cardiac surgery patients. *Anesth Analg* 1999;88(5):1011–1016.
191. Losser MR, Bernard C, Beaudeux JL, et al. Glucose modulates hemodynamic, metabolic, and inflammatory responses to lipopolysaccharide in rabbits. *J Appl Physiol* 1997;83(5): 1566–1574.
192. Hammarqvist F, Wernerman J, Ali R, et al. Addition of glutamine to total parenteral nutrition after elective abdominal surgery spares free glutamine in muscle, counteracts the fall in muscle protein synthesis, and improves nitrogen balance. *Ann Surg* 1989;209(4):455–461.
193. Stehle P, Zander J, Mertes N, et al. Effect of parenteral glutamine peptide supplements on muscle glutamine loss and nitrogen balance after major surgery. *Lancet* 1989;1(8632):231–233.
194. Daly JM, Reynolds J, Thom A, et al. Immune and metabolic effects of arginine in the surgical patient. *Ann Surg* 1988;208(4): 512–523.
195. Barbul A. Arginine: biochemistry, physiology, and therapeutic implications. *JPEN J Parenter Enteral Nutr* 1986;10(2): 227–238.
196. Souba WW, Herskowitz K, Austgen TR, et al. Glutamine nutrition: theoretical considerations and therapeutic impact. *JPEN J Parenter Enteral Nutr* 1990;14(5 Suppl):237S–243S.
197. Gianotti L, Alexander JW, Pyles T, et al. Arginine-supplemented diets improve survival in gut-derived sepsis and peritonitis by modulating bacterial clearance. The role of nitric oxide. *Ann Surg* 1993;217(6):644–653, discussion 653–654.
198. Barbul A. Arginine and immune function. *Nutrition* 1990;6(1): 53–58, discussion 59–62.

199. Rudolph FB, Kulkarni AD, Schandle VB, et al. Involvement of dietary nucleotides in T lymphocyte function. *Adv Exp Med Biol* 1984;165(Pt B):175–178.
200. Fanslow WC, Kulkarni AD, Van Buren CT, et al. Effect of nucleotide restriction and supplementation on resistance to experimental murine candidiasis. *JPEN J Parenter Enteral Nutr* 1988;12(1):49–52.
201. Wan JM, Teo TC, Babayan VK, et al. Invited comment: lipids and the development of immune dysfunction and infection. *JPEN J Parenter Enteral Nutr* 1988;12(6 Suppl):43S–52S.
202. Endres S, Ghorbani R, Kelley VE, et al. The effect of dietary supplementation with n-3 polyunsaturated fatty acids on the synthesis of interleukin-1 and tumor necrosis factor by mononuclear cells. *N Engl J Med* 1989;320(5):265–271.
203. Kinsella JE, Lokesh B, Broughton S, et al. Dietary polyunsaturated fatty acids and eicosanoids: potential effects on the modulation of inflammatory and immune cells: an overview. *Nutrition* 1990;6(1):24–44, discussion 59–62.
204. Humes HD, Cieslinski DA, Coimbra TM, et al. Epidermal growth factor enhances renal tubule cell regeneration and repair and accelerates the recovery of renal function in postischemic acute renal failure. *J Clin Invest* 1989;84(6):1757–1761.
205. Miller SB, Martin DR, Kissane J, et al. Hepatocyte growth factor accelerates recovery from acute ischemic renal injury in rats. *Am J Physiol* 1994;266(1 Pt 2):F129–134.
206. Miller SB, Martin DR, Kissane J, et al. Insulin-like growth factor I accelerates recovery from ischemic acute tubular necrosis in the rat. *Proc Natl Acad Sci U S A* 1992;89(24):11876–11880.
207. Clark R, Mortensen D, Rabkin R. Recovery from acute ischaemic renal failure is accelerated by des-(1-3)-insulin-like growth factor-1. *Clin Sci (Lond)* 1994;86(6):709–714.
208. Schramm L, Heidbreder E, Schmitt A, et al. Role of L-arginine-derived NO in ischemic acute renal failure in the rat. *Ren Fail* 1994;16(5):555–569.
209. Edelstein CL, Ling H, Wangsiripaisan A, et al. Emerging therapies for acute renal failure. *Am J Kidney Dis* 1997;30(5 Suppl 4):S89–S95.
210. Burke TJ, Arnold PE, Gordon JA, et al. Protective effect of intrarenal calcium membrane blockers before or after renal ischemia. Functional, morphological, and mitochondrial studies. *J Clin Invest* 1984;74(5):1830–1841.
211. Siegel NJ, Glazier WB, Chaudry IH, et al. Enhanced recovery from acute renal failure by the postischemic infusion of adenine nucleotides and magnesium chloride in rats. *Kidney Int* 1980; 17(3):338–349.
212. Siegel NJ, Gaudio KM, Katz LA, et al. Beneficial effect of thyroxin on recovery from toxic acute renal failure. *Kidney Int* 1984;25(6):906–911.
213. Paller MS, Hoidal JR, Ferris TF. Oxygen free radicals in ischemic acute renal failure in the rat. *J Clin Invest* 1984;74(4): 1156–1164.
214. Linas SL, Shanley PF, White CW, et al. O2 metabolite-mediated injury in perfused kidneys is reflected by consumption of DMTU and glutathione. *Am J Physiol* 1987;253(4 Pt 2): F692–F701.
215. Baines AD, Shaikh N, Ho P. Mechanisms of perfused kidney cytoprotection by alanine and glycine. *Am J Physiol* 1990;259 (1 Pt 2):F80–F87.
216. Weinberg JM, Buchanan DN, Davis JA, et al. Metabolic aspects of protection by glycine against hypoxic injury to isolated proximal tubules. *J Am Soc Nephrol* 1991;1(7):949–958.
217. Kribben A, Wieder ED, Wetzels JF, et al. Evidence for role of cytosolic free calcium in hypoxia-induced proximal tubule injury. *J Clin Invest* 1994;93(5):1922–1929.
218. Neumayer HH, Wagner K. Prevention of delayed graft function in cadaver kidney transplants by diltiazem: outcome of two prospective, randomized clinical trials. *J Cardiovasc Pharmacol* 1987;10(Suppl 10):S170–S177.
219. Neumayer HH, Kunzendorf U, Schreiber M. Protective effects of calcium antagonists in human renal transplantation. *Kidney Int Suppl* 1992;36:S87–S93.
220. Edelstein CL, Wieder ED, Yaqoob MM, et al. The role of cysteine proteases in hypoxia-induced rat renal proximal tubular injury. *Proc Natl Acad Sci U S A* 1995;92(17):7662–7666.
221. Edelstein CL, Yaqoob MM, Alkhunaizi AM, et al. Modulation of hypoxia-induced calpain activity in rat renal proximal tubules. *Kidney Int* 1996;50(4):1150–1157.
222. Yu L, Gengaro PE, Niederberger M, et al. Nitric oxide: a mediator in rat tubular hypoxia/reoxygenation injury. *Proc Natl Acad Sci U S A* 1994;91(5):1691–1695.
223. Noiri E, Peresleni T, Miller F, et al. In vivo targeting of inducible NO synthase with oligodeoxynucleotides protects rat kidney against ischemia. *J Clin Invest* 1996;97(10):2377–2383.
224. Kudsk KA. Enteral versus parenteral feeding in critical illness. In: Vincent JL, ed. *From nutrition support to pharmacologic nutrition in the ICU.* Berlin: Springer-Verlag, 2000:115–124.
225. Kirby DF, Kudsk KA. Obtaining and maintaining access for nutrition support. In: Vincent JL, ed. *From nutrition support to pharmacologic nutrition in the ICU.* Berlin: Springer-Verlag, 2000:125–137.
226. Hadfield RJ, Sinclair DG, Houldsworth PE, et al. Effects of enteral and parenteral nutrition on gut mucosal permeability in the critically ill. *Am J Respir Crit Care Med* 1995;152(5 Pt 1):1545–1548.
227. Moore FA, Feliciano DV, Andrassy RJ, et al. Early enteral feeding, compared with parenteral, reduces postoperative septic complications. The results of a meta-analysis. *Ann Surg* 1992; 216(2):172–183.
228. Schroeder D, Gillanders L, Mahr K, et al. Effects of immediate postoperative enteral nutrition on body composition, muscle function, and wound healing. *JPEN J Parenter Enteral Nutr* 1991;15(4):376–383.
229. Levine GM, Deren JJ, Steiger E, et al. Role of oral intake in maintenance of gut mass and disaccharide activity. *Gastroenterology* 1974;67(5):975–982.
230. Lo CW, Walker WA. Changes in the gastrointestinal tract during enteral or parenteral feeding. *Nutr Rev* 1989;47:193–198.
231. Ford WD, Boelhouwer RU, King WW, et al. Total parenteral nutrition inhibits intestinal adaptive hyperplasia in young rats: reversal by feeding. *Surgery* 1984;96(3):527–534.
232. Buchman AL, Moukarzel AA, Bhuta S, et al. Parenteral nutrition is associated with intestinal morphologic and functional changes in humans. *JPEN J Parenter Enteral Nutr* 1995;19(6): 453–460.
233. Hirschberg R, Kopple JD. Enteral nutrition and renal disease. In: Roumbeau JL, Caldwell MD, ed. *Clinical nutrition: enteral and tube feeding.* Philadelphia: WB Saunders, 1990:400–415.
234. Strife CF, Quinlan M, Mears K, et al. Improved growth of three uremic children by nocturnal nasogastric feedings. *Am J Dis Child* 1986;140(5):438–443.
235. Terzi F, Dartois AM, Kleinknecht C, et al. Management of chronic renal failure during the first year of life: A European perspective. *J Ren Nutrition* 1993;3:120–129.
236. Shike M. Enteral feeding. In: Shils ME, Olson JA, Shike M, eds. *Modern nutrition in health and disease.* Philadelphia: Williams & Wilkins, 1999:1643–1656.
237. Driscoll DF. Formulation of parenteral and enteral admixtures. In: Vincent JL, ed. *From nutrition support to pharmacologic nutrition in the ICU.* Berlin: Springer-Verlag, 2000:138–150.
238. Powell-Tuck J, Goldhill DR. Monitoring nutritional support in the intensive care unit. In: Vincent JL, ed. *From nutrition*

support to pharmacologic nutrition in the ICU. Berlin: Springer-Verlag, 2000:191–208.

239. Shils ME. Parenteral nutrition. In: Shils ME, Olson JA, Shike M, eds. *Modern nutrition in health and disease.* Philadelphia: Williams & Wilkins, 1999:1657–1688.
240. Freeman JB, Fairfull-Smith RJ. Physiologic approach to peripheral parenteral nutrition. In: Fischer JE, ed. *Surgical nutrition.* Boston: Little, Brown, 1983:703–717.
241. Shils ME, Wright WL, Turnbull A, et al. Long-term parenteral nutrition through an external arteriovenous shunt. *N Engl J Med* 1970;283(7):341–344.
242. Zager RA, Venkatachalam MA. Potentiation of ischemic renal injury by amino acid infusion. *Kidney Int* 1983;24(5):620–625.
243. Zager RA, Johannes G, Tuttle SE, et al. Acute amino acid nephrotoxicity. *J Lab Clin Med* 1983;101(1):130–140.
244. Malis CD, Racusen LC, Solez K, et al. Nephrotoxicity of lysine and of a single dose of aminoglycoside in rats given lysine. *J Lab Clin Med* 1984;103(5):660–676.
245. Andrews PM, Bates SB. Dietary protein prior to renal ischemia and postischemic kidney function. *Kidney Int Suppl* 1987;22: S76–S80.
246. Weinberg JM. The effect of amino acids on ischemic and toxic injury to the kidney. *Semin Nephrol* 1990;10(5):491–500.
247. Kaltenbach JP, Ganote CE, Carone FA. Renal tubular necrosis induced by compounds structurally related to D-serine. *Exp Mol Pathol* 1979;30(2):209–214.
248. Vieth R, Pinto TR, Reen BS, et al. Vitamin D poisoning by table sugar. *Lancet* 2002;359(9307):672.
249. Gunda S, Kwan JT, Sampson S. Hypercalcaemia and acute renal failure. *Nephrol Dial Transplant* 2001;16(2):425–426.
250. Alkhunaizi AM, Chan L. Secondary oxalosis: a cause of delayed recovery of renal function in the setting of acute renal failure. *J Am Soc Nephrol* 1996;7(11):2320–2326.

31

NUTRITIONAL MANAGEMENT OF PATIENTS TREATED WITH CONTINUOUS RENAL REPLACEMENT THERAPY

RINALDO BELLOMO

The treatment of critically ill patients with severe acute renal failure (ARF) is one of the major challenges for the nephrologist and critical care physician. This is because ARF-related mortality remains high and because ARF affects the most severely ill patients in the intensive care unit (ICU). The management of these patients requires careful and frequent physiologic assessment, continuous monitoring, broad medical expertise, and detailed and assiduous attention to every detail of treatment. A particularly complex and controversial aspect of the care of these patients is the area of nutritional support. The type of renal replacement therapy significantly affects such nutritional support. Indeed, in the modern ICU, there are several approaches to providing artificial renal replacement therapy (RRT). They include peritoneal dialysis and conventional intermittent hemodialysis (IHD), which remain common, as well as frequent or daily long, slow hemodialysis and CRRT. In fact, the use of CRRT has become more widespread and in some countries, such as Australia, it is now the treatment of choice for more than 95% of patients in the ICU (1). If the nephrologist or the intensivist wishes to prescribe nutritional support to patients receiving CRRT they need to make themselves familiar with the nutritional implications of this type of therapy. This chapter seeks to summarize the available evidence and to offer a possible approach to nutritional support in patients undergoing CRRT.

PRINCIPLES OF NUTRITIONAL SUPPORT FOR PATIENTS RECEIVING CONTINUOUS RENAL REPLACEMENT THERAPY

A clinician faced with prescribing nutritional support to patients receiving CRRT should be guided by some general principles that help define the broad goals of nutrition in these patients. The first principle of nutritional support for CRRT patients is this: the presence of ARF should not cause inadequate nutritional support.

If a patient has a serum urea nitrogen (SUN) of 80 mg/dL and nitrogen-rich nutritional support would increase urea concentrations to levels requiring further dialytic support, such nutrition should still be given and the intensity of CRRT should be adjusted promptly to prevent uremia. Thus, a patient with ARF will either be able to receive full nutritional support with conventional levels of CRRT or he/she will need to have his/her CRRT intensity increased to receive adequate nutrition without uncontrolled azotemia. Whatever the situation, adequate nutrition should be given.

The second principle of nutritional support in these patients is that the nitrogen catabolism induced by multiorgan failure with ARF overwhelms any catabolic effects of ARF. The corollary of this insight is that the nutrition of critically ill patients with ARF should be, in general, no different from that of other patients with multiorgan failure.

The third principle of nutritional support in these patients is that the effect of CRRT on catabolism is small. The corollary of this principle is that CRRT should be applied early and aggressively without fear that it will significantly increase protein breakdown.

With regard to these three principles, it is understood that, in patients receiving CRRT, there are no randomized controlled trials that demonstrate major clinical advantages of a particular approach to nutritional support. It also is understood that there is controversy as to what represents the "best" uremic control of ARF. As will be argued in this chapter, these principles represent a rational response to the available evidence, however flawed it might be.

METABOLIC CHANGES WITH ACUTE RENAL FAILURE

To understand what might be logical nutritional support during CRRT, one needs to understand the effects that

ARF has on metabolism. This subject is discussed more extensively in Chapter 29. The effects of ARF on metabolism have been well studied in animals. Several experimental studies show that inducing ARF by removing both kidneys from mammals leads to a catabolic state with negative nitrogen balance, insulin resistance, increased gluconeogenesis, increased ureagenesis, and imbalances in plasma amino acid concentrations (2–4). Such imbalances in the plasma aminogram appear to occur in humans. In subjects with ARF, for example, the plasma concentrations of cystine, methionine, and sometimes phenylalanine are markedly elevated, whereas the concentrations of valine and leucine are relatively low (5). It is unclear, however, how ARF-specific these findings are because similar findings have been reported in patients with severe sepsis (6). Accordingly, in critically ill patients, it is doubtful whether the presence of ARF significantly exacerbates catabolism beyond the effect of the illness itself.

Extrapolations from relatively stable patients with chronic or end-stage renal failure also have been used to draw conclusions about metabolic changes in ARF (7–9). Their relationship to what we see in severe ARF of critical illness is questionable. Finally, the effects of the decreased intake of protein (10), which is seen spontaneously in acutely ill patients who do not receive artificial nutritional support, represent yet another confounding factor in our ability to discern any truly ARF-specific metabolic changes in humans.

Thus, no persuasive evidence exists that critically ill patients with ARF have metabolic needs that clearly differ in a clinically significant way from those of similarly ill patients who do not have ARF. Equally, much evidence exists that the metabolic needs of patients with ARF are similar to patients with critical illness of similar severity but without ARF.

Energy and Micronutrient Requirements

Caloric requirements in critically ill patients with ARF are determined mostly by the severity of the accompanying illness, whereas in ward patients with uncomplicated ARF (e.g., radiocontrast-induced ARF) energy requirements are generally normal (11). This means that in critically ill patients with ARF, as in other patients with the multiorgan dysfunction syndrome (MODS), calorie expenditure will approximate 25 to 30 kcal/kg/day or 120 to 160 kjoule/kg/day.

Determining how such energy should be provided in terms of the carbohydrates/lipids ratio is controversial. Most clinicians traditionally prescribe about 50% to 80% of energy intake as carbohydrates. However, lipids provide not only energy, but also essential fatty acids. The type of lipids and fatty acids that should be administered to critically ill patients has been the subject of much investigation (12). Several randomized controlled studies using enteral preparations enriched with ω-3 or ω-6 polyunsaturated fatty acids have shown decreased morbidity and reduced hospital stay (13–16) in general populations of medical and surgical ICU patients. Furthermore, another recent randomized controlled trial in patients with acute respiratory distress syndrome showed a more rapid improvement in gas exchange among patients treated with a preparation rich in γ-linolenic acid, eicosapentaenoic acid, and medium-chain triglycerides. With this preparation, most of the calories were administered in the form of lipids rather than carbohydrates (17). Unfortunately, no ARF-specific information is available to tell us whether these preparations have a beneficial effect on renal recovery or how they may affect renal patients differently. However, it is likely that patients receiving CRRT would benefit from these preparations in the same way other patients do.

The dose of micronutrients (i.e., vitamins and trace minerals) that should be administered to critically ill patients is unknown. The same observation is true of patients receiving CRRT. In the absence of controlled studies, it would seem reasonable to provide at least the recommended dietary allowance (RDA) of trace minerals and vitamins. This statement should be adjusted for potential losses of trace elements and vitamins during RRT.

In fact, there is only a modest amount of information on the effect of IHD on micronutrients and carbohydrate or lipid losses in patients in the ICU. However, there have been several careful studies in critically ill patients treated with CRRT (18–20).

The first of these studies (18) demonstrated that there are no lipid losses during CRRT. This is not surprising because CRRT can remove only water-soluble molecules and not lipid-soluble metabolites. This study also demonstrated that, if a glucose rich peritoneal dialysis fluid is used as the dialysate for CRRT, there is glucose movement from dialysate to patient, resulting in the administration of about 500 kcal/day of carbohydrates at a dialysate flow rate of 1 L/hr. If the dialysate flow rate is increased or the concentration of glucose in dialysate in increased, the carbohydrate administration increases proportionately. If one of the new commercially available preparations is used, however, little glucose exchange takes place because glucose concentration is similar on both sides of the dialyzer membrane (glucose in commercial dialysate fluid or replacement fluid: 10 mmol/L). However, some caloric intake occurs if continuous veno-venous hemofiltration (CVVH) is performed and the replacement fluid contains lactate as a buffer. The lactate administered can be expected to add further to energy intake, depending on the rate and site of fluid replacement administration. Such lactate balance, of course, will vary according to the site of replacement fluid delivery (prefilter or postfilter), according to whether the lactated solution is used as dialysate, and according to the acid-base status of the patients. These observations also apply to the administration of trisodium citrate as a combined buffer and anticoagulant. No studies yet have sought to quantify the overall calorie contribution of lactate or citrate under these operating circumstances.

The second study (19) demonstrated that trace elements are not lost in significant amounts in the ultrafiltrate during CVVH. This is because the amount on nonprotein–bound trace elements is low and because only "free" trace elements can be filtered. Therefore, there is no justification for supplemental administration of such trace elements in patients undergoing CRRT beyond what is considered adequate for the illness itself. It is worth noting, however, that the serum concentrations of antioxidant trace elements such as selenium and zinc are low in these patients (19). This finding suggests that there may be increased oxidant activity and depletion of natural antioxidants in ARF. It is possible that aggressive supplementation of antioxidants may improve patient outcome (21). Similarly, there was no loss of lipid-soluble vitamins during CVVH and only minute losses of vitamin B_1 and B_2. There was, however, some loss of vitamin C at amounts equal to its RDA. Accordingly, we supplement our patients with at least 100 mg of vitamin C/day during treatment with CRRT.

A third study (20) has provided evidence of significant losses of folate and vitamin B_6 during CRRT. Thus, we consider it advisable that additional amounts of folate and vitamin B_6 be administered to patients treated with CRRT.

As is the case with antioxidant trace elements, there is depletion of antioxidant vitamins (vitamin E and C) in critically ill patients with severe ARF. Once again, it may be desirable to correct this imbalance by the more aggressive supplementation of vitamin E and C in these patients because vitamin E, selenium, and other antioxidant deficiencies have been shown to decrease the rate of renal recovery in experimental renal failure (22,23). However, because vitamin C supplements increase serum oxalate levels in individuals with chronic renal failure, caution should be exercised with regard to giving large vitamin C doses.

Nitrogen Administration During Continuous Renal Replacement Therapy

Nitrogen administration is fundamental to the preservation of body protein. In severe sepsis, daily nitrogen losses can exceed 40 g/day with or without ARF (24–26), and the net rate of protein degradation (protein catabolism minus protein synthesis) can be extraordinary and has been reported to be greater than 150 g/day (27–29).

The presence or absence of ARF does not appear to have a major effect on these changes in metabolism (30,31). In patients with ARF treated with conventional IHD and in the absence of adequate protein supplementation (e.g., administration of only 0.5 g of amino acids/kg/day or less), protein balance has been reported (28,32) to reach negative values of 1.5 to 2.3 kg over a 2-week period. Such negative nitrogen balance represents the loss of about one-third of all noncollagenous protein mass in the average 70-kg man (33). Losses of this magnitude are likely to contribute to mortality because protein malnutrition has been identified as an independent predictor of outcome in patients with MODS (25,34). Accordingly, the first goal of artificial protein administration is to prevent or minimize the negative nitrogen balance of critical illness (35–37).

Several studies of protein nitrogen metabolism and protein nitrogen balance have been performed in critically ill patients with ARF receiving either IHD or CRRT (25, 27–29,32,34,38–46). In our opinion, they clearly demonstrate the following points:

1. Protein nitrogen catabolism can be extraordinary (net rate of protein degradation >150 g/day) in patients with ARF and MODS.
2. Protein restriction (less than 0.5 g/kg/day) in such patients often results in a highly (>70 g/day) negative protein balance.
3. Some protein/amino acid administration is better than no protein/amino acid administration and may increase survival.
4. Increasing protein administration from 0.5 to 2.5 g/kg/day improves nitrogen balance in an almost linear fashion.
5. Protein/amino acid administration at 2.5 g/kg/day achieves a positive nitrogen balance in approximately 50% of cases and a slightly negative (1.6 to 2.4 g/day) overall mean nitrogen balance.
6. Standard protein/amino acid administration (1.0 to 1.5 g/kg/day) achieves a positive nitrogen balance in about 30% of cases and a moderately negative (3.2 to 4.0 g/day) overall mean nitrogen balance.
7. During total parenteral nutrition (TPN) and dialytic therapy, amino acids are lost into the effluent dialysate. Such amino acid losses are about 10% to 12% of administered dose, although the percentage losses of individual amino acids may be greater.
8. There are no clinically important differences in amino acid losses during IHD versus CRRT.
9. Increasing protein or amino acid administration increases the protein catabolic rate and the urea generation rate, thus requiring more intensive dialytic therapy to achieve azotemic control.
10. Excellent azotemic control can be achieved with CRRT even when protein intake is 2.5 g/kg/day. This is impossible with conventional (3 to 4 hrs × 3 times/week) IHD.
11. CRRT, unlike conventional IHD, removes virtually any limitation on protein or amino acid administration.
12. The composition of amino acid solutions administered does not appear to influence nitrogen balance as long as solutions of standard amino acid composition are used.
13. There is no perceptible advantage from the administration of essential amino acids over a mixture of essential

TABLE 31.1. CHANGES IN AMINOGRAM DURING ACUTE RENAL FAILURE WITH VARIABLE REGIMENS OF AMINO ACID SUPPLEMENTATION

Amino Acid	Feinstein (27)	Druml (5)	Davies (39)	Frankenfield (41)	Hynote (40)	Kihara (44)
Histidine	Low	Normal	Normal	Normal	Normal	Normal
Isoleucine	Low	Normal	Low	High	Normal	High
Leucine	Low	Low	Normal	High	Normal	Normal
Lysine	Low	Normal	Normal	High	High	High
Methionine	High	High	High	High	High	High
Phenylalanine	High	High	High	High	High	High
Threonine	Low	Normal	Normal	High	Normal	Normal
Valine	Low	Low	Normal	High	Normal	High
Alanine	Low	Normal	Normal	Normal	Normal	Normal
Arginine	Low	Normal	Normal	Normal	Normal	Normal
Aspartate	High	Normal	Normal	Low	High	[a]
Glutamate	Normal	Normal	High	Normal	Normal	[a]
Asparagine	Low	Normal	Normal	Low	[a]	Normal
Glutamine	Low	Normal	Low	Normal	Low	Normal
Glycine	Normal	Normal	Normal	High	High	Normal
Proline	[a]	Normal	[a]	High	Normal	Normal
Serine	Low	Normal	Low	Normal	Normal	Normal
Ornithine	Low	Normal	[a]	High	[a]	[a]
Taurine	[a]	Normal	Low	Low	Low	Normal
Tyrosine	Low	Normal	Normal	Normal	Normal	Normal
Cystine	Normal	High	[a]	Normal	[a]	Low

[a]The amino acid in question was not measured.

and nonessential amino acids in a catabolic critically ill patient, and large doses of only the essential amino acids (i.e., ≥ 0.5g/kg/day) may be hazardous (see Chapter 29).

14. The administration of supplemental solutions with standard composition of amino acids appears to decrease selective disturbances in the serum aminogram that are seen in the absence of such nutritional support (Table 31.1).
15. The amount and type of amino acid supplementation has a greater impact on the serum aminogram than the effect of ARF per se (Figs. 31.1 and 31.2).

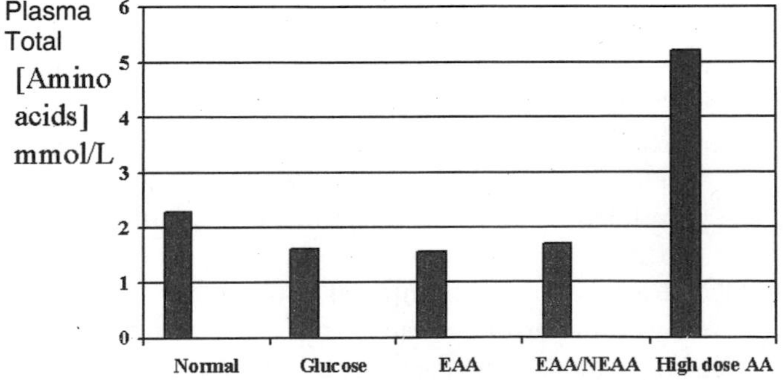

FIGURE 31.1. Histogram representing the changes in total serum amino acid concentration in normal patients and in patients with acute renal failure with different regimens of nutritional support including essential amino acids (EAA), a mixture of essential and nonessential amino acids (EAA/NEAA), and high-dose amino acids.

In our opinion, the clinical implications of the findings of the previously mentioned studies in critically ill patients with severe ARF and MODS are the following:

1. The practice of restricting protein/amino acid intake is physiologically undesirable, clinically unnecessary, and a potential contributor to increased mortality.
2. If CRRT is used for renal replacement, there is virtually no technical limitation on protein or amino acid that can be administered (Fig. 31.3).
3. There is no justification for the administration of so-called "Nephro" preparations or other allegedly "renal failure–specific" nutritional preparations.
4. There is no case for the administration of essential amino acids in preference to mixtures of essential and nonessential amino acids.

The decision of what is a reasonable nutritional prescription, which best takes into account the advantages and disadvantages of intensive protein/amino acid administration, and what are the additional costs associated with the administration of further amounts of amino acids is a matter of judgment. Such clinical judgment also must take into account experimental evidence that excessive amounts of given amino acids may have a nephrotoxic effect (47–49) as well as contrary evidence in experimented animals that such administration, in fact, may expedite renal recovery (50).

Studies comparing the effect of high nitrogen intake to low nitrogen intake on the rate and time to renal recovery in patients with ARF are limited in the numbers of subjects

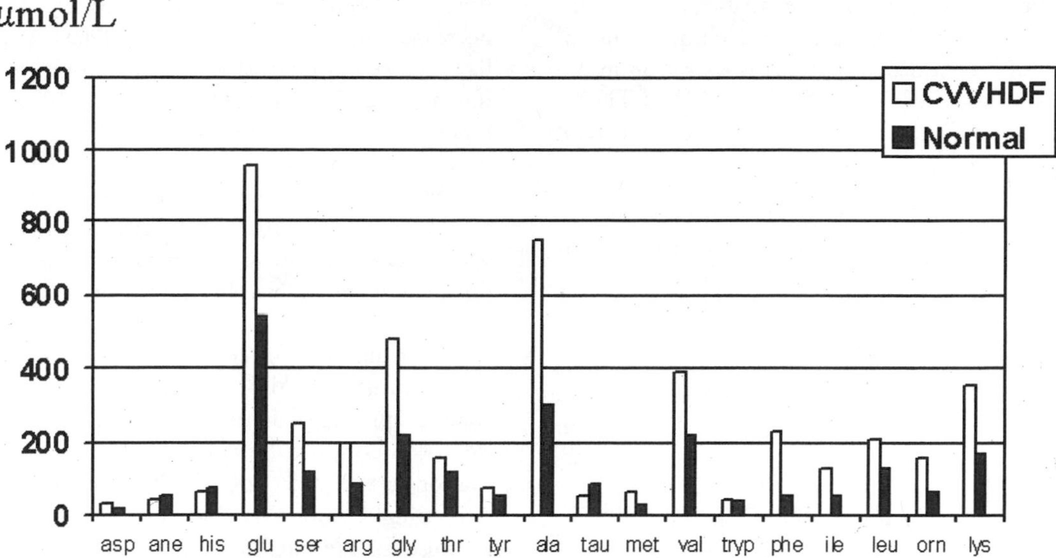

FIGURE 31.2. Histogram representing the effect of intensive amino acid supplementation on the aminogram during continuous renal replacement therapy (CRRT) compared to normal concentrations.

studied and do not give clear answers (27,28). Thus, in the absence of suitably large randomized controlled trials, it is impossible to make firm recommendations. Also, no firm recommendations can be made about the need to administered supplemental amounts of glutamine (51) until preliminary findings have been confirmed by larger clinical trials.

Monitoring of Nitrogen Balance

In individual patients, it may be helpful to monitor the impact of the chosen nutritional strategy on nitrogen metabolism. If such monitoring is contemplated, several equations are helpful to the clinician.

The first equation describes all measurable urea nitrogen outputs:

$$\text{UNA} = \text{urine UN} + \text{dialysate or ultrafiltrate UN} + \text{UN of other lost body fluids} + \text{change in body content of UN}$$

where UN stands for urea nitrogen and UNA stands for urea nitrogen appearance.

Calculation of UNA requires measurement of [urea] in all the fluids in the previous equation and multiplication of the obtained amount by the fraction of the molecular weight (MW) of urea represented by nitrogen. In some laboratories the value of urea may be reported already as urea nitrogen.

The change in body urea nitrogen is approximated as serum urea nitrogen concentration [SUN] $\times$ 0.6 of body weight at time 1 $-$ [SUN] $\times$ 0.6 of body weight at time 0 (time 0 being the beginning of the observation period and time 1 the end of such period). This approximation is derived from the view that total body water represents the estimated volume of distribution of urea. However, UNA only represents a fraction (although the largest) of TNA (total nitrogen appearance):

$$\text{TNA} = \text{UNA} + \text{appearance of other nitrogen}$$

Instruments that directly measure total nitrogen (18) can be used to measure TNA. TNA also can be calculated by measuring total body changes and losses of amino acids, uric acid, creatinine, and total protein. This procedure, however, is laborious and imprecise. Because the direct mea-

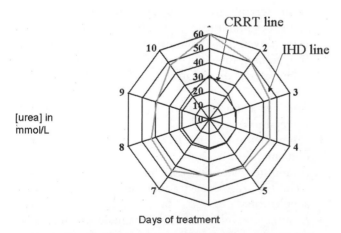

FIGURE 31.3. Diagram demonstrating the superiority of continuous renal replacement therapy (CRRT) in terms of uremic control. The inner line contour shows the daily mean urea levels in a cohort of patients receiving CRRT compared to a similar cohort of patients receiving IHD (*outer line perimeter*). Uremic control is almost twice as good despite more intensive nitrogen administration, with a mean level around 20 mmol/L during CRRT versus around 40 mmol/L during conventional IHD.

surement of nitrogen is not widely available, another approach is to use formulas that provide a clinically useful approximation of TNA (31). From our observation in patients with ARF, UNA represents 65% to 75% of TNA.

Once TNA is known, it is possible to calculate total nitrogen losses:

$$\text{Total nitrogen losses} = \text{TNA} + \text{skin losses of nitrogen} + \text{fecal losses of nitrogen}$$

In patients receiving TPN, fecal losses of nitrogen typically are absent and skin nitrogen losses can be approximated as 15 to 20 mg/kg/day.

If total nitrogen losses are known and nitrogen intake is known, then nitrogen balance can be calculated for a given period:

$$\text{Nitrogen balance} = \text{nitrogen intake} - \text{nitrogen losses}$$

Because nitrogen makes up about 16% of the molecular weight of proteins, protein balance can be calculated by multiplying all nitrogen measurements by 6.25. This operation allows the clinician to estimate the protein equivalent of total nitrogen appearance (PNA).

$$\text{PNA} = (\text{TNA} + \text{fecal nitrogen} + \text{skin nitrogen loss}) \times 6.25$$

These equations allow the clinician to monitor the effectiveness of nitrogen therapy on nitrogen balance and to appreciate the need to adjust, if necessary, the dose of nitrogen administered to minimize the negative nitrogen balance typical of MODS and ARF.

Hormonal Impact of Continuous Renal Replacement Therapy and Hormonal Manipulation

There has been concern over the possible impact of CRRT on the serum concentration of hormones. It has been feared that the continuous removal of hormones such as insulin, catecholamines, cortisol, testosterone, and thyroid hormones may adversely affect the metabolic state of patients with ARF. However, several recent investigations have demonstrated that insulin losses, even during continuous insulin infusion, are negligible (<1% to 2% of total dose) (52). Equally, losses of catecholamines, testosterone, cortisol, parathyroid hormone, and thyroid hormones are minute in relation to daily production or administration (53).

It has been suggested (4) that to achieve a positive nitrogen balance on most, if not all, days of nutritional support in critically ill patients with severe ARF more nitrogen administration will not suffice and hormonal manipulation will be needed. In this regard, the two hormones that have come under attention are growth hormone (GH) and insulinlike growth factor-I (IGF-I). Both of these agents have a significant anabolic effect, and the catabolism of critical illness has been, in part, attributed to resistance to GH and decreased production and action of IGF-I. Recent studies have suggested that the administration of recombinant human growth hormone (rhGH) (at 10 to 20 times the replacement dose) in a variety of patients with acute injury improves nitrogen balance (54) and that IGF-I accelerates recovery in experimental renal failure (55). It, therefore, would have been rational to believe that the use of such agents holds promise as adjunctive nutritional management during critical illness. However, two recent randomized controlled trials (56) have demonstrated clearly that rhGH increases mortality in critically ill patients. The same may apply to rhIGF-I. Also, two further randomized controlled trials in surgical patients with postoperative renal dysfunction or in critically ill patients with ARF have shown minimal or absent effects of IGF-I on renal function (57,58). Accordingly, both GH and IGF-I currently do not offer promise for the nutritional management of ARF.

A Suggested Approach to Nutrition in Critically Ill Patients Undergoing Continuous Renal Replacement Therapy

In light of the evidence presented in this chapter, the growing concern about increased mortality with the use of TPN (59), and the possible beneficial effects of full and early enteral nutrition (60) and immunonutrition (61), we suggest the following approach to nutritional support during CRRT:

1. Institute enteral nutrition early after admission to ICU.
2. Start enteral nutrition at full dose immediately.
3. Consider a preparation rich in ω-3 fatty acids.
4. If during nasogastric (NG) feeding 6-hr gastric residual is greater than 300 mL, introduce motility-enhancing agents (erythromycin 200 mg intravenously [IV] qid or metoclopramide at 10 to 20 mg IV qid).
5. If motility agents are not successful, insert nasojejunal (NJ) feeding tube and start NJ feeding.
6. Administer approximately 1.5 to 2.5 g/kg of protein per day.
7. Administer approximately 120 to 160 kJoule/kg/day of energy intake.
8. Administer at least the RDA for all vitamins and trace elements.
9. Administer twice the RDA for folate, vitamin B_6, and vitamin C. Also consider additional zinc and selenium supplementation.
10. Control azotemia at all times (maintain serum urea between 10 to 20 mmol/L) by adjusting the intensity of CRRT as necessary.

With this approach we have been able to decrease TPN use to less than 5% of patients with severe ARF. We also have been able to achieve nitrogen balances approximating neutral values in most patients. We recognize that no elements of this suggested approach are supported by randomized controlled trials or have been shown to have an impact on morbidity and mortality. However, when faced with clinical situations, physicians still must make judgments about what is a logical and rational treatment at the present time until further evidence emerges to either confirm or contradict available data and expert opinion.

Therapeutic nihilism is often the consequence of lack of appreciation of the quality of available evidence. Furthermore, the belief that absence of randomized controlled evidence equates absence of any evidence is unreasonable. It is also unreasonable to believe that any treatment or even lack of treatment is equal to a treatment plan generated by thoughtful consideration of the data available. Therefore, we believe that the approach outlined here is logical, physiologically sound, and supported by available animal experiments and limited human studies.

REFERENCES

1. Cole L, Bellomo R, Silvester W, et al. A prospective multicenter study of the epidemiology, management and outcome of severe acute renal failure in a closed ICU system. Am *J Respir Crit Care Med* 2000;162:191–196.
2. Flugel-Link RM, Salusky IB, Jones MR, et al. Protein and amino acid metabolism in the posterior hemicorpus of acutely uremic rats. *Am J Physiol* 1983;244:615–623.
3. Lacy WW. Effect of acute uremia on amino acid uptake and urea production by perfused rat liver. *Am J Physiol* 1969;216: 1300–1305.
4. Druml W. Protein metabolism in acute renal failure. *Miner Electrolyte Metab* 1998;24:47–54.
5. Druml W, Burger U, Kleinberger G, et al. Elimination of amino acids in acute renal failure. *Nephron* 1986;40:261–290.
6. Siegel JH, Cerra FB, Coleman B, et al. Physiological and metabolic correlations in human sepsis. *Surgery* 1979;86(2):163–193.
7. DeFronzo RA, Smith D, Alverstrand A. Insulin action in uremia. *Kidney Int* 1983;24(Suppl 16):S102–S114.
8. Mitch WE, May RC, Maroni BJ, et al. Protein and amino acid metabolism in uremia: influence of metabolic acidosis. *Kidney Int* 1989;36(suppl 27):S205–S207.
9. May RC, Kelly RA, Mitch WE. Mechanisms for defects in muscle protein metabolism in rats with chronic uremia: the influence of metabolic acidosis. *J Clin Invest* 1987;79:1099–1103.
10. Baliga R, George VT, Ray PE, et al. Effects of reduced renal function and dietary protein on muscle protein synthesis. *Kidney Int* 1991;39:831–835.
11. Schneeweiss B, Graninger W, Stockenhuber F, et al. Energy metabolism in acute and chronic renal failure. *Am J Clin Nutr* 1990; 52:596–601.
12. Zaloga G. Dietary lipids: ancestral ligands and regulators of cell signaling pathways. *Crit Care Med* 1999;27:1646–1648.
13. Zaloga G. Immune-enhancing enteral diets: where's the beef? *Crit Care Med* 1998;26:1143–1146.
14. Daly JM, Lieberman MD, Goldfine J, et al. Enteral nutrition with supplemental arginine, RNA, and omega-3 fatty acids in patients after operation: immunologic, metabolic and clinical outcome. *Surgery* 1992;112:56–67.
15. Bower RH, Cerra FB, Bershadsky B, et al. Early enteral administration of a formula (Impact) supplemented with arginine, nucleotides, and fish oil in intensive care unit patients: results of a multicenter, prospective, randomized, clinical trial. *Crit Care Med* 1995;23:436–449.
16. Atkinson S, Sieffert E, Bihari D. A prospective randomized, double-blind controlled clinical trial of enteral immunonutrition in the critically ill. Guy's Hospital Intensive Care Group. *Crit Care Med* 1998;26:1164–1172.
17. Gadek JE, De Michele SJ, Karlstad MD, et al. Effect of enteral feeding with eicosapentaenoic acid, γ-linolenic acid, and antioxidants in patients with acute respiratory distress syndrome. *Crit Care Med* 1999;27:1409–1420.
18. Bellomo R, Martin H, Parkin G, et al. Continuous arterio-venous hemofiltration in the critically ill. Influence on major nutrients. *Intensive Care Med* 1991;17:399–402.
19. Story D, Ronco C, Bellomo R. A prospective, controlled study of trace element and vitamin concentrations and losses in critically ill patients treated with continuous veno-venous hemofiltration. *Crit Care Med* 1999;27:220–223.
20. Fortin MC, Amyot SL, Geadah D, et al. Serum concentrations and clearances of folic acid and pyridoxal-5-phosphate during veno-venous continuous renal replacement therapy. *Intensive Care Med* 1999;25:594–598.
21. Opal SM. Selenium replacement in severe systemic inflammatory response syndrome. *Crit Care Med* 1999;27:2042–2043.
22. Nath KA, Paller MS. Dietary deficiency of anti-oxidants exacerbates ischemic injury in the rat kidney. *Kidney Int* 1990;38: 1109–1117.
23. Joannidis M, Bonn G, Pfaller W. Lipid peroxidation—an initial event in experimental acute renal failure. *Renal Physiol Biochem* 1989;12:47–55.
24. Radrizzani D, Iapichino G, Cambisano M, et al. Peripheral, visceral and body nitrogen balance in catabolic patients, without and with parenteral nutrition. *Intensive Care Med* 1988;14:212–216.
25. Bartlett RH, Mault JR, Deckert RE, et al. Continuous arteriovenous hemofiltration: improved survival in surgical acute renal failure? *Surgery* 1986;100:400–408.
26. Bartlett RH. Energy metabolism in acute renal failure. In: Sieberth HG, Mann H, eds. *Continuous arteriovenous hemofiltration (CAVH).* Basel: Karger, 1985:194–203.
27. Feinstein EI, Blumenkrantz MJ, Healy M, et al. Clinical and metabolic responses to parenteral nutrition in acute renal failure. A controlled double-blind study. *Medicine* 1981;60:124–137.
28. Feinstein EI, Kopple JD, Silberman H, et al. Total parenteral nutrition with high or low nitrogen intakes in patients with acute renal failure. *Kidney Int* 1983;24(Suppl 16):S319–S323.
29. Leonard CD, Luke RG, Siegel RR. Parenteral essential amino acids in acute renal failure. *Urology* 1975;6:154–157.
30. Kierdorf HP. The nutritional management of acute renal failure in the intensive care unit. *New Horizons* 1995;3:699–707.
31. Kopple JD. The nutritional management of the patient with acute renal failure. *JPEN J Parenter Enteral Nutr* 1996;20:3–12.
32. Bouffard Y, Viale JP, Annat G, et al. Energy expenditure in the acute renal failure patient mechanically ventilated. *Intensive Care Med* 1987;13:401–404.
33. Cahill GF Jr. Starvation in man. *N Engl J Med* 1970;282: 668–675.
34. Mault JR, Bartlett RH, Deckert RE, et al. Starvation: a major contributing factor to mortality in acute renal failure. *Trans Am Soc Artif Intern Organs* 1983;29:390–394.
35. Rennie MJ. Muscle protein turnover and the wasting due to injury and disease. *Br Med Bull* 1985;41:257–264.
36. Bessey PQ. Nutritional support in critical illness. In: Deitch EA, ed. *Multiple organ failure.* Stuttgart, Germany: Thieme, 1990: 126–149.
37. Bellomo R. Nutrition in acute renal failure. In: Bellomo R, Ronco C, eds. *Acute renal failure in the critically ill.* Heidelberg, Germany: Springer-Verlag, 1995:164–180.

38. Abel RM, Beck CH, Abbott WM, et al. Improved survival from acute renal failure after treatment with intravenous essential l-amino acids and glucose. *N Engl J Med* 1973;288:695–699.
39. Davies SP, Reaveley DA, Brown EA, et al. Amino acid clearances and daily losses in patients with acute renal failure treated by continuous arteriovenous haemodialysis. *Crit Care Med* 1991; 19(12):1510–1515.
40. Hynote ED, McCamish MA, Depner TA, et al. Amino acid losses during hemodialysis: Effects of high-solute flux and parenteral nutrition in acute renal failure. *JPEN J Parenter Enteral Nutr* 1995;19(1):15–21.
41. Frankenfield DC, Badellino MM, Reynolds HN, et al. Amino acid loss and plasma concentration during continuous hemodiafiltration. *JPEN J Parenter Enteral Nutr* 1993;17(6):551–561.
42. Davenport A, Roberts NB. Amino acid losses during haemofiltration. *Blood Purif* 1989;7:192–196.
43. Wolfson M, Jones MR, Kopple JD. Amino acid losses during hemodialysis with infusion of amino acids and glucose. *Kidney Int* 1982;21:500–506.
44. Kihara M, Ikeda Y, Fujita H, et al. Amino acid losses and nitrogen balance during diurnal hemodialysis in critically ill patients with renal failure. *Intensive Care Med* 1997;23:110–113.
45. Bellomo R, Seacombe J, Daskalakis M, et al. A prospective comparative study of moderate versus high protein intake for critically ill patients with acute renal failure. *Renal Failure* 1997;19: 111–120.
46. Kierdorf H, Stehle P, Behrend W, et al. Influence of anew amino acid (AA)–solution with increased amount of essential and branched-chain AA on protein catabolism in acute renal failure and multiple organ failure (MOF). *J Clin Nutr* 1991;10(Suppl 2):57–58.
47. Malis CD, Racusen LC, Solez K, et al. Nephrotoxicity of lysine and of a single dose of aminoglycosides in rats given lysine. *J Lab Clin Med* 1984;103:660–676.
48. Zager RA, Venkatachalam MA. Potentiation of ischemic renal injury by amino acid infusion. *Kidney Int* 1983;24:620–625.
49. Zager RA, Johannes G, Tuttle SE, et al. Acute amino acid nephrotoxicity. *J Lab Clin Med* 1983;130–140.
50. Toback GF. Amino acid enhancement of renal regeneration after acute tubular necrosis. *Kidney Int* 1977;12:193–198.
51. Houdijk APJ, Rijnsburger ER, Jansen J, et al. Randomised trial of glutamine-enriched enteral nutrition on infectious morbidity in patients with multiple trauma. *Lancet* 1998;352:772–776.
52. Bellomo R, Colman PG, Caudwell J, et al. Acute continuous hemofiltration with dialysis: effect on insulin concentrations and glycemic control in critically ill patients. *Crit Care Med* 1992; 20:1672–1676.
53. Bellomo R, McGrath B, Boyce N. The impact of continuous veno-venous hemofiltration with dialysis on hormone and catecholamine clearance in critically ill patients with acute renal failure. *Crit Care Med* 1994;22:833–837.
54. Ziegler TR, Rombeau JL, Young LS, et al. Recombinant human growth hormone enhances the metabolic efficacy of parenteral nutrition: a double-blind, randomized, controlled study. *J Clin Endocrinol Metab* 1992;74:865–873.
55. Hirschberg R, Adler S. Insulin-like growth factor system and the kidney: physiology, pathophysiology, and therapeutic implications. *Am J Kidney Dis* 1998;31:901–919.
56. Takala J, Ruokonen E, Webster N, et al. Increased mortality associated with growth hormone treatment in critically ill adults. *N Engl J Med* 1999;341:785–792.
57. Franklin C, Moulton M, Sicard G, et al. Insulin-like growth factor I preserves renal function post-operatively. *Am J Physiol* 1997;272:F257–F259.
58. Kopple J, Hirschberg R, Guler H, et al. Lack of effect of recombinant human insulin-like growth factor I (IGF-I) in patients with acute renal failure. *J Am Soc Nephrol* 1996;7:1375 (abstract).
59. Heyland DK, MacDonald S, Keefe L, et al. Total parenteral nutrition in the critically ill. A meta-analysis. *JAMA* 1998;280: 2013–2019.
60. Taylor SJ, Fettes SB, Jewkes C, et al. Prospective, randomized, controlled trial to determine the effect of early enhanced enteral nutrition on clinical outcome in mechanically ventilated patients suffering head injury. *Crit Care Med* 1999;27:2525–2531.
61. Beale RJ, Bryg DJ, Bihari DJ. Immunonutrition in the critically ill: a systematic review of clinical outcome. *Crit Care Med* 1999; 27:2799–2805.

32

THERAPEUTIC USE OF GROWTH FACTORS IN RENAL DISEASE

RALPH RABKIN

Protein-energy malnutrition, manifested as loss of muscle mass and reduced serum albumin, prealbumin, and transferrin levels, is relatively common in patients with advanced kidney failure (occurring in 20% to 50% of these patients) (1). Protein-energy malnutrition is also common in patients with severe acute renal failure. Because of the greater morbidity and mortality rates in malnourished patients with renal failure, there is a pressing need to develop more effective treatments to enhance the nutritional status of these patients (2,3). One such approach is the use of recombinant growth factors and anabolic steroids for malnourished patients refractory to standard nutritional therapy (4). Recombinant growth factors also may have a place in promoting recovery of renal function after acute tubular injury (5) and for increasing renal function in advanced chronic renal failure (CRF) (6). Finally, growth hormone has been very effective in promoting body growth in children with stunted body growth as a result of renal failure.

Before considering the therapeutic use of growth factors for the management of malnourished patients with renal disease, it should be kept in mind that some basic steps often are sufficient to prevent or correct malnutrition in many patients, and it is important to institute these measures before considering more complicated regimens (3). First, it is essential to provide the appropriate amounts of calories and proteins to meet the patient's daily needs. Although this may appear straightforward, it is not always easily carried out in anorexic, seriously ill patients. Next, providing oral bicarbonate supplements—or for patients receiving renal replacement therapy, increasing the dialysate bicarbonate concentration—may suppress protein breakdown in acidotic subjects. It turns out that acidosis stimulates muscle proteolysis (7). Any coexistent or superimposed diseases such as diabetes or infection need to be effectively treated; increasing dialysis to provide a Kt/V above 1.2 is another essential step in preventing and correcting malnutrition (8). This general approach may need to be modified for the individual patient according to the etiology of the malnourished state. This falls into two major categories: inadequate food intake, usually resulting from a loss of appetite, and increased catabolism, often with impaired net protein synthesis (1,7). These categories usually overlap.

It is important that the clinician recognize that several of the common parameters used to evaluate the nutritional state of patients with end-stage renal disease (ESRD), such as the serum transferrin, prealbumin, and albumin levels, are severely affected by chronic inflammation, a common event in patients receiving renal replacement therapy (1,9). It has been shown that prolonged subclinical inflammation, detectable by measurement of the serum C-reactive protein and amyloid A levels, is a frequent cause of low serum albumin levels in patients undergoing dialysis and that this is the result of a decrease in protein synthesis (10). This effect is induced by proinflammatory cytokines, such as tumor necrosis factor α and certain interleukins, and in some patients these cytokines may be the cause of refractory malnutrition. Although it is established that malnutrition and chronic inflammation adversely affect the patient's long-term outcome, it is now evident that both conditions are separately predictive of an increase in morbidity, and treatment should be directed accordingly (3,11).

Aggravating the negative effects of protein-calorie malnutrition in patients with renal failure are the endocrine changes that occur as renal function declines (12); these may be worsened further by malnutrition, chronic inflammation, and acidosis (13,14). In addition to the alterations in the production, secretion, and metabolism of hormones that occur in uremia, an especially important endocrine change is insensitivity to the action of hormones such as insulin, growth hormone (GH), and insulinlike growth factor-1 (IGF-1) (12). Although the mechanisms of resistance are not fully understood, in the case of insulin it appears to be the result of a defect in postreceptor signal transduction (15). With respect to GH, resistance largely has been attributed to insensitivity to IGF-1 (12). Expression of this growth factor is regulated by GH and mediates many of the actions of GH. However, the situation may be more complex because, as discussed later, GH-mediated receptor signal transduction via the JAK/STAT (Janus kinase/signal transducer and activator of transcription) pathway also is impaired in uremia (16). In contrast to insulin and GH, resistance to IGF-1 mainly is caused by increased sequestration of IGF-1 by circulating high-affinity IGF-binding proteins (IGFBPs) that increase in concentration in renal failure (17), although post-IGF-1 receptor signaling defect also may be present (18). Compounding the adverse effects of uremia on the GH–IGF-1 axis are the suppressive effects of protein-calorie malnutrition and chronic inflammation. Malnutrition, even in the absence of uremia, causes a depression of IGF-1 production, and serum IGF-1 levels decrease (13,14). The GH–IGF-1 axis also is depressed by acidosis and potassium depletion (14,19). Thus, when managing severely malnourished patients with renal failure, these endocrine changes must be taken into account and any underlying causes should be corrected whenever possible. Also, given that GH therapy is effective in promoting body growth in children with renal failure (20–23), it would seem reasonable to administer GH or IGF-1 to malnourished patients with renal failure who are unresponsive to standard therapy, so as to promote anabolism.

THERAPEUTIC USE OF GROWTH FACTORS IN RENAL DISEASE

Several recent clinical studies have begun to address the potential use of growth hormone and IGF-1 as well as anabolic steroids in the management of wasting in uremia. Although not generally thought of as growth factors, anabolic steroids also have shown promise in the management of uremic wasting. Insulin, essential for normal growth, is also potently anabolic, but because of its hypoglycemic action, it generally is reserved for the management of the patient with diabetes. The following discussion reviews the use of growth factors in the management of wasting in renal failure and the potential use of growth factors to augment renal function in advanced CRF and to enhance recovery from acute tubular necrosis.

GROWTH FACTORS IN THE MANAGEMENT OF WASTING IN RENAL DISEASE

Growth Hormone

One of the most successful therapeutic applications of a recombinant growth factor in clinical nephrology has been in the treatment of growth failure in children with CRF. The other is treatment of anemia with erythropoietin. Encouraging results also have been obtained in several small studies examining the use of growth hormone in the management of wasting in malnourished adults with ESRD (24–30). Before going into details regarding the therapeutic usage of GH in renal disease, however, a brief description of the physiology of the GH–IGF-1 system and the changes that occur in renal failure will be provided.

Growth Hormone Physiology and Perturbations in Renal Failure

Growth hormone is a 22-kD, 191-amino acid protein synthesized in the pituitary gland and released into the circulation in a pulsatile manner (Fig. 32.1). These processes are regulated largely by two hypothalamic hormones: somatostatin, which is inhibitory, and growth hormone–releasing hormone, which is stimulatory (31–33). In addition, other factors that influence GH production and secretion include the peptide hormone ghrelin, produced in the stomach and hypothalamus; leptin; neuropeptide Y; and fatty acids and other nutrients. Together these factors appear to coordinate GH secretion and metabolism. Nutrient intake regulates GH secretion in a manner that tends to preserve lean body mass during energy restriction. Fasting increases pulsatile GH secretion in humans (31,33). Oral or intravenous glucose loads acutely decrease serum GH levels by increasing the release of somatostatin. Insulin-induced acute hypoglycemia increases GH secretion by decreasing somatostatin release. Arginine, and potentially other amino acids, intravenously infused or taken as a high-protein meal, strongly increases GH secretion. Free fatty acids also reduce GH secretion by a direct suppressive effect on the pituitary gland.

Apart from its action to promote longitudinal bone growth, GH induces amino acid uptake and protein synthesis in muscle, resulting in a positive nitrogen balance (31). GH also has lipolytic effects on fat and muscle that leads to increased fat mobilization and a decrease in body fat. This, together with its action on protein synthesis, leads to an increase in lean body mass. It also modulates carbohydrate, fluid, and electrolyte balance and influences the immune system. In addition, GH regulates the expression of IGF-1, IGFBPs, and the acid-labile subunit that binds with IGF-1 and IGFBP-3. Many, but not all, of the actions of GH are mediated through the action of IGF-1, including essentially all of the anabolic effects of IGF-1 (31,32).

In patients with CRF, fasting plasma GH levels usually are normal or even elevated, depending on the severity of the renal failure (21,34). Generally, GH production is decreased, although in some prepubertal children it actually may be increased (34–36), and adults with ESRD have an exaggerated release of GH in response to GH-releasing hormone (37). Because GH largely is cleared from the circulation through the kidney, its metabolic clearance rate is reduced in CRF (38), and this accounts for the normal or elevated plasma GH levels in CRF, even in the presence of reduced GH production (39). Despite these normal or elevated GH levels, children with CRF have retarded body growth and require large doses of GH to promote body growth (39,40). Resistance to GH also has been demonstrated in the uremic rat (41–43). Although the mechanism of GH resistance is not fully understood, there is evidence of resistance to IGF-1 action (18,44) and possibly a defect in GH-receptor expression (41,43).

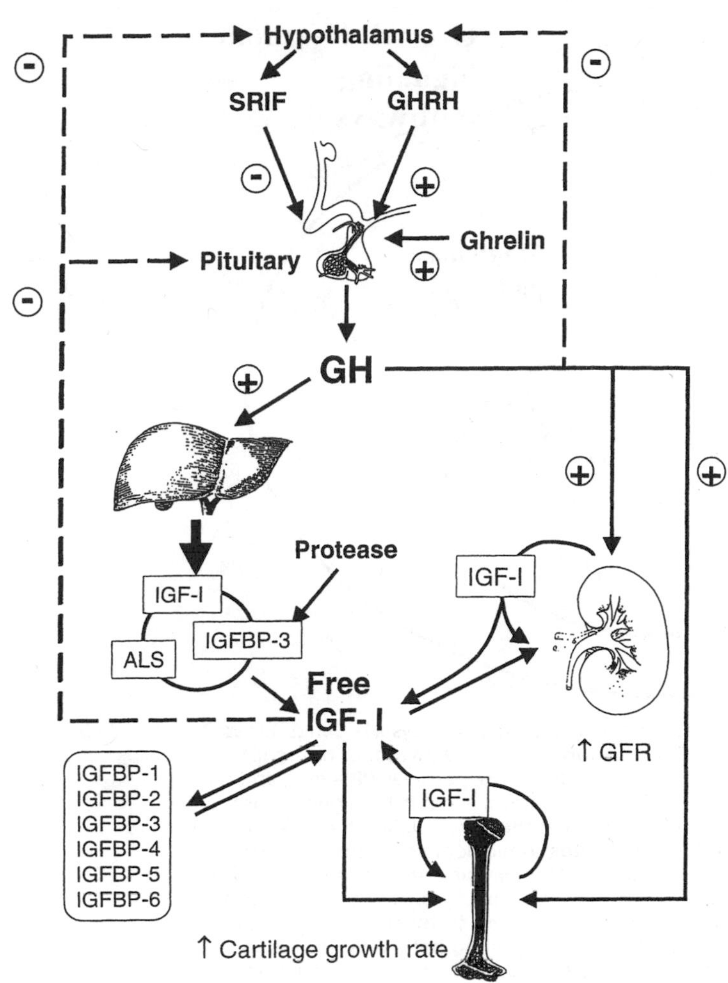

FIGURE 32.1. The growth hormone (GH)–insulin-like growth factor-1 (IGF-1) axis. The synthesis and release of GH from the pituitary are controlled by the hypothalamic hormones, growth hormone–releasing hormone (GHH) and somatostatin (SRIF), which in turn are regulated by feedback (*dashed lines*) from blood GH and IGF-1 concentrations. The recently discovered endogenous GH-releasing peptide, called ghrelin, also stimulates GH release. Circulating GH acts directly on many organs to stimulate IGF-1 production, with IGF-1 production in the liver providing the main source of blood IGF-1. Most of the IGF-1 in the circulation is bound to IGF-binding protein-3 (IGFBP-3) in a ternary complex with acid-labile subunit (ALS); a smaller fraction is bound to the five other IGFBPs. A small fraction of the total IGF-1 in blood is in a bioactive-free fraction. In the kidney, IGF-1 increases renal plasma flow and GFR, whereas on bone it acts on the epiphysial plate, which leads to longitudinal bone growth. As illustrated, GH also has direct effects on many organs, including kidney and cartilage, which can be independent of IGF-1 action. (From Roelfsema V, Clark RG. The growth hormone and insulin-like growth factor axis: its manipulation for the benefit of growth disorders in renal failure. *J Am Soc Nephrol* 2001; 12:1297–1306, with permission.)

The growth hormone receptor, a transmembrane glycoprotein, is distributed in tissues throughout the body including liver, heart, kidney, intestine, lung, muscle, pancreas, brain, and testes (31,45). Each GH molecule binds two receptors, inducing receptor dimerization. This is followed by receptor signal transduction that is mediated through the receptor intracellular domain (see Carter-Su and Smit [45] and Carter-Su et al. [46] for a review). A truncated variant of GH known as the growth hormone–binding protein (GHBP) is present in the circulation and also binds GH with relatively high affinity (47). In humans GHBP is generated largely by proteolytic cleavage of the GH receptor. The expression of the intact GH receptor appears to be regulated by GH; chronically elevated GH levels increase GH binding in liver, whereas acute increases in GH tend to downregulate GH receptor expression (13). Nutrients also influence GH receptor and GHBP abundance. In humans the GHBPs bind approximately 50% of the circulating GH, slowing its clearance and reducing its bioavailability. Circulating GHBP levels in humans are believed to reflect tissue GH receptor abundance and are used as an indirect measurement of GH number, although the validity of this assumption has not been tested rigorously (47).

There are several reports of low GHBP levels in patients with CRF (48–50), and this has been taken to indicate that cellular GH levels are reduced in renal failure, although there is no direct evidence to support this conclusion. In contrast, a recent study of 69 children with CRF failed to show low GHBP levels (51). However, this interpretation requires caution because the controls used for comparison were from an older study. Some support for a defect at the level of the GH receptor is provided from studies with uremic rats that show reduced hepatic GH receptor messenger RNA (mRNA) levels and reduced growth plate GH receptor protein levels (41,43). However, there are studies that indicate that hepatic GH receptor protein levels are unaltered by uremia (16,52) and that reduced food intake is the main cause of reduced GH receptor expression (41,52).

Another potential cause of GH resistance is a defect in the postreceptor signaling pathway at one or more sites. In a 2001 study of uremic rats, we demonstrated a convincing defect in a pathway that involves the tyrosine kinase janus kinase 2 (JAK2), which in turn phosphorylates and activates members of a protein family that serve as both signal transducers and activators of transcription (STAT) (16). This signaling pathway is illustrated in Fig. 32.2. In our study

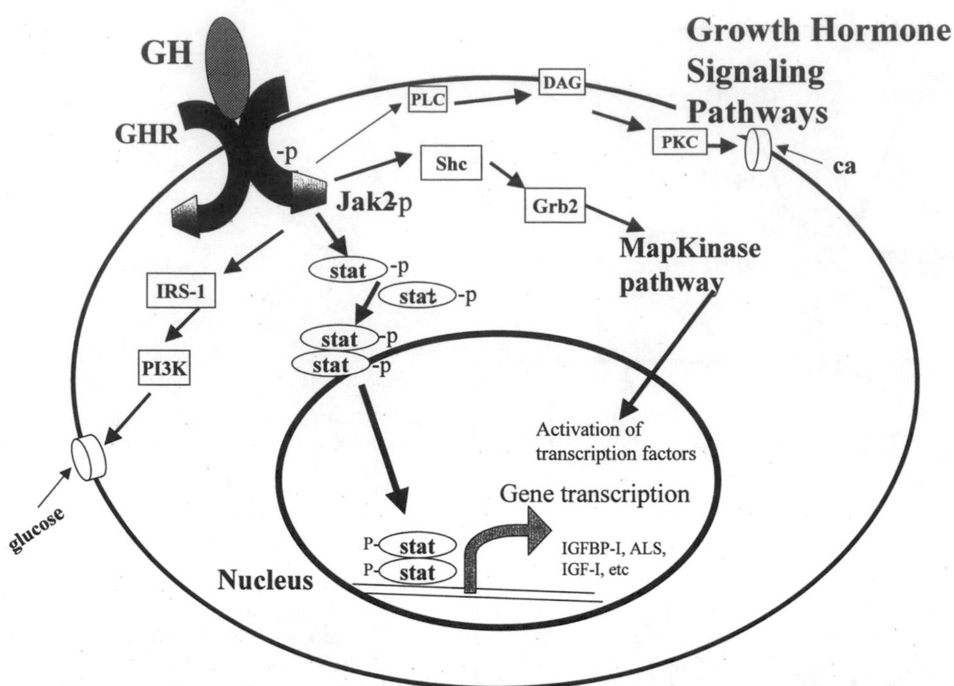

FIGURE 32.2. Growth hormone (GH) activates several signaling pathways via Janus kinase2 (JAK2), including the recently described JAK/STAT (signal transducer and activator of transcription) pathway, the insulin receptor substrate-phosphatidyl-inositol-3-kinase pathway (IRS-PI-3), and the mitogen-activated protein (MAP) kinase pathway (45,46). The earliest event in GH signal transduction is the binding of GH to its receptor, which in turn activates the enzyme JAK2 tyrosine kinase. The activated JAK2 phosphorylates both itself and the cytoplasmic domain of the GH receptor on tyrosine residues. Proteins bound to the GH receptor–JAK2 complex are phosphorylated by JAK2, leading to their activation and interaction with other signaling proteins. Alternatively, recruitment to the complex alone may be sufficient for some proteins to function in signal transduction. These initial activation steps in turn activate several signaling pathways, including the GH-activated STAT pathway. This latter pathway involves STAT 1a, 3, 5a, and 5b—members of a larger family of latent cytoplasmic transcription factors. These particular STATs are recruited to the activated GH receptor–JAK2 complex where they are tyrosine phosphorylated, after which they translocate to the nucleus where they bind to specific DNA sequences and activate their target genes. Ablation of STAT5 expression leads to retarded body growth. In renal failure phosphorylation of JAK2 and the downstream signaling molecules STAT5, STAT3, and STAT1 are impaired as is the level of phosphorylated STAT proteins (16). This may be one cause of resistance to GH that occurs in uremia. (Adapted from Carter-Su C, Smit L. Signaling via JAK tyrosines kinases: growth hormone receptor as a model system. *Recent Prog Horm Res* 1998;53:61–82.)

we found that although GH receptor binding and the levels of the downstream proteins—namely, JAK2, STAT5, 3, and 1—were unaffected by uremia, tyrosine phosphorylation of these proteins was depressed. Because activation of STAT5 is required for normal growth, we concluded that this defect in JAK-STAT phosphorylation contributes to the GH-resistant state and hence the stunted body growth and wasting seen in uremia. An acquired defect in GH receptor-JAK2/STAT signaling also has been described in inflammatory conditions, and, although somewhat different to that seen in uremia, this may account for GH resistance in patients with ESRD with underlying chronic inflammation (53). It also should be recognized that malnutrition alone impairs GH-stimulated IGF-1 gene transcription and translation (13); thus, malnutrition in uremia may worsen the resistance to GH. Finally, there is evidence that in uremia resistance to GH is to a large part caused by insensitivity to the action of IGF-1, its major mediator (17,18,21).

Therapeutic Use of Growth Hormone to Promote Growth in Children and to Improve the Nutritional State in Adults

The most effective use of a growth factor in clinical nephrology has been in the treatment of growth failure in children with CRF (20–23). Administration of GH in pharmacologic doses induces significant catchup body growth in these children, and with long-term treatment and commencing treatment at a sufficiently early age, most children are able to attain normal adult height albeit at the lower level of normal (20) (Fig. 32.3). This treatment also stimulates body protein synthesis and has an antilipolytic effect. These ac-

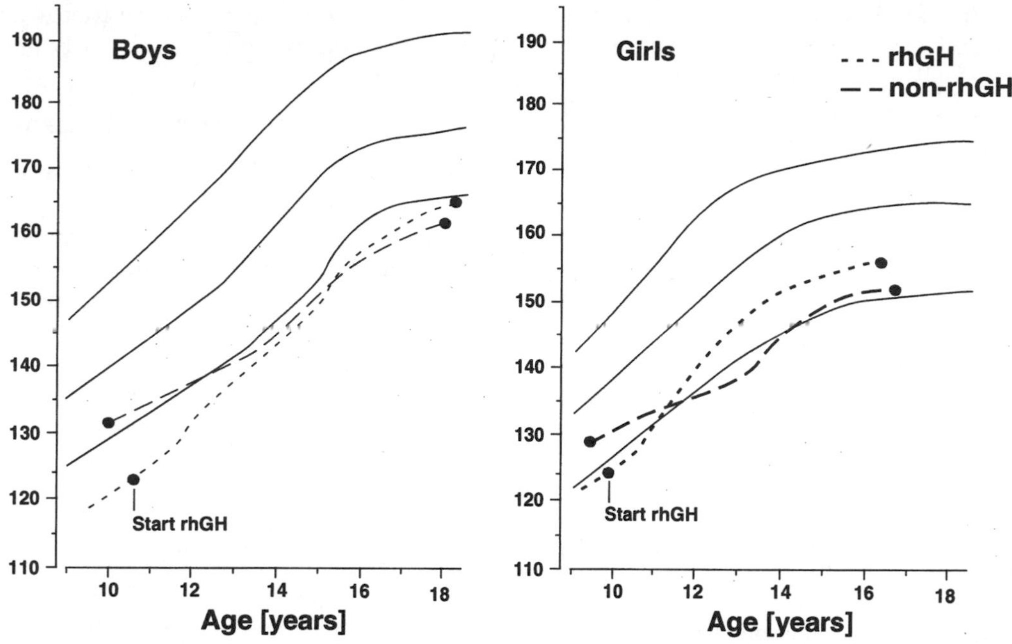

FIGURE 32.3. Synchronized mean growth curves during growth hormone (GH) treatment for 38 children (32 boys and six girls) with chronic renal failure, as compared with 50 control children with chronic renal failure not treated with GH, according to sex. Of the GH-treated children, 65% attained normal adult height. Normal values are indicated by the 3rd, 50th, and 97th percentiles. The circles indicate the time of the first observation (the start of GH treatment in the treated children) and the end of the pubertal growth spurt. (From Haffner D, Schaefer F, Nissel R, et al. Effect of growth hormone treatment on the adult height of children with chronic renal failure. German Study Group for Growth Hormone Treatment in Chronic Renal Failure. *N Engl J Med* 2000;343:923–930, with permission. © 2001 Massachusetts Medical Society.)

tions lead to a change in body composition with a decrease in body fat and an increase in lean body mass (54). Growth hormone now is approved in the United States and Europe for the treatment of growth retardation in children with uremia. Side effects have been minor and mainly limited to the induction of hyperinsulinemia; there has been no evidence of accelerated renal failure (20–23).

Several investigators have studied the use of GH to improve the nutritional status of adults with ESRD, and although the studies were limited in respect to the number of patients studied, the duration of study, and the presence or absence of malnutrition, the results have been encouraging (24). In a preliminary study, Kopple et al. administered GH daily to severely malnourished patients undergoing maintenance dialysis for 17 ± 2 days (55). Four patients developed a strong anabolic response as evidenced by a sustained increase in serum IGF-1, a decrease in serum urea nitrogen (SUN), and an increase in positive nitrogen balance. However, two patients, who were acutely ill during the study, generated only a slight increase in serum IGF-1 and a limited increase in the positive nitrogen balance. Ziegler et al. (25), studying five adequately nourished patients undergoing regular hemodialysis, showed that GH administered three times a week for 14 days induced an anabolic response. The predialysis SUN levels fell by 25%, and the urea generation and net protein catabolic rates fell significantly. Serum IGF-1 and serum phosphate levels also fell. Schulman et al. (26) studied the effect of GH together with intradialytic parenteral nutrition in seven malnourished patients hemodialyzed with a Kt/V of 1.03. Although intradialytic parenteral nutrition alone had no positive effect on nutritional parameters, the addition of GH therapy induced a significant increase in serum albumin, transferrin, and IGF-1 levels.

In a prospective crossover designed study of GH therapy in patients maintained with peritoneal dialysis in which the patients served as their own controls, Ikizler et al. (27,28) showed that even 1 week of daily GH therapy was efficacious. Over this short period GH reduced the total urea nitrogen appearance as evidenced by a fall in SUN levels and daily nitrogen excretion; serum IGF-1 and IGFBP-3 levels increased. They also showed that GH caused a significant decrease in plasma and dialysate essential amino acid levels. This suggested that the net anabolic response induced by GH reflects a shift in amino acid metabolism toward muscle. This positive response to GH therapy also suggests that GH also may be of value in managing or preventing malnutrition in patients with acute renal failure.

In a rigorous self-controlled crossover study of six chronically wasted malnourished patients hemodialyzed regularly with a Kt/V of 1.26, Garibotto et al. (29) demonstrated that GH administered three times a week over a 6-week period induced a strongly positive anabolic response. There was a significant increase in protein synthesis, the negative protein balance observed in the postabsorptive state fell, and arm-muscle area increased. Serum IGF-1 and IGFBP-3 levels rose significantly. The net reduction in protein catabolism was attributed to an increase in free serum IGF-1. In a randomized control study of GH in 17 malnourished adults receiving maintenance hemodialysis or peritoneal dialysis, Iglesias et al. (56) showed that daily GH therapy for 4 weeks had a salutary nutritional effect. Body weight and serum IGF-1 and transferrin levels increased, whereas SUN levels fell, despite a constant food intake.

A long-term double-blind randomized controlled study of 31 malnourished adults undergoing maintenance hemodialysis was conducted by Hansen et al. (30). Twenty subjects completed the 6-month study. GH treatment administered three times per week induced an increase in lean body mass and a decrease in fat mass, especially truncal, whereas total body mass remained unchanged. The effect of GH on cardiac function also was examined in these subjects (57). GH caused a significant increase in left ventricular mass without any effect on ejection fraction and maximal work capacity. No changes in blood pressure or pulse rate were noted. In 1999 Johannsson et al. reported on a 6-month double-blind placebo-controlled study of GH treatment of 20 elderly subjects undergoing regular maintenance hemodialysis (58). The average age was 74 years. GH given three times each week produced an increase in lean body mass and serum albumin levels that was not observed in the placebo-treated group. In addition to the positive anabolic effects, GH treatment improved muscle function as measured by handgrip strength. Two of the elderly subjects in the GH treatment group died of undefined causes. The authors concluded that these deaths were consistent with the expected mortality in the age group studied.

In summary, several investigators have shown that in adults with CRF, short-term GH therapy lasting up to 6 weeks has been effective in decreasing net urea generation, improving dietary amino acid and protein utilization, and increasing protein synthesis. Serum albumin levels and arm-muscle area increased. In more prolonged studies lasting 6 months, treatment with GH caused a decrease in fat mass and an increase in lean body mass; muscle function also improved. Of note, it also has been reported that GH treatment enhances erythropoietin secretion in patients with anemia and CRF (59). Taken together, these preliminary studies are encouraging and point to the need for more extensive and prolonged studies in adult patients with advanced renal failure and in those receiving dialysis. However, before GH can be recommended as a therapeutic agent in the adult patient with kidney failure, it will be essential to establish not only that it is positively anabolic, but also that it improves the patient's functional capacity, reduces morbidity, and has an acceptable safety profile.

Safety of Growth Hormone Therapy

Growth hormone has been used for the treatment of malnutrition and wasting in several disease states other than renal failure. These include acquired immunodeficiency syndrome (AIDS), severe burns, cirrhosis, and chronic obstructive pulmonary disease (59–63). Because growth hormone has been effective and relatively safe in treating wasting in patients with AIDS (59), the short-term use of GH for this specific indication has been approved in the United States. However, because the cost of GH therapy is very high, its use has been restricted.

Adverse effects may occur in adults treated with GH. These effects include arthralgias, myalgias, carpal tunnel syndrome, hypertension, fluid retention, a flulike syndrome, hyperinsulinemia, and hyperglycemia (61). These side effects are infrequent and appear to be dose dependent; lowering the GH dose can diminish them. Of concern is the multicenter European studies carried out by Takala et al. in 1999 (63) that described not only an increase in morbidity but also a twofold increase in mortality in critically ill patients treated with GH. In this double-blind placebo-controlled study, critically ill patients in intensive care units (ICU) were treated with GH for up to 3 weeks with the objective of diminishing the catabolic response to injury, surgery, and sepsis. Most of the patients had undergone cardiac or abdominal surgery or suffered multiple traumas. On entry into the study almost all the patients had respiratory failure, and about one-fourth of them had some element of acute renal failure. Subjects with CRF were excluded from the study. Most of the deaths were attributed to uncontrolled infection, septic shock, or multiple organ failure. The pathogenesis of the increase in morbidity and mortality in the GH-treated group has not been established but may be related to a GH-mediated metabolic or proinflammatory properties (62). High-dose GH therapy may induce a state of hypermetabolism and a deficit in energy substrate. For example, although GH increases muscle protein synthesis, it decreases glutamine production, which is needed for immune cell and intestinal mucosal cell proliferation (64). Nevertheless, it is important to note that trials of GH therapy in patients with severe burns or trauma have not resulted in an increase in the mortality rate (62). In these studies pulmonary failure on entry was uncommon, and GH was effective in promoting wound healing and maintaining lean body mass (62,65).

With respect to children with renal failure, GH has been administered safely to those with pre-ESRD, those receiving maintenance dialysis, and to renal transplant recipients to promote body growth. Despite concerns that GH might accelerate the progression of renal disease, increase the rate of transplant rejection, or induce diabetes, there is no evidence that such adverse effects occur (22,66). Hyperinsulinemia and altered lipids are frequent findings, however, and the potential long-term adverse effects on the cardiovascular system need to be monitored (66,67).

The Growth Hormone Research Society (67) has issued a statement on the safety of GH since its commercial introduction in 1985 and concluded that "The extensive data, collected on a large number of children and adults treated with GH indicate that for current approved indications GH is safe." The Society recommended against initiating GH therapy in adult patients in the ICU and stated that ongoing pharmacologic GH treatment should be stopped if such a patient becomes critically ill. Finally, they concluded that this ICU trial should not discourage new studies of GH therapy in subjects that may benefit from GH. In this regard, because GH therapy appears to be safe for the long-term treatment of children with chronic kidney failure, more extensive and prolonged trials should be carried out in adult patients with ESRD to evaluate its efficacy in treating malnutrition and muscle wasting refractory to standard therapeutic regimens.

Insulinlike Growth Factor-1

Because the growth-promoting and anabolic actions of GH are mediated mainly by IGF-1, there has been considerable interest in determining whether IGF-1 treatment is more efficacious and safer than GH in the management of wasting in patients with ESRD. Before reviewing these studies a brief description of IGF-1 physiology and the impact of uremia thereon follows.

Insulinlike Growth Factor-1 Physiology and Perturbations in Renal Failure

Normally, IGF-1 is produced in tissues throughout the body, including kidney, muscle, and bone, under the influence of GH and nutrients (Fig. 32.1) (13,14,17,31,32,68). IGF-1 has general growth-promoting and anabolic properties (31). Although liver is the major source of circulating IGF-1, and bone, muscle, and kidney are three of its endocrine targets, locally produced IGF-1 is also important in promoting body growth (31). Circulating IGF-1 is bound mostly to high-affinity IGFBPs, especially IGFBP-3, that together with an acid-labile subunit forms a 150 kD complex (17,32,68). A lesser amount of IGF-1 circulates bound to IGFBP-1, -2, -4, and -6, and normally less than 2% is freely bioavailable. In general, IGFBPs inhibit IGF-1 action; however, some IGFBPs may enhance IGF-1 activity in certain tissues. Seven major IGFBPs have been described (members of an IGFBP superfamily) and are expressed in different patterns in tissues throughout the body (68). Serum IGF-1 levels are normal in well-nourished adults receiving dialysis and reduced in poorly nourished adults receiving dialysis and have been used as a marker of malnutrition (14). However, serum IGF-1 decreases or increases so rapidly as nutrient intake varies that serum IGF-1 levels are not good indicators of visceral protein mass or body composition. Children with CRF have normal or low-normal IGF-1 levels (21). In all subjects with CRF, the serum IGFBP profile is altered (17,21,40). In uremic rats, IGF-1 mRNA levels are reduced in liver, muscle, and long bone growth plate; this is the result of resistance to GH (16) and reduced nutrient intake (41,69). This decrease in IGF-1 in the presence of normal or elevated GH levels contributes to growth retardation. Whether tissue IGF-1 expression is reduced in uremic humans remains to be established.

Resistance to IGF-1 in patients with CRF has been attributed largely to the accumulation of circulating low–molecular-weight IGFBPs (21,39,70). Circulating IGFBP-1, -2, -4, and -6 levels are elevated, and it has been suggested that these IGFBPs might reduce IGF-1 bioavailability and account for the resistance to IGF-1. Immunoreactive IGFBP-3 levels also are increased in ESRD, but this increase is largely the result of accumulation of immunoreactive fragments with reduced IGF-1 affinity, a consequence of reduced renal clearance (32,71); intact IGFBP-3 levels are not elevated. Animal studies suggest that IGF-1 resistance in uremia also may be the result of an end-organ insensitivity caused by a postreceptor signaling defect (18), although the exact site of the defect is controversial (72). Tissue resistance also may arise because of altered local IGFBP production.

It is interesting that, unlike the metabolic clearance of GH that is largely renal and thus impaired in CRF, the metabolic clearance rate of IGF-1 is unaffected (73,74). However, because of the increase in several serum IGFBPs in the vascular compartment the volume of distribution of IGF-1 is decreased, and higher serum levels of IGF-1 are achieved in patients with CRF after the administration of IGF-1.

Insulinlike Growth Factor-1 in Nutritional Management

Early studies of small groups of patients receiving continuous ambulatory peritoneal dialysis or maintenance hemodialysis therapy indicated that IGF-1 has an anabolic effect in these patients, although they are resistant to IGF-1 as compared to normal subjects (44). Despite this resistance, administration of pharmacologic doses of recombinant human IGF-1 induces a more anabolic state. Fouque et al. administered rhIGF-1 (100 to 200 μg/kg/day) for 20 days to six malnourished patients undergoing chronic peritoneal dialysis who ingested a constant diet and underwent a constant peritoneal dialysis regimen (75). The patients had a body weight of 88% of desirable body weight and a serum albumin level averaging 2.8 g/dL. After starting IGF-1 treatment, serum IGF-1 rose dramatically. All patients showed a strong and sustained increase in nitrogen balance during the entire IGF-1 treatment period, from −0.06 g of nitrogen a day during baseline to approximately +1.9 g/day during the entire 20-day treatment period. The SUN and the nitrogen content of the dialysate fell during treatment. Both phenomena became evident within the first 24 hours of treatment. Another potentially more effective approach to treating wasting is combined treatment with GH and IGF-1. There is evidence indicating that combined treatment of hypocaloric, hypercatabolic volunteers who are free of renal disease induces an even stronger anabolic action than that attained with GH alone (32,76). In conclusion, it would seem that further studies are required to evaluate whether long-term IGF-1 treatment, either alone or together with GH, can improve the nutritional status, body composition, quality of life, morbidity, and mortality of malnourished patients with ESRD. Furthermore, it will be important to determine the safety profile of IGF-1 (see Section B).

Androgenic Steroids

Testosterone, the male steroid hormone, is essential for normal sexual differentiation, growth and development, and maintenance of secondary sexual characteristics (77). It primarily is synthesized in the Leydig cells of the testes; lesser amounts are produced by the adrenal gland and small amounts by the ovary (78). Besides its androgenic actions, testosterone and its active metabolites have important anabolic actions, such as promoting nitrogen retention and increasing muscle mass and body weight (77,78). Testosterone circulates in plasma largely bound to proteins; in advanced renal failure testosterone levels fall. Indeed, in about two-thirds of the males with ESRD, plasma testosterone levels are low, and it has been suggested that this contributes to the muscle wasting of uremia (79).

In view of its anabolic properties and its value in other wasting diseases such as AIDS (60), there has been interest in using androgens in the management of the wasted renal failure patient. This seems to be a reasonable approach, especially in males with low testosterone levels. Unfortunately, prolonged use of testosterone and several of its analogues carries the risk of significant side effects. These include disturbances in liver function, hepatocellular adenoma and carcinoma, altered plasma lipids, skin changes, and virilization (in females) (77). However, several small studies suggest that the non-17α-alkylated androgen, nandrolone, may be safer to use and that it is effective in improving weight gain and serum protein levels in patients with ESRD (77,80).

In a 1999 report Johansen et al. (81) described the results of a randomized double-blind, placebo-controlled trial in which they administered nandralone decanoate or saline by weekly intramuscular injection for 6 months to patients receiving maintenance peritoneal dialysis or hemodialysis therapy. Fourteen patients received androgens and 15 received saline. Compared to placebo-treated controls, the nandralone-treated subjects showed a significant increase in lean body mass and serum creatinine levels, suggesting that muscle mass had increased. Also, after 3 months of nandralone treatment, walking and stair-climbing times improved. However, after 6 months of treatment there was no significant difference between groups. Hematocrit was unaffected. The nandralone was well tolerated with only minimal side effects. In view of these encouraging findings and the low cost of treatment, further carefully controlled prolonged studies with special attention to the impact of nandralone on liver function and lipid profile are needed to establish whether androgens truly have a role in the management of wasting in uremia. It should be noted that in addition to their potential benefit in the management of malnutrition, androgens also may enhance the response to erythropoietin, and in some centers androgens are used for this reason to reduce the cost of anemia management (80).

USE OF GROWTH FACTORS TO AUGMENT RENAL FUNCTION IN CHRONIC RENAL FAILURE: GROWTH HORMONE AND INSULINLIKE GROWTH FACTOR-1

It has been known for many years that GH affects kidney size and function (68). This is best illustrated in patients with acromegaly. These patients have renal hypertrophy and an increase in glomerular filtration rate (GFR) and renal plasma flow (RPF) (82). These measures decrease after successful treatment of the acromegalic state. Conversely, renal function is low in GH-deficient states. In normal adults, one single intramuscular GH injection induces a 30% increase in GFR, which is delayed by about 20 hours and occurs in temporal association with an increase in serum IGF-1 levels (83). In contrast, IGF-1 administration causes a more similar but more rapid response, and by 6 hours after the injection GFR and RPF are increased (84). Taken together, this indicates that the GH-induced increase in renal function is mediated through the release of IGF-1. In rats, an intravenous IGF-1 infusion increases the GFR within 20 minutes, and these effects are mediated through an increase in RPF and the glomerular ultrafiltration coefficient (85). Renal tubular function also is affected by GH or IGF-1 administration; renal tubular phosphate and, to a lesser extent, sodium reabsorption increases (84). Retention of sodium and water is a side effect of chronic high-dose GH or IGF-1 treatment in adults (86). Some evidence supports a modest stimulatory effect of IGF-1 on sodium reabsorption in healthy adults (84).

Both recombinant GH and IGF-1 have been administered to patients with CRF. When adult patients with advanced CRF (20 mL/min/1.73 m^2 or lower) were treated with growth hormone for 3 days, GFR did not increase (87). In contrast, healthy volunteers displayed a modest 11% increase in GFR in response to GH. It is interesting that after GH administration, serum IGF-1 levels increased to three to four times baseline levels in both the patients with CRF and the normal subjects. Hepatic resistance to GH therefore cannot explain the absence of an increase in GFR in the CRF group. It is possible that the GH-induced increase in IGF-1 responsible for the modest increase in GFR observed in healthy subjects may not have been sufficient to induce a significant response in the patients with CRF. Similarly, GH treatment had no significant effect on renal function in children with CRF (66).

In contrast to GH, administration of IGF-1 to adults with CRF repeatedly has been shown in small studies to augment renal function (6). The earliest study of IGF-1 therapy, conducted by O'Shea et al. (88), was carried out with four patients with GFRs of 22 to 55 mL/min/1.73 m^2. IGF-1 was given subcutaneously twice a day for 3 days and induced a 41% to 71% increase in inulin clearance with a similar increase in para-ammohippurate clearance. Renal function declined to baseline within days after therapy was discontinued. The same group carried out a more prolonged study in subjects with more severe renal functional impairment (89). Five subjects with GFRs averaging 14 $\pm$ 2 mL/min/1.73 m^2 were treated with IGF-1, 100 μg/g subcutaneously twice a day. This resulted in a 28% increase in GFR on day 4, which subsequently decreased with time. Because of untenable side effects that included Bell's palsy, gingival hyperplasia, and pericarditis, only one patient completed the 28-day study protocol. The mechanism of the acquired resistance to the renal actions of the high-dose IGF-1 therapy was unclear but may be related to changes in the circulating IGFBP profile (6). IGF-1 administration causes a decrease in IGFBP-3 and an increase in the low–molecular-weight IGFBP-1 and -2 in patients with CRF (71,89). The net effect may be to decrease IGF-1 bioavailability because IGF-1 bound to the lower molecular weight IGFBPs is cleared more rapidly from the vascular compartment.

Ike et al. (71), using a lower dose of IGF-1, 60 μg/Kg twice a day, studied the renal response in six subjects with GFR averaging 16 mL/min/1.73 m^2 (71). Over a 28-day study period there was a modest increase in GFR of 14% that approached statistical significance ($p < 0.051$). Side effects attributable to IGF-1 were mild and included mild fluid retention responsive to diuretics, headache, and palpitations that resolved with lower IGF-1 dosage. Renal function returned to baseline after discontinuing the IGF-1 therapy. In a randomized double-blind placebo-controlled trial in 1999, Vijayen et al. (90) treated 10 patients with advanced CRF, GFR 8 $\pm$ 0.4 mL/min/1.73 m^2, for 31 days with an intermittent low IGF-1 dose schedule and followed them for 45 days. The patients received IGF-1 (50 μg/day) on 4 consecutive days followed by three treatment-free days. On days 17, 31, and 45, the inulin clearances were increased significantly by about 45%. Serum IGFBPs were not significantly different, and there was no evidence of tachyphylaxis. No patient required discontinuation of treatment because of adverse effects. One patient chose to continue therapy, and her renal function remained above baseline for about 1.5 years. Taken together, these studies indicate that IGF-1 can produce a sustained increase in renal function in patients with advanced renal failure without troubling side effects.

Although the adverse events reported in the last two studies were relatively minor and easily managed, concern has been expressed that long-term IGF-1 therapy might induce malignancies or accelerate the progression of kidney disease. The question of whether IGF-1 therapy can accelerate the progression arises from the observation that GH treatment worsens experimental kidney disease (91) and that GH transgenic mice develop glomerulosclerosis (92). In contrast, IGF-1 transgenic mice do not develop glomerulosclerosis (92). Furthermore, prolonged GH treatment of children with CRF does not lead to more rapid progression of renal failure, although the serum IGF-1 levels are increased (22). Concern regarding neoplasia has been based on recent epidemiologic studies that reported increases in the serum levels of IGF-1 in subjects who had, or who eventually developed, prostate or premenopausal breast cancer (93). Whether the elevated serum IGF-1 levels are related causally to an increase cancer risk has not been established. Because the proposed use of IGF-1 in the management of renal failure is likely to be limited in duration, and given the high morbidity and mortality of patients with ESRD, the use of IGF-1 for delaying the need for dialysis would seem reasonable. In many instances, this might allow for the placement and maturation of a permanent vascular access. However, before this point is reached, extensive long-term double-blind placebo-controlled studies are required to establish whether IGF-1 safely can induce a clinically significant increase in renal function in the patients with advanced CRF.

CONCLUSIONS

Although growth factors and anabolic steroids offer the potential for improving nutritional status, body composition, and even the motor function of malnourished patients with renal failure, further large-scale and prolonged studies are required before these agents can be used in clinical practice. The research should include an assessment of the impact of growth factors on body composition, functional ability, quality of life, and morbidity and mortality. In the meantime, much can be done to improve the nutritional status of the patient with kidney failure. This includes ensuring that the patient is receiving and ingesting needed nutrients sufficient to improve lean body mass, even if this requires tube feeding, parenteral nutrition, or intradialytic parenteral nutrition. It is also important to correct acidemia when present, to eliminate any source of chronic inflammation, and to establish that the patient with ESRD receives optimal dialysis therapy. Finally, for the patient with pre-ESRD, the potential of improving renal function by administering IGF-1, although encouraging, requires far more extensive evaluation before being considered for clinical use.

REFERENCES

1. Riella MC. Malnutrition in dialysis: malnourishment or uremic inflammatory response? *Kidney Int* 2000;57:1211–1232.
2. Ikizler TA, Hakim RM. Nutrition in end-stage renal disease. *Kidney Int* 1996;50:343–357.
3. Kopple JD. Therapeutic approaches to malnutrition in chronic dialysis patients: the different modalities of nutritional support. *Am J Kidney Dis* 1999;33:180–185.
4. Chen Y, Fervenza FC, Rabkin R. Growth factors in the treatment of wasting in kidney failure. *J Ren Nutr* 2001;11:62–66.
5. Hirschberg R. Biologically active peptides in acute renal failure: recent clinical trials. *Nephrol Dial Transplant* 1997;12: 1563–1566.
6. Vijayan A, Behrend T, Miller SB. Clinical use of growth factors in chronic renal failure. *Curr Opin Nephrol Hypertens* 2000;9: 5–10.
7. Mitch WE, Maroni BJ. Factors causing malnutrition in patients with chronic uremia. *Am J Kidney Dis* 1999;33:176–179.
8. Ikizler TA, Wingard RL, Hakim RM. Interventions to treat malnutrition in dialysis patients: the role of the dose of dialysis, intradialytic parenteral nutrition, and growth hormone. *Am J Kidney Dis* 1995;26:256–265.
9. Stenvinkel P, Heimburger O, Lindholm B, et al. Are there two types of malnutrition in chronic renal failure? Evidence for relationships between malnutrition, inflammation and atherosclerosis (MIA syndrome). *Nephrol Dial Transplant* 2000;15:953–960.
10. Kaysen GA. Inflammation, nutritional state and outcome in end stage renal disease. *Miner Electrolyte Metab* 1999;25:242–250.
11. Ikizler TA, Wingard RL, Harvell J, et al. Association of morbidity with markers of nutrition and inflammation in chronic hemodialysis patients: a prospective study. *Kidney Int* 1999;55: 1945–1951.
12. Rabkin R. Growth factor insensitivity in renal failure. *Ren Fail* 2001;23:291–300.
13. Thissen J, Ketelslegers J, Underwood L. Nutritional regulation of the insulin-like growth factors. *Endo Rev* 1997;15:80–101.
14. Rabkin R. Nutrient regulation of IGF-1. *Miner Electrolyte Metab* 1997;23:157–160.
15. Alvestrand A. Carbohydrate and insulin metabolism in renal failure. *Kidney Int* 1997;52:S48–S52.
16. Schaefer F, Chen Y, Tsao T, et al. Impaired JAK-STAT signal transduction contributes to growth hormone resistance in chronic uremia. *J Clin Invest* 2001;108:467–475.
17. Hirschberg R, Adler S. Insulin-like growth factor system and the kidney: physiology pathophysiology, and therapeutic implications. *Am J Kidney Dis* 1998;31:901–919.
18. Ding H, Gao X-L, Hirschberg R, et al. Impaired actions of IGF-I on protein synthesis and degradation in skeletal muscle of rats with CRF. *J Clin Invest* 1996;97:1064–1075.
19. Kuemmerle N, Krieg R, Latta K, et al. Growth hormone and insulin-like factor in non-uremic acidosis and uremic acidosis. *Kidney Int* 1997;51:5102–5105.
20. Haffner D, Schaefer F, Nissel R, et al. Effect of growth hormone treatment on the adult height of children with chronic renal failure. German Study Group for Growth Hormone Treatment in Chronic Renal Failure. *N Engl J Med* 2000;343:923–930.
21. Tönshoff B, Blum W, Mehls O. Derangements of the somatotropic hormone axis in chronic renal failure. *Kidney Int* 1997; 51:S106–S113.
22. Fine RM. Growth hormone treatment of children with chronic renal insufficiency and endstage renal disease following renal transplantation. *J Pediatr Endocrinol Metab* 1997;10:361–370.
23. Hokken-Koelega AC, Stijnen T, de Muinck K, et al. Placebo-controlled, double-blind, cross-over trial of growth hormone treatment in prepubertal children with chronic renal failure. *Lancet* 1991;338:585–590.
24. Iglesias P, Diez JJ. Recombinant human growth hormone therapy in adult dialysis patients. *Int J Artif Organs* 2000;23:802–804.
25. Ziegler TR, Lazarus JM, Young LS, et al. Effects of recombinant human growth hormone in adults receiving maintenance hemodialysis. *J Am Soc Nephrol* 1991;2:1130–1135.
26. Schulman G, Wingard RL, Hutchison RI, et al. The effects of recombinant human growth hormone and intradialytic parenteral nutrition in malnourished hemodialysis patients. *Am J Kidney Dis* 1993;21:527–534.
27. Ikizler TA, Wingard RL, Breyer JA, et al. Short-term effects of recombinant human growth hormone in CAPD patients. *Kidney Int* 1994;46:1178–1183.
28. Ikizler TA, Wingard RL, Flakoll PJ, et al. Effects of recombinant human growth hormone on plasma and dialysate amino acid profiles in CAPD patients. *Kidney Int* 1996;50:229–234.
29. Garibotto G, Barreca A, Russo R, et al. Effects of recombinant human growth hormone on muscle protein turnover in malnourished hemodialysis patients. *J Clin Invest* 1997;99:97–105.
30. Hansen TB, Gram J, Jensen PB, et al. Influence of growth hormone on whole body and regional soft tissue composition in adult patients on hemodialysis. A double-blind, randomized, placebo-controlled study. *Clin Nephrol* 2000;53:99–107.
31. Butler AA, Le Roith D. Control of growth by the somatropic axis: Growth hormone and the insulin-like growth factors have related and independent roles. *Annu Rev Physiol* 2001;63: 141–164.
32. Roelfsema V, Clark RG. The growth hormone and insulin-like growth factor axis: Its manipulation for the benefit of growth disorders in renal failure. *J Am Soc Nephrol* 2001;12:1297–1306.
33. Pombo M, Pombo CM, Garcia A, et al. Hormonal control of growth hormone secretion. *Horm Res* 2001;55:11–16 (Suppl 1).
34. Schaefer F, Veldhuis JD, Stanhope R, et al. Alterations in growth hormone secretion and clearance in peripubertal boys with chronic renal failure and after renal transplantation. *J Clin Endocrinol Metab* 1994;78:1298–1306.
35. Schaefer F, Hamill G, Stanhope R. Pulsatile growth hormone secretion in peripubertal patients with chronic renal failure. *J Pediatr* 1991;119:568–577.
36. Tönshoff B, Veldhuis JD, Heinrich U, et al. Deconvolution analysis of spontaneous nocturnal growth hormone secretion in prepubertal children with preterminal chronic renal failure and with end-stage renal disease. *Pediatr Res* 1995;37:86–93.
37. Ramirez G, Bercu BB, Bittle PA, et al. Response to growth hormone-releasing hormone in adult renal failure patients on hemodialysis. *Metabolism* 1990;39:764–768.
38. Haffner D, Schaefer F, Girard J. Metabolic clearance of recombinant human growth hormone in health and chronic renal failure. *J Clin Invest* 1994;93:1163–1171.
39. Blum WF, Ranke B, Kietzmann D, et al. Growth hormone resistance and inhibition of somatomedin activity by excess of IGF binding protein in uremia. *Ped Nephrol* 1991;5:539–544.
40. Zadik Z, Frishberg Y, Drukker A, et al. Excessive dietary protein and suboptimal caloric intake have a negative effect on the growth of children with chronic renal disease before and during growth hormone therapy. *J Clin Endocrinol Metab* 1998;47:264–268.
41. Chan W, Valerie KC, Chan JCM. Expression of insulin-like

growth factor-1 in uremic rats: growth hormone resistance and nutritional intake. *Kidney Int* 1993;43:790–795.

42. Mak RHK, Pak YK. End-organ resistance to growth hormone and IGF-I in epiphyseal chondrocytes of rats with chronic renal failure. *Kidney Int* 1996;50:400–406.
43. Edmondson SR, Baker NL, Oh J, et al. Growth hormone receptor abundance in tibial growth plates of uremic rats: GH/IGF-I treatment. *Kidney Int* 2000;58:62–70.
44. Fouque D, Peng S, Kopple JD. Impaired metabolic response to recombinant insulin-like growth factor 1 in dialysis patients. *Kidney Int* 1995;47:876–883.
45. Carter-Su C, Smit L. Signaling via JAK tyrosines kinases: growth hormone receptor as a model system. *Recent Prog Horm Res* 1998; 53:61–82.
46. Carter-Su C, Rui L, Herrington J. Role of the tyrosine kinase JAK2 in signal transduction by growth hormone. *Pediatr Nephrol* 2000;14:550–557.
47. Baumann G. Growth hormone binding protein. *J Pediatr Endocrinol Metab* 2001;14:355–375.
48. Postel-Vinay MC, Tar A, Crosnier H, et al. Plasma growth hormone-binding activity is low in uraemic children. *Pediatr Nephrol* 1991;5:545–547.
49. Bauman G. Growth hormone binding protein and free growth hormone in chronic renal failure. *Pediatr Nephrol* 1996;10: 328–330.
50. Tonshoff B, Cronin MJ, Reichert M, et al. Reduced concentration of serum growth hormone (GH)-binding protein in children with chronic renal failure: correlation with GH insensitivity. The European Study Group for Nutritional Treatment of Chronic Renal Failure in Childhood. The German Study Group for Growth Hormone Treatment in Chronic Renal Failure. *J Clin Endocrinol Metab* 1997;82:1007–1013.
51. Powell D, Liu F, Baker B, et al. Modulation of growth factors by growth hormone in children with chronic renal failure. *Kidney Int* 1997;51:1970–1979.
52. Villares S, Goujon L, Maniar S, et al. Reduced food intake is the main cause of low GH expression in uremic rats. *Mol Cell Endocrinol* 1994;106:51–56.
53. Mao Y, Ling PR, Fitzgibbons TP, et al. Endotoxin-induced inhibition of growth hormone receptor signaling in rat liver *in vivo*. *Endocrinology* 1999;140:5505–5515.
54. Johnson VL, Wang J, Kaskel FJ, et al. Changes in body composition of children with chronic renal failure on growth hormone. *Pediatr Nephrol* 2000;14:695–700.
55. Kopple JD. The rationale for the use of growth hormone or insulin-like growth factor 1 in adult patients with renal failure. *Miner Electrolyte Metab* 1992;18:269–275.
56. Iglesias P, Diez JJ, Fernandez-Reyes MJ, et al. Recombinant human growth hormone therapy in malnourished dialysis patients: *Am J Kidney Dis* 1998;32:454–463.
57. Jensen PB, Ekelund B, Nielsen FT, et al. Changes in cardiac muscle mass and function in hemodialysis patients during growth hormone treatment. *Clin Nephrol* 2000;53:25–32.
58. Johannsson G, Bengtsson BA, Ahlmen J. Double-blind, placebo-controlled study of growth hormone treatment in elderly patients undergoing chronic hemodialysis: Anabolic effect and functional improvement. *Am J Kidney Dis* 1999;33:709–717.
59. Sohmiya M, Ishikawa K, Kato Y. Stimulation of erythropoietin secretion by continuous subcutaneous infusion of recombinant human GH in anemic patients with chronic renal failure. *Eur J Endocrinol* 1998;138:302–307.
60. Corcoran C, Grinspoon S. Treatments for wasting in patients with the acquired immunodeficiency syndrome. *New Engl J Med* 1999;340:1740–1750.
61. Vance ML, Mauras N. Growth hormone therapy in adults and children. *N Engl J Med* 1999;341:1206–1216.
62. Demling R. Growth hormone therapy in critically ill patients. *N Engl J Med* 1999;341:837–839.
63. Takala J, Ruokonen E, Webster NR, et al. Increased mortality associated with growth hormone treatment in critically ill adults. *N Engl J Med* 1999;341:785–792.
64. Biolo G, Iscra F, Bosutti A, et al. Growth hormone decreases muscle glutamine production and stimulates protein synthesis in hypercatabolic patients. *Am J Physiol Endocrinol Metab* 2000; 279:E323–E332.
65. Jeschke MG, Barrow RE, Herndon DN. Recombinant human growth hormone treatment in pediatric burn patients and its role during the hepatic acute phase response. *Crit Care Med* 2000; 28:1578–1584.
66. Haffner D, Nissel R, Wuhl E, et al. Metabolic effects of long-term growth hormone treatment in prepubertal children with chronic renal failure and after kidney transplantation. The German Study Group for Growth Hormone Treatment in Chronic Renal Failure. *Pediatr Res* 1998;43:209–215.
67. Consensus. Critical evaluation of the safety of recombinant human growth hormone administration: Statement from the Growth Hormone Research Society. *J Clin Endocrinol Metab* 2001;86:1868–1870.
68. Feld S, Hirschberg R. Growth hormone, the insulin-like growth factor system, and the kidney. *Endocrine Rev* 1996;17:423–480.
69. Hanna J, Santos F, Foreman J, et al. Insulin-like growth factor-1 gene expression in the tibial epiphyseal growth plate of growth hormone-treated uremic rats. *Kidney Int* 1995;47:1374–1382.
70. Powell DR, Liu F, Baker BK, et al. Effect of chronic renal failure and growth hormone therapy on the insulin-like growth factors and their binding proteins. *Pediatr Nephrol* 2000;14:579–583.
71. Ike J, Fervenza F, Hintz R, et al. Early experience with extended use of IGF-I in the treatment of advanced chronic renal failure. *Kidney Int* 1997;51:840–849.
72. Tsao T, Fervenza FC, Friedlaender M, et al. Effect of prolonged uremia on insulin-like growth I autophosphorylation and tyrosine kinase activity in muscle. *Exp Nephrol* 2002;10:285–292.
73. Rabkin R, Fervenza FC, Maidment H, et al. Pharmacokinetics of insulin-like growth factor-1 in advanced chronic renal failure. *Kidney Int* 1996;49:1134–1140.
74. Fouque D, Peng SC, Kopple JD. Pharmacokinetics of recombinant human insulin-like growth factor-1 in dialysis patients. *Kidney Int* 1995;47:869–875.
75. Fouque D, Peng SC, Shamir E, et al. Recombinant human insulin-like growth factor-1 induces an anabolic response in malnourished CAPD patients. *Kidney Int* 2000;57:646–654.
76. Kupfer SR, Underwood LE, Baxter RC, et al. Enhancement of the anabolic effects of growth hormone and insulin-like growth factor 1 by use of both agents simultaneously. *J Clin Invest* 1993; 91:391–396.
77. Navarro JF, Mora C. In-depth review effect of androgens on anemia and malnutrition in renal failure: implications for patients on peritoneal dialysis. *Perit Dial Int* 2001;21:14–24.
78. Urban RJ. Effects of testosterone and growth hormone on muscle function. *J Lab Clin Med* 1999;134:7–10.
79. Handelsman DJ. Hypothalamic-pituitary gonadal dysfunction in renal failure, dialysis and renal transplantation. *Endocr Rev* 1985; 6:151–182.
80. Johnson CA. Use of androgens inpatients with renal failure. *Semin Dial* 2000;13:36–39.
81. Johansen KL, Mulligan K, Schambelan M. Anabolic effects of nandrolone decanoate in patients receiving dialysis: a randomized controlled trial. *JAMA* 1999;281:1275–1281.
82. Ikkos D, Ljunggren R, Luft R. Glomerular filtration rate and renal plasma flow in acromegaly. *Acta Endocrinol (Copenh)* 1957; 21:226–236.
83. Hirschberg R, Rabb H, Bergamo R, et al. The delayed effect of

growth hormone on renal function in humans. *Kidney Int* 1989; 35:865–870.
84. Hirschberg R, Brunori G, Kopple JD, et al. Effects of insulin-like growth factor 1 on renal function in normal men. *Kidney Int* 1993;43:387–397.
85. Hirschberg R, Kopple JD, Blantz RC, et al. Effect of recombinant human insulin-like growth factor 1 on glomerular dynamics in the rat. *J Clin Invest* 1991;87:1200–1206.
86. Biglieri EG, Watlington CO, Forsham PH. Sodium retention with human growth hormone and its subfractions. *J Clin Endocrinol Metab* 1961;21:361–370.
87. Haffner D, Zacharewicz S, Mehls O, et al. The acute effect of growth hormone on GFR is obliterated in chronic renal failure. *Clin Nephrol* 1989;32:266–269.
88. O'Shea MH, Miller SB, Hammerman MR. Effects of IGF-1 on renal function in patients with chronic: renal failure. *Am J Physiol* 1993;264:F917–F922.
89. Miller SB, Moulton M, O'Shea MH, et al. Effects of IGF-1 on renal function in end-stage chronic renal failure. *Kidney Int* 1994; 46:201–207.
90. Vijayan A, Franklin SC, Behrend T, et al. Insulin-like growth factor I improves renal function in patients with end-stage chronic renal failure. *Am J Physiol* 1999,276:R929–R934.
91. Trachtman H, Futterweit S, Schwob N, et al. Recombinant human growth hormone exacerbates chronic puromycin aminonucleoside nephropathy in rats. *Kidney Int* 1993;44:1281–1288.
92. Doi T, Striker LJ, Quaife C, et al. Progressive glomerulosclerosis develops in transgenic mice chronically expressing growth hormone and growth hormone releasing factor but not in those expressing insulin growth factor-1. *Am J Pathol* 1988;131: 398–403.
93. Cohen P, Clemmons DR, Rosenfeld RG. Does the GH–IGF axis play a role in cancer pathogenesis? *Growth Horm IGF Res* 2000;10:297–305.

33

DRUG–NUTRIENT INTERACTIONS IN RENAL FAILURE

RAIMUND HIRSCHBERG

Foods and nutrients and prescribed or over-the-counter medicines can interact in multiple ways. Such interactions may result in reduced or increased drug effects or in (often subtle) nutritional deficiencies. Drug efficacy may be reduced as a result of food-induced delayed or decreased absorption from the gastrointestinal tract. Diet or nutrients may induce drug-metabolizing enzymes or increase or decrease the rate of metabolism of a given drug. The rate of excretion of the drug or of active or toxic metabolites also may be altered by dietary effects.

The most commonly observed drug–food interaction is altered drug absorption from the gastrointestinal tract, usually a decrease in the rate of absorption. Less commonly, the drug absorption rate may be increased if taken concurrently with foods. Drugs also can induce certain specific nutrient deficiencies, particularly for vitamins and minerals.

In patients with chronic renal failure or end-stage renal disease (ESRD), drug–nutrient interactions may lead to overt nutritional deficiencies, particularly when the general nutritional status is poor or specific subclinical nutritional deficiencies exist. In this chapter, drug–nutrient interactions that may result from those medicines or food supplements that commonly or occasionally are used in patients with chronic renal failure or ESRD will be reviewed. The possible underlying mechanisms will be elucidated.

EFFECT OF FOOD INTAKE ON DRUG ABSORPTION

The intestinal absorption of many drugs is slowed when administered concurrently with food, either because of delayed gastric emptying or because of dilution of the drug in the intestinal contents. Certain medications, such as central $\alpha 2$-adrenergic drugs, can reduce gastrointestinal motility and delay the emptying of the stomach and, hence, increase the oral–fecal transit time (1). In contrast, calcium channel blockers do not appear to affect gastrointestinal motility (2). Captopril-induced increased gastric motility was observed in *in vitro* experiments, but data in humans are lacking, and the clinical importance of the *in vitro* findings is questionable (3). Table 33.1 lists several drugs that may be prescribed to patients with renal failure and that may interfere with the gastric emptying rate. Table 33.2 lists drugs that commonly or occasionally are prescribed to patients with renal failure and that are absorbed more slowly when given concurrently with meals. To optimize drug absorption, these medicines should be given 1 hour before or 2 hours after meals. However, there are a few commonly administered oral medicines that will undergo more effective absorption when administered with foods (Table 33.3).

In most circumstances the food-dependent increase in drug absorption may enhance drug efficacy. However, serious toxic side effects may arise, such as when lithium or cyclosporine are given with foods. Thus, for each of these prescribed medicines, patients should be advised as to whether to take them with or without meals.

Subclinical or overt iron deficiency commonly is observed in patients with advanced chronic renal failure or ESRD. Low or empty iron stores may be caused by reduced nutrient intakes and, hence, iron intakes as well as subtle iron losses. Iron deficiency is the most common reason for resistance to erythropoietin in patients with renal failure. Experimental studies have shown that administration of the phosphate binder calcium carbonate ($CaCO_3$) with foods reduces the bioavailability of iron from oral iron sulfate (4). Apparently, in the presence of calcium, iron is taken up normally into the gut mucosa, but the transfer through mucosal cytoplasm and/or basolateral membranes is reduced. In experimental animals with iron-deficiency anemia, coadministration of $CaCO_3$ reduces the ability to replete iron stores (4).

In normal subjects, calcium carbonate reduces the absorption of nonheme iron from foods by about two-thirds. However, in these iron-replete normal individuals, long-term oral ingestion of supplemental calcium does not change hematologic indices (5). In lactating women, oral calcium supplements also do not reduce serum ferritin levels (6). There is no systematic study in patients with chronic renal failure or in patients undergoing dialysis to examine

TABLE 33.1. DRUGS AFFECTING THE GASTRIC EMPTYING RATE

Increase GER	Decrease GER
Metoclopramide	Anticholinergics
Reserpine	Atropine
Sodium bicarbonate	Amitriptyline
	Imipramine
	Analgesics
	Morphine
	Pentazocine
	Isoniazid
	Chloroquine
	Phenytoin
	Aluminum hydroxide
	Phenothiazines
	Chlorpromazine
	Diphenylhydramine
	Promethazine
	Sympathomimetics
	Levodopa
	Amantadine

GER, gastric emptying rate.
From Nimmo W. Drugs, disease and altered gastric emptying. *Clin Pharmacolinet* 1976;1:189–203, with permission; and Prescott L. Gastric emptying and drug absorption. *Br J Clin Pharmacol* 1974; 1:189–190, with permission.

whether the interference of calcium with iron absorption can cause iron depletion. Given relatively poor dietary intakes in some patients with renal failure and additional blood losses that occur through the gastrointestinal tract and with hemodialysis and blood draws, it is not unlikely that oral $CaCO_3$ contributes to iron deficiency and anemia.

TABLE 33.2. DRUGS UNDERGOING REDUCED OR DELAYED ABSORPTION IF ADMINISTERED WITH FOOD

Acetaminophen	Erythromycin	Nifedipine
Amoxicillin	Ferrous sulfate[b]	Norfloxacin
Ampicillin	Fosinopril	Ofloxacin
Aspirin	Furosemide	Oxacillin
Atenolol	Glipizide	Oxytetracycline[b]
Captopril	Hydralazine[c]	Penicillamine
Cephalexin	Ibuprofen	Provastatin
Cephrodine	Indomethacin	Ramipril
Cephaclor	Isoniazid	Rifampin
Enalapril	Ketoconazole	Simvastatin
Cimetidine[a]	Ketoprofen	Spironolactone
Ciprofloxacin[a]	Levodopa	Sulindac
Clindamycin	Levothyroxine[c]	Tetracycline[b]
Demeclocycline	Methotrexate	Zidovudine
Digoxin	Misoprostol	Zinc salts
Doxycycline	Nicardipine	

[a]Concurrent administration with caffeine-containing foods may increase caffeine uptake.
[b]Mainly dairy products.
[c]Particularly enteral formulas.

TABLE 33.3. DRUGS THAT ARE ABSORBED MORE EFFECTIVELY IF GIVEN WITH FOOD

Buspirone	Griseofulvin
Carbamazepine	Isradipine
Cefpodoxime	Labetolol
Cefuroxime	Lithium salts
Chlorothiazide	Metoprolol
Cyclosporine	Morphine
Diazepam	Nitrofurantoin
Dicumarol	Propaphenone
Diltiazem	Propranolol
Etretinate	Quinidine
Famotidine	Sertraline
Felodipine	Triclopidine

EFFECTS OF NUTRIENTS ON DRUG METABOLISM

Dietary Protein and Lipids

The hepatic clearance of some drugs is reduced in renal failure (7). Drugs that are metabolized by oxidation, conjugation, or both processes may be predisposed to decreased hepatic clearance in chronic renal failure. Anderson et al. examined the effects of high-protein diets on the activity of cytochrome P-450–dependent mixed function oxidases (8). These investigators found that the metabolic clearance of theophylline and antipyrine were increased in six normal men fed a high-protein diet, but the volume of distribution of both drugs was unaffected. These two drugs are substrates for the mixed function oxidases and commonly are used to assess the activity of this oxidative system in clinical studies. Juan et al. compared the effects of high- and low-protein diets on the metabolism of theophylline, caffeine, and aminopyrine (9). Eleven subjects were fed the respective diets for periods of at least 12 days each with a 2-week washout period in between. When fed the high-protein diet, theophylline clearance and caffeine metabolism were enhanced by about 50% and 30%, respectively. In another study in six healthy volunteers, a high-protein diet induced an increase in the metabolic clearance of theophylline and propranolol by about 28% and 60%, respectively (10).

Low-protein diets also reduce the activity of xanthine oxidase (11) and increase the plasma levels of allopurinol and oxypurinol. The renal clearance of oxypurinol also was reduced in this study, suggesting that a low-protein-diet–induced reduction in the glomerular filtration rate (GFR) may contribute to the increased plasma levels (11). Because oxypurinol accounts for some of the adverse effects of allopurinol, the concurrent prescription of low-protein diets and allopurinol may increase the likelihood of allopurinol toxicity.

The prescription of low-protein diets to patients with chronic renal failure also may reduce the sulfate conjugation of some drugs, although clinical studies directly examining this question in patients or normal subjects are lacking. Drug sulfation depends on the availability of sulfur-containing amino acids and the possible release of sulfur in the gut by the action of intestinal sulfatases (12).

Cruciferous Vegetables and Drug Metabolism

Drug metabolism can be affected by other compounds derived from certain foods. For example, various indoles that originate from cruciferous vegetables, such as cabbage and Brussels sprouts, enhance oxidation and increase the metabolic clearance rate of medicines. Such foods also may enhance drug glucuronidation in healthy subjects (e.g., for acetaminophen) (13,14). Diet-derived compounds may affect the activity of the P-450 enzyme species, and such substances can compete as substrates for the P-450–dependent monooxygenase system (15). For example, indole-3-carbinol and related compounds that are present in cruciferous vegetables, particularly Brussels sprouts, are potent inducers of the intestinal P-450 IA1 and hepatic P-450 IA1 and IA2 isoenzymes (16).

Nutrients and Cytochrome P-450–Dependent Drug Metabolism

Increased dietary protein augments hepatic microsomal cytochrome P-450 content (17). Furthermore, studies in cultured liver cells as well as *in vivo* in animals indicate that tryptophan and sulfur amino acids induce the mixed function oxidase system (18,19). Thus, these *in vitro* and *in vivo* studies suggest that high-protein intakes increase the activity of cytochrome P-450–dependent enzymes and substantially enhance oxidative drug metabolism. In contrast, the activity of this enzyme system is reduced by low-protein, high-carbohydrate, or high-fat diets; flavonoids (i.e., contained in citrus fruits); and large doses of riboflavin and possibly during total parenteral nutrition (15).

The cytochrome P-450-IIE1 isoenzyme is induced by dietary lipids (20). This isoenzyme participates in the metabolism of acetaminophen, enflurane, and halothane (15). Moreover, the P-450 IIE1 isoenzyme also is activated by fasting (21) and thiamin deficiency (22). Several other alterations in the micronutrient status can affect the oxidative metabolism of drugs (Table 33.4).

Cytochrome P-450 Isoenzyme Activity and Citrus Juice Compounds

Flavonoids, such as naringin, are present in rather large amounts in citrus fruits and citrus juices. The related aglycone, naringenin, is readily formed in humans from its precursor. This compound, like other flavonoids, inhibits the cytochrome P-450 3A4 isoenzyme. Grapefruit juice, which is perhaps the food most potently inhibiting CYP3A4, contains naringenin but also contains psoralen derivatives, which are thought to inhibit this isoenzyme (23). *In vitro* studies identified several compounds that were extracted from grapefruit juice and inhibit CYPIIIA4 with half-maximal rate of inactivation as low as 0.13 μM (24). These include furanocoumarin monomers and dimers. In clinical studies in normal subjects, naringin was found to inhibit metabolism of the CYP3A4 substrates nisoldipine only moderately, giving rise to the importance of other compounds in grapefruit juice as inhibitors of this cytochrome P-450 isoenzyme (25,26). Although the effect of these grapefruit juice compounds on CYP3A4 may be clinically more important, they also tend to inhibit several other cytochrome P-450 isoenzymes such as CYP1A2, CYP2C9, CYP2C19, and CYP2D6 (24).

CYP3A4 is present in relatively large concentrations in the wall of the small intestine, where it contributes to the first pass metabolism of several drugs and limits the amount of active drug that reaches the bloodstream. The inhibition of CYP3A4 by compounds in grapefruit juice and other citrus fruit juices is clinically important because this isoenzyme plays a major role in the metabolism of drugs that commonly are used in patients with chronic renal failure or ESRD. These include cyclosporine A; the dihydropyridine calcium channel blockers nifedipine, nimodipine, felodipine, nitrendipine, and nisoldipine; the calcium channel blocker verapamil; saquinavir; diazepam; midazolam; triazolam; terfenadine; and lovastatin (23,25–27). The bioavailability of these drugs is increased by coadministration with grapefruit juice and, perhaps, even more so in subjects con-

TABLE 33.4. EFFECTS OF VITAMIN AND TRACE ELEMENT ALTERATIONS ON OXIDATIVE DRUG METABOLISM

Vitamin A deficiency	↓ P-450 ↓ Metabolism of aminopyrine, coumarin
Vitamin A, high dose	↑ Metabolism of coumarin
Niacin deficiency	↓ Metabolism of anesthetics
Riboflavin deficiency	↓ NADPH: P-450 reductase ↑ Aminopyrine metabolism
Vitamin C deficiency	↓ P-450 ↓ NADPH: P-450 reductase ↓ Monooxigenase activities
Folic acid deficiency	↓ Induction of P-450 IIB1 by barbiturates
Aluminum, high dose	↓ Hepatic P-450
Selenium deficiency	↓ Induction of P-450 by phenobarbital
Zinc deficiency	↓ Phenobarbital and aminopyrine metabolism

NADPH, reduced form of nicotinamide adenine dinucleotide.
From Yang C, Brady J, Hong J. Dietary effects on cytochromes P-450, xenobiotic metabolism, and toxicity. *FASEB J* 1992;6:737–744, with permission.

suming large amounts of citrus juices chronically. For example, ingestion of diazepam, 5 mg, with 250 mL of grapefruit juice as compared to water increases the diazepam area under the curve 3.2-fold (28).

Bailey et al. examined the effects of grapefruit juice on nisoldipine and felodipine pharmacokinetics in normal subjects (25,26). Compared to water, grapefruit juice increased the maximum concentration of nisoldipine after a single dose about fourfold and the area under the plasma concentration time curve about twofold, both with considerable individual variability. Similarly, felodipine peak plasma concentration was increased, on average, about twofold and the area under the curve was increased about 1.7-fold.

This drug–nutrient interaction between compounds in citrus juices and dihydropyridine calcium channel blockers has significant clinical implications. First, the increased plasma levels of the drugs may increase the incidence of adverse effects. Second, in patients with hypertension treated with dihydropyridines, sporadic concomitant ingestion of grapefruit juice may cause symptomatic hypotension. Third, the combination of a dihydropyridine antihypertensive with grapefruit juice can increase the therapeutic efficacy. This has been illustrated in a published case report (29). However, larger clinical trials are lacking.

Cytochrome P-450 3A3, 4, 5, and 7 isoenzymes also are inhibited by cimetidine, rifampicin, barbiturates, and other drugs (30). However, detailed discussion of drug–drug interactions is not the subject of this chapter.

Effects of Vitamins and Trace Elements on Cytochrome P-450 Activity

Some vitamin deficiencies also can reduce the rate of oxidative metabolism of drugs in humans and can impair the mixed-function oxidase system in laboratory animals. Ascorbic acid deficiency in guinea pigs results in reduced metabolic rates of oxidative drugs, reduced cytochrome P-450 levels, and reduced activities of most associated enzymes (31). Some studies in patients demonstrate a reduced metabolic clearance of antipyrine, an indicator of reduced oxidative drug metabolism, that correlates with the leucocyte vitamin C levels (32). In contrast, other studies have not confirmed that mild to moderate ascorbic acid deficiency reduces oxidative drug metabolism (33,34).

Large doses of vitamin C given as nutritional supplements to patients without ascorbic acid deficiency may increase the rate of oxidative drug metabolism (35). High vitamin C intakes also can reduce the rate of sulfate conjugation of drugs, such as acetaminophen, by competing for the available sulfate (36). Dietary supplementation with large doses of pyridoxine may increase the metabolism and decrease the therapeutic efficacy of levodopa because this vitamin is a cofactor for the dopa decarboxylase (37).

Nutrients and Drug Glucuronidation and Urinary Excretion

The deficiency in some trace elements such as iron, zinc, copper, and selenium has been shown to influence the mixed-function oxidase system in experimental animals, but for most such elements, studies in humans are not available. Moreover, even marked iron deficiency in humans does not appear to affect oxidative drug metabolism (38).

In chronic renal failure the half-life of drugs that primarily are metabolized by hepatic glucuronidation may be prolonged (39–41). Although it is possible that fasting, malnutrition or specific nutrient deficiencies may alter the hepatic glucuronidation of some drugs, the literature at present does not provide data that would clearly indicate this.

The urinary excretion of certain drugs or of bioactive or toxic metabolites depends on the degree of renal failure (i.e., GFR or creatinine clearance) as well as on urinary pH (42). In patients with normal renal function and even in patients with moderate or advanced chronic renal failure, urinary pH depends largely on dietary intakes, at least during the postabsorptive period. A low-protein diet produces a more alkaline urine; conversely, a high-protein diet results in more acidic urine. Drugs or drug metabolites that are weak bases are excreted more efficiently in acidic urine, whereas more alkaline urine will promote the excretion of drugs or metabolites that are weak acids. Foods that potentially acidify the urine include meats, fish, eggs, cheese, bread, cranberries, plums, and prunes. More alkaline urine can be caused by milk, various fruit, and all vegetables except corn and lentils (43).

INTERACTIONS OF FOOD SUPPLEMENTS WITH DRUGS

Patients with advanced chronic renal failure and those undergoing maintenance dialysis often are prescribed food supplements, such as vitamins and iron preparations, or phosphate binders. Specific interactions between certain drugs and these food supplements have been described that not only may reduce the blood levels of the drug but may reduce the drug efficacy. Thus, it may be necessary to separate the timing of the intake of the food supplement from that of the drug. In general, the drug should be taken 1 hour before or 2 hours after the supplement, but in some circumstances this period should be even longer.

There is evidence that the intake of certain vitamins above the levels occurring in normal diets can lower the blood levels of some drugs with which these supplements interact. In this setting the desired therapeutic effects of the medicine may not occur. Supplemental folic acid decreases the blood levels of phenobarbital (44) and may lead to breakthrough seizures. Pyridoxine (vitamin B_6), when given in large dosages (400 mg/day), also can reduce the serum levels of phenobarbital (45), possibly by increasing the activity of pyridoxal phosphate-dependent enzymes. In animal experiments, large doses of pyridoxine may reduce the activity of isonicotinic acid against tuberculosis. Pyridoxine appears to form a Schiff base with isonicotinic acid, which then is excreted in the urine or removed during dialysis (46). Concomitant therapy with pyridoxine and L-dopa in patients with Parkinson's disease reduces the efficacy of the latter drug and worsens the disease symptoms (47). The formation of a Schiff base between L-dopa and pyridoxine may prevent the delivery of L-dopa to the brain (48).

Excess intake of vitamin E can induce a hemorrhagic state in laboratory animals caused by vitamin K deficiency (49,50). Patients on coumarin therapy are at risk for developing hemorrhages that result from unwarranted further suppression of the vitamin K–dependent clotting factors by concomitant intake of vitamin E. It has been suggested that megadoses of vitamin C (approximately 1g/day) may lead to vitamin B_{12} deficiency, apparently by destruction of vitamin B_{12} by vitamin C when it is taken together with vitamin B_{12}. However, Newmark et al. have questioned the importance of this interaction, and its clinical significance is unclear (51,52).

Clinically important interactions occur between iron supplements or phosphate binders and fluoroquinolone antibiotics. Golper et al. reported on the effects of antacids on the pharmacokinetics of oral ciprofloxacin in patients treated with continuous ambulatory peritoneal dialysis (53). These authors found a decrease in the bioavailability of ciprofloxacin if the drug was coadministered with aluminum hydroxide–containing phosphate binders. Other investigators confirmed these findings and demonstrated that magnesium hydroxide as well as aluminum hydroxide reduce the bioavailability of ciprofloxacin by as much as 90% when given concomitantly or within less than 0.5 hours, and a lesser but still significant reduction occurs when the drug is given within up to 4 hours after the antacid (54, 55). Similar reductions in the bioavailability occur for other fluoroquinolone antibiotics, such as norfloxacin, ofloxacin, and enoxacin, when administered up to 4 hours after intake of aluminum-, magnesium-, or calcium-containing phosphate binders (56). A significant decrease in the bioavailability of fluoroquinolones also was described by several authors to occur on coadministration with several oral iron supplement preparations such as ferrous sulfate, fumarate, or gluconate. Calcium-containing phosphate binders or antacids also have been shown to reduce the bioavailability of tetracyclines (57,58). The reduction of iron absorption from diet or ferrous sulfate as a result of coadministration of calcium-containing phosphate binders was discussed earlier in this chapter.

DRUG-INDUCED NUTRITIONAL DEFICIENCIES

Several prescribed or over-the-counter medicines may reduce appetite and food intake. In patients with chronic renal failure or receiving maintenance dialysis, this may aggravate an already poor nutritional status and may contribute to frank malnutrition. However, of greater concern are more specific interactions of prescribed drugs with micronutrients, mainly with certain vitamins and minerals.

Drug-Induced Vitamin Deficiencies

Vitamin metabolism and requirements in renal disease and renal failure are described in Chapter 20. Thiamin deficiency may be caused or aggravated by chronic alcoholism. The literature, at present, does not suggest that specific short-term or long-term drug therapies may cause vitamin B_1 deficiency. However, thiamin deficiency may occur in severely ill patients who undergo parenteral nutrition (59–62). Thiamin is a coenzyme for pyruvate dehydrogenase, and thiamin deficiency may cause the acute onset of unexplained, severe lactic acidosis (59–63). Riboflavin deficiency can be caused or aggravated by long-term administration of chlorpromazine or amitriptyline. Pyridoxine deficiency may be caused by long-term treatment with isoniazid. It is recommended that vitamin B_6 supplements (10 to 15 mg/day) should be prescribed for the entire time that isoniazid is taken. Vitamin B_6 deficiency also may be caused by hydralazine and penicillamine (37). High doses of pyridoxine hydrochloride reduce the serum levels of anticonvulsants and may reduce the clinical seizure control. Chronic vitamin B_{12} deficiency may develop during long-term treatment with colchicine or cimetidine (64,65).

Several drugs antagonize folic acid and may cause megaloblastic anemia. These include phenytoin, phenobarbital, sulfasalazine, triamterene, trimethoprim, trimetrexate, and methotrexate (66–69). However, folate supplementation may interact with these medicines and reduce their clinical efficacy. Daily dosages of folate of more than 5 mg reduces the plasma levels of phenytoin and phenobarbital and may reduce their therapeutic efficacy (70). A risk for the development of niacin deficiency may exist when treatment with isoniazid is prescribed. During such treatment, concurrent administration of niacin (100 mg/day) may be advisable. Retinoids and possibly retinol increase the blood cyclosporine levels (71). Vitamin A supplements should be avoided in renal patients. In addition to coumarin anticoagulants, there are a number of drugs that can cause vitamin K deficiency and that may induce or enhance severe bleeding. This has been described particularly with the administration of moxalactam, cefotetan, cefamandole, cefoperazone, and other cephalosporins that contain the methylthiotetrazole side chain. Vitamin K supplements should be administered concurrently with these antibiotics (72,73). Weaker antivitamin K effects have been shown with tetracycline and cholestyramine (74). Ingestion of megadoses of vitamin E can cause vitamin K deficiency and should be avoided (49, 50).

Drug-induced osteomalacia can be the result of chronic intake of anticonvulsants, isoniazid, and possibly cimetidine. Anticonvulsant therapy with phenytoin, phenobarbital, or carbamazepine results in reduced levels of 24,25-dihydroxyvitamin D_3, and this may play a role in the anticonvulsant-induced osteomalacia (75). In patients with chronic renal failure, this drug-induced risk for osteomalacia may be additive to the increased risk of renal bone disease. Patients undergoing chronic dialysis therapy often are supplemented with 1,25-dihydroxycholecalciferol. However, in patients with moderate chronic renal failure not receiving 1,25-dihydroxycholecalciferol, vitamin D supplements should be given concurrently with the above listed drug treatments.

Drug-Induced Mineral and Trace Element Deficiencies

As a rule, the intakes of many minerals such as sodium, potassium, magnesium, calcium, and phosphate correlate with the intake of nitrogen (76). Mineral and trace element deficiencies may develop because of poor nutritional intakes, and elderly patients are at greater risk. Mineral depletion can occur as a result of poor gastrointestinal absorption and/or enhanced renal excretion, the latter mainly in patients with lesser degrees of chronic renal failure. Both reduced absorption and enhanced excretion of minerals can be caused by drug therapy. Potassium, calcium, magnesium, iron, and zinc are the most common minerals that become depleted in patients with chronic renal failure. Drug-induced potassium deficiency in patients with chronic renal failure most commonly results from diuretic therapy and can be caused by both thiazide and loop diuretics. With diuretic therapy, magnesium deficiency also may develop.

Concurrent intake of aminoglycosides and cephalosporin antibiotics can be interactive and cause potassium (and magnesium) depletion, particularly when intakes of these minerals are low, which may occur with ingestion of low-protein diets. Hypokalemia also can occur with gentamycin toxicity and during treatment with amphotericin B (77). Potassium deficiency also may be caused by laxative abuse with resulting potassium losses through the gastrointestinal tract. Lithium carbonate and levodopa can contribute to potassium deficiency (78). Hypokalemia and potassium depletion worsen blood pressure levels in patients with hypertension and may contribute to the thiazide-induced carbohydrate intolerance (79,80).

Calcium deficiency can be caused by poor dietary intake, primary malabsorption, vitamin D deficiency–induced malabsorption, or drug-induced hypercalciuria. Primary calcium malabsorption can result from enteropathy caused by neomycin, colchicine, methotrexate, and corticosteroids (81). Aluminum and magnesium hydroxide may reduce calcium absorption. Phenytoin and phenobarbital may interfere with vitamin D metabolism, as described earlier. Loop diuretics, such as furosemide and ethacrynic acid, can cause hypocalcemia secondary to hypercalciuria (82). In patients with chronic renal failure, combined treatments with drugs that interfere with calcium metabolism are not uncommon.

Hypercalcemia in patients with chronic renal failure may result in soft-tissue calcification and nephrocalcinosis that may contribute to the progression of renal disease or may in itself cause chronic renal failure. The long-term combined intakes of large amounts of calcium carbonate and (vitamin D-fortified) milk can lead to severe chronic hypercalcemia and nephrocalcinosis, causing chronic renal failure, the so-called milk-alkali syndrome (83,84). In chronic renal failure, hypercalcemia may result from the intake of calcium-containing phosphate binders and/or vitamin D derivatives.

Hyperoxalemia and hyperoxaluria can be caused or aggravated by vitamin C supplementation, even at moderate doses (i.e., 500 mg/day) (83,85). Patients who eat relatively large amounts of foods that generate oxalate (e.g., green salads) and take moderate or megadoses of vitamin C have an increased risk to develop hyperoxalemia-associated illnesses (83,85).

Zinc deficiency may be caused or worsened by total parenteral nutrition without adequate zinc intake (86). Administration of penicillamine or corticosteroids also has been associated with zinc deficiency (87). Zinc depletion causes or contributes to clinical symptoms that often are observed in patients with chronic renal failure, such as loss of appetite and altered taste and smell sensation. Loss of taste or smell may lead to reduced food intake and, hence, malnutrition. Aspirin, indomethacin, and other nonsteroidal antiinflammatory drugs may cause occult gastrointestinal bleeding and contribute to iron losses (88). Iron depletion and anemia also may be caused by poor food intake or reduced bioavailability from nonheme iron in foods such as resulting from concomitant calcium-containing phosphate binders. There are not sufficient data to indicate whether there are important drug interactions with other trace elements, such as selenium, molybdenum, chromium, manganese, rubidium, and others.

TAURINE AND ANGIOTENSIN CONVERTING ENZYME INHIBITOR EFFECTS

Angiotensin I converting enzyme (ACE) inhibitors are among the most commonly used drugs in patients with chronic renal failure or in patients undergoing chronic dialysis. ACE inhibitors are potent antihypertensives. They reduce cardiac afterload, cardiac hypertrophy, and fibrosis and may reduce macrovascular and microvascular sclerosis as well as the rate of progression of chronic renal failure in patients with various chronic progressive renal diseases, most notably diabetic nephropathy. These latter effects of ACE inhibitors are a result of reducing profibrogenic activity of angiotensin II. However, even with high-dose ACE inhibitor therapy, angiotensin II levels are not blocked completely but tend to rebound with prolonged treatment. This is the basis for combination therapy with ACE inhibitors and AT1-blockers.

The amino acid taurine also blocks actions of angiotensin II by inhibiting cellular calcium uptake and angiotensin II signaling (89). In experimental *in vitro* and *in vivo* studies taurine food supplements were found to have renal antifibrogenic effects comparable to those of ACE inhibitors (90).

Serum and blood cell taurine levels tend to be lower in patients with diabetes compared to normal subjects, and taurine food supplements can normalize taurine levels (91). Foods rich in taurine include seafood, particularly crustaceans and mollusks, and lesser amounts are present in beef, pork, and lamb (92). Taurine-containing food supplements are available over the counter. Whether increased dietary taurine will indeed reduce the progression of renal disease and/or reduce the cardiovascular mortality in patients undergoing chronic dialysis is unknown as a result of the lack of respective clinical trials. Nevertheless, this may be an example of collaborative, beneficial drug–nutrient interactions.

INTERACTIONS OF CYCLOSPORINE A WITH NUTRIENTS

Treatment with cyclosporine A is the mainstay of most immunosuppressive regimens that are used in kidney transplantation. Cyclosporine inhibits the interleukin-2-dependent proliferation of activated T-cells. The drug has several side effects, including nephrotoxicity, hepatotoxicity, hypertrichosis, gingival hyperplasia, hyperuricemia, and gout (7% of patients); gout occurs particularly when used together with loop diuretics (93). Cyclosporine is absorbed incompletely from the gastrointestinal tract, and administration of the drug with foods tends to increase absorption. Oral administration of cyclosporine A together with food and bile salts increases the bioavailability of the drug apparently because of improved absorption. However, coadministration of cyclosporine with bile salts alone does not raise the cyclosporine blood levels (94). The incomplete absorption of intact cyclosporine is caused, in part, by metabolism in the small bowel wall (95). Cyclosporine is metabolized by oxidation in liver microsomes through the cytochrome P-450 3A isoenzyme system (30,96). This enzyme system also is expressed in the small bowel wall, which explains the first-pass metabolism of cyclosporine A (95,97).

There is great variation in the bioavailability of cyclosporine between patients. Because of this variability and because of the narrow therapeutic window, it is necessary to monitor cyclosporine therapy with frequent blood level measurements (93).

Cyclosporine A is a highly lipid-soluble drug, and about 40% of cyclosporine in plasma is bound to lipoproteins. Thus, it is reasonable to speculate that dietary fat intakes or the fat content of meals may raise the gastrointestinal absorption and plasma levels of cyclosporine A. Menon et al. examined this question in 15 renal transplant recipients with stable renal function who were treated with cyclosporine A for at least 3 months (98). Subjects received cyclosporine A with a meal containing either 73% or 12% of the calories as fat. No difference in blood cyclosporine levels was observed, suggesting that the meal fat content does not increase the rate of absorption of the drug.

Evidence from clinical studies indicates that the absorption of cyclosporine A is enhanced by concomitant administration of a water-soluble form of vitamin E, d-α-tocopheryl-polyethylene-glycol-succinate (25 mg/kg/day). This has been shown primarily in children after liver transplantation (99,100). Whether this is specific to liver transplant recipients or whether this effect of the water-soluble vitamin E is also present in patients after renal transplantation remains to be determined. Dietary or supplemental vitamin E (α-tocopherol) does not appear to exert an effect on cyclosporine absorption (101).

An increase in blood cyclosporine levels was observed in a patient with renal failure who was treated concomitantly with cyclosporine A and the retinoid etretinate (71). *In vitro* studies using a human liver microsomal system indicate that vitamin A retinoids inhibit cyclosporine metabolism, which may cause the observed increase in blood cyclosporine levels in patients receiving etretinate (71). This combination therapy sometimes is used in the treatment of severe psoriasis. Webber and Back, however, could not confirm this effect of etretinate on cyclosporine A metabolism, using a similar *in vitro* microsomal system (102). Whether a clinically important interaction between dietary or supplemental vitamin A and cyclosporine metabolism and blood levels exists remains unclear. As indicated earlier, citrus juices, particularly grapefruit juice, reduce the metabolic rate of cyclosporine and increase its blood levels (103), possibly through the inhibitory effects of flavonoids and other compounds on cytochrome P-450 3A enzymes (23,30). Brunner et al. examined the interaction between grapefruit juice and the steady-state pharmacokinetics of cyclosporine in stable renal transplant recipients in an open-label, crossover study (104). In this study grapefruit juice significantly increased the area under the curve and caused an increase in the 24-hour trough cyclosporine level.

There are also several drugs that affect blood cyclosporine levels. Some drugs increase the drug levels by decreasing the cytochrome P-450 3A enzyme activity or by competing with

TABLE 33.5. DRUGS THAT INCREASE BLOOD CYCLOSPORINE A LEVELS AS A RESULT OF INHIBITION OF OR COMPETITION WITH CYTOCHROME P-450 IIIA ISOENZYMES

Verapamil	Diltiazem
Nicardipine	Ketoconazole
Fluconazole	Itraconazole
Erythromycin	Ceftazidime
Imipenem	Norfloxacin
Sulfamethoxazole	Ponsinomycin[a]
Cimetidine	Ranitidine
Omeprazole	

[a]Couet W, Istin B, Sinata P, et al. Effect of ponsinomycin on cyclosporin pharmacokinetics. *Eur J Clin Pharmacol* 1990;39:165–167.
Adapted from Danovitch G. Immunosuppressive medications and protocols for kidney transplantation. In: Danovitch G, ed. *Handbook of kidney transplantation*. Boston: Little, Brown and Co., 1992:67–103, with permission.

this metabolic pathway (Table 33.5). Other drugs induce this enzyme system and, hence, decrease the blood cyclosporine levels as a result of enhanced metabolism (Table 33.6).

ENTERAL TUBE FEEDING AND ORAL DRUG ADMINISTRATION

Enteral tube feeding may be a necessary or desirable mode of nutrient delivery in some patients with chronic renal failure or ESRD, either transiently during periods of acute, severe illness or for longer periods. In such patients, drugs may be administered preferably by intravenous routes, but enteral drug administration sometimes may be necessary because many medicine preparations are not available for intravenous infusion.

Several considerations should be taken into account when giving oral drug preparations through enteral feeding tubes. First, oral medicines should be delivered into the stomach to ensure proper preparation for subsequent drug absorption in the jejunum. Second, drugs should be used in liquid form rather than as crushed tablets. Third, slow-release or enteric-coated tablets should not be crushed at all. Fourth, drugs may not be compatible with the tube feeding formula. Fifth, the osmolality of some liquid drug preparations may be very high and may add to the osmolality of the formula. When significant amounts of hyperosmolar solutions reach the small bowel, large electrolyte and water fluxes into the gut lumen may occur and cause osmotic diarrhea. In this setting neither nutrients nor drugs will be absorbed efficiently (105). A complete list of commercially available liquid preparations of commonly used drugs has been published elsewhere (106).

Only a few studies have examined the bioavailability of drugs when administered with enteral formulas, and this information is not available for most medicines. Phenytoin bioavailability, for example, is much reduced when given with enteral formulas as compared to a similar dose given orally (107,108). Scott examined the potassium admixture to a milk-based enteral formula and found that an effervescent potassium tablet preparation caused marked coagulation of the enteral formula, whereas potassium chloride or gluconate solutions were compatible (109). Administration of aluminum-containing phosphate binders with some enteral formulas can lead to precipitation of formula proteins with the aluminum salts and gastrointestinal plug formation can occur (110,111). Case reports have suggested that enteral tube feeding reduces the efficacy of warfarin (110,112). Apparently, this results from the antagonistic effect of vitamin K that is present in enteral formulas (106). In patients undergoing treatment with warfarin, a formula with a lesser vitamin K content should be used and will improve the response to warfarin.

Little is known about interactions of many other drugs that may be used in patients with renal failure undergoing tube feeding. Hence, close monitoring of the plasma drug levels, treatment response, and compatibility with the formula are necessary.

TABLE 33.6. DRUGS THAT DECREASE BLOOD CYCLOSPORINE A LEVELS AS A RESULT OF INDUCTION OF CYTOCHROME P-450 IIIA ISOENZYMES

Rifampicin	Isoniazid
Barbiturates	Phenytoin
Carbamazepinl	Benzodiazepines
Valproic acid	Nafcillin
Trimethoprim	Cephalosporins

Adapted from Danovitch G. Immunosuppressive medications and protocols for kidney transplan-tation. In: Danovitch G. ed. *Handbook of kidney transplantation*. Boston: Little, Brown and Co., 1992:67–103, with permission.

REFERENCES

1. Nagata M, Osumi Y. Central alpha-2-adrenoreceptor-mediated inhibition of gastric motility in rats. *Jpn J Pharmacol* 1993;62: 329–330.
2. Baba T, Ishizaki T. Recent advances in pharmacological management of hypertension in diabetic patients with nephropathy. Effects of antihypertensive drugs on kidney function and insulin sensitivity. *Drugs* 1992;43:464–489.
3. Rani R, Rao K. Enhanced contractility of rat stomach during suppression of angiotensin converting enzyme by captopril *in vitro*. *Br J Pharmacol* 1991;102:827–830.
4. Wienk KJ, Marx JJ, Lemmens AG, et al. Mechanism underlying the inhibitory effect of high calcium carbonate intake on iron bioavailability from ferrous sulphate in anaemic rats. *Br J Nutr* 1996;75(1):109–120.
5. Minihane AM, Fairweather-Tait SJ. Effect of calcium supple-

mentation on daily nonheme-iron absorption and long-term iron status. *Am J Clin Nutr* 1998;68(1):96–102.
6. Kalkwarf HJ, Harrast SD. Effects of calcium supplementation and lactation on iron status. *Am J Clin Nutr* 1998;67(6): 1244–1249.
7. Touchette M, Slaughter R. The effect of renal failure on hepatic drug clearance. *DICP* 1991;25:1214–1224.
8. Anderson K, Conney A, Kappas A. Nutrition and oxidative drug metabolism in man: Relative influence of dietary lipids, carbohydrates, and protein. *Clin Pharmacol Ther* 1979;26: 493–501.
9. Juan D, Worwag E, Schoeller D, et al. Effects of dietary protein on theophylline pharmacokinetics and caffeine and aminopyrine breath tests. *Clin Pharmacol Ther* 1986;40:187–194.
10. Fagan T, Walle T, Oexmann M, et al. Increased clearance of propranolol and theophylline by high-protein compared with high-carbohydrate diet. *Clin Pharmacol Ther* 1987;41: 402–406.
11. Berlinger W, Park G, Spector R. The effect of dietary protein on the clearance of allopurinol and oxypurinol. *N Engl J Med* 1985;313:771–776.
12. George C. Drug metabolism by the gastrointestinal mucosa. *Clin Pharmacokinet* 1981;6:259–274.
13. Pantuck E, Pantuck C, Garland W, et al. Stimulatory effect of brussels sprouts and cabbage on human drug metabolism. *Clin Pharmacol Ther* 1979;25:88–95.
14. Pantuck E, Pantuck C, Anderson K, et al. Effect of brussels sprouts and cabbage on drug conjugation. *Clin Pharmacol Ther* 1984;35:161–169.
15. Yang C, Brady J, Hong J. Dietary effects on cytochromes P-450, xenobiotic metabolism, and toxicity. *FASEB J* 1992;6:737–744.
16. Vang O, Jensen M, Autrup H. Induction of cytochrome P450 1A1 in rat colon and liver by indole-3-carbinol and 5,6-benzoflavone. *Carcinogenesis* 1990;11:1259–1263.
17. Campbell T, Hayes J. The role of nutrition in the drug-metabolizing enzyme system. *Pharmacol Rev* 1974;26:171–197.
18. Evarts R, Mostafa M. Effects of indole and tryptophane on cytochrome P-450, dimethylnitrosamine demethylase, and arylhydrocarbon hydroxylase activities. *Biochem Pharmacol* 1981; 30:517–522.
19. Paine A. Effects of amino acids and inducers on the activity of microsomal monooxygenase system in rat liver cell culture. *Chem Biol Interact* 1976;13:307–315.
20. Yoo J, Hong J, Ning S, et al. Roles of dietary corn oil in the regulation of cytochromes P-450 and glutathione S-transferases in rat liver. *J Nutr* 1990;120:1718–1726.
21. Hong J, Pan J, Gonzalez F, et al. The induction of a specific form of cytochrome P-450 (P-450j) by fasting. *Biochem Biophys Res Commun* 1987;142:1077–1083.
22. Yoo J, Park H, Ning S, et al. Effects of thiamine deficiency on hepatic cytochromes P450 and drug-metabolizing enzyme activities. *Biochem Pharmacol* 1990;39:519–525.
23. Fuhr U. Drug interactions with grapefruit juice. Extent, probable mechanism and clinical relevance. *Drug Safety* 1998;18(4): 251–272.
24. Tassaneeyakul W, Guo LQ, Fukuda K, et al. Inhibition selectivity of grapefruit juice components on human cytochromes P450. *Arch Biochem Biophys* 2000;378(2):356–363.
25. Bailey DG, Arnold JM, Munoz C, et al. Grapefruit juice—felodipine interaction: mechanism, predictability, and effect of naringin. *Clin Pharmacol Ther* 1993;53(6):637–642.
26. Bailey DG, Arnold JM, Strong HA, et al. Effect of grapefruit juice and naringin on nisoldipine pharmacokinetics. *Clin Pharmacol Ther* 1993;54(6):589–594.
27. Guengerich F, Kim D. *In vitro* inhibition of dihydropyridine oxidation and aflatoxin B1 activation in human liver microsomes by naringenin and other flavonoids. *Carcinogenesis* 1990; 11:2275–2279.
28. Ozdemir M, Aktan Y, Boydag BS, et al. Interaction between grapefruit juice and diazepam in humans. *Eur J Drug Metab Pharmacokinet* 1998;23(1):55–59.
29. Pisarik P. Blood pressure-lowering effect of adding grapefruit juice to nifedipine and terazosin in a patient with severe renovascular hypertension. *Arch Fam Med* 1996;5(7):413–416.
30. Guengerich F. Characterization of human cytochrome P450 enzymes. *FASEB J* 1992;6:745–748.
31. Holloway D, Peterson F. Ascorbic acid in drug metabolism. In: Roe D, Campbell T, eds. *Drug and nutrients: The interactive effects.* New York: Marcel Dekker Inc, 1984:225–295.
32. Ginter E, Vejmolova J. Vitamin C status and pharmacokinetics profile of antipyrine in man. *Br J Clin Pharmacol* 1981;12: 256–258.
33. Holloway D, Hutton S, Peterson F, et al. Lack of effect of subclinical ascorbic acid deficiency upon antipyrine metabolism in man. *Am J Clin Nutr* 1982;35:917–924.
34. Trang J, Blanchard J, Conrad K, et al. The effect of vitamin C on the pharmacokinetics of caffeine in elderly men. *Am J Clin Nutr* 1982;35:487–494.
35. Houston J. Effect of vitamin C supplement on antipyrine disposition in man. *Br J Clin Pharmacol* 1977;4:236–239.
36. Houston L, Levy G. Modification of drug biotransformation by vitamin C in man. *Nature* 1975;255:78–79.
37. Shigetomi S, Kuchel O. Defective 3,4-dihydroxyphenylalanine decarboxylation to dopamine in hydralazine-treated hypertensive patients may be pyridoxine remedial. *Am J Hypertension* 1993;6:33–40.
38. O'Malley K, Stevenson I. Iron deficiency anemia and drug metabolism. *J Pharm Pharmacol* 1973;25:339–340.
39. Brater D. Clinical pharmacology of loop diuretics in health and disease. *Eur Heart J* 1992;13(Suppl G):10–14.
40. Fillastre J, Montay G, Bruno R, et al. Pharmacokinetics of sparfloxacin in patients with renal impairment. *Antimicrob Agents Chemother* 1994;38:733–737.
41. Verpooten G, Genissel P, Thomas J, et al. Single-dose pharmacokinetics of perindopril and its metabolites in hypertensive patients with various degrees of renal insufficiency. *Br J Clin Pharmacol* 1991;32:187–192.
42. Lamy P. Effects of diet and nutrition of drug therapy. *J Am Geriatr Soc* 1982;30(Suppl):S99–S112.
43. Roe D. Therapeutic significance of drug–nutrient interactions in the elderly. *Pharmacol Rev* 1984;36:109S–122S.
44. Botez M, Botez T, Ross-Chouinard A, et al. Thiamine and folate treatment in chronic epileptic patients: A controlled study with the Wechsler IQ scale. *Epilepsy Res* 1993;16:157–163.
45. Hansson O, Sillanpaa M. Pyridoxine and serum concentrations of phenytoin and phenobarbitone. *Lancet* 1976;1:256 (letter).
46. McCune R, Deuschle K, McDermott W. The delayed appearance of isoniazid antagonism by pyridoxine in-vivo. *Ann Rev Tuberc* 1957;76:1106–1109.
47. Jemeson H. Pyridoxine for levodopa-induced dystonia. *JAMA* 1970;211:1700.
48. Evered DF. L-dopa as a vitamin-B6 antagonist. *Lancet* 1971; 1(7705):914.
49. Kappus H, Diplock A. Tolerance and safety of vitamin E: A toxicological position report. *Free Radical Biol Med* 1992;13: 55–74.
50. March B, Wong E, Seier I, et al. Hypervitaminosis E in the chick. *J Nutr* 1973;103:371–377.
51. Herbert V, Jacob E. Destruction of vitamin B12 by ascorbic acid. *JAMA* 1974;230:241–242.
52. Newmark H, Scheiner J, Marcus M, et al. Stability of vitamin

B12 in the presence of ascorbic acid. *Am J Clin Nutr* 1976;29: 645–649.
53. Golper T, Hartstein A, Morthland V, et al. Effects of antacids and dialysis dwell times on multiple-dose pharmacokinetics of oral ciprofloxacin in patients on continuous ambulatory peritoneal dialysis. *Antimicrob Agents Chemother* 1987;31: 1787–1790.
54. Hoeffken G, Borner K, Glatzel P, et al. Reduced enteral absorption of ciprofloxacin in the presence of antacids. *Eur J Clin Microbiol* 1985;3:345.
55. Nix D, Watson W, Lerner M, et al. Effects of aluminum and magnesium antacids and ranitidine on the absorption of ciprofloxacin. *Clin Pharmacol Therapeut* 1989;46:700–705.
56. Redandt J, Marchbanks C, Dudley M. Interactions of fluoroquinolones with other drugs: Mechanisms, variability, clinical significance and management. *Clin Infect Dis* 1992;14:272–284.
57. Toothaker R, Welling P. The effect of food on drug bioavailability. *Ann Rev Pharmacol Toxicol* 1980;20:173–199.
58. Deppermann K, Lode H. Fluoroquinolones: Interaction profile during enteral absorption. *Drugs* 1993;45(Suppl 3):65–72.
59. Kitamura K, Takahashi T, Tanaka H, et al. Two cases of thiamine deficiency-induced lactic acidosis during total parenteral nutrition. *Tohoku J Exp Med* 1993;171:129–133.
60. Klein G, Probst S, Kessler P, et al. Thiamine deficiency as a cause of life threatening lactic acidosis in total parenteral nutrition. *Klin Wochenschr* 1991;69(Suppl 26):193–195.
61. Naito E, Ito M, Takeda E, et al. Molecular analysis of abnormal pyruvate dehydrogenase in a patient with thiamine-responsive congenital lactic acidosis. *Pediatr Res* 1994;36:340–346.
62. Sanz París A, Albero Gamoa R, Acha Pérez FJ, et al. Thiamine deficiency associated with parenteral nutrition: apropos of a new case. *Nutricion Hospitalaria* 1994;9(2):110–113.
63. Hamalatha S, Kerr D, Wexler I, et al. Pyruvate dehydrogenase complex deficiency due to a point mutation (P188L) within the thiamine pyrophosphate binding loop of the E1 alpha subunit. *Hum Mol Gen* 1995;4:315–318.
64. Palopoli J, Waxman J. Recurrent aphthous stomatitis and vitamin B12 deficiency. *South Med J* 1990;83:475–477.
65. Force R, Nahata M. Effect of histamine H2-receptor antagonists on vitamin B12 absorption. *Ann Pharmacother* 1992;26: 1283–1286.
66. Carl G, Smith M. Phenytoin-folate interaction: Differing effects of the sodium salt and the free acid of phenytoin. *Epilepsia* 1992;33:372–376.
67. Casserly C, Stange K, Chren M. Severe megaloblastic anemia in a patient receiving low dose methotrexate for psoriasis. *J Am Acad Dermatol* 1993;29:477–480.
68. Elmazar M, Nau H. Trimetoprim potentiates valproic acid-induced neural tube defects in mice. *Reprod Toxicol* 1993;7: 249–254.
69. Joosten E, Pelemans W. Megaloblastic anemia in the elderly patient treated with triamterene. *Neth J Med* 1991;38:209–211.
70. Baylis E, Crowley J, Preece J, et al. Influence of folic acid on blood phenytoin levels. *Lancet* 1971;1:62–64.
71. Shah I, Whiting P, Omar G, et al. The effects of retinoids and terbinafine on the human microsomal metabolism of cyclosporine. *Br J Dermatol* 1993;129:395–398.
72. Kaiser C, McAuliffe J, Barth R, et al. Hypoprothrombinemia and hemorrhage in a surgical patient treated with cefotetan. *Arch Surg* 1991;126:524–525.
73. Kikuchi S, Ando A, Minato K. Acquired coagulopathy caused by administration of parenteral broad spectrum antibiotics. *Jpn J Clin Pathol* 1991;39:83–90.
74. Westphal J, Vetter D, Brogard J. Hepatic side-effects of antibiotics. *J Antimicrob Chemother* 1994;33:387–401.
75. Zerwekh J, Homan R, Tindall R, et al. Decreased serum 24, 25-dihydroxyvitamin D concentration during long-term anticonvulsant therapy in adult epileptics. *Ann Neurol* 1982;12: 184–186.
76. Kopple J, Hirschberg R. Nutrition and peritoneal dialysis. In: Mitch W, Klahr S, eds. Nutrition and the kidney. Boston: Little, Brown and Company, 1993:290–313.
77. Drutz D, Tai T, Cheng T, et al. Hypokalemic rhabdomyolysis and myoglobinuria following amphotericin B therapy. *JAMA* 1970;211:824–826.
78. Shirley D, Singer D, Sagnella G, et al. Effect of a single test dose of lithium carbonate on sodium and potassium excretion in man. *Clin Sci* 1991;81:59–63.
79. Murphy M, Lewis P, Kohner E, et al. Glucose intolerance in hypertensive patients treated with diuretics. A 14 year follow-up. *Lancet* 1982;2:1293–1295.
80. Hoskins B, Jackson C. Mechanism of chlorothiazide-induced carbohydrate intolerance. *J Pharmacol Exp Ther* 1978;206: 423–430.
81. Race T, Paes I, Faloon W. Intestinal malabsorption induced by oral colchicine: comparison with neomycin and cathartic agents. *Am Med Sci* 1981;259:32–41.
82. Eknoyan G, Suki W, Martinez-Maldonato M. Effect of diuretics on urinary excretion of phosphate, calcium and magnesium in thyroparathyroidectomized dogs. *J Lab Clin Med* 1970;76: 257–266.
83. Ono K. Secondary hyperoxalemia caused by vitamin C supplementation in regular hemodialysis patients. *Clin Nephrol* 1986; 26:239–243.
84. Newmark K, Nugent P. Milk-alkali syndrome: A consequence of chronic antacid abuse. *Postgrad Med* 1993;93:149–150,156.
85. Mitwalli A, Oreopoulos D. Hyperoxaluria and hyperoxalemia: One more concern for the nephrologist. *Int J Artific Org* 1985; 8:71–74.
86. Chen W, Chiang T, Chen T. Serum zinc and copper during long-term parenteral nutrition. *J Formosan Med Assoc* 1991;90: 1075–1080.
87. Milanino R, Frigo A, Bambara L, et al. Copper and zinc status in rheumatoid arthritis: Studies of plasma, erythrocytes, and urine and their relationship to disease activity markers and pharmacological treatment. *Clin Exp Rheumat* 1993;11:271–281.
88. Goldwasser P, Koutelos T, Abraham S, et al. Serum ferritin, hematocrit and mean corpuscular volume in hemodialysis. *Nephron* 1994;67:30–35.
89. Schaffer SW, Lombardini JB, Azuma J. Interaction between the actions of taurine and angiotensin II. *Amino Acids* 2000;18(4): 305–318.
90. Cruz CI, Ruiz-Torres P, del Moral RG, et al. Age-related progressive renal fibrosis in rats and its prevention with ACE inhibitors and taurine. *Am J Physiol Renal Physiol* 2000;278(1): F122–129.
91. Franconi F, Bennardini F, Mattana A, et al. Plasma and platelet taurine are reduced in subjects with insulin-dependent diabetes mellitus: effects of taurine supplementation. *Am J Clin Nutr* 1995;61(5):1115–1119.
92. Zhao X, Jia J, Lin Y. Taurine content in Chinese food and daily intake of Chinese men. *Adv Exp Med Biol* 1998;442(5): 501–505.
93. Danovitch G. Immunosuppressive medications and protocols for kidney transplantation. In: Danovitch G, ed. *Handbook of kidney transplantation.* Boston: Little, Brown and Company, 1992:67–103.
94. Lindholm A, Henriccson S, Dahlqvist R. The effect of food and bile acid administration on the relative bioavailability of cyclosporine. *Br J Clin Pharmacol* 1990;29:541–548.
95. Kolars J, Awni W, Merion R, et al. First-pass metabolism of cyclosporine by the gut. *Lancet* 1991;338:1488–1490.

96. Fahr A. Cyclosporine clinical pharmacokinetics. *Clin Pharmacokinet* 1993;24:472–495.
97. Christians U, Sewing K. Cyclosporine metabolism in transplant patients. *Pharmacol Ther* 1993;57:291–345.
98. Menon S, Walker R, Duggin G, et al. Cyclosporine A blood levels are not influenced by dietary alterations in lipids. *Res Commun Chem Pathol Pharmacol* 1991;72:203–212.
99. Bodreaux J, Heyes D, Mizrahi S, et al. Use of water-soluble liquid vitamin E to enhance cyclosporine absorption in children after liver transplantation. *Transpl Proc* 1993;25:1875.
100. Sokol E, Johnson K, Karrer F, et al. Improvement of cyclosporine absorption in children after liver transplantation by means of water-soluble vitamin E. *Lancet* 1991;338:212–214.
101. de Lorgeril M, Boissonnat P, Salen P, et al. The beneficial effect of dietary antioxidant supplementation on platelet aggregation and cyclosporine treatment in heart transplant recipients. *Transpl* 1994;58:193–195.
102. Webber I, Back D. Effect of etretinate on cyclosporine metabolism in-vitro. *Br J Dermatol* 1993;128:42–44.
103. Herlitz H, Edgar B, Hedner T, et al. Grapefruit juice: A possible source of variability in blood concentrations of cyclosporine A. *Nephr Dial Transpl* 1993;8:375.
104. Brunner LJ, Munar MY, Vallian J, et al. Interaction between cyclosporine and grapefruit juice requires long-term ingestion in stable renal transplant recipients. *Pharmacotherapy* 1998;18(1):23–29.
105. Dickerson R, Melnik G. Osmolality of oral drug solutions and suspensions. *Am J Hosp Pharm* 1988;45:832–834.
106. Melnik G. Pharmacologic aspects of enteral nutrition. In: Rombeau J, Coldwell M, eds. *Clinical nutrition: enteral and tube feeding.* Philadelphia: W.B. Saunders Company, 1990: 472–509.
107. Worden J, Wood C, Workman C. Phenytoin and nasogastric feedings. *Neurology* 1994;34:132.
108. Au Yeung SC, Ensom MH. Phenytoin and enteral feedings: does evidence support an interaction? *Ann Pharmacother* 2000; 34(7–8):896–905.
109. Scott D. Addition of potassium supplements to mild-based tube feedings. *J Hum Nutr* 1980;34:85–90.
110. Howard P, Hannaman K. Warfarin resistance linked to enteral nutrition products. *J Am Diet Assoc* 1985;85:713–715.
111. Valli C, Schultheiss H, Asper R, et al. Interaction of nutrients with antacids: A complication during enteral tube feeding. *Lancet* 1986;1:747–748.
112. Lee M, Schwartz R, Sharifi R. Warfarin resistance and vitamin K. *Ann Intern Med* 1981;94:140–141.
113. Nimmo W. Drugs, disease and altered gastric emptying. *Clin Pharmacokinet* 1976;1:189–203.
114. Prescott L. Gastric emptying and drug absorption. *Br J Clin Pharmacol* 1974;1:189–190.
115. Couet W, Istin B, Sinuta P, et al. Effect of ponsinomycin on cyclosporine pharmacokinetics. *Eur J Clin Pharmacol* 1990;39: 165–167.

34

REHABILITATIVE EXERCISE TRAINING IN PATIENTS UNDERGOING DIALYSIS

RICHARD CASABURI

Although dialysis prolongs the lives of patients with chronic renal failure, these patients frequently have a low level of physical function (1). More than one-third of patients undergoing hemodialysis are unable to perform the normal activities of daily living without assistance (1). Only a small proportion of patients undergoing chronic dialysis therapy who are less than 65 years of age are employed (2). Depression is highly prevalent (3); these patients tend to withdraw from the world and become homebound and isolated. Poor functioning is associated with lower quality of life (4) and decreased survival (5) in this population. Rehabilitation programs for patients receiving dialytic therapy are surprisingly scarce (2,6); yet it might be suspected that the patient undergoing dialysis might be a good candidate for rehabilitation. By the nature of their requirement for regular dialysis, these patients are identified easily by health care providers. Seeing them on a regular basis simplifies the evaluation of their rehabilitative needs.

Programs of rehabilitation generally are multifaceted and multidisciplinary. Common components include disease education, psychosocial support, nutritional advice, family involvement, and patient support groups (7,8). These components tend to help patients accept their disease and optimize their function. An *exercise program* is almost universally used, based on solid evidence of effectiveness in almost all chronic disease states (9).

Exercise programs potentially have two distinct benefits: psychologic and physiologic. The psychologic benefits of exercise are beginning to be understood; exercise programs generally have a marked antidepressant effect (10). One antidepressant mechanism is that people who master something that they perceive to be difficult (e.g., exercise) experience positive psychologic feedback that improves their self-confidence and their ability to cope with everyday problems (11). Another mechanism of improvement is that patients socially interacting in an exercise program in a group setting in the presence of trained medical personnel lose their unrealistic fear of activity. An additional mechanism of psychologic benefit of exercise is desensitization. This often occurs if the patient can be distracted from the unpleasant sensations that exercise elicits. Providing distractions —interacting with staff and other patients or listening to music—often can yield better tolerance of exercise. The latter two mechanisms likely explain why home exercise programs are generally less successful than programs organized in a rehabilitation center. Exercise programs that focus on reaping these psychologic benefits are often successful in improving exercise tolerance and quality of life. In contrast to exercise programs designed to yield physiologic benefits, the design of these programs does not have to adhere to specific design features.

If physiologic gains are to be obtained from an exercise program, more careful attention to design features is required. This review seeks to summarize those design features relevant to patients with chronic renal failure. It draws on the large body of literature defining successful strategies for exercise training in *healthy* subjects. There also is a substantial literature defining specific factors that contribute to exercise intolerance in patients undergoing dialysis therapy. A small but growing number of studies have documented the effectiveness of physiologically sound exercise training programs in patients with chronic renal failure.

PHYSIOLOGIC TRAINING PRINCIPLES IN HEALTHY SUBJECTS

Morphologic and Functional Changes Induced by Training

The human machine adapts differently to two distinct training strategies (12). Strength training improves the ability to perform explosive tasks, such as weightlifting or sprinting (13). Endurance training improves the tolerance of sustained tasks, such as walking or stair climbing. These latter tasks generally are felt to be more relevant to day-to-day activities, so rehabilitative exercise programs usually focus on endurance training.

This focus may change in the future as the benefits of strength training become better defined. Strength training has been considered particularly important for patients who are debilitated because decline in muscle mass and strength has been related to physical frailty, falls (with consequent bone fracture), and functional decline (14–16). Strength-training programs have the effect of inducing selective fiber hypertrophy and thus increasing muscle mass. The muscle thereby increases its ability to generate more tension.

Endurance activities require a sustained supply of bioenergetic substrate. Skeletal muscle utilizes ATP (adenosine triphosphate) to initiate and sustain contraction (17). ATP generation is a central focus of muscle biochemistry. Nutrients (mainly fats and carbohydrates) are metabolized to yield CO_2 and water. The energy yield of this process is stored in the form of ATP and other high-energy phosphate compounds. Efficient ATP generation requires an adequate supply of oxygen to the exercising muscle. Therefore, it is an important design criterion for the exercising muscles (and for the body as a whole) that oxygen delivery be promoted. When oxygen requirements of an exercise task outstrip oxygen supply (i.e., when *aerobic* metabolism is inadequate), a supplementary backup mechanism is available. *Anaerobic* metabolism requires no oxygen but operates at a much less efficient ATP yield. Further, the side product of anaerobic metabolism is lactic acid accumulation. This acidifies the cellular environment, depletes the body's buffer supply (lowering blood bicarbonate levels), and ultimately contributes to muscle fatigue (18).

Skeletal muscle is composed of two types of contractile cells (19). Type I fibers (also known as slow-twitch or oxidative) are designed for prolonged, repetitive contraction. Type II fibers (fast-twitch or glycolytic) contract rapidly but rely on anaerobic metabolism at relatively low rates of work. Although the distribution of fiber types within a muscle essentially is fixed (20,21), other aspects of muscle structure and biochemistry change dramatically after an effective program of endurance exercise training. Type IIb fibers, which have a low capacity for oxidative metabolism, remodel into type IIa fibers (22), which are more similar to type I fibers. In type I fibers, the mitochondria (the principal site of ATP production) increase in size and number with endurance exercise training (19). The concentration of the enzymes that facilitate oxidative metabolism increase, often by 100% or more (23). Another key adaptation is the proliferation of muscle capillaries (19). The number of capillaries increases out of proportion to the increase in fiber diameter. This decreases the distance oxygen must diffuse from the capillary to the site of utilization in the mitochondria. As a result, oxygen extraction from the capillary blood can be more complete.

The cardiovascular system also undergoes changes as a result of an endurance training program (24–26). The heart's ventricular walls thicken, and chamber size increases. Peak cardiac output is higher. At a given level of exercise, stroke volume is higher and heart rate is lower; but cardiac output is approximately unchanged. Both systolic and diastolic pressures are generally lower after training, especially in the individual with hypertension (27).

Body composition changes often are seen after a program of endurance training (28,29), although these are not nearly as great as those seen after a strength-training program. Muscle mass increases, but only in the muscles that participate in the training exercises. Body fat decreases. The net effect on body weight is variable and largely depends on dietary intake during the training program.

Cardiopulmonary exercise testing, which includes ventilatory, gas exchange, and heart rate measurements (30), is a tool that can be used to define the beneficial changes induced by a training program. If a healthy subject performs a progressively increasing work rate test on a cycle ergometer, the peak oxygen uptake (and the peak work rate) increases after an effective program of exercise training (29). Increases in peak oxygen uptake on the order of 10% to 15% are common. In such a test, it is possible to use oxygen uptake and CO_2 output responses to define the oxygen uptake at which lactic acid accumulation in the blood begins (17,31) (i.e., the lactic acidosis threshold, also known as the anaerobic threshold). After training, better oxygen supply to the muscle mitochondria forestalls the onset of lactic acidosis and the lactic threshold can increase by 25% to 35% (32).

Responses to submaximal exercise also are altered after a training program; these changes mainly are seen at work rates above the lactic acidosis threshold (32,33). After endurance training, better oxygen delivery yields lower blood lactate levels at a given level of submaximal exercise. Oxygen uptake is mildly lower at high work rates and is well correlated with the fall in blood lactate (32). The decrease in CO_2 output is related to the decrease in CO_2 generated as bicarbonate buffers lactic acid. Pulmonary ventilation is substantially lower at higher work rates, both because ventilation is linked to CO_2 output and less CO_2 needs to be exhaled and also because of decreased acid stimulation of the carotid bodies. Heart rate is lower at all work rates, related to the shift toward higher stroke volumes mentioned earlier. Sympathetic tone falls, leading to lower blood epinephrine and norepinephrine levels (32–34). Finally, ratings of perceived exertion for a given work rate are generally lower after a program of endurance training (35).

Characteristics of an Effective Exercise Training Program

Rational design of endurance exercise training programs is hampered by our lack of knowledge of the specific stimulus-response relationships that mediate the structural and biochemical changes that occur in the exercising muscles.

Clearly, tropic substances must be secreted that mediate these changes. The discovery of vascular endothelial growth factor (VEGF) and the description of its ability to increase capillarity of muscle tissue (36) may be one step toward understanding the cellular signals linking exercise and muscle growth. Because training-induced changes occur only in the muscles involved in the training exercise (the specificity principle) (25,37), at least some portion of the mediation must involve local events. Some evidence favors the concept that repetitive stretch, in itself, initiates both hypertrophy and hyperplasia (38). Hormonal control of muscle growth seems likely. Considerable attention has been focused on the possibility that anabolic hormones may play at least a facilitating role. However, the two anabolic hormonal systems that are best defined seem to produce changes in muscle that resemble strength, not endurance, training responses in that hypertrophy and not adaptations facilitating aerobic function are prominent. Recent evidence has shown that testosterone administration increases muscle strength and bulk in healthy men (39,40). There is evidence that secretion of growth hormone by the pituitary is increased modestly by bouts of endurance exercise (41–43); this increases the circulating level of insulinlike growth factor-1 (IGF-1), which mediates growth hormone's anabolic effects on muscle. It seems possible that stimulation of intracellular increases in IGF-1 may mediate muscle hypertrophic responses from a number of stimuli.

Because we are unsure of the stimulus-response relationships mediating the training response, we must rely on empiric evidence when considering how to design training programs. This empiric evidence is difficult to obtain (the training response takes weeks to develop), and it is difficult to be sure that findings can be extrapolated from one group of subjects to another.

Nevertheless, much is known about what constitutes an effective training program. Further, the basic considerations found valid for healthy subjects have been found to apply (with some quantitative adjustments) to a variety of patient groups (44). The following are the recognized determinants of the effectiveness of a training program.

Exercise Intensity

Exercise intensity prescription has two major tenets. It is believed that there is a threshold intensity below which no training effect will be obtained (a "critical training intensity") no matter how rigorous the other training program characteristics (45). It also is believed that if the work rate is above this critical intensity, the total work per session is the primary determinant of the training response (29,45).

These tenets are not beyond challenge, however. For example, it has been demonstrated that exercise intensities generally felt to be below the "critical training intensity" can yield a physiologic training effect (46). A major problem in prescribing exercise intensity is deciding which physiologic variable to use to monitor intensity. Because exercise tolerance often differs markedly among individuals presenting for a training program, work rate itself cannot be used directly as a training intensity guide without some normalizing procedure. Several normalizing approaches have been proposed.

Heart Rate

The heart rate variable has the virtue of being easy to measure. Also, peak heart rate does not vary markedly with fitness among healthy subjects, although it does vary with age. In healthy subjects, exercise that induces a heart rate greater than 70% of the predicted maximum heart rate (often calculated as 220 − age) has been asserted to be a good training target (25,45). However, in patients with chronotropic disorders, in situations where changes in circulating blood volume can alter the relation between heart rate and work rate, in patients taking certain medications (e.g., beta blockers), and in cases where noncardiac limitations to exercise exist, the use of heart rate as an exercise intensity guide can be problematic.

Oxygen Uptake (VO_2)

To utilize oxygen uptake as a training intensity guide, a preliminary incremental exercise test is performed, preferably using the mode of exercise to be used in the training program. A training intensity is prescribed as the work rate corresponding to a fixed percentage of the measured peak VO_2. An often-quoted definition of the critical training intensity for healthy subjects is the work rate corresponding to 50% of the observed peak VO_2 (45), although distinct training effects have been documented using work rates below this target (46–48).

Blood Lactate

Work rates associated with lactic acidosis place more stress on the exercising muscle in terms of local acidosis and hypoxia, as well as accelerated substrate utilization. It has been hypothesized that these factors have at least an indirect relationship to the actual training stimulus (33,49,50). Credence is lent to the use of the lactic acidosis threshold as a critical training intensity because it generally occurs at roughly 50% of peak VO_2 in healthy subjects (51). However, the validity of using blood lactate levels to select exercise intensities has been challenged: healthy subjects have developed physiologic evidence of training from exercise programs using work rates below the lactic acidosis threshold (46). Also, patients with chronic obstructive pulmonary disease who are unable to sustain work rates associated with lactic acidosis during training have nonetheless manifested a physiologic training effect (52).

Ratings of Perceived Exertion

Scales for rating exertion have been developed (53), either as visual analogue scales (anchored on each end by descriptions of minimal and maximal symptom intensities) and numeric scales (with numbers corresponding to progressively increasing symptoms, such as the Borg scale) (54). However, the perception of sensations is only moderately reproducible and is clearly subject to psychologic modification (10). It is inadvisable to use ratings of perceived exertion as the sole training intensity assessment, particularly in research studies.

Training Session Frequency

There is consensus that training three to five times per week is desirable (29,45,55). A discernibly smaller, but still distinct, training effect can be obtained from sessions held twice a week. There is little evidence that sessions held more than five times per week are of additional benefit (29).

Training Session Duration

Training sessions of 30 to 60 minutes duration seem to be optimal (29,56); 45 minutes seems to be a reasonable target. Sessions 10 to 20 minutes in duration yield significantly smaller effects. It should be mentioned that the specificity principle dictates that sessions composed of short segments of exercise involving different muscle groups (e.g., arm cranking and treadmill walking) may not yield a substantial training effect, even if the total exercise time is in the 30 to 60 minute range.

Training Program Duration

If the training work rate is kept constant in a well-designed training program, measures of the training effect approach a new steady state exponentially, with a half-time of roughly 10 days (57,58). Therefore, after about 3 to 4 weeks no further changes are seen (57–59). Because in most settings the training work rate is advanced as the program proceeds, a program of longer duration will yield further benefits.

Mode of Exercise

Suitable activities are those that involve the large muscle groups and cause a substantial increase in metabolic rate (29,60). These activities include running, rapid walking, stair climbing, swimming, bicycling, and arm cranking (45).

Other Factors

Potential for improvement of performance is greater, when expressed as a percent increase, in sedentary subjects as compared to the very fit (29,55,61). Training programs can be effective in older subjects as well as younger subjects (62–65). Training work rates are generally lower in the elderly (predicted peak VO_2 decreases roughly 10% per decade between the age of 20 and 60 years) (66). Because the lactic acidosis threshold is a slightly higher fraction of peak O_2 in older subjects (17), if training intensity is assigned in terms of a percentage of peak VO_2, a slightly higher target is advisable for healthy older subjects.

Although most investigations of training program effectiveness have involved male subjects, available evidence indicates that women adapt to endurance training in a manner similar to men (29). Infrequently, women with low body fat undergoing very rigorous training experience menstrual irregularity or infertility (67).

Maintenance Programs

Once a training program has been started, participants must be advised to continue for life. If sedentary behavior is resumed, the benefits recede roughly as fast as they were achieved (i.e., within a few weeks) (29,45,68,69). It seems likely that once a given level of fitness has been established, a modest decrease in the frequency of sessions and session duration will not yield a discernible decrease in fitness (70, 71). However, a decrease in training intensity seems to result in a gradual decrease in fitness (72).

CAUSES OF EXERCISE INTOLERANCE IN PATIENTS WITH CHRONIC RENAL FAILURE

Patients undergoing long-term dialysis therapy generally have substantially reduced exercise tolerance (73–75). As can be seen in Tables 34.1 and 34.2, peak oxygen uptake is most often in the range of 15 to 22 mL/kg/min, which is little more than half the predicted levels of healthy subjects of similar characteristics. Further, the lactic acidosis threshold, a measure of the ability to sustain endurance activities, clearly is reduced in both adults (76,77) and children (78) undergoing dialysis therapy. Among the identified factors that yield decreased exercise tolerance in patients with chronic renal failure are deconditioning, low muscle mass and malnutrition, anemia, cardiovascular dysfunction, myopathy, and low levels of anabolic hormones.

Deconditioning

Deconditioning is the physiologic change that occurs in the body as a result of physical inactivity. Primarily from experiments in which healthy subjects have undergone prolonged periods of bedrest, a constellation of changes in the muscle have been identified that result from deconditioning. Muscle mass declines. The activity of enzymes involved in aerobic energy production along with mitochondrial density decreases. The number of capillaries surrounding each muscle fiber is lower, increasing diffusion distance for oxygen transport. There is a transformation among type II fibers: type IIa fibers remodel into type IIb fibers, and this lowers aerobic capacity. All of these structural and

TABLE 34.1. SELECTED REPORTS OF THE EFFECTS OF ERYTHROPOIETIN TREATMENT ON EXERCISE TOLERANCE IN PATIENTS UNDERGOING HEMODIALYSIS

Reference	Mayer et al. (1988) (93)	MacDougall et al. (1990) (94)	Canadian Erythropoietin Study Group (1990) (95)	Grunze et al. (1990) (96)	Robertson et al. (1990) (97)	Braumann et al. (1991) (98)	Lundin et al. (1991) (99)	Metra et al. (1991) (100)	Davenport et al. (1991) (101)	Barany et al. (1993) (102)	Lewis et al. (1993) (103)	Marrades et al. (1993) (104)
Number of subjects (# male)	8 (4)	10 (6)	78 (45)	8 (6)	19 (11)	12 (10)	10 (7)	10 (8)	11(7)	21 (11)	9 (5)	8 (8)
Age (y)	35	43	44	43	47 ± 13	22–57	44 ± 8	29 ± 11	34	39 ± 12	36	24 ± 5
Initial VO_2max (mL/kg/min)	16 ± 3	19 ± 7	—	1.2 ± 0.3 L/min	15 ± 5	—	15 ± 5	21 ± 4	—	20 ± 5	19 ± 4	25 ± 5
Treatment duration	9 weeks	12 months	6 months	6 months	10 months	10 and 30 weeks	3 ± 2 months	3 months	13.5 weeks	12 months	5 ± 8 months	7 ± 5 months
Treatment dose (U/kg/wk)	300	240	226	150	450–900 initially	147	450	150 ng/kg/wk	80	90–450	120	93 ± 21
Initial hemoglobin (g/dL)	5.9 ± 6.1	6.4 ± 0.6	7.0	7.3	—	7.3 ± 1.2	7.1 ± 1.4	5.9 ± 1.2	6.0	7.3 ± 1.0	7.0 ± 1.2	7.5 ± 1.0
Final hemoglobin (g/dL)	10.9 ± 0.6	10.8 ± 0.7	11.0	10.4	—	11.9 ± 1.5	9.8 ± 1.2	9.9 ± 1.4	11.0	10.4 ± 1.4	11.1 ± 1.1	12.5 ± 1.0
Initial hematocrit (%)	17 ± 1	20 ± 2	—	—	21 ± 4	20 ± 3	21 ± 5	17 ± 3	18	—	—	—
Final hematocrit (%)	33 ± 3	33 ± 1	—	—	35 ± 3	31 ± 3	32 ± 5	31 ± 5	33	—	—	—
Exercise testing modality	Cycle	Treadmill	Treadmill	Cycle	Cycle	Cycle	Treadmill	Cycle	Cycle	Cycle	Treadmill	Cycle
Magnitude of the exercise performance increase	45% VO_2max, 39% anaerobic threshold	19% VO_2max, 19% anaerobic threshold	24% treadmill time	15% VO_2max, 25% anaerobic threshold	17% VO_2max	—	50% O_2max	24% VO_2max, 13% anaerobic threshold	20% maximum work rate	35% VO_2max	34% VO_2max, 18% lactate threshold	29% VO_2max
Other physiologic changes	Heart rate lower at rest and during exercise	Decreased left ventricular mass	9% increase in 6-min walk distance	Decreased heart rate at 50 watts	Decreased heart rate, ventilation at constant work rate, increased quadriceps strength	Work rate at heart rate of 130 increased 35%. Work rate at lactate = 2 mmol/L increased	Decrease in ventilation and R at submaximal work rate	—	—	—	—	Decreased ventilation, lactate, and leg blood flow at submaximal work rate

TABLE 34.2. PUBLISHED RESULTS OF EXERCISE TRAINING PROGRAMS FOR PATIENTS UNDERGOING DIALYSIS IN THE PRE-ERYTHROPOIETIN ERA

Reference	Zabetakis et al. (1982) (151)	Shalom et al. (1984) (152)	Harter and Goldberg 1985) (153)	Painter et al. (1986) (154)	Lennon et al. (1986) (155)	Stephens (1991) (156)	Moore et al. (1993) (108)
Number of subjects (# male)	5 (gender not stated)	7 (4)	13 (8)	14 (60% male)	10(5)	10 (9)	11 (10)
Number in control group	4	7	12	7	None	Unclear	None
Age (y)	45 ± 4	46 ± 13	40 ± 4	42 ± 10	48 ± 21	52 ± 13	Not stated
Dialysis type	Hemodialysis	5 hemodialysis, 2 CAPD	Hemodialysis	Hemodialysis	4 hemodialysis, 6 CAPD	Hemodialysis	Hemodialysis
Initial VO_2max (mL/kg/min)	18.9 ± 3.6	15.4 ± 5.8	22 ± 2	19.6 ± 4.1	18.5 ± 5.9	—	14.8 ± 3.0
Initial hematocrit (%)	23 ± 5	27 ± 4	24 ± 3	24 ± 5	27 ± 8	27 ± 4	—
Initial hemoglobin (gm/dL)	7.3 ± 1.8	—	8.3 ± 0.8	—	—	8.8 ± 1.3	9.8 ± 2.2
Supervised vs. home program	Supervised	Supervised	Supervised	Supervised	Home	Home	Supervised
Training modality	Treadmill	Bicycle, walk, jog	Bicycle, walk, jog	Bicycle	Bicycle	Mostly walking	Bicycle
Program duration	10 weeks	12 weeks	12 ± 1 months	6 months	8 weeks	8 months	12 weeks
Session frequency	3 days/week	3 days/week	3 days/week	3 days/week	3 days/week	5 ± 2 days/week	3 days/week
Session duration	25–45 min	45 min	Up to 45 min	30 min	Unclear	26 ± 8 minutes	30–60 minutes
Exercise intensity	At lactic acidosis threshold	75%–80% heart rate max	50%–80% VO_2max	65%–85% VO_2max monitored by heart rate and perceived exertion	40%–55% VO_2max	11 ± 2 on perceived exertion scale	>70% heart rate max, 6/10 on perceived exertion scale
Exercise testing modality	Treadmill	Treadmill	Treadmill	Treadmill	Cycle ergometer	None	Cycle ergometer
Exercise endurance increase	13% VO_2max; 19% lactic acidosis threshold	42% VO_2max	17 ± 4% VO_2max	23% VO_2max	−9% VO_2max	—	13% VO_2max
Other physiologic changes	No changes in hematocrit, hemoglobin, or 2–3 DPG	No changes in LV ejection fraction, hematocrit, use of antihypertensive drugs	Better blood pressure control, better lipid profiles, improved carbohydrate metabolism, increased hemoglobin and hematocrit	Better blood pressure control, no change in hematocrit or cholesterol profile	No changes in resting cholesterol or lipids	No change in hematocrit, triglycerides, or cholesterol	Lower heart rate submaximal work rates, no histologic or enzymatic changes in muscle
Quality-of-life changes	—	No change	Decreased depression and anxiety	—	—	—	—

CAPD, continuous ambulatory peritoneal dialysis; DPG, diphosphoglycerate; LV, left ventricular.

biochemical changes reduce the capacity of muscle to perform exercise aerobically. As a result, both maximal oxygen uptake and the lactic acidosis threshold decrease. A number of other physiologic changes are seen, including declines in cardiovascular function, alterations in body composition, deterioration in central nervous system function, and decreases in the levels of anabolic hormones (79).

As with patients with many chronic diseases, there is evidence that most patients undergoing hemodialysis have a very sedentary lifestyle (80). The conclusion is unavoidable that the physiologic changes associated with deconditioning contribute to exercise intolerance in many patients with chronic renal failure. However, review of the morphologic changes seen in the muscles of patients undergoing chronic hemodialysis (see later in this chapter) reveals some features not seen in studies of otherwise healthy deconditioned individuals. Selective type II fiber atrophy, abnormal myofilament and mitochondrial structure, and evidence of peripheral neuropathy are not seen in individuals who are merely deconditioned. It seems fair to conclude that deconditioning produces some, but not all, of the muscle abnormalities seen in patients receiving hemodialysis. How completely muscle architecture reverts toward normal after reversal of the deconditioned state remains an issue of importance.

Low Muscle Mass and Malnutrition

Body composition studies have shown that even patients with chronic renal failure who are free of intercurrent illness have reduced lean body mass (81–85). The depletion of lean tissue is particularly pronounced in the limbs (81–83). In a survey of 180 stable patients undergoing hemodialysis, male patients had severe reductions in muscle mass compared with a healthy population, with 50% falling below the 10th percentile of normal (84). There is agreement that protein malnutrition in patients receiving hemodialysis is associated with increased morbidity and mortality (82–89). Among all laboratory variables, protein malnutrition, as reflected by the serum albumin level, is the best predictor of survival (89,90), days of hospitalization (91), and symptoms of fatigue (84).

Anemia

Anemia reduces exercise tolerance by decreasing oxygen delivery to the exercising muscle. Hemoglobin carries the vast majority of oxygen to the tissues; oxygen delivery is reduced in approximate proportion to the decrease in hemoglobin concentration. Because peak cardiac output is low in patients undergoing hemodialysis (92), peak oxygen delivery to the muscles during exercise is reduced considerably.

There is a substantial literature documenting the effect of increasing hemoglobin levels in patients undergoing dialysis. The chief cause of low hemoglobin levels in these patients is reduced erythropoietin stimulation of the bone marrow. Erythropoietin normally is secreted by the kidney; in the last 15 years recombinant erythropoietin has become routinely available in clinical practice.

A number of clinical trials, many of them randomized and controlled, have been performed that investigate the effect of a course of erythropoietin on exercise tolerance and other variables in patients undergoing chronic hemodialysis. Table 34.1 describes the design and results of a majority of these studies. A total of 204 patients (about 60% male) underwent erythropoietin treatment in these 12 studies. The average age of participants was 40 years, although individuals in their third through sixth decade of life were well represented. Before therapy, exercise tolerance, measured in incremental exercise tests using either the treadmill or cycle ergometer, was in the range of 15 to 20 mL/min/kg in most participants in the nine studies in which it was measured (it might be noted that maximum O_2 uptake averages roughly 10% less in cycle ergometer tests than in treadmill tests, because of the smaller group of muscles participating in the exercise) (17). This corresponds to moderate to severe exercise intolerance.

In these studies, erythropoietin was administered for periods varying from 2½ to 12 months; the magnitude of the treatment effect did not vary noticeably with treatment duration. Average hemoglobin concentration rose from 6.9 to 11.3 g/dL as a result of erythropoietin treatment—a 64% increase in oxygen-carrying capacity. Increases in exercise tolerance were found in each of these studies; VO_2max increases averaged 29% in the nine studies in which it was measured. This is a large increase indeed, given that a rigorous program of exercise training generally results in an increase in VO_2max of no more than 15% to 20%.

The improvements seen in this effort-dependent measure are likely to stem from better motivation or practice at the task. Lactic acidosis threshold, an effort-independent measure, increased by an average of 22% in the five studies in which it was assessed. In several studies, physiologic responses to submaximal tasks were measured (93,96–99, 104); decreased levels of pulmonary ventilation, heart rate, and blood lactate were seen, consistent with an improved physiologic ability to perform exercise. In the study by Park et al. (105), magnetic resonance spectroscopy showed that the capacity for mitochondrial oxidative phosphorylation (i.e., the energy reserve) of the skeletal muscles was improved by erythropoietin treatment. Isolated muscle mitochondria were studied by Barany et al. (106) before and after correction of anemia with erythropoietin. An abnormally high rate of ATP production (likely a sign of chronically decreased O_2 transport) normalized after erythropoietin treatment. Cardiac chamber volumes (107) and left ventricular mass (94) have been reported to decrease, most likely as a result of reversal of the hyperdynamic state associated with chronic anemia.

The recent study of Marrades et al. (104) sheds considerable light on the effects of erythropoietin therapy on muscle function in patients with chronic renal failure. Eight patients performed incremental exercise testing with arterial and femoral venous catheters in place before and after erythropoietin therapy. With this arrangement, the time course of leg blood flow and oxygen extraction could be measured. Although hemoglobin increased 69% as a result of erythropoietin administration, peak VO_2 increased only 33%, most likely because peak leg blood flow was lower after erythropoietin therapy. Muscle oxygen conductance was found to be reduced, limiting oxygen extraction at maximal exercise to 70%. This study defines intrinsic muscle abnormalities and explains why erythropoietin therapy fails to normalize exercise tolerance.

Although erythropoietin therapy clearly produces substantial functional benefits in patients undergoing hemodialysis, the findings of Marrades et al. (104) and of others investigators (108–110) show that other factors besides reduced hemoglobin levels limit exercise tolerance.

Cardiovascular Dysfunction

Several factors dictate suboptimal cardiac function in patients with chronic renal failure and particularly those undergoing maintenance dialysis. The myopathy that affects skeletal muscle might affect cardiac muscle as well. The chronotropic response to exercise is limited (peak heart rate was 77% of predicted in a recent study) (92), thus decreasing peak cardiac output. This occurs despite higher than normal circulating levels of epinephrine and norepinephrine at a given level of exercise (111). Further, a persistent elevation in cardiac work tends to lead to myocardial hypertrophy. Hypertension is common in patients undergoing dialysis, in part because of fluid overload and the increased cardiac output necessitated by anemia (112). Left ventricular hypertrophy and increases in left ventricular end diastolic and end systolic volumes are common (107). Negative inotropic factors commonly include hypocalcemia, hypermagnesemia, hyperkalemia, and acidemia (113,114). Myocardial oxygen supply tends to be decreased by low coronary artery blood oxygen content as a result of anemia. Finally, the arteriovenous fistula commonly used for chronic dialysis acts as a shunt increasing cardiac output requirements and directing blood flow away from the exercising muscles.

Therapy for the cardiovascular dysfunction that occurs with chronic renal failure includes good pharmacologic control of blood pressure, avoidance of chronic fluid overload, and correction of electrolyte abnormalities. Correction of anemia with erythropoietin therapy can cause regression of cardiac hypertrophy and cause chamber volumes to normalize.

Myopathy

Patients with chronic renal failure, whether predialytic or undergoing chronic dialysis therapy, suffer from a constellation of muscle structure and function abnormalities collectively known as "uremic myopathy." In some patients, this syndrome manifests as profound proximal muscle weakness (predominantly of the legs) (115–117); in others the symptoms are more generalized and subtle. A number of muscle biopsy studies have demonstrated a unique set of abnormalities. Fiber atrophy is present that predominantly involves the type II fibers (115–121) (particularly the type IIb fibers [119]). The fibers exhibit abnormal morphology, including whorling and inclusion bodies (118). Electron microscopy shows a variety of changes consistent with mitochondrial damage and myofilament abnormalities (118,119). In children, fiber atrophy, lipidosis, glycogen depletion, and mitochondrial proliferation are seen (120). Other alterations include low concentrations of aerobic enzymes (122–124), loss of capillarity (108,109), and lowered levels of contractile proteins (116), although these changes may conceivably be, in part, the result of deconditioning (see earlier). Electromyographic studies reveal evidence of denervation, consistent with peripheral neuropathy (115,116,125).

Innovative studies from a group in Barcelona and their colleagues (126,127) have helped to define the mechanisms of muscle dysfunction in chronic renal failure. Mitochondrial oxidative capacity appears not to be a limiting factor. Rather, low muscle oxygen conductance, perhaps in part related to poor capillarity, appears to be the factor limiting aerobic performance. Further, lower intracellular pH at a given level of exercise impairs cellular bioenergetics.

The cause of muscle dysfunction in chronic renal failure is not known with certainty. The following have been suggested as contributing factors.

1. There is diminished oxygen supply resulting from anemia and altered muscle blood flow (119). Somewhat similar changes are seen in skeletal muscle of patients with peripheral vascular disease.
2. There is evidence for insulin resistance, leading to a reduced utilization of glucose as an energy source (128).
3. Abnormalities in vitamin D metabolism are present and there is an excess of parathyroid hormone, which may interfere with excitation–contraction coupling (106, 116,124).
4. Peripheral neuropathy, possibly combined with denervation, may lead to fiber atrophy and degeneration (116).
5. Animal models of renal insufficiency have demonstrated impaired muscle metabolism of amino acids (129,130).
6. Magnetic resonance spectroscopy studies suggest limitation of exchange of metabolites between muscle and blood because of dissociation between capillary supply and myocyte need (presumably secondary to decreased capillary density) (109,131).
7. It has been hypothesized (but not conclusively proven) that metabolic products that are not effectively cleared by dialysis ("middle molecules") accumulate and are toxic to the muscles (122). These "uremic toxins" may play a role in exercise intolerance.

8. Skeletal muscle protein degradation is increased and synthesis may be impaired (147).
9. Abnormalities in carnitine metabolism may contribute to muscle dysfunction. Carnitine facilitates the transfer of activated long-chain fatty acids into the mitochondria (124,132,133). There is a somewhat confusing literature concerning deficiencies of carnitine in blood and muscle of patients receiving regular hemodialysis. Clinical trials of carnitine supplementation in patients undergoing dialysis have failed, in general, to yield consistent improvements in exercise tolerance (e.g., 134–136).

Low Levels of Anabolic Hormones

A substantial majority of men with end-stage renal disease undergoing hemodialysis have testosterone levels in the hypogonadal range (137–143). Sex hormone–binding globulin levels are not low (141,142), so free testosterone levels also are reduced (137,138,144). Although plasma clearance rates of testosterone are increased during hemodialysis (145, 146), the loss of testosterone is relatively small. The primary cause of low testosterone levels in patients receiving hemodialysis is decreased testosterone production (137,138). Gynecomastia, impotence, testicular dysfunction, and infertility are common in men receiving hemodialysis (143); these disorders might be manifestations of low androgen levels in some of these men.

Evidence has been presented, from studies in animals, that renal insufficiency is associated with resistance to the effects of IGF-1 on the muscle (147). Therefore, the growth hormone axis is less effective in stimulating muscle anabolism.

EXERCISE TRAINING PROGRAMS IN PATIENTS WITH CHRONIC RENAL FAILURE

Several recent studies have provided information regarding the logistics and safety of vigorous exercise training in patients undergoing dialysis. Many patients undergoing dialysis are subject to arrhythmias, but physical training has been shown to augment cardiac vagal activity and decrease vulnerability to arrhythmias (148). A study of responses to exercise performed during dialysis sessions shows that during the first 2 hours of treatment, exercise is well tolerated. After 3 hours, decreasing cardiac output and blood pressure inhibit exercise capacity (149). Exercise during dialysis therapy actually increases the rebound of solute concentrations, apparently as a result of increased perfusion of the skeletal muscles (150).

It is useful to divide studies of exercise training in patients undergoing dialysis into two groups: studies performed before erythropoietin therapy became available and those in which patients were on a stable dose of erythropoietin. Table 34.2 summaries the published literature concerning the response to exercise programs in patients undergoing chronic dialytic therapy in the preerythropoietin era. At the outset, it is striking that only seven investigations involving only a total of 70 patients were performed (108,151–156). Despite the modest size of this literature, several well-performed studies give insight into the potential benefits of exercise training. The characteristics of participants are fairly typical of patients undergoing chronic dialysis therapy. The average age is 45 years, and the majority received hemodialysis three times weekly. Initial VO_2max averaged 18.5 mL/kg/min in the six studies in which it was measured, indicating moderate exercise intolerance. Hematocrit averaged 26%, consistent with the anemia expected in renal failure.

Most characteristics of the exercise programs summarized in Table 34.2 seem likely to contribute to the elicitation of a physiologic training effect. Exercise sessions generally were held three times per week, and the target session durations were 25 to 60 minutes. Program duration ranged from 8 weeks to 12 months—more than adequate for a training effect to develop. Exercise intensity prescriptions, however, varied markedly among studies. Three studies used intensity targets based on percentages of observed VO_2max (153–155), two used a percentage of the observed maximum heart rate (108,152), one used the lactic acidosis threshold (151) as the intensity target, and two principally used perceived exertion ratings (108,156). This disparity reflects genuine uncertainty as to how to design intensity prescriptions for patients with chronic disease. In patients with chronic renal failure, heart rate targets may be problematic because of variation in fluid status and sympathetic dysfunction (157). Perceived exertion ratings, although recommended by some authorities, seem inadequate to use as a sole target. Basing target intensity on a percentage of observed VO_2max (or, because VO_2 is not generally measured during training sessions, on percentages of peak work rate achieved in an incremental test) is likely the most desirable procedure. However, choosing the optimal percentage to be used is problematic, and whether targets considering the VO_2 at which the lactic acidosis threshold occurs improves the ability to specify the target intensity remains to be determined.

In six of seven studies, responses to these training programs were assessed in terms of VO_2max (Table 34.2). We must consider whether measured VO_2max may have been influenced by better motivation and familiarity with the exercise task at the end of the training program. However, the consistent (and rather large) increases in VO_2max in five of the six studies suggest a training effect. Further, Zabetakis et al. (151,158) reported an increased lactic acidosis threshold, and Moore et al. (108) reported a lower heart rate at a given submaximal work rate, both clear signs of a physiologic training effect. Only two studies failed to yield improvements (155,156). It is important to note that these were the two studies in which exercise was performed at home and was not supervised by health care professionals. In view of the concerns that some authors have expressed as to the compliance of patients receiving hemodialysis with an exercise program (80,159), supervised programs are to be recommended.

In each of these studies, the investigators sought evidence of benefits other than improvements in exercise tolerance. Both Goldberg's group (153,160–164) and Painter's group (154) found that blood pressure control improved and that some patients were able to decrease the number or dose of antihypertensive medications. However, several other benefits were described by Goldberg's group in a series of reports on the responses of 13 patients receiving hemodialysis to exercise training; other investigators to date have failed to reproduce these findings. Improvements in cholesterol and triglyceride profiles (153,160,161,163–165), risk factors for coronary artery disease (a common complication in patients undergoing chronic hemodialysis), were observed. An apparent decrease in insulin resistance was detected (153, 160–165), and hemoglobin levels increased (153, 160–164). Further, distinct improvements in the quality of life were documented, with decreased depression and anxiety scores noted on standardized tests (153,161,163,164, 166). It is difficult to understand this disparity in results; the parameters of the exercise program described by Harter and Goldberg (153) were not markedly different from other programs (although the program duration was mildly longer). Whether the broad-based benefits observed by Goldberg's group can be expected routinely from programs of exercise training for patients with chronic renal failure remains to be determined.

Table 34.3 summarizes reports of exercise training programs for patients receiving dialytic therapy in the post-erythropoietin era. In these four studies, hematocrit values averaged about 33% (versus 26 in the pre-erythropoietin studies). Initial maximum oxygen uptake was generally in the same range as the studies displayed in Table 34.2. Although there were appreciable differences among studies, these reports suggest that exercise training is capable of improving exercise tolerance and quality of life in patients

TABLE 34.3. PUBLISHED RESULTS OF EXERCISE TRAINING PROGRAMS FOR PATIENTS UNDERGOING DIALYSIS IN THE POST-ERYTHROPOIETIN ERA

Reference	Akiba et al. (1995) (167)	Lo et al. (1998) (168)	Kouidi et al. (1998) (169)	Painter et al. (2000) (170)
Number of subjects (# male)	9 (2)	13 (6)	7 (5)	143 (61)
Number in control group	6	7	None	143 (49)
Age (y)	38 ± 10	47 ± 13	44 ± 17	56 ± 15
Dialysis type	Hemodialysis	Peritoneal dialysis	Hemodialysis	Hemodialysis
Initial VO_2max (mL/kg/min)	19	17.2 ± 5.2	17.7 ± 5.0	—
Initial hematocrit (%)	—	28 ± 8	31 ± 4	34 ± 5
Initial hemoglobin (gm/dL)	11.5 ± 1.3	—	—	—
Supervised vs. home program	Supervised	Supervised	Supervised	8 weeks home, 8 weeks supervised
Training modality	Cycle	Treadmill, bike, arm ergometer	Calisthenics, swimming, resistance exercise	Cycle
Program duration	12 weeks	12 weeks	6 months	16 weeks
Session frequency	3/week	3/week	3/week	3/week
Session duration	20 minutes	30 minutes	50 minutes	30 minutes
Exercise intensity	RPE < 12	70%–85% of peak heart rate	"Progressed gradually"	Perceived exertion
Exercise testing modality	Cycle	Treadmill	Treadmill	Gait speed, sit-to-stand test, 6-minute walk
Exercise endurance increase	Peak work rate increased 22%, no increase in VO_2max and LAT	VO_2max increased 16.2%	VO_2max increased 48%	Not evaluated (few patients completed postintervention 6-minute walk)
Other physiologic changes	—	Ambulatory systolic blood pressure increased	Muscle biopsy: increased fiber size and capillarity and increased strength	Modest improvements in gait speed and sit-to-stand test
Quality-of-life changes	—	Improved kidney disease quality-of-life scores	—	Improved Short-form 36 scores

RPE, rating of perceived exertion; LAT, lactic acidosis threshold.

undergoing dialysis receiving erythropoietin. It is worth contrasting the studies of Painter et al. (170) with that of Kouidi et al. (169). Painter's group conducted an ambitious multicenter trial of 286 subjects. However, the exercise intensity guidelines were based on perceived exertion and the outcome measures included simple but highly effort-dependent measures (gait speed, sit-to-stand test, and 6-minute walk). Although the results are clouded by the large number of participants who failed to complete postintervention testing, only modest improvements in only a subset of these measures were detected. In contrast, Kouidi et al. (169) studied only a small number of subjects and did not include a control group. However, this 6-month training program used thrice weekly 50-minute aerobic training sessions. Peak oxygen uptake increase averaged a remarkable 48%. Moreover, vastus lateralis muscle biopsies performed before and after the program confirmed that substantial improvements in muscle structure had taken place. Mean muscle fiber area increased by 29%. Abnormalities in muscle architecture, observed both on light microscopy and electron microscopy, resolved. Specifically, improvements in the structure and number of capillaries and mitochondria were seen. Contrasting the results of these two studies emphasizes the value of rigorous exercise training and effort-independent outcome measures.

ADJUNCTIVE ANABOLIC THERAPIES

Pharmacologic agents capable of improving muscle function might be useful additions to programs of exercise training in patients receiving dialysis therapy. A few reports have appeared studying the response to growth hormone (or similar drugs) or to anabolic steroids. Recent improvements in our understanding of the mechanism of action of these drugs suggests that these agents produce changes in the muscle similar to strength, not endurance, training. Therefore, outcome measures including muscle mass and strength would be of particular interest in these studies.

Several clinical trials have evaluated the effects of growth hormone or IGF-1 in patients undergoing dialysis (171–178). In a 6-month randomized, placebo-controlled trial, growth hormone treatment increased muscle mass, albumin concentration, and handgrip strength and improved performance in a walking test (171). Growth hormone treatment of malnourished patients increased muscle protein synthesis (174,175,178). Short-term administration of IGF-1 induced nitrogen retention in malnourished patients receiving chronic ambulatory peritoneal dialysis (172).

Anabolic steroids do not consistently improve sexual dysfunction in men with chronic renal failure (179). This is not surprising because sexual dysfunction is often multifactorial and not simply the result of androgen deficiency. Before the advent of erythropoietin therapy, testosterone commonly was used to treat anemia in patients undergoing dialysis (179–188). Testosterone increases red cell production by stimulating erythropoietin, by augmenting erythropoietin action, and by its direct effects on marrow stem cells. Johansen et al. (189) conducted a randomized, placebo-controlled 6-month trial of weekly injections of nandrolone decanoate, an anabolic steroid, in men undergoing dialysis. In the nandrolone group, average lean body mass increased by 4.5 kg and fat mass decreased by 2.4 kg. Treadmill exercise tests, performed only in a minority of patients, showed no improvements in the nandrolone group. Handgrip strength also showed no improvement.

In summary, exercise training programs for patients with chronic renal failure, if designed on a firm physiologic basis, can yield substantial benefits that improve but do not normalize exercise tolerance. Further research is needed into the nature of, and the therapy for, the myopathy associated with chronic renal failure. Anabolic pharmacologic agents deserve attention for their potential to amplify the benefits of exercise training programs.

EXERCISE PRESCRIPTION RECOMMENDATIONS FOR PATIENTS UNDERGOING CHRONIC DIALYSIS

Although further research may modify these recommendations, certain principles seem likely to apply.

1. Before initiating a vigorous exercise program, patients should undergo formal exercise testing, preferably featuring gas exchange measurements and 12 lead electrocardiogram monitoring (17). A test of this type must be used to rule out severe cardiovascular disease and serve as the basis for exercise intensity prescription.
2. If an exercise program directed at achieving a physiologic training effect is not deemed possible, then a less formal program should be pursued. It seems likely that encouraging a less sedentary lifestyle can be of psychologic benefit.
3. If a formal program is pursued, it seems reasonable that exercise sessions should be scheduled either during (154) or near the time of dialysis. Exercise sessions should be held in group settings, preferably supervised by a rehabilitation therapist.
4. The principal mode of exercise should involve large muscle groups. Cycle ergometer and treadmill exercise are suitable indoor activities. Rapid walking, running, bicycling, and swimming can be pursued if outdoor activities are practical.
5. Exercise intensity recommendations must be tentative. If cardiopulmonary exercise testing results are available, an intensity moderately above the lactic acidosis threshold (perhaps 25% of the difference between the lactic acidosis threshold and the peak VO_2) might be a practical target. If exercise is to be performed on a calibrated

ergometer, this target can be expressed as a work rate. If not, then the heart rate corresponding to this intensity target can be used, with the understanding that changes in autonomic and volume status, cardiovascular disease, and certain medications can alter the relation between exercise intensity and heart rate. Training intensities based on perceived exertion alone are unlikely to be adequate. In any case, the exercise target should be progressively advanced by the rehabilitation therapist as the exercise program proceeds.

6. A reasonable design is to hold sessions three times per week and to have sessions feature 45 minutes of exercise. The formal exercise program should be at least 5 to 8 weeks in duration.
7. The formal exercise training program should be followed by a maintenance program, preferably in a group setting.
8. Although strength-training programs have been shown to be of value in patients with other chronic diseases (190), no reports have appeared involving patients receiving dialysis. However, a recent report of Castaneda et al. (191) demonstrated that a strength-training program was of substantial benefit in patients with renal insufficiency not yet receiving dialysis therapy. Presumably, strength training can elicit improvements in muscle mass and strength in patients receiving dialysis therapy as well, but exercise prescription guidelines cannot be specified at this time. In designing strength-training programs for this patient population, risk factors for bone fracture (e.g., osteoporosis) and tendon rupture (192) should be considered.

REFERENCES

1. Ifudu O, Paul H, Mayers J, et al. Pervasive failed rehabilitation in center-based maintenance hemodialysis patients. *Am J Kidney Dis* 1994;23:394–400.
2. Gutman R, Stead W, Robinson R. Physical activity and employment status of patients on maintenance dialysis. *N Engl J Med* 1981;304:309–313.
3. Kimmel PL, Peterson RA, Weihs KL, et al. Multiple measurements of depression predict mortality in a longitudinal study of chronic hemodialysis outpatients. *Kidney Int* 2000;57: 2093–2098.
4. Churchill D, Torrance G, Taylor D, et al. Measurement of quality of life in end-stage renal disease: The time trade-off approach. *Clin Invest Med* 1987;10:14–20.
5. DeOreo P. Hemodialysis patient-assessed functional health status predicts continued survival, hospitalization, and dialysis-attendance compliance. *Am J Kidney Dis* 1997;30:204–212.
6. Blagg CR. The socioeconomic impact of rehabilitation. *Am J Kidney Dis* 1994;24(Suppl 1):S17–S21.
7. Casaburi R, Petty TL, eds. *Principles and practice of pulmonary rehabilitation.* Philadelphia: WB Saunders, 1993.
8. Pulmonary rehabilitation—1999. American Thoracic Society. *Am J Respir Crit Care Med* 1999;159(5 Pt 1):1666–1682.
9. Ries AL, Carlin BW, Carrieri-Kohlman V, et al. Pulmonary rehabilitation: evidence based guidelines. *Chest* 1997;112: 1363–1396.
10. Haas F, Salazar-Schicchi J, Axen K. Desensitization to dyspnea in chronic obstructive pulmonary disease. In: Casaburi R, Petty TL, eds. *Principles and practice of pulmonary rehabilitation.* Philadelphia: WB Saunders, 1993:241–251.
11. Bandura A. Self-efficacy: Towards a unifying theory of behavioral change. *Psychol Rev* 1977;2:191–215.
12. Lamb DR. Physiology of exercise. *Responses and adaptations*, 2nd ed. New York: Macmillan, 1984.
13. Baechle TR. *Essentials of strength training and conditioning.* Champaign, IL: Human Kinetics Publishers, 1996.
14. Fiatarone MA, O'Neill EF, Ryan ND, et al. Exercise training and nutritional supplementation for physical frailty in very elderly people. *N Engl J Med* 1994;330:1769–1775.
15. Hakkinen K, Hakkinen A. Muscle cross-sectional area, force production, and relaxation characteristics in women of different ages. *Eur J Appl Physiol* 1991;62:410–414.
16. Larsson L, Karlsson J. Isometric and dynamic endurance as a function of age and skeletal muscle characteristics. *Acta Physiol Scand* 1978;104:129–136.
17. Wasserman K, Hansen JE, Sue DY, et al. *Principles of exercise testing and interpretation*, 3rd ed. Philadelphia: Lippincott, Williams and Wilkins, 1999.
18. Metzger JM, Fitts RH. Role of intracellular pH in muscle fatigue. *J Appl Physiol* 1987;62:1392–1397.
19. Saltin B, Gollnick PD. Skeletal muscle adaptability: significance for metabolism and performance. In: Peachey LD, ed. *Handbook of physiology. Skeletal muscle.* Washington, DC: *American Physiology Society* 1986;555–631.
20. Komi PV, Viitasalo JHT, Havu M, et al. Skeletal muscle fibers and muscle enzyme activities in monozygous and dizygous twins of both sexes. *Acta Physiol Scand* 1977;100:385–392.
21. Gollnick PD, Armstrong RB, Saltin B, et al. Effect of training on enzyme activity and fiber composition of human skeletal muscle. *J Appl Physiol* 1973;34:107–111.
22. Anderson P, Henriksson J. Training induced changes in the subgroups of human type II skeletal muscle fibers. *Acta Physiol Scand* 1977;99:123–125.
23. Holloszy JO. Adaptation of skeletal muscle to endurance exercise. *Med Sci Sports* 1975;7:155–164.
24. Clausen JP, Klausen K, Rasmussen B, et al. Central and peripheral circulatory changes after training of the arms or legs. *Am J Physiol* 1973;225:675–682.
25. McArdle WD, Katch FI, Katch VL. *Exercise physiology. Energy, nutrition and human performance.* Philadelphia: Lea and Febiger, 1986.
26. Saltin B. Cardiovascular and pulmonary adaptation to physical activity. In: Bouchard C, Shephard RJ, Stephens T, et al., eds. *Exercise, fitness and health. A consensus of current knowledge.* Champaign, IL: Human Kinetics, 1990:187–203.
27. Hagberg JM. Exercise, fitness and hypertension. In: Bouchard C, Shephard RJ, Stephens T, et al., eds. *Exercise, fitness and health. A consensus of current knowledge.* Champaign, IL: Human Kinetics, 1990:455–466.
28. Pollock ML, Miller HS, Janeway R, et al. Effects of walking on body composition and cardiovascular function of middle-aged men. *J Appl Physiol* 1971;30:126–130.
29. Pollock ML, Wilmore JH. *Exercise in health and disease*, 2nd ed. Philadelphia: WB Saunders, 1990.
30. Casaburi, R. Use of pulmonary function and cardiopulmonary exercise laboratories for diagnostic testing. In: Rippe JM, ed. *Lifestyle medicine.* Cambridge: Blackwell, 1999;446–459.
31. Sue DY, Wasserman K, Moricca RB, et al. Metabolic acidosis during exercise in patients with chronic obstructive pulmonary disease. *Chest* 1988;94:931–938.
32. Casaburi R, Storer TW, Ben-Dov I, et al. Effect of endurance

training on possible determinants of O_2 during heavy exercise. *J Appl Physiol* 1987;62:199–207.
33. Casaburi R, Storer TW, Wasserman K. Mediation of reduced ventilatory response to exercise after endurance training. *J Appl Physiol* 1987;63:1533–1538.
34. Winder WW, Hickson RC, Hagberg JM, et al. Training-induced changes in hormonal and metabolic responses to submaximal exercise. *J Appl Physiol* 1979;46:766–771.
35. Hill DW, Cureton KJ, Grisham SC, et al. Effect of training on the rating of perceived exertion at the ventilatory threshold. *Eur J Appl Physiol* 1987;56:206–211.
36. Gustafsson T, Kraus WE. Exercise-induced angiogenesis-related growth and transcription factors in skeletal muscle, and their modification in muscle pathology. *Frontiers in Bioscience* 2001; 6:D75–89.
37. Henriksson J. Training induced adaptation of skeletal muscle and metabolism during submaximal exercise. *J Physiol* 1977; 270:661–675.
38. Vandenburgh HH, Hatfaludy S, Karlisch P, et al. Skeletal muscle growth is stimulated by intermittent stretch-relaxation in tissue culture. *Am J Physiol* 1989;256:C674–C682.
39. Bhasin S, Storer TW, Berman N, et al. The effects of supraphysiological doses of testosterone on muscle size and strength in normal men. *N Engl J Med* 1996;335:1–7.
40. Bhasin S, Woodhouse L, Casaburi R, et al. Testosterone dose-response relationships in healthy young men. *Am J Physiol Endocrinol Metab* 2001;E1172–E1181.
41. Kozlowski S, Chwalbinska-Moneta J, Viga M, et al. Greater serum GH response to arm than to leg exercise performed at equivalent oxygen uptake. *Eur J Appl Physiol* 1983;52:131–135.
42. Van Helder WP, Casey K, Goode RC, et al. Growth hormone regulation in two types of aerobic exercise of equal oxygen uptake. *Eur J Appl Physiol* 1986;55:236–239.
43. Van Helder WP, Casey K, Randomski MW. Regulation of growth hormone during exercise by oxygen demand and availability. *Eur J Appl Physiol* 1987;56:628–632.
44. Casaburi R, Patessio A, Ioli F, et al. Reductions in exercise lactic acidosis and ventilation as a result of exercise training in patients with obstructive lung disease. *Am Rev Respir Dis* 1991;143: 9–18.
45. American College of Sports Medicine Position Stand. The recommended quantity and quality of exercise for developing and maintaining cardiorespiratory and muscular fitness in healthy adults. *Med Sci Sports Exerc* 1990;22:265–274.
46. Casaburi R, Storer TW, Sullivan CS, et al. Validity of blood lactate level as an intensity criterion for endurance exercise training. *Med Sci Sports Exerc* 1995;27:852–862.
47. Gaesser GA, Rich RG. Effects of high- and low-intensity exercise training on aerobic capacity and blood lipids. *Med Sci Sports Exerc* 1984;16:269–274.
48. Shephard RJ. Intensity, duration and frequency of exercise as determinants of the response to a training regime. *Int Zangew Physiol* 1968;26:272–278.
49. Kindermann W, Simon G, Keul J. The significance of the aerobic-anaerobic transition for the determination of work load intensities during endurance training. *Eur J Appl Physiol* 1979; 42:25–34.
50. Katch V, Weltman A, Sady S, et al. Validity of the relative percent concept for equating training intensity. *Eur J Appl Physiol* 1978;39:219–227.
51. Hansen JE, Sue DY, Wasserman K. Predicted values for clinical exercise testing. *Am Rev Respir Dis* 1984;129(Suppl):S49–S55.
52. Casaburi R, Porszasz J, Burns MR, et al. Physiologic benefits of exercise training in rehabilitation of severe COPD patients. *Am J Respir Crit Care Med* 1997;155:1541–1551.
53. Killian KJ. Dyspnea: implications for rehabilitation. In: Casaburi R, Petty TL, eds. *Principles and practice of pulmonary rehabilitation.* Philadelphia, WB Saunders, 1993:103–114.
54. Borg GAV. Psychophysical bases of perceived exertion. *Med Sci Sports Exerc* 1982;14:377–381.
55. Wenger HA, Bell GJ. The interactions of intensity, frequency and duration of exercise training in altering cardiorespiratory fitness. *Sports Med* 1986;3:346–356.
56. Davies CTM, Knibbs AV. The training stimulus. *Int Zangew Physiol* 1971;29:299–305.
57. Gaesser GA, Poole DC. Blood lactate during exercise: time course of training adaptation in humans. *Int J Sports Med* 1988; 9:284–288.
58. Hickson RC, Hagberg JM, Ehsani AA, et al. Time course of the adaptive responses of aerobic power and heart rate to training. *Med Sci Sports Exerc* 1981;13:17–20.
59. Poole DC, Gaesser GA. Response of ventilatory and lactate thresholds to continuous and interval training. *J Appl Physiol* 1985;58:1115–1121.
60. Pollock ML, Dimmick J, Miller HS, et al. Effects of mode of training on cardiovascular function and body composition of middle-aged men. *Med Sci Sports Exerc* 1977;7:139–144.
61. Pollock ML. The quantification of endurance training programs. *Exerc Sports Sci Rev* 1973;1:155–188.
62. Hagberg JM, Graves JE, Limacher M, et al. Cardiovascular responses of 70- to 79-yr-old men and women to exercise training. *J Appl Physiol* 1989;66:2589–2594.
63. Makrides L, Heigenhauser JF, Jones NL. High-intensity endurance training in 20- to 30- and 60- to 70-yr old healthy men. *J Appl Physiol* 1990;69:1792–1798.
64. Seals DR, Hurley BF J, Schultz J, et al. Endurance training in older men and women II. Blood lactate response to submaximal exercise. *J Appl Physiol* 1984;57:1030–1033.
65. Tzankoff SP, Robinson S, Pyke FS, et al. Physiological adjustments to work in older men as affected by physical training. *J Appl Physiol* 1972;33:346–350.
66. Cunningham DA, Patterson DH. Discussion: Exercise, fitness and aging. In: Bouchard C, Shephard RJ, Stephens T, et al., eds. *Exercise, fitness and health. A consensus of current knowledge.* Champaign, IL: Human Kinetics, 1990:699–704.
67. Prior JC. Reproduction: exercise-related adaptations and the health of women and men. In: Bouchard C, Shephard RJ, Stephens T, et al., eds. *Exercise, fitness and health. A consensus of current knowledge.* Champaign, IL: Human Kinetics 1990; 661–675.
68. Coyle EF, Martin WH, Bloomfield SA, et al. Effects of detraining on responses to submaximal exercise. *J Appl Physiol* 1985;59:853–859.
69. Coyle EF, Martin WH, Sinacore DR, et al. Time course of loss of adaptations after stopping prolonged intense endurance training. *J Appl Physiol* 1984;57:1857–1864.
70. Hickson RC, Kanakis C, Davis JR, et al. Reduced training duration effects on aerobic power, endurance and cardiac growth. *J Appl Physiol* 1982;53:225–229.
71. Hickson RC, Rosenkoetter MA. Reduced training frequencies and maintenance of increased aerobic power. *Med Sci Sports Exerc* 1981;13:13–16.
72. Hickson RC, Foster CC, Pollock ML, et al. Reduced training intensities and loss of aerobic power, endurance and cardiac growth. *J Appl Physiol* 1985;58:492–499.
73. Johansen KL. Physical functioning and exercise capacity in patients on dialysis. *Adv Ren Replace Ther* 1999;141–148.
74. Capodaglio EM, Villa G, Jurisic D, et al. Levels of sustainable aerobic workload in dialysis patients. *Int J Artif Organs* 1998; 21:391–397.
75. Sietsema KE, Hiatt WR, Esler A, et al. Clinical and demo-

graphic predictors of exercise capacity in end-stage renal disease. *Am J Kidney Dis* 2002;39:76–85.
76. Barnea N, Drory Y, Iaina A, et al. Exercise tolerance in patients on chronic hemodialysis. *Isr J Med Sci* 1980;16:17–21.
77. Parrish AE. The effect of minimal exercise on blood lactate in azotemic subjects. *Clin Nephrol* 1981;16:35–39.
78. Zanconato S, Baraldi E, Montini G, et al. Exercise tolerance in end-stage renal disease. *Child Nephrol Urol* 1990;10:26–31.
79. Casaburi R. Deconditioning. In: Fishman AP, ed. *Pulmonary rehabilitation. Lung biology in health and disease series.* New York: Marcel Dekker, 1996:213–230.
80. Painter PL. Exercise in end-stage renal disease. *Exer Sports Sci Reviews* 1988;16:305–339.
81. Woodrow G, Oldroyd B, Turney J, et al. Whole body and regional body composition in patients with chronic renal failure. *Nephrol Dial Transplant* 1996;11:1613–1618.
82. Pollock C, Allen B, Warden R, et al. Total body nitrogen by neutron activation in maintenance hemodialysis. *Am J Kidney Dis* 1990;16:38–45.
83. Coles G. Body composition in chronic renal failure. *QJM* 1972; 41:25–47.
84. Williams AJ, McArley A. Body composition, treatment time, and outcome in hemodialysis patients. *J Renal Nutr* 1999;9: 157–162.
85. Kopple JD. Nutritional status as a predictor of morbidity and mortality in maintenance dialysis patients. *Asaio Journal* 1997; 43:246–250.
86. Hakim R, Levin N. Malnutrition in hemodialysis patients. *Am J Kidney Dis* 1993;21:125–137.
87. Lazarus J. Nutrition in hemodialysis patients. *Am J Kidney Dis* 1993;21:99–105.
88. Kopple J. Effect of nutrition on morbidity and mortality in maintenance dialysis patients. *Am J Kidney Dis* 1994;24: 1002–1009.
89. Lowrie E, Lew N. Death risk in hemodialysis patients: the predictive value of commonly measured variables and an evaluation of death rate difference between facilities. *Am J Kidney Dis* 1990; 15:458–482.
90. Owen WF, Lew NL, Liu Y, et al. The urea reduction ratio and serum albumin concentrations as predictors of mortality in patients undergoing hemodialysis. *N Engl J Med* 1993;329: 1001–1006.
91. Blake PG, Flowerdew G, Blake RM, et al. Serum albumin in patients on continuous ambulatory peritoneal dialysis—predictors and correlations with outcomes. *J Am Soc Nephrol* 1993; 3:1501–1507.
92. Moore GE, Brinker KR, Stray-Gundersen J, et al. Determinants of VO_2 peak in patients with end-stage renal disease: on and off dialysis. *Med Sci Sports Exerc* 1993;25:18–23.
93. Mayer G, Thum J, Cada EM, et al. Working capacity is increased following recombinant human erythropoietin treatment. *Kidney Int* 1988;34:525–528.
94. MacDougall IC, Lewis NP, Saunders MJ, et al. Long-term cardiorespiratory effects of amelioration of renal anaemia by erythropoietin. *Lancet* 1990;335:489–493.
95. Canadian Erythropoietin Study Group. Association between recombinant human erythropoietin and quality of life and exercise capacity of patients receiving haemodialysis. *Br Med J* 1990; 300:573–578.
96. Grunze M, Kohlmann M, Mulligan M, et al. Mechanisms of improved physical performance of chronic hemodialysis patients after erythropoietin treatment. *Am J Nephrol* 1990;10:15–23.
97. Robertson HT, Haley NR, Guthrie M, et al. Recombinant erythropoietin improves exercise capacity in anemic hemodialysis patients. *Am J Kidney Dis* 1990;4:325–332.
98. Braumann KM, Nonnast-Daniel B, Boning D, et al. Improved physical performance after treatment of renal anemia with recombinant erythropoietin. *Nephron* 1991;58:129–134.
99. Lundin AP, Akerman MJH, Chesler RM, et al. Exercise in hemodialysis patients after treatment with recombinant human erythropoietin. *Nephron* 1991;58:315–319.
100. Metra M, Cannella G, La Canna G, et al. Improvement in exercise capacity after correction of anemia in patients with end-stage renal failure. *Am J Cardiol* 1991;68:1060–1066.
101. Davenport A, Will EJ, Khanna K, et al. Blood lactate is reduced following successful treatment of anaemia in haemodialysis patients with recombinant human erythropoietin both at rest and after maximal exertion. *Am J Nephrol* 1992;12:357–362.
102. Barany P, Freyschuss U, Pettersson E, et al. Treatment of anaemia in haemodialysis patients with erythropoietin: long-term effects on exercise capacity. *Clin Sci* 1993;84:441–447.
103. Lewis NP, MacDougall IC, Willis N, et al. Effects of the correction of renal anaemia by erythropoietin on physiological changes during exercise. *Eur J Clin Invest* 1993;23:423–427.
104. Marrades RM, Roca J, Campistol JM, et al. Effects of erythropoietin on muscle O_2 transport during exercise in patients with chronic renal failure. *J Clin Invest* 1996;2092–2100.
105. Park JS, Kim SB, Park SK, et al. Effect of recombinant human erythropoietin on muscle energy metabolism in patients with end-stage renal disease: A ^{31}P-nuclear magnetic resonance spectroscopic study. *Am J Kidney Dis* 1993;21:612–618.
106. Barany P, Wibom R, Hultman E, et al. ATP production in isolated muscle mitochondria from haemodialysis patients: effects of correction of anaemia with erythropoietin. *Clin Sci* 1991;81:645–653.
107. Low I, Grutzmacher P, Bergmann M, et al. Echocardiographic findings in patients on maintenance hemodialysis substituted with recombinant human erythropoietin. *Clin Nephrol* 1989; 31:26–30.
108. Moore GE, Parsons DB, Stray-Gundersen J, et al. Uremic myopathy limits aerobic capacity in hemodialysis patients. *Am J Kidney Dis* 1993;22:277–287.
109. Moore GE, Bertocci LA, Painter PL. ^{31}P-Magnetic resonance spectroscopy assessment of subnormal oxidative metabolism in skeletal muscle of renal failure patients. *J Clin Invest* 1993;91: 420–424.
110. Diesel W, Noakes TD, Swanepoel C, et al. Isokinetic muscle strength predicts maximum exercise tolerance in renal patients on chronic hemodialysis. *Am J Kidney Dis* 1990;16:109–114.
111. Kettner A, Goldberg A, Hagberg J, et al. Cardiovascular and metabolic responses to submaximal exercise in hemodialysis patients. *Kidney Int* 1984;26:66–71.
112. Capell JP, Kasparian H. Cardiac work demands and left ventricular function in end-stage renal disease. *Ann Int Med* 1977;86: 261–267.
113. Painter P, Zimmerman SW. Exercise in end-stage renal disease. *Am J Kidney Dis* 1986;7:386–394.
114. Ayus JC, Frommer JP, Young JB. Cardiac and circulatory abnormalities in chronic renal failure. *Semin Nephrol* 1981;1: 112–120.
115. Floyd M, Ayyar DR, Barwick DD, et al. Myopathy in chronic renal failure. *Q J Med* 1974;43:509–524.
116. Lazaro RP, Kirshner HS. Proximal muscle weakness in uremia. *Arch Neurol* 1980;37:555–558.
117. Bautista J, Gil-Necija E, Castilla J, et al. Dialysis myopathy. *Acta Neuropathol* 1983;61:71–75.
118. Ahonen RE. Light microscopic study of striated muscle in uremia. *Acta Neuropathol* 1980;49:51–55.
119. Bradley JR, Anderson JR, Evans DB, et al. Impaired nutritive skeletal muscle blood flow in patients with chronic renal failure. *Clin Sci* 1990;79:239–245.
120. do Prado LB, do Prado GF, Oliveira ACB, et al. Histochemical

study of the skeletal muscle in children with chronic renal failure in dialysis treatment. *Arq Neuropsiquiatr* 1998;56(3-A): 381–387.
121. Diesel W, Emms M, Knight BK, et al. Morphologic features of the myopathy associated with chronic renal failure. *Am J Kidney Dis* 1993;22:677–684.
122. Metcoff J, Lindeman R, Baxter D, et al. Cell metabolism in uremia. *Am J Clin Nutr* 1978;31:1627–1634.
123. Nakao T, Fujiwara S, Isoda K, et al. Impaired lactate production by skeletal muscle with anaerobic exercise in patients with chronic renal failure. *Nephron* 1982;31:111–115.
124. Brautbar N. Skeletal myopathy in uremia: Abnormal energy metabolism. *Kidney Int* 1983;24(Suppl 16):S81–S86.
125. Wanic-Kossowska M, Grzegorzewska A, Plotast H, et al. Does calcitriol therapy improve muscle function in uremic patients? *Perit Dial Int* 1996;16(1):S305–S308.
126. Marrades RM, Alonso J, Roca J, et al. Cellular bioenergetics after erythropoietin therapy in chronic renal failure. *J Clin Invest* 1996;97(9):2101–2110.
127. Sala E, Noyszewski EA, Campistol JM, et al. Impaired muscle oxygen transfer in patients with chronic renal failure. *Am J Physiol Regul Integr Comp Physiol* 2001;280:R1240–R1248.
128. De Fronzo RA, Alvestrand A, Smith D, et al. Insulin resistance in uremia. *J Clin Invest* 1981;67:563–568.
129. Garber AJ. Skeletal muscle protein and amino acid metabolism in experimental chronic uremia in the rat. Accelerated alanine and glutamine formation and release. *J Clin Invest* 1978;61: 623–632.
130. Harter HR, Karl IE, Klahr S, et al. Effects of reduced renal mass and dietary protein intake on amino acid release and glucose uptake by rat muscle in vivo. *J Clin Invest* 1979;64: 513–523.
131. Durozard D, Pimmel P, Baretto S, et al. ^{31}P NMR spectroscopy investigation of muscle metabolism in hemodialysis patients. *Kidney Int* 1993;43:885–892.
132. Wanner C, Hörl WH. Carnitine abnormalities in patients with renal insufficiency. *Nephron* 1988;50:89–102.
133. Golper TA, Ahmad S. L-Carnitine administration to hemodialysis patients: Has its time come? *Semin Dial* 1992;5:94–98.
134. Rogerson ME, Rylance PB, Wilson R, et al. Carnitine and weakness in haemodialysis patients. *Nephrol Dial Transplant* 1989; 4:366–371.
135. Fagher B, Cederblad G, Eriksson M, et al. L-Carnitine and haemodialysis: double blind study on muscle function and metabolism and peripheral nerve function. *Scand J Clin Lab Invest* 1985;45:169–178.
136. Ahmad S, Robertson HT, Golper TA, et al. Multicenter trial of L-carnitine in maintenance hemodialysis patients. II. Clinical and biochemical effects. *Kidney Int* 1990;38:912–918.
137. Handelsman DJ. Hypothalamic–pituitary gonadal dysfunction in renal failure, dialysis, and renal transplantation. *Endocrine Rev* 1985;6:151–182.
138. Handelsman DJ, Dong Q. Hypothalamo-pituitary gonadal axis in chronic renal failure. *Endocrinol Metab North Am* 1993;22: 145–159.
139. Guevara A, Vidt D, Hallberg MC, et al. Serum gonadotropins and testosterone levels in uremic males undergoing intermittent dialysis. *Metabolism* 1969;18:1062.
140. Holdsworth J, Atkins RC, Deketser DM. The pituitary–testicular axis in men with chronic renal failure. *N Engl J Med* 1977; 296:1245–1249.
141. Sawin CT, Langcope C, Schmidt GW, et al. Blood levels of gonadotropins and gonadal hormones in gynecomastia associated with chronic hemodialysis. *J Clin Endocrinol Metab* 1973; 36:988–994.
142. Gomez F, De LA Cueva R, Wauters J, et al. Endocrine abnormalities in patients undergoing long term hemodialysis. *Am J Med* 1985;65:522–529.
143. Handelsman DJ, Liu PY. Androgen therapy in chronic renal failure. In: Bhasin S, ed. *Clinical endocrinology and metabolism.* London: Bailliere's Tindall, 1998:485–500.
144. De Vries CP, Gooren LJG, Oe PL. Hemodialysis and testicular function. *Int J Androl* 1984;7:97–102.
145. Van Kammen E, Thijssen JHH, Schawrtz F. Sex hormones in male patients with chronic renal failure, I. The production of testosterone and of androstenedione. *Clin Endocrinol (Oxf)* 1987;8:7–15.
146. Stewart-Bentley M, Gan D, Horton R. Regulation of gonadal function in uremia. *Metabolism* 1974;23:1065–1075.
147. Ding H, Gao XL, Hirschberg R, et al. Impaired actions of insulin-growth factor 1 on protein synthesis and degradation in skeletal muscle of rats with chronic renal failure. *J Clin Invest* 1996;97:1064–1075.
148. Diligiannis A, Kouidi E, Tourkantonis A. Effects of physical training on heart rate variability in patients on hemodialysis. *Am J Cardiol* 1999;84:197–202.
149. Moore GE, Painter PL, Brinker KR, et al. Cardiovascular response to submaximal stationary cycling during hemodialysis. *Am J Kidney Dis* 1998;31(4):631–637.
150. Kong CH, Tattersall JE, Greenwood RN, et al. The effect of exercise during haemodialysis on solute removal. *European Renal Association–European Dialysis and Transplant Association* 1999; 2927–2931.
151. Zabetakis PM, Gleim GW, Pasternack FL, et al. Long-duration submaximal exercise conditioning in hemodialysis patients. *Clin Nephrol* 1982;18:17–22.
152. Shalom R, Blumenthal JA, Williams RS, et al. Feasibility and benefits of exercise training in patients on maintenance dialysis. *Kidney Int* 1984;25:958–963.
153. Harter HR, Goldberg AP. Endurance exercise training. *Med Clin North Am* 1985;69:159–175.
154. Painter PL, Nelson-Worel JN, Hill MM, et al. Effects of exercise training during hemodialysis. *Nephron* 1986;43:87–92.
155. Lennon DLF, Shrago E, Madden M, et al. Carnitine status, plasma lipid profiles, and exercise capacity of dialysis patients: effects of a submaximal exercise program. *Metabolism* 1986;35: 728–735.
156. Stephens R, Williams A, McKnight T, et al. Effects of self-monitored exercise on selected blood chemistry parameters of end-stage renal disease patients. *Am J Phys Med Rehabil* 1991; 70:149–153.
157. Hanson P, Ward A, Painter P. Exercise training for special patient populations. *J Cardiopulmonary Rehabil* 1986;6: 104–112.
158. Greene MC, Zabetakis PM, Gleim GW, et al. Effect of exercise on lipid metabolism and dietary intake in hemodialysis patients. *Proc Dialysis Transplant Forum* 1979;9:80–85.
159. Painter P. The importance of exercise training in rehabilitation of patients with end-stage renal disease. *Am J Kidney Dis* 1994; 24(Suppl 1):S2–S9.
160. Goldberg AP, Hagberg J, Delmez JA, et al. The metabolic and psychological effects of exercise training in hemodialysis patients. *Am J Clin Nutr* 1980;33:1620–1628.
161. Goldberg AP, Hagberg J, Delmez JA, et al. Metabolic effects of exercise training in hemodialysis patients. *Kidney Int* 1980; 18:754–761.
162. Hagberg JM, Goldberg AP, Ehsani AA, et al. Exercise training improves hypertension in hemodialysis patients. *Am J Nephrol* 1983;3:209–212.
163. Goldberg AP, Geltman EM, Hagberg JM, et al. Therapeutic benefits of exercise training for hemodialysis patients. *Kidney Int* 1983;24(Suppl 16):S303–S309.

164. Goldberg AP, Geltman EM, Gavin JR, et al. Exercise training reduces coronary risk and effectively rehabilitates hemodialysis patients. *Nephron* 1986;42:311–316.
165. Goldberg AP, Hagberg JM, Delmez JA, et al. Exercise training improves abnormal lipid and carbohydrate metabolism in hemodialysis patients. *Trans Am Soc Artif Intern Organs* 1979;25: 431–437.
166. Carney RM, McKevitt PM, Goldberg AP, et al. Psychological effects of exercise training in hemodialysis patients. *Nephron* 1983;33:179–181.
167. Akiba T, Matsui N, Shinohara S, et al. Effects of recombinant human erythropoietin and exercise training on exercise capacity in hemodialysis patients. *Artif Organs* 1995;19(12):1262–1268.
168. Lo C, Li L, Lo W, et al. Benefits of exercise training in patients on continuous ambulatory peritoneal dialysis. *Am J Kidney Dis* 1998;32(6):1011–1018.
169. Kouidi E, Albani M, Natsis K, et al. The effects of exercise training on muscle atrophy in haemodialysis patients. *Nephrol Dial Transplant* 1998;13:685–699.
170. Painter P, Carlson L, Carey S, et al. Physical functioning and health-related quality-of-life changes with exercise training in hemodialysis patients. *Am J Kidney Dis* 2000;35(3):482–492.
171. Jahannsson G, Bengtsson BA, Ahlmen J. Double-blind, placebo-controlled study of growth hormone treatment in elderly patients undergoing chronic hemodialysis: anabolic effect and functional improvement. *Am J Kidney Dis* 1999;33:709–717.
172. Fouque D, Peng SC, Shamir E, et al. Recombinant human insulin-like growth factor-1 induces an anabolic response in malnourished CAPD patients. *Kidney Int* 2000;57:646–654.
173. Garibotto G, Barreca A, Russo R, et al. Effects of recombinant human growth hormone on muscle protein turnover in malnourished hemodialysis patients. *J Clin Invest* 1997;99:97–105.
174. Mehls O, Ritz E, Hunziker E-B, et al. Improvement of growth and food utilization by human recombinant growth hormone in uremia. *Kidney Int* 1988;33:45–52.
175. Ziegler TR, Lazarus JM, Young LS, et al. Effects of recombinant human growth hormone in adults receiving maintenance hemodialysis. *J Am Soc Nephrol* 1991;2:1130–1135.
176. Tonshoff B, Loelega AC, Stinjen T, et al. Growth-stimulating effect of recombinant human growth hormone in children with end-stage renal disease. *J Pediatr* 1990;116:561–566.
177. Iglesias P, Diez JJ, Fernández-Reyes MJ, et al. Recombinant human growth hormone therapy in malnourished dialysis patients: a randomized controlled study. *Am J Kidney Dis* 1998; 32(3):454–463.
178. Garibotto G, Barreca A, Sofia A, et al. Effects of growth hormone on leptin metabolism and energy expenditure in hemodialysis patients with protein-calorie malnutrition. *J Am Soc Nephrol* 2000;11(11):1–12.
179. Handelsman DJ. Hypothalamic-pituitary gonadal dysfunction in renal failure, dialysis, and renal transplantation. *Endocrine Rev* 1985;6:151–182.
180. Ballal SH, Domoto DT, Polack DC, et al. Androgens potentiate the effects of erythropoietin in the treatment of anemia of end stage renal disease. *Am J Kidney Dis* 1991;17:29–33.
181. Barton CH, Marahmadi MK, Vaziri ND. Effects of long term testosterone administration on pituitary-testicular axis in end-stage renal failure. *Nephron* 1982;31:61–64.
182. Berns JS, Rudnick MR, Cohen RM. A controlled trial of recombinant erythropoietin and nandrolone decanoate in the treatment of anemia in patients on chronic hemodialysis. *Clin Nephrol* 1992;37:264–267.
183. Buchwald D, Argyres S, Easterling RE, et al. Effect of nandrolone decanoate on the anemia of chronic hemodialysis patients. *Nephron* 1977;18:232–238.
184. Hendler ED, Goffinet JA, Ross S, et al. Controlled study of androgen therapy in anemia of patients on maintenance hemodialysis. *N Engl J Med* 1974;291:1046–1051.
185. Jones RWA, El Bishti MM, Bloom SR, et al. The effects of anabolic steroids on growth, body composition, and metabolism in boys with chronic renal failure on regular hemodialysis. *J Pediatr* 1980;97:559–566.
186. Kassmann K, Rappaport R, Broyer M. The short term effect of testosterone on growth in boys on hemodialysis. *Clin Nephrol* 1992;37:148–154.
187. Neff MS, Goldberg J, Slifkin RF, et al. A comparison of androgens for anemia in patients on hemodialysis. *N Engl J Med* 1981;304:871–875.
188. Teruel JL, Marcen R, Navarro-Antolin J, et al. Androgen versus erythropoietin for the treatment of anemia in hemodialysis patients: a prospective study. *J Am Soc Nephrol* 1996;7:140–144.
189. Johansen KL, Mulligan K, Schambelan M. Anabolic effects of nandrolone decanoate in patients receiving dialysis. *JAMA* 1999;281:1275–1281.
190. Casaburi R, Storer TW. Special considerations for exercise training in chronic lung disease. *ACSM's resource manual for guidelines for exercise testing and prescription*, 4th edition. Baltimore: Williams and Wilkins, 2001:346–352.
191. Castaneda C, Gordon PL, Uhlin KL, et al. Resistance training to counteract the catabolism of a low-protein diet in patients with chronic renal insufficiency. A randomized controlled trial. *Ann Intern Med* 2001;135:965–976.
192. Ryuzaki M, Konishi K, Kauga A, et al. Spontaneous rupture of the quadriceps tendon in patients on maintenance hemodialysis: Report of three cases with clinicopathological observations. *Clin Nephrol* 1989;32:144–148.

35

NUTRITIONAL FACTORS IN HYPERTENSION*

KEVIN C. ABBOTT
GEORGE L. BAKRIS

Whereas previous discussions of the role of diet in hypertension primarily focused on dietary excess (salt, calories, etc.) (1), more recent findings emphasized the role of dietary deficiency, particularly intrauterine malnutrition, which may have a host of profound and delayed effects resulting in adult hypertension; type II diabetes; cardiovascular complications; and, paradoxically, obesity (2). Although each of the following factors has been investigated in isolation, the dietary approaches that most effectively treat or prevent hypertension consistently have been combined and balanced diets, such as the DASH (Dietary Approaches to Stop Hypertension) diet and the Mediterranean diet.

SALT

Diets with high sodium content consistently have been cited as a cause of hypertension, confirmed in both animal (3,4) and human studies (5,6). A reduction in salt intake to less than 4 g/day reduces elevated blood pressure (7). The findings of the initial DASH trial (8) were incorporated into the reports of the Sixth Joint National Committee on Prevention, Detection, Evaluation and Treatment of High Blood Pressure (JNC-VI) (9) and the American Heart Association (10). Salt sensitivity, independent of blood pressure and other factors, has been identified as a risk factor for mortality (11). The INTERSALT trial demonstrated that blood pressure response to changes in sodium intake could be observed in patients considered normotensive (12). Although there was concern over "excessive" (less than 3 g/day) restriction of salt intake (13), it now is established through reanalysis of the DASH trial that dietary sodium restriction and the DASH diet (which is rich in vegetables, fruits, and low-fat dairy products) both lower blood pressure substantially, more in combination than singly (Fig. 35.1) (14,15). This benefit was seen in patients with blood pressures higher than 120/80 mm/Hg, including patients with stage I hypertension. Patients who had high-normal blood pressures (130 to 135 systolic) on a conventional high sodium–intake diet (141 to 144 mmol/day as measured) had mean systolic blood pressures 8.9 mm/Hg lower on a low sodium–intake DASH diet (64 to 67 mmol/day). Diastolic blood pressures also were lowered. Adherence to the DASH diet, at the same level of sodium intake, lowered systolic blood pressure significantly, although more at high sodium intake than at low sodium intake (Fig. 35.1). These reductions are comparable to those achieved through the use of antihypertensive medications. The benefits of dietary sodium restriction are greater in older people, in people with hypertension, in African Americans, and with long-term interventions (16–20). In addition to its benefits as a "nonpharmacologic therapy," it is also clear that sodium restriction improves the effect of antihypertensive medications (21–23). With the completion of the Human Genome Project, the medical community now is focused on the genetic and acquired basis of the heterogeneity of sodium sensitivity in human hypertension (24).

Previous objections to very–low-sodium diets (less than 3 g/day) have focused on the difficulty of adhering to this diet, given the high level of sodium in processed foods in the United States (25), and possibly deleterious effects based on hormonal changes (13). However, the appeal of low-salt foods appears to increase after 8 to 12 weeks of sodium restriction (26). Other public health issues also must be balanced against the benefits of low-sodium diets, among them the current linkage of iodine with salt supplements (27). Thus, interventions such as the Mediterranean diet in cardiovascular disease (28) and the DASH diet in hypertension are likely to be more effective (and better tolerated) than any single nutritional intervention.

* The opinions are solely those of the authors and do not represent an endorsement by the Department of Defense or the National Institutes of Health. This is a U.S. Government work. There are no restrictions on its use.

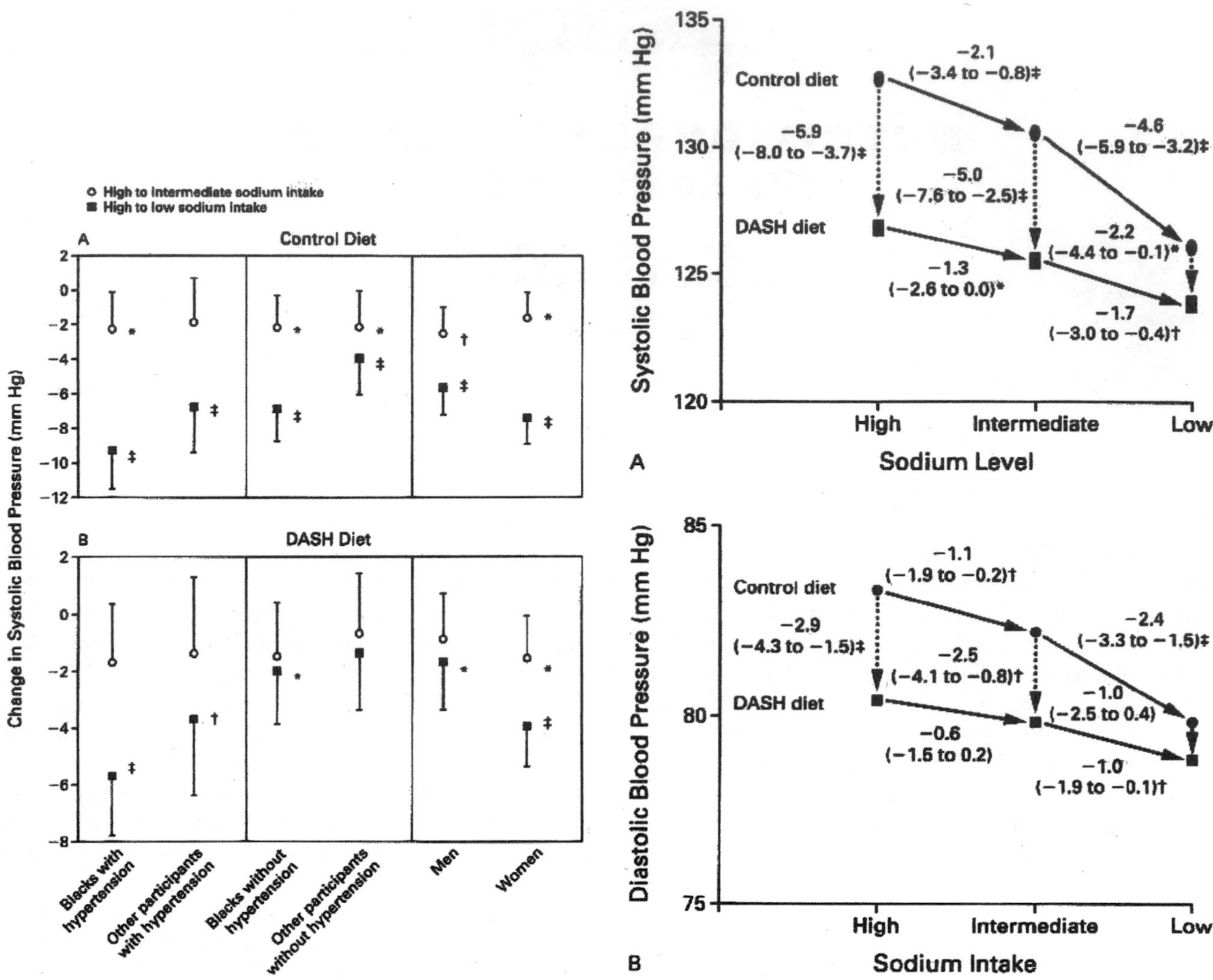

FIGURE 35.1. The relationship between the DASH (Dietary Approaches to Stop Hypertension) diet, salt intake, and both systolic and diastolic blood pressure (14). The effects of the DASH diet and reduced sodium intake were synergistic, achieving levels of blood pressure reduction comparable to antihypertensive therapy. The effects of dietary sodium reduction were more marked in patients on the DASH diet than for patients on the control diet.

OBESITY

The World Health Organization has declared an "epidemic of obesity," especially in the young (29,30). Obesity, when defined as a body mass index (BMI) equal to or greater than 30 kg/m^2, was present in 20% of men and 25% of women in a sample of the U.S. population from 1988 to 1994 (31) and increased by 49% between 1991 and 1998 (32). The greatest increases occurred among the youngest age group and those of Hispanic ethnicity, but the trend was universal (32). Although diet clearly is important in the development of obesity, the generally decreasing levels of physical activity in industrialized nations may be just as important (33). Obesity in the general population is associated with higher rates of hypertension, as well as diabetes, cardiac disease, and premature death (34,35). Because the prevalence of obesity is increasing so rapidly worldwide, it legitimately could be considered the most rapidly increasing risk factor for hypertension in the world. Weight loss has been associated with reductions in blood pressure both as monotherapy (although in a diet with "recommended" levels of sodium) (36) and more consistently as part of combined therapy (for example, the placebo arm of the Treatment of Mild Hypertension [TOMHS] study) (37). In the TOMHS study, even modest weight loss (6.6 pounds), in concert with a 10% reduction in sodium intake, was associated with substantial (almost 9 mm/Hg) reductions in systolic blood pressure, along with reduced left ventricular mass. In a more recent study, a weight loss of 5% (in addition to general lifestyle changes, including increased physical activity) resulted in a significantly lower risk of several undesirable outcomes, including diabetes and hypertension (5 mm Hg reduction in both systolic and diastolic blood pressure) (38).

It generally is recognized that in the general population the relationship between BMI and mortality follows a "J"-shaped curve in men and a "U"-shaped curve in women, at least among nonsmokers (Fig. 35.2) (39). Thus, risk for mortality increases at the extreme low end (<18.5 kg/m^2) as well as the high end of BMI. This relationship does not hold for patients with end-stage renal disease (ESRD) (40), particularly for cardiovascular causes of death (Abbott et al., unpublished data), where risk is entirely segregated with lower levels of BMI in men and African Americans. This relationship is also uncertain in the elderly (41,42) and for African Americans in the general population and with ESRD (43,44), who have significantly higher BMI and weight than whites with or without ESRD (45,46). It should be noted that after renal transplantation, obesity again becomes a significant risk factor for poor outcomes (47,48), although an association with worsened hypertension has not been shown.

In contrast to the relationship of obesity with hypertension seen in adults, hypertension manifesting in adulthood appears to be related to low BMI and low weight at birth. Brenner et al. suggested that reduced nephron number at birth could contribute to adult hypertension (49). Barker et al. suggested that low birthweight predisposes to multiple complications of adulthood, including hypertension (2). A case control study by Lackland et al. demonstrated a reverse "J"-shaped curve between birthweight and adjusted risk for

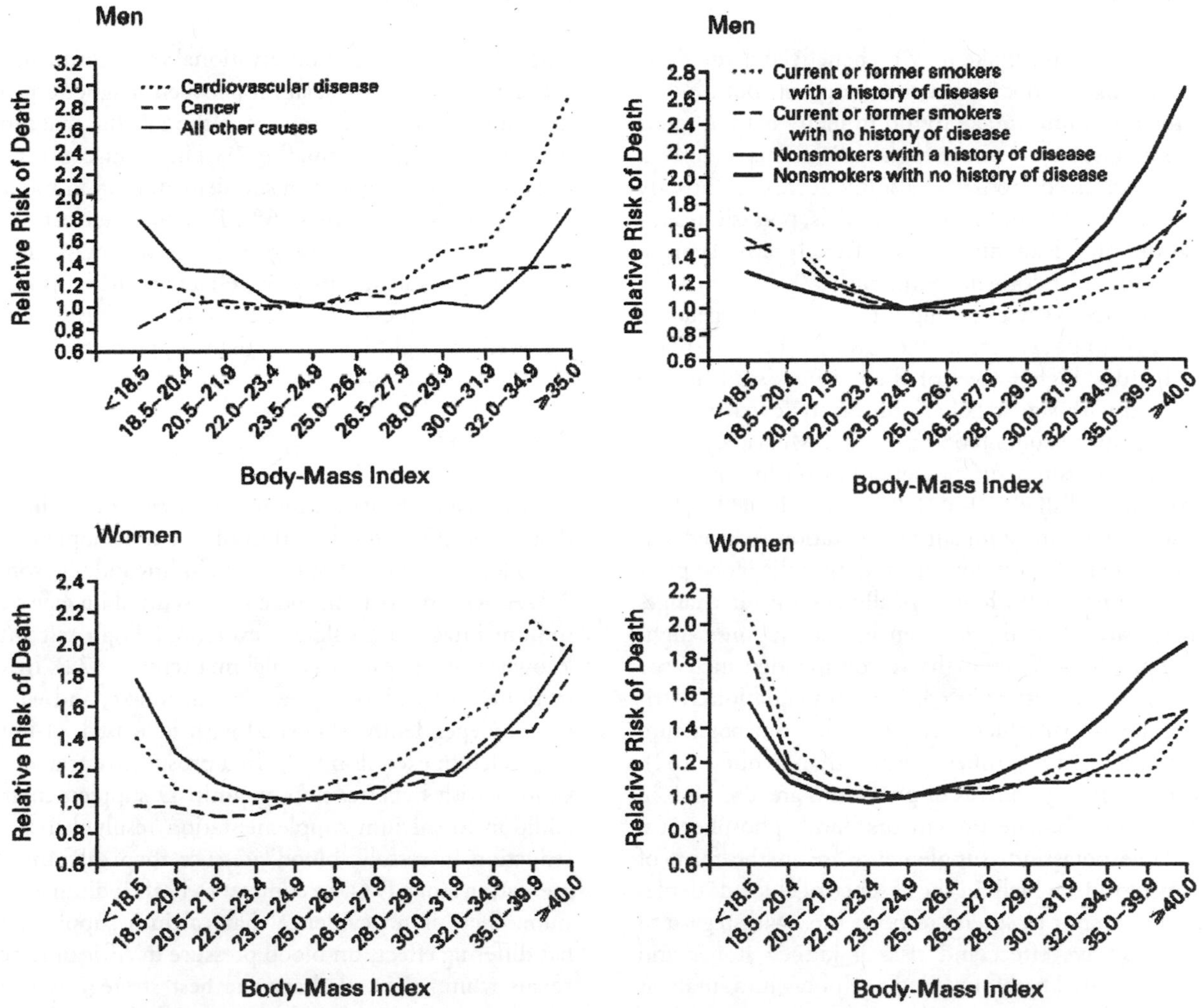

FIGURE 35.2. The relationship between body mass index (BMI) and differing causes of mortality in the general population. The adverse impact of obesity on survival is magnified in nonsmokers with no history of disease. However, in smokers or nonsmokers with a history of disease, low BMI had a greater adverse impact. In nonsmokers, obesity was most associated with increased risk of cardiovascular death, although in women this risk was matched closely by cancer-related death. (From Calle EE, Thun MJ, Petrelli JM, et al. Body-mass index and mortality in a prospective cohort of U.S. adults. N Engl J Med 1999;341:1097–1105, with permission.)

renal failure resulting from hypertension (50). Eriksson et al. found that after birth, low birthweight persons gained weight more rapidly and caught up with their contemporaries by age 7 (51). They suggested that the rapid weight gain and growth during childhood contributed to the risk for hypertension. In fact, people with low birthweight eventually may develop higher BMIs than their normal birthweight counterparts, suggesting a link with adult obesity (52). Animal models have suggested the mechanism for this relationship is fewer glomeruli in animals subjected to intrauterine malnutrition, with subsequent glomerular hypertrophy and hyperfiltration (53). These findings may have enormous implications not only for health care but for public policy as well (54).

POTASSIUM

Lower dietary sodium intake may be beneficial through its effects on raising the body potassium content, both by increasing the potassium intake found in many natural foods ingested as an alternative to the high sodium intake derived from eating processed foods and also by decreasing urinary potassium excretion (55). In animal models, potassium supplementation may lead directly to arterial vasodilatation (56) and improve endothelial function (57). Many of the benefits associated with a diet high in fruits and vegetables may be related to potassium intake (58). In the Rotterdam Study, a 1-g/day higher level of dietary potassium intake was associated with statistically significantly lower levels of diastolic, but not systolic, blood pressure. Metaanalyses on the effects of potassium supplementation on hypertension also have been published (59–61). The analysis by Whelton et al. showed that potassium supplementation reduced systolic blood pressure by 4.4 mm/Hg and diastolic blood pressure by 2.4 mm/Hg, both statistically significant changes (59). The greatest benefit was seen in patients on a high-salt diet. The JNC-VI report has recommended increased potassium intake as part of its core recommendations. African Americans in particular derive benefit from potassium supplementation (three times greater than whites) (62). Whereas most dietary sources of potassium are also high in bicarbonate, bicarbonate precursors, and phosphorous, most available potassium supplements are in the form of potassium chloride, which, in the absence of chloride depletion, may be inferior in several respects (i.e., with regard to its antihypertensive effect and risk of kidney stones and osteoporosis) (63). Therefore, adequate potassium intake is best achieved through proper diet rather than potassium chloride supplements.

Prevention of hypokalemia should be distinguished from potassium repletion. Most instances where potassium repletion is needed occur in a setting of chloride depletion (diuretic use, vomiting, or nasogastric drainage) (64). As mentioned, dietary potassium most often is coupled with bicarbonate and phosphorous, which will be less effective in these situations; therefore potassium chloride supplements are indicated (64). Patients who need diuretic therapy for hypertension also should receive the lowest dose of diuretics necessary along with potassium-sparing medications, such as potassium-sparing diuretics (although caution is advised with the use of triamterene because it is a well-described cause of acute renal failure from acute interstitial nephritis and also can lead to triamterene stone deposition) (65,66), angiotensin converting enzyme inhibitors, angiotensin receptor blockers, or beta blockers. Repletion of hypokalemia should consist of dietary supplementation, use of salt substitutes, or use of prescription potassium supplements (64).

MAGNESIUM

A 1998 metaanalysis of observational trials confirmed a significantly negative association between magnesium supplementation and blood pressure, although the magnitude of benefit was relatively small (67). This is in contrast to the clear benefit of magnesium supplementation in blood pressure control in pregnancy (68). Perhaps the clearest role of magnesium is as a necessary adjunct to potassium intake because hypokalemia may be refractory in the presence of coexisting magnesium deficiency (69). This is also best achieved through diet rather than supplementation.

CALCIUM

After initial enthusiasm, more recent experience has shown that the antihypertensive effect of calcium supplementation is modest and not without risk, including kidney stones (70, 71). As with potassium, there is substantial linkage between sodium intake and calcium excretion. High salt intake is known to increase urinary calcium excretion (72). In a cross-sectional survey, blood pressure, salt intake, and white race were independently associated with increased 24-hour urinary calcium excretion (73). In a prospective trial of elderly women with hypertension, vitamin D supplementation in addition to calcium supplementation resulted in a greater reduction in systolic blood pressure than calcium supplementation alone (74). In contrast to both sodium and potassium, there is no evidence that calcium supplementation has differing effects on blood pressure in African Americans versus whites (75). Perhaps the best strategy is to ensure adequate dietary intake of calcium and vitamin D while on a diet of low saturated fat and low sodium (which necessarily reduces consumption of dairy products). Based on available evidence, postmenopausal women likely would benefit most from calcium and possibly vitamin D supplementation for prevention of hypertension. It has been suggested that increasing calcium intake to equal the dietary calcium requirements may lower blood pressure, whereas increasing calcium intake above the dietary requirements has no further blood pressure–lowering effect (76). Further studies are needed to confirm this.

ALCOHOL

Moderate alcohol consumption (less than 1 ounce of ethanol per day) does not increase the prevalence of hypertension. Excessive use of alcohol is associated with hypertension and has been called the most common cause of reversible hypertension (77). Moderate alcohol use has a well-publicized association with a lower risk of coronary heart disease (78), although this benefit may be limited to people with specific genetic backgrounds (79). A factor often neglected in the public enthusiasm for the consumption of "moderate" amounts of alcohol is the frequency of alcohol–drug interactions. For example, the combined consumption of alcohol and α1 blockers may cause severe hypotension, especially in people of Oriental descent (80). The possibility of other alcohol–drug interactions, just as drug–drug interactions, always should be considered before recommending moderate alcohol intake.

DIETARY SUPPLEMENTS

A diet rich in fresh fruits, vegetables, and fiber, in combination with sodium restriction, clearly is associated with improved blood pressure (14). Unfortunately, the "more is better" and reductionist philosophies have led to the proliferation of dietary supplements that are purported to improve a wide variety of ills, including hypertension, without substantial clinical proof. The use of these supplements has grown in recent years, fueled by claims on the World Wide Web. Few well-performed clinical trials support the efficacy of dietary supplements, other than potassium, on lowering blood pressure in humans (81,82,83). For example, a meta-analysis of trials of garlic concluded it had modest effects on hyperlipidemia and cardiovascular disease but insignificant effects on blood pressure (84). In contrast, many widely used over-the-counter supplements have hypertension as a side effect. The most notorious among these are ephedrine (available as Ma Huang, "Ripped Fuel," and others), yohimbine, and Siberian (but apparently not American) ginseng (85). There is no evidence to support the superiority of any specific dietary supplement over the DASH diet for the prevention and treatment of hypertension.

CONCLUSIONS

Efforts to raise public awareness of the risk of high dietary fat and cholesterol intake have been tremendously successful. However, public awareness of the importance of dietary sodium and other factors important in the development of hypertension has suffered in comparison. It will take a concerted effort to generate public demand to reduce sodium concentrations in processed food to achieve further gains in blood pressure control (25). Many cultural and societal pressures will have to be overcome to turn the tide against the epidemic of obesity, and temptations for potentially toxic "easy fixes" will need to be rejected (33). The issue of intrauterine malnutrition in the development of adult complications should underscore the importance of proper maternal nutrition (50). To be effective, changes in diet must be permanent. For this reason, balanced diets such as the DASH diet and the Mediterranean diet are to be preferred over isolated restriction or supplementation of any one dietary substance.

REFERENCES

1. Braunwald E, ed. *Heart disease. A textbook of cardiovascular medicine*, 6th ed. Philadelphia: WB Saunders, 2001:977.
2. Barker DJ, Hales CN, Fall CH, et al. Type 2 (non-insulin-dependent) diabetes mellitus, hypertension and hyperlipidaemia (syndrome X): relation to reduced fetal growth. *Diabetologia* 1993; 36:62–67.
3. Tobian L. Salt and hypertension. Lessons from animal models that relate to human hypertension. *Hypertension* 1991 Jan;17(1 Suppl):152–158.
4. Denton D, Weisinger R, Mundy NI, et al. The effect of increased salt intake on blood pressure of chimpanzees. *Nat Med* 1995;1: 1009–1016.
5. He J, Klag MJ, Whelton PK, et al. Migration, blood pressure pattern, and hypertension: the Yi Migrant Study. *Am J Epidemiol* 1991;134:1085–1101.
6. Froment A, Milar H, Grovier C. Relationship of sodium intake and arterial hypertension: contribution of geographical epidemiology. *Rev Epidemiol Sante Publique* 1979;27:437–454.
7. Dyer AR, Stamler R, Elliott P, et al. Dietary salt and blood pressure. *Nat Med* 1995;1:994–996.
8. Appel LJ, Moore TJ, Obarzanek E, et al. A clinical trial of the effects of dietary patterns on blood pressure. DASH Collaborative Research Group. *N Engl J Med* 1997;336:1117–1124.
9. The sixth report of the Joint National Committee on Prevention, Detection, Evaluation, and Treatment of High Blood Pressure. *Arch Intern Med* 1997;157:2413–2446.
10. Krauss RM, Eckel RH, Howard B, et al. AHA Dietary Guidelines: revision 2000: A statement for healthcare professionals from the Nutrition Committee of the American Heart Association. *Stroke* 2000;31:2751–2766.
11. Weinberger MH, Fineberg NS, Fineberg SE, et al. Salt sensitivity, pulse pressure, and death in normal and hypertensive humans. *Hypertension* 2001;37:429–432.
12. Stamler J, Rose G, Elliot P, Dyer A, et al. Findings of the international cooperative INTERSALT study. *Hypertension* 1991;17: 9–15.
13. Graudal N, Galloe A. Should dietary salt restriction be a basic component of antihypertensive therapy? *Cardiovasc Drugs Ther* 2000;14:381–386.
14. Sacks FM, Svetkey LP, Vollmer WM, et al. Effects on blood pressure of reduced dietary sodium and the Dietary Approaches to Stop Hypertension (DASH) diet. DASH-Sodium Collaborative Research Group. *N Engl J Med* 2001;344:3–10.

15. Greenland P. Beating high blood pressure with low-sodium DASH. *N Engl J Med* 2001;344:53–55.
16. Alam S, Johnson AG. A meta-analysis of randomised controlled trials (RCT) among healthy normotensive and essential hypertensive elderly patients to determine the effect of high salt (NaCl) diet of blood pressure. *J Hum Hypertens* 1999;13:367–374.
17. Midgley JP, Matthew AG, Greenwood CM, et al. Effect of reduced dietary sodium on blood pressure: a meta-analysis of randomized controlled trials. *JAMA* 1996;275:1590–1597.
18. Cutler JA, Follmann D, Allender PS. Randomized trials of sodium reduction: an overview. *Am J Clin Nutr* 1997;65: 643S–651S.
19. Lenfant C, Roccella EJ. A call to action for more aggressive treatment of hypertension. *J Hypertens Suppl* 1999;17:S3–7.
20. Bakris GL, Weir MR. Salt intake and reductions in arterial pressure and proteinuria. Is there a direct link? *Am J Hypertens* 1996; 9:200S–206S.
21. Abbott KC, Bakris G. Renal effects of antihypertensive medications: an overview. *J Clin Pharmacol* 1993;33:392–399.
22. Heeg JE, de Jong PE, van der Hem GK, et al. Efficacy and variability of the antiproteinuric effect of ACE inhibition by lisinopril. *Kidney Int* 1989;36:272–279.
23. Smith AC, Abbott KC, Bakris GL. Sodium intake determines the degree of albuminuria with certain calcium antagonists. *J Am Soc Nephrol* 1995;6:650 (Abstract).
24. Weinberger MH. Salt and blood pressure. *Curr Opin Cardiol* 2000;15:254–257.
25. Nestel PJ. Controlling coronary risk through nutrition. *Can J Cardiol* 1995;11:96–146.
26. Mattes RD. The taste for salt in humans. *Am J Clin Nutr* 1997; 65:692S–697S.
27. van der Haar F. The challenge of the global elimination of iodine deficiency disorders. *Eur J Clin Nutr* 1997;51 Suppl 4:S3–8.
28. de Lorgeril M, Salen P, Martin JL, et al. Mediterranean diet, traditional risk factors, and the rate of cardiovascular complications after myocardial infarction: final report of the Lyon Diet Heart Study. *Circulation* 1999;99:779–785.
29. Obesity: preventing and managing the global epidemic. Report of a WHO consultation. *WHO Tech Rep Ser* 2000;894:i–xii, 1–253.
30. Visscher TL, Seidell JC. The public health impact of obesity. *Annu Rev Public Health* 2001;22:355–375.
31. Allison DB, Saunders SE. Obesity in North America: an overview. *Med Clin North Am* 2000;84:305–332.
32. Mokdad AH, Serdula MK, Dietz WH, et al. The spread of the obesity epidemic in the United States, 1991–1998. *JAMA* 1999; 282:1519–1522.
33. Franklin BA. The downside of our technological revolution? An obesity-conducive environment. *Am J Cardiol* 2001;87: 1093–1095.
34. Ramos F, Baglivo HP, Ramirez AJ, et al. The metabolic syndrome and related cardiovascular risk. *Curr Hypertens Rep* 2001;3: 100–106.
35. Obesity epidemic increases dramatically in the United States. Center for Disease Control. National Center for Chronic Disease Prevention and Health Promotion. *http://www.cdc.gov/nccdphp/dnpa/obesity-epidemic.htm*. Accessed May 2, 2003.
36. Metz JA, Stern JS, Kris-Etherton P, et al. A randomized trial of improved weight loss with a prepared meal plan in overweight and obese patients: impact on cardiovascular risk reduction. *Arch Intern Med* 2000;160:2150–2158.
37. Neaton JD, Grimm RH Jr, Prineas RJ, et al. Treatment of mild hypertension study. Final results. Treatment of Mild Hypertension Study Research Group. *JAMA* 1993;270:713–724.
38. Tuomilehto J, Lindstrom J, Eriksson JG, et al. Prevention of type 2 diabetes mellitus by changes in lifestyle among subjects with impaired glucose tolerance. *N Engl J Med* 2001;344: 1343–1350.
39. Calle EE, Thun MJ, Petrelli JM, et al. Body-mass index and mortality in a prospective cohort of U.S. adults. *N Engl J Med* 1999;341:1097–1105.
40. Wong JS, Port FK, Hulbert-Shearon TE, et al. Survival advantage in Asian American end-stage renal disease patients. *Kidney Int* 1999;55:2515–2523.
41. Stevens J, Cai J, Pamuk ER, et al. The effect of age on the association between body-mass index and mortality. *N Engl J Med* 1998;338:1–7.
42. Heiat A, Vaccarino V, Krumholz HM. An evidence-based assessment of federal guidelines for overweight and obesity as they apply to elderly persons. *Arch Intern Med* 2001;161:1194–1203.
43. Sanchez AM, Reed DR, Price RA. Reduced mortality associated with body mass index (BMI) in African Americans relative to Caucasians. *Ethn Dis* 2000;10:24–30.
44. Stevens J. Obesity and mortality in Africans-Americans. *Nutr Rev* 2000;58:346–353.
45. Brown CD, Higgins M, Donato KA, et al. Body mass index and the prevalence of hypertension and dyslipidemia. *Obes Res* 2000; 8:605–619.
46. Kimm SY, Barton BA, Obarzanek E, et al. Racial divergence in adiposity during adolescence: the NHLBI Growth and Health Study. *Pediatrics* 2001;107:E34.
47. Meier-Kriesche HU, Vaghela M, Thambuganipalle R, et al. The effect of body mass index on long-term renal allograft survival. *Transplantation* 1999;68:1294–1297.
48. Pischon T, Sharma AM. Obesity as a risk factor in renal transplant patients. *Nephrol Dial Transplant* 2001;16:14–17.
49. Brenner BM, Garcia DL, Anderson S. Glomeruli and blood pressure. Less of one, more the other? *Am J Hypertens* 1988;1: 335–347.
50. Lackland DT, Bendall HE, Osmond C, et al. Low birth weights contribute to high rates of early-onset chronic renal failure in the Southeastern United States. *Arch Intern Med* 2000;160: 1472–1476.
51. Eriksson J, Forsen T, Tuomilehto J, et al. Fetal and childhood growth and hypertension in adult life. *Hypertension* 2000;36: 790–794.
52. Jackson AA, Langley-Evans SC, McCarthy HD. Nutritional influences in early life upon obesity and body proportions. *Ciba Found Symp* 1996;201:118–129.
53. Lucas SRR, Miraglia SM, Zaladek F, Coimbra TM. Intrauterine food restriction as a determinant of nephrosclerosis. *Am J Kidney Dis* 2001;37:467–476.
54. Luft FT. Food intake and the kidney: the right amounts at the right times. *Am J Kidney Dis* 2001;37:629–631.
55. Cohn JN, Kowey PR, Whelton PK, et al. New guidelines for potassium replacement in clinical practice: a contemporary review by the National Council on Potassium in Clinical Practice. *Arch Intern Med* 2000;160:2429–2436.
56. Zhou MS, Kosaka H, Yoneyama H. Potassium augments vascular relaxation mediated by nitric oxide in the carotid arteries of hypertensive Dahl rats. *Am J Hypertens* 2000;13:666–672.
57. Ishimitsu T, Tobian L. High potassium diets reduce endothelial permeability in stroke-prone spontaneously hypertensive rats. *Clin Exp Pharmacol Physiol* 1996;23:241–245.
58. Ascherio A, Hennekens C, Willett WC, et al. Prospective study of nutritional factors, blood pressure, and hypertension among US women. *Hypertension* 1996;27:1065–1072.
59. Whelton PK, He J, Cutler JA, et al. Effects of oral potassium on blood pressure. Meta-analysis of randomized controlled clinical trials. *JAMA* 1997;277:1624–1632.
60. Cutler JA. The effects of reducing sodium and increasing potas-

sium intake for control of hypertension and improving health. *Clin Exp Hypertens* 1999;21:769–783.
61. Whelton PK, He J. Potassium in preventing and treating high blood pressure. *Semin Nephrol* 1999;19:494–499.
62. Langford HG. Dietary potassium and hypertension: epidemiologic data. *Ann Intern Med* 1983;98:770–772.
63. Morris RC Jr, Schmidlin O, Tanaka M, et al. Differing effects of supplemental KCl and KHCO3: pathophysiological and clinical implications. *Semin Nephrol* 1999;19:487–493.
64. Gennari FJ. Hypokalemia. *N Engl J Med* 1998;339:451–458.
65. Sica DA, Gehr TW. Triamterene and the kidney. *Nephron* 1989; 51:454–461.
66. Perazella MA. Crystal-induced acute renal failure. *Am J Med* 1999;106:459–465.
67. Mizushima S, Cappuccio FP, Nichols R, et al. Dietary magnesium intake and blood pressure: a qualitative overview of the observational studies. *J Hum Hypertens* 1998;12:447–453.
68. Rudnicki M, Frolich A, Pilsgaard K, et al. Comparison of magnesium and methyldopa for the control of blood pressure in pregnancies complicated with hypertension. *Gynecol Obstet Invest* 2000;49:231–235.
69. Rude RK. Physiology of magnesium metabolism and the important role of magnesium in potassium deficiency. *Am J Cardiol* 1989;63:316–346.
70. Griffith LE, Guyatt GH, Cook RJ, et al. The influence of dietary and nondietary calcium supplementation on blood pressure: an updated metaanalysis of randomized controlled trials. *Am J Hypertens* 1999;12:84–92.
71. Allender PS, Cutler JA, Follmann D, et al. Dietary calcium and blood pressure: a meta-analysis of randomized clinical trials. *Ann Intern Med* 1996;124:825–831.
72. Cappuccio FP, Kalaitzidis R, Duneclift S, et al. Unraveling the links between calcium excretion, salt intake, hypertension, kidney stones and bone metabolism. *J Nephrol* 2000;13:169–177.
73. Blackwood AM, Sagnella GA, Cook DG, et al. Urinary calcium excretion, sodium intake and blood pressure in a multi-ethnic population: results of the Wandsworth Heart and Stroke Study. *J Hum Hypertens* 2001;15:229–237.
74. Pfeifer M, Begerow B, Minne HW, et al. Effects of a short-term vitamin D(3) and calcium supplementation on blood pressure and parathyroid hormone levels in elderly women. *J Clin Endocrinol Metab* 2001;86:1633–1637.
75. Freudenheim JL, Russell M, Trevisan M, et al. Calcium intake and blood pressure in blacks and whites. *Ethn Dis* 1991;1: 114–122.
76. Hajjar IM, Grim CE, Kotchen TA. Dietary calcium lowers age-related rise in blood pressures in the United States: the NHANES III survey. *J Clin Hypertens (Greenwich)* 2003;5(2):122–126.
77. Aguilera MT, de la Sierra A, Coca A, et al. Effect of alcohol abstinence on blood pressure: assessment by 24-hour ambulatory blood pressure monitoring. *Hypertension* 1999;33:653–657.
78. Glaser JH. Why mortality from heart disease is low in France. Wine consumption clearly correlates with residual differences in mortality. *BMJ* 2000;320:250.
79. Hines LM, Stampfer MJ, Ma J, et al. Genetic variation in alcohol dehydrogenase and the beneficial effect of moderate alcohol consumption on myocardial infarction. *N Engl J Med* 2001;344: 549–555.
80. Kawano Y, Abe H, Kojima S, et al. Interaction of alcohol and an alpha1-blocker on ambulatory blood pressure in patients with essential hypertension. *Am J Hypertens* 2000;13:307–312.
81. Silagy CA, Neil HA. A meta-analysis of the effect of garlic on blood pressure. *J Hypertens* 1994;12:463–468.
82. Hodgson JM, Puddey IB, Beilin LJ, et al. Effects of isoflavonoids on blood pressure in subjects with high-normal ambulatory blood pressure levels: a randomized controlled trial. *Am J Hypertens* 1999;12:47–53.
83. Rimm EB, Katan MB, Ascherio A, et al. Relation between intake of flavonoids and risk for coronary heart disease in male health professionals. *Ann Intern Med* 1996;125:384–389.
84. Ackermann RT, Mulrow CD, Ramirez G, et al. Garlic shows promise for improving some cardiovascular risk factors. *Arch Intern Med* 2001;161:813–824.
85. Nelson L, Perrone J. Herbal and alternative medicine. *Emerg Med Clin North Am* 2000;18:709–722.

36

ACHIEVING PATIENT ADHERENCE TO DIET THERAPY

JERRILYNN D. BURROWES
DAVID B. COCKRAM

Dietary management is becoming increasingly important in the prevention and treatment of a variety of chronic disorders. However, it is difficult for people to make and maintain dietary changes (1,2). Successful adherence to diet therapy depends on the individual's willingness to accept and ability to maintain the required behaviors. Adherence is a complex and incompletely understood behavioral process that is strongly influenced by the environment in which people live, the social and cultural aspects of their life, the quality of the patient–health care provider relationship, the complexity and duration of the diet recommendations, patient attitudes about the benefits of the diet, and the techniques used to counsel and teach the patient. Although adherence often is conceptualized as a dichotomous variable (i.e., adherent versus nonadherent), it is actually a spectrum of behaviors (3). This is particularly true for a diet in which day-to-day and seasonal fluctuations in intake are substantial (4). Adherence to a treatment regimen is not influenced by age, sex, race, income, occupation, social status, level of education, or any other readily determinable factor (5–8).

Dietary interventions are an integral component of successful medical management in people with kidney disease. However, dietary management may fail for a number of reasons. First, patient lifestyle, support systems, and attitude toward their disease all affect adherence. Second, the health practitioner may have limited technical and conceptual knowledge of the dietary principles or the patient's food habits and practices or beliefs. Third, necessary counseling skills to educate the patient may be lacking. Fourth, the patient may not be ready to change his or her behavior. For patients to achieve and maintain adherence to diet therapy, the practitioner must understand the factors that influence adherence, how to measure dietary adherence, and the strategies used to achieve adherence. This chapter reviews factors influencing dietary adherence and biologic markers that may be used to monitor adherence, describes the strategies used to achieve dietary adherence, and reviews the tools that can be used to help patients maintain long-term dietary adherence.

DEFINITIONS

Both adherence and compliance refer to the extent that a person's behavior coincides with medical advice or recommendations (9,10). Although the terms frequently are used interchangeably, their meanings have a subtle difference (9). Adherence is used in this chapter because of its less judgmental and more collaborative connotation. Dietary change requires a great deal of collaboration by the patient, and adherence, with its implication of active participation, seems more appropriate in this context.

Adherence

Adherence connotes an active partnership between provider and patient, a partnership in which both provider and patient strive to ensure that the patient will become as self-sufficient as possible in managing his or her condition. In this context, the patient who is adherent makes a voluntary and active decision to follow a regimen that he or she thinks is sensible and contributes to management of the condition (9).

Compliance

Compliance connotes a passive role with the patient faithfully following the advice and directions of the health care provider (8,9). The term noncompliance incorporates an evaluative concept that may imply a negative or prejudicial attitude toward the patient and often presumes that failure to comply is the patient's fault (11).

MEASURES OF ADHERENCE TO DIET THERAPY

It is difficult to determine the level of adherence to diet therapy (Fig. 36.1) because (a) adherence may be conceptualized in several ways; (b) the criteria for defining adher-

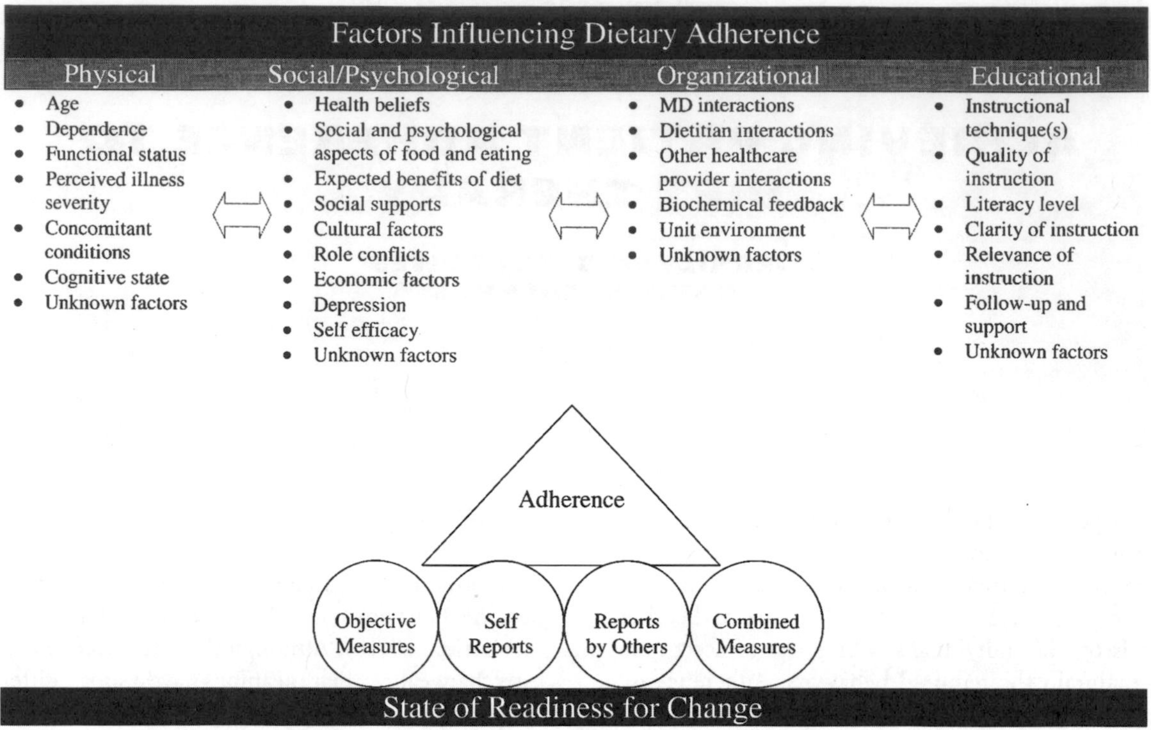

FIGURE 36.1. Adherence is a multifaceted phenomenon with many poorly understood relationships between factors. Patient instruction must consider numerous known and unknown factors that can influence dietary adherence and the patient's readiness for behavioral change. Observed adherence with diet is a behavioral continuum that is affected both by the complex interaction of these factors from the patient's perspective and by the methods used to measure adherence.

ence differs across studies; (c) adherence rates vary widely from one situation to another, depending on the context; (d) adherence may be assessed by very different methods, and each method has its own inherent strengths and weaknesses; and (e) there have been few well-controlled, prospective, randomized trials evaluating methods to achieve or assess adherence. In general, dietary adherence in renal disease may be assessed using subjective assessments (e.g., patient self reports, diet records, and caregiver evaluations), relatively objective techniques (e.g., biochemical markers—such as serum albumin, protein nitrogen appearance [PNA], blood urea nitrogen [BUN], serum potassium, and serum phosphate—interdialytic weight gain, dialysis session attendance, shortening of dialysis sessions, or percentage of total prescribed dialysis time received), or combinations of these objective and subjective markers (8). For some aspects of dietary adherence, such as determining dietary energy or fluid intake, only subjective measures requiring patient input (e.g., diet records/recalls) are clinically practical despite their limitations.

Biochemical Markers of Dietary Adherence

Biochemical markers are useful in assessing dietary adherence in some clinical conditions. For example, hemoglobin A_{1C} is a useful (i.e., relatively sensitive and specific) indicator of dietary compliance in people with diabetes. However, the natural history of renal disease and the effectiveness of the treatment regimen make biologic markers relatively nonspecific and insensitive indicators of dietary adherence in most people with kidney disease. Yet in some instances, biochemical markers of adherence to the renal diet may be useful. For example, adherence to dietary protein intake may be measured with the PNA, assuming the patient is approximately in nitrogen balance (12). Less specific biochemical indicators such as serum albumin, serum potassium, serum phosphate, BUN, and interdialytic fluid weight gain are affected by other factors (e.g., hydration status, medications, and catabolism) in people with kidney disease (8).

RATES OF ADHERENCE TO DIET THERAPY

Adherence to diet therapy in chronic disease is usually poorer and more subjective than other types of medical adherence, such as taking medications or attending scheduled appointments. This is because dietary changes need to be sustained indefinitely and may be complicated further by serial changes in the diet as the underlying renal disease process progresses. In addition, changes in lifestyle imposed by diet therapy frequently have more social consequences than is the case with other medical interventions (8,13, 14–16). Educational techniques that focus primarily on imparting knowledge are likely to be less effective in promoting long-term adherence than those incorporating education as well as problem-solving and behavioral change techniques (13).

Methods used to assess adherence also may influence conclusions about adherence rates. Although some authors advocate use of objective methods over subjective approaches, no consensus or gold standard currently exists (8). The relationship between subjective and objective adherence measures is generally weak, and identifiable demographic and social factors typically explain only a small fraction of the variance in objective measures (8,9). Whereas educational approaches may need individualization to optimize adherence, techniques used to assess adherence probably also require individualization depending on which factors limit adherence.

Nonadherence may take many different forms, including both intentional and unintentional behavior. Nonadherence to diet therapy may lead to unnecessary diagnostic tests, emergency care, alternative treatments, increased doses of or additional medications, hospitalization, short- and long-term degenerative changes, premature initiation of dialysis for people with chronic renal failure, increased time on the machine for people undergoing dialysis, exacerbation of renal bone disease, hypertension, and/or acidosis. Nonadherence even may lead to increased morbidity and mortality and an inability to establish and evaluate the efficacy of a therapeutic regimen (11). Table 36.1 lists patient, treatment, and relationship variables relating to treatment nonadherence.

TABLE 36.1. FACTORS RELATED TO TREATMENT NONADHERENCE

Patient variables
Characteristics of the individual
Sensory disabilities
Forgetfulness
Lack of understanding
Inappropriate or conflicting health benefits
Competing sociocultural and ethnic concepts of disease and treatment
Apathy and pessimism
Failure to recognize that one is ill or in need of treatment
Previous or present history of nonadherence with other regimen
Health beliefs
Dissatisfaction with practitioner or treatment
Characteristics of individual's social situation
Lack of social supports
Environment that supports nonadherent behavior
Competing or conflicting demands or other pressing demands (e.g., poverty, unemployment)
Lack of resources (e.g., transportation, money, time)
Treatment variables
Characteristics of treatment setting
Adherence of continuity of care
Inadequate supervision by health care professionals
Complexity of treatment recommendations
Degree of behavioral change
Inconvenience
Expense
Characteristics of treatment
Relationship variables: patient–health care provider interaction
Inadequate communication
Poor rapport
Attitudinal or behavioral faults on the part of either health care provider or patient
Failure of health care provider to elicit negative feedback about problems with treatment regimen
Inconsistencies in the message among health care providers
Patient's dissatisfaction
Inadequate supervision

FACTORS INFLUENCING DIETARY ADHERENCE

Adherence to dietary advice is a multidimensional phenomenon; any assessment of adherence must consider the impact of numerous influences on an individual's behavior (Table 36.1 and Fig. 36.1). These include patient variables, such as health beliefs and cultural and social factors, and treatment variables, such as complexity of the diet, duration of the disease, and the patient's knowledge of his or her illness. To optimize adherence, clinicians must understand how these factors influence each patient and design educational strategies to equip each patient with the knowledge and techniques necessary for a variety of social, physiologic, and psychologic conditions. Sustaining dietary change is extremely challenging because multiple modifications of long-standing behaviors typically are required, and food frequently plays a central role in many social situations (13).

Patient Variables

Patient Beliefs

The health belief model was developed to predict the effect of preventive health behaviors (17) and was modified (18) to study compliance with prescribed health regimens. A patient's readiness to adhere to a prescribed regimen is explained by a general motivation toward health, the perceived threat of the illness, the value of reducing that threat, the expected outcomes of the proposed health action, and the perceived barriers to taking the proposed action. The state of readiness interacts with modifying variables, such as complexity of the diet and social support, to determine the likelihood of compliance (19). Situational factors that modify a patient's readiness to adhere include characteristics of the regimen, interactions between the patient and the health care providers, and interactions with family and social groups.

Culture

An individual's cultural background influences his or her beliefs, language, values, and relationships (20). Culture also plays a significant role in food choices, perceptions about food and food preparation, and relationship between diet and health. These factors, in turn, may influence adherence with diet therapy. The literature suggests that while people of all cultural heritages can adhere to diets, the issues and barriers to adherence differ for people with different backgrounds (13,21–23). Assessing cultural issues surrounding food and food behaviors, and addressing them, may help improve adherence (23).

Social

Individuals exist in a social environment consisting of oneself, their community, and a wider society (24). The impact of this social environment on adherence must be considered at each level, with strategies developed to address barriers to adherence (4,24). Patients may perceive their dietary needs as incompatible with the preferences of their family members. Preparation of two sets of meals may be viewed as excessively time-consuming and expensive, and selection of dietetic foods can be difficult, necessitating a thorough review and understanding of food labels.

Adherence with dietary needs may be challenged during holidays and special occasions where food frequently plays an important social role. People who are dependent on others for food procurement, preparation, or both, face further challenges in adhering to dietary recommendations. Clinicians must assess the patient's social support and, if limited, identify practical ways to increase support for the patient. Perceptions of support from a spouse, family members, friends, and health care professionals, depending on the outcome parameter, can affect dietary adherence. People with strong social support typically are better able to cope with the demands of the disease and dietary management. Therefore, diet adherence may be improved. Including family members and friends in the process (as appropriate) may improve adherence by heightening awareness of the seriousness of the disease and the central role of nutritional interventions in medical management and prevention of long-term consequences. Specific educational materials (e.g., meal plans and shopping lists) incorporating social and cultural preferences developed at appropriate reading levels (e.g., menus versus exchange lists) may be helpful in enhancing adherence (25). Improving social interaction skills, such as negotiation or self-assertion, has been advocated (4,13).

Knowledge of Illness

Traditional hospital-based nutrition education has several limitations: (a) patients with recent onset of a chronic condition may not be receptive to diet instruction or ready to make behavioral changes; (b) the time to perform instruction typically is limited; and (c) ongoing education and support after discharge may be lacking. Because of these issues, inpatient education frequently tends to be a unidirectional disgorgement of facts from caregiver to patient rather than an individualized process designed to address lifestyle issues and competing demands from the patient's perspective. Providing relevant information at an appropriate rate and educational level and correcting misinformation the patient may acquire are key components for future dietary adherence (4,26).

Achieving diet adherence is substantially different and more challenging than most other aspects of medical management (4,13). For example, unlike "bad habits" such as alcohol abuse, illicit drug use, or smoking, eating is essential to life and, therefore, cannot be categorically discouraged. Because most foods can fit into a renal diet with appropriate education, effort, and planning, achieving long-term adherence requires patients to be empowered. Providing patients with problem-solving skills will enable them to continue to enjoy the nutritional, psychologic, and social functions of food without compromising disease management.

Psychologic

Personality traits have not been identified as clear predictors of dietary nonadherence. However, certain psychologic characteristics may influence adherence (e.g., depression and anxiety), although the data are not definitive (27). Depression appears to be a barrier to adherence to medical and dietary management in people with kidney disease, especially end-stage renal disease (ESRD). Although adherence rates are generally constant over time within individuals, people with depression typically have poorer adherence based on adherence to prescribed total dialysis time (8). Research in people with diabetes also suggests that diet adherence is poorer and health costs are higher with increasing depression (28). Care must be taken in interpreting adherence measures, such as interdialytic weight gain and serum potassium or phosphate levels, in people with depression because levels in the desirable "range" may be the result of insufficient nutrient intake and not dietary adherence.

Age and Dependence

Historically, the elderly have been suggested to exhibit better adherence with medical interventions than younger people, although the validity of this conclusion has been questioned because individuals who were expected to be nonadherent frequently were excluded from many studies (29). Although age can be thought of in a chronologic sense, from an adherence standpoint it is more useful to consider aging from a psychosocial perspective. This view considers aging as a process, addressing age-related health beliefs, stresses, cognitive abilities, physical functioning, environmental considerations, competing role demands, dependency, literacy level, change in health status over time, treatment burden, polypharmacy, and social factors (29). Because people with kidney disease cover the spectrum for each of these variables, adherence strategies for the elderly need to consider these factors and the interventions must be individualized to address each person's unique needs, recognizing that their needs will change over time.

Many elderly people with renal disease are dependent on others to some extent for various aspects of their care. Although dependence does not imply lower levels of expected adherence to diet, the nature of the renal dietitian's educational and motivational tasks will change. In situations where someone other than the patient procures or prepares foods and when either separate food preparation or a change in the diet of others is necessary, educating this person on the role of diet in disease management and the expected benefits can be helpful in facilitating adherence.

Economics

The relationship between socioeconomic status and adherence to nutritional recommendations is unclear. Higher educational levels and employment, which are associated with socioeconomic status, are often, but not always, associated with better adherence. People of greater means tend not to have economic barriers to compliance (i.e., they can afford to change their diet) and may be highly adherent in the presence of strong social support. These individuals also may participate in more social situations that make sustained adherence to the renal diet more challenging. In contrast, people with less education may be more influenced by caregiver expectations and face financial barriers in making changes in food choices. Careful evaluation of an individual's economic and social support is warranted when counseling patients.

Treatment Variables

As medical therapy becomes more complex, inconvenient, expensive, or lengthy, the expected rate of long-term adherence becomes poorer (7,11,30).

Complexity of the Diet

The renal diet is complex. The diet can be made less complex by prioritizing the regimen (i.e., address hyperkalemia first versus hyperphosphatemia), breaking the dietary plan into sequentially implemented stages, and minimizing inconvenience by tailoring the dietary regimen to the patient's culture and lifestyle as much as possible. Nutritional counseling should be preceded by careful assessment of the patient to assure that extraneous instructions are minimized or eliminated and the focus of the counseling is appropriate for the readiness of the patient to implement dietary change. The diet should be as liberal as possible, given concomitant conditions and the patient's history, to minimize its intrusiveness. Clinicians should attempt to balance the desire for a liberal diet with safety and tolerance of longer dialysis regimens and presence of any residual renal function in people receiving dialysis.

Intrusiveness

The patient's feelings about the nature of his or her illness and the impact of his or her medical condition(s) on current and future well-being are significant factors influencing the burden of disease. People who are depressed are more likely to have higher disease burdens and, thus, generally have lower levels of dietary adherence. In contrast, people who view their condition as a challenge to manage and are able to appropriately modify their lifestyle to incorporate necessary behavioral changes are more likely to feel a lower disease burden and exhibit higher levels of dietary adherence.

Duration

Once established, chronic renal disease tends to progress toward ESRD in most individuals, necessitating a series of lifelong changes in dietary habits. Dietary adherence tends to decrease with increasing duration of the disease (6). The challenges facing the renal dietitian initially are to determine the patient's state of readiness for behavioral change and to provide appropriate information to assist the patient in the change process. Because dietary changes need to be sustained, both tasks must continue indefinitely. The challenges for the patient are to assimilate the information, implement behavioral changes, and acquire problem-solving skills to assist with maintenance of long-term adherence. These tasks are more difficult in people with renal disease because the dietary restrictions required for each stage of the disease change during the progression from chronic renal insufficiency to ESRD. Dietary changes may continue to evolve further as residual renal function is lost once ESRD is diagnosed, dialysis modality changes, or kidney transplantation occurs.

Organizational Issues

The health care team and system are potent influences on dietary management of renal disease. Of concern is the effect of the dialysis setting itself on influencing adherence, an area that has not been well studied. A cheerful, supportive environment—in which experienced staff members and patients interact positively and creatively with each other and clinicians are readily available to address questions or provide information and work collaboratively to assist in individualized problem-solving—may help limit disease burden and facilitate adherence. However, providing this environment and individualized support may be difficult or impossible in dialysis units with high patient to dietitian ratios (i.e., greater than 150 to 1) (12). As a result, adherence may be lower and clinical outcomes may be poorer.

Prescription of multiple regimens, complex regimens, or both; lack of consistency in health care providers; care provider behavior toward patients; inadequacy of diet instruction; and inconvenience of the regimen are factors under the control of the provider that are likely to lead to patient nonadherence (27). Unintended communications from health care providers that imply that dietary management or lifestyle components of the self-management regimen are not important also contribute to nonadherence.

STAGES OF CHANGE

Although there are several behavior change models, most have common themes (9). Implicit in each is the notion that patients make rational decisions regarding future events and, given the appropriate skills, can establish goals and modify or regulate behavior to achieve these goals (9). The stages of change model of behavior (31–33) suggests that behavioral change is a process that occurs gradually, with the individual moving through a series of fairly predictable stages (Table 36.2). These levels reflect a process of change—from precontemplation (not considering change) to motivation to change (contemplation)—before making a commitment to change (preparation) and actually making the change (action). Although relapses occur, they become part of the process of working toward lifelong change (31). The implication for clinicians is that each patient's readiness to embrace change must be assessed and the message must be tailored appropriately (Table 36.2). Initially, the focus may be on assisting patients in moving along the progression to the action stage with relatively little emphasis on specific dietary goals, whereas later interactions may be more supportive during the maintenance or relapse stages.

STRATEGIES TO ACHIEVE DIETARY ADHERENCE

Strategies for improving adherence fall into three broad categories: behavioral, educational, and organizational.

Behavioral Strategies

Behavioral strategies focus on the behaviors involved in adherence. These include (a) attempts to reduce barriers to adherence such as cost of treatment or inconvenience, (b) cues to stimulate adherence, and (c) rewards or reinforcement for adherence (30). Behavioral strategies attempt to influence specific behaviors directly using techniques such as reminders, self-monitoring, and reinforcement, with information and instruction playing a secondary role (34). These strategies are particularly effective in the elderly because they address the problem of declining cognitive and physical function, as well as a lack of social support and financial resources for many. Various mechanisms or aids, such as charts and menus that remind elders to limit high potassium foods or to consume adequate amounts of dietary energy and protein each day, are effective for improving

TABLE 36.2. STAGES OF CHANGE MODEL AND IMPLICATIONS FOR NUTRITIONAL COUNSELING

Stage of Change	Patient Characteristics	Nutritional Counseling Implications
Precontemplation	Not thinking about change; lack of control; denial or resignation common; not yet convinced of seriousness of condition	Relationship building key, educate about the underlying disease process; put minimal emphasis on specific dietary changes; focus on overcoming individual barriers and benefit to addressing them
Contemplation	Considering advantages and disadvantages of changing behavior	Educate about long-term complications of disease, role of diet in medical management, expected benefits; begin to establish a timeline for change
Preparation	Tentative steps to change behavior	Initial simplified diet instruction; begin to set goals and encourage self-management/self-monitoring behaviors; reinforce initial successful behavioral changes; build self-efficacy
Action	Significant steps to change behavior	Use progressive nutrition education to develop self-management skills; offer continued reinforcement for successful incorporation of new behavior into patient's lifestyle; develop goal-setting and self-monitoring skills
Maintenance	Sustained incorporation of new behaviors into lifestyle	Self-management and coping skills; skills for managing diet in new/difficult social situations; build self-management, goal-setting, and monitoring skills
Relapse	Experiencing normal part of process of change; usually feels demoralized	Reinforce self-management skills and develop social supports; address factors associated with relapse; build self-efficacy and self-monitoring skills; emphasize what can be learned from relapse versus focusing on failure

adherence (35). Although behavioral approaches to adherence tend to support change in the short term (34), they fail to maintain consistent change in the long term (36). Patients must take responsibility for regulating their own change process to maintain behavioral change (37).

Contracting

Contracting enables patients, with assistance from the health care provider, to identify specific behaviors they will perform between counseling visits. The behaviors typically are composed of a series of small, manageable steps leading toward the patient's goals. This process helps shape patient behaviors and enhances commitment to follow the regimen. Key components of contracting include (a) focusing on the behaviors leading to the goal, rather than focusing on the end goal; (b) identifying small steps the patient believes can be achieved realistically between counseling visits; (c) describing a set of steps that are unique to, or tailored to, the patient; (d) identifying an end goal that is important to the patient over a period of contracts; (e) identifying how patient behaviors will be recorded; and (f) identifying a reward that the patient values, if rewards are part of the contract (38).

One of the primary goals of contracting is to keep the patient in care and to increase the opportunity for successful management of his or her condition. Even when progress is not made toward the desired behavioral change, patients should be provided with support for trying (if appropriate) and encouraged in their continuing efforts. When patients are able to master these behaviors, they move closer to the end goals that provide the clinician the opportunity to acknowledge and reinforce progress.

Self-Management

Self-management emphasizes behavior modification principles and the individual as a decisionmaker. It includes problem-solving skills necessary to deal with issues arising from the prescribed regimen and the condition itself. The patient also uses knowledge and experience to increase his or her flexibility in applying the principles underlying the dietary regimen rather than only following the specifics of the regimen.

The theoretic model of self-management is based on three assumptions. First, several factors predispose an individual to manage a disease. These include interpersonal factors, such as knowledge, feelings, and beliefs, and external factors, such as role models and social support. Second, the patient learns which strategies are effective (and which are not) in manipulating situations to reduce the impact of disease on daily life. Last, self-management is a means to reduce symptoms and other clinical manifestations of disease, improve function, reduce side effects, and improve quality of life (39). The health care provider encourages patients as they select, evaluate, and adjust their goals and strategies for behavioral change (37).

Self-Monitoring

Self-monitoring is a process of observing and recording one's dietary intake that can help promote dietary change. Recordkeeping is a form of self-monitoring used to engage patients more actively in adherence (40,41). Self-monitoring may be strengthened with the following interventions: (a) the patient is motivated to change; (b) the behavior being observed is easy to discriminate; (c) recordkeeping materials are easy to use; (d) the patient is instructed on how to self-monitor; (e) recording occurs in close time proximity to the behavior; (f) feedback is provided; and (g) the patient knows the record will be checked for accuracy (34). Participants in the Modification of Diet in Renal Disease (MDRD) study (5,37) recorded, or "self-monitored," the protein content of all foods consumed on a daily basis throughout the study; some monitored the phosphorus, sodium, or energy content of foods as well. Most MDRD study subjects rated self-monitoring a very useful technique in helping them achieve their diet goals (37). Self-monitoring also provides an opportunity for the health care provider to give positive reinforcement to patients for their efforts.

Goal Setting

Contracting and goal setting are conceptually similar methods of shaping behavior by having the patient set and achieve a series of iterative steps designed to reach the desired endpoint. There are four steps for successful goal setting with adults. These include recognizing a need for change, establishing a goal for change, monitoring progress toward achieving that goal, and rewarding attainment of the goal (42).

Educational Strategies

There is abundant information on educational strategies designed to alter dietary behavior. Nutrition education is a necessary first step in achieving dietary change. However, in most cases, education alone is not sufficient to achieve long-term dietary adherence and sustain behavioral change. Educational interventions to promote dietary adherence rely on transmission and dissemination of information about a disease and instruction as a means of changing behavior. The information may (or may not) be presented in a motivational format. The immediate objectives of these educational strategies are patient knowledge and attitudes (30). Health care providers should use innovative techniques to improve quality of patient education and promote dietary adherence (16,43).

Communication

Good communication between the health care provider and patient is fundamental for dietary adherence. Dietary advice should be simplified to the extent possible and specific to the needs of the patient. Providers also are encouraged to reveal their human side to patients, describing their own approach to dietary change and exhibiting awareness, interest, and empathy. Revealing one's own efforts or problems in achieving dietary adherence is a technique used to help build rapport with the patient, increase communication, and encourage the patient to talk openly and honestly without fear of a negative reaction (44). Use of this technique may support behavioral change.

Health care professionals involved in teaching patients need to develop skills that promote adherence. Table 36.3 lists strategies and tactics that can help to improve the likelihood that patients will apply what they learn (45). Interpersonal skills help build trust and rapport. Essential teaching functions, such as assessment and feedback, are strategies that form a framework for teaching. Adherence counseling skills are necessary for effectiveness, and presentation skills improve efficiency in education. Ongoing communication among the renal care team is essential to optimize patient care and promote adherence.

Nutrition Counseling

Nutrition counseling that includes motivational interviewing techniques establishes an environment of trust and understanding with the patient (46). Motivational interviewing is a directive, patient-centered counseling style to help patients examine and resolve ambivalence about behavior change, reduce resistance, and enhance long-term adherence. This approach may help a patient be more receptive to traditional educational approaches, such as diet tips, menus, and recipes, which may overwhelm someone who is ambivalent about changing behavior (47).

The key elements in motivational interviewing are empa-

TABLE 36.3. ADHERENCE STRATEGIES, TACTICS, AND CONSIDERATIONS FOR THE RENAL CARE TEAM

Strategy	Tactic or Consideration
Focus on critical issues first; follow up with less pressing factors and barriers to adherence	Begin with complications of hyperkalemia and inadequate intake of dietary protein and energy. Follow up with phosphorus, calcium, fluid, cholesterol, vitamin/mineral intake, etc., sequentially as appropriate. Let people know priorities may change over time. Minimize presentation of extraneous information.
Individualize	Address key issues from patient's perspective when suggesting changes. Age, culture, personality, finances, etc. all affect adherence (Table 36.1).
Use body language; develop communication skills	People respond to subtleties such as good eye contact, sitting rather than standing, obvious enthusiasm, and nonverbal encouragement (such as a nod in response to comments).
Interact rather than pontificate	Use open-ended questions. Ask patients to tell you what they expect from adhering to the diet. Ask them to summarize your discussion and encourage questions. Solicit feedback.
Focus on concrete steps to overcoming specific barriers and what can be learned rather than dwelling on nonadherence	If behavioral change does not occur, repeating the same instructions, extracting promises for improvement, confrontation, or speaking loudly to people with poor language skills tends to emphasize a patient's shortcomings and they may withdraw. Show concern. Determine specific barriers to change. Educate in manageable steps, addressing specific issues impeding adherence. When successful, compliment patients liberally. If less than successful, focus on the lessons to be learned from the experience rather than emphasizing failure/nonadherence.
Use a variety of people to reinforce your messages	Use the renal care team to reinforce the importance of dietary adherence. Consider group sessions so patients can help each other work through issues. Include the patient's family, caregiver, etc. as appropriate.
Use educational materials	Advice should be reinforced with the use of educational materials tailored to the needs of the patient. Use well-designed, high-quality educational materials (e.g., color, clean copies) to present a professional image and to show the importance of the information communicated. Consider using the patient's own grocery receipts and menus/recipe books as a basis for instruction.
Use educational techniques designed for individual patients	Be prepared; present an outline of what is to be presented initially and summarize what was presented. Use a variety of educational techniques and media. Consider how each individual learns (e.g., visual or verbal), and select instructional techniques accordingly. Be sensitive to educational levels and cultural and social issues during instruction. Personalized instruction is likely to be more effective than mediated instruction (i.e., videos). Quality of instruction or instructional method is more important than quantity.

thy, collaboration between practitioner and patient, encouragement for the patient to be active in decision-making and problem-solving, and acknowledgment of the patient's autonomy. Patients are able to explore their motivation and commitment for change and their plans for movement toward the desired behaviors with assistance from the practitioner (47).

The patient-centered counseling model provides an effective approach for intervening with patients to promote dietary change and long-term adherence (48). This model facilitates change by assessing patient needs and tailoring the intervention to the patient's stage in the process of change, goals, and challenges. The objectives of the patient-centered counseling model for dietary change are (a) to increase awareness of diet-related risks, (b) to increase nutrition knowledge, (c) to promote confidence in the patient's ability to make dietary changes, and (d) to enhance skills needed for long-term adherence to dietary change.

Self-Efficacy

Self-efficacy refers to the patient's belief that he or she can modify behavior as required to produce particular outcomes. Self-efficacy has been shown to predict the ability to initiate and maintain changes in a variety of health-related behaviors (2). The most critical components to enhance self-efficacy for long-term adherence include relapse prevention and problem-solving skills. Patients should be provided with new skills and knowledge on an ongoing basis to promote confidence in their ability to maintain behavioral change. Furthermore, encouraging patients to regard setbacks in dietary adherence as opportunities to avoid future lapses is a key component in education. Clinicians also should encourage patients to believe they can adhere if they want to and that the decision to do so (or not) is solely up to them.

Organizational Strategies

Support Groups

Small groups are an effective way to provide some patients with both educational and emotional support and to help identify and overcome barriers to adherence (25). Self-management of a chronic disease requires mastery of specific skills to control the condition, in addition to emotional adjustment to follow the treatment regimen and lifestyle changes. Small groups help patients share insights and feelings about their disease and adjust to and manage their condition (38). However, for most elderly people, individualized one-to-one educational sessions that are flexible are more effective than structured group approaches (35).

Key issues to consider when developing small groups include the following:

- What will the patient receive from the group relative to his or her needs for information, peer contact, support, and self-management?
- What impact will the patient have on the group? Will he or she bring the ability to share information, attention, support, and experience that will aid others?
- Will the patient help provide a good mix of group participants? It is important that the group have at least a few members who have acknowledged their disease and have reevaluated their priorities. These group members are helpful in assisting others to adjust to their condition and confront situations.
- Is the person emotionally able to participate in group activities?

Social Support

Social support is an important aspect of self-management that plays a role in influencing dietary adherence. Social support is especially important in long-term treatment plans that require continuous action on the part of the patient (49). Family members, significant others, or both can influence the commitment and ability of patients to manage their condition (38). The effect of interactions between the patient and his or her social network also determines whether a person will adhere to a dietary regimen (1).

Social support is a key factor in facilitating diet adherence in studies of other chronic conditions (50–53). It is recommended that family members or significant others attend dietary counseling sessions with the patient to learn more about the patient's condition and dietary management. Family members can provide support by encouraging the patient's efforts, witnessing behavioral contracts, and helping to facilitate management of his or her disease such as meal planning. The goal of social support is to help the patient reduce roadblocks, increase confidence in self-management, and provide positive feedback for success.

TOOLS TO FACILITATE DIETARY ADHERENCE

Table 36.3 summarizes strategies, tactics, and considerations that can be used to facilitate dietary adherence. The specific techniques and tools selected should take into account the patient, his or her learning needs, the environment, and his or her stage of readiness to implement change. These include assessment techniques to help determine the individual's ability to change, counseling techniques, educational materials, and a variety of behavioral change strategies.

SUMMARY

There is no gold standard for measuring dietary adherence in renal disease. The absence of a reliable, valid, clinically sensitive indicator of adherence is important because adherence can affect the patient's outcome. Although educational and behavioral strategies may promote dietary adherence, no one strategy is completely effective. In addition, because diet is highly variable day-to-day but is required for survival and has numerous psychosocial roles, the need to measure the continuum of diet adherence is important to optimize clinical outcomes. Individualized assessment, considering the patient, his or her roles, functional and cognitive status, educational level, psychosocial aspects, and readiness to implement behavioral changes, is the first step. The next step is to design educational approaches that present the knowledge needed in a simple, concise, stepwise approach. Sustained behavioral change requires more than knowledge. Therefore, the third step is to provide individualized behavioral change strategies. Finally, ongoing support is necessary to achieve long-term adherence to diet change.

REFERENCES

1. Brownell KD, Cohen LR. Adherence to dietary regimens. 2: Components of effective interventions. *Behav Med* 1995;20:155–164.
2. McCann BS, Bovbjerg VE. Promoting dietary change. In: Shumaker SA, Schron EB, Ockene JK, et al., eds. *The handbook of health behavior change.* New York: Springer Publishing Company, 1998:166–188.
3. Vitolins MZ, Rand CS, Rapp SR, et al. Measuring adherence to behavioral and medical interventions. *Control Clin Trials* 2000;21:188S–194S.
4. Sherman AM, Bowen DJ, Vitolins M, et al. Dietary adherence: characteristics and interventions. *Control Clin Trials* 2000;21:206S–211S.
5. Milas NC, Nowalk MP, Akpele L, et al. Factors associated with adherence to the dietary protein intervention in the Modification of Diet in Renal Disease Study. *J Am Diet Assoc* 1995;95:1295–1300.
6. Kouris A, Wahlqvist ML, Worsley A. Characteristics that enhance adherence to high-carbohydrate/high-fiber diets by persons with diabetes. *J Am Diet Assoc* 1988;88:1422–1425.
7. Haynes RB. A critical review of the "determinants" of patient compliance with therapeutic regimens. In: Sacket DL, Haynes RB, eds. *Compliance with therapeutic regimens.* Baltimore: Johns Hopkins University Press, 1976:26–39.
8. Kaveh K, Kimmel PL. Compliance in hemodialysis patients: multidimensional measures in search of a gold standard. *Am J Kidney Dis* 2001;37:244–266.
9. Brawley LR, Culos-Reed SN. Studying adherence to therapeutic regimens: overview, theories, recommendations. *Control Clin Trials* 2000;21:156S–163S.
10. Hulka BS. Patient-clinician interactions and compliance. In: Haynes RB, Taylor DW, Sacket DL, eds. *Compliance in health care.* Baltimore: Johns Hopkins University Press, 1979:63–73.
11. Meichenbaum D, Turk DC. *Facilitating treatment adherence: a practitioner's guidebook.* New York: Plenum Press, 1987.
12. Clinical practice guidelines for nutrition in chronic renal failure. K/DOQI, National Kidney Foundation. *Am J Kidney Dis* 2000;35:S1–140.
13. Kumanyika SK, Ewart CK. Theoretical and baseline considerations for diet and weight control of diabetes among blacks. *Diabetes Care* 1990;13:1154–1162.
14. Sacket DL. The magnitude of compliance and noncompliance. In: Sacket DL, Haynes RB, eds. *Compliance with therapeutic regimens.* Baltimore: Johns Hopkins University Press, 1976:9–25.
15. Anderson JW, Gustafson NJ. Adherence to high-carbohydrate, high-fiber diets. *Diabetes Educ* 1989;15:429–434.
16. Eckerling L, Kohrs MB. Research on compliance with diabetic regimens: applications to practice. *J Am Diet Assoc* 1984;84:805–809.
17. Rosenstock I. Historical origins of the health belief model. *Health Educ Monogr* 1974;2:328–335.
18. Becker MH, Maiman LA. Sociobehavioral determinants of compliance with health and medical care recommendations. *Med Care* 1975;13:10–24.
19. Hume MR. Factors influencing dietary adherence as perceived by patients on long-term intermittent peritoneal dialysis. *Nurs Pap* 1984;16:38–54.
20. Charonko CV. Cultural influences in "noncompliant" behavior and decision making. *Holist Nurs Pract* 1992;6:73–78.
21. Connett JE, Stamler J. Responses of black and white males to the special intervention program of the Multiple Risk Factor Intervention Trial. *Am Heart J* 1984;108:839–848.
22. Auslander WF, Thompson S, Dreitzer D, et al. Disparity in glycemic control and adherence between African-American and Caucasian youths with diabetes. Family and community contexts. *Diabetes Care* 1997;20:1569–1575.
23. Fitzgerald JT, Anderson RM, Funnell MM, et al. Differences in the impact of dietary restrictions on African Americans and Caucasians with NIDDM. *Diabetes Educ* 1997;23:41–47.
24. Kidd KE, Altman DG. Adherence in social context. *Control Clin Trials* 2000;21:184S–187S.
25. El Kebbi IM, Bacha GA, Ziemer DC, et al. Diabetes in urban African Americans. V. Use of discussion groups to identify barriers to dietary therapy among low-income individuals with non-insulin-dependent diabetes mellitus. *Diabetes Educ* 1996;22:488–492.
26. Williamson AR, Hunt AE, Pope JF, et al. Recommendations of dietitians for overcoming barriers to dietary adherence in individuals with diabetes. *Diabetes Educ* 2000;26:272–279.
27. Dunbar-Jacob JM, Schlenk EA, Burke LE, et al. Predictors of patient adherence: Patient characteristics. In: Shumaker SA, Schron EB, Ockene JK, et al., eds. *The handbook of health behavior change.* New York: Springer Publishing Company, 1998:491–511.
28. Ciechanowski PS, Katon WJ, Russo JE. Depression and diabetes: impact of depressive symptoms on adherence, function, and costs. *Arch Intern Med* 2000;160:3278–3285.
29. Anderson RT, Ory M, Cohen S, et al. Issues of aging and adherence to health interventions. *Control Clin Trials* 2000;21:171S–183S.
30. Haynes RB. Strategies for improving compliance: A methodologic analysis and review. In: Sacket DL, Haynes RB, eds. *Compliance with therapeutic regimens.* Baltimore: Johns Hopkins University Press, 1976:69–82.
31. Zimmerman GL, Olsen CG, Bosworth MF. A 'stages of change' approach to helping patients change behavior. *Am Fam Physician* 2000;61:1409–1416.
32. Prochaska J, DiClemente C. Stages and processes of self-change of smoking: Toward an integrative model of change. *J Consult Clin Psychol* 1983;51:390–395.
33. Prochaska J, Johnson S, Lee P. The transtheoretical model of behavior change. In: Schumaker SA, Schron EB, Ockene J, et al., eds. *The handbook of health behavior change.* New York: Springer Publishing Company, 1998:59–84.
34. Dunbar JM, Marshall GD, Howell MF. Behavioral strategies for improving compliance. In: Haynes RB, Taylor DW, Sacket DL,

eds. *Compliance in health care.* Baltimore: Johns Hopkins University Press, 1979:174–190.
35. Murdaugh CL. Problems with adherence in the elderly. In: Shumaker SA, Schron EB, Ockene JK, et al., eds. *The handbook of health behavior change.* New York: Springer Publishing Company, 1998:357–376.
36. Leventhal H, Cameron L. Behavioral theories and the problem of compliance. *Patient Educ Counsel* 1987;10:117–138.
37. Gillis BP, Caggiula AW, Chiavacci AT, et al. Nutrition intervention program of the Modification of Diet in Renal Disease Study: a self-management approach. *J Am Diet Assoc* 1995;95: 1288–1294.
38. US Department of Health and Human Services, Public Health Service, Centers for Disease Control, Center for Health Promotion and Education. *Strategies to promote self-management of chronic disease.* Chicago: American Hospital Association, 1982.
39. Clark NM, Becker MH. Theoretical models and strategies for improving adherence and disease management. In: Shumaker SA, Schron EB, Ockene J, et al., eds. *The handbook of health behavior change.* New York: Springer Publishing Company, 1998:5–32.
40. Snetselaar L. Counseling skills. In: Snetselaar L, ed. *Nutrition counseling skills: assessment, treatment, and evaluation.* Rockville, MD: Aspen Systems Corp., 1975:55–88.
41. Kanfer FH. Self-monitoring: Methodological limitations and clinical applications. *J Consult Clin Psychol* 1979;35:148–152.
42. Cullen KW, Baranowski T, Smith SP. Using goal setting as a strategy for dietary behavior change. *J Am Diet Assoc* 2001;101: 562–566.
43. Bartlet EE. Forum: Patient education. *Prevent Med* 1985;14: 667–669.
44. Hauenstein DJ, Schiller MR, Hurley RS. Motivational techniques of dietitians counseling individuals with type II diabetes. *J Am Diet Assoc* 1987;87:37–42.
45. Roach RR, Pichert JW, Stetson BA, et al. Improving dietitians' teaching skills. *J Am Diet Assoc* 1992;92:1466–1470,1473.
46. Rollnick S, Miller WR. What is motivational interviewing? *Behav Cogn Psychother* 1995;23:325–334.
47. Windhauser MM, Ernst DB, Karanja NM, et al. Translating the Dietary Approaches to Stop Hypertension diet from research to practice: dietary and behavior change techniques. DASH Collaborative Research Group. *J Am Diet Assoc* 1999;99:S90–S95.
48. Rosal MC, Ebbeling CB, Lofgren I, et al. Facilitating dietary change: the patient-centered counseling model. *J Am Diet Assoc* 2001;101:332–341.
49. Becker MH. Patient adherence to prescribed therapies. *Med Care* 1985;23:539–555.
50. McCann BS, Retzlaff BM, Dowdy AA, et al. Promoting adherence to low-fat, low-cholesterol diets: review and recommendations. *J Am Diet Assoc* 1990;90:1408–1414, 1417.
51. Schlenk EA, Hart LK. Relationship between health locus of control, health value, and social support and compliance of persons with diabetes mellitus. *Diabetes Care* 1984;7:566–574.
52. Shenkel RJ, Rogers JP, Perfetto G, et al. Importance of "significant others" in predicting cooperation with diabetic regimen. *Int J Psychiatry Med* 1985;15:149–155.
53. Wilson W, Ary DV, Biglan A, et al. Psychosocial predictors of self-care behaviors (compliance) and glycemic control in non-insulin-dependent diabetes mellitus. *Diabetes Care* 1986;9: 614–622.
54. Prochaska JO, DiClemente CC, Norcross JC. In search of how people change. Applications to addictive behaviors. *The American Psychologist*, 1992;47:1102–1114.

37

NUTRITION PLANS, MEAL PATTERNS, AND SUPPLEMENTS FOR ACUTE AND CHRONIC RENAL FAILURE

LINDA M. McCANN

Medical nutrition therapy is a complex but essential component of successful treatment for kidney disease. The thrust of nutrition care for renal disease in the 1970s was authoritarian, with strict nutrient levels, standard diets, and lists of "forbidden" foods. Renal nutrition care today has evolved into a process of matching nutrition care to the individual. Although some standard guidelines are used, the individual needs and preferences of each patient are considered and incorporated into nutrition care plans. A team approach, including the patient, provides the best likelihood for successful, individualized dietary modification in renal disease.

A thorough nutrition assessment forms the foundation for the development of a diet prescription, nutrition care plan, and treatment goals. The patient's ability and willingness to adhere to diet modifications can be enhanced by assessing and evaluating the following patient-specific factors:

1. Knowledge of kidney disease and dietary modifications including review of previous instruction and assessment of individual education and literacy levels (1)
2. Usual dietary intake and meal patterns
3. Special needs and preferences—medical, cultural, educational, religious, financial, and psychosocial
4. Personal goals of the patient

Recommended nutrient levels are defined in a diet prescription, which must be translated into an individualized meal pattern and daily food choices. One widely used method of creating individualized meal plans is to provide food choice lists such as those established through the collaboration of the American Diabetes Association, American Dietetic Association, and the United States Public Health Service in 1950. These "exchange" lists allowed greater variety in the diet and enhanced its palatability. Similar "food choice lists" were established for patients with renal disease by the American Dietetic Association Renal Practice Group and the National Kidney Foundation Council on Renal Nutrition in 1993 (2). These lists, similar to exchange lists, group foods according to their content of protein, sodium, potassium, and phosphorus. The National Renal Diet (NRD) provides two groups of choice lists—one for those without the need to restrict carbohydrate and one for individuals who have diabetes. The food choice list averages can be found in Table 37.1. While the National Renal Diet food choice lists were revised in 2002, 1993 food choice lists are used in this chapter because the tighter range of nutrients is more amenable to the development of standard meal patterns. The complexities of renal diet modifications lend themselves well to the concept of food choice lists. These lists allow the patient to eat a variety of foods while preserving the consistency of daily nutrient levels. With the current focus on dietary individualization, food choice lists provide the maximum flexibility and eliminate the need for extensive "forbidden food" lists. Ideally, exchange lists are tailored specifically to the patient—including foods that the patient eats in the appropriate food choice lists and eliminating those foods that are not eaten. However, tailoring exchange lists to that degree may be difficult with limited dietetic resources.

Renal food choice lists easily can be used for all stages of kidney disease and renal replacement therapies. Because average nutrient contents are used in the food choice lists, standard meal patterns can be developed (Table 37.2) and then individualized for a specific patient, and they even can be adapted to cultural preferences and religious customs (Table 37.3). They can be simplified (Fig. 37.1), illustrated in pictures, or expanded for increased flexibility. Because exchange lists are based on averages, it is important for the patient to eat a variety of foods and ensure that the nutrients balance out over several days of intake.

Food choice lists and meal patterns can be used to provide written guidance and nutrient goals for patients while

TABLE 37.1. 1993 NATIONAL RENAL DIET FOOD CHOICE LIST NUTRIENT VALUES

	Nondiabetic					Diatbetic					
Food Group	Kcal	Protein (g)	Na^+ (mg)	K^+ (mg)	P (mg)	kcal	Cholesterol	Protein	Na	K	P
Milk	120	4.0	80	185	110	100	8.0	4.0	80	185	110
Milk substitute	140	0.5	40	80	30	140	12.0	0.5	40	80	30
Meat	65	7.0	25	100	65	65	—	7.0	25	100	65
Starches	90	2.0	80	35	35	80	15	2.0	80	35	35
Vegetable											
Low potassium	25	1.0	15	70	20	25	5	1.0	15	70	20
Medium potassium	25	1.0	15	150	20	25	5	1.0	15	150	20
High potassium	25	1.0	15	270	20	25	5	1.0	15	270	20
Fruit											
Low potassium	70	0.5	Trace	70	15	60	15	0.5	Trace	70	15
Medium potassium	70	0.5	Trace	150	15	60	15	0.5	Trace	150	15
High potassium	70	0.5	Trace	270	15	60	15	0.5	Trace	270	15
Fats	45	—	55	10	5	45	—	—	55	10	5
High calorie	100	Trace	15	20	5	60	15	Tr	15	20	5
Beverage	Varies	—	Varies	Varies	Varies	Varies	Varies	Varies	Varies	Varies	Varies
Salt choices	—	—	250	—	—	—	—	—	250	—	—

From McCann L, ed. *Pocket guide to nutrition assessment of the renal patient*, 3rd ed. New York: National Kidney Foundation Council on Renal Nutrition, 2001, with permission.

allowing them to eat as normally as possible. Recognizing the significant incidence of malnutrition in patients with chronic kidney disease and renal failure undergoing dialysis, most renal clinicians strive to minimize dietary restrictions. This does not eliminate the responsibility for giving the patient guidelines and goals. A meal pattern and food choice list can provide those guidelines and goals in a practical format. However, the clinician must avoid merely presenting lists, forms, and other documents in a way that removes the patient from the process. Direct patient involvement in the development of the nutrition care plan provides the foundation for adherence and success. The initial success can be very important to long-term success because of the multitude of challenges that patients with kidney disease face.

Many cookbooks and sample menus are available to patients with kidney disease. However, it has been observed that many people who are advised to follow a special diet

TABLE 37.2. MEAL PATTERNS (BASED ON NONDIABETIC EXCHANGE VALUES OF THE 1993 NATIONAL RENAL DIET)

Grams of Protein Food Groups	40 Servings	60 Servings	60 Servings	80 Servings	100 Servings
Milk	0	0	1	1	1
Milk substitute	2	1	0	0	0
Meat	4	6	6	8	11
Starch	4	6	6	8	8
Veg, low K^+	0	1	0	1	0
Veg, med K^+	0	1	1	0	1
Veg, high K^+	2	1	1	1	0
Fruit, low K^+	1	0	1	0	0
Fruit, med K^+	1	1	1	1	1
Fruit, high K^+	2	2	1	1	1
Fats	8	8	8	8	6
High calorie	5	4	3	2	1
Beverage	3	2	3	3	2
Salt choices	4	3	3	2	2

Meal patterns contain approximately 2,100 kcal, 2 g Na^+, $<$2.5 g K^+, $<$15 mg P/g protein. Servings can be adjusted or added to change calories or other nutrients.
From McCann L, ed. *Pocket guide to nutrition assessment of the renal patient*, 2nd ed. New York: National Kidney Foundation Council on Renal Nutrition, 1998, with permission.

TABLE 37.3. SAMPLE MENUS CONTAINING 60 GRAMS OF PROTEIN FOR SPECIFIC ETHNIC GROUPS OR REGIONS

Meals	White American	Mexican American	Native American	Asian American	East Indian
Breakfast	1 egg 1 slice toast 2 tsp. margarine 1/2 cup orange juice 1 cup coffee 2 tsp. sugar	Pan dulce 1/2 cup applesauce 2 cup coffee with 2 T whitener	1/2 cup corn meal gruel 1/2 cup nondairy cream 2 tsp. margarine 1 sweet roll 1 cup tea 2 tsp. honey	1/2 cup milk 1/2 cup rice gruel 1 tsp. sugar 1 doughnut 1 small star fruit 1 cup tea	1 slice wheat toast 1 cup pear nectar 1/2 cup yogurt (lassi) 3 tsp. margarine 1 cup tea 2 T molasses
Lunch	2 slices white bread 2 oz. chicken 2 tsp. mayonnaise Lettuce leaf 1/2 medium pear 1 can regular soda	2 tortillas 1 oz. pork 1/4 cup frijoles 1/4 cup salsa fresca 1/2 cup cabbage 2 T oil 1 cup diet soda 1 cup jello	1 portion fry bread 2 eggs 2 oz. sausage 2 tsp. margarine 1/2 cup nopales 1 cup regular soda 1/2 cup cherries	2 oz. soy curd 1/2 cup chicken broth 1/2 cup winter melon 2 oz. chicken 1/2 cup rice 2 T oil 1/2 cup pears 1 cup tea	2 oz. pork 1/4 cup chickpeas 1/2 cup rice 1/2 cup bamboo shoots 3 fig bars 3 T peanut oil 1 cup coffee 2 tsp. sugar
Dinner	3 oz. ground beef 1/2 cup rice 1/2 cup broccoli Small salad 2 T dressing 1 T olive oil Dinner roll 3 tsp. margarine 1/2 medium apple	4 oz. grilled beef 1/2 cup Spanish rice 1/2 cup yellow squash 1 tortilla Lettuce wedge 3 T oil 1/2 small papaya	3 oz. salmon 1/2 cup wild rice 1 cup summer squash 2 tsp. margarine 1 cup lemonade	3 oz. steamed fish 1 cup rice 1/2 cup summer squash 1/2 cup mushrooms 2 T sesame oil 1/2 cup regular soda	3 oz. lamb curry 1/2 cup rice 1/2 cup cabbage 1 slice bread 3 tsp. margarine 1 cup lemonade
Snacks	1/2 cup ice cream 1/2 cup strawberries	1/2 cup strawberries	1 cup blueberries	1 small pear-apple	15 grapes

These meal patterns were developed with food choice list averages for a 60-g protein diet. They subsequently were analyzed with Mosby's Nutritrac©, Mosby, Inc, 1998. Each of the menus was found to have between 58 and 63 g of protein, 1,925–2,070 calories, 1,957–2,106 mg potassium, and <16 mg phosphorus/g of protein. When specific foods were not found, those closest in nutrient content were substituted in the computer analysis.

do not significantly change what they have eaten throughout their lives. They treasure family recipes and favorite foods. One of the challenges for the renal dietitian is to help patients accommodate their favorite foods in the diet, usually with some limitations on frequency and portion size. In addition, it may be important to help the patient identify some acceptable "prepared meals" to use when time or physical limitations preclude meal preparation (3).

Meal patterns, food choice lists, and sample menus provide tools to incorporate a variety of foods and recipes into the overall nutrient prescription. Whereas some patients follow their nutrition guidelines closely, others refer to them primarily in times of nutrient imbalance or abnormal serum chemistries. Routine follow-up and reports of progress help reinforce the importance of nutrition and diet modification for the patient with renal disease.

Ideally, patients with chronic kidney disease or those on renal replacement therapy will be able to meet their nutrient goals with conventional foods. When they are unable to meet their needs with conventional foods, there are a number of options that can be used progressively to enhance nutrient intake. These options include oral and enteral products used as supplements or as the sole source of nutrition (orally or in tube feedings). Other more aggressive nutrition support alternatives are discussed in Chapters 26 and 27.

Oral modular supplements contain individual macronutrients. They are combined with conventional foods, beverages, or other supplements for additional protein or calories. Some examples can be found in Table 37.4. Milano et al. found that modular energy supplements increased patients' fatty tissue but did not improve their nutrition status (4). The clinician must monitor the patient for nutrient imbalance when supplementing a single nutrient. Oral essential amino acid supplements are also safe and effective for people with kidney disease. They have been used successfully to enhance the efficacy of low-protein diets in pre-end-stage renal disease and to treat hypoalbuminemia in patients with renal disease, but they are not recommended as the sole source of nutrition. Oral essential amino acid products are listed in Table 37.5 (5,6).

Oral supplements, containing a complete balance of nutrients, are used frequently in patients with chronic kidney disease and renal failure. These medical nutrition products (MNPs) may be consumed with or between meals, but if possible the patient is encouraged to eat conventional foods

FOOD GROUP	#SERVS	SERVING SIZE	FOODS TO AVOID
Milk 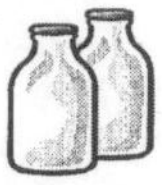		½ cup milk, yogurt, ice cream, milk substitute; 2 Tbsp sour cream or cream	Check with your dietitian before using buttermilk
Meat 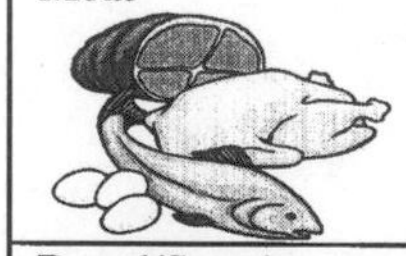		1 ounce beef, chicken, turkey, lamb, veal, or pork; ¼ cup tuna or cottage cheese; 1 egg; 1 ounce cheese; 2 Tbsp peanut butter.	Processed meats like hot dogs, corned beef, lunch meats; canned or salted meats and fish, nuts Limit cheese and peanut butter to occasional use.
Bread/Starch 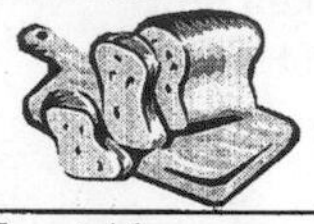		1 slice bread; ½ bun or muffin; ½ cup cooked cereal, rice, pasta, potato, or noodles; ¾ cup dry cereal	Salted crackers, pretzels, potato chips, or highly salted snack foods.
Vegetables 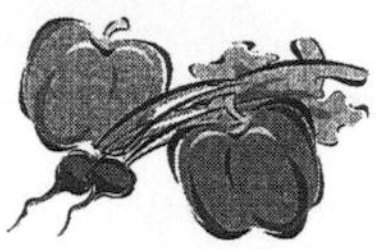		½ cup cooked or raw; 1 cup raw cabbage or lettuce. If cooked, use ample water. LIMIT TO ONE SMALL SERVING PER DAY: Deep green/dark yellow/orange vegetables, tomato or potato	Dried beans (kidney, pinto, navy, etc.) lentils, pickles, sauerkraut, and avocado. Check with your dietitian about using an occasional, small serving of baked or French fried potatoes.
Fruits 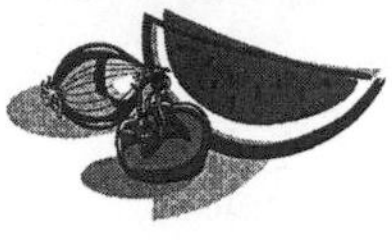		½ cup canned fruit or juice: fresh fruit; 15 grapes, cherries, berries; ½ grapefruit; LIMIT TO ONE SMALL SERVING PER DAY: Citrus fruits/juices, banana, melons	Dried fruits LIMIT FRESH FRUIT TO ONE SERVING PER DAY
Fats 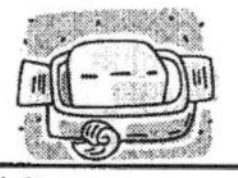		1 teaspoon margarine, mayonnaise, or oil; 1 Tablespoon salad dressing or non-dairy liquid creamer	Salt pork, olives LIMIT CREAM OR CHEESE BASED SALAD DRESSINGS
Fluids 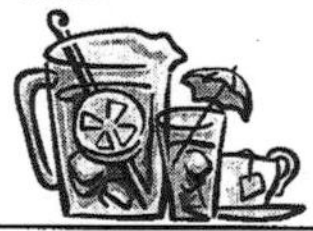		1 cup coffee, tea, soda, lemonade, instant powdered drinks, water LIMIT coffee, tea, cola to _____ cup(s) per day.	Orange soda
Other: 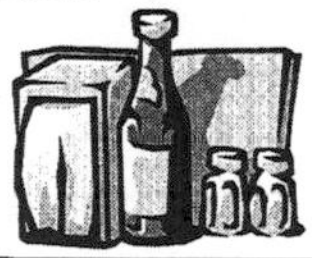			CHECK WITH YOUR DIETITIAN BEFORE USING: salt, seasoned salts, soy sauce, MSG, soups, sauces, frozen dinners, instant or convenience foods.

FIGURE 37.1. Simple meal pattern.

TABLE 37.4. MODULAR PRODUCTS (ADDED TO OTHER SOURCES OF NUTRITION)

Product	Amount	Kcal	Carbohydrate g	Protein g	Fat g	Na^+ mg	K^+ mg	P mg	Ca^{++} mg	Use
Casec® Dry	100 g	380	0	90	2.0	100	10	800	1,400	Protein
Moducal® Dry	100 g	380	95	0	0	70	NA	NA	NA	Carbohydrate/kcal
Polycose® Dry	100 g	380	94	0	0	110	10	12	30	Carbohydrate/kcal
Polycose® Liquid	100 mL	200	50	0	0	70	6	3	20	Carbohydrate/kcal
ProCel®	1 scoop	28	<0.4	5.3	<0.5	<10	<30	<23	<30	Protein
Promod®	6.6 g	28	0.67	5	0.6	25	45	33	65	Protein

From McCann L, ed. *Pocket guide to nutrition assessment of the renal patient*, 3rd ed. New York: National Kidney Foundation Council on Renal Nutrition, 2001, with permission.

TABLE 37.5. ORAL AMINO ACID PRODUCTS

Product	Amino Acid Content	Form	Manufacturer/ Distributor
Aminess-N®	Each table contains 720 mg of amino acid and 88 mg of nitrogen (= to 0.55 g protein)	Tablets	Recip AB, Stockholm
Nutramine T™	3.5 g UPS grade amino acid in 1 packet	Powder/granules to be used with foods/liquid to make chewable "candy," custard, beverage, etc.	Calwood Nutritionals, Inc.

From McCann L, ed. *Pocket guide to nutrition assessment of the patient with chronic kidney disease*, 3rd ed. New York: National Kidney Foundation Council on Renal Nutrition, 2002, with permission.

and meals in addition to the supplement. There are a number of factors that must be considered when selecting an MNP for use in a patient with renal disease. These include:

Willingness of the patient to consume the supplement
Kidney function or method of renal replacement therapy
Tolerance for fluids and electrolytes
Integrity of the gastrointestinal tract
Nutritional requirements

It is also necessary to identify and eliminate potential barriers to the use of supplements, such as lack of financial resources, need for home delivery, gastrointestinal side effects, taste fatigue, and lack of storage capability. The choices of renal-specific MNPs have expanded greatly in the last decade. These are typically more concentrated for fluid control, have higher macronutrient content, and have a lower electrolyte content. Analogous to diet modification, the individual needs of the patient must be considered to identify the most appropriate supplement.

MNPs fall into broad product categories that help clinicians make patient-specific recommendations. Historically, these products were formulated to mimic the standard American diet for healthy individuals. Currently, many available products are formulated to meet the requirements of compromised individuals with specific medical needs. Those that commonly are used in patients with renal disease can be found in Table 37.6. Specialty MNPs such as cookies, bars, and puddings are listed in Table 37.7. Formulas are categorized as polymeric, peptide-based, or elemental, depending on the degree of digestibility required prior to absorption. Polymeric formulas contain intact proteins,

TABLE 37.6. MEDICAL NUTRITION PRODUCTS (LIMITED TO THOSE THAT ARE MOST APPROPRIATE FOR RENAL PATIENTS)

Product	Amount	Kcal	Carbohydrate g	Protein g	Fat g	Na^+ mg	K^+ mg	P mg	Ca^{++} mg	Uses
Boost Plus	8 oz	360	45	14	14	170	380	310	330	C, V, O, HC, HP
Choice DM	8 oz	220	24	9	10	200	430	310	330	C, S, DM, F
Enlive	8 oz	300	65	10	0	65	40	20	60	HC, clear liquid
Ensure Hi Pro	8 oz	230	31	12	6	290	500	250	300	C, O, S, HP, V
Glucerna Shake	8 oz	220	29	10	8.5	210	370	250	250	C, DM, O
Magnacal Renal	8 oz	470	47	17.7	24	190	300	189	240	C, O, T, renal
Nepro	8 oz	475	52.8	16.7	22.7	200	250	165	325	C, O, T, renal
Novasource Renal	8 oz	475	47.3	17.4	24.1	210	192	154	308	C, HC, V, O, T
NuBasics Coffee	2 scoops	125	18.8	6.25	28	210	227	80	88	C, S
NuBasics Juice	1 box	163	34	6.5	0.1	50	50	166	83	S, O
NuBasics Soup	3 scoops	250	33	9.5	9.2	490	310	165	150	S, O
NutriRenal	8 oz	500	51.2	17.5	26	185	314	175	350	C, S, O, HP/HC
ReNeph	4 oz	250	31	8	11	120	15	45	10	S
ReNeph Reduced Sugar	4 oz	230	23	9	11	125	20	60	10	S, DM
Resource Diabetic	8 oz	250	23.4	15	11.1	290	320	260	260	DM, F, O
Resource Fruit Beverage	8 oz	250	53.5	9.0	0	<80	<20	160	10	S, fat free

C, complete; V, volume restricted; O, appropriate for oral; HC, high calorie; HP, high protein; S, supplement to food; DM, appropriate for persons with diabetes mellitus; F, added fiber; T, appropriate for tube; LR, low residue; NA, information not available.
Due to frequent changes, clinicians are encouraged to update the information regularly.
From Manufacturer's information, Internet, 2003.

TABLE 37.7. SPECIALTY MEDICAL NUTRITION PRODUCTS

Nutrition Bars and Cookies	Amount	Kcal	Carbohydrate	Protein	Fat	Na^+	K^+	P	Ca^{++}	Use Code
ChoiceDM bar	1.23 oz.	140	19	6	4.5	80	105	110	133	DM, S, V
Ensure bar		130	21	6	3	115	200	150	80	C, S, V
Glucerna Snack bar	1 bar	140	24	6	4	65–120	40–150	150	250	C, DM, F, V
Puddings	**Amount**	**Kcal**	**Carbohydrate**	**Protein**	**Fat**	Na^+	K^+	**P**	Ca^{++}	**Use Code**
Boost pudding	5 oz.	240	33	7	9	125	250	200	250	O, V, S
Ensure Nutrition and Energy Bar	1 bar	230	35	9	6	135	150	300	300	C, S, O, V
Sustacal pudding	5 oz.	240	32	7	9	120	320	220	220	O, S, V

S, supplement to food; V, volume restricted; DM, appropriate for persons with diabetes mellitus; C, complete; F, added fiber; O, appropriate for oral; NA, no information available.

complex carbohydrates, and significant amounts of calories from long-chain fats. Peptide and amino acid–based supplements differ primarily in nitrogen sources. MNPs have been shown to be an effective sole source of nutrition in patients undergoing hemodialysis, and disease-specific formulations seem to have advantages over standard formulas for biochemical balance (7). However, it is possible to deplete blood electrolyte levels using a renal-specific MNP as the sole source of nutrition. Once again, close consultation and follow-up with the patient are critical for success.

If a patient is unable to meet specific nutrition requirements with traditional foods and/or supplements, the aggressiveness of intervention must be increased. The next step in the hierarchy of nutrition interventions is tube feeding. Although this intervention is used commonly in the hospital or long-term care setting and in children with renal disease, it has not been widely embraced in the adult outpatient dialysis population. Tube feeding care for patients who receive outpatient dialysis usually is administered by a home health agency or the staff of the long-term care facility. Common tube feeding products are listed in Table 37.8. Many of these products have special characteristics such as lower osmolality (isotonic), increased fiber for normal bowel function, high calorie or nitrogen for increased metabolic needs or fluid restriction, low carbohydrate levels for glucose control, freedom from lactose for lactose intolerance, or hydrolyzed protein sources for malabsorption or radiation treatment. The availability of specially formulated products allows the renal clinician to closely tailor the feeding to the needs of the patient.

There have been reports of successful tube feeding in patients receiving peritoneal dialysis using percutaneous endoscopic gastrostomy feeding (8) and a retroperitoneal feeding tube (9). These case reports identified potential side effects that require close monitoring, such as hypokalemia and hypophosphatemia (resulting from refeeding syndrome or the use of low electrolyte supplements). There is also the burden of yet another medical procedure for the patient. In general, tube feedings with moderate protein and electrolyte levels and added fiber may be best for patients with renal disease. Too much protein can add risk for dehydration, hypernatremia, hyperchloremia, and azotemia, especially in the elderly patient or anyone with compromised kidney function. Concentrated formulas minimize the fluid load but should be administered at a slower speed. The fluid load can also be minimized by limiting the volume of fluid used to flush the tube. Close monitoring of laboratory values allows the clinician to make timely, appropriate adjustments in the choice of MNP or medications. Methods of tube feeding administration are listed in Table 37.9, and common tube feeding sites are listed in Table 37.10.

Today's limited resources and minimal funding for nutri-

TABLE 37.8. COMPOSITION OF COMMON TUBE FEEDINGS PER LITER

Product	Kcal	Carbohydrate g	Protein g	Fat g	Na^+ mg	K^+ mg	P mg	Ca^{++} mg
Comply	1,500	180	60	61	1,200	1,850	1,200	1,200
Criticare HN	1,060	220	38	5.3	630	1,310	530	530
Isocal	1,060	135	34	44	530	1,320	530	630
Isocal HN	1,060	124	44	45	930	1,610	850	850
Jevity 1 Cal	1,060	154.7	44.3	34.7	930	1,570	760	910
Nutren 1.0	1,000	127	40	38	876	1,248	668	668
Osmolite 1.2 Cal	1,200	157	55	39.3	1,420	1,940	1,200	1,200
Osmolite HN	1,060	143.9	44.3	34.7	930	1,570	760	760
Two-cal HN	2,000	219	83.5	90.5	1,460	2,450	1,055	1,055
UltraCal HN+	1,200	156	54	40	1,350	1,850	1,000	1,000

From Manufacturer's information, Internet, 2003.

TABLE 37.9. METHODS OF TUBE FEEDING ADMINISTRATION

Feeding	Description	Advantages	Disadvantages
Continuous	Pump is used to deliver feeding at a regulated rate	May reach goals more quickly, enhanced patient tolerance, nutrient absorption is maximized	Requires pump, more costly, decreased mobility
Bolus or gravity drip	Given in specific volumes every 3 to 8 hours	Mobility, less costly, less equipment	Fullness, discomfort, reflux requires more caregiver time
Cyclic	Feeding the patient continuously via pump over only part of the day (usually 12–16 hours)	Frees patient during the day, decreased fullness, smoother transition to full oral intake	Need for higher infusion rate or formula concentration to meet needs, requires larger water volume, requires a pump

From McCann L, ed. *Pocket guide to nutrition assessment of the patient with chronic kidney disease*, 3rd ed. National Kidney Foundation Council on Renal Nutrition, 2002, with permission.

TABLE 37.10. COMMON TUBE FEEDING SITES

Site	Characteristics
Intragastric	Tube through nose or mouth into stomach; used for short-term with functional gastrointestinal tract; easily inserted; risk for aspiration pneumonia; potential discomfort; remains in place between meals; bolus or pumped
Nasoduodenal or nasojejunal	Short-term enteral feeding; may allow feeding after gastric surgery; difficult to place and maintain
PEG (percutaneous endoscopic gastrostomy)	Used for long-term tube feedings into stomach of patients with functional gastrointestinal tract; often used for alterations in swallowing; less discomfort than nasogastric; can be inserted at bedside with local anesthesia; risk of skin breakdown around tube; contraindicated in peritonitis, ascites, morbid obesity, obstruction, esophageal obstruction, or reflux; formula can be given at night as intermittent or pumped
Jejunostomy or PEG-J	Direct access to jejunum when stomach must be bypassed; potential for dumping syndrome/diarrhea; lower risk of aspiration; pumped with slow infusion working up to volume needed to meet nutritional needs of the patient

From Rombeau J, Caldwell M. *Clinical nutrition: enteral and tube feeding*. Philadelphia: W.B. Saunders, 1990, with permission; and McCann L, ed. *Pocket guide to nutrition assessment of the patient with chronic kidney disease*, 3rd ed. National Kidney Foundation Council on Renal Nutrition, 2002, with permission.

tion interventions, such as oral supplementation, enteral feeding, intradialytic parenteral nutrition, and intraperitoneal nutrition, thwart renal clinicians' attempts to nourish compromised or at-risk patients. Chima et al. showed that compromised nutrition status is associated with higher hospital length of stay, increased hospitalization costs, and discharge status of patients on medicine service (10). Strong evidence relating compromised nutrition status to morbidity and mortality in patients with renal disease (11–15) has failed to affect funding for the continuum of nutrition support and hinders its efficacy. Options for nutrition intervention have expanded, but funding has been static or even decreased in some areas. Counseling for patients with chronic kidney disease by renal dietitians will be enhanced by the Medical Nutrition Therapy Act (16,17). Oral, enteral, and other more aggressive nutrition interventions, as well as monitoring and administration techniques, continue to improve, but to be fully effective financial support must be expanded.

Renal nutrition is recognized as a specialty by the American Dietetic Association (Certified Specialist in Renal Nutrition). There are many complex biochemical and medical implications of kidney failure. A successful renal nutrition care plan requires careful translation of the multifaceted, individualized diet modifications into practical day-to-day meal patterns and menus. Patients need nutrition guidance and goals to help them succeed at each stage of kidney disease and renal replacement therapy. A hierarchy of progressive nutrition interventions must be used to maintain nutrition status and minimize morbidity and mortality. Innovation, dedication, and patient advocacy are important qualities for renal dietitians. From intense nutritional counseling, to supplementation, to oral or enteral feedings, to parenteral nutrition, the dietitian is the expert resource on the renal care team.

REFERENCES

1. Wilson BM. Matching instructional methods to renal patients' learning abilities: the effect on knowledge and compliance with fluid restriction. *J Renal Nutr* 1991;1(4):173–181.
2. National Renal Diet: Professional Guide. Washington, DC: American Dietetic Association, 1993.
3. Fagen A, Scheidler J. Meals to go. *J Renal Nutr* 2000;10(4): 215–230.

4. Milano MC, Cusumano MD, Navaro ET, et al. Energy supplementation in chronic hemodialysis patients with moderate and severe malnutrition. *J Renal Nutr* 1998;8(4):212–217.
5. Eustace JA, Coresh J, Kutchey C, et al. Randomized double-blind trial of oral essential amino acids for dialysis-associated hypoalbuminemia. *Kidney Int* 2000;57(6):2527–2538.
6. Aparicio M, Chauveau P, De Precigout V, et al. Nutrition and outcome on renal replacement therapy of patients with chronic renal failure treated by a supplemented very low protein diet. *J Am Soc Nephrol* 2000;11(4):708–716.
7. Cockram DB, Hensley MK, Rodriguez M, et al. Safety and tolerance of medical nutritional products as sole sources of nutrition in people on hemodialysis. *J Renal Nutr* 1998;8(1):25–33.
8. Patel MG, Raftery MJ. Successful percutaneous endoscopic gastrostomy feeding in continuous ambulatory peritoneal dialysis. *J Renal Nutr* 1997;7(4):208–211.
9. Kramer M, Koolpe H, Goldstein S, et al. Retroperitoneal feeding tube for peritoneal dialysis patients. *Am Soc Artif Intern Organs* 1989;XXXV:593–595.
10. Chima CS, Barco K, DeWitt MLA, et al. Relationship of nutritional status to length of stay. *J Am Diet Assoc* 1997;97(9): 975–978.
11. Gotch FA, Sargent JA. A mechanistic analysis of the National Cooperative Dialysis Study (NCDS). *Kidney Int* 1985;28: 526–534.
12. Lowrie EG, Huang WH, Lew NL. Death risk prediction among peritoneal and hemodialysis patients: a preliminary comparison. *Am J Kidney Dis* 1995;26:220–228.
13. Leavey SF, Strawderman RL, Jones CA, et al. Simple nutritional indicators as independent predictors of mortality in hemodialysis patients. *Am J Kidney Dis* 1998;31:997–1006.
14. Foley RN, Parfrey PS, Hartnett JD, et al. Hypoalbuminemia, cardiac morbidity, and mortality in end-stage renal disease. *J Am Soc Nephrol* 1996;7:728–736.
15. Canada-USA Peritoneal Dialysis Study Group. Adequacy of dialysis and nutrition in continuous peritoneal dialysis: Association with clinical outcomes. *J Am Soc Nephrol* 1996;7:198–207.
16. Sheils JF, Rubin R, Stapleton DC. The estimated costs and savings of medical nutrition therapy: The Medicare population. *J Am Diet Assoc* 1999;99(4):428–435.
17. Johnson RK. The Lewin Group Study—What does it tell us and why does it matter? *J Am Diet Assoc* 1999;99(4):426–427.
18. McCann L, ed. *Pocket guide to nutrition assessment of the patient with chronic kidney disease*, 3rd ed. New York: National Kidney Foundation Council on Renal Nutrition, 2002.
19. Mosby's Nutritrac©. St. Louis: Mosby, Inc. 1998.

SUBJECT INDEX

Page numbers followed by f refer to figures; page numbers followed by t refer to tables.

Q

R